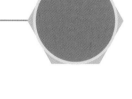

Neuromuscular Disorders:
Treatment and Management

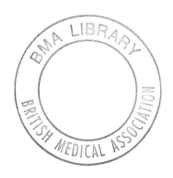

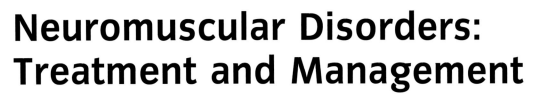

Neuromuscular Disorders:
Treatment and Management

Tulio E. Bertorini, MD

Professor of Neurology and Pathology
University of Tennessee, Center for the Health Sciences, Memphis
Chief of Neurology, Methodist University Hospital
Director, Wesley Neurology Clinic and Muscular Dystrophy and ALS Clinic
Memphis, Tennessee

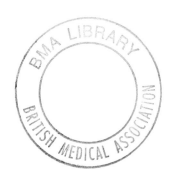

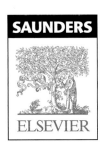

SAUNDERS

ELSEVIER

SAUNDERS
ELSEVIER

1600 John F. Kennedy Boulevard
Suite 1800
Philadelphia, PA 19103-2899

NEUROMUSCULAR DISORDERS: TREATMENT AND MANAGEMENT   ISBN: 978-1-4377-0372-6

Notices

Knowledge and best practice in this field are constantly changing. As new research and experience broaden our understanding, changes in research methods, professional practices, or medical treatment may become necessary.

Practitioners and researchers must always rely on their own experience and knowledge in evaluating and using any information, methods, compounds, or experiments described herein. In using such information or methods they should be mindful of their own safety and the safety of others, including parties for whom they have a professional responsibility.

With respect to any drug or pharmaceutical products identified, readers are advised to check the most current information provided (i) on procedures featured or (ii) by the manufacturer of each product to be administered, to verify the recommended dose or formula, the method and duration of administration, and contraindications. It is the responsibility of practitioners, relying on their own experience and knowledge of their patients, to make diagnoses, to determine dosages and the best treatment for each individual patient, and to take all appropriate safety precautions.

To the fullest extent of the law, neither the Publisher nor the authors, contributors, or editors, assume any liability for any injury and/or damage to persons or property as a matter of products liability, negligence or otherwise, or from any use or operation of any methods, products, instructions, or ideas contained in the material herein.

Library of Congress Cataloging-in-Publication Data
Neuromuscular disorders: treatment and management / [edited by] Tulio E. Bertorini. —1st ed.
      p. ; cm.
   Includes bibliographical references.
   ISBN 978-1-4377-0372-6
   1. Neuromuscular diseases. I. Bertorini, Tulio E.
   [DNLM: 1. Neuromuscular Diseases—therapy. WE 550 N49443 2010]
   RC925.5.N474   2011
   616.7'44—dc22

                                                2010010083

Acquisitions Editor: Adrianne Brigido
Developmental Editor: Taylor Ball
Design Direction: Lou Forgione

Working together to grow
libraries in developing countries

www.elsevier.com | www.bookaid.org | www.sabre.org

ELSEVIER   BOOK AID International   Sabre Foundation

Printed in China

Last digit is the print number: 9 8 7 6 5 4 3 2 1

This work is dedicated to the members of my loving family: to my father,
Nicolas; the memory of my mother, Enriqueta; my wife, Emma; my daughter,
Paola and her husband Jason; my sons, Tulio and Francisco, and their girlfriends,
Stacy and Paulinha; as well as my grandson, Nicolas.
Also, I want to dedicate this book to the families of my collaborators and particularly to the
memory of my friend, excellent clinician and researcher,
Lisa Krivickas, MD, who collaborated in this book and who recently passed away.

Preface

Recent advances in the understanding of the genetics and basic mechanisms of neuromuscular diseases have been both rapid and spectacular. Furthermore, these advances have resulted in an expansion of the methods used for diagnosis—from routine clinical histologic and electrophysiologic tests to more specific techniques, such as biochemical and Western Blot analysis, and, most important, molecular genetic testing. These modern techniques have begun to replace more costly and painful procedures for some patients.

Innovations in the field of molecular genetics have led to the identification of certain protein deficiencies and thus to the design of replacement therapy for some conditions. Examples include enzyme replacement with recombinant alpha-glucosidase for Pompe disease and agalsidase for Fabry disease. Another important advance in the understanding of neuromuscular disorders has been the recognition of the pathways of the cascade of immune mechanisms of autoimmune diseases. This understanding allows us to treat these disorders with newer immunosuppressants and selective monoclonal antibodies that target specific molecules of this cascade. These treatments hold promise for better patient care, but more knowledge of possible adverse effects is needed. At times monoclonal antibodies have been found to cause autoimmune disorders, further complicating therapy.

Although the goal of our specialty is to find cures or effective treatments for neuromuscular disorders, the management of symptoms to improve quality of life is still paramount. The control of pain in the treatment of dysautonomic symptoms and the management of muscle hyperactivity in the myotonias are examples.

Ambulation and survival can be prolonged with well-planned rehabilitation programs, orthopaedic surgery, and proper early management of cardiac, respiratory, and gastrointestinal complications, particularly in patients with motor neuron diseases and muscular dystrophy. Prolonged survival has changed the care of these patients. For example, in the past patients with Duchenne muscular dystrophy generally died of respiratory failure before they developed symptomatic cardiac disease; now they are living longer and require aggressive treatment of their cardiac complications to further prolong their lives.

Many excellent textbooks and treatises dedicated to the understanding of the basic mechanisms of clinical and laboratory diagnoses of neuromuscular diseases also include discussions of treatment but this information is not comprehensive. In this text we aim to cover the current treatment and management of these subjects and to discuss promising experimental therapies. Also included are discussions of the prevention and treatment of neuromuscular complications of medical conditions and surgery.

The introductory chapter is a brief overview of the approach to diagnosis and treatment in patients with neuromuscular disease—information that we hope will be helpful to young clinicians. The next several chapters discuss complications of neuromuscular disorders and their general management, such as rehabilitation, orthopaedic surgery, and cardiac, gastrointestinal, and respiratory care, as well as the treatment of painful neuropathy and dysautonomia. The balance of the chapters cover specific diseases as well as the basic mechanisms of these disorders.

The information in each chapter is intended to complement that in others, although occasionally there are minor repetitions. When possible, evidence-based treatment recommendations are given, particularly for the more common conditions, though we emphasize that the treatment of all patients should be individualized. For less common disorders, for which controlled trials have not yet been published, recommendations are based on published information and the authors' experience.

I am honored and grateful for the collaboration of an excellent group of renowned specialists. They have generously contributed their time and expertise to make what we hope is a textbook that is useful for all physicians who care for patients with neuromuscular disorders.

Tulio E. Bertorini, MD

Acknowledgments

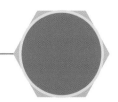

For their untiring editorial assistance, I want to express my sincere appreciation to Rachel Young, RN, BS, BSN, my research coordinator, and to Kay Daugherty, medical editor of the Campbell Foundation.

I thank Mariallen Shadle for her work on the excellent histologic slides and Cindy Culver for transcription of the manuscripts.

The compilation of my Introduction was completed with the help of Rachel Young, Mariallen Shadle, and Kay Daugherty.

Recognition is extended to Taylor Ball and Adrianne Brigido of Elsevier and to Peggy Gordon of P. M. Gordon Associates.

My appreciation is also extended to Wesley Neurology Clinic, Methodist Hospitals of Memphis, and The University of Tennessee Health Science Center for continuous support.

I wish in particular to express my gratitude to the authors and collaborators of the various chapters of this work, with a special thanks to their families, as they have sacrificed their time together to participate in the preparation of this book. I also wish to thank Drs. Genaro Palmieri, Abbas Kitabchi, and Cesar Magsino for their insightful comments regarding Chapter 20, on endocrine disorders.

Finally, to all of our patients, whom we hope will benefit from the knowledge we continue to gain.

Tulio E. Bertorini, MD

Contributors

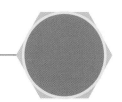

Bassam A. Bassam, MD
Professor of Neurology
Director of Neuromuscular and EMG Laboratory
University of South Alabama
College of Medicine
Attending and Professor of Neurology
University of South Alabama Medical Center
Mobile, Alabama
Chapters 10 and 20

Tulio E. Bertorini, MD
Professor of Neurology and Pathology
University of Tennessee, Center for the Health Sciences, Memphis
Chief of Neurology, Methodist University Hospital
Director, Wesley Neurology Clinic and Muscular Dystrophy
   and ALS Clinic
Memphis, Tennessee
Chapters 1, 7, 10, and 20

William W. Campbell, Jr., MD
Professor and Chairman
Uniformed Services University of Health Sciences
Chief, Clinical Neurophysiology
Walter Reed Army Medical Center
Bethesda, Maryland
Chapter 16

Vinay Chaudhry, MD
Professor of Neurology
Vice Chair, Clinical Affairs
Johns Hopkins University School of Medicine
Baltimore, Maryland
Chapter 13

Marinos C. Dalakas, MD
Professor, Clinical Neurosciences
Chief, Neuromuscular Diseases Service
Imperial College, London
Hammersmith Hospital Campus
London, England
Chief, Neuroimmunology Unit
Department of Pathophysiology
University of Athens Medical School
Athens, Greece
Chapter 21

Marcus Deschauer, MD
Neurologische Klinik
Universitat Halle-Wittenberg
Halle, Germany
Chapter 22

Diana M. Escolar, MD
Associate Professor of Neurology
John Hopkins School of Medicine
Center for Genetic Muscle Disorders
Kennedy Krieger Institute
Baltimore, Maryland
Chapter 19

Christopher H. Gibbons, MD, MMSc
Assistant Professor of Neurology
Harvard Medical School
Staff Neurologist
Beth Israel Deaconess Medical Center
Director, Diabetic Neuropathy Clinic
Joslin Diabetes Center
Boston, Massachusetts
Chapter 5

Daniel M. Goodenberger, MD
Professor and Chairman
Department of Medicine
University of Nevada School of Medicine
Las Vegas, Nevada
Chapter 2

Nivia Hernandez-Ramos, MD
Neuromuscular Medicine Program
Division of Neurology
University of Puerto Rico School of Medicine
San Juan, Puerto Rico
Chapter 15

Susan T. Iannaccone, MD
Jimmy Elizabeth Westcott Distinguished Chair
  in Pediatric Neurology
Professor of Neurology and Pediatrics
University of Texas Southwestern Medical Center
Director of Pediatric Neurology
Children's Medical Center
Chair, Section on Child Neurology
American Academy of Neurology
Dallas, Texas
Chapter 12

Cristian Ionita, MD
Assistant Professor of Pediatrics
University of Arkansas for Medical Sciences
Director of Neuromuscular Diagnostic Clinic
Arkansas Children's Hospital
Little Rock, Arkansas
Chapter 12

Mohammad K. Ismail, MD
Program Director
Gastroenterology Fellowship and Training
University of Tennessee, Memphis
Chief of Gastroenterology
Methodist University Hospital
Memphis, Tennessee
Chapter 4

Lisa S. Krivickas, MD[†]
Associate Professor of Physical Medicine and Rehabilitation
Harvard Medical School
Associate Chair of Academic Affairs
Associate Chief of Physical Medicine and Rehabilitation
Massachusetts General Hospital
Boston, Massachusetts
Chapter 8

Robert T. Leshner, MD
Professor of Neurology and Pediatrics
Children's National Medical Center
George Washington University
Washington, DC
Chapter 19

Yingjun David Li, MD
Consulting Neurologist
Methodist Le Bonheur Healthcare
Memphis, Tennessee
Chapter 10

Thomas E. Lloyd, MD, PhD
Assistant Professor
Department of Neurology
The Johns Hopkins School of Medicine
Baltimore, Maryland
Chapter 13

Catherine Lomen-Hoerth, MD, PhD
Associate Professor of Neurology
University of California, San Francisco
San Francisco, California
Chapter 11

Carlos A. Luciano, MD
Professor of Neurology
Director, Neuromuscular Medicine Program
Division of Neurology
University of Puerto Rico School of Medicine
San Juan, Puerto Rico
Chapter 15

Daniel L. Menkes, MD
Director of Clinical Neurophysiology
University of Connecticut Health Center
Farmington, Connecticut
Chapter 6

Christopher W. Mitchell, MD
Neurologist
West Tennessee Neurosciences
Jackson, Tennessee
Chapters 7 and 10

Pushpa Narayanaswami, MD
Instructor of Neurology
Division of Neuromuscular Diseases
Department of Neurology
Harvard Medical School
Beth Israel Deaconess Medical Center
Boston, Massachusetts
Chapter 17

Peter O'Carroll, MD
Fellow, Clinical Neurophysiology
The University of Tennessee Health Science Center
Memphis, Tennessee
Chapter 19

Shin J. Oh, MD
Distinguished Professor of Neurology
Department of Neurology and Pathology
University of Alabama at Birmingham
Birmingham, Alabama
Chapter 18

Nicholas J. Silvestri, MD
Assistant Professor of Neurology
State University of New York at Buffalo School of Medicine
Staff Neurologist
Erie County Medical Center
Buffalo, New York
Chapter 5

[†]Deceased

Zachary Simmons, MD
Professor of Neurology
The Pennsylvania State University School of Medicine
Director, Neuromuscular Program and ALS Center
Penn State Hershey Medical Center
Hershey, Pennsylvania
Chapter 14

Christopher F. Spurney, MD
Assistant Professor of Pediatrics
Division of Cardiology
Children's National Heart Institute
Children's National Medical Center
Washington, DC
Chapter 3

Matthias Vorgerd, MD
Associate Professor of Neurology
Bergmannsheil GmbH
Department of Neurology, Ruhr-University Bochum
Neuromuscular Center
Bochum, Germany
Chapter 22

William C. Warner, Jr., MD
Professor, Department of Orthopaedic Surgery
University of Tennessee Center for the Health Sciences
LeBonheur Children's Medical Center
Campbell Clinic, Inc.
Memphis, Tennessee
Chapter 9

Dorothy Weiss, MD, EdM
Clinical Fellow, Physical Medicine and Rehabilitation
Chief Resident, Spaulding Rehabilitation Hospital
Harvard Medical School
Boston, Massachusetts
Chapter 8

Contents

PART I:

General Principles in the Treatment and Management of Neuromuscular Disorders

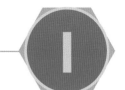

Tulio E. Bertorini, MD

Introduction: Evaluation of Patients with Neuromuscular Disorders

This book is dedicated to the treatment of neuromuscular disorders (NMDs), which include those that affect the anterior horn cells, nerve roots, plexi, peripheral nerves, neuromuscular junction, and muscles (Fig. 1-1).[1] These disorders may be caused by genetic defects or may be acquired, as in autoimmune diseases; they also may be secondary to general medical conditions or may arise as complications of surgery. To make therapeutic decisions about these disorders, clinicians should be able to recognize their clinical presentation and characteristics. This chapter provides a brief introduction to the evaluation of patients with NMDs.

Medical History and Symptoms

The evaluation should include obtaining detailed medical and family histories as well as identifying possible complicating factors. In children, information should be obtained on the prenatal period and delivery, especially if the patient was a "floppy baby," and details of the patient's developmental milestones should be recorded.[1,2]

Identifying general medical problems is important because some NMDs are associated with other conditions, such as, for example, endocrine and connective tissue diseases. Medications also should be considered, because many are known to produce neurologic complications.

Muscle weakness is a common symptom, except in patients with sensory or autonomic neuropathy or in some radiculopathies and entrapment syndromes. The rate of progression varies, and in some conditions, such as Guillain-Barré syndrome (GBS), electrolyte imbalance, toxic neuropathy, and myopathy associated with rhabdomyolysis, it is rapid (Box 1-1). In disorders of neuromuscular transmission, such as myasthenia gravis (MG), weakness fluctuates during the day. In periodic paralysis, weakness is recurrent,[3] whereas in other disorders, such as muscular dystrophies, or in hereditary and some autoimmune neuropathies, it is subacute or chronic (Box 1-2).[3,4]

The distribution of weakness also is important in diagnosis; for example, it is proximal in spinal muscular atrophies and most myopathies, except for some rare disorders in which it is more distal. In myopathies, weakness usually is symmetric, although asymmetry can be seen in some cases, as in fascioscapulohumeral dystrophy. In polyneuropathies, this characteristically begins in the legs, but may initially manifest more prominently in the upper extremities, as in multifocal neuropathy, brachial plexopathies, and cervical spinal canal disorders as well as in amyotrophic lateral sclerosis (ALS). This follows the territory of roots or nerves in radiculopathies and focal neuropathies.[4]

Dysphagia, diplopia, and droopy eyelids also help to identify NMDs because they occur in some myopathies and also in disorders of neuromuscular transmission, such as MG. Symptoms of respiratory difficulty should be recognized and treated promptly because this can be the first manifestation of a disorder such as MG, GBS, ALS, and myopathies, such as acid maltase deficiency, whereas in other disorders, it appears at later stages.[4,5]

Difficulty combing the hair and placing objects in high cabinets commonly occurs in patients with shoulder-girdle weakness, whereas difficulty writing and grasping objects indicates involvement of the forearm and hand muscles, as in ALS and inclusion body myositis. Weakness of the hip extensors usually causes inability to rise from a low chair or a toilet seat, whereas difficulty ascending stairs indicates dysfunction of the hip flexors and quadriceps muscles. More severe weakness of the quadriceps muscles occurs in inclusion body myositis, causing difficulty descending stairs.[3,6] When the distal muscles are affected, foot drop may cause a steppage gait and difficulty negotiating curves or changing courses, as seen in polyneuropathies, distal dystrophies, and ALS.

Muscle stiffness, tightness, and spasms occur as a result of spasticity in disorders affecting the upper motor neuron, but these also occur in patients with motor unit hyperactivity, such as "stiff-person" and Isaac syndromes or the myotonias. Those with inflammatory myopathies, polymyalgia rheumatica, fasciitis, and hypothyroidism also complain of stiff limbs. Cramping at rest or during exercise is a prominent symptom of cramp-fasciculation syndrome[7] and also some neuropathies. In metabolic myopathies, this usually occurs during or after exercise, or after fasting in some cases. Fatigue is common in disorders of neuromuscular transmission, such as Eaton-Lambert syndrome (ELS) and MG, but also in myopathies, even though weakness is the major symptom. In ELS, there may be temporary improvement after brief exercise.

Numbness and decreased sensation as well as paresthesias and neuropathic pain are symptoms of peripheral neuropathies.[8] These symptoms are localized in the affected areas in those with radiculopathies, plexopathies, and entrapment neuropathies. Autonomic dysfunction can occur in some neuropathies and also in ELS.

Physical Examination

A careful general physical examination is essential to arrive at a diagnosis, and the clinician should assess cardiac and lung function, examine the eyes for cataracts and retinal disease, and check for hearing loss,

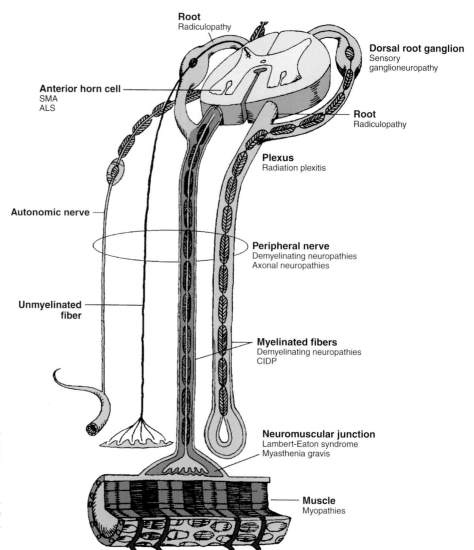

Root
Radiculopathy

Dorsal root ganglion
Sensory
ganglioneuropathy

Anterior horn cell
SMA
ALS

Root
Radiculopathy

Plexus
Radiation plexitis

Autonomic nerve

Peripheral nerve
Demyelinating neuropathies
Axonal neuropathies

Unmyelinated
fiber

Myelinated fibers
Demyelinating neuropathies
CIDP

Neuromuscular junction
Lambert-Eaton syndrome
Myasthenia gravis

Muscle
Myopathies

Figure 1-1 Anatomic elements of the peripheral nervous system and related neurologic disorders. ALS, amyotrophic lateral sclerosis; CIDP, chronic inflammatory demyelinating polyneuropathy; SMA, spinal muscular atrophy. (Adapted from Bertorini TE: Overview and classification of neuromuscular disorders. In Bertorini TE, ed: *Clinical Evaluation and Diagnostic Tests for Neuromuscular Disorders*, Woburn, MA, 2002, Butterworth-Heinemann, pp 1–13.)

Box 1-1 Neuromuscular Disorders That May Present with Acute Generalized Weakness

Motor Neuron Diseases

Poliomyelitis
Amyotrophic lateral sclerosis (rarely)

Neuropathies

Guillain-Barré syndrome and variants
Porphyria, particularly acute intermittent
Dinoflagellate toxins
Diphtheria
Arsenic poisoning and other acute toxic neuropathies

Disorders of Neuromuscular Transmission

Botulism and other biologic toxins (black widow spider bites, snake bites)
Organophosphate poisoning
Eaton-Lambert myasthenic syndrome
Hypermagnesemia
Myasthenia gravis

Myopathies

Rhabdomyolysis (from various causes, including metabolic, toxic, and infectious)
Polymyositis/dermatomyositis
Infectious myositis (e.g., trichinosis, toxoplasmosis)
Electrolyte imbalance (e.g., hypohyperkalemia, hypermagnesemia, hypocalcemia, hypercalcemia, hypophosphatemia)
Hyperthyroidism
Toxins
Intensive care myopathy (after immobilization with paralyzing agents and steroids in the intensive care unit)

Box 1-2 Examples of Conditions That Present with Progressive Subacute or Chronic Proximal Muscle Weakness

Progressive spinal muscular atrophy
Bulbospinal muscular atrophy (Kennedy disease)
Amyotrophic lateral sclerosis (sometimes)
Chronic inflammatory demyelinating neuropathy
Eaton-Lambert myasthenic syndrome
Myasthenia gravis
Endocrine diseases (e.g., hypothyroidism, Cushing disease, hyperparathyroidism)
Drugs (e.g., steroids, cholesterol-lowering agents, zidovudine, colchicine, chloroquine)
Toxins (e.g., alcoholic myopathy)
Electrolyte imbalance
Congenital myopathies (usually of earlier onset)
Muscular dystrophies
Polymyositis and dermatomyositis
Inclusion body myositis
Adult "nemaline" or "rod" myopathy
Mitochondrial myopathy
Juvenile and adult forms of acid maltase deficiency
Carnitine deficiency

which is often seen in mitochondrial disorders. Visceromegaly and skin changes are present in some patients with neuropathies, for example, those with POEMS (polyneuropathy, organomegaly, endocrinopathy, monoclonal gammopathy, skin changes) syndrome. Skin abnormalities can also be seen in connective tissue disorders, whereas patients with dermatomyositis have a characteristic rash.[4]

Intellectual function should be assessed because it could be impaired in some diseases, such as in some cases of ALS and in myotonic dystrophy. During the neurologic examination, posture and muscle strength should be evaluated to determine, for example, whether there is hyperlordosis with proximal atrophy in myopathies or distal atrophy in neuropathies, whether it is symmetric (Fig. 1-2) or focal (Fig. 1-3), or whether it affects the upper or lower extremities more prominently (see Fig. 1-2). The clinician should examine the patient for muscle hypertrophy, which is seen in some dystrophies and disorders of neuromuscular hyperactivity. Examination of muscle tone also is important to determine whether there is focal or generalized hypotonia, particularly in infants (Fig. 1-4 and Box 1-3). Gait analysis includes observation for the characteristic waddling of myopathies, the circumduction of spasticity, the steppage gait of peripheral neuropathy and distal dystrophies, and the ataxic gait in

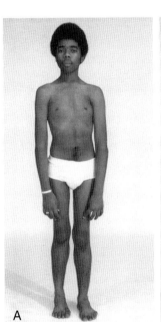
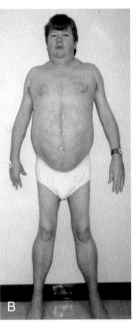
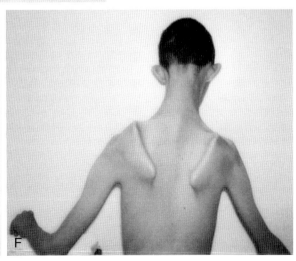
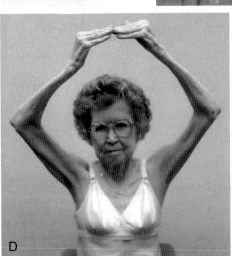
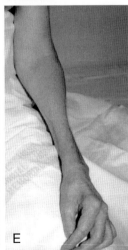
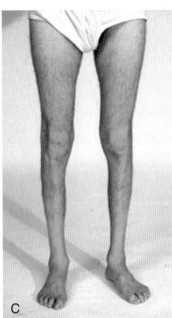

Figure 1-2 A, Patient with juvenile spinal muscular atrophy showing hyperpronation of the arms with atrophy of the pectoralis and quadriceps muscles and mild calf hypertrophy. **B,** Lordosis, calf hypertrophy, and atrophy of the thigh muscles in a patient with Becker muscular dystrophy. **C,** Patient with peripheral neuropathy showing distal leg wasting. **D,** Forearm and hand atrophy in a patient with inclusion body myositis. **E,** Prominent forearm wasting and wrist extensor weakness in a patient with Welander muscular dystrophy. **F,** Patient with congenital myotonic dystrophy with prominent winging and inward rotation of both scapulae. (**A–D,** From Bertorini TE: *Neuromuscular Case Studies,* Philadelphia, 2008, Butterworth-Heinemann, pp 273, 477, 29; **E** and **F,** From Bertorini TE: Clinical evaluation and clinical diagnostic tests. In Bertorini TE, ed: *Clinical Evaluation and Diagnostic Tests for Neuromuscular Disorders,* Woburn, MA, 2002, Butterworth-Heinemann, pp 15–97.)

A

B

C

D

E

F

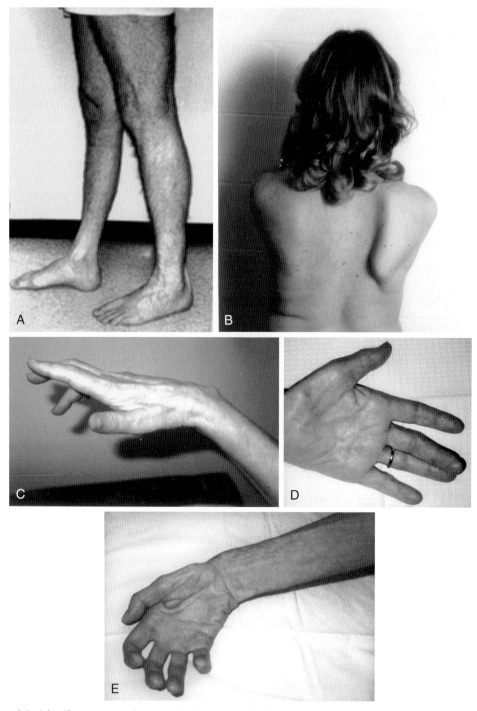

Figure 1-3 A, Wasting of the left calf in a patient with postmyelopathy amyotrophy from a cornus medullaris lesion involving the anterior horn cells of L5 to S1 segments with chronic denervation on electromyography. **B,** Patient with brachial plexopathy and serratus anterior weakness causing winging of the scapula and medial deviation of the bone. **C,** Patient with ulnar neuropathy attempting hand and finger extension, showing partial flexion of the last two digits and atrophy of the first dorsal interosseous muscle. **D,** Median neuropathy causing thenar atrophy. **E,** Claw hand and atrophy of the median and ulnar innervated muscles. (**A–C,** From Bertorini TE: *Neuromuscular Case Studies*, Philadelphia, 2008, Butterworth-Heinemann, pp 247, 145, 125; **D** and **E,** From Bertorini TE: Clinical evaluation and clinical diagnostic tests. In Bertorini TE, ed: *Clinical Evaluation and Diagnostic Tests for Neuromuscular Disorders*, Woburn, MA, 2002, Butterworth-Heinemann, pp 15–97.)

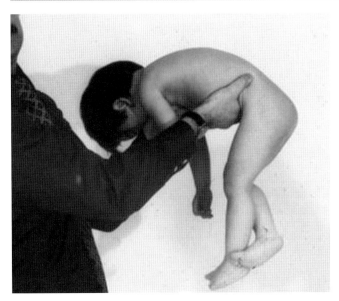

Figure 1-4 Floppy infant with infantile acid maltase deficiency. Note how the limbs hang loosely and the chest is arched when the examiner holds the patient by the thorax. (From Bertorini TE: *Neuromuscular Case Studies*, Philadelphia, 2008, Butterworth-Heinemann, p 537.)

Box 1-3 Causes of Floppy Infants

Central Nervous System Disorders

Cerebral palsy
Mental retardation from primary metabolic disorders

Mixed (Central and Peripheral)

Metachromatic leukodystrophy and other lipidosis
Neuroaxonal atrophy
Giant axonal neuropathy
Merosin-deficient muscular dystrophy, other congenital muscular
    dystrophies (e.g., Fukuyama type)

Anterior Horn Cell Diseases

Infantile spinal muscular atrophy

Neuropathies

Charcot-Marie-Tooth disease, particularly types 3 and 4

Diseases of the Neuromuscular Junction

Congenital myasthenic syndromes
Infantile botulism
Neonatal transient autoimmune myasthenia gravis

Myopathies

Infantile metabolic myopathies (e.g., acid maltase deficiencies or
    Pompe disease, infantile phosphorylase deficiency)
Congenital muscular dystrophy
Other congenital myopathies (e.g., central core disease, myotubular
    myopathy, nemaline myopathy)
Congenital myotonic dystrophy
Myopathy from electrolyte and endocrine abnormalities

those with spinal cerebellar degeneration[4] or neuropathies causing prominent proprioceptive deficits that could also cause a positive Romberg test.

Examination of the eyelids and eye movements is helpful to diagnose acute paralysis in diabetic ophthalmoplegia and Miller-Fisher syndrome or chronic paralysis in mitochondrial myopathy and oculopharyngeal dystrophy (Fig. 1-5). Fluctuating ophthalmoplegia and ptosis are seen in MG (Fig. 1-6).[9] Assessment of the pupils

determines the presence of Horner syndrome (Fig. 1-7), whereas poorly reactive pupils may be seen in some neuropathies.[4,5]

Prominent facial weakness occurs in GBS, but also in MG and some dystrophies. A decreased or hyperactive gag reflex, as in ALS, not only might provide help in the diagnosis, but also might determine the risk of aspiration. Tongue atrophy and fasciculations are characteristically seen in motor neuron diseases, whereas a typical forked tongue occurs in MG (Fig. 1-8). Examination of the neck muscles helps to identify neck extensor muscle weakness causing head drop (Fig. 1-9 and Box 1-4).[10]

Manual muscle testing with proper grading helps to determine the distribution and degree of involvement, assess the progression of the disease, and diagnose segmental neurologic disorders. The examination should also include observation for fasciculations, which are more common in motor neuron disorders, but also are seen in some neuropathies, such as multifocal motor neuropathy. Increased reflexes with the presence of the Babinski sign indicate involvement of the corticospinal tracts, as in ALS, whereas generalized hypo- or areflexia is seen in peripheral neuropathies and some neuromuscular transmission disorders, such as ELS and botulism. Distal reflexes are lost early in neuropathies and are preserved until the later stages in myopathies (Table 1-1). The examiner also should observe the patient for myotonia (Fig. 1-10), myoedema, and slow relaxation of the ankle reflexes, as seen in hypothyroidism.

The sensory examination helps to determine the type and distribution of deficits to determine whether they are distal, symmetric, or follow the dermatomes of nerve roots or individual nerves, and whether they affect more severely the large myelinated axons (proprioceptive deficits), the unmyelinated axons (dysautonomia, pain, and temperature deficits), or both.[5,8,11,12]

Diagnostic Tests

Laboratory studies should include a complete chemistry profile, which can help in the diagnosis of several disorders; for example, low or high potassium is seen in the periodic paralyses, whereas hypocalcemia and hypomagnesia are associated with tetany. Hypercalcemia could lead to the diagnosis of hyperparathyroidism. Elevated blood sugar levels could indicate diabetes as a cause of peripheral neuropathy and, if blood sugar levels are normal and the diagnosis is suspected, this testing should be followed by measurement of 2-hour postprandial blood sugar and glycosylated hemoglobin levels. A complete blood count also is helpful to assess for anemia, as seen in connective tissue diseases, and for leukocytosis, indicating infection or leukopenia from medication effects. An elevated erythrocyte sedimentation rate implies an inflammatory process, although it has low specificity, and increased mean corpuscular volume could suggest pernicious anemia or folate deficiency.[13] Testing for serum muscle enzymes is important, particularly serum creatine, aspartate aminotransferase, alanine aminotransferase, and aldolase, which are elevated in myopathies and sometimes in motor neuron disorders[14] and hypothyroidism. Elevated levels of alanine aminotransferase and aspartate aminotransferase alone suggest liver disease, and when this is considered, gamma glutamyl transpeptidase should be measured because it is affected only in liver disease. A very high creatine level with myoglobulin in plasma and urine is characteristic of rhabdomyolysis.[4,15]

Assessment of autoimmune myopathies and neuropathies also should include measurement of complement, lupus serology, and cryoglobulins.[16] SSA and SSB antibodies should be tested when Sjögren syndrome is suspected as the cause of ganglioneuritis and myositis.

Figure 1-5 A, Patient with diabetic third-nerve palsy with ptosis of the left eye (*left*). Limitation of adduction of the same eye (*right*). **B,** Ophthalmoplegia and ptosis in a patient with Miller-Fisher syndrome. **C,** Ptosis and symmetric limitation of gaze in a patient with mitochondrial myopathy. **D,** Astronomer's posture in a patient with oculopharyngeal dystrophy showing ptosis and contraction of the frontalis muscle to compensate for the ptosis. (**A, C,** and **D,** From Bertorini TE: Clinical evaluation and clinical diagnostic tests. In Bertorini TE, ed: *Clinical Evaluation and Diagnostic Tests for Neuromuscular Disorders*, Woburn, MA, 2002, Butterworth-Heinemann, pp 15–97; **B,** From Bertorini TE: *Neuromuscular Case Studies*, Philadelphia, 2008, Butterworth-Heinemann, p 288.)

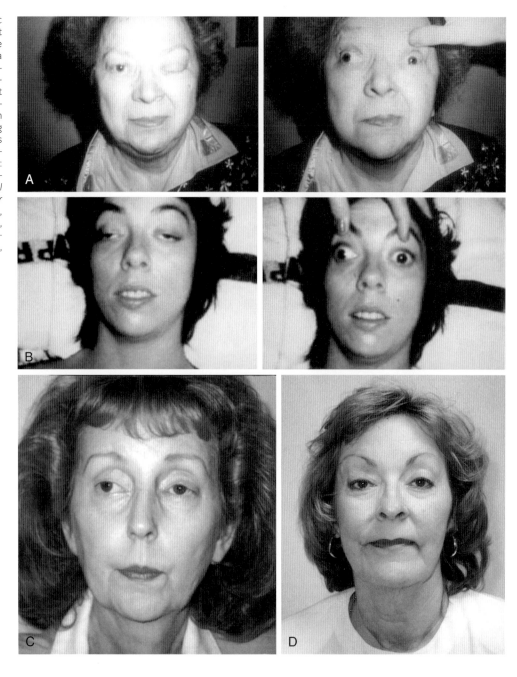

Figure 1-6 A, Patient with myasthenia gravis. **B,** Development of ptosis on sustained upward gaze. (From Bertorini TE: *Neuromuscular Case Studies*, Philadelphia, 2008, Butterworth-Heinemann.)

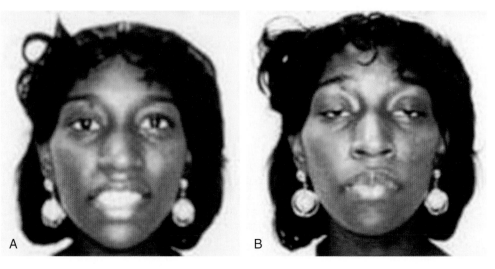

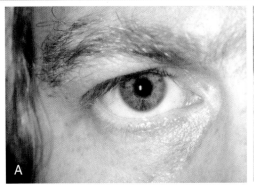

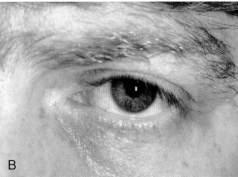

Figure 1-7 Horner syndrome of the left eye (**B**) in a patient with lymphoma of the lower brachial plexus showing ptosis and a smaller pupil in the affected eye compared with the normal eye (**A**). (From Bertorini TE: *Neuromuscular Case Studies,* Philadelphia, 2008, Butterworth-Heinemann, p 150.)

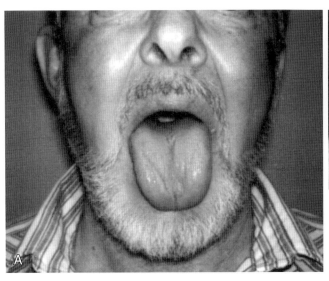

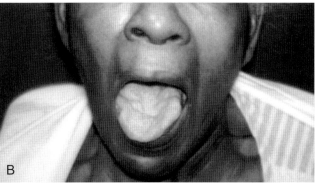

Figure 1-8 A, Patient with myasthenia gravis with a forked, triple furrowed tongue. **B,** Amyotrophic lateral sclerosis with tongue atrophy. (From Bertorini TE: Clinical evaluation and clinical diagnostic tests. In Bertorini TE, ed: *Clinical Evaluation and Diagnostic Tests for Neuromuscular Disorders,* Woburn, MA, 2002, Butterworth-Heinemann, pp 15–97.)

Measurement of a number of other antibodies is helpful in the diagnosis. These include, for example, those against myelin-associated glycoprotein, GM1, and other gangliosides, as well as Hu antibodies in autoimmune neuropathies, and those against acid decarboxylase and antiphysin antibodies in stiff person syndrome. Assessment of acetylcholine receptor and MuSK antibodies helps in those suspected of having MG, whereas elevation of voltage-gated

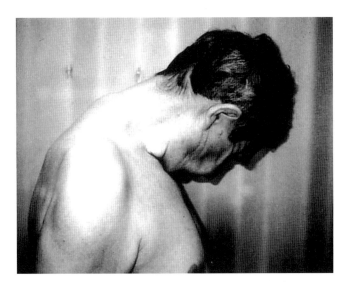

Figure 1-9 Head drop in a patient with amyotrophic lateral sclerosis as a result of neck extensor weakness. (From Bertorini TE: *Neuromuscular Case Studies,* Philadelphia, 2008, Butterworth-Heinemann, p 229.)

Box 1-4 Conditions Associated with Cervical Paraspinal Weakness and Dropped Head Syndrome

Prominent, Early Paraspinal Weakness in Generalized Processes

Amyotrophic lateral sclerosis
Myasthenia gravis
Polymyositis/dermatomyositis

Isolated Paraspinal Muscle Weakness

Isolated neck extensor myopathy
Bent spine syndrome
Benign focal amyotrophy

Other Diseases Associated with Paraspinal Weakness, Atrophy, or Both

Chronic inflammatory demyelinating polyneuropathy
Eaton-Lambert myasthenic syndrome
Inclusion body myositis
Facioscapulohumeral dystrophy
Nemaline myopathy
Proximal myotonic myopathy
Mitochondrial myopathy
Acid maltase deficiency
Carnitine deficiency
Hypokalemic myopathy
Hyperparathyroidism

Disorders That Mimic Dropped Head Syndrome

Cervical dystonia (anterocollis)
Fixed skeletal deformities of the spine

From Narayanaswami P, Bertorini T: The dropped head syndrome. *J Clin Neuromusc Dis* 2:106–112, 2000.

Table 1-1 Neuromuscular Disease: Clinical Evaluation

Clinical Parameter	Motor Neuron Disease	Polyneuropathy	Myopathy	Diseases of Neuromuscular Junction
Pattern of weakness	Variable, symmetric in most, often asymmetric in ALS	Distal > proximal	Proximal > distal; fluctuates; often involves extraocular muscles	Proximal distal in most
Fasciculations	Yes	Sometimes	No	No
Muscle stretch reflexes	Variable, decreased in most, increased in ALS	Decreased or absent	Normal in postsynaptic disorders (myasthenia gravis), decreased in presynaptic disorders (Eaton-Lambert syndrome and botulism)	Normal initially, may be decreased in later stages (ankle reflexes often preserved until very late)
Sensory loss	No	Usually present	No	No

ALS, amyotrophic lateral sclerosis.

From Bertorini TE, ed: *Clinical Evaluation and Diagnostic Tests for Neuromuscular Disorders*, Woburn, MA, 2002, Butterworth-Heinemann.

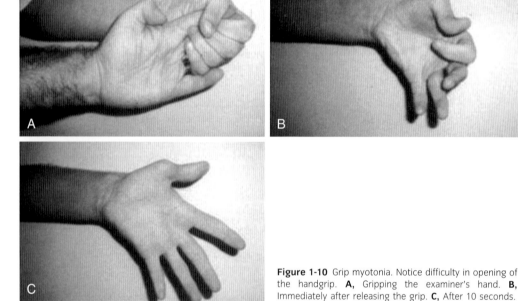

Figure 1-10 Grip myotonia. Notice difficulty in opening of the handgrip. **A,** Gripping the examiner's hand. **B,** Immediately after releasing the grip. **C,** After 10 seconds.

calcium antibodies is seen in patients with ELS and those against voltage-gated potassium channels[17-20] are elevated in Isaac syndrome. JO antibodies are elevated in some patients with myositis and interstitial lung disease.[21] These tests are discussed in detail in Chapters 14, 17, 18, and 21.

Other studies that may be appropriate, depending on the presentation, include measurement of vitamin B_{12}, folic acid, and if pernicious anemia is suspected, methylmalonic acid and homocysteine levels. Measurement of copper levels and thyroid function testing, as well urinary arsenic, porphyrins,[22,23] and serum and urine immunoelectrophoresis testing, are helpful for the evaluation of polyneuropathies.

Spinal fluid analysis is not always necessary; however, it can help to identify high protein levels in acquired demyelinating neuropathies or an elevated number of lymphocytes in those with human immunodeficiency virus, for whom serologic testing should be performed.

Electrophysiologic Tests

Nerve conduction studies help to identify diseases affecting sensory or motor nerves, or both,[24,25] assisting in the differentiation of axonal from demyelinating neuropathies, and can also localize focal entrapments.[25] Measurement of latencies of proximal responses, such as the H-reflex and F-waves, helps to show more proximal demyelination. Significant conduction velocity slowing and prolonged or absent F-waves and H-reflexes are seen in acquired demyelinating neuropathies, such as GBS and chronic inflammatory demyelinating polyneuropathy, in which there also are conduction blocks (Fig. 1-11) and temporal dispersion of the compound muscle action potential (CMAP), whereas uniform slowing occurs in most hereditary demyelinating neuropathies.[5] Somatosensory-evoked responses also help in the diagnosis of disorders involving central pathways, such as pernicious anemia.[26]

The blink reflex is another test applied in the diagnosis of proximal demyelination and disorders that affect the facial and trigeminal

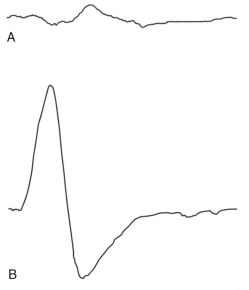

Figure 1-11 **A,** Conduction block (500 µV/10 msec) in a patient with acquired demyelinating polyneuropathy. **B,** Musculocutaneous compound muscle action potential from the axilla and at Erb point stimulation. (From Bertorini TE: *Neuromuscular Case Studies*, Philadelphia, 2008, Butterworth-Heinemann, p 326.)

nerves,[27] whereas autonomic function should be tested in those with autonomic dysfunction and small-fiber polyneuropathies.[28]

The repetitive stimulation test is used for the evaluation of neuromuscular transmission defects, particularly MG, showing the characteristic decrement of the CMAP at slow stimulation rates,[29,30] whereas in ELS, the CMAP is of low amplitude, which increases (facilitation) after a tetanic contraction or during fast stimulation[31] (see Chapter 18). A double response of the CMAP is seen in some congenital myasthenic syndromes, such as slow-channel syndrome (Fig. 1-12), and in overmedication with anticholinesterase drugs or organophosphate poisoning.[29]

Needle electromyography assesses the presence of spontaneous activity and its distribution, helping in the diagnosis.

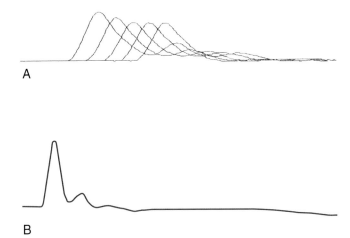

Figure 1-12 **A,** Compound muscle action potential of the abductor digiti minimi muscle during repetitive stimulation of the ulnar nerve at 2 Hz in a patient with slow-channel myasthenic syndrome showing a decrement of the CMAP during repetitive stimulation (2 mV/2 msec). **B,** Characteristics after discharge (second wave) of the CMAP (2 mV/5 msec). (From Bertorini TE: Neurological evaluation and diagnostic tests. In Bertorini TE, ed: *Neuromuscular Case Studies*, Philadelphia, 2008, Butterworth-Heinemann, pp 27–76.)

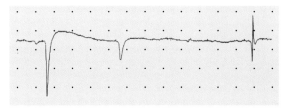

Figure 1-13 Two positive sharp waves and one fibrillation potential (200 µV/10 msec). (From Bertorini TE: Neurological evaluation and diagnostic tests. In Bertorini TE, ed: *Neuromuscular Case Studies*, Philadelphia, 2008, Butterworth-Heinemann, pp 27–76.)

Fasciculations, which are spontaneous depolarizations of the motor unit, are more commonly seen in motor neuron diseases, but as discussed earlier, could also occur in some neuropathies and metabolic disorders, and even in healthy persons. Myokymic discharges are seen, particularly in radiation plexopathies and GBS. Fibrillations and positive sharp waves are denervation potentials originating from individual denervated muscle fibers (Fig. 1-13). These are observed in neurogenic disorders (Table 1-2), but can also occur in the myopathies, causing membrane instability, such as polymyositis (Fig. 1-14), and some muscular dystrophies. Myotomal distribution of fibrillations or positive waves helps to localize segmental neurologic disorders, such as mononeuropathies and radiculopathies (Table 1-3).[32–34]

The characteristic waxing and waning myotonic discharges (Fig. 1-15) accompanied by clinical myotonia are seen in chloride and some sodium channelopathies, whereas electrical myotonia not accompanied by clinical myotonia can sometimes be found in some myopathies, such as polymyositis and acid maltase deficiency. Neuromyotonia and myokymic discharges are present diffusely in Isaac syndrome. Doublets, triplets, or multiplex potentials can be observed in motor neuron diseases, but are characteristic of tetany. Complex repetitive discharges occur in disorders of peripheral nerves, but also in myopathies (Fig. 1-16).

Analysis of motor unit action potentials (MUAPs) is valuable in diagnosis because large MUAPs with decreased recruitment are observed in chronic neuropathies and can be seen in motor neuron diseases (Fig. 1-17), whereas in myopathies, MUAPs are small and their recruitment is increased for the level of effort. In both types of disorders, MUAPs could be polyphasic, but small, polyphasic MUAPs of decreased recruitment are seen during early reinnervation (Fig. 1-18).[32] Satellite potentials occur in both neurogenic and myopathic disorders, whereas MUAPs of amplitude variability are characteristic of neuromuscular transmission diseases, but can also be seen in ALS.

Single-fiber electromyography is a more sophisticated technique that is used in the diagnosis of neuromuscular transmission disorders (Fig. 1-19). This test has high sensitivity, but low specificity, because increased "jitter" (increased variability of firing of individual muscle fiber potentials in relation to others of the same motor unit) and blocking occur in motor neuron diseases. However, when there is no evidence of other abnormalities on routine electromyography, increased jitter and blocking are diagnostic of neuromuscular transmission defects.[35]

Histologic Tests

Muscle biopsy is a valuable diagnostic tool that uses frozen sections for histochemistry (Fig. 1-20),[36] electromicroscopy, Western blot analysis, and biochemistry,[37] and in some mitochondrial disorders,

Table 1-2 Neuromuscular Disease: Laboratory Evaluation

Test	Motor Neuron Disease	Polyneuropathy	Myopathy	Disease of Neuromuscular Junction
Serum "muscle" enzymes	Normal or mild elevation	Normal	Increased	Normal
Nerve conduction studies	Normal or low-amplitude CMAPs, normal SNAPs	Usually slow nerve conduction velocities or low-amplitude CMAPs and SNAPs	Normal	Normal
Electromyography	Decreased number of MUAPs, evidence of denervation and reinnervation (large MUAPs)	Decreased number of motor units, evidence of denervation and reinnervation (large MUAPs)	Normal number of MUAPs that are of short duration and low amplitude, frequently polyphasic	Normal or small MUAPs, variability of motor unit size and shape
Repetitive nerve stimulation test	Usually normal; decremental responses of CMAPs can occur	Normal	Normal	Decrement of CMAPs at low rate of stimulation, increment at fast rates in presynaptic disorders
Muscle biopsy	Denervation (atrophic angular and target fibers, fiber type grouping, group atrophy)	Denervation (atrophic angular and target fibers, fiber type grouping)	"Myopathic" (necrosis, storage material inflammation)	Normal or some type II muscle fiber atrophy

CMAPs, compound muscle action potentials; SNAPs, sensory nerve action potentials; MUAPs, motor unit action potentials.
From Bertorini TE, ed: *Clinical Evaluation and Diagnostic Tests for Neuromuscular Disorders*, Woburn, MA, 2002, Butterworth-Heinemann.

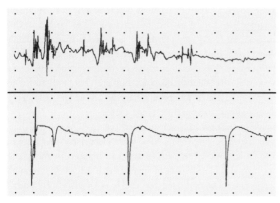

Figure 1-14 Electromyography study of the deltoid muscle in a patient with polymyositis. Note the small polyphasic motor units (*top*) and tracing showing positive sharp wave (100 μV/10 msec). (From Bertorini TE: Neurological evaluation and diagnostic tests. In Bertorini TE, ed: *Neuromuscular Case Studies*, Philadelphia, 2008, Butterworth-Heinemann, pp 27–76.)

also for DNA analysis. The biopsy specimen should always be obtained from a mildly affected muscle, likely opposite those in which electromyographic abnormalities are present. Biopsy from an end-stage muscle might not provide an accurate diagnosis, and specimens should not be taken close to a tendon, because the findings might resemble changes seen in chronic myopathies. In patients with muscle pain, fascia biopsy helps to diagnose fasciitis.[36,38]

Many histologic findings are characteristic of some conditions; for example, atrophic angular fibers that stain dark with nonspecific esterase, target fibers, fiber type grouping, and group atrophy are indicative of neurogenic disorders (Fig. 1-21 and Tables 1-2 and 1-4).[39] Inflammation and perifascicular atrophy are diagnostic of dermatomyositis, and ragged red fibers are characteristic of mitochondrial disorders, whereas enzyme deficiencies and lipid or

glycogen accumulation are found in metabolic myopathies (examples of other myopathies are seen in Fig. 1-22). Otherwise, in most myopathies, the biopsy specimen may show hypertrophy and atrophy, internalized nuclei, and proliferation of interstitial connective tissue and fat.[36,39]

Muscle biopsy can be avoided in some diseases. For example, in patients who present as a floppy baby with a positive family history and in whom spinal muscular atrophy is suspected, direct DNA testing may be diagnostic, and in those with suspected acid maltase deficiency, a definite diagnosis can be made by enzyme measurement in blood cells. In dystrophinopathies with characteristic phenotypes or patients with a positive family history, direct DNA testing may also be diagnostic. However, in a small group of patients, this testing is uninformative, and for these patients, biopsy for Western blot analysis is still necessary.

Nerve biopsy is used less frequently than muscle biopsy but can help in the evaluation of significant axonal degeneration or demyelination and the onion bulbs in chronic demyelination (Table 1-5).[36,40–43] Nerve biopsy might also provide findings that are diagnostic of some disorders, such as leprosy, hereditary neuropathy with liability to pressure palsy and storage diseases, such as amyloidosis, and vasculitis (Fig. 1-23),[44] for which simultaneous muscle biopsy is recommended to increase the diagnostic yield.[45]

Imaging has become increasingly valuable, particularly in focal conditions; for example, magnetic resonance imaging of the spine, which is performed in patients suspected of having ALS, helps to diagnose cervical spondylosis or compressive root disease.[46] Ultrasound and magnetic resonance imaging of muscle help to determine the distribution of atrophy and localize the muscle for biopsy.[47,48] Ultrasound of nerves and magnetic resonance neurography are helpful in focal peripheral neuropathies.[47]

Molecular diagnostic tests help to arrive at a specific diagnosis when analyzing for deletions, duplications, point mutations,

Table 1-3 Clinical and Laboratory Descriptions of Segmental Neurologic Disorders

	Mononeuropathy	Plexopathy	Radiculopathy
Muscle strength and reflexes	Weakness, decreased reflexes in muscles innervated by single nerves	Weakness or decreased reflexes in muscles innervated from affected plexus nerves	Weakness in muscles innervated by same root but different nerves
Sensory deficit	Follows a single nerve dermatome	Follows a plexus sensory territory	Follows dermatomes of affected roots
Limb needle electromyography	Signs of denervation in the myotome of one nerve	Signs of denervation in multiple nerves involved in affected plexus area (e.g., lower trunk = hand muscles of ulnar, median nerves)	Signs of denervation in muscles innervated by same roots, but different nerves
Paraspinal needle	No paraspinal muscle denervation	No paraspinal muscle denervation	Paraspinal muscle denervation is common
Motor nerve	Slow in affected nerve; CMAP amplitude could be decreased when stimulating the affected nerve; conduction block could be seen	Normal (CMAP amplitude could be decreased when stimulating nerves whose axons travel through affected plexus), slowing across Erb's point (brachial plexus)	Normal (CMAP amplitude could be decreased when stimulating nerves whose axons originate in affected roots)
Sensory-evoked potentials	Low-amplitude or prolonged-latency SNAP	Low-amplitude SNAPs in nerves whose axons travel through affected plexus area	Normal SNAPs
Proximal responses	Could be slow or absent in affected nerves	Could be slow or absent in nerves from affected plexus area	Could be slow or absent in nerves from affected roots

CMAP, compound muscle action potential; SNAPs, sensory nerve action potentials.
Reprinted with permission from Bertorini TE, ed: *Clinical Evaluation and Diagnostic Tests for Neuromuscular Disorders*, Woburn, MA, 2002, Butterworth-Heinemann.

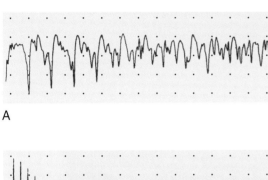

A

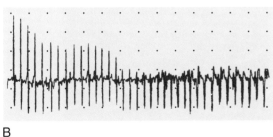

B

Figure 1-15 Myotonic discharges waxing and waning in amplitude: **A,** 100 µV/10 msec; **B,** 200 µV/20 msec. (From Bertorini TE: Neurological evaluation and diagnostic tests. In Bertorini TE, ed: *Neuromuscular Case Studies*, Philadelphia, 2008, Butterworth-Heinemann, pp 27–76.)

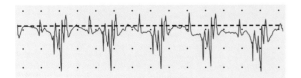

Figure 1-16 Complex but uniform waveforms that do not change in size or shape (100 µV/20 msec). (From Bertorini TE: Neurological evaluation and diagnostic tests. In Bertorini TE, ed: *Neuromuscular Case Studies*, Philadelphia, 2008, Butterworth-Heinemann, pp 27–76.)

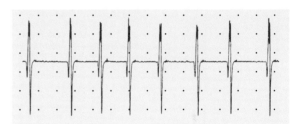

Figure 1-17 Electromyography in a patient with previous poliomyelitis showing very large motor unit action potentials firing at an increased rate of 20 Hz without recruiting a second motor unit (1 mV/20 msec). (From Bertorini TE: Neurological evaluation and diagnostic tests. In Bertorini TE, ed: *Neuromuscular Case Studies*, Philadelphia, 2008, Butterworth-Heinemann, pp 27–76.)

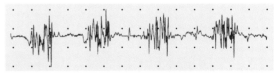

Figure 1-18 Nascent motor unit action potential in the deltoid muscle of a patient with radiculopathy and early reinnervation. Firing occurs at a rate of 20 Hz without recruiting a second motor unit (100 µV/10 msec). (From Bertorini TE: Neurological evaluation and diagnostic tests. In Bertorini TE, ed: *Neuromuscular Case Studies*, Philadelphia, 2008, Butterworth-Heinemann, pp 27–76.)

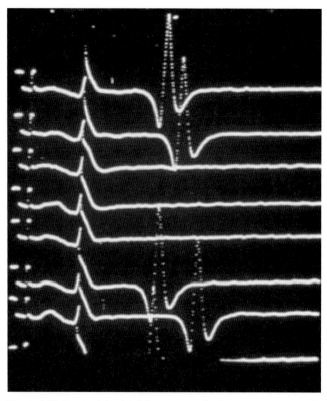

Figure 1-19 A potential pair of the extensor digitorum communis muscle; jitter and blocking are seen in a patient with myasthenia gravis (200 µV/ 0.5 msec). (From Bertorini TE: Neurological evaluation and diagnostic tests. In Bertorini TE, ed: *Neuromuscular Case Studies*, Philadelphia, 2008, Butterworth-Heinemann, pp 27–76.)

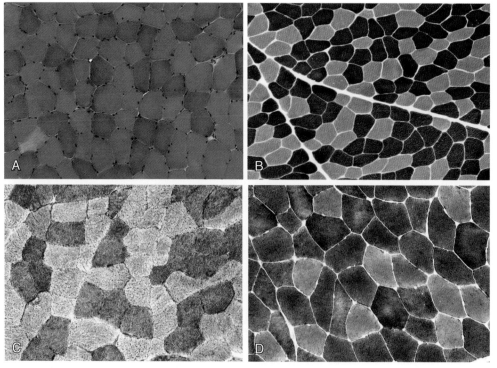

Figure 1-20 Normal muscle histochemistry, **A,** Hematoxylin and eosin stain (×200), **B,** Adenosine triphosphatase stain at pH 9.4 (×100), **C,** Nicotinamide adenine dinucleotide-tetrazolium stain (×200), **D,** Phosphorylase stain (×200).

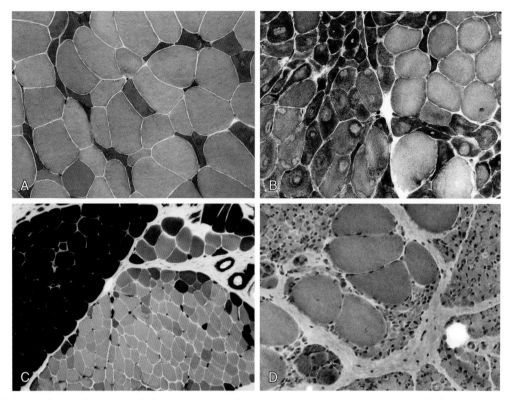

Figure 1-21 Muscle biopsy showing characteristic findings in neurogenic diseases. **A,** Atrophic angular denervated muscle fibers staining dark with nonspecific esterase stain (×200). **B,** Nicotinamide adenine dinucleotide-tetrazolium stain showing atrophic and "target" fibers (×200). **C,** Fiber type grouping in chronic disease with adenosine triphosphatase stain at pH 4.6 (×100). **D,** Group atrophy in infantile spinal muscular atrophy with trichrome stain (×200). In this disease, the atrophic denervated fibers are round rather than angulated, and most of the large fibers are type I on oxidative stains.

Table 1-4 Histologic Changes in Muscle Biopsy Found Predominantly in Neurogenic Disease and Myopathies*

Neurogenic Disease	Myopathy
Atrophic, esterase-positive angular fibers	Necrosis, phagocytosis
Targets, targetoids	Regenerating fibers
Large fiber-type grouping	Round atrophic and hypertrophic fibers (variation in fiber size), fiber splitting
Group atrophy	Internalized nuclei and capillaries, lobulated fibers
Pyknotic nuclei[†]	Specific fiber abnormalities (e.g., ragged red fibers, storage, inflammation, vacuoles, protein deficiencies)

*Some of these can be seen in both myopathies and neurogenic diseases; the prominence of the findings would suggest one or the other.
[†]Can be prominent in some myopathies as well (e.g., myotonic dystrophy).

or increased repeat expansions. For these, blood testing is performed, but in some mitochondrial disorders, muscle biopsy is necessary.[49,50]

Polymerase chain reaction (Fig. 1-24), Southern blot (Fig. 1-25), and particularly multiplex polymerase chain reaction testing is now standard. DNA sequencing, however, sometimes is necessary to detect point mutations that cannot be found with other tests.[51,52] Recent techniques for sequencing, such as emulsion polymerase chain reaction and ligation-based sequencing, are very sensitive.

Genetic tests should be considered in those who have features of a disease, even if they lack the complete phenotype; for example, patients with Kennedy disease might have bulbar spinal atrophy without systemic manifestations, and DNA testing allows for diagnosis of a more benign disorder than ALS as well as proper counseling. Also, in those with familial ALS, Cu/Zn superoxide dismutase gene mutations allow a diagnosis to be made in suspected cases.

In some conditions, a definitive diagnosis can be made only with molecular diagnostic tests; for example, in limb-girdle dystrophy caused by mutations of the sarcoglycan genes, an individual deficiency cannot be identified histologically, but genetic testing determines a specific sarcoglycogen gene mutation. Also, limb-girdle muscular dystrophy 2-I, a disease that might manifest similarly to Duchenne dystrophy or have milder phenotypes, is caused by mutations of the fukutin-related protein gene that can be diagnosed only by mutation analysis and not by histologic study or Western blot.

Another consideration is that molecular diagnosis may sometimes provide inconclusive data, for example, when there are borderline numbers of CTG repeats in suspected myotonic dystrophy I. Also,

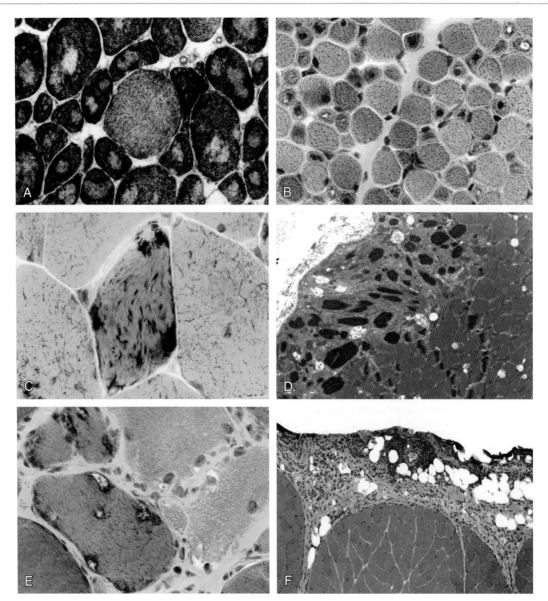

Figure 1-22 Examples of muscle biopsy findings in some myopathies. **A,** Central core disease showing a central core devoid of oxidative staining with nicotinamide adenine dinucleotide-tetrazolium (×400). **B,** Myotubular myopathy showing small fibers with centrally located nuclei with trichrome stain (×200). **C,** Nemaline rod myopathy showing the characteristic rods in the muscle fibers with trichrome stain (×400). **D,** EM showing the characteristic nemaline rods (×9000). **E,** Rimmed vacuoles in inclusion body myositis with trichrome stain (×400). **F,** Fasciitis and perimyositis showing lymphocytes in the fascia and perimysium with hematoxylin and eosin (×100). Examples of findings in other myopathies are seen in other chapters.

Table 1-5 Biopsy Findings That Indicate Axonal Degeneration or Demyelination*

Axonal Degeneration	Demyelination
May affect myelinated and unmyelinated fibers	Affects primarily myelinated fibers
Axonal degeneration of myelinated fibers seen on semithin plastic sections, teased nerve preparations (large ovoids)	Segmental demyelination
Axonal atrophy, inclusions	Large axons with thin myelin
Denervated Schwann cell subunits	Onion-bulb formations
Flattened, unmyelinated axons	Some tiny ovoids with variation in internodal length may be seen on teased nerve preparations
Bands of Büngner†	
Regenerating clusters of myelinated fibers	
Schwann cell processes with increased numbers of small unmyelinated axons	

*These changes are not definitive for diagnosis and in many neuropathies could show evidence of both axonal degeneration and demyelination, with the diagnosis based on the predominance of one or the other to determine whether the process is primarily demyelinating or an axonopathy.
†Groups of Schwann cell processes that were previously associated with myelinated axons.

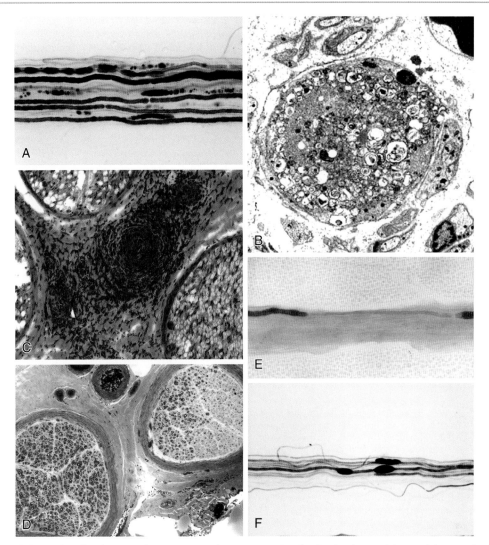

Figure 1-23 Examples of abnormalities found on nerve biopsy. **A,** Teased nerve preparation showing the characteristic axonal degeneration in the form of myelin ovoids (×400). **B,** Electromicroscopy showing an example of large degenerated axons. Small unmyelinated axons appear normal (×4000). **C,** Vasculitic neuropathy showing lymphocytes in the vessel wall. Hematoxylin and eosin stain (×200). **D,** Plastic-embedded sections from a patient with vasculitis. Toluidine blue staining of the fascicle on the top right showing a focal area with axons lacking myelin (×400). **E,** Teased nerve preparation of a nerve biopsy specimen from a patient with an acquired demyelinating polyneuropathy showing a demyelinated axon (×200). **F,** Tomaculae seen on a teased nerve preparation of a biopsy of a patient with hereditary neuropathy with liability to pressure palsy. (From Bertorini TE: Neurological evaluation and diagnostic tests. In Bertorini TE, ed: *Neuromuscular Case Studies*, Philadelphia, 2008, Butterworth-Heinemann, pp 27–76.)

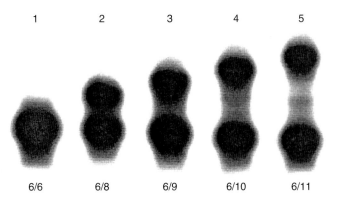

Figure 1-24 Molecular analysis of the poly (A)-binding protein 2 (*PABP2*) gene trinucleotide repeat. Polymerase chain reaction analysis with primers flanking with GCTGN repeat in five patients referred for diagnostic testing for oculopharyngeal muscular dystrophy. The numbers denote GCG sizes. The patient in lane 1 is homozygously normal for two alleles carrying six GCG repeats. Patients in lanes 2 through 5 carry expanded alleles (GCG8–11) within the *PABP2* gene. Alleles in this size range are associated with the clinical manifestations of oculopharyngeal muscular dystrophy. (Courtesy of Dr. Nicholas Potter, Department of Medical Genetics, University of Tennessee Medical Center, Knoxville. From Bertorini TE: Neurological evaluation and diagnostic tests. In Bertorini TE, ed: *Neuromuscular Case Studies*, Philadelphia, 2008, Butterworth-Heinemann, pp 27–76.)

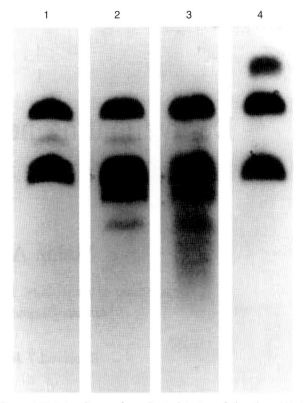

Figure 1-25 Autoradiogram from direct detection of the Charcot-Marie-Tooth type 1A (*CMT1A*) mutation and the hereditary neuropathy with liability to pressure palsies (HNPP) mutation by restriction endonuclease digestion and Southern blot analysis of pulse-field gel electrophoresed genomic DNA. Lane 1 is a normal control subject, lanes 2 and 3 are positive for *CMT1A*, and lane 4 is a control subject with HNPP, respectively. (From Almasaddi M, Bertorini TE, Seltzer WK: Demyelinating neuropathy in a patient with multiple sclerosis and genotypical HMSN-1. *Neuromusc Disord* 8:87–89, 1998.)

a diagnosis cannot be made in all cases of facioscapulohumeral dystrophy because some patients do not have the known genetic defects. Finally, with some disorders, such as limb-girdle dystrophies and Charcot-Marie-Tooth disease, many patients do not have the recognizable mutations as studied by commercial laboratories. For these patients, proper clinical and routine laboratory studies remain important. However, genetic testing technology is improving rapidly, and the cost of such testing is diminishing, so it is hoped that in the future many of these tests can be offered to families even when they do not have a known mutation for the disease. The utility of this has been demonstrated in a recent study in which whole-genome sequencing identified the responsible mutated allele in a family with Charcot-Marie-Tooth disease.[53]

More detailed descriptions of specific diagnostic tests for various NMDs are discussed in detail in other chapters of this book.

References

1. Dubowitz V: Diagnosis and classification of the neuromuscular disorders. In Dubowitz V, editor: *Muscle Disorders in Childhood*, Philadelphia, 1996, Saunders, pp 1–33.
2. Brooke M: Clinical evaluation of patients with neuromuscular disease. In Shapira AHV, Griggs RC, editors: *Muscle Diseases*, Boston, 1999, Butterworth-Heinemann, pp 1–30.
3. Brooke M: A Clinician's view of neuromuscular diseases. In Brooke M, editor: *The Symptoms and Signs of Neuromuscular Disease*, Baltimore, 1986, Williams & Wilkins, pp 1–33.
4. Bertorini TE: Clinical evaluation and clinical laboratory tests. In Bertorini TE, editor: *Clinical Evaluation and Diagnostic Tests for Neuromuscular Disorders*, Woburn, MA, 2002, Butterworth-Heinemann, pp 15–97.
5. Bertorini TE: Neuromuscular evaluation and ancillary tests. In Bertorini TE, editor: *Neuromuscular Case Studies*, Philadelphia, 2008, Butterworth-Heinemann, pp 27–76.
6. Griggs R, Mendell J, Miller R: Evaluation of the patient with myopathy. In Griggs R, Mendell J, Miller R, editors: *Evaluation and Treatment of Myopathies. Contemporary Neurology Series*, Philadelphia, 1995, FA Davis, pp 17–78.
7. Masland RL: Cramp-fasciculation syndrome, *Neurology* 42(2):466, 1992.
8. Ochoa JL: Positive sensory symptoms in neuropathy. Mechanisms and aspects of treatment. In Asbury AK, Thomas PK, editors: *Peripheral Nerve Disorders*, Oxford, UK, 1995, Butterworth-Heinemann, pp 44–58.
9. Barton JJ, Fouladvand M: Ocular aspects of myasthenia gravis, *Semin Neurol* 20(1):7–10, 2000.
10. Narayanaswami P, Bertorini TE: The dropped head syndrome, *J Clin Neuromuscul Disord* 2(2):106–112, 2000.
11. Reese BN, Lovelace-Chandler V, Soderberg GL: *Muscle and Sensory Testing*, Philadelphia, 1999, Saunders.
12. Haerer AF, DeJong RN: *DeJong's: The Neurologic Examination*, Philadelphia, 1992, Lippincott-Raven.
13. Pruthi RK, Tefferi A: Pernicious anemia revisited, *Mayo Clin Proc* 69(2):144–150, 1994.
14. Welch KM, Goldberg DM: Serum creatine phosphokinase in motor neuron disease, *Neurology* 22(7):697–701, 1972.
15. Bertorini TE: Myoglobinuria, malignant hyperthermia, neuroleptic malignant syndrome and serotonin syndrome, *Neurol Clin* 15(3):649–671, 1997.
16. Agnelio V: Mixed cryoglobulinemia and hepatitis C virus infection, *Hosp Pract* 32:80–85, 1995.
17. Narayanaswami P: Autoantibody testing. In Bertorini T, editor: *Clinical Evaluation and Diagnostic Tests for Neuromuscular Disorders*, Woburn, MA, 2002, Butterworth-Heinemann, pp 99–130.
18. Solimena M, Folli F, Denies-Donini S, et al: Autoantibodies to glutamic acid decarboxylase in a patient with stiff-man syndrome, epilepsy and type I diabetes mellitus, *N Engl J Med* 318:1012–1020, 1988.
19. Quarles RH, Weiss MD: Autoantibodies associated with peripheral neuropathy, *Muscle Nerve* 11(7):800–822, 1999.
20. Archelos JJ, Hartung HP: Pathogenic role of autoantibodies in neurologic disease, *Trends Neurosci* 23:317–327, 2000.
21. Sherer Y, Livneh A, Levy Y, et al: Dermatomyositis and polymyositis associated with the antiphospholipid syndrome—a novel overlap syndrome, *Lupus* 9:42–46, 2000.
22. Albers J: Porphyria neuropathy in the diagnosis and management of peripheral nerve disorders. In Mendell JR, Kissel JT, Cornblath PR, editors: *Contemporary Neurology Series*, New York, 2001, Oxford University Press, pp 344–366.
23. Moore MR: Biochemistry of porphyria, *Int J Biochem* 25(10):1353–1368, 1993.
24. Bertorini TE: Sensory nerve conduction studies. In Kimura J, editor: *Handbook of Clinical Neurophysiology*, Vol 7, Amsterdam, 2006, Elsevier, pp 155–176.
25. Oh SJ: Nerve conduction velocity tests: their clinical applications. In Bertorini TE, editor: *Clinical Evaluation and Diagnostic Tests for Neuromuscular Disorders*, Woburn, MA, 2002, Butterworth-Heinemann, pp 141–207.
26. Menkes DL: Proximal conduction techniques: Somatosensory evoked potentials, magnetic stimulation, root stimulation. In Bertorini TE, editor: *Clinical Evaluation and Diagnostic Tests for Neuromuscular Disorders*, Woburn, MA, 2002, Butterworth-Heinemann, pp 209–238.
27. Luciano CA: Other useful electrodiagnostic techniques: Blink reflex, massiter reflex, and silent periods. In Bertorini TE, editor: *Clinical Evaluation and Diagnostic Tests for Neuromuscular Disorders*, Woburn, MA, 2002, Butterworth-Heinemann, pp 239–256.
28. Wang AK, Kaufmann H: Autonomic function testing. In Bertorini TE, editor: *Clinical Evaluation and Diagnostic Tests for Neuromuscular Disorders*, Woburn, MA, 2002, Butterworth-Heinemann, pp 281–294.
29. Ciafaloni E, Massey JM: Repetitive stimulation tests. In Bertorini TE, editor: *Clinical Evaluation and Diagnostic Tests for Neuromuscular Disorders*, Woburn, MA, 2002, Butterworth-Heinemann, pp 281–294.

30. Oh SJ, Eslami N, Mishihira T, et al: Electrophysiological and clinical correlation in myasthenia gravis, *Ann Neurol* 12:348–354, 1982.

31. Oh SJ, Kurokawa K, Clauseen GC, Ryan HF Jr, : Electrophysiological diagnostic criteria of Lambert-Eaton myasthenic syndrome, *Muscle Nerve* 32(4):15–20, 2005.

32. Kimura J: Routine needle electromyographyin. In Bertorini TE, editor: *Clinical Evaluation and Diagnostic Tests in Neuromuscular Disorders*, Woburn, MA, 2002, Butterworth-Heinemann, pp 331–364.

33. Dumitru D, King JC, Rogers WE, Stegeman DF: Positive sharp wave and fibrillation potential modeling, *Muscle Nerve* 22:242–251, 1999.

34. Daube Jr, Rubin DI: Electrodiagnostics of muscle disorders. In Engel AG, Franzini-Armstrong C, editors: *Myology*, 3rd ed, New York, 2004, McGraw-Hill, pp 619–654.

35. Trontelj JV, Stalberg A: Single fiber and macro electromyography. In Bertorini T, editor: *Clinical Evaluation and Diagnostic Tests for Neuromuscular Disorders*, Woburn, MA, 2002, Butterworth-Heinemann, pp 417–447.

36. Bertorini TE, Horner LH: Histology and histochemistry of muscle and nerve. In Bertorini TE, editor: *Clinical Evaluation and Diagnostic Tests for Neuromuscular Disorders*, Woburn, MA, 2002, Butterworth-Heinemann, pp 595–692.

37. DiMauro S, Shanske S, Naini A, Krishna S: Biochemical evaluation of metabolic myopathies. In Bertorini TE, editor: *Clinical Evaluation and Diagnostic Tests for Neuromuscular Disorders*, Woburn, MA, 2002, Butterworth-Heinemann, pp 535–564.

38. Bertorini TE: Inflammatory myopathies (polymyositis, dermatomyositis, inclusion body myositis), *Compr Ther* 24:494–502, 1998.

39. Dubowitz V: Definitions of changes seen in muscle biopsies. In Dubowitz V, editor: *Muscle Biopsy. A Practical Approach*, 2nd ed, London, 1985, Bailliere Tindall, pp 82–128.

40. Dyck PJ, Lofgren EP: Nerve biopsy: choice of nerve, method, symptoms and usefulness, *Med Clin North Am* 52:885–893, 1968.

41. Midroni G, Balbao JM: Peripheral neuropathy and the role of nerve biopsy. In Midroni G, Bilbao JM, Cohen SM, editors: *Biopsy Diagnosis of Peripheral Neuropathy*, Woburn, MA, 1995, Butterworth-Heinemann, pp 1–12.

42. Dyck PJ, Lais AC, Ohta M, et al: Chronic inflammatory polyradiculoneuropathy, *Mayo Clin Proc* 50:631–637, 1975.

43. Krendel DA, Parks HP, Anthony DC, et al: Sural nerve biopsy in chronic inflammatory demyelinating polyradiculoneuropathy, *Muscle Nerve* 12:257–264, 1989.

44. Midroni G, Bilbao JM, Cohen SM: *Vasculitis Neuropathy. Biopsy Diagnosis of Peripheral Neuropathy*, Boston, 1995, Butterworth-Heinemann, pp 241–262.

45. Claussen G, Thomas D, Goyne CH, et al: Diagnostic value of nerve and muscle biopsy in suspected vasculitis cases, *J Clin Neuromuscul Disord* 1:117–123, 2000.

46. Halford H, Graves A: Imaging techniques. In Bertorini TE, editor: *Clinical Evaluation and Diagnostic Tests for Neuromuscular Disorders*, Woburn, MA, 2002, Butterworth-Heinemann, pp 565–593.

47. Zuberi SM, Matta N, Nawaz S, et al: Muscle ultrasound in the assessment of suspected neuromuscular disease in childhood, *Neuromuscul Disord* 9(4):203–207, 1999.

48. Reimers CD, Schedel H, Fleckenstein JL, et al: Magnetic resonance imaging of skeletal muscles in idiopathic inflammatory myopathies of adults, *J Neurol* 241:306–314, 1994.

49. Gorospe JR, Hoffman EP: Basic medical genetics and molecular diagnostics. In Bertorini TE, editor: *Clinical Evaluation and Diagnostic Tests for Neuromuscular Disorders*, Woburn, MA, 2002, Butterworth-Heinemann, pp 693–836.

50. Pulst S-M: Introduction to medical genetics. In Pulst S-M, editor: *Neurogenetics*, New York, 2000, Oxford University Press, pp 1–24.

51. Mendell JR, Buzin CH, Feng J, et al: Diagnosis of Duchenne dystrophy by enhanced detection of small mutations, *Neurology* 57:645–650, 2001.

52. Flanigan KM, von Niederhausern A, Dunn DM, et al: Rapid direct sequence analysis of the dystrophin gene, *Am J Hum Genet* 72:931–939, 2003.

53. Lupski JR, Reid JG, Gonzaga-Jaureguil C, et al: Whole-genome sequencing in a patient with Charcot-Marie-Tooth neuropathy, *N Engl J Med* 2010; 362:1181–1191.

Daniel M. Goodenberger, MD

2

Respiratory Complications in Neuromuscular Disorders

Respiratory management of patients with neuromuscular diseases has been highly successful in reducing morbidity and extending survival. The monitoring and therapy described subsequently will be based on the available literature. In areas in which a scientific basis for management is insufficient, conflicting, or nonexistent, recommendations will be based on the author's more than 21 years of experience in the area and his position as the only pulmonary consultant in this field at a major medical center. In the penultimate 6 years at this center, the author was involved in the ongoing care of 170 patients with amyotrophic lateral sclerosis (ALS) and 134 other patients with neuromuscular disease, principally muscular dystrophies. Thus, many recommendations are derived from that experience; in instances in which the recommendations are different from those of other authors, the reasoning will be outlined.

Management of Neuromuscular Diseases Resulting in Chronic Respiratory Failure

The evaluation of patients with neuromuscular diseases that result in chronic respiratory failure does not usually involve a primary diagnosis. Most patients presenting to a pulmonologist with these disorders already have a diagnosis that has been made or verified by a referring neurologist. Detailed descriptions of the initial presentation and evaluation of these diseases are provided elsewhere in this book and will not be repeated here except to make illustrative points about therapy that may differ by disease process.

Bilateral Diaphragm Paralysis

Exceptions are patients who present with dyspnea as a result of diaphragmatic weakness or paralysis and do not yet have a diagnosis or etiology. This condition may be caused by muscle weakness as a result of metabolic (hypothyroidism[1]), inflammatory (systemic lupus erythematosus; vanishing lung syndrome[2]), or myopathic (Pompe disease[3,4]) causes. It may also be caused by phrenic nerve injury as a result of cardiac surgery[5] (a common current cause), trauma, inflammation (neuralgic amyotrophy[6]), hereditary neuropathy (Charcot-Marie-Tooth or Dejerine-Sottas, spinal muscular atrophy), or motor neuron disease presenting first in this way.[7]

Patients with unilateral diaphragm paralysis are rarely symptomatic unless there is underlying lung disease. Symptoms that should lead the clinician to suspect bilateral diaphragm paralysis include profound orthopnea, with which the patient is unable to lie completely flat for more than a few seconds. The patient may have mild to moderate dyspnea at rest that is severely exacerbated by bending sharply at the waist, as when tying the shoes. The patient will invariably describe an inability to submerge in water above the waist, which results in profound dyspnea. This results from interference with a primary compensatory mechanism. These individuals have learned to function by using their abdominal expiratory muscles to force the diaphragm upward to a level below functional residual capacity; during inspiration, the muscles are relaxed and the abdominal viscera pull the diaphragm down by gravity, augmenting inspiration. The buoyant effect of the water prevents this, resulting in a feeling that patients call "suffocating." Physical examination shows the use of accessory muscles in the neck, and the patient generally ensures that the upper extremities are supported to provide mechanical advantage. Expiratory use of abdominal muscles may be detected. In the supine position, the patient invariably has paradoxical motion, with the abdomen moving in rather than out with inspiration. Careful percussion of the chest may show failure of normal diaphragmatic excursion.

The general history and physical examination should focus on possible underlying disease processes that may produce diaphragm paralysis. Neuralgic amyotrophy is a brachial plexitis that results in severe shoulder pain preceding the onset of dyspnea. Patients with adult Pompe disease may have associated proximal muscle weakness. Primary respiratory-onset ALS may be associated with pathologic reflexes and fasciculations. Primary underlying diseases, such as lupus, hypothyroidism, and previous trauma, including surgery, should be sought.

The first test conducted to confirm the diagnosis is the "sniff" test, during which the patient forcefully sniffs through the nose while chest fluoroscopy is performed. This test is excellent for confirming the diagnosis of unilateral paralysis; the unaffected diaphragm descends rapidly and normally, and the affected diaphragm rises while the mediastinal structures move toward the unaffected side. However, if performed while the patient is upright, it may miss bilateral paralysis; as described earlier, passive fall of the diaphragm during inspiration may confound the examiner and result in a report of normal diaphragmatic function.[8] To be effective, fluoroscopy must be performed with the patient supine; in this position, paradoxical diaphragmatic excursion will be seen. Ultrasound may also be used to assess diaphragmatic movement.[9]

Confirmatory tests include pulmonary function tests, measurement of diaphragmatic pressure generation, and electrodiagnostic studies. Spirometry generally shows a reduction in forced vital capacity (FVC) of approximately 50%. Lung volumes are restrictive, with a pattern that the majority of reduced lung volumes are in the voluntary portion of spirometry. Residual volume is generally preserved. Characteristically, FVC is reduced by an additional 40% or more in the supine position.

Maximum inspiratory pressure, achieved by asking the patient to inhale with greatest force from residual volume against a manometer, is typically reduced from normal and can be measured in the pulmonary function laboratory. Occasionally, an otherwise healthy patient can generate surprisingly high pressures, approaching normal. Maximum expiratory pressure (measured from total lung capacity) is generally preserved. Maximum transdiaphragmatic pressure, or P_{DImax} (the difference between esophageal pressure and gastric pressure, which requires balloon manometry in both organs), is always reduced, usually less than 30 cm H_2O. Reproducibility is improved by using a sniff technique.[10] This technique is beyond the capacity of most clinical pulmonary function test laboratories and is seldom necessary. Similarly, nerve conduction studies of the phrenic nerves and diaphragmatic electromyograms may be performed, but are seldom necessary for clinical diagnosis. When they are believed to be required, they are best performed in a laboratory with substantial experience with the techniques.

Because of their profound orthopnea, these patients are generally sleeping in a chair at presentation. Therapy is indicated at the time of diagnosis. Most patients can be treated successfully with nocturnal noninvasive ventilation,[11] which is initiated as described later.

Diaphragmatic pacing is not indicated in these patients; this procedure requires both intact phrenic nerves and normal muscle function, and it is generally limited to patients with high spinal cord injuries and intact phrenic nerves and patients with central alveolar hypoventilation.[12]

Assessment and Management of the Patient with an Established Neurologic Diagnosis

Most patients seen by a pulmonologist as outpatients fall into one of two groups: those with muscular dystrophy and those with motor neuron disease. The approach to these patients is discussed separately because their monitoring and care are different. Depending on local referral patterns, ventilator-dependent patients with spinal cord injury and those with post-polio syndrome requiring ventilatory support may also be seen and will be discussed briefly. Other diseases that may have respiratory involvement include inflammatory myopathies, critical illness polyneuropathy, myasthenia gravis, Eaton-Lambert syndrome, intoxications, Guillain-Barré syndrome, botulism, and porphyria. However, these diseases do not generally result in chronic respiratory failure and will be discussed in the section of the chapter on management of acute respiratory failure.

Muscular Dystrophies

The most common of the hereditary neuromuscular disorders requiring chronic mechanical ventilation is Duchenne muscular dystrophy. The young men with this disease have a relatively similar course, being wheelchair-bound by roughly 12 years of age and having respiratory failure by the late teens or occasionally as late as the early 20s. Occasionally, the first manifestation is acute respiratory failure after a lower respiratory tract infection or surgical procedure. More often, the onset is insidious. The patients do not often have dyspnea as the primary symptom; presumably this is because by this point they are invariably bed- and wheelchair-bound, the latter being driven by electric motors. Occasionally, the presentation is weight loss, which seems to be caused by postprandial dyspnea, or occasionally by early satiety because of very slow eating. Often, patients have evidence of sleep disturbance or nocturnal hypoventilation, with daytime sleepiness, morning headaches, and nightmares that may involve smothering. The headaches are characteristic, being present on awakening and clearing within 1 hour or less without intervention, and are caused by nocturnal hypercapnea. Sleep abnormalities are common in Duchenne muscular dystrophy before the onset of frank respiratory failure, and a polysomnogram may be necessary to identify the nocturnal disturbances.[13] This appears to have become more common after the widespread prescription of corticosteroids, which may result in substantial weight gain. It is not uncommon to have hypoventilation with hypercapnea and secondary hypoxemia, particularly during rapid eye movement sleep. Occasionally, nocturnal hypoventilation is sufficiently severe by the time of evaluation to result in right heart failure out of proportion to left ventricular function; this is less common now because most such individuals are followed by neuromuscular specialists who are alert to respiratory dysfunction and refer patients earlier than in the past.

The second most common muscular dystrophy requiring ventilatory support is myotonic dystrophy. There is not a characteristic age of onset because the severity of the symptoms is influenced by the length of the responsible CTG trinucleotide repeats. Because of trinucleotide expansion from generation to generation ("anticipation"), a physician caring for several generations of the same family can expect onset of respiratory failure a decade or more earlier in each successive generation. Sleep apnea is common in myotonic dystrophy, and a substantial minority of patients has excessive daytime sleepiness, even without respiratory failure. As a consequence, polysomnography should be performed in sleepy patients, even if they have normal gas exchange. Earlier studies attributing hypoventilation to abnormal respiratory drive were based on ventilatory response to carbon dioxide; the interpretation of the results was confounded by muscle weakness reducing minute ventilation, the measured variable. Later studies using inspiratory pressure during the first 100 msec of inspiration ($P_{0.1}$) suggest normal ventilatory response.[14] Myotonia of the diaphragm is undoubtedly present, but of uncertain significance in the development of respiratory symptoms.

A less common X-linked muscular dystrophy also caused by a dystrophin mutation is Becker muscular dystrophy. These patients follow a course very similar to that of Duchenne muscular dystrophy, but with each milestone, including the development of respiratory failure, delayed in onset by approximately a decade.

Other hereditary muscular dystrophies (limb-girdle, facioscapulohumeral, Emery-Dreifuss) are less likely to result in respiratory failure, but may do so on occasion.

All symptomatic patients should be evaluated. At a minimum, pulmonary function tests, including FVC, lung volumes, maximum inspiratory and expiratory pressures, oximetry, and arterial blood gases on room air, should be performed. A baseline chest x-ray will be helpful in evaluating subsequent respiratory infections, particularly if there are baseline abnormalities in heart size, spinal structure or hardware, pulmonary parenchyma, or diaphragm placement.

Symptoms of sleep apnea should prompt a sleep study. Symptomatic dysphagia or recurrent pneumonias suggesting aspiration (uncommon in muscular dystrophy in my experience) may be evaluated by modified barium swallow or fiberoptic evaluation of swallowing by a speech pathologist.[15] All patients should have appropriate influenza and pneumococcal vaccinations. If the individual has significant dysphagia or evidence of aspiration, or more commonly, weight loss associated with dyspnea, gastric tube placement should be considered. Although there is no direct evidence that improved nutrition results in better respiratory outcome, it seems reasonable to prevent muscle loss attributable to malnutrition. Moreover, weight loss may lead to loss of soft tissue on the buttocks and back, making both bed and wheelchair use very uncomfortable. As described later, we prefer gastric tube insertion by interventional radiology, not least because it allows respiratory support more readily than percutaneous endoscopic gastric tube placement.

Monitoring of patients who are asymptomatic is arbitrary, particularly given the evidence that prophylactic or early initiation of ventilatory support is not helpful and appears to be harmful, at least in Duchenne muscular dystrophy.[16] When FVC is 50% or less than predicted, it is reasonable to follow handheld spirometry in the neuromuscular clinic and refer patients for formal evaluation to obtain the formal pulmonary function testing described earlier. If the patient is asymptomatic, repeat visits and evaluations are scheduled at 6- to 12-month intervals, depending on status and gestalt. Because of the possibility of life-threatening complications of even apparently minor respiratory infections (discussed later), patients and their caregivers are told to seek care promptly at onset.

Pulmonary function tests in these muscular dystrophies characteristically show restriction, with normal flow rates (normal ratio of forced expiratory volume in 1 second to FVC and normal midexpiratory flow). In contrast to the restriction seen in pulmonary fibrosis, however, the majority of volume reduction occurs in the voluntary, spirometric components that depend on muscle strength. Thus, FVC and its subdivisions are much more reduced than functional residual capacity or residual volume, whereas in fibrosis, all components are reduced more or less proportionately (Fig. 2-1). Most of the reduction is probably the result of muscle weakness, although there is some evidence that chronic breathing at low lung volumes reduces pulmonary compliance. Some of this is likely caused by microatelectasis and surfactant loss, but some appears to be the result of poorly understood reductions in chest wall compliance.[17,18] As a result, functional residual capacity (determined by the relative

elasticity of the lungs and chest wall) may be mildly reduced. Residual volume may appear increased because weak expiratory muscles may reduce the expiratory reserve volume, used to calculate residual volume after functional residual capacity is determined.

Maximum inspiratory and expiratory pressures have the advantage that they are easily measured with a handheld manometer and nose clips. The disadvantage is that there is a wide range of normal values, as determined by multiple studies, affected by age, sex, ability to form and maintain a tight mouth seal, and general health. Normal maximum expiratory pressure, measured from residual volume after a full exhalation, is roughly -120 cm H_2O for men and approximately -90 cm H_2O for women, with a broad range. Corresponding values for maximal expiratory pressure, measured from total lung capacity after a full inhalation, are approximately $+230$ cm H_2O for men and $+150$ cm H_2O for women. Values of less than 30 cm for maximum inspiratory pressure are often accompanied by hypercapneic respiratory failure. Because this test adds little or nothing to spirometry and arterial blood gases, which are repeated at every routine visit, I do not routinely follow these tests.

Respiratory management of patients with muscular dystrophy is the subject of strongly held opinion but a relative paucity of evidence based on controlled clinical trials.

Inspiratory muscle training has been suggested to build respiratory muscle strength and improve respiratory status. There is little evidence to support this, however. Moreover, initiation of noninvasive ventilation in hypercarbic patients invariably results in reduction in daytime P_{CO_2}, suggesting that these damaged muscles are fatigued and benefit from rest. As a result, resistive training is not part of our regimen. Similarly, we do not use theophylline as a respiratory muscle "tonic."

Because expiratory muscles are weak, some practitioners routinely use a mechanical in-exsufflator to improve sputum removal.[19,20] These devices, based on the original Coughalator (J.H. Emerson Co., Cambridge, MA; now Philips Respironics, Murrysville, PA), rapidly inflate and then deflate the lungs, generating high airway velocities. Pressures are gradually increased as tolerated to achieve maximum pressures of approximately 40 cm H_2O for both the inspiratory and expiratory components. Controlled data supporting the use of this device in patients with stable muscular dystrophy are lacking. In our experience, these patients have normal (but often small) airways and do not clinically have excess mucus production in the uninfected state. As a consequence, use of this device has not been a routine part of management for our patients. Cough assistance can, however, provide substantial benefit for these patients when they have a lower respiratory infection (discussed later).

Evidence of respiratory failure or serious nocturnal hypoventilation is generally considered an indication for initiation of ventilatory support.[21] These factors include daytime hypercapnea and nocturnal hypoventilation (demonstrated by sleep study or recording nocturnal oximetry, particularly when accompanied by the symptoms described earlier). Although there is virtually no evidence of benefit rising to the level of controlled clinical trials, the longitudinal experience of multiple groups is unequivocal in showing that noninvasive positive pressure ventilation (NPPV) improves symptoms, quality of life, and longevity,[22,23] compared with studies that showed very poor survival in the absence of ventilatory support once vital capacity is less than 1 L or once nocturnal hypoxemia and daytime hypercapnea occur.[24,25]

Although individual groups have been using mouthpiece NPPV for many years,[26,27] the most common devices used for noninvasive ventilation until the mid-1980s were negative pressure ventilators.[28]

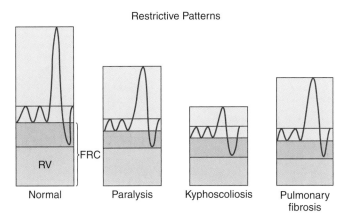

Restrictive Patterns

RV

FRC

Normal   Paralysis   Kyphoscoliosis   Pulmonary fibrosis

Figure 2-1 Patterns of restriction. FRC, functional residual capacity; RV, residual volume.

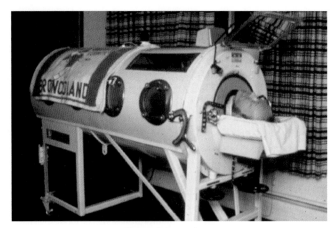

Figure 2-2 Iron lung.

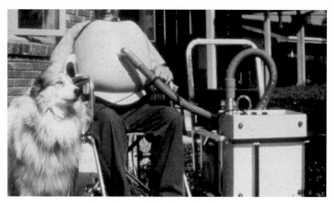

Figure 2-4 Cuirass ventilator with user.

The Drinker respirator (iron lung) was in wide use in the United States and abroad during the polio epidemics in the mid-20th century. The patient lies on a padded platform that slides into the cylinder, with an airtight seal achieved via a gasket around the neck (Fig. 2-2). Intracylinder negative pressure was generated by a piston, which in turn resulted in thoracic expansion and inspiration. Respiratory rate and tidal volume were regulated by piston stroke frequency and stroke length, respectively. In those with normal thoracic cages, adequate tidal volumes were generated by pressures of -12 to -25 cm H_2O. For those with significant deformity, as in the case of severe kyphoscoliosis, higher negative pressures were required. Tidal volumes may be measured with a Wright spirometer. These ventilators continued to be used by polio patients requiring respiratory assistance and were adapted for use by patients with chest wall deformities and neuromuscular disease. However, they were cumbersome and difficult to enter for patients with neuromuscular disorders, caused soreness around the neck, made routine hygiene needs difficult, and worsened sleep apnea in patients with neuromuscular failure.[29,30]

Fiberglass cuirass ventilators worked on the same principle, but were less effective, had a limited number of sizes, and could not be used on those with thoracic deformities (Figs. 2-3 and 2-4). Poncho (raincoat) ventilators used a frame that could accommodate variations in body habitus and was covered by fabric with seals at the neck, wrists, and pelvis (Fig. 2-5). However, it could be used only in the supine position, leading to discomfort, and it was drafty because of

air leaks. Because of inefficiencies in thoracic expansion, each of these required greater negative pressures, typically -20 to -40 cm H_2O.

Other respiratory assist devices included the rocking table and pneumobelt. The rocking table rotated from the head up to the head down position and back at a variable rate. This allowed the abdominal viscera to participate in diaphragmatic movement and assist respiration (Fig. 2-6). The pneumobelt functions in much the same way that the abdominal expiratory muscles do in diaphragmatic paralysis, inflating during expiration to force the diaphragm and abdominal viscera cephalad, with passive fall on inhalation (Figs. 2-7 and 2-8). The patient must be sitting or standing for this to be effective. Pressures required are generally 30 to 50 cm H_2O.[31]

These devices are largely of historical interest, and descriptions of these kinds of treatments can be expected to disappear over the next decade. They are included in this discussion because occasional patients may be seen who continue to use these in various combinations (iron lung or rocking bed at night, pneumobelt in the daytime). Most of these patients have used these devices since their bout of acute poliomyelitis or required resumption of ventilatory support as a result of post-polio syndrome.

Alba and colleagues[32] have used NPPV by mouthpiece for decades. This ventilatory modality was revolutionized by the introduction of positive pressure by nasal mask in the mid-1980s.[33,34]

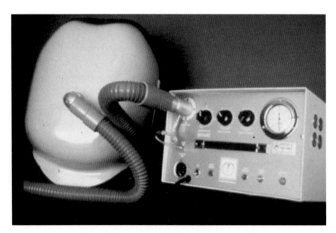

Figure 2-3 Cuirass ventilator ("turtle shell").

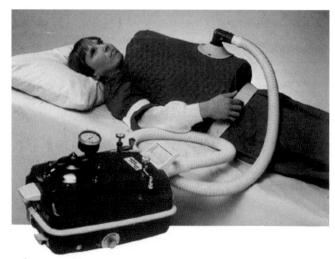

Figure 2-5 Poncho ventilator.

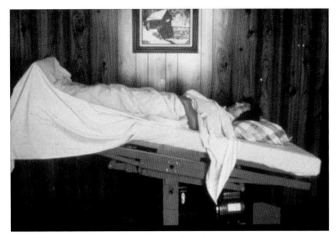

Figure 2-6 Rocking bed.

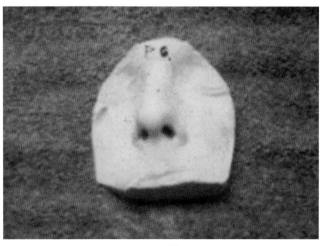

Figure 2-9 Facial mold for custom mask.

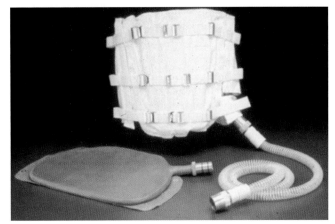

Figure 2-7 Pneumobelt.

The vast majority of NPPV is now delivered by nasal interface, although some patients require or benefit from oronasal masks or mouthpieces.

Initiation of nasal positive pressure ventilation is best done in the hospital; mask fit, ventilator education, selection of ventilator settings, family education, and troubleshooting can often be accomplished in a 36- to 48-hour admission encompassing 2 nights.

Mask selection is a matter of individual choice and comfort. The original masks, designed for continuous positive airway pressure, were more likely to cause erosions and breakdown at the nasal bridge and maxillary spine. Early on, this led some of us to seek out prosthodontists to make custom masks based on facial impressions (Fig. 2-9). However, newer-generation masks with softer silicone (Silastic; Dow Corning, Midland, MI) seals and gel cushioning have reduced the discomfort (Fig. 2-10). Nevertheless, some patients tolerate intranasal interfaces (pillows) better (Fig. 2-11), and interchange of the two kinds of devices may allow continuous use until the nasal skin or mucosa becomes more resistant to injury.[35–37]

Continuous positive airway pressure and bilevel positive airway pressure masks are designed with holes for air leak. Combined with

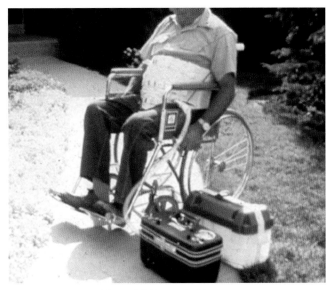

Figure 2-8 Pneumobelt in use.

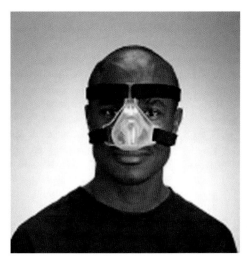

Figure 2-10 Softfit Ultra mask (Puritan Bennett, Boulder, CO).

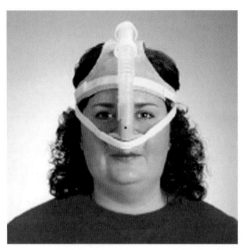

Figure 2-11 ADAM circuit (nasal pillows) (Puritan Bennett, Boulder, CO).

expiratory positive pressure, the holes minimize CO_2 rebreathing. If volume ventilation is used, these masks must be modified or they cannot be used. If assist-control ventilation is used with a nasal mask leak, the patient may find it impossible to trigger the ventilator, or rapid autocycling may occur. Home respiratory therapists, accustomed to bilevel positive airway pressure, are unfamiliar with this and may be resistant to change; they must be instructed carefully.

In the beginning, most ventilation was performed with volume-controlled portable home ventilators. Bilevel positive airway pressure devices, originally designed for more comfortable treatment of sleep apnea, have evolved into more sophisticated ventilators and have largely supplanted volume ventilators for noninvasive treatment, both in the United States and in Europe.[38,39] This likely has its genesis in the near-simultaneous development of pressure support ventilation, the familiarity of large numbers of pulmonologists with these devices compared with the much smaller numbers familiar with portable volume ventilators, and aggressive marketing of these machines by manufacturers and durable medical equipment companies; they are substantially less expensive and are amortized more quickly. In one instance, a durable medical equipment company refused to provide a volume ventilator for a patient without a tracheostomy, citing nonexistent Medicare regulations. Interactions with the company suggested that this refusal sprang from financial motives. There is no evidence of difference in outcomes supporting the choice of one mode over the other,[40–42] although there is some suggestion that patients find pressure mode more comfortable. Models include BiPAP ST-D and related devices (Respironics), GoodKnight 425ST (Nellcor Puritan Bennett, Boulder, CO), and VPAP ST (Resmed, Poway, CA).

If pressure mode is chosen, pressures necessary to provide adequate tidal volume and rest the respiratory muscles must be chosen. There is good evidence that inspiratory pressure of approximately 15 cm H_2O is necessary to silence the diaphragmatic electromyogram.[43] (Some authors have suggested that it may be necessary to start at lower pressures and increase them gradually; that has not been my experience when ventilation is initiated in the hospital and pressures are based on tidal volume and minute ventilation.) The most frequent reason for unsatisfactory results from pressure ventilation in my experience is inadequate inspiratory pressures; it is not uncommon to find patients referred for a second opinion with settings of inspiratory positive airway pressure/expiratory positive airway pressure of 8/4 to 10/5. On the occasions when I use bilevel positive pressure ventilation, inspiratory pressure is set to achieve a

tidal volume of approximately 10 mL/kg, and the backup rate is set to achieve a minute ventilation of approximately 100 mL/kg. Expiratory pressure is not used as external positive end-expiratory pressure, but is used solely for the purpose of purging carbon dioxide from the mask; 4 to 5 cm H_2O is generally adequate.

I use volume ventilation nearly exclusively in patients with muscular dystrophy. First, episodes of acute respiratory failure superimposed on the chronic state are most often precipitated by infection. Typically, these infections are viral and accompanied by nasal congestion. As a result, when patients need additional ventilatory support, they get less; the increased nasal resistance reproducibly results in lower tidal volumes and minute ventilation. Moreover, increased lower airway secretions result in substantial variations in airway resistance and relatively wide swings in minute ventilation over short periods. Second, many of these patients transition to tracheostomy ventilation over a decade or so. When they do, they and their families are already fully familiar with the ventilator they will use.

Originally, I followed a fairly intensive protocol for initiation, adjusting respiratory rate and tidal volume based on arterial blood gases.[44] Over time, it became apparent that this was ineffective and unnecessary. Currently, tidal volumes and respiratory rates are initially chosen based on the patient's size and weight, to achieve tidal volumes and minute ventilation in the range described earlier. These are adjusted by well-trained respiratory therapists overnight based on comfort and compliance. Results are reviewed the next morning, and further adjustments are made under direct observation during the day. The second night is usually more successful than the first, and after teaching and troubleshooting, the patient is discharged. The ventilator mode is usually assist-control, although intermittent mandatory ventilation with pressure support is a comfortable alternative. Oxygen administration during this process is less likely to cause problems in this group of patients than in those with ALS, but should be avoided (discussed later).

Common problems during initiation and thereafter include mask air leak, which may result in eye irritation and exposure keratitis; skin breakdown; nasal congestion and dryness; and stomach bloating. The mask leak can usually be corrected with strap adjustment and appropriate support of ventilator tubing (Fig. 2-12). This

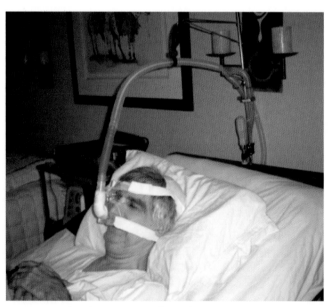

Figure 2-12 Ventilator tubing support.

in turn will reduce eye irritation; early on, it may be necessary to provide eye lubricant. Skin irritation and breakdown can be helped with padding, application of moleskin, and alternating between mask and nasal pillows. Gastric distention may be treated with simethicone, but it usually abates on its own over the first 2 weeks.

In-hospital initiation allows observation for oral leaks. If they occur, they may be corrected with a chinstrap. If initiation occurs on an outpatient basis and results are suboptimal, nocturnal family observation or recording oximetry may show ineffective ventilation.

Home care arrangements are crucial. If possible, the home respiratory team should meet with the patient and physician in the hospital so that expectations and instructions are fully understood by both parties. Family instruction is equally important.

The patient is seen and evaluated after 3 to 4 weeks. With few exceptions, daytime P_{CO_2} will have diminished to less than 50 mm Hg, regardless of the starting point. The mechanisms remain uncertain; reduction of chronic muscle fatigue likely plays a part, but a significant role may be played by "resetting" central chemoreceptors to new, lower levels of nighttime P_{CO_2}.[45]

Thereafter, the patient is seen regularly at intervals of 3 to 6 months. Early on, increases in daytime P_{CO_2} are often caused by reductions in nocturnal use and will respond to increases. Over several years, it will be necessary to increase duration of ventilation to achieve the same results. This may be conveniently applied during an afternoon nap. Over the ensuing years, the required duration increases, and often over a decade or so, continuous ventilation becomes necessary. Many patients can be ventilated comfortably and successfully with nasal ventilation, but as the ability to tolerate ventilator-free time decreases, ventilator failure or mask displacement becomes increasingly hazardous. Nevertheless, some choose to continue NPPV indefinitely. Previous generations of portable ventilators (LP-10, Nellcor Puritan Bennett; PLV-100, Respironics) required modifications of wheelchairs to accommodate daytime use, with a platform on the back that increased turning radius and could interfere with van transport. More modern ventilators, such as the LTV-900 or -1000 (Pulmonetics, now Cardinal Health, Dublin, OH) and Puritan Bennett 540 (Nellcor Puritan Bennett), are small enough to be suspended from the back of the wheelchair in a hanging bag, which is much more convenient (Figs. 2-13 and 2-14).

Some experts believe that noninvasive ventilation is preferable to tracheostomy ventilation at all costs, using daytime mouthpiece ventilation mounted via gooseneck on the wheelchair and nighttime mask or oronasal interface.[46] I am not of that persuasion. At the

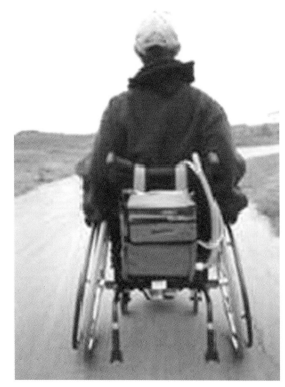

Figure 2-14 LTV-900 ventilator (Pulmonetics, now Cardinal Health, Dublin, OH) on wheelchair.

point at which the patient requires continuous ventilation, I prefer tracheostomy. In the event of ventilator failure, ventilation may be continued much more safely and conveniently with an Ambu bag. At least some of the reluctance to this approach is an incorrect belief that tracheostomy is incompatible with speech and normal oral intake.

When a mutual decision is reached to undertake tracheostomy, elective admission is arranged. In the postoperative period, a cuffed tracheostomy tube is used; the air leak associated with an uncuffed tube may result in subcutaneous emphysema, pneumomediastinum, and pneumothorax. This is continued for 7 to 10 days, until the tissue planes are sealed. During this time, communication may be maintained with an electrolarynx. After healing, the cuffed tube is exchanged for an uncuffed tube. This should be sized to allow adequate exhalation with the tube plugged; this may require endoscopic evaluation. Fenestrated tubes should be avoided: no matter how carefully they are sized, the fenestration will rub on the anterior tracheal wall at the stoma and result in the formation of granulation tissue; unfenestrated tubes virtually never do so.

Although it is possible for a patient to produce speech while ventilated with an uncuffed tube alone, the speech pattern is noncontinuous and occurs during inspiration, a nonintuitive process. The use of a one-way valve in-line with the ventilator (Passy-Muir speaking valve; Passy-Muir Inc., Irvine, CA) allows normal speech (Figs. 2-15 and 2-16). As a beneficial side effect, speech is often stronger because greater tidal volumes are delivered. Aspiration is uncommon; severe dysphagia is unusual in the muscular dystrophies, and most patients can continue oral intake after becoming accustomed to the tracheostomy and having a confirmatory swallowing evaluation. Moreover, the positive pressure exhalation helps to clear perilaryngeal secretions. The instructions for the Passy-Muir valve call for removal at night.

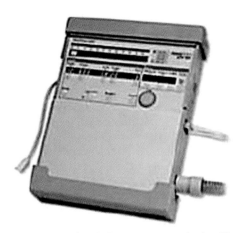

Figure 2-13 LTV-900 ventilator (Pulmonetics; now Cardinal Health, Dublin, OH).

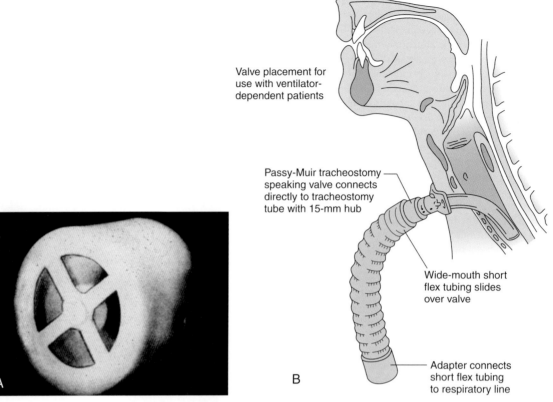

Valve placement for use with ventilator-dependent patients

Passy-Muir tracheostomy speaking valve connects directly to tracheostomy tube with 15-mm hub

Wide-mouth short flex tubing slides over valve

Adapter connects short flex tubing to respiratory line

A

B

Figure 2-15 Passy-Muir speaking valve (Passy-Muir Inc., Irvine, CA).

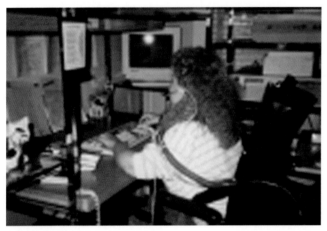

Figure 2-16 Telemarketing with Passy-Muir speaking valve (Passy-Muir Inc., Irvine, CA).

I know of no practical reason for this, and routinely continue to ventilate the patient at night with a cuffless tube and speaking valve. This greatly improves nocturnal communication with caregivers.

Tracheostomy impairs the ability to cough, and suctioning is necessary. Family members must be taught the proper technique. Long experience shows that clean technique is adequate; inner cannulae may be cleaned with soap, water, and hydrogen peroxide and reused. There is no need for routine tracheostomy changes; they may be changed for wear and tear, signs of irritation, or infection. Inhaled adrenergic bronchodilator drugs are virtually never needed and should be avoided in those patients with underlying cardiomyopathy. The prolonged survival

in patients with Duchenne muscular dystrophy in particular has greatly increased cardiomyopathy-induced dysrhythmias as a cause of death, leading to increased use of beta-adrenergic blockers and, on occasion, automated implantable cardiac defibrillators.

Nutrition is not usually an issue. Those who have been able to eat preoperatively are generally able to continue after a suitable interval and appropriate swallowing evaluation. Those who have been fed by gastric tube because of dyspnea and weight loss may be able to resume oral feedings; given the normal expiratory flow allowed by a one-way valve, aspiration risk is reduced.

Spinal Cord Injury

Spinal cord injury above C4 often is associated with paralyzed diaphragms as well as paralysis of the scalene, intercostal, and abdominal muscles; sternocleidomastoid innervation remains intact. As a result, 40% of those with C3 injury remain ventilator-dependent, as do all or nearly all of those with higher lesions. Very high lesions may leave the phrenics intact but nonfunctional, with the potential for electrical stimulation later. Lesions below C5 leave the neck accessories and diaphragms intact, but lower intercostals and abdominals are nonfunctional. All patients eventually become ventilator-independent, but because of impaired cough and secretion clearance, they may have problems with major atelectasis, most often in the left lower lobe. This may result in short-term respiratory failure.

For patients with permanent ventilator dependence, tracheostomy ventilation with ventilator speech, as described earlier, represents the best choice, but not all experts agree.[47] For patients with very high lesions and demonstrable phrenic function by nerve conduction studies and diaphragmatic electromyogram, electrophrenic respiration may be an option.

Persistent Polio Disability and Post-Polio Syndrome

A relatively small number of patients who had polio in the 1950s with an ongoing need for ventilatory support remain. They may continue to use the noninvasive modalities described earlier, including rocking beds, pneumobelts, and negative pressure ventilators. Others have converted to NPPV or may have an interest in doing so.

An increasing number of patients with recurrent symptoms resembling their original poliomyelitis began to be seen in the 1980s. The latent period appeared to be 20 to 30 years. Gradually progressive weakness was seen in the distribution of the original symptoms; patients requiring ventilatory assistance were generally those who had required mechanical ventilation during the original illness. These patients can be managed in a way similar to those with muscular dystrophy. Because the polio epidemics ended with the widespread administration of the Salk polio vaccine more than 50 years ago, it can be assumed that few additional cases will be seen.

Motor Neuron Diseases
Spinal Muscular Atrophy

The most common form of spinal muscular atrophy, and the most common type to cause respiratory dysfunction and the need for ventilatory support, is type II, with onset in early childhood and slowly progressive motor dysfunction. The age at which ventilatory support is needed varies, but it is often in the 20s. It is not uncommon for respiratory function to plateau for variable periods. Without intervention, scoliosis is common and adds to the respiratory dysfunction. Ventilatory management is similar to that for the muscular dystrophies.

Amyotrophic Lateral Sclerosis

ALS, a disease of both upper and lower motor neurons, differs from the muscular dystrophies in several important aspects that affect respiratory management. The course of the disease is much more rapid: average time from onset to death is approximately 3 years. Although approximately 80% of patients have onset in an extremity and 20% have initial bulbar involvement, all eventually have bulbar incompetence, leading to dysphagia, trouble handling oral secretions, and aspiration, if they live long enough. Finally, in contrast to the muscular dystrophies, all patients eventually lose the power of speech, in addition to having quadriplegia, and ultimately have great difficulty communicating by any mode.

The treating neurologist should follow the vital capacity and refer patients for pulmonary evaluation when it approaches 50% predicted. Performance of the vital capacity is dependent on adequate seal around the mouthpiece and so is susceptible to inaccuracy with bulbar involvement. In that case, sniff nasal inspiratory force may be used to follow the patient.[48] A value of less than 40 cm H_2O is associated with nocturnal hypoxemia and a median 6-month survival rate of 50%. Blood gases should also be obtained when it is not possible to follow vital capacity, when there is dyspnea or orthopnea, or when there is hypoxemia on pulse oximetry.

The American Academy of Neurology consensus guidelines recommend consideration of noninvasive ventilation when one of the following is present: FVC less than 50%, orthopnea, stiff nasal pressure less than −40 cm, or MIP less than −60 cm.[49] This recommendation is based on a single randomized controlled trial comparing noninvasive ventilation to standard care in a total of 41 patients with orthopnea and NIP less than 60% predicted or symptomatic daytime hypercapnia.[50] The study design and results do not permit extrapolation to asymptomatic individuals or to those earlier in the disease course. Survival and quality of life were improved in patients without severe bulbar dysfunction. Other nonrandomized studies have shown improved survival and quality of life in those without bulbar involvement who could tolerate NPPV.[51,52]

My own practice is to outline ventilatory support options at the patient's first visit, regardless of the stage of respiratory involvement. The guidelines for patient information outlined by the American Academy of Neurology are followed, and ample time is allowed for questions. The subject is addressed at each subsequent visit. The option of withdrawal of support under patient control and with comfort measures is made explicit; that is, patients clearly understand that, having decided on tracheostomy ventilation, their rescinding that decision will not be met by opposition or legal action on the part of the treating physician.[53–56] Using this approach, and with information presented uniformly by a single physician expert, my experience with the most recent 170 patients has been that fewer than 6% opt for tracheostomy ventilation and fewer than 30% wish noninvasive ventilation. The rest of the patients opt for supportive care. Quality of life appears to be improved for patients who are offered NPPV after respiratory symptoms develop.[57] The quality of life of caregivers for patients using NPPV does not appear to be negatively affected, in contrast to tracheostomy ventilation.[58,59] Patients undergoing tracheostomy ventilation may be satisfied with that mode, although experience is more mixed.[60] Those choosing NPPV undergo initiation in the hospital in much the same way as those with muscular dystrophy. As with patients with muscular dystrophy, these patients have modest or no alveolar–arterial gradient. Hypoxemia is generally caused by hypercapnea. Before the initiation of ventilatory support, many of these patients have substantial nocturnal hypercapnea and hypoxemia. In the early stages of noninvasive ventilation, this will persist. The night nursing staff must understand that they must not give patients oxygen without direct physician involvement because it may result in severe hypercapnea, even on mask ventilation.[61] Despite these precautions, unordered nocturnal oxygen administration has resulted in hypercapneic coma detected on morning bedside rounds; nursing notes recorded that the patient "slept comfortably." These patients can usually be revived without endotracheal intubation, using full-face mask ventilation under the supervision of the attending physician at the bedside for 1 hour or more.

Attempts at NPPV in patients with bulbar involvement, even with full-face masks, are nearly uniformly unsuccessful. Those without bulbar involvement can often be supported successfully as long as that condition obtains, sometimes for up to several years. These are the exceptions, and the usual course is more rapid deterioration. Dysphagia and aspiration predispose patients to respiratory infections that may result in acute respiratory failure. Patients should understand that this is likely to be the case.

Tracheostomy ventilation is initiated, for those desiring it, in a way similar to that described for muscular dystrophy. Because most have bulbar dysfunction, risk of aspiration, and loss of speech, ventilation with a cuffed tracheostomy tube is usually appropriate. The cuff should be inflated using minimal leak technique, and cuff pressure should be measured. Ideally, cuff pressure should be 15 to 20 mm Hg and always less than 25 mm Hg. Monitoring by caregivers at home may help to reduce the incidence of tracheomalacia and tracheoesophageal fistula, which is already very low, in my experience, in these patients whose ventilator pressures are usually low. Tracheostomy tubes may be changed on an as-needed basis, when the balloon fails. It is not necessary to change the tube on a scheduled basis because balloon failure does not generally result in significant difficulty ventilating patients with normal compliance for short periods. Ideally, the caregiver should be taught to change the tube, but it may also be changed in the clinic or emergency room. A spare inner cannula should be kept on hand and cleaned as described earlier.

Recent reports have suggested that diaphragmatic pacing may be useful in patients with ALS.[62,63] Evidence of efficacy is offered by comparing rates of decline in FVC before and after laparoscopic placement of electrodes after mapping. Given the highly variable rates of respiratory decline over time in the same patient, it seems prudent to await the results of controlled, appropriately randomized clinical trials before adopting this as standard therapy.

Adjuncts that may increase comfort and forestall complications are available. Control of sialorrhea may reduce microaspiration. A variety of anticholinergic agents may be used (I prefer glycopyrrolate and hyoscyamine liquids because they are easily titratable. Having an oropharynx that is too dry is nearly as bad as one that is too wet). Salivary injection of botulinum toxin has been used by some, although concerns remain that this may result in worsening of the underlying disease; parotid radiation may be used as a last resort. Portable suction is also useful. Gastric tube placement allows nutrition without aspiration on swallowing (although reflux aspiration may still occur). Percutaneous endoscopic gastrostomy tube placement should be done while FVC is more than 50%. I prefer to have the tube placed with interventional radiology because it avoids esophageal intubation, reduces the need for sedation, and allows noninvasive respiratory support during the procedure.

For those desiring only symptomatic care, comfort is usually achievable. Home nursing services or home hospice care can assist the patient's family.[64] Oxygen may be given without regard to Medicare guidelines. Opioids are generally effective in relieving dyspnea and may be administered by a variety of routes. Transdermal fentanyl beginning at 25 μg every 72 hours may be titrated upward as needed. Liquid morphine may be administered orally or via gastric tube. Morphine may also be effective for dyspnea when administered via nebulizer. Benzodiazepines are effective at relieving anxiety.

Management of Neuromuscular Diseases Resulting in Acute Respiratory Failure

Acute respiratory failure in patients with neuromuscular disease generally falls into one of two categories. First are the patients with an acute illness, such as Guillain-Barré syndrome, which results in respiratory failure as part of its natural history, and which, with appropriate care, is reversible, with return to normal respiratory function. Second are patients with chronic neuromuscular disease with respiratory involvement who have a crisis requiring initiation or extension of ventilatory support, such as ALS or one of the muscular dystrophies discussed earlier.

Guillain-Barré Syndrome

Guillain-Barré syndrome is the most common neuropathy precipitating respiratory failure. The typical case is marked by paresthesias, ascending paralysis, and loss of deep tendon reflexes. Between 15% and 30% of patients ultimately require mechanical ventilation. Poor prognostic factors include rapid progression, bulbar dysfunction, bilateral facial weakness, and autonomic dysfunction.[65,66] Patients with these characteristics should be admitted to an intensive care unit, with frequent neurologic and respiratory monitoring. Vital capacity should be measured with a bedside spirometer, and maximum inspiratory pressures should be monitored.[67]

Factors associated with the development of respiratory failure and portending the need for mechanical ventilation include vital capacity of less than 20 mL/kg, maximal inspiratory pressure of less than 30 cm H_2O, maximal expiratory pressure of less than 40 cm H_2O, or a reduction of more than 30% in vital capacity, maximal inspiratory pressure, and maximal expiratory pressure.[68] Other factors that predict the need for mechanical ventilation include severely impaired cough and inability to clear secretions and weakness so profound that the patient cannot raise the arms or head.[69] Oximetry and blood gases should be monitored.

When the course strongly predicts the need for mechanical ventilation, endotracheal intubation should be performed before the patient is in crisis. The procedure can be done electively and in a controlled fashion. Orotracheal intubation is preferred to nasotracheal intubation because it allows a larger tube size and avoidance of nosocomial sinusitis. NPPV is not often successful because the need for ventilation is frequently for 2 weeks or longer and because of bulbar dysfunction, secretions, and autonomic instability.

Care from that point is supportive. The duration of need for mechanical ventilation may be shortened by plasmapheresis or intravenous immunoglobulin.

Liberation from mechanical ventilation is the norm, although prolonged ventilation may be required. Standard weaning parameters are followed by T-tube or pressure support ventilation trials, depending on the preference of the critical care team. If mechanical ventilation exceeds 10 to 14 days, particularly if there is little progress, tracheostomy will improve the patient's comfort and nursing care.

Myasthenia Gravis

Myasthenia gravis does not ordinarily require long-term respiratory support. However, abrupt deterioration (myasthenic crisis) may precipitate respiratory failure. This may be caused by infection, a surgical procedure (a number of anesthetic agents and neuromuscular blockers may exacerbate myasthenia gravis), or reduction of immunosuppressive therapy. It may also occur after administration of any of a large number of drugs that may interfere with neuromuscular transmission. The best known are the aminoglycoside antibiotics; however, a large number of other antibiotics, beta-adrenergic blockers, anticonvulsants, and antipsychotics may also cause deterioration. The medication list of the deteriorating patient should be reviewed carefully and compared with one of the widely available contraindicated drug lists. In earlier times, cholinergic crisis as a result of anticholinesterase therapy was a serious part of the differential diagnosis. The increasing role of immunosuppression and avoidance of high-dose anticholinesterase administration has made this much less common. As a result, edrophonium administration (Tensilon test) for differentiation is no longer used routinely.

Patients with progressive and significant weakness should be admitted to an intensive care unit. Vital capacity and maximum inspiratory pressure (also known as negative inspiratory force) should be measured frequently.[70]

The goal is to avoid uncontrolled emergency intubation as well as to anticipate the need in a way that allows a controlled, elective procedure. Orotracheal intubation should be considered if the vital capacity falls to 15 to 20 mL/kg, maximum inspiratory pressure is less than 25 to 30 cm H_2O, the patient has bulbar dysfunction interfering with secretion and airway control, or the patient is in significant respiratory distress. Oximetry and blood gases should be monitored.[71]

In general, noninvasive ventilation is not appropriate because of bulbar involvement. Once mechanical ventilation is required, anticholinesterase medication is discontinued and therapy with either plasmapheresis or intravenous immunoglobulin is begun, depending on local capabilities and preference. After this therapy, anticholinesterase medication may be resumed and high-dose steroids may be initiated or resumed. Liberation from mechanical ventilation follows standard ventilatory parameters and weaning protocols.

Miscellaneous Conditions

A wide variety of medical conditions may rarely precipitate acute respiratory failure through involvement of the neurologic system in various ways, including botulism, acute attack porphyrias, Eaton-Lambert syndrome, anticholinesterase intoxication, severe phosphate deficiency, and periodic paralysis. Respiratory care is supportive and similar to that described earlier. The principal challenges are making the diagnosis and instituting appropriate specific therapies.

Acute Exacerbations of Chronic Neuromuscular Respiratory Failure

The first recognition of respiratory involvement in a patient with a neuromuscular disease is sometimes occasioned by acute respiratory failure. This is almost invariably precipitated by a respiratory infection. It need not be pneumonia; bronchitis will suffice. The reason is fundamentally mechanical. Resistance to linear airflow through a tube is an inverse fourth-power function. That is to say, if the diameter is reduced by half, the resistance increases 16 times. The small airway edema and mucus accumulation may result in substantial increases in respiratory work. This accounts for the chest tightness felt by the otherwise healthy patient with a lower respiratory infection, but in all but the most severe cases, there is an abundance of respiratory reserve. However, if a neuromuscular disease has reduced function by 60% to 70%, the additional work of breathing may be unsupportable, and acute respiratory failure may occur rapidly.

If the underlying disease is ALS, the patient may not yet have a diagnosis. If the patient has a muscular dystrophy, the diagnosis may be known, but the respiratory involvement may be unevaluated or unprepared for. In these cases, the patient often presents in respiratory crisis, and endotracheal intubation and mechanical ventilation ensue.

The patient who is fortunate enough to present more subacutely is monitored in a way similar to that described earlier, after spirometry, static inspiratory pressures, oximetry, and arterial blood gases are measured, with a decision to intubate and initiate mechanical ventilation based on similar parameters. Noninvasive ventilation may be attempted, but may not be successful if the patient has no experience or has bulbar involvement, difficulty with secretions, or altered consciousness.[72]

Mechanical ventilatory support is generally necessary until the infection subsides. With the first episode, the patient may wean from ventilation successfully after standard protocols. If that is not possible, extubation to noninvasive ventilatory support may be attempted. This should be undertaken when all variables are favorable: the patient's general status and strength are improved, infection is under control, secretions are minimal, and the patient is fully alert. If this is not successful, a decision about long-term support and tracheostomy must be made. This does not preclude subsequent attempts to convert to noninvasive ventilation, which may be successful.[73]

If the patient is already successfully receiving NPPV, the chance of noninvasive management is greatly increased. Over approximately 16 years, no patient with muscular dystrophy in my cohort who was already being managed in this way and who had acute respiratory failure as a result of infection required endotracheal intubation. After admission to the hospital, nasal ventilation is increased to 24 hours daily for the duration of the illness, which is treated with antibiotics and supportive care. The experience in patients with ALS who were successfully treated was similar, largely because virtually all had intact bulbar function and were doing well with noninvasive support. However, if the patient's condition is deteriorating, endotracheal intubation may be lifesaving. It is very important to discuss and finalize decisions about these kinds of interventions before the onset of an acute illness, particularly for those with ALS.

References

1. Martinez FJ, Bermudez-Gomez M, Celli BR: Hypothyroidism. A reversible cause of diaphragmatic dysfunction, *Chest* 96:1059–1063, 1989.
2. Laroche CM, Mulvey DA, Hawkins PN, et al: Diaphragm strength in the shrinking lung syndrome of systemic lupus erythematosus, *Q J Med* 71:429–439, 1989.
3. Rosenow EC, Engel AG: Acid maltase deficiency in adults presenting as respiratory failure, *Am J Med* 64:485–491, 1978.
4. Moufarrej NA, Bertirini TE: Respiratory insufficiency in adult-type acid maltase, *South Med J* 86:560–567, 1993.
5. Chandler KW, Rozas CJ, Kory RC, et al: Bilateral diaphragmatic paralysis complicating local cardiac hypothermia during open heart surgery, *Am J Med* 77:243–249, 1984.
6. Cape CA, Fincham RW: Paralytic brachial neuritis with diaphragmatic paralysis. Contralateral recurrence, *Neurology* 15:191–193, 1965.
7. Fromm GB, Wisdom PJ, Block AJ: Amyotrophic lateral sclerosis presenting with respiratory failure, *Chest* 71:612–614, 1977.
8. Loh L, Goldman M, Newsom Davis J: The assessment of diaphragm function, *Medicine* 56:165–169, 1977.
9. Ambler R, Gruenewald JE: Ultrasound monitoring of diaphragm activity in bilateral diaphragmatic paralysis, *Arch Dis Child* 60:170–172, 1985.
10. Miller JM, Moxham J, Green M: The maximal sniff in the assessment of diaphragm function in man, *Clin Sci* 69:91–96, 1985.
11. Celli B, Rassulo J, Corral R: Ventilatory muscle dysfunction in patients with bilateral idiopathic diaphragmatic paralysis: Reversal by intermittent negative pressure ventilation, *Am Rev Respir Dis* 136:1276–1278, 1987.
12. Glenn WWL, Brouillette RT, Dentz G, et al: Fundamental considerations in pacing of the diaphragm for chronic ventilatory insufficiency: a multicenter study, *Pacing Clin Electrophysiol* 11:2121–2127, 1988.
13. Redding GJ, Okamoto GA, Guthrie RD, et al: Sleep patterns in nonambulatory boys with Duchenne muscular dystrophy, *Arch Phys Med Rehabil* 66:818–821, 1985.
14. Baydur A: Respiratory muscle strength and control of ventilation in patients with neuromuscular disease, *Chest* 99:330–338, 1991.
15. Finder JD, Birnkrant D, Carl J, et al: Respiratory care of the patient with Duchenne muscular dystrophy: ATS consensus statement, *Am J Respir Crit Care Med* 170:456–465, 2004.
16. Raphael JC, Chevret S, Chastang C, et al: Randomised trial of preventive nasal ventilation in Duchenne muscular dystrophy. French Multicentre Cooperative Group on Home Mechanical Ventilation Assistance in Duchenne de Boulogne Muscular Dystrophy, *Lancet* 343(8913):1600–1604, 1994.
17. De Troyer A, Borenstein S, Cordier R: Analysis of lung volume restriction in patients with respiratory muscle weakness, *Thorax* 35:602–610, 1980.
18. Estenne M, Heilporn A, Delhez L, et al: Chest wall stiffness in patients with chronic respiratory muscle weakness, *Am Rev Respir Dis* 128:1002–1007, 1983.
19. Bach JR: Mechanical insufflation-exsufflation. Comparison of peak expiratory flows with manually assisted and unassisted coughing techniques, *Chest* 104:1553–1562, 1993.
20. Vianello A, Corrado A, Arcaro G, et al: Mechanical insufflation-exsufflation improves outcomes for neuromuscular disease patients with respiratory tract infections, *Am J Phys Med Rehabil* 84:83–88, 2005.
21. Ward S, Chatwin M, Heather S, et al: Randomised controlled trial of noninvasive ventilation (NIV) for nocturnal hypoventilation in neuromuscular and chest wall disease patients with daytime normocapnia, *Thorax* 60:1019–1024, 2005.
22. Meyer TJ, Hill NS: Noninvasive positive pressure ventilation to treat respiratory failure, *Ann Intern Med* 120:760–770, 1994.
23. Gomez-Merino E, Bach JR: Duchenne muscular dystrophy: prolongation of life by noninvasive ventilation and mechanically assisted coughing, *Am J Phys Med Rehabil* 81:411–415, 2002.

24. Phillips MF, Smith PE, Carroll N, et al: Nocturnal oxygenation and prognosis in Duchenne muscular dystrophy, *Am J Respir Crit Care Med* 161:675–676, 2000.

25. Vianello A, Bevilacqua M, Salvador V, et al: Long-term nasal intermittent positive pressure ventilation in advanced Duchenne's muscular dystrophy, *Chest* 105:445–448, 1994.

26. Bach JR, Alba AS, Saporito LR: Intermittent positive pressure ventilation via the mouth as an alternative to tracheostomy for 257 ventilator users, *Chest* 103:174–182, 1993.

27. Toussaint M, Steens M, Wasteels G, et al: Diurnal ventilation via mouthpiece: survival in end-stage Duchenne patients, *Eur Respir J* 28:549–555, 2006.

28. Garay SM, Turino GM, Goldring RM: Sustained reversal of chronic hypercapnia in patients with alveolar hypoventilation syndromes. Long-term maintenance with noninvasive nocturnal mechanical ventilation, *Am J Med* 70:269–274, 1981.

29. Bach JR, Penek J: Obstructive sleep apnea complicating negative-pressure ventilatory support in patients with chronic paralytic/restrictive ventilatory dysfunction, *Chest* 99:1386–1393, 1991.

30. Hill NS, Redline S, Carskadon MA, et al: Sleep-disordered breathing in patients with Duchenne muscular dystrophy using negative pressure ventilators, *Chest* 102:1656–1662, 1992.

31. Bach JR, Alba AS: Intermittent abdominal pressure ventilator in a regimen of noninvasive ventilatory support, *Chest* 99:630–636, 1991.

32. Bach JR, Alba AS, Saporito LF: Intermittent positive pressure ventilation via the mouth as an alternative to tracheostomy for 257 ventilator users, *Chest* 103:174–182, 1993.

33. Ellis ER, Bye PT, Bruderer JW, et al: Treatment of respiratory failure during sleep in patients with neuromuscular disease. Positive-pressure ventilation through a nose mask, *Am Rev Respir Dis* 135:148–152, 1987.

34. Kerby GR, Mayer LS, Pingleton SK: Nocturnal positive pressure ventilation via nasal mask, *Am Rev Respir Dis* 135:738–740, 1987.

35. Leger SS, Leger P: The art of interface. Tools for administering noninvasive ventilation, *Med Klin (Munich)* 94:35–39, 1999.

36. Hess DR: Noninvasive ventilation in neuromuscular disease: equipment and application, *Respir Care* 51:896–911, 2006.

37. Navalesi P, Fanfulla F, Frigerio P, et al: Physiologic evaluation of noninvasive mechanical ventilation delivered with three types of masks in patients with chronic hypercapnic respiratory failure, *Crit Care Med* 28:1785–1790, 2000.

38. Lloyd-Owen SJ, Donaldson GC, Ambrosino N, et al: Patterns of home mechanical ventilation use in Europe: results from the Eurovent survey, *Eur Respir J* 25:1025–1031, 2005.

39. Janssens JP, Derivaz S, Breitenstein E, et al: Changing patterns in long-term noninvasive ventilation: a 7-year prospective study in the Geneva Lake area, *Chest* 123:67–79, 2003.

40. Meecham Jones DJ, Wedzicha JA: Comparison of pressure and volume preset nasal ventilator systems in stable chronic respiratory failure, *Eur Respir J* 6:1060–1064, 1993.

41. Schonhofer B, Sonneborn M, Haidl P, et al: Comparison of two different modes for noninvasive mechanical ventilation in chronic respiratory failure: volume versus pressure controlled device, *Eur Respir J* 10:184–191, 1997.

42. Chadda K, Clair B, Orlikowski D, et al: Pressure support versus assisted controlled noninvasive ventilation in neuromuscular disease, *Neurocrit Care* 1:429–434, 2004.

43. Carrey Z, Gottfried SB, Levy RD: Ventilatory muscle support in respiratory failure with nasal positive pressure ventilation, *Chest* 97:150–158, 1990.

44. Spessert C, Weilitz P, Goodenberger D: A protocol for initiation of nasal positive pressure ventilation, *Am J Crit Care* 2:54–60, 1993.

45. Annane D, Quera-Salva MA, Lofaso F, et al: Mechanisms underlying effects of nocturnal ventilation on daytime blood gases in neuromuscular diseases, *Eur Respir J* 13:157–162, 1999.

46. Bach JR: Tracheostomy for advanced neuromuscular disease. Con, *Chron Respir Dis* 4:239–241, 2007.

47. Bach JR: Alternative methods of ventilatory support for the patient with ventilatory failure due to spinal cord injury, *J Am Paraplegia Soc* 14:158–174, 1991.

48. Morgan RK, McNally S, Alexander M, et al: Use of sniff nasal-inspiratory force to predict survival in amyotrophic lateral sclerosis, *Am J Respir Crit Care Med* 171:269–274, 2005.

49. Miller RG, Jackson CE, Kasarskis EJ, et al: Practice parameter update: the care of the patient with amyotrophic lateral sclerosis: drug, nutritional, and respiratory therapies (an evidence-based review), *Neurology* 73:1218–1226, 2009.

50. Bourke SC, Tomlinson M, Williams TI, et al: Effects of noninvasive ventilation on survival and quality of life in patients with amyotrophic lateral sclerosis, *Lancet Neurol* 5:140–147, 2006.

51. Aboussouan LS, Khan SU, Meeker DP, et al: Effect of noninvasive positive-pressure ventilation on survival in amyotrophic lateral sclerosis, *Ann Intern Med* 127:450–453, 1997.

52. Farrero E, Prats E, Povedano M, et al: Survival in amyotrophic lateral sclerosis with home mechanical ventilation: the impact of systematic respiratory assessment and bulbar involvement, *Chest* 127:1879–1882, 2005.

53. Goldblatt D, Greenlaw J: Starting and stopping the ventilator for patients with amyotrophic lateral sclerosis, *Neurol Clin* 7:789–806, 1989.

54. Position statement: certain aspects of the care and management of profoundly and irreversibly paralyzed patients with retained consciousness and cognition. Report of the Ethics and Humanities Subcommittee of the American Academy of Neurology, *Neurology* 43:222–223, 1993.

55. Moss AH, Oppenheimer EA, Casey P, et al: Patients with amyotrophic lateral sclerosis receiving long-term mechanical ventilation. Advance care planning and outcomes, *Chest* 110:249–255, 1996.

56. Borasio GD, Voltz R. Discontinuation of mechanical ventilation in patients with amyotrophic lateral sclerosis. *J Neurol.* 245:717–722, 199.

57. Lyall RA, Donaldson N, Fleming T, et al: A prospective study of quality of life in ALS patients treated with noninvasive ventilation, *Neurology* 57:153–156, 2001.

58. Mustfa N, Walsh E, Bryant V, et al: The effect of noninvasive ventilation on ALS patients and their caregivers, *Neurology* 66:1211–1217, 2006.

59. Rabkin JG, Albert SM, Tider T, et al: Predictors and course of elective long-term mechanical ventilation: A prospective study of ALS patients, *Amyotroph Lateral Scler* 7:86–95, 2006.

60. Cazzoli PA, Oppenheimer EA: Home mechanical ventilation for amyotrophic lateral sclerosis: nasal compared to tracheostomy-intermittent positive pressure ventilation, *J Neurol Sci* 139(Suppl):123–128, 1996.

61. Gay PC, Edmonds LC: Severe hypercapnia after low-flow oxygen therapy in patients with neuromuscular disease and diaphragmatic dysfunction, *Mayo Clin Proc* 70:327–330, 1995.

62. Onders RP, Carlin AM, Elmo M, et al: Amyotrophic lateral sclerosis: the Midwestern surgical experience with the diaphragm pacing stimulation system shows that general anesthesia can be safely performed, *Am J Surg* 197:386–390, 2009.

63. Onders RP, Elmo M, Khansarinia S, et al: Complete worldwide operative experience in laparoscopic diaphragm pacing and differences in spinal cord injured patients and amyotrophic lateral sclerosis patients, *Surg Endosc* 23:1433–1440, 2009.

64. O'Brien T, Kelly M, Saunders C: Motor neurone disease: a hospice perspective, *BMJ* 304(6825):471–473, 1992.

65. Lawn ND, Fletcher DD, Henderson RD, et al: Anticipating mechanical ventilation in Guillain-Barré syndrome, *Arch Neurol* 58:893–898, 2001.

66. Sharshar T, Chevret S, Bourdain F, et al: Early predictors of mechanical ventilation in Guillain-Barré syndrome, *Crit Care Med* 31:278–283, 2003.

67. Hughes RA, Wijdicks EF, Benson E, et al: Supportive care for patients with Guillain-Barré syndrome, *Arch Neurol* 62:1194–1198, 2005.

68. Lawn ND, Fletcher DD, Henderson RD, et al: Anticipating mechanical ventilation in Guillain-Barré syndrome, *Arch Neurol* 58:893–898, 2001.

69. Sharshar T, Chevret S, Bourdain F, et al: Early predictors of mechanical ventilation in Guillain-Barré syndrome, *Crit Care Med* 31:278–283, 2003.

70. Rabinstein AA, Wijdicks EF: Warning signs of imminent respiratory failure in neurological patients, *Semin Neurol* 23:97–104, 2003.

71. Juel VC: Myasthenia gravis: management of myasthenic crisis and perioperative care, *Semin Neurol* 24:75–81, 2004.

72. Vianello A, Bevilacqua M, Arcaro G, et al: Non-invasive ventilatory approach to treatment of acute respiratory failure in neuromuscular disorders. A comparison with endotracheal intubation, *Intensive Care Med* 26:384–390, 2000.

73. Goodenberger D, Couser J, May J: Successful discontinuation of ventilation via tracheostomy by substitution of nasal positive pressure ventilation, *Chest* 102:1277–1279, 1992.

Christopher F. Spurney, MD

3

Cardiac Complications of Neuromuscular Disorders

Cardiac disease has a significant association with neuromuscular diseases (Table 3-1). In all cases, early recognition of the neuromuscular diagnosis can improve timely recognition of forthcoming cardiac disease. The extent and severity of cardiac disease can vary significantly within and between specific neuromuscular disorders. In some cases, cardiac disease is the presenting symptom, long before skeletal muscle symptoms develop. In other cases, where skeletal muscle weakness occurs first, the signs and symptoms of cardiac failure can be masked by limitations in the patient's mobility and may not become apparent until cardiac failure is severe. Quality of life and longevity in some patients with muscular dystrophy are more dependent on disease of the cardiovascular system than on disease of the musculoskeletal system. Over the past 50 years, a more complete understanding of cardiac involvement in these patients has evolved. However, the specific etiologies and mechanisms of cardiac damage remain unclear. Although more data continue to emerge and improve the understanding of cardiac disease in these patients, there are still significant gaps in the etiology and best treatment practices. This chapter discusses the neuromuscular disorders most associated with cardiac disease and the current understanding of the proper diagnosis and treatment of these disorders.

Duchenne Muscular Dystrophy

Cardiac involvement in Duchenne muscular dystrophy (DMD) occurs in all patients older than 18 years old. In a large study of 328 patients with DMD by Nigro et al, cardiac involvement was found in 26% of patients younger than 6 years old, 62% of patients 6 to 10 years old, 81% of patients 10 to 14 years old, 95% of patients 14 to 18 years old, and 100% of patients older than 18 years.[1] Cardiac symptoms are unrelated to the severity of skeletal muscle disease, and one study showed that patients with stronger skeletal muscles were even more likely to die of cardiac disease than those with weaker muscles.[2]

Despite frequent myocardial involvement, most patients are free of cardiovascular symptoms. Diagnosis of cardiac dysfunction is often difficult because patients are less active and do not have early clinical symptoms (i.e., exercise intolerance).[3] As treatment of the skeletal and respiratory muscle systems improves, more patients with DMD are developing symptomatic heart disease. Approximately 72% of patients younger than 18 years were asymptomatic, but only 57% of patients older than 18 years old were symptomatic, even though all patients at this age were affected.[1] Gulati et al studied 30 patients older than 6 years, and only 10% had symptoms or signs suggestive of heart failure. However, one third had cardiomegaly, 93% had electrocardiographic (ECG) abnormalities, and left ventricular ejection fraction (LVEF) was less than 55% in 64% of patients and less than 50% in 18% of patients (normal range is 55%–65%).[4] Other studies also found that only 15% to 22% of patients with DMD and cardiac disease reported symptoms.[5,6]

Recognition of cardiomyopathy in DMD requires active cardiac evaluation because signs and symptoms of cardiac dysfunction may be vague and nonspecific. These include fatigue, weight loss, vomiting, sleep disturbance, inability to tolerate the daily regimen, and orthopnea. However, the development of cardiomyopathy usually precedes any symptoms and requires routine follow-up to identify early disease and start treatment.[7]

Becker Muscular Dystrophy

In contrast to DMD, cardiac involvement in Becker muscular dystrophy (BMD) is frequently out of proportion to the skeletal muscle involvement and can be the main clinical problem.[6] Cardiomyopathy is rare before 16 years of age, but it increases progressively with age, eventually affecting more than 70% of patients older than 40 years.[8] There is significant variability, both within and between families, in the onset, severity, and progression of cardiac disease, as is true for skeletal muscle involvement.[9] One concern about the increased incidence of cardiac disease is the increased long-term workload on the heart because of slower progression of skeletal muscle weakness compared with DMD.[10]

Dilated cardiomyopathy (DCM) can sometimes be the main pathologic finding in BMD. Despite the high proportion of DCM in BMD, only one third of patients are symptomatic. Patients with BMD and severe DCM can undergo cardiac transplantation with good results.[11] Hoogerwaard et al studied 27 patients with a mean age of 37.5 years and a mean follow-up of 12.5 years. Only 5 of 27 patients (19%) had completely normal heart evaluations. ECG abnormalities increased from 44% to 71%, and 63% of the patients showed progression of cardiac abnormalities. The presence of

Table 3-1 Summary of Cardiac Diseases Related to Specific Neuromuscular Disorders

Diagnosis	Age of Onset of Cardiac Disease	Cardiac Symptoms	Electrocardiographic Findings	Echocardiographic Findings	Prognosis
DMD	Preclinical disease presents at 6–8 years Clinical disease presents at 10–18 years	Asymptomatic CHF	Tall R waves in V1, V2 Q waves BBB PACs, PVCs	DCM RWMA MR	Death of cardiac or respiratory complications in the 20s to 30s
BMD	Preclinical disease presents at 10 to 20s Clinical disease rare in children, progresses with age, prevalent after 40 years	Asymptomatic CHF	Q waves Tall R waves BBB	DCM MR/MVP RV dilation RWMA	Heart failure in the 40s Poor prognosis once heart failure is present Heart transplant (eval)
DMD/BMD carrier	Preclinical disease presents at 10 to 20s Clinical disease presents at 30 to 50s	Asymptomatic CHF	Tall R waves	Normal DCM	Can have normal life expectancy Heart transplant (eval) in severe cases
XL-DCM	Clinical disease presents at 20 to 50s	Asymptomatic CHF	Q waves ST/T wave changes	DCM	Poor survival after symptomatic Heart transplant (eval)
LGMD (types 1B, 2C, 2D, 2E, 2F, 2I)	Clinical disease mild and varies with diagnosis	Asymptomatic CHF	Tall R waves Q waves 1°, 2°, 3° AVB	Normal DCM RWMA	Variable, depending on diagnosis Heart transplant (eval)
Myotonic dystrophy	Clinical disease presents in adulthood	Asymptomatic Syncope Sudden death	1°, 2°, 3° AVB Afib/Aflutter VT/VF	Normal DCM rare	Progressive cardiac involvement, death in 50s Sudden death
EDMD	Arrhythmias in 30s to 40s; can be earlier in XL-EDMD	Presyncope/syncope CHF (mostly AD-EDMD)	Sinus bradycardia 1°, 2°, 3° AVB Afib/Aflutter Atrial standstill VT/VF	Normal DCM Atrial thrombus	Pacemaker placement at 30 to 40s Heart transplant (eval) Sudden death
FSHMD	Arrhythmias in adulthood	Presyncope/syncope	1°, 2°, 3° AVB SVT/VT	Normal	Minimal cardiac involvement
Friedreich ataxia	Uncommon in children; increases with age	Asymptomatic	LVH Repolarization abnormalities Arrhythmias	HCM with LVOTO	Death occurs in 30s to 40s
Barth syndrome	Clinical symptoms present at 3–6 months	CHF	LVH with strain LAD Prolonged QTc Arrhythmias	DCM HCM LV noncompaction	Improvement with cardiac medications Heart transplant (eval)
Pompe disease	Clinical symptoms have infantile onset	CHF	Marked LVH Short PR interval	HCM	Death usually occurs by 1 year
Mitochondrial disorders	Variable onset, depending on diagnosis	CHF Syncope	ST/T wave abnormalities 1°, 2°, 3° AVB Arrhythmias	DCM HCM	Variable, depending on diagnosis
Congenital myopathies	Variable onset, depending on diagnosis	Asymptomatic CHF	Tall R wave Q waves	DCM	Usually more dependent on skeletal and respiratory function Heart transplant (eval)

AD-EDMD, autosomal dominant Emery-Dreifuss muscular dystrophy; Afib, atrial fibrillation; Aflutter, atrial flutter; AVB, atrioventricular block; BBB, bundle branch block; BMD, Becker muscular dystrophy; CHF, congestive heart failure; DCM, dilated cardiomyopathy; DMD, Duchenne muscular dystrophy; EDMD, Emery-Dreifuss muscular dystrophy; FSHMD, facioscapulohumeral muscular dystrophy; HCM, hypertrophic cardiomyopathy; LAD, left axis deviation; LGMD, limb-girdle muscular dystrophy; LV, left ventricular; LVH, left ventricular hypertrophy; LVOTO, left ventricular outflow tract obstruction; MR, mitral regurgitation; MVP, mitral valve prolapse; PACs, premature atrial contractions; PVCs, premature ventricular contractions; RV, right ventricular; RWMA, regional wall motion abnormalities; SVT, supraventricular tachycardia; VF, ventricular fibrillation; VT, ventricular tachycardia; XL-DCM, X-linked dilated cardiomyopathy; XL-EDMD, X-linked Emery-Dreifuss muscular dystrophy.

DCM increased from 15% to 33% over the 12 years. Five of the patients died during the follow-up period, and four of these deaths were the result of congestive heart failure. Three of these patients were able to walk at the time of death. The mean age of death in these four patients was 42 years.[9]

Melacini et al studied 28 patients with BMD ranging in age from 6 to 48 years with subclinical or benign skeletal muscle disease. Nineteen of these patients showed myocardial involvement, but only two were symptomatic.[12] Nigro et al reviewed the clinical history of 68 patients and found preclinical cardiac involvement in 67% of patients younger than 16 years of age. Clinically evident cardiomyopathy was found in 15% of patients younger than 16 years, increasing to 73% in patients older than 40 years.[8] These studies show a high incidence of myocardial involvement among patients with mild or subclinical skeletal muscle symptoms that progresses with time.

Carriers of Duchenne Muscular Dystrophy and Becker Muscular Dystrophy

A small percentage of female carriers of DMD and BMD can also have DCM that can progress to heart failure and even lead to heart transplantation.[13,14] Politano et al found preclinical or clinical evidence of myocardial involvement in 84% of DMD ($n = 152$) and BMD ($n = 45$) carriers. This increased with age, and 90% of carriers older than 16 years were affected. There were no statistically significant differences between DMD and BMD carriers. Only 11% of carriers were reported as having DCM, yet clinical symptoms were not reported.[15] Hoogerwaard et al studied 129 DMD and BMD carriers. ECG abnormalities were found in 47%, but DCM was found in 7 DMD carriers (8%) and no BMD carriers.[14] This agreed with the study of Grain et al that found a 7% incidence of DCM in carriers.[16] In these patients, DCM often occurs without any skeletal muscle symptoms.

X-Linked Dilated Cardiomyopathy

X-linked DCM (XL-DCM) is a rare cardiomyopathy associated with increased serum creatine kinase levels, but an absence of significant skeletal muscle weakness. Berko and Swift first described a group of affected males and their mothers. The patients presented with DCM at 15 to 21 years and survived only 5 to 12 months after diagnosis. The mothers presented in their 40s with atypical chest pain and slowly progressing heart failure.[17] Towbin et al found mutations in the dystrophin gene of patients with XL-DCM who had normal dystrophin levels in skeletal muscle.[18] These patients can have mild myopathic changes on skeletal muscle biopsy, but have complete loss of dystrophin in cardiac muscle.[19,20]

Limb-Girdle Muscular Dystrophy

Limb-girdle muscular dystrophy (LGMD) is a heterogeneous group of diseases with variable cardiac involvement. Cardiac presentation can be similar to that of DMD because of the loss of the dystrophin-associated glycoproteins that stabilize the dystrophin complex. There is currently no evidence of cardiomyopathy in LGMD types 1A (caveolin), 1C (myotilin), 2A (calpain), 2B (dysferlin), 2G

(telethonin), 2H (TRIM32), or 2J (titin).[21] However, cardiac involvement can be severe in the LGMD types 1B (lamin A/C), 2C (gamma), 2D (alpha), 2E (beta), 2F (delta), and 2I (fukutin-related protein).

Politano et al studied patients with sarcoglycanopathy, and 11 of 20 patients had evidence of cardiac involvement. Patients with gamma and delta sarcoglycan deficiency had DCM, and patients with alpha and beta deficiency had preclinical involvement.[22] Melacini et al studied patients with alpha, beta, and gamma sarcoglycan deficiency, and mild cardiac abnormalities were seen in 30% of patients who had severe skeletal muscle dystrophy. Four of 13 patients showed ECG abnormalities and 2 showed wall motion abnormalities on echocardiography. Patients were asymptomatic, and only one had a decreased LVEF of 43%. No correlation was found between the presence of cardiac abnormalities and the type of mutation or sarcoglycan gene involved.[23] Barresi et al described two patients with beta sarcoglycan deficiency who had severe cardiomyopathy. One died at 18 years and the other died at 26 years of age.[24] Calvo et al showed 10 patients with LGMD 2C who had ECG and echocardiographic abnormalities, especially of the right ventricle. Only one patient had decreased left ventricular function.[25]

The 1B type of LGMD (lamin A/C) is an autosomal dominant disease associated with conduction defects. Chrestian et al described a large French-Canadian family in which three of seven carriers of the gene had atrioventricular (AV) conduction blocks.[26] Ben Yaou et al described 13 patients with LGMD 1B who had conduction defects and arrhythmias. Seven of these patients needed a pacemaker or an implantable cardiac defibrillator, and two underwent heart transplantation.[27] Van der Kooi et al studied 26 patients with autosomal dominant LGMD 1B, and 12 showed ECG abnormalities, including 6 cases of AV conduction block, 4 requiring pacemakers. Six patients also showed echocardiographic abnormalities, including DCM.[28]

The 2I type of LGMD is related to defects in fukutin-related protein and is significantly associated with cardiac disease. Wahbi et al studied 23 patients with an average age of 32 years and found that 60% had decreased left ventricular function, 8% of which were severely decreased. None of the patients had significant arrhythmias, and no sudden death was recorded.[29] Poppe et al studied 38 patients with LGMD 2I who were 10 to 61 years old. Overall, 55% of patients had cardiac involvement, which was defined as decreased shortening fraction, left ventricular wall motion abnormalities, or ECG abnormalities. There was a tendency for cardiomyopathy to develop in patients with more severe skeletal muscle phenotypes, but 88% of patients with cardiac disease could still ambulate. Of 19 patients with a known clinical course, 8 had symptomatic cardiac failure at 18 to 67 years of age.[30] An earlier study by the same group described 16 patients 11 to 53 years old. They found symptomatic cardiac failure in three patients at ages 28, 39, and 51 years and asymptomatic left ventricular systolic dysfunction in three patients at 38, 57, and 58 years.[31] The possibility of severe cardiac disease was shown by D'Amico et al, who described the case of an 8-year-old boy who presented with severe cardiomyopathy and LGMD 2I. He required heart transplantation and is doing well, with no clinical skeletal muscle weakness.[32] Murakami et al identified six patients in four families with fukutin gene mutations who had DCM with no significant skeletal muscle involvement. One patient died of congestive heart failure at 12 years and one patient received a heart transplant at 18 years. The other patients had cardiomyopathy at 17, 27, 30, and 46 years.[33]

These studies show that cardiac disease is significantly involved in some forms of LGMD, and a specific muscle diagnosis is required to best anticipate cardiac complications.

Myotonic Dystrophy

Myotonic dystrophy (DM) is an autosomal dominant disorder that presents in adulthood with myotonia and weakness of the skeletal muscles. There are two major subtypes: DM type I is caused by increased CTG repeats and DM type II is caused by increased CCTG repeats. The severity of cardiac disease in these patients is unrelated to the severity of skeletal muscle disease. Groh et al studied 406 patients with confirmed DM type I with abnormal CTG repeat sequences. Ninety-six of these patients had evidence of non-sinus rhythm, prolonged QRS duration (>120 msec), or heart block. These patients were older, had more CTG repeats, and had more severe muscular disease. Twenty-nine of the patients with ECG abnormalities had atrial tachyarrhythmias, but only four had ventricular tachyarrhythmias, and of the patients with initially normal ECG findings ($n = 310$), 69 patients developed severe abnormalities. During follow-up, 81 (20%) of the 406 patients died: 27 (33%) died suddenly, 32 (40%) died of respiratory failure, and 5 (6%) died of other cardiac causes. Ventricular tachyarrhythmias were commonly observed in patients who died suddenly. The presence of a severe ECG abnormality had a sensitivity of 74% for predicting sudden death.[34]

In DM type II, patients can have DCM and arrhythmias. Schoser et al described four patients with DM type II who had sudden death. Three of the patients were asymptomatic, and one had symptoms of heart failure. All of the patients had DCM, and fibrosis of the conduction system was found in two of them.[35]

Patients with DM require careful cardiac monitoring to recognize abnormal heart rhythms and provide appropriate treatment options.

Emery-Dreifuss Muscular Dystrophy

Emery-Dreifuss muscular dystrophy (EDMD) is related to loss of the nuclear membrane protein emerin in X-linked (XL) inheritance (in the *STA* gene) and loss of lamin A/C in autosomal dominant (AD) inheritance. In XL-EDMD, muscle disease is milder and progresses more slowly than in AD-EDMD. In many patients, the severity of skeletal muscle disease is not significant, and the initial presentation is secondary to cardiac disease. It tends to start as sinus bradycardia and first-degree heart block and can evolve into third-degree (complete) heart block and atrial arrhythmias that lead to atrial paralysis. Left ventricular dysfunction can occur after the development of arrhythmias. The long-term prognosis of these patients depends significantly on the severity of cardiac involvement.

Boriani et al studied 18 patients with EDMD as a result of both emerin and lamin deficiencies. Arrhythmias were found in 15 patients, including all of the patients with emerin deficiency. Only one patient had significant heart failure and presented with atrial flutter and AV block necessitating a pacemaker. This patient did not improve and eventually required heart transplantation. One patient had right-sided heart failure as a result of AV block that resolved with pacemaker implantation, and three other patients had mild to moderate left ventricular dysfunction with limited or no impairment in daily activities.[36]

Buckley et al described three patients with XL-EDMD. The first presented at 19 years with atrial tachycardia and variable AV conduction. At 24 years of age, he was noted to have atrial standstill and junctional bradycardia of 37 beats per minute. A pacemaker was implanted at 29 years because of periods of atrial tachycardia

and atrial arrest with junctional escape beats. The patient was then free of cardiac symptoms. His nephew was found to have junctional bradycardia at 17 years. No tachyarrhythmias were noted, and a pacemaker was implanted. He had atrial fibrillation at 22 years, with a history of brief episodes of visual disturbances. Anticoagulants were administered and continued with intermittent atrial fibrillation. This patient's brother had junctional bradycardia at 15 years and had a pacemaker implanted. He remained asymptomatic after the pacemaker was placed.[37]

Sanna et al studied 10 patients with AD-EDMD. The average age at the first evidence of cardiac disease was 18.3 ± 9.7 years. ECG findings were abnormal in 8 of 10 patients, showing atrial fibrillation, atrial standstill, and AV conduction abnormalities. Holter recordings showed five patients with both atrial and ventricular arrhythmias, four associated with AV conduction abnormalities. Five patients had nonsustained ventricular tachycardia. On echocardiography, only one patient had a mild reduction in LVEF. One patient showed mild left ventricular dilation with normal function, and another patient showed right ventricular enlargement with a ventricular filling pattern consistent with a restrictive cardiomyopathy. Pacemakers were implanted in three patients. One patient who had a pacemaker because of atrial fibrillation with a slow ventricular response died suddenly at 48 years. Four patients had various degrees of left ventricular dysfunction.[38]

Brodsky et al described a single family found to have a lamin A/C mutation transmitted in an autosomal dominant pattern in 5 of 14 members. The five affected family members had minimal skeletal muscle weakness, but two had severe cardiomyopathy, AV block, and ventricular tachycardia. One of these patients received a heart transplant, and the second had sudden death.[39]

Fatkin et al studied 85 members of five families with EDMD and found 44 with lamin A/C mutations, 39 with cardiovascular disease. The mean age of disease onset was 38 years (range, 19–53 years) and often the diagnosis was based on asymptomatic ECG changes. Progressive abnormalities developed with increasing age. In all, 34 of 39 had sinus node dysfunction or AV conduction disease and 23 affected members had atrial fibrillation or flutter. Twenty-one patients had pacemakers implanted, and 25 of 39 had DCM. Heart transplant was required in six members because of rapid progression of heart failure, and 11 of the 25 died suddenly between the ages of 30 and 59 years.[40]

Based on these reports, the long-term survival of patients with EDMD is dependent on early diagnosis and proper treatment of cardiac arrhythmias.

Facioscapulohumeral Dystrophy

Facioscapulohumeral muscular dystrophy (FSHMD) does not appear to be a major cause of myocardial disease but is associated with conduction defects. Laforet et al studied 100 patients with FSHMD and found 5 with AV conduction defects or arrhythmias (supraventricular tachycardia, ventricular tachycardia), but no structural or functional cardiac defects.[41] De Visser et al found no evidence of cardiac changes in 31 patients with FSHMD.[42] Stevenson et al studied 30 patients with well-documented FSHMD. ECG abnormalities were present in 60% of patients, and abnormal electrophysiologic findings were present in 27% of patients. Atrial flutter or fibrillation was induced in 10 of 12 patients during electrophysiologic studies and sinus node function was abnormal in 3 patients.[43]

Other Neuromuscular Disorders

Friedreich Ataxia

Friedreich ataxia is an autosomal recessive disorder caused by mutations in the frataxin gene. Patients usually have ataxia with significant, but variable, progression over time. Patients have hypertrophic cardiomyopathy and show abnormal repolarization and arrhythmias on ECG findings. In a study by Casazza and Morpurgo, 50 of 66 patients diagnosed with Friedreich ataxia showed left ventricular hypertrophy. Ten of these patients had decreased cardiac function during the follow-up period. Only 1 of the 16 patients with a normal-sized heart had decreased function.[44]

Barth Syndrome

Barth syndrome is an X-linked disorder caused by mutations in the taffazin gene that result in abnormal mitochondria. Patients have a spectrum of symptoms, including skeletal muscle weakness, neutropenia, growth delay, and cardiomyopathy. Cardiac disease associated with Barth syndrome has a variable presentation unrelated to neurologic symptoms. In a study by Spencer et al, 90% of patients had a history of cardiomyopathy, with a mean age of 5.5 months at diagnosis. More than half of these patients had abnormal left ventricular morphology (increased trabeculations or noncompaction) on echocardiography.[45]

Pompe Disease

Pompe disease is a rare autosomal recessive disorder caused by a deficiency in acid alpha-glucosidase, a lysosomal enzyme that degrades glycogen. Symptoms can begin at 2 months of age in the infantile-onset form, and approximately 88% of these patients have hypertrophic cardiomyopathy.[46] Death often occurs before 12 months, but juvenile- and adult-onset forms have different prognoses and cardiac disease is rare.

Mitochondrial Disorders (Myoclonus Epilepsy with Ragged-Red Fibers, Mitochondrial Encephalomyopathy with Lactic Acidosis and Stroke-like Episodes, Kearns-Sayre Syndrome, and Leigh Syndrome)

Mitochondrial disorders, most often maternally inherited, are caused by specific defects in the mitochondrial respiratory transport chain or oxidative phosphorylation. Because of the high energy requirements of cardiac tissue, the heart is affected in these disorders. Cardiac manifestations include DCM and hypertrophic cardiomyopathy, AV conduction disturbances, and arrhythmias.[47]

Congenital Muscular Dystrophies

Congenital muscular dystrophies constitute a heterogeneous group of disorders with varying degrees of cardiac involvement. Ceviz et al found decreased cardiac function in patients with merosin-positive congenital muscular dystrophy.[48] Nakanishi et al showed increasing cardiac dysfunction as a function of age in Fukuyama-type congenital muscular dystrophy.[49] In these disorders, the prognosis is usually more dependent on skeletal and respiratory muscle weakness than on cardiac disease.

Diagnosis and Evaluation

History and Physical Examination

It is of vital importance to obtain a complete history of the type of muscular dystrophy and current treatments, if known. Special attention should be given to the family history, especially in cases of undiagnosed dystrophies. Two or more affected males in a single family should raise concern about a familial inheritance pattern, as is seen with XL-DCM, especially if there is no significant history of muscle weakness. Also, a family history of sudden death should raise suspicion for inherited cardiomyopathies.

Because these patients are inactive and often do not have significant exertional symptoms, it is important for the physician to ask specifically about changes in the activities of daily living. Is there increased fatigue? Does a child now use two pillows to sleep instead of one? Are there any changes in appetite, or has there been weight loss? These are subtle changes that patients and caregivers may not recognize. Has the patient had any episodes of palpitations or dizziness? Arrhythmias are usually symptomatic in young patients, but because of conduction abnormalities associated with some muscular dystrophies, they can occur with normal or even low ventricular rates, causing patients to remain asymptomatic.[36,50]

On physical examination, cardiac findings can be nonspecific but may provide initial clues to the presence and extent of cardiac disease. Vital signs can include tachycardia in patients with DMD and increased blood pressure as a result of steroid use. On examination of the neck, cannon A waves in the jugular venous pulse are suggestive of AV conduction disease and loss of A waves can be related to atrial fibrillation or atrial standstill. Increased jugular venous distention can be present in heart failure. During palpation of the chest, displacement of the point of maximal impulse to the left and inferolaterally is caused by an enlarged left ventricle. The point of maximal impulse can also be displaced secondary to scoliosis. On auscultation, there is usually a regular rhythm, with normal S1 and S2. Irregular rhythms are associated with atrial fibrillation. A midsystolic click secondary to mitral valve prolapse is sometimes appreciated in BMD. An S3 gallop can be heard during acute congestive heart failure and an S4 gallop can be heard secondary to left ventricular dysfunction. Systolic ejection murmurs can be associated with DMD, and systolic regurgitant murmurs, often as a result of mitral regurgitation, can be heard in BMD.[10] Gilroy et al found systolic ejection murmurs with grade I to II intensity in approximately 10% of patients with DMD.[3] In Friedreich ataxia, systolic ejection murmurs can be present as a result of subaortic stenosis from left ventricular hypertrophy. Hepatomegaly can be found on abdominal examination but can be difficult to palpate because of positioning and scoliosis. Examination of the extremities often shows dependent edema when heart failure develops.

Electrocardiography

An ECG is an important tool for the diagnosis of arrhythmias, and muscular dystrophies often have subtle early ECG changes. A 12-lead ECG examination provides noninvasive assessment of cardiac rhythm, ventricular axis, chamber enlargement, and conduction abnormalities or arrhythmias. The tracing speed can be increased (to 50 mm/sec) to aid in the diagnosis of conduction abnormalities.

Sinus tachycardia is found in most patients with DMD, even when these patients are immobile.[3,5,51] This tachycardia occurs in childhood and persists into adulthood. In an early study of DMD, Gilroy et al presented findings in 139 patients with DMD who were 4 to 35 years old. The most common clinical finding was sinus tachycardia, present in 124 cases (89%). The tachycardia was labile and appeared with minimal stimulation (e.g., raising the bed).[3] In another study, sinus tachycardia was seen in 78% of patients with DMD.[52] The exact cause is unknown, but possible etiologies include compensatory tachycardia secondary to ventricular dysfunction, autonomic dysregulation, or fibrosis of the sinoatrial node and conduction system.

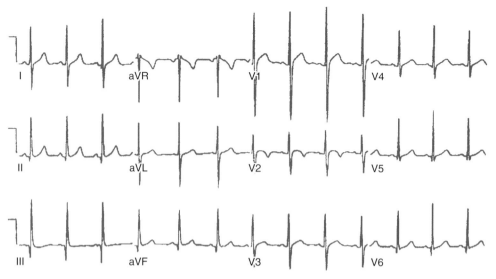

Figure 3-1 Electrocardiogram from a 16-year-old boy with Duchenne muscular dystrophy (DMD). This tracing shows common features of DMD including sinus tachycardia with a heart rate of more than 100 beats per minute; large R waves in leads V1, V2, and V3; and Q waves in the lateral and inferior leads (II, III, aVF, V5, and V6).

Another common ECG finding is tall R waves in both DMD and BMD (Fig. 3-1). Abnormally tall R waves in leads V1 to V3 were found in a study of patients with DMD.[3] Saito et al also showed prominent R waves in V1 in 88% of patients with DMD and 47% of patients with BMD.[10] Other studies confirmed the prominent R waves in patients with DMD and BMD.[5,12,53] These forces represent a loss of posteriorly directed forces because of selective scarring of the posterobasal portion of the left ventricle that is common in dystrophic myocardium. This correlation was pathologically confirmed in a previous study.[54]

This myocardial scarring can also extend laterally and produce large Q waves on surface ECG findings (see Fig. 3-1). Q waves are most frequently seen in the lateral leads (I, aVL, V6) and less frequently in the inferior (II, III, aVF) or anterior leads (V1–V4).[53–55] Lateral lead Q waves were seen in 73% of patients with DMD and 37% of those with BMD.[10] In DMD, lateral Q waves were present in 54% of patients compared with inferior Q waves in 30% of patients.[52] Hoogerwaard et al studied patients with BMD and found 33% with Q waves in the lateral leads and 11% with Q waves in the inferior leads.[9]

Arrhythmias and conduction defects can also be present. Premature atrial contractions are common in DMD.[55] Other atrial arrhythmias, including flutter and fibrillation, and premature ventricular contractions are also seen in DMD (Fig. 3-2).[56] Corrado et al found ventricular arrhythmias in 32% of patients with DMD who were studied.[57] Melacini et al found arrhythmias on ECG tracings in patients with BMD, including benign, isolated, monomorphic, and polymorphic premature ventricular contractions. Ventricular arrhythmias were documented in one patient who died suddenly.[12] Conduction defects are also frequent. Many patients with DMD and BMD are found to have bundle branch block patterns, but heart block is rarely seen.[3,9,12]

An ECG examination is most important in other muscular dystrophies where conduction defects are more prevalent. In LGMD 1B, AV conduction defects are seen. These defects initially begin as a prolonged PR interval but become progressively more severe over time and can develop into complete heart block. Atrial fibrillation with a variable ventricular response is seen.[26–28] In LGMD 2C and 2I, along with AV conduction defects, abnormal findings include dysmorphic notched P waves, tall R waves, Q waves, inverted T waves, and ectopic beats.[25,30,31] MD types I and II and EDMD, both XL and AD, are significantly associated with progressive AV conduction defects. Often these are the first and only presenting symptoms because muscular weakness has not developed. Atrial fibrillation and flutter are present in approximately 25% of patients with MD type I.[34–40,50] Atrial standstill can develop in patients with MD (Fig. 3-3).

The ECG results can show many other pathologic changes that indicate myocardial damage. These include ST segment and T wave changes, shortened PQ interval, increased cardiomyopathy index (QT/PQ), prolonged QTc, and increased QT dispersion.[1,3,52,53,58] Repolarization abnormalities are common in Friedreich ataxia. In a study by Child et al, 79% of patients showed ST/T wave abnormalities.[59]

Holter Monitors

Holter monitoring can provide additional important information in muscular dystrophies. As noted, depending on the type of dystrophy, the goals of Holter monitoring may differ. However, extending monitoring of the cardiac rhythm can provide greater detail of sporadic abnormalities that are not seen on the brief electrocardiogram. It is also a necessity in muscular dystrophies associated with conduction delay and heart block.

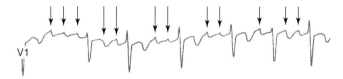

Figure 3-2 Rhythm strip from a 17-year-old boy with Duchenne muscular dystrophy. The strip shows atrial flutter with the *arrows* pointing to visible flutter waves at a rate of approximately 300 beats per minute. The atrioventricular node has variable conduction, with a ventricular rate of approximately 80 to 110 beats per minute.

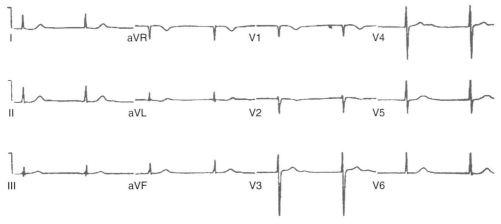

Figure 3-3 Electrocardiogram from a 19-year-old man with myotonic dystrophy type I. The tracing shows atrial standstill. There are no P waves evident, and there is a junctional rhythm at approximately 45 beats per minute.

In DMD, Holter monitoring can show variations in heart rate. Autonomic dysregulation has always been evident in patients with DMD. Kirchmann et al reported that Holter monitoring in DMD showed sinus tachycardia in 26% of patients, deprivation of circadian rhythm in 31% of patients, and reduced heart rate variability in 51% of patients.[6] D'Orsogna et al described labile abrupt sinus tachycardia in 11 of 18 cases.[5] Yotsukura et al also found a higher ratio of sympathetic to parasympathetic activity in patients with DMD compared with normal control subjects.[58,60] Similarly, Lanza et al showed impairment of cardiac autonomic function with an increased ratio of sympathetic activity.[61] These Holter results could reflect disturbances in the cardiac autonomic nervous system as a result of focal degeneration of the conduction system or adaptation to heart failure in patients with DMD. Autonomic dysfunction is also reported in BMD.[62]

Holter monitoring can also capture arrhythmias (Fig. 3-4). D'Orsogna et al reported 4 of 18 patients with DMD who had high-grade ventricular ectopy.[5] Kirchmann et al found premature ventricular beats in 9% of patients with DMD.[6] Corrado et al found more than six premature ventricular beats per hour in 32% and ventricular tachycardia in 7% of patients with DMD who were monitored.[57] There are less frequent arrhythmias seen in BMD. Kirchmann et al found normal sinus rhythm with normal mean frequency in BMD, and only 1 in 17 patients had premature

ventricular contractions.[6] Hoogerwaard et al reported only one arrhythmia (atrial fibrillation) in 21 patients with BMD who had Holter monitors.[9]

For patients who might benefit from longer monitoring or who have infrequent symptoms, implantable loop recorders are a consideration. However, unfortunately, normal ECG and Holter monitoring findings do not exclude the possibility of sudden death.

Echocardiography

Echocardiography is an important diagnostic tool for cardiomyopathy in muscular dystrophies. As noted, many patients have few or no symptoms because of limitations in ambulation. Echocardiography provides a noninvasive assessment of cardiac structure and function that can direct therapy and future follow-up. However, standard two-dimensional echocardiography can be limited by poor imaging windows secondary to scoliosis, lung hyperinflation, and chest wall deformities, and alternative methods for the early detection of cardiac abnormalities continue to be studied.

Most patients with muscular dystrophy have normally structured hearts. Once dilation of the left ventricle occurs, patients can have mitral regurgitation and left atrial enlargement. Saito et al showed that the left ventricular end diastolic dimension was significantly larger in patients with BMD (5.2 ± 0.7 cm) compared with those

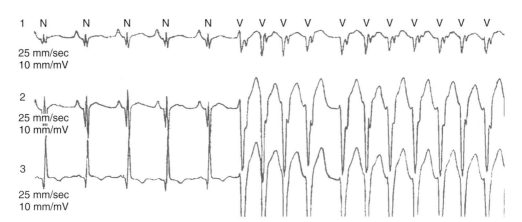

Figure 3-4 Holter monitor tracing from an 18-year-old man with Duchenne muscular dystrophy. The tracing shows a sustained run of ventricular tachycardia at a rate of approximately 160 beats per minute. The patient was asymptomatic throughout the recording. N, normal sinus beat; V, abnormal ventricular beat.

with DMD (4.2 ± 0.7) and healthy control subjects (4.2 ± 0.7). The mitral annulus was also larger in patients with BMD, and the frequency of mitral regurgitation was significantly higher in patients with BMD (28%) compared with patients with DMD (9.3%).[10] Atrial enlargement can also be seen in patients with atrial arrhythmias. Atrial flutter, fibrillation, or standstill can be associated with atrial thrombi, usually in the left atrial appendage. This should be excluded, usually with transesophageal echocardiography, before restoration of normal sinus rhythm.[36]

A decrease in left ventricular systolic function is the gold standard for the diagnosis of cardiomyopathy (Fig. 3-5). Kirchmann et al showed that the median age of onset of decreased fractional shortening (FS) (<25%; normal is 30%–40%) was 16.8 years in DMD and 30.4 years in BMD.[6] Corrado et al found decreased left ventricular systolic function to be a strong predictor of mortality in DMD during a 10-year follow-up period.[57] Associated with decreased systolic function, two-dimensional echocardiography can also delineate DMD-related regional wall motion abnormalities. In a study by de Kermadec et al, 72% of patients with DMD had at least one segment with wall motion abnormality. The most commonly involved segments were the inferior basal and inferior apical segments. Involvement of the anterior and lateral walls was usually limited to diffuse areas of hypokinesis.[63] Sasaki et al also showed wall motion abnormalities in the inferior, lateral, and apical segments of patients with DMD.[64] Hoogerwaard et al also found hypokinesis of the inferolateral wall and global hypokinesis without dilation in patients with BMD.[9]

However, the more important function of echocardiography is identifying preclinical cardiac disease. Markham et al showed that patients younger than 15 years old with normal cardiac function had abnormal indices of diastolic function for ventricular relaxation and ventricular compliance at the initial visit.[65] Evaluation of diastolic function is becoming one of the most important aspects of the cardiac evaluation. These abnormalities precede losses in systolic function and may provide quantifiable measures for treatment initiation and evaluation. Meune et al showed that despite normal echocardiographic and radionucleotide ventriculography-derived systolic function, tissue Doppler-derived strain rates showed systolic and diastolic myocardial dysfunction in BMD.[66]

Using myocardial strain imaging (MSI), Ogata et al showed that 10 of 13 patients with DMD, 11 to 20 years old with normal left ventricular function, had negative strain values in the outer layer of the posterolateral wall in the parasternal short axis. In 5 of these 10 patients, the timing to peak systolic velocity at the inferoposterior wall was delayed more than 60 msec.[67] Mori et al measured myocardial radial strain in the left ventricle in 25 patients with DMD who were 14.8 ± 3 years with normal left ventricular shortening fraction. Results showed significantly decreased peak systolic strain of the left ventricular posterior wall in patients with DMD compared with normal control subjects. Peak strain did not differ in the interventricular septum.[68] Thus, MSI can detect early changes in myocardial function before the onset of cardiomyopathy.

Hypertrophic cardiomyopathy is associated with some neuromuscular disorders, and many patients with DMD pass through a

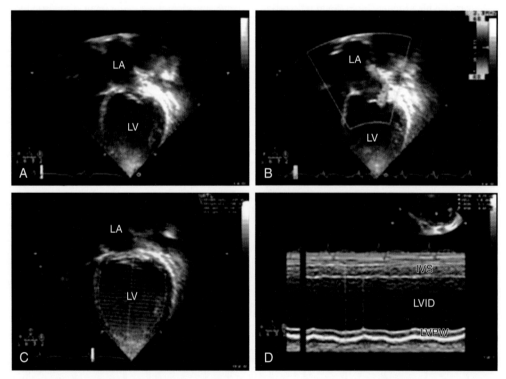

Figure 3-5 Echocardiographic images of a 20-year-old man with Duchenne muscular dystrophy and cardiomyopathy. **A,** Two-dimensional apical four-chamber view of a dilated left ventricle (LV) and normal-sized left atrium (LA). **B,** Color Doppler image in the same view as **A,** showing mitral regurgitation as a blue jet of color extending into the left atrium (LA) from the plane of the mitral valve. **C,** Measurement of ejection fraction in the apical four-chamber view. The endocardial border of the left ventricle (LV) is shown traced in diastole and the percent volume difference between systole and diastole is calculated. The ejection fraction in this image is 29% (normal, 55%–65%). **D,** M-mode image of the left ventricle showing decreased movement of both the interventricular septum (IVS) at the top of the image and the left ventricular posterior wall (LVPW) at the bottom of the image. The distance between the septum and the posterior wall, the left ventricular internal diameter (LVID), is measured in systole and diastole, and the percent fractional shortening is derived. This image shows fractional shortening of 8% (normal, 28%–40%).

hypertrophic stage before DCM develops. As noted, infantile Pompe disease is associated with severe hypertrophic cardiomyopathy.[46] Patients with Friedreich ataxia also have a thickened left ventricle, and echocardiogram shows concentric left ventricular hypertrophy or asymmetrical septal hypertrophy. Some of these patients go on to have decreased systolic function and DCM.[59,69]

Echocardiography is also used in evaluation of the right ventricle and pulmonary pressure. Right ventricular abnormalities were seen early in 64% of asymptomatic patients with BMD, including right ventricular enlargement in 18 patients.[12] In LGMD 2C, echocardiography showed 8 of 10 patients with right ventricular dilation, right ventricular free wall hypertrophy, and no evidence of increased pulmonary artery pressure. This was accompanied by abnormal right ventricle relaxation using tissue Doppler imaging.[25] Right ventricular dilation was also seen in two patients with alpha-sarcoglycan deficiency.[23]

Magnetic Resonance Imaging

Magnetic resonance imaging (MRI) is another imaging modality that can provide clues to preclinical cardiac dysfunction. MRI is useful for looking at myocardial fibrosis and thickness, thrombi, and the ventricular apices. In a study by Ashford et al, 13 patients with DMD, mean age 10.6 years and without apparent heart disease, underwent cardiac MRI in a 1.5-T clinical scanner. These patients showed normal left ventricular volume and ejection fraction, but manifested reduced midventricular and basal cross-sectional global circumferential strain compared with control subjects. These alterations also appeared in segmental analysis of the septal, anterior, lateral, and inferior walls.[70] A study by Silva et al used delayed myocardial enhancement to show early myocardial fibrosis in DMD, even in patients younger than 10 years old.[71] In LGMD 2I, MRI showed decreased cardiac function with fatty replacement and fibrosis of the myocardium.[29] In another study of patients with 2I LGMD, 8 of 9 patients showed cardiac involvement with cardiac MRI compared with only 2 patients using echocardiography.[72] Thus, MRI may become an important early imaging modality during preclinical cardiac disease.

Cardiac Catheterization

There is limited use for cardiac catheterization in the diagnosis of known dystrophy-related cardiomyopathy because the structure of the heart and coronary arteries is normal. In cases of cardiomyopathy with absent or minimal skeletal muscle disease (i.e., XL-DCM), catheterization can confirm normal coronary angiography and endomyocardial biopsy can be performed for pathologic analysis and dystrophin staining. Cardiac catheterization can also be used during acute cardiac decompensation for the placement of assistance devices to provide systolic function support to the failing myocardium.

Electrophysiologic Testing

Invasive electrophysiologic (EP) studies are indicated when certain abnormalities are present. These include pauses greater than 2.5 seconds, sinus bradycardia less than 40 bpm, first-degree AV block greater than 240 msec, second- or third-degree AV block, and documented atrial or ventricular arrhythmias.[73] DM and EDMD are known to affect the cardiac conduction system. EP testing can play a role in the diagnosis of conduction abnormalities. However, Lazarus et al studied 83 patients with DM and primarily with asymptomatic conduction abnormalities using invasive electrophysiologic testing.

AV conduction disturbances were common. Atrial arrhythmias were inducible in 41% of cases, and ventricular arrhythmias were induced in 18% of cases. However, no relationship between ECG findings and EP testing abnormalities was found and the predictive value for sudden death was unclear.[74] Negri et al presented a case of BMD with recurrent wide complex tachycardia found to have a bundle branch re-entrant ventricular tachycardia during EP testing. This pathway was treated successfully with radiofrequency ablation.[75]

Pathology

Cardiomyopathy is referred to as a "final common pathway" because many etiologies lead to a dilated, poorly functioning heart. However, pathologic specimens show specific differences in dystrophy-related cardiomyopathies. Gilroy et al showed in DMD that the myocardium varied from areas of well-preserved fibers with slightly or moderately enlarged nuclei to areas of extensive replacement by connective tissue. Also, no inflammatory or granulation tissue was present.[3] Most myocardiocytes were atrophic, with loss of striations and nuclear fragmentation, and there was selective scarring of the posterobasal portion of the left ventricle.[76] The fibrosis appears to especially involve the outer half of the posterior left ventricular free wall, often in a band-like distribution.[77] In BMD, pathology shows marked damage in the lateral wall, consistent with the lateral ECG findings.[10] In dystrophies significantly associated with arrhythmias, progressive fibrosis of the sinoatrial node, AV node, and Purkinje conduction fibers is prominent.[35,40,50] These differences underscore the need to further understand the specific pathways and mechanisms affected by muscular dystrophy so that more directed therapy can be developed.

Treatment

The treatment of cardiac disease in neuromuscular disorders depends on the skeletal muscle diagnosis and stage of progression. As noted, DMD and BMD are dominated by myocardial dysfunction and decreased cardiac function and disease progression is treated with an increasing amount of medical therapy (Fig. 3-6 and Table 3-2). EDMD and DM are dominated by conduction system disease, and progressive disease requires pacemaker implantation (Fig. 3-7). A discussion of the benefits of specific medical and device therapies for cardiac complications in neuromuscular disease follows.

Corticosteroids

The gold standard for treatment of dystrophic skeletal muscle disease is steroid therapy. However, long-term cardiovascular effects of steroid treatment include obesity, hypertension, and cardiac hypertrophy.[78] The effects of steroid treatment on cardiac function have also been studied. Markham et al looked at patients with DMD who were 7.5 to 12 years old and were treated with either prednisone or deflazacort ($n = 14$) or with no steroids at all ($n = 23$). The FS decreased from 35.5% to 26.0% in the untreated group, whereas it remained unchanged (36%–34%) in the steroid-treated group. The steroid-treated patients' hearts also did not dilate as much as those of untreated patients. There were no significant differences in blood pressure between the two groups. Thus, steroids, started before there was any evidence of decreased cardiac function, delayed the onset of ventricular dysfunction in these patients.[79] In an earlier study by the same group, untreated subjects 10 years old or younger were 4.4 more

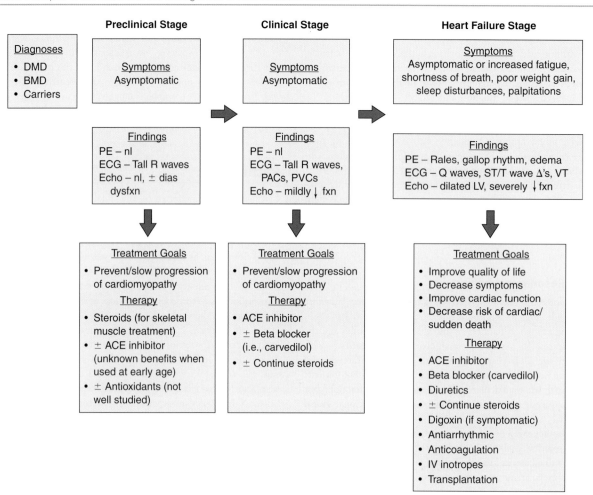

Figure 3-6 Progressive stages and treatment of cardiomyopathy in Duchenne muscular dystrophy and Becker muscular dystrophy. ACE, angiotensin-converting enzyme; dias, diastole; dysfxn, dysfunction; ECG, electrocardiogram; Echo, echocardiogram; fxn, function; IV, intravenous; LV, left ventricular; nl, normal; PAC, premature atrial contraction; PE, physical examination; PVC, premature ventricular contraction; VT, ventricular tachycardia.

Table 3-2 Recommended Dosages for Cardiac Medications Used in the Treatment of Duchenne Muscular Dystrophy–Related Cardiomyopathy

Cardiac Medication	Pediatric Dosing	Adult Dosing
Angiotensin-converting Enzyme Inhibitors		
Captopril	0.3–0.5 mg/kg/dose; max dose 6 mg/kg/day	25–100 mg/day divided BID
Enalapril	0.1–0.5 mg/kg/day divided BID	5–20 mg/day divided BID
Perindopril	2–4 mg once daily	4–8 mg once daily
Beta Blockers		
Carvedilol	0.05 mg/kg/dose BID; increase as tolerated to max dose of 0.4 mg/kg/dose BID	3.125 mg BID; increase as tolerated to max dose of 25 mg BID
Propranolol	2–4 mg/kg/day divided TID	40–320 mg/day divided TID
Atenolol	1–2 mg/kg/day	25–50 mg daily
Diuretics		
Furosemide	1 mg/kg/dose BID	20–40 mg daily
Spironolactone	1–3 mg/kg/day divided BID	25–50 mg daily
Digoxin	10 μg/kg/day divided BID	125–250 μg daily
Diltiazem	1.5–2 mg/kg/day divided TID; max 3.5 mg/kg/day	180–420 mg/day extended-release capsule form
Amiodarone	Loading dose of 10 mg/kg/day divided BID for 4–14 days, followed by maintenance dose of 5 mg/kg/day once daily	800–1600 mg/day divided BID for 1–3 weeks, decrease to 600–800 mg/day for 4 weeks, followed by maintenance dose of 400 mg/day once daily

BID, twice daily; max, maximum; TID, three times daily.

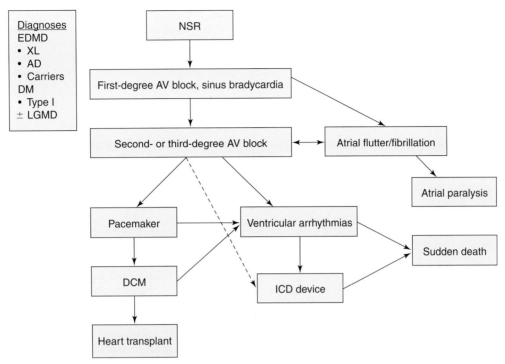

Figure 3-7 Progression and treatment of heart rhythm abnormalities in EDMD, DM type I, and limb-girdle muscular dystrophy. AD, autosomal dominant; AV, atrioventricular; DCM, dilated cardiomyopathy; ICD, implantable cardioverter–defibrillator; NSR, normal sinus rhythm; XL, X-linked.

times likely to have FS of less than 28%. Untreated subjects older than 10 years were 15.2 times more likely to have decreased FS compared with steroid-treated subjects. There was no difference in FS between the prednisone and deflazacort groups (see also Chapter 19).

Data also suggest that the beneficial effect of steroids may persist. In patients for whom treatment was discontinued secondary to side effects, steroids appear to have helped to preserve cardiac function up to 6 years after discontinuation.[80] Silversides et al studied patients with DMD between the ages of 10 and 18 years. Patients receiving deflazacort for at least 3 years had better FS (33% vs. 21%), and only 5% of patients taking deflazacort had an LVEF of less than 45% compared with 58% for untreated subjects. Patients also showed improvement in pulmonary and skeletal muscle strength.[81] These results support a beneficial effect of steroids on cardiac function in the short term. Further understanding of the long-term effects of steroids on cardiac size and function are not yet known.

Other Pharmacologic Therapy

In recent years, there has been some success in treating DMD-related cardiomyopathy. Currently, there is no specific treatment for cardiomyopathy secondary to muscular dystrophies, but treatments used for other forms of cardiomyopathy have proven useful. Once decreased systolic cardiac function is found, pharmacologic therapy is recommended to slow the progression of cardiomyopathy. The main focus of medical therapy has included angiotensin-converting enzyme inhibitors (ACEis) and beta blockers, and this has led to some success in improving DMD-related cardiomyopathy (see Fig. 3-6 and Table 3-2).

Angiotensin-Converting Enzyme Inhibitors and Beta Blockers

In an important study, Duboc et al studied 57 children with DMD, 9.3 to 13.0 years old, with LVEF of greater than 55%. In the initial phase, 27 children were treated with the ACEi perindopril (2–4 mg/day) and 29 children received placebo for 3 years. After this

period, all patients ($n = 51$) received perindopril for 2 years. There were no significant differences at the start or the end of the initial 3 years. The mean ejection fraction in the treated group was 60.7% versus 64.4% in the untreated group. One patient in each group had an ejection fraction of less than 45%. However, at the completion of the second phase, the LVEF was 58.6% in the initially treated group versus 56% in the initially untreated group. Eight patients in the initially untreated group had an LVEF of less than 45% compared with one patient in the treated group.[82] The same group published results after 10 years of follow-up. Even though all patients started with normal cardiac function, 93% of the initially treated group were alive versus only 66% of the untreated group.[83] These studies showed that early treatment delayed the onset and progression of left ventricular dysfunction and led to lower mortality rates in DMD. Ramaciotti et al also showed a benefit from ACEi treatment. In a retrospective analysis of 50 patients with DMD who were 10 to 20 years old, 10 of 27 patients with systolic dysfunction returned to normal function after treatment with the ACEi enalapril.[84]

Jefferies et al followed patients with DMD ($n = 62$) and BMD ($n = 7$) with a mean age of 12.9 years and 13.7 years, respectively. After the first abnormal echocardiogram (LVEF < 55%), patients were treated with an ACEi (enalapril, captopril, or lisinopril). If no improvements in the ACEi group were seen at 3 months, beta blockers (carvedilol or metoprolol) were added. ACEi was the single therapy in 42% of patients, and combination therapy was required in 58% of patients. The mean age of onset for ACEi therapy was 14.1 years in BMD and 16.1 years in DMD. Beta blockers were initiated at a mean age of 16.0 years old in BMD and 18.1 years old in DMD. ACEi or beta blocker therapy improved cardiac function in 27 of 29 patients.[85] Ishikawa et al also reported a reduction in neuroendocrine activity and left ventricular dilatation in patients with DMD taking ACEi and beta blockers, and Kajimoto et al showed that combination therapy with carvedilol and an ACEi for 2 years resulted in a significant increase in FS in a mixed muscular dystrophy cohort.[86,87]

The beta blocker carvedilol was studied by Rhodes et al in patients with DMD who were 14 to 46 years old and had DCM and LVEF of less than 50%. Carvedilol was administered for 6 months and was associated with a modest but statistically significant improvement in cardiac MRI-derived LVEF (41%–43%). There were also trends toward improved FS and diastolic function. Carvedilol also decreased the incidence of ventricular tachycardia seen in two patients.[88]

Because these patients are at high risk for cardiomyopathy, additional studies are required to better understand the benefits of early initiation of cardiac "preventive" therapy with ACEi and beta blockers and any potential interactions with concomitant steroid therapy.

Heart Failure

Management of symptomatic heart failure related to dystrophic cardiomyopathy is the same as that recommended by the American Heart Association for other forms of heart failure.[89] Diuretics (furosemide), aldosterone antagonists (spironolactone), and salt restriction are indicated in patients with fluid retention. Beta blockers, especially carvedilol, long-acting metoprolol, and bisoprolol, blunt the sympathetic nervous system and reduce mortality rates in heart failure. An ACEi, as noted previously, modulates the renin-angiotensin-aldosterone system and improves cardiac remodeling. Drugs that adversely affect patients, including most antiarrhythmics and calcium channel blockers, should be avoided. Digoxin is most beneficial as an adjunctive therapy in patients who remain symptomatic while receiving the previously mentioned therapies. Initiation and maintenance dosing of these medications requires a cardiologist's expertise and close monitoring of blood pressure, electrolyte levels, and renal function.

Anticoagulation

Oral anticoagulation therapy can be used in cases of severe cardiac dysfunction to prevent intracardiac thrombus formation; however, the efficacy of this treatment remains unclear.[89] Anticoagulation should be used in cases of atrial fibrillation and flutter or if there is any history of an embolic event. A goal international normalized ratio of 2.0 to 2.5 should be maintained. Boriani et al showed that 4 of 11 patients with atrial fibrillation or flutter in EDMD had an embolic stroke. Unfortunately, stroke was the initial presentation in three of these cases. Earlier diagnosis and anticoagulation might have prevented this outcome.[36] EDMD is also associated with atrial standstill, and even with a pacemaker, these patients are still at risk for thrombus formation and should be treated with anticoagulants.[90]

Arrhythmias

The treatment of arrhythmias in muscular dystrophy and other neuromuscular disorders depends on the type of disorder and associated arrhythmia. Physicians must consider the proarrhythmic side effects of these drugs. Conversion of atrial arrhythmias may be attempted with medical therapy, including propafenone and ibutilide. If ventricular arrhythmias are present, treatment with amiodarone, sotalol, or carvedilol can be effective. Standard monitoring of thyroid, liver, and pulmonary function is required for prolonged use of amiodarone. Drugs that can slow cardiac conduction are contraindicated in heart block and progressive bradyarrhythmias, including digoxin, beta blockers, and calcium channel blockers.

Cardioversion

Synchronized cardioversion is a potential treatment for stable atrial flutter or fibrillation or stable ventricular tachycardia. Imaging studies should confirm the absence of atrial thrombi, especially in the left atrial appendage. If a thrombus is present, anticoagulation therapy should be started and conversion of the rhythm delayed. Once the rhythm has been converted to sinus, medical therapy should be considered to decrease the likelihood of recurrent arrhythmias.

Pacemaker Implantation

Some neuromuscular diseases are a class I indication for pacemaker implantation because of acquired AV block. These include forms of DM, Kearns-Sayre syndrome, and LGMD. This indication includes both symptomatic and asymptomatic patients because of the unpredictable progression of AV conduction disease in these patients.[91] The placement of devices can be limited by kyphoscoliosis and muscle wasting.

Lazarus et al studied patients with DM and a prolonged His bundle–ventricular muscle interval. These patients, even if asymptomatic, received pacemakers. During EP testing, complete AV block, sinoatrial block, and atrial or ventricular tachyarrhythmias were found. Unfortunately, pacemakers did not prevent all deaths. Ten deaths occurred during the study, and four of these deaths were sudden. Pacemaker interrogation showed no arrhythmias in two of the patients with sudden death, and the other two patients did not have an interrogation performed. Other deaths were related to respiratory failure, and two deaths were related to embolic events.[92] There are other reports of patients with DM who die suddenly despite functioning pacemakers.[93]

Boriani et al studied patients with EDMD, and pacemakers were required for symptomatic bradyarrhythmias in seven with XL-EDMD and three with AD-EDMD. These patients were treated successfully, and complications occurred in 3 of these 10 cases, including lead displacements and lead fractures. One of the patients with EDMD had a pacemaker for 24 years and was 67 years old when the report was published. This shows that, with careful monitoring, pacemaker implantation is successful and survival can be long.[36]

The effective use of biventricular pacing for the treatment of DCM in muscular dystrophy is not well studied.

Implantable Cardioverter–Defibrillator Implantation

The benefits of implantable cardioverter–defibrillator (ICD) implantation compared with pacemaker implantation remain under evaluation. Golzio et al described the case of a 20-year-old woman who initially had first-degree AV block. She was diagnosed with EDMD at 41 years and required pacemaker implantation because of the new diagnosis and low ventricular rate response atrial fibrillation on Holter monitoring. She had palpitations, and Holter monitoring showed nonsustained ventricular tachycardia. The pacemaker was replaced with an ICD device. Nine months later, during a febrile illness, the patient experienced three discharges from the ICD. Interrogation of the device showed three appropriate discharges for fast polymorphic ventricular tachycardia that deteriorated into ventricular fibrillation. This life-saving discharge argues for ICD placement with concern that a stressful event, such as a febrile illness, could incite lethal arrhythmias in this susceptible population.[94]

In an earlier study, Meune et al prospectively offered ICDs to patients with EDMD who were referred for cardiac pacemakers. The indication for pacemaker implantation was progressive conduction block or sinus block, and no evidence of previous ventricular arrhythmias was required. The study involved 19 patients, and during a mean follow-up period of 34 months, 8 patients received appropriate ICD discharges. Six patients had ventricular fibrillation and two had rapid ventricular tachycardia. One patient received an inappropriate shock. No other factors, including LVEF, spontaneous or inducible ventricular tachycardia, or drug therapy, were related to the occurrence of ventricular arrhythmias in this population.[95]

Walker et al described a 42-year-old woman and manifesting carrier of EDMD who presented with palpitations secondary to premature ventricular beats. Seven years later, she had atrial fibrillation with slow ventricular response and required pacemaker implantation. She had normal ventricular function. Later, she developed heart failure secondary to progressive DCM and also developed ventricular tachycardia. A biventricular ICD was placed without complication. The patient improved clinically and had appropriate antitachycardia pacing function. She did not have any ICD discharges (appropriate or inappropriate). This scenario should make ICD placement at initial presentation a consideration.[96]

Cardiac Transplantation

Cardiac transplantation is a viable option in muscular dystrophy when the cardiac component presents earlier and with more severity than the skeletal muscle disease. Complete evaluation of skeletal muscle disease and respiratory function is important. Previous concerns about transplantation in this group included higher perioperative risk and potential cardiomyopathy in the transplanted heart, but these concerns are now minimal. It is an effective therapy in patients with BMD and maternal carriers of dystrophin gene mutations.[13,97,98] Transplantation has also been reported in patients with LGMD 2I and EDMD.[32,33,40] In a recent review, 27 patients with DMD ($n = 3$), BMD ($n = 19$), carrier status ($n = 3$), or XL-DCM ($n = 2$) underwent cardiac transplantation. Those with DMD underwent transplantation at ages 12, 24, and 31 years. All patients with BMD were younger than 33 years at the time of transplant except one 45-year-old.[73] Ruiz-Cano et al reported five patients with muscular dystrophy who underwent transplantation at a mean age of 38 years with no significant differences in hospital course or long-term complications compared with control subjects.[99] These studies show that cardiac transplantation is a potentially successful therapy for significant heart failure in many muscular dystrophies, although there are no uniform criteria for its use.

Preoperative Assessment

A complete cardiac evaluation should be performed before major surgical procedures. Medical therapy must be optimized before surgery, and there are specific concerns in patients with muscular dystrophy. Intraoperative monitoring and anesthesia performed by anesthesiologists experienced in cardiac dysfunction and muscular dystrophy is recommended. Schmidt et al reported a case of acute heart failure in an 11-year-old boy with DMD and normal cardiac function during elective thoracolumbar stabilization.[100] Patients with DMD are known to be at high risk for anesthesia-associated malignant hyperthermia. Complications have also occurred in patients with BMD and in carriers.[101–103] Breucking et al found that sudden cardiac arrest during anesthesia in DMD and BMD occurred in 6 of 221 patients, but all 6 had undiagnosed muscular dystrophy at the time. No events occurred in patients with a known diagnosis.[104] These cases show how major surgical procedures should be performed in tertiary care centers using subspecialty services familiar with muscular dystrophies. This is also discussed in Chapter 10.

Experimental Therapies

Because of the lack of current specific cardiac treatments for neuromuscular disorders, pharmaceutical agents are continuously tested in animal models and human clinical trials. Antioxidant therapies, including coenzyme Q10 and idebenone, were studied in DMD and BMD and Friedreich ataxia and showed some improvements in cardiac disease.[105–108]

Several studies have investigated genotype–phenotype correlation in cardiac disease as a possible technique to predict disease severity or treatment response. Jefferies et al used DNA analysis in 47 cases and found a significant association between DCM and mutations in exons 12 and 14 to 17. There was also possible protection against DCM by mutations at exon 51 to 52 and a trend toward an association between the onset of DCM and mutations in exons 31 to 42.[85] However, Ramaciotti et al could not find a specific mutation that was associated with response to enalapril or predictive of systolic dysfunction.[84] Nigro et al studied 284 patients and showed that cardiac involvement was related to deletions in exons 48 to 49 in 38% of patients with DMD and BMD. Patients with DMD who had this deletion died 3 years earlier than those with other deletions.[109] Melacini et al did not show a significant relationship between specific gene mutations and the development of cardiomyopathy in BMD.[12] With further testing, genotype may become a useful clinical tool to personalize cardiac therapy.

Other experimental therapies are under development. Cell-based therapy involves stem cell delivery and myoblast transplant into the heart.[110] Gene-based therapy involves the use of viral vectors to deliver new genetic material or exon skipping and read through therapies to repair the reading frame of the gene.[111,112] Growth factor modulation is another potential modality that focuses on muscle cell growth by increasing insulin-like growth factor-1 stimulation and myostatin inhibition.[113,114]

Monitoring

Routine monitoring of cardiovascular disease in muscular dystrophy is important. As noninvasive methods for the quantification of cardiac function improve, certain treatments may begin at earlier ages. Two committees have recommended general guidelines for the routine follow-up of the cardiovascular system in muscular dystrophy: the American Academy of Pediatrics Section on Cardiology and Cardiac Surgery and the 107th European Neuromuscular Centre international workshop on the management of cardiac involvement in muscular dystrophy and MD.[7,90] A brief summary of these recommendations follows and is found in Table 3-3. Once cardiac disease is identified, these recommendations no longer apply, and follow-up is dictated by the type and severity of cardiac disease. Also, evaluation with more sophisticated tools for detection of preclinical abnormalities at tertiary care centers is recommended.

Duchenne Muscular Dystrophy

A complete initial evaluation should be performed at the time of diagnosis. This evaluation should include history and physical examination, electrocardiogram, and echocardiogram. Consideration should be given to further testing, including Holter monitoring and MRI (especially if the patient has poor imaging on transthoracic echocardiography). For DMD, patients should have a complete cardiac evaluation at least every 2 years until age 10 years and then complete evaluations should occur annually.[6] Evaluations should also be performed before any scheduled surgery.

Table 3-3 Summary of Follow-up Recommendations for Cardiac Diseases Present in Neuromuscular Disorders

Diagnosis	Cardiology Evaluation	Electrocardiogram	Echocardiogram	Holter Monitor	Other
DMD	At initial diagnosis Once every 1–2 years until 10 years old Every year after 10 years old Based on clinical disease	At every visit Monitor R/Q waves, conduction intervals, arrhythmias	Complete evaluation at every visit, including assessment of diastolic function	At every visit Look for arrhythmias, heart rate variability	Cardiac MRI (especially if poor echocardiogram images)
BMD	At initial diagnosis or at 10 years of age Every 2–5 years afterward Based on clinical disease	At every visit Monitor R/Q waves, conduction intervals, arrhythmias	Complete evaluation at every visit, including assessment of diastolic function	At every visit Look for arrhythmias, heart rate variability	Cardiac MRI (especially if poor echocardiogram images) Consider transplant evaluation when appropriate
DMD/BMD carrier	Initial evaluation at 25–30 years old Every 5 years	At every visit Monitor R/Q waves, conduction intervals, arrhythmias	Complete evaluation at every visit, including assessment of diastolic function	At every visit Look for arrhythmias, heart rate variability	Cardiac MRI (especially if poor echocardiogram images) Consider transplant evaluation when appropriate
LGMD (1B, 2C, 2D, 2E, 2F and 2I)	At initial diagnosis Once every 1–2 years until 10 years old Every year after 10 years old	At every visit Monitor R/Q waves, conduction intervals, arrhythmias	Complete evaluation at every visit, including assessment of diastolic function	At every visit Look for arrhythmias, heart rate variability	Cardiac transplant dependent on skeletal myopathy
DM	At initial diagnosis Yearly	At initial diagnosis Yearly Monitor for AV conduction intervals, arrhythmias (especially atrial)	At initial diagnosis Every few years	At initial diagnosis Yearly Monitor for arrhythmias and heart block	EP testing Pacemaker placement if progressive delays
EDMD (XL and AD)	At initial diagnosis Yearly	At initial diagnosis Yearly Monitor for AV conduction intervals, arrhythmias	At initial diagnosis Every few years	At initial diagnosis Yearly Monitor for arrhythmias and heart block	EP testing Pacemaker/?ICD placement when progressive disease present
Friedreich ataxia	At initial diagnosis Yearly	At initial diagnosis Yearly Monitor for Q waves, ventricular hypertrophy, and repolarization abnormalities	At initial diagnosis Yearly Monitor for hypertrophic cardiomyopathy with outflow obstruction and dilated cardiomyopathy	As needed based on ECG findings	Genetic evaluation of GAA repeats because longer repeats are associated with more severe cardiac disease

AD, autosomal dominant; AV, atrioventricular; BMD, Becker muscular dystrophy; DM, myotonic dystrophy; DMD, Duchenne muscular dystrophy; EDMD, Emery-Dreifuss muscular dystrophy; EP, electrophysiologic; ICD, implantable cardioverter–defibrillator; LGMD, limb-girdle muscular dystrophy; MRI, magnetic resonance imaging; XL, X-linked.

Data from American Academy of Pediatrics Section on Cardiology and Cardiac Surgery: Cardiovascular health supervision for individuals affected by Duchenne or Becker muscular dystrophy. *Pediatrics* 116:1569–1573, 2005, and Hunt SA, Abraham WT, Chin MH, et al: ACC/AHA 2005 Guideline Update for the Diagnosis and Management of Chronic Heart Failure in the Adult: a report of the American College of Cardiology/American Heart Association Task Force on Practice Guidelines (Writing Committee to Update the 2001 Guidelines for the Evaluation and Management of Heart Failure): developed in collaboration with the American College of Chest Physicians and the International Society for Heart and Lung Transplantation: endorsed by the Heart Rhythm Society. *Circulation* 112:e154–e235, 2005.

Becker Muscular Dystrophy

A complete cardiac evaluation should be performed at the time of diagnosis or no later than 10 years of age and should continue every 2 to 5 years if asymptomatic. Once significant cardiac disease is diagnosed, cardiac transplantation is a viable treatment option, and referral to a cardiac transplant center is recommended.

Carriers of Duchenne Muscular Dystrophy or Becker Muscular Dystrophy

Known carriers should be referred for cardiac evaluation in late adolescence or early adulthood. The patient must be informed of the risks of cardiac disease and the signs and symptoms of heart failure. Carriers should be screened with a complete evaluation at 25 to 30 years and every 5 years thereafter.

Limb-Girdle Muscular Dystrophy

An initial or occasional cardiac evaluation may be useful in LGMD not associated with cardiac disease (LGMD 1A, 1C, 2A, 2B, 2G, 2H, and 2J). LGMD 1B, 2C, 2D, 2E, 2F, and 2I can be associated with severe cardiac disease and should be monitored with the same intensity as DMD. Complete evaluations, including ECG testing, echocardiography, Holter monitoring, and additional testing as indicated, is recommended. Because of different skeletal muscle manifestations, cardiac transplantation may be indicated in selected patients.

Myotonic Dystrophy

A complete cardiac evaluation, including ECG examination, echocardiogram, and Holter monitoring, should be performed at diagnosis. Annual ECG testing should be performed after diagnosis, with echocardiography performed less frequently, depending on arrhythmias or symptoms. Holter monitors should be placed if any progressive changes are seen on ECG findings. Referral to a tertiary cardiac center for EP testing may further elucidate AV conduction abnormalities. Treatment with a pacemaker is indicated when a progressive arrhythmia is detected, even if it is asymptomatic. The value of ICD use is not clear at this time. Although cardiac disease is seen in DM type II, there are no current recommendations, but evaluation similar to that for DM type I is likely prudent.

X-Linked Emery-Dreifuss Muscular Dystrophy

The major cardiac defect in XL-EDMD is AV conduction defect. Complete cardiac evaluation, including ECG examination, echocardiogram, and Holter monitoring, should be performed at diagnosis. ECG testing and Holter monitoring should be performed annually. Referral to a tertiary cardiac center for EP testing may further elucidate AV conduction abnormalities. Treatment with a pacemaker is indicated when a progressive arrhythmia is detected, even if asymptomatic. The value of ICD use is not clear at this time. DCM is less frequent, and echocardiograms are not required on a yearly basis. Follow-up for EDMD carriers is not clear.

Autosomal Dominant Emery-Dreifuss Muscular Dystrophy

In patients with AD-EDMD, the concerns are similar to those with XL-EDMD; however, there is stronger evidence of progressive cardiac involvement and DCM. Complete cardiac evaluation, including ECG examination, echocardiogram, and Holter monitoring, should be completed at diagnosis and annually. Referral to a tertiary cardiac center for EP testing may help to further elucidate AV conduction abnormalities. Treatment with a pacemaker is indicated when a progressive arrhythmia is detected. Sudden death is also seen, even after pacemaker implantation, so ICD may be a more appropriate device in these patients.

Friedreich Ataxia

There is significant variation in the degree of cardiac involvement in Friedreich ataxia. Most patients are asymptomatic, but cardiac hypertrophy can become severe enough to obstruct blood flow out of the left ventricle. Patients can also progress from a hypertrophic cardiomyopathy to a DCM. Cardiac evaluation should be performed at diagnosis and yearly to monitor for progression of disease. Genetic testing may be valuable because studies have shown increased cardiac hypertrophy with a larger number of GAA repeats.[69,115]

Summary

Outcomes for neuromuscular disease vary significantly, and some patients present early in the course of disease with cardiac complications. However, in many cases, the severity of cardiac disease is mild and secondary to skeletal muscle disease. Yet, with improvements in the recognition and treatment of skeletal and respiratory muscle systems, cardiac disease will account for a greater proportion of morbidity and mortality in these cases. It seems logical that early diagnosis and treatment of cardiac disease will lead to improved patient quality of life and outcomes. Unfortunately, there are limited studies and conflicting evidence to completely support this theory. Although some studies have shown benefits of early treatment in DMD and BMD, the sample sizes are small and the treatment paradigms varied. As the ability to diagnose preclinical changes in myocardial function improves with echocardiography, MRI, and other modalities, the benefits of different pharmacologic therapies will require further investigation. Corrado et al showed that even after following ECG findings, ventricular late potentials, and ventricular arrhythmias in DMD patients, only the late finding of decreased ventricular systolic function was a significant predictor of outcome.[57] Recently, Connuck et al studied outcomes in DMD and BMD cardiomyopathy and found a significantly worse mortality rate in DMD compared with BMD and other forms of cardiomyopathy. More importantly, the authors also found a lower rate of medical therapy with ACEi and beta blockers in DMD.[11] Thus, to improve outcomes, further study of early diagnosis and the benefits of early treatment are needed.

For muscular dystrophies significantly associated with AV conduction block and arrhythmias, there is clear benefit from early diagnosis and treatment. These patients benefit from pacemaker implantation and show improved quality of life and prognosis. Unfortunately, even with the use of ICDs, these measures cannot prevent sudden death in these patients.[92,93]

Conclusion

Neuromuscular disorders are significantly associated with cardiac disease. Early recognition of cardiac dysfunction or abnormal electrical conduction can have a profound effect on the long-term prognosis of these patients. With improved imaging techniques, a more complete understanding of myocardial dysfunction may help to reduce morbidity and mortality rates. However, to improve the diagnosis and treatment of cardiac disease in muscular dystrophy, further multi-institutional studies with specific treatment protocols are required to better establish revised guidelines using evidence. These studies, combined with continued advances in genotyping and new experimental therapies, will lead to improved treatment and outcomes for patients.

References

1. Nigro G, Comi LI, Politano L, Bain RJ: The incidence and evolution of cardiomyopathy in Duchenne muscular dystrophy, *Int J Cardiol* 26:271–277, 1990.
2. Brooke MH, Fenichel GM, Griggs RC, et al: Duchenne muscular dystrophy: patterns of clinical progression and effects of supportive therapy, *Neurology* 39:475–481, 1989.
3. Gilroy J, Cahalan JL, Berman R, Newman M: Cardiac and pulmonary complications in Duchenne's progressive muscular dystrophy, *Circulation* 27 (4 Pt 1):484–493, 1963.
4. Gulati S, Saxena A, Kumar V, Kalra V: Duchenne muscular dystrophy: prevalence and patterns of cardiac involvement, *Indian J Pediatr* 72:389–393, 2005.
5. D'Orsogna L, O'Shea JP, Miller G: Cardiomyopathy of Duchenne muscular dystrophy, *Pediatr Cardiol* 9:205–213, 1988.
6. Kirchmann C, Kececioglu D, Korinthenberg R, Dittrich S: Echocardiographic and electrocardiographic findings of cardiomyopathy in Duchenne and Becker-Kiener muscular dystrophies, *Pediatr Cardiol* 26:66–72, 2005.

7. American Academy of Pediatrics Section on Cardiology and Cardiac Surgery: Cardiovascular health supervision for individuals affected by Duchenne or Becker muscular dystrophy, *Pediatrics* 116:1569–1573, 2005.

8. Nigro G, Comi LI, Politano L, et al: Evaluation of the cardiomyopathy in Becker muscular dystrophy, *Muscle Nerve* 18:283–291, 1995.

9. Hoogerwaard EM, de Voogt WG, Wilde AA, et al: Evolution of cardiac abnormalities in Becker muscular dystrophy over a 13-year period, *J Neurol* 244:657–663, 1997.

10. Saito M, Kawai H, Akaike M, et al: Cardiac dysfunction with Becker muscular dystrophy, *Am Heart J* 132:642–647, 1996.

11. Connuck DM, Sleeper LA, Colan SD, et al: Characteristics and outcomes of cardiomyopathy in children with Duchenne or Becker muscular dystrophy: a comparative study from the Pediatric Cardiomyopathy Registry, *Am Heart J* 155:998–1005, 2008.

12. Melacini P, Fanin M, Danieli GA, et al: Myocardial involvement is very frequent among patients affected with subclinical Becker's muscular dystrophy, *Circulation* 94:3168–3175, 1996.

13. Melacini P, Fanin M, Angelini A, et al: Cardiac transplantation in a Duchenne muscular dystrophy carrier, *Neuromuscul Disord* 8:585–590, 1998.

14. Hoogerwaard EM, van der Wouw PA, Wilde AA, et al: Cardiac involvement in carriers of Duchenne and Becker muscular dystrophy, *Neuromuscul Disord* 9:347–351, 1999.

15. Politano L, Nigro V, Nigro G, et al: Development of cardiomyopathy in female carriers of Duchenne and Becker muscular dystrophies, *JAMA* 275:1335–1338, 1996.

16. Grain L, Cortina-Borja M, Forfar C, et al: Cardiac abnormalities and skeletal muscle weakness in carriers of Duchenne and Becker muscular dystrophies and controls, *Neuromuscul Disord* 11:186–191, 2001.

17. Berko BA, Swift M: X-linked dilated cardiomyopathy, *N Engl J Med* 316:1186–1191, 1987.

18. Towbin JA, Hejtmancik JF, Brink P, et al: X-linked dilated cardiomyopathy. Molecular genetic evidence of linkage to the Duchenne muscular dystrophy (dystrophin) gene at the Xp21 locus, *Circulation* 87:1854–1865, 1993.

19. Muntoni F, Cau M, Ganau A, et al: Brief report: deletion of the dystrophin muscle-promoter region associated with X-linked dilated cardiomyopathy, *N Engl J Med* 329:921–925, 1993.

20. Muntoni F, Ferlini A, Sewry C, et al: Dilated cardiomyopathy and muscular dystrophies: which lesson can be learned? *Cardiologia* 44(Suppl 1 Pt 1):209–211, 1999.

21. Muntoni F: Cardiac complications of childhood myopathies, *J Child Neurol* 18:191–202, 2003.

22. Politano L, Nigro V, Passamano L, et al: Evaluation of cardiac and respiratory involvement in sarcoglycanopathies, *Neuromuscul Disord* 11:178–185, 2001.

23. Melacini P, Fanin M, Duggan DJ, et al: Heart involvement in muscular dystrophies due to sarcoglycan gene mutations, *Muscle Nerve* 22:473–549, 1999.

24. Barresi R, Di Blasi C, Negri T, et al: Disruption of heart sarcoglycan complex and severe cardiomyopathy caused by beta sarcoglycan mutations, *J Med Genet* 37:102–107, 2000.

25. Calvo F, Teijeira S, Fernandez JM, et al: Evaluation of heart involvement in gamma-sarcoglycanopathy (LGMD2C). A study of ten patients, *Neuromuscul Disord* 10:560–566, 2000.

26. Chrestian N, Valdmanis PN, Echahidi N, et al: A novel mutation in a large French-Canadian family with LGMD1B, *Can J Neurol Sci* 35:331–334, 2008.

27. Ben Yaou R, Becane HM, Demay L, et al: [Autosomal dominant limb-girdle muscular dystrophy associated with conduction defects (LGMD1B): a description of 8 new families with the LMNA gene mutations], *Rev Neurol (Paris)* 161:42–54, 2005.

28. van der Kooi AJ, de Voogt WG, Barth PG, et al: The heart in limb girdle muscular dystrophy, *Heart* 79:73–77, 1998.

29. Wahbi K, Meune C, Hamouda el H, et al: Cardiac assessment of limb-girdle muscular dystrophy 2I patients: an echography, Holter ECG and magnetic resonance imaging study, *Neuromuscul Disord* 18:650–655, 2008.

30. Poppe M, Bourke J, Eagle M, et al: Cardiac and respiratory failure in limb-girdle muscular dystrophy 2I, *Ann Neurol* 56:738–741, 2004.

31. Poppe M, Cree L, Bourke J, et al: The phenotype of limb-girdle muscular dystrophy type 2I, *Neurology* 60:1246–1251, 2003.

32. D'Amico A, Petrini S, Parisi F, et al: Heart transplantation in a child with LGMD2I presenting as isolated dilated cardiomyopathy, *Neuromuscul Disord* 18:153–155, 2008.

33. Murakami T, Hayashi YK, Noguchi S, et al: Fukutin gene mutations cause dilated cardiomyopathy with minimal muscle weakness, *Ann Neurol* 60:597–602, 2006.

34. Groh WJ, Groh MR, Saha C, et al: Electrocardiographic abnormalities and sudden death in myotonic dystrophy type 1, *N Engl J Med* 358:2688–2697, 2008.

35. Schoser BG, Ricker K, Schneider-Gold C, et al: Sudden cardiac death in myotonic dystrophy type 2, *Neurology* 63:2402–2404, 2004.

36. Boriani G, Gallina M, Merlini L, et al: Clinical relevance of atrial fibrillation/flutter, stroke, pacemaker implant, and heart failure in Emery-Dreifuss muscular dystrophy: a long-term longitudinal study, *Stroke* 34:901–908, 2003.

37. Buckley AE, Dean J, Mahy IR: Cardiac involvement in Emery Dreifuss muscular dystrophy: a case series, *Heart* 82:105–108, 1999.

38. Sanna T, Dello Russo A, Toniolo D, et al: Cardiac features of Emery-Dreifuss muscular dystrophy caused by lamin A/C gene mutations, *Eur Heart J* 24:2227–2236, 2003.

39. Brodsky GL, Muntoni F, Miocic S, et al: Lamin A/C gene mutation associated with dilated cardiomyopathy with variable skeletal muscle involvement, *Circulation* 101:473–476, 2000.

40. Fatkin D, MacRae C, Sasaki T, et al: Missense mutations in the rod domain of the lamin A/C gene as causes of dilated cardiomyopathy and conduction-system disease, *N Engl J Med* 341:1715–1724, 1999.

41. Laforet P, de Toma C, Eymard B, et al: Cardiac involvement in genetically confirmed facioscapulohumeral muscular dystrophy, *Neurology* 51:1454–1456, 1998.

42. de Visser M, de Voogt WG, la Riviere GV: The heart in Becker muscular dystrophy, facioscapulohumeral dystrophy, and Bethlem myopathy, *Muscle Nerve* 15:591–596, 1992.

43. Stevenson WG, Perloff JK, Weiss JN, Anderson TL: Facioscapulohumeral muscular dystrophy: evidence for selective, genetic electrophysiologic cardiac involvement, *J Am Coll Cardiol* 15:292–299, 1990.

44. Casazza F, Morpurgo M: The varying evolution of Friedreich's ataxia cardiomyopathy, *Am J Cardiol* 77:895–898, 1996.

45. Spencer CT, Bryant RM, Day J, et al: Cardiac and clinical phenotype in Barth syndrome, *Pediatrics* 118:e337–e346, 2006.

46. Kishnani PS, Hwu WL, Mandel H, et al: A retrospective, multinational, multicenter study on the natural history of infantile-onset Pompe disease, *J Pediatr* 148:671–676, 2006.

47. Marin-Garcia J, Goldenthal MJ: Mitochondrial cardiomyopathy: molecular and biochemical analysis, *Pediatr Cardiol* 18:251–260, 1997.

48. Ceviz N, Alehan F, Alehan D, et al: Assessment of left ventricular systolic and diastolic functions in children with merosin-positive congenital muscular dystrophy, *Int J Cardiol* 87:129–133, 2003 discussion 133–134.

49. Nakanishi T, Sakauchi M, Kaneda Y, et al: Cardiac involvement in Fukuyama-type congenital muscular dystrophy, *Pediatrics* 117:e1187–e1192, 2006.

50. Groh WJ, Lowe MR, Zipes DP: Severity of cardiac conduction involvement and arrhythmias in myotonic dystrophy type 1 correlates with age and CTG repeat length, *J Cardiovasc Electrophysiol* 13:444–448, 2002.

51. Oguz D, Olgunturk R, Gucuyener K, et al: A comparison between MUGA and echocardiography in patients with muscular dystrophy in the early detection of cardiac involvement, *Pediatr Cardiol* 19:150–154, 1998.

52. Bhattacharyya KB, Basu N, Ray TN, Maity B: Profile of electrocardiographic changes in Duchenne muscular dystrophy, *J Indian Med Assoc* 95:40–42, 47, 1997.

53. Steare SE, Dubowitz V, Benatar A: Subclinical cardiomyopathy in Becker muscular dystrophy, *Br Heart J* 68:304–308, 1992.

54. Perloff JK, Roberts WC, de Leon AC Jr, O'Doherty D: The distinctive electrocardiogram of Duchenne's progressive muscular dystrophy. An electrocardiographic-pathologic correlative study, *Am J Med* 42:179–188, 1967.

55. Ishikawa K: Cardiac involvement in progressive muscular dystrophy of the Duchenne type, *Jpn Heart J* 38(2):163–180, 1997.

56. Akita H, Matsuoka S, Kuroda Y: Predictive electrocardiographic score for evaluating prognosis in patients with Duchenne's muscular dystrophy, *Tokushima J Exp Med* 40:55–60, 1993.

57. Corrado G, Lissoni A, Beretta S, et al: Prognostic value of electrocardiograms, ventricular late potentials, ventricular arrhythmias, and left ventricular systolic dysfunction in patients with Duchenne muscular dystrophy, *Am J Cardiol* 89:838–841, 2002.

58. Yotsukura M, Sasaki K, Kachi E, et al: Circadian rhythm and variability of heart rate in Duchenne-type progressive muscular dystrophy, *Am J Cardiol* 76:947–951, 1995.

59. Child JS, Perloff JK, Bach PM, et al: Cardiac involvement in Friedreich's ataxia: a clinical study of 75 patients, *J Am Coll Cardiol* 7:1370–1378, 1986.

60. Yotsukura M, Fujii K, Katayama A, et al: Nine-year follow-up study of heart rate variability in patients with Duchenne-type progressive muscular dystrophy, *Am Heart J* 136:289–296, 1998.

61. Lanza GA, Dello Russo A, Giglio V, et al: Impairment of cardiac autonomic function in patients with Duchenne muscular dystrophy: relationship to myocardial and respiratory function, *Am Heart J* 141:808–812, 2001.

62. Ducceschi V, Nigro G, Sarubbi B, et al: Autonomic nervous system imbalance and left ventricular systolic dysfunction as potential candidates for arrhythmogenesis in Becker muscular dystrophy, *Int J Cardiol* 59:275–279, 1997.

63. de Kermadec JM, Becane HM, Chenard A: Prevalence of left ventricular systolic dysfunction in Duchenne muscular dystrophy: an echocardiographic study, *Am Heart J* 127:618–623, 1994.

64. Sasaki K, Sakata K, Kachi E, et al: Sequential changes in cardiac structure and function in patients with Duchenne type muscular dystrophy: a two-dimensional echocardiographic study, *Am Heart J* 135(6 Pt 1):937–944, 1998.

65. Markham LW, Michelfelder EC, Border WL, et al: Abnormalities of diastolic function precede dilated cardiomyopathy associated with Duchenne muscular dystrophy, *J Am Soc Echocardiogr* 19:865–871, 2006.

66. Meune C, Pascal O, Becane HM, et al: Reliable detection of early myocardial dysfunction by tissue Doppler echocardiography in Becker muscular dystrophy, *Heart* 90:947–948, 2004.

67. Ogata H, Nakatani S, Ishikawa Y, et al: Myocardial strain changes in Duchenne muscular dystrophy without overt cardiomyopathy, *Int J Cardiol* 115:190–195, 2007.

68. Mori K, Hayabuchi Y, Inoue M, et al: Myocardial strain imaging for early detection of cardiac involvement in patients with Duchenne's progressive muscular dystrophy, *Echocardiography* 24:598–608, 2007.

69. Dutka DP, Donnelly JE, Nihoyannopoulos P, et al: Marked variation in the cardiomyopathy associated with Friedreich's ataxia, *Heart* 81:141–147, 1999.

70. Ashford MW Jr, Liu W, Lin SJ, et al: Occult cardiac contractile dysfunction in dystrophin-deficient children revealed by cardiac magnetic resonance strain imaging, *Circulation* 112:2462–2467, 2005.

71. Silva MC, Meira ZM, Gurgel Giannetti J, et al: Myocardial delayed enhancement by magnetic resonance imaging in patients with muscular dystrophy, *J Am Coll Cardiol* 49:1874–1879, 2007.

72. Gaul C, Deschauer M, Tempelmann C, et al: Cardiac involvement in limb-girdle muscular dystrophy 2I: conventional cardiac diagnostic and cardiovascular magnetic resonance, *J Neurol* 253:1317–1322, 2006.

73. Finsterer J, Stollberger C: The heart in human dystrophinopathies, *Cardiology* 99:1–19, 2003.

74. Lazarus A, Varin J, Ounnoughene Z, et al: Relationships among electrophysiological findings and clinical status, heart function, and extent of DNA mutation in myotonic dystrophy, *Circulation* 99:1041–1046, 1999.

75. Negri SM, Cowan MD: Becker muscular dystrophy with bundle branch reentry ventricular tachycardia, *J Cardiovasc Electrophysiol* 9:652–654, 1998.

76. James TN: Observations on the cardiovascular involvement, including the cardiac conduction system, in progressive muscular dystrophy, *Am Heart J* 63:48–56, 1962.

77. Frankel KA, Rosser RJ: The pathology of the heart in progressive muscular dystrophy: epimyocardial fibrosis, *Hum Pathol* 7:375–386, 1976.

78. Bushby K, Muntoni F, Urtizberea A, et al: Report on the 124th ENMC International Workshop. Treatment of Duchenne muscular dystrophy; defining the gold standards of management in the use of corticosteroids. 2–4 April 2004, Naarden, The Netherlands, *Neuromuscul Disord* 14:526–534, 2004.

79. Markham LW, Kinnett K, Wong BL, et al: Corticosteroid treatment retards development of ventricular dysfunction in Duchenne muscular dystrophy, *Neuromuscul Disord* 18:365–370, 2008.

80. Markham LW, Spicer RL, Khoury PR, et al: Steroid therapy and cardiac function in Duchenne muscular dystrophy, *Pediatr Cardiol* 26:768–771, 2005.

81. Silversides CK, Webb GD, Harris VA, Biggar DW: Effects of deflazacort on left ventricular function in patients with Duchenne muscular dystrophy, *Am J Cardiol* 91:769–772, 2003.

82. Duboc D, Meune C, Lerebours G, et al: Effect of perindopril on the onset and progression of left ventricular dysfunction in Duchenne muscular dystrophy, *J Am Coll Cardiol* 45:855–857, 2005.

83. Duboc D, Meune C, Pierre B, et al: Perindopril preventive treatment on mortality in Duchenne muscular dystrophy: 10 years' follow-up, *Am Heart J* 154:596–602, 2007.

84. Ramaciotti C, Heistein LC, Coursey M, et al: Left ventricular function and response to enalapril in patients with Duchenne muscular dystrophy during the second decade of life, *Am J Cardiol* 98:825–827, 2006.

85. Jefferies JL, Eidem BW, Belmont JW, et al: Genetic predictors and remodeling of dilated cardiomyopathy in muscular dystrophy, *Circulation* 112:2799–2804, 2005.

86. Ishikawa Y, Bach JR, Minami R: Cardioprotection for Duchenne's muscular dystrophy, *Am Heart J* 137:895–902, 1999.

87. Kajimoto H, Ishigaki K, Okumura K, et al: Beta-blocker therapy for cardiac dysfunction in patients with muscular dystrophy, *Circ J* 70:991–994, 2006.

88. Rhodes J, Margossian R, Darras BT, et al: Safety and efficacy of carvedilol therapy for patients with dilated cardiomyopathy secondary to muscular dystrophy, *Pediatr Cardiol* 29:343–351, 2008.

89. Hunt SA, Abraham WT, Chin MH, et al: ACC/AHA 2005 Guideline Update for the Diagnosis and Management of Chronic Heart Failure in the Adult: a report of the American College of Cardiology/American Heart Association Task Force on Practice Guidelines (Writing Committee to Update the 2001 Guidelines for the Evaluation and Management of Heart Failure): developed in collaboration with the American College of Chest Physicians and the International Society for Heart and Lung Transplantation: endorsed by the Heart Rhythm Society, *Circulation* 112:e154–e235, 2005.

90. Bushby K, Muntoni F, Bourke JP: 107th ENMC International Workshop: The Management of Cardiac Involvement in Muscular Dystrophy and Myotonic Dystrophy. 7–9 June 2002, Naarden, The Netherlands, *Neuromuscul Disord* 13:166–172, 2003.

91. Gregoratos G, Abrams J, Epstein AE, et al: ACC/AHA/NASPE 2002 Guideline Update for Implantation of Cardiac Pacemakers and Antiarrhythmia Devices—summary article: a report of the American College of Cardiology/American Heart Association Task Force on Practice Guidelines (ACC/AHA/NASPE Committee to Update the 1998 Pacemaker Guidelines), *J Am Coll Cardiol* 40:1703–1719, 2002.

92. Lazarus A, Varin J, Babuty D, et al: Long-term follow-up of arrhythmias in patients with myotonic dystrophy treated by pacing: a multicenter diagnostic pacemaker study, *J Am Coll Cardiol* 40:1645–1652, 2002.

93. Grigg LE, Chan W, Mond HG, et al: Ventricular tachycardia and sudden death in myotonic dystrophy: clinical, electrophysiologic and pathologic features, *J Am Coll Cardiol* 6:254–256, 1985.

94. Golzio PG, Chiribiri A, Gaita F: 'Unexpected' sudden death avoided by implantable cardioverter defibrillator in Emery Dreifuss patient, *Europace* 9:1158–1160, 2007.

95. Meune C, Van Berlo JH, Anselme F, et al: Primary prevention of sudden death in patients with lamin A/C gene mutations, *N Engl J Med* 354:209–210, 2006.

96. Walker S, Levy T, Rex S, Paul VE: Biventricular implantable cardioverter defibrillator use in a patient with heart failure and ventricular tachycardia secondary to Emery-Dreifuss syndrome, *Europace* 1:206–209, 1999.

97. Piccolo G, Azan G, Tonin P, et al: Dilated cardiomyopathy requiring cardiac transplantation as initial manifestation of Xp21 Becker type muscular dystrophy, *Neuromuscul Disord* 4:143–146, 1994.

98. Rees W, Schuler S, Hummel M, Hetzer R: Heart transplantation in patients with muscular dystrophy associated with end-stage cardiomyopathy, *J Heart Lung Transplant* 12:804–807, 1993.

99. Ruiz-Cano MJ, Delgado JF, Jimenez C, et al: Successful heart transplantation in patients with inherited myopathies associated with end-stage cardiomyopathy, *Transplant Proc* 35:1513–1515, 2003.

100. Schmidt GN, Burmeister MA, Lilje C, et al: Acute heart failure during spinal surgery in a boy with Duchenne muscular dystrophy, *Br J Anaesth* 90:800–804, 2003.

101. Kelfer HM, Singer WD, Reynolds RN: Malignant hyperthermia in a child with Duchenne muscular dystrophy, *Pediatrics* 71:118–119, 1983.

102. Kerr TP, Duward A, Hodgson SV, et al: Hyperkalaemic cardiac arrest in a manifesting carrier of Duchenne muscular dystrophy following general anaesthesia, *Eur J Pediatr* 160:579–580, 2001.

103. Sethna NF, Rockoff MA, Worthen HM, Rosnow JM: Anesthesia-related complications in children with Duchenne muscular dystrophy, *Anesthesiology* 68:462–465, 1988.

104. Breucking E, Reimnitz P, Schara U, Mortier W: [Anesthetic complications. The incidence of severe anesthetic complications in patients and families with progressive muscular dystrophy of the Duchenne and Becker types], *Anaesthesist* 49:187–195, 2000.

105. Buyse GM, Van der Mieren G, Erb M, et al: Long-term blinded placebo-controlled study of SNT-MC17/idebenone in the dystrophin deficient mdx mouse: cardiac protection and improved exercise performance, *Eur Heart J* 30:116–124, 2009.

106. Folkers K, Vadhanavikit S, Mortensen SA: Biochemical rationale and myocardial tissue data on the effective therapy of cardiomyopathy with coenzyme Q10, *Proc Natl Acad Sci U S A* 82:901–904, 1985.

107. Hausse AO, Aggoun Y, Bonnet D, et al: Idebenone and reduced cardiac hypertrophy in Friedreich's ataxia, *Heart* 87:346–349, 2002.

108. Lodi R, Hart PE, Rajagopalan B, et al: Antioxidant treatment improves in vivo cardiac and skeletal muscle bioenergetics in patients with Friedreich's ataxia, *Ann Neurol* 49:590–596, 2001.

109. Nigro G, Politano L, Nigro V, et al: Mutation of dystrophin gene and cardiomyopathy, *Neuromuscul Disord* 4:371–379, 1994.

110. Gussoni E, Soneoka Y, Strickland CD, et al: Dystrophin expression in the mdx mouse restored by stem cell transplantation, *Nature* 401:390–394, 1999.

111. Gregorevic P, Blankinship MJ, Allen JM, et al: Systemic delivery of genes to striated muscles using adeno-associated viral vectors, *Nat Med* 10:828–834, 2004.

112. Yin H, Lu Q, Wood M: Effective exon skipping and restoration of dystrophin expression by peptide nucleic acid antisense oligonucleotides in mdx mice, *Mol Ther* 16:38–45, 2008.

113. Barton ER, Morris L, Musaro A, et al: Muscle-specific expression of insulin-like growth factor I counters muscle decline in mdx mice, *J Cell Biol* 157:137–148, 2002.

114. Bogdanovich S, Krag TO, Barton ER, et al: Functional improvement of dystrophic muscle by myostatin blockade, *Nature* 420:418–421, 2002.

115. Isnard R, Kalotka H, Durr A, et al: Correlation between left ventricular hypertrophy and GAA trinucleotide repeat length in Friedreich's ataxia, *Circulation* 95:2247–2249, 1997.

Mohammad K. Ismail, MD

Gastrointestinal Complications of Neuromuscular Disorders

4

The gastrointestinal tract is an extremely dynamic organ, with extensive muscle that is regulated not only by the enteric nervous system but also by the central and autonomic nervous systems, as well as by humoral factors. Therefore, it is not surprising that many neuromuscular diseases affect the gastrointestinal tract.[1] Gastrointestinal symptoms occur commonly in neurologic diseases, usually as transfer or oropharyngeal dysphagia, nausea, early satiety, constipation, or incontinence (Box 4-1).[2,3]

Pharynx and Esophagus

Impairment of Deglutition (Dysphagia)

Dysphagia is one of the most disabling conditions arising from neuromuscular disorders, causing high morbidity, mortality, and cost.[4,5] Dysphagia typically refers to difficulty in eating as a result of disruption in the swallowing process. It is a subjective sensation that suggests the presence of an organic abnormality in the passage of liquids or solids from the oral cavity to the stomach. Patients' complaints range from the inability to initiate a swallow to the sensation of solids or liquids being hindered during their passage through the esophagus into the stomach.

Dysphagia can be classified as either oropharyngeal or esophageal. Oropharyngeal dysphagia, also called transfer dysphagia, arises from disorders that affect the function of the oropharynx, larynx, and upper esophageal sphincter. Neurogenic and myogenic disorders as well as oropharyngeal tumors are the most common underlying causes of oropharyngeal dysphagia. Esophageal dysphagia arises within the body of the esophagus, the lower esophageal sphincter, or cardia, and is most commonly the result of mechanical causes or a motility disturbance. Some neuromuscular disorders, however, such as inflammatory myopathies, also affect the esophagus.

Normal swallowing consists of three phases (oral, pharyngeal, and esophageal), which are usually performed effortlessly up to 600 times daily. A total of five cranial nerves (V, VII, IX, X, and XII) and 26 muscle groups are involved in coordinating the act of swallowing. In the oral phase, the food is chewed and the bolus is pushed to the pharynx under voluntary control. In the pharyngeal phase, the nasopharynx closes to prevent the entry of food into the nasal passages. The vocal cords approximate and the epiglottis tilts downward to prevent the entry of food into the airway. With the relaxation of the upper esophageal sphincter, progressive waves of muscular contraction propel the food bolus into the esophagus. In the esophageal phase, peristalsis moves the food bolus through the esophagus and lower esophageal sphincter into the stomach.

Pathogenesis
Oropharyngeal dysphagia can arise from abnormalities of the oral or pharyngeal phases of swallowing. A variety of disorders related to neurologic and muscular diseases affecting the strength and coordination of orofacial muscles can lead to disrupted swallowing. As described earlier, coordinated neuromuscular events in the pharyngeal phase are required for successful transit of bolus in the esophagus and any disruption caused by neuromuscular disease can lead to failure of swallowing and result in dysphagia (Box 4-2).

Clinical Manifestations
As with any other medical conditions, a detailed history is useful in elucidating the cause of dysphagia.

Patients affected with dysphagia often present with subjective complaints of either choking on solids or inability to swallow food. Associated symptoms, including coughing, choking, nasal regurgitation, and dysarthria, are suggestive of oropharyngeal dysphagia.

Dysphagia in Motor Neuron Disorders

Dysphagia as a result of bulbar or pseudobulbar palsy occurs in up to 25% of patients with amyotrophic lateral sclerosis (ALS) at the onset of disease.[6] Eventually, almost all patients with ALS have at least some degree of dysphagia.[7] In motor neuron disease (MND), weakness of the orolingual and pharyngeal muscles leads to swallowing difficulties. Weakness of the pharyngeal constrictor muscles results in choking or coughing during or immediately after swallowing. Sialorrhea (drooling) is common and results from impaired pharyngeal clearance and weakness of the oral muscles rather than an increase in salivation. Progression of dysphagia results in weight loss as a result of the patient's inability to maintain adequate caloric intake with oral feedings alone.

Dysphagia in Primary Muscular Disorders

Dysphagia in myopathies arises from impairment of the pharyngeal and esophageal phases.[8]

Unlike neurogenic disorders (neuropathies and MND) and disorders of neuromuscular transmission, there is usually no significant impairment of mastication. However, to avoid aspiration, patients may spend a long time chewing their food. Nasal regurgitation and dysarthria are also less frequent.[9]

Box 4-1 Gastrointestinal Manifestations of Neuromuscular Diseases

Dysphagia
Dyspepsia
Gastroparesis
Chronic intestinal pseudo-obstruction
Bacterial overgrowth
Weight loss
Constipation
Incontinence

Box 4-2 Neurologic and Neuromuscular Etiologies of Dysphagia

Neurogenic Disorders, Central and Peripheral	Neuromuscular Transmission Disorders, Myopathies
Stroke	Connective tissue disorders
Head injury	Dermatomyositis
Brain stem tumor	Oculopharyngeal dystrophy
Cerebral palsy	Muscular dystrophy
Guillian-Barré syndrome	Polymyositis
Huntington disease	Sarcoidosis
Polio	Myasthenia gravis
Postpolio syndrome	Paraneoplastic syndromes
Amyotrophic lateral sclerosis	
Parkinson disease	
Multiple sclerosis	
Tardive dyskinesia	
Dementia	
Metabolic encephalopathy	

Although, in theory, any muscular disorder may present with impairment of swallowing, abnormalities of deglutition tend to predominate in some types of muscle disease. These include certain muscular dystrophies, such as oculopharyngeal muscular dystrophy (OPMD),[10] myotonic dystrophy (DM), and advanced stages of Duchenne muscular dystrophy (DMD) and facioscapulohumeral myopathy.[8,11–13] Inflammatory disorders such as polymyositis, dermatomyositis, and inclusion body myositis (IBM) can affect the muscles of deglutition. Metabolic myopathies, particularly mitochondrial myopathies, may present with impairment of swallowing as well.[14] Some patients have cricopharyngeal achalasia with associated impairment of the function of the cricopharyngeal muscle and its ability to relax, which can manifest with oropharyngeal dysphagia. Recently, some authors have suggested that a combined myopathic and neuropathic etiology could provide a more satisfactory explanation for the pharyngoesophageal symptoms of DM, but this remains speculative.[15] Marked atrophy of the esophageal striated muscles, but only small changes in the smooth muscle, were observed in one study.[13] In another study, Ludatscher et al used electron microscopy to detect mild degenerative changes with disoriented filaments of the smooth muscle.[16]

The most common adult-onset form of muscular dystrophy is DM. There is frequent dysarthria and dysphagia as a result of weakness of the palatal and pharyngeal muscles.[4] Different studies have reported a prevalence of dysphagia ranging from 25% to 80% in DM.[17–19]

The autosomal dominant disorder OPMD manifests as bilateral symmetrical ptosis, external ophthalmoparesis, and dysphagia.[10] Dysphagia is frequent and may be the presenting symptom, with impairment mainly of the pharyngeal phase, although the lingual and oral phases can also be affected. Patients usually have symptoms between the fourth and fifth decades. In one study, retroflexion of the head because of ptosis was noted to worsen preexisting dysphagia in patients with OPMD. Subjective and objective reduction of swallowing problems was noted when patients were instructed to eat and drink with a slightly flexed head position.[20] Complications, including dysphonia and aspiration, can develop after years of progression.

In DMD, there is some involvement of the oropharyngeal muscles.[8] Macroglossia further complicates the oral phase of swallowing. Difficulty in bringing food to the mouth, difficulty chewing, and malocclusion have been observed in patients with DMD, including tongue bite as a result of macroglossia.

Dysphagia in Inflammatory Myopathies and Neuromuscular Junction Disorders

Among inflammatory myopathies, the polymyositis associated with connective tissue disease and IBM are most likely associated with dysphagia.[21,22] Dysphagia occurs primarily as a result of involvement of the striated muscles, but in some cases, the upper third of the esophagus may be affected. In one study of 62 patients with systemic sclerosis or related disorders who were referred for evaluation of upper gastrointestinal symptoms, dysphagia was present in 61%.[23] Dysphagia is often an early presenting symptom in older patients affected with inflammatory myopathy. Disorders affecting the neuromuscular junction, including myasthenia gravis, can present with intermittent swallowing and are often associated with oculomotor abnormalities, including diplopia, and facial muscle weakness. Clinical symptoms include problems while chewing food or moving it in the mouth and problems related to the pharyngeal phase. Involvement of the pharyngeal muscles in Lambert-Eaton syndrome has been described, and only a small number of patients develop dysphagia.

Dysphagia in Peripheral Neuropathy

Peripheral neuropathy seldom involves the pharyngeal muscles. However, polyradiculoneuropathies, both acute (Guillain-Barré syndrome), involving the cranial nerves, and rarely, chronic inflammatory demyelinating neuropathy, can lead to pharyngeal and cervical muscle weakness.

Weight Loss

Failure to gain weight and associated weight loss are commonly associated with feeding and nutritional problems in patients with neuromuscular diseases. Feeding difficulties have been reported in approximately 30% of patients with DMD who are younger than 25 years.[24] Weight loss is also a common symptom in ALS,[25–27] and it usually relates to the progression of dysphagia, resulting in the inability to maintain adequate caloric intake with oral feedings alone.[28] Weight loss also may occur in patients with and without bulbar involvement because of generalized fatigue, poor appetite, and associated depression.[29] Malnutrition is a poor prognostic factor and correlates with increased risk of death; therefore, once the patient has lost 5% to 10% of normal body weight, physicians should consider enteric feeding and discuss options with the patient and caregivers. Assessment of the patient's nutrition status should involve referral to a nutrition specialist soon after diagnosis to facilitate careful monitoring of caloric intake and body mass.

Malnutrition can be indicated by triceps skin fold and arm muscle circumference measurements that are below the 30th percentile; measurements below the 24th percentile indicate severe malnutrition.[26] The upper extremity anthropometrics of mid-arm circumference, triceps skin fold thickness, and mid-arm muscle circumference are argued to be precise indicators of nutritional status.[27,30] A combination of body composition measures (body weight, dietary history, body mass index, biochemical tests, anthropometry) is recommended to achieve accurate assessment of nutritional status. Assessments of lean body mass by dual-energy x-ray absorptiometry and bioelectrical impedance analysis are useful, but cost and feasibility in the clinical practice are the limiting factors. Laboratory values for hemoglobin, hematocrit, serum iron, transferrin, glucose, blood urea nitrogen, creatinine, lipids, and protein stores of albumin and transthyretin (prealbumin) should be evaluated and monitored. Given the evidence showing a direct relationship between survival and nutritional status, early nutritional intervention should be a standard component of care in the patient with neuromuscular disease.[25]

Diagnosis and Evaluation of Dysphagia

Modified barium swallow with videofluoroscopy in conjunction with oropharyngeal examination by a speech pathologist can provide a more objective measurement of swallowing.[31] Videofluoroscopy involves swallowing a barium suspension of varying consistency, fluid and semisolid. An analysis of the various stages of swallowing is made, and laryngeal penetration can be detected reliably by videofluoroscopy (Figs. 4-1 and 4-2).

Videofluoroscopy can also help to guide decisions about feeding regimens and estimate the patient's risk of respiratory complications from oral feeding. Videofluoroscopy could be used to assess the risk of aspiration. The presence of laryngeal penetration on videofluoroscopy in the setting of clinical dysphagia indicates a high risk of aspiration pneumonia. Cineradiographic studies of the pharynx in patients with DM have shown abnormalities, such as weak and asymmetrical contractions of the pharynx and cricopharynx, myotonia of the tongue and pharynx with stasis and pooling of contrast in the pyriform sinuses, and valleculae. A combined technique

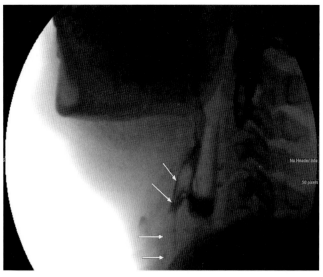

Figure 4-2 Modified barium swallow with aspiration: on the lateral image, *arrows* show abnormal spillover with aspiration.

of videofibrolaryngoscopy and videofluoroscopy can be the best method for evaluating dysphagia.

Manometry is useful to detect motility disturbances, which show in the form of asymmetric contractions of the pharynx and weak contractions of the upper esophageal sphincter. In the esophageal body, significant decreases in peristaltic amplitude or simultaneous waves have often been reported in patients with myotonic dystrophy.[4,15,18,32–34] Manometric findings, however, are not significantly different between symptomatic and asymptomatic patients, or in patients with different degrees of striated muscular involvement. Eleven patients with an established diagnosis of OPMD were studied by Castell et al.[35] Nine of these patients showed abnormal upper esophageal sphincter and pharyngeal manometrics, with the most common abnormalities found in the pharynx (upper esophageal sphincter and pharyngeal incoordination, prolonged pharyngeal contraction, low pharyngeal pressure, and low pharyngeal contraction rate). Another procedure that has been used for the evaluation of dysphagia in patients with MND is electromyographic techniques.

Routine endoscopy is not helpful in most patients unless underlying esophageal inflammation with complications related to reflux needs endoscopic evaluation.

Treatment and Management

The initial management of dysphagia includes modification of food and fluid consistency and coaching by a speech pathologist.[36] The use of thicker liquids, semisolid foods with a high water content, such as gelatin, can help to alleviate aspiration.[37] In relation to liquids, drinking through straws can help with swallowing.[38]

Patients are usually advised to eat more slowly, take smaller bites, and alternate bites of solid food with sips of liquid to ensure adequate oral and pharyngeal clearing. In this regard, involvement of a speech and language therapist in assessing the patient and providing advice on the consistency and quantity of food and fluid in the diet, with the use of various positioning techniques (e.g., chin tuck) to improve swallowing, is helpful. If these initial measures fail, then evaluation for an alternative route for nutrition is warranted. Enteral nutrition can be achieved through various means, including a nasogastric or nasoenteric tube, a percutaneous endoscopic (or radiologically placed) gastrostomy (PEG/PRG) tube, or a jejunostomy tube.

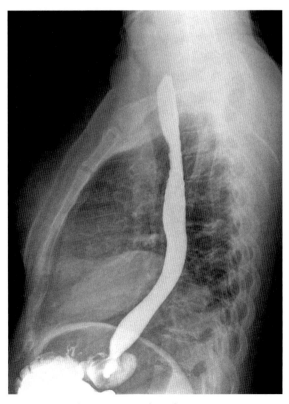

Figure 4-1 Normal esophagogram.

These tubes are inserted into the stomach (gastrostomy) through the abdominal wall, or into the intestine (jejunostomy).[39] Nasoenteric feeding tubes are commonly used for short-term nutritional support, and can be placed more reliably using endoscopic or fluoroscopic guidance.[40] PEG tube placement is the recommended choice for long-term maintenance of good nutrition in patients with myopathies[41–43] and patients with MND/ALS and pronounced dysphagia.[12,44–46]

The timing of PEG/PRG tube placement is based on an individual approach, taking into account bulbar symptoms, malnutrition (weight loss > 10%), respiratory function, and the patient's general condition. Thus, an early operation is highly recommended.[38,46]

The literature specifies a number of factors that influence the timing of PEG tube placement: forced vital capacity (FVC), accelerated weight loss, and dysphagia symptoms. According to the U.S. clinical guidelines reported by Miller at al, there are insufficient data to support or refute specific timing of PEG tube insertion in patients with ALS; but patients with dysphagia may be exposed to less risk if the PEG tube is placed when the FVC is above 50% of predicted.[46,47] Specifically, PEG tube placement is indicated when patients with ALS have symptomatic dysphagia with accelerated weight loss as a result of insufficient caloric intake, dehydration, or ending meals prematurely because of dysphagia or choking on food. Although a barium swallow study may provide supportive evidence of dysphagia,[48] the indication for PEG tube placement in ALS depends on the presence of inadequate oral intake and diminished quality of life as a result of choking rather than the result of a swallowing study.

Because PEG tube insertion typically employs procedural sedation, knowledge of a patient's respiratory capacity and monitoring of oxygen saturation are essential.[49,50] A novel use of noninvasive positive pressure ventilation to provide respiratory support during sedation for percutaneous placement has been described for patients with neuromuscular disease.[51–53]

Endoscopic placement requires upper endoscopy, usually under conscious sedation, and includes inspection of the stomach and identification of the placement site using transillumination and finger indentation. Safe placement depends on adequate transillumination of the anterior abdominal wall with a gastroscope light. Inability to transilluminate the anterior abdominal wall optimally is a common cause of failure of endoscopic gastrostomy tube placement. In some patients with ALS, because of intrinsic weakness of the diaphragm, the stomach migrates high under the costal margin, which can make placement difficult.

In patients with ALS, PRG techniques have been used successfully when endoscopic tube placement was not feasible.[54] In PRG, gastropexy with T-fasteners is used to fix the anterior wall of the stomach to the anterior abdominal wall, which stabilizes the anterior wall of the stomach and allows safe dilation of the gastrostomy tract. T-fastener gastropexy enables routine use of larger gastrostomy tubes and ready replacement of a displaced tube, even before the development of a mature tract. Because PRG does not involve passage of a scope through the pharynx, local anesthesia of the pharynx is not needed. This may be safer in patients with borderline respiratory status who require less sedation. Multiple case series of uncomplicated PEG tube placement with noninvasive positive pressure ventilation assistance have been reported in patients with advanced ALS with FVC of less than 50%.[50,51]

Contraindications to PEG Tube Placement

Absolute contraindications to PEG tube placement include inability to bring the gastric wall in opposition to the abdominal wall, pharyngeal or esophageal obstruction, and uncontrolled coagulopathy. Previous gastric resection, ascites, hepatomegaly, and obesity are conditions that may impede gastric transillumination and subsequent PEG tube placement. PEG tube placement should not be used for nutritional support when a gastrointestinal tract obstruction is present. Relative contraindications to PEG tube placement include neoplastic, inflammatory, or infiltrative diseases of the gastric or abdominal wall.[55]

Although nutritional goals and hydration can be achieved successfully with PEG tube placement, this does not prevent aspiration. Therefore, prevention of aspiration pneumonia is not an indication for PEG tube placement. Recognized risk factors for aspiration include a history of aspiration pneumonia alone, evidence of reflux esophagitis at the time of endoscopy, older age, male sex, diabetes, and infection.[40,56,57]

Patients undergoing PEG tube placement are often at high risk for complications caused by associated comorbidity. Minor complications associated with PEG tube placement occur in 13% to 43% of patients and include tube occlusion, maceration from leakage of gastric contents around the tube, and peristomal pain. Major complications, reported in 0.4% to 8.4% of procedures, include transient laryngeal spasm (7.2%), localized infection (6.6%), gastric hemorrhage (1%–4%), failure of placement because of technical difficulties (1%–9%), necrotizing fasciitis, aspiration, bleeding, perforation, ileus, injury of internal organs, and death as a result of respiratory arrest (1.9%), with a 30-day mortality rate of 6.7% to 26.0%. This may be due, in part, to patients' underlying comorbidities.[58–60]

The most common complication is wound infection. Antimicrobial prophylaxis is recommended because it may reduce the frequency of peristomal wound infection and it is cost-effective. Parenteral cefazolin (or an antibiotic with equivalent coverage) should be administered to all patients 30 minutes before they undergo PEG tube placement. Such prophylaxis is necessary only in patients who are not already receiving appropriate antibiotic treatment at the time of PEG tube insertion.[61–63]

A mature fistulous tract is required to replace a percutaneous gastrostomy tube or button safely. Nonendoscopic replacement of a dislodged tube or button is contraindicated in the absence of a mature tract. Pneumoperitoneum occurs commonly after PEG tube placement and is of no clinical significance unless accompanied by signs and symptoms of peritonitis.[64]

Gastrostomy in Children

Since its first use in children in 1980 by Gauderer et al,[65] studies of those with neurodevelopmental disorders have shown that receiving nutrition through a gastrostomy tube can improve clinical outcome and quality of life. Two major groups of feeding-related problems before gastrostomy were identified among children with muscular dystrophies and other neuromuscular disorders. The most common group presented primarily with poor growth and nutrition, and the second group had swallowing difficulties that resulted in aspiration. After gastrostomy, improvement in growth velocity was marked for weight and height. The procedure was well tolerated, with minimal postoperative complications. It also seemed to improve quality of life.[41,42,66] It is, however, difficult to know whether gastrostomy feeding will have a similar effect in patients with severe congenital myopathy, severe gastroesophageal reflux, severe respiratory insufficiency that requires intensive care, or a poor short-term prognosis with a high risk of death.

Survival after PEG Tube Placement

In one study, the frequency of PEG tube placement among patients with ALS was 11%, with a mean duration of disease of approximately 24 months. Median survival after PEG tube insertion was

146 days. The 1-month mortality rate after gastrostomy was 25%.[49] However, other studies, including PEG tube, have reported a lower 30-day mortality, around 6.3% to 9.6%.[50] A positive effect of PEG tube placement was noted in 79% of patients who underwent PEG tube placement.[67] The best evidence to date, based on controlled prospective cohort studies, suggests an advantage for survival in all patients with ALS or MND, but these conclusions are tentative.[68]

Enteral Nutrition

Enteral formulas (Box 4-3) are generally nutritionally complete emulsions of macronutrients and micronutrients that consist of intact protein, glucose polymers, and a mixture of long-chain and medium-chain triglycerides. Methods of administration of the formula include bolus, gravity, and continuous feeding. In bolus feeding, 300 to 400 mL is infused with a syringe through a feeding tube over 5 to 10 minutes several times daily. Gravity, especially continuous feeding, provides intermittent and more controlled delivery of feeding and is recommended when a reduction in the risk of gastroesophageal reflux and aspiration is needed.

Cricopharyngeal Myotomy

Cricopharyngeal myotomy,[69] a surgical procedure in which the cricopharyngeal muscle (the major contributor to the upper esophageal sphincter) is severed, may be useful in selected patients. It is best suited when there is documented dysfunction at the pharyngoesophageal junction but adequate laryngeal/hyoid elevation and pharyngeal propulsion are present.[5]

This procedure is found to benefit patients with OPMD, IBM, and ALS. In surgical series, the overall mortality rate after cricopharyngeal myotomy was 1.6%.[70] In one series, oropharyngeal symptoms improved in 75% of patients. Cricopharyngeal myotomy was performed in 139 patients who had dysphagia secondary to OPMD, and complications were noted in 16 patients. Four of these, all with respiratory distress syndrome, eventually died of lung infection. Permanent tracheostomy with laryngeal exclusion was required in two patients with muscular dystrophy, because of infection. Pulmonary infection was the most common complication after cricopharyngeal myotomy in patients with muscular dystrophy.

Box 4-3 Commonly Used Enteral Feeding Formulas
Polymeric
1.0 kcal/mL
Nutren 1.0
Ensure
Resource
2.0 kcal/mL
Magnacal
TwoCal HN (high nitrogen)
Fiber-containing
Jevity
Small peptide–based
Peptamen
Specialty
Nutra-Hep (hepatic)
Pulmocare (pulmonary)
Amin-Aide (renal)
Glucerna, Diabeta Source (glucose intolerance)

Stomach and Duodenum

Dyspepsia and Gastric Emptying Issues

Patients with DM frequently experience dyspeptic symptoms, such as early satiety, nausea, vomiting, and epigastric pain. Rare cases of gastric bezoar and retention have also been reported.[71]

Gastric emptying delay, gastroparesis, and acute gastrointestinal dilation have been shown to characterize the clinical course of DM.[9] The delayed gastric emptying in muscular dystrophy can be explained by the muscular disease, with associated fatty infiltration and dystrophy of smooth muscle; however, histologic evidence is limited. Malfunctioning electromechanical control of gastric activity may be the cause of slow gastric emptying.[72] Abnormalities have been noted on electrogastrography in patients with DM compared with control subjects, and studies have shown partial deregulation of the gastrointestinal endocrine system in patients with DM, with decreased postprandial secretion of motilin and glucagon-like peptide-1.[17,73] Similar problems of gastric emptying have been reported in patients with DMD and BMD. Delayed gastric emptying for solids has been shown in patients with ALS and was attributed to subclinical involvement of the autonomic nervous system.[3,74,75]

Diagnosis and Evaluation

Patients with dyspepsia, nausea, and vomiting usually require radiologic and endoscopic evaluation to exclude peptic ulcer disease and gastric outlet obstruction, followed by a gastric emptying study. Routine laboratory testing is not useful for the diagnosis of gastric stasis itself, although it may help to identify diseases that are associated with delayed gastric emptying or to exclude other disorders and related electrolyte disturbances. The most widely available and robust technique to confirm the presence of postprandial gastric stasis is scintigraphic gastric emptying. Consensus standards for performing and reporting gastric emptying scintigraphy have been published by the American Neurogastroenterology and Motility Society and the Society of Nuclear Medicine.[76] This involves consumption of a low-fat, egg white meal labeled with technetium (TC)-99m sulfur colloid, with imaging performed 0, 1, 2, and 4 hours after meal ingestion, providing standardized information about normal and delayed gastric emptying. Gastric residue of more than 10% at 4 hours is most accurate for detecting delayed gastric emptying. A scintigraphic study by Rönnblom et al indicated delayed emptying of the stomach in patients with DM who had dyspeptic symptoms, although patients without dyspeptic symptoms may have delayed gastric emptying as well.[73] In addition, there is no significant difference in gastric emptying between patients with different degrees of skeletal muscle involvement.[17,73] Similar gastric motor abnormalities were shown in a group of children with a recent diagnosis of muscular dystrophy, both DMD and BMD, at the initial phases of the disease. Worsening of gastric motor activity parallels progressive derangement of neuromuscular function during the 3-year follow-up.[77] Abnormalities have been noted on electrogastrography in patients with DM compared with control subjects; however, testing is limited to research purposes.[78]

Treatment and Management

Different drugs, particularly prokinetics, have been proposed to treat dyspeptic symptoms and motor disturbances in patients with muscular dystrophy. In a small series of 16 patients with delayed gastric emptying of solids and liquids, Horowitz et al showed that oral administration of metoclopramide 10 mg three times daily can improve solid gastric emptying.[79] Its mechanism of action involves local release of acetylcholine. Patients should be informed of extrapyramidal side effects and the risk of tardive dyskinesia, which although rare, can be irreversible.

Cisapride stimulates 5-hydroxytryptamine-4 receptors, resulting in the release of acetylcholine from the neurons in the myenteric plexus. It has also been reported to improve gastric emptying and digestive symptoms, such as nausea, vomiting, early satiety, abdominal distention, and pain.[80] Availability in the United States is severely restricted because of significant drug interactions (e.g., macrolide antibiotics, antifungals, and phenothiazines) that have caused cardiac arrhythmias and death.[81] However, it remains available in several other countries. In the United States, prescriptions for the drug can only be filled directly through the manufacturer, and documentation is required as to the need for the drug and assessment of risk factors for cardiac arrhythmias in the individual patient.

Use of erythromycin in small doses (100 mg, twice daily orally) in dyspeptic patients with DM over a period of 4 weeks minimally improved nausea and early satiety, and some patients noted marked improvement in diarrhea.[73] Its clinical effect lies in its agonistic action on the motilin receptors, inducing high-amplitude gastric propulsive contractions. Although no trials using intravenous erythromycin are available in patients with myopathic gastroparesis, in these patients, it can be used to improve gastric emptying in acute episodes of gastric stasis when oral intake is not tolerated.

Domperidone has been used in patients with gastroparesis. It is not approved for use by the U.S. Food and Drug Administration, but it is available in Canada and other countries. The U.S. Food and Drug Administration encourages physicians who would like to prescribe domperidone for their patients with severe gastrointestinal disorders that are refractory to standard therapy to open an investigational new drug application. QT prolongation has been reported with domperidone, which may also increase the risk of cardiac arrhythmias.

Gastric pacing using a gastric electrical stimulator received humanitarian device exemption approval for the treatment of refractory diabetic and idiopathic gastroparesis. However, the use of this technology in patients with gastroparesis secondary to other conditions is not well known.

Small Intestine

Chronic Intestinal Pseudo-Obstruction

Chronic intestinal pseudo-obstruction (CIPO) is a severe digestive syndrome characterized by derangement of gut propulsive motility that resembles mechanical obstruction, in the absence of obstructive process.[19,82,83]

There are various etiologies of intestinal pseudo-obstruction,[84,85] and it is usually secondary to an underlying disorder affecting neuromuscular function, although rare familial cases have been described. Based on tissue examination, CIPO can be classified into three major entities: neuropathies, "enteric mesenchymopathies," and myopathies.[86]

Inflammatory neuropathies related to several diseases, including paraneoplastic syndrome, infectious diseases (Chagas disease), and idiopathic causes, are characterized by dense lymphocytic and plasma cell infiltrates involving myenteric plexus and axons of the enteric nervous system. Degenerative noninflammatory neuropathies occur secondary to damage or loss of enteric neurons. This can be familial, a primary idiopathic form, or acquired as a result of radiation injury, diabetes, vinca alkaloids, and amyloidosis. The typical neuropathologic findings include neuronal damage and hypoganglionosis.

Enteric mesenchymopathies are associated with alteration in the interstitial cells of the Cajal network.[87]

Myopathic etiologies include primary visceral myopathy, muscular dystrophies, polymyositis,[88] and scleroderma. Primary visceral myopathy, including familial visceral myopathy, is characterized by degeneration and fibrosis of the smooth muscle layer of the gastrointestinal system.[89] The gastrointestinal system shows marked dilation of the entire digestive tract, especially the duodenum (megaduodenum), and this has been reported in hollow visceral myopathy as well.[90] Adult patients with spinal motor atrophy can also have CIPO.[91] In scleroderma, altered function of enteric neurons and progressive loss of smooth muscle, with fibrosis of the gastrointestinal tract, leads to impaired motility, intestinal stasis, and secondary bacterial overgrowth. In both DM and DMD, marked damage to enteric smooth muscle cells has been described.[83,92] Histopathologic analysis of the enteric muscle layer may show muscular abnormalities of the circular and longitudinal layers in patients with primary visceral myopathy. Gastrointestinal smooth muscle involvement, manifested pathologically as muscle cell hypereosinophilia, nuclear pyknosis, and cell fragmentation, was reported in three cases of DMD.[93]

The typical clinical manifestation of CIPO depends on whether functional derangement affects the upper gastrointestinal tract, in which case nausea and vomiting with abdominal pain are predominant, or a more distal segment of the gut, in which case abdominal distention and constipation are more likely. Diarrhea and steatorrhea can occur as a result of small bowel bacterial overgrowth.[94]

Chronic intestinal pseudo-obstruction and ophthalmoplegia, described as MNGIE (mitochondrial neurogastrointestinal encephalomyopathy) and also known as POLIP (polyneuropathy, ophthalmoplegia, leukoencephalopathy, and intestinal pseudo-obstruction) or MEPOP (mitochondrial encephalomyopathy, polyneuropathy, ophthalmoplegia, and pseudo-obstruction) syndrome, is a condition characterized by moderate to severe sensorimotor polyneuropathy, ophthalmoplegia, and severe, sometimes fatal, gastrointestinal dysmotility.[95,96] The initial presentation is usually of gastrointestinal symptoms that include dyspepsia, bloating, eructation, cramps, intolerance of large meals, and episodic vomiting and diarrhea. The disease usually presents before the age of 20 years, ranging from 2.5 to 32.0 years. Esophageal motility is variably affected, the smooth muscle of the small intestine does not function normally, and intestinal pseudo-obstruction is the rule. Upper gastrointestinal manometric studies show diminished amplitude of contractions in the small bowel during the fasting and fed states.[14] Skeletal muscle biopsy shows abnormalities of the mitochondria (see Chapter 22). Helpful screening tests include elevated serum lactate-to-pyruvate ratios that result from relative excess of reduced nicotinamide adenine dinucleotide and lack of nicotinamide adenine dinucleotide. Glucose loading may unmask hyperlactatemia and give rise to a paradoxical increase in ketone bodies.[97–99]

Diagnosis and Evaluation

The diagnosis of CIPO is mainly clinical, and diagnostic tests in patients with suspected CIPO are necessary to exclude mechanical occlusion. Plain abdominal films usually show signs of intestinal occlusion, such as distended bowel loop with air-fluid levels, and small bowel barium studies or computed tomography enterography is necessary to exclude organic lesions. Endoscopic evaluation, based on symptoms and the findings on radiologic evaluation, may be indicated to exclude mechanical occlusions. Intestinal biopsy can be performed to exclude inflammatory bowel disease and celiac sprue.[100] Diagnosis may require determination of small bowel transit studies using scintigraphy.[101] Small bowel manometry is usually not required when associated with known conditions, but it is helpful in selected cases, although it is not widely available.[102] Manometric findings described in the myopathic form consist of normally coordinated motor patterns with low amplitude. In neuropathic CIPO, contractions are uncoordinated, although they have normal amplitude.

In a recent study of 115 patients with CIPO who underwent full-thickness jejunal biopsy, 24% showed absent or reduced α-actin staining in the circular muscle of the jejunum, in the absence of other structural abnormalities of muscle and nerve, compared with control subjects.[103]

Treatment and Management
Medical therapy for CIPO in patients with neuromuscular disease is aimed at controlling symptoms and avoiding complications.[104] The use of antiemetics, antisecretory agents, antispasmodics, prokinetics,[105] laxatives, or antidiarrheals, based on dominant symptoms and in addition to analgesic drugs, may be necessary. Bacterial overgrowth should be treated with antibiotics.[106] Alternating cycles with metronidazole and tetracycline is sometimes necessary to reduce the chance of resistance. Octreotide is a long-acting somatostatin analog that increases intestinal motor activity and has been shown to decrease bacterial overgrowth. It can be used in selected cases.[107]

Gastrostomy for gastric decompression, along with feeding jejunostomy,[108] may be helpful in patients with recurrent hospitalization because of vomiting and abdominal distention and may be an option in patients who can be fed by enteral nutrition. Most patients with CIPO require nutritional support, and some may require total parenteral nutrition.[109]

Large Intestine and Anal Sphincter

Constipation

Constipation, defined as infrequent, incomplete evacuation or the passage of excessively hard stools, is a common complication of neuromuscular diseases, especially as the disease progresses. Various abnormalities, including megacolon, loss of haustration, absence of segmental contractions, loss of peristaltic activity, sigmoid volvulus, and segmental narrowing, have been reported in patients with muscular dystrophy.[110,111] Light microscopy showed atrophy of the individual muscle fibers, similar to what is seen in skeletal muscle.[93]

Constipation is common in patients with ALS and plays an important role in malnutrition because it can exacerbate appetite loss. In this disease, it results from limited physical exercise, weakness of the abdominal and pelvic muscles, diet lacking in fiber, dehydration, and the use of certain medical treatments that slow colonic transit. There has been evidence of autonomic dysfunction in patients with ALS that might be associated with gastrointestinal symptoms.[112] A study using radio-opaque markers to measure colonic transit time showed markedly delayed colonic transit time in patients with ALS compared with control subjects.[113]

Treatment and Management
Treatment is generally supportive, and close attention should be paid to medications commonly prescribed to these patients, such as scopolamine in patients with ALS (reduces excessive salivation but may exacerbate constipation). Management suggestions include the use of osmotic laxatives (e.g., lactulose), bulk-forming laxatives (e.g., methyl cellulose), suppositories, enemas, and the augmentation

of fluid and fiber intake.[114] However, in patients with poor colonic transit, excessive bulking of stools may have the opposite effect of worsening constipation or increasing obstruction potential. Additionally, psyllium-based supplements are degraded by colonic bacteria, which can lead to a worsening of bloating and flatus. For severe constipation, newer polyethylene glycol solutions can be used. The use of newer agents, including lubiprostone (Amitiza, Sucampo), a locally acting chloride channel activator that enhances a chloride-rich intestinal fluid secretion, and prucalopride, a selective, high-affinity 5-hydroxytryptamine-4 receptor agonist, has been shown to be effective for the treatment of chronic idiopathic constipation in adults.[115,116] These have not been studied in patients with neuromuscular diseases, but thus far, they appear to be a relatively safe and effective option in the general population.

Fecal Incontinence

In healthy individuals, the internal anal sphincter normally contributes approximately 80% of the manometrically determined resting pressure. The most burdensome and disabling problem affecting patients with DM may be fecal incontinence as a result of sphincter involvement. Up to 66% of patients with DM have occasional fecal incontinence, and more than 10% report fecal incontinence one or more times a week.[117]

Studies using manometry report a decrease in both resting pressure (based on the tonic activity of the internal anal sphincter) and squeezing pressure (exerted by the phasic activity of the external anal sphincter).[18,118] Pudendal nerve terminal motor latencies are normal in these patients, confirming the absence of a neurogenic lesion.[119] Eckardt et al studied the external anal sphincter using electromyography and found myopathic potentials with myotonia.[120] Herbaut et al reported decreased duration and amplitude of the motor units in the external anal sphincter and puborectalis muscle of patients with DM and fecal incontinence.[117] A study using electron microscopy to evaluate the anal sphincter in two siblings with DM found that the external anal sphincter was atrophic in both patients, with marked fibrosis and a high variation in the diameter of the fibers. In addition, the striated muscle was almost entirely substituted by smooth muscle cells derived from the internal sphincter.[118] In ALS, the Onufrowicz nucleus in the medial sacral spinal cord, which innervates the sphincter and pelvic floor muscles, is spared; therefore, urinary and bowel incontinence is not a feature of even advanced cases.[121]

Treatment and Management
Medical treatment with procainamide (300 mg twice daily) has been reported in a case report for fecal incontinence in patients with DM.[122]

Rehabilitation, involving a combination of volumetric rehabilitation, electroanal stimulation, kinesitherapy, and biofeedback, can be effective in patients without severe damage to the pelvic floor muscle.[123–126]

Peripheral Neuropathy and the Gastrointestinal System

Most generalized peripheral polyneuropathies are accompanied by clinical or subclinical autonomic dysfunction. In these cases, autonomic dysfunction affecting gut motility is the most prominent manifestation.

Diabetic autonomic neuropathy is characterized by gastrointestinal reflux, gastric emptying problems with gastroparesis, abnormal small bowel motility, constipation, diarrhea, and fecal incontinence.[125–128]

The diarrhea is watery and painless, occurs at night, and may be associated with fecal incontinence. The prevalence is estimated at 8% to 22%.[129,130] Therapy is usually directed toward the predominant symptoms. Diarrhea is usually treated with antidiarrheal drugs (loperamide and diphenoxylate). The use of antibiotics to treat small bowel bacterial overgrowth and the use of octreotide (50–75 μg subcutaneously two to three times daily) have been found to be somewhat helpful in the treatment of diabetic diarrhea.[131,132]

Autonomic dysfunction is present in patients with Guillain-Barré syndrome, amyloidosis, and hepatic porphyrias with peripheral neuropathy. MNGIE, which was discussed earlier, is associated with peripheral neuropathy with severe visceral neuropathy and secondary gastrointestinal dysfunction.

Conclusion

Gastrointestinal involvement is frequently observed in patients with neuromuscular diseases, and digestive symptoms may be the first sign of the disease. Problems with swallowing and motility disorders are the two main gastrointestinal manifestations usually observed in these patient groups. Collaboration between gastroenterologists and neurologists is essential for appropriate understanding, diagnosis, and management.

After exclusion of intrinsic mucosal disease of the gut, the presence of these symptoms in patients with established neurologic disorders suggests that the underlying condition is responsible for the symptoms. Recognition of these complications is imperative, and early intervention with hydration and nutritional support, including appropriate timing of feeding tube placement, is necessary. Principles of management also include the treatment of the neurologic disease itself, suppression of bacterial overgrowth, correction of dysmotility with medical therapy, and a multidisciplinary approach toward the management of these patients.

References

1. Chaudhry V, Umapathi T, Ravich WJ: Neuromuscular diseases and disorders of the alimentary system, *Muscle Nerve* 25:768–784, 2002.
2. Tieleman AA, van Vliet J, Jansen JB, et al: Gastrointestinal involvement is frequent in myotonic dystrophy type 2, *Neuromuscul Disord* 18:646–649, 2008.
3. Toepfer M, Folwaczny C, Klauser A, et al: Gastrointestinal dysfunction in amyotrophic lateral sclerosis, *Amyotroph Lateral Scler Other Motor Neuron Disord* 1:15–19, 1999.
4. Costantini M, Zaninotto G, Anselmino M, et al: Esophageal motor function in patients with myotonic dystrophy, *Dig Dis Sci* 41:2032–2038, 1996.
5. Janzen VD, Rae RE, Hudson AJ: Otolaryngologic manifestations of amyotrophic lateral sclerosis, *J Otolaryngol* 17:41–42, 1988.
6. Caroscio JT, Mulvihill MN, Sterling R, Abrams B: Amyotrophic lateral sclerosis. Its natural history, *Neurol Clin* 5:1–8, 1987.
7. Leighton SE, Burton MJ, Lund WS, Cochrane GM: Swallowing in motor neurone disease, *J R Soc Med* 87:801–805, 1994.
8. Jaffe KM, McDonald CM, Ingman E, Haas J: Symptoms of upper gastrointestinal dysfunction in Duchenne muscular dystrophy: case-control study, *Arch Phys Med Rehabil* 71:742–744, 1990.
9. Bellini M, Biagi S, Stasi C, et al: Gastrointestinal manifestations in myotonic muscular dystrophy, *World J Gastroenterol* 12:1821–1828, 2006.
10. Tiomny E, Khilkevic O, Korczyn AD, et al: Esophageal smooth muscle dysfunction in oculopharyngeal muscular dystrophy, *Dig Dis Sci* 41:1350–1354, 1996.
11. Wohlgemuth M, de Swart BJ, Kalf JG, et al: Dysphagia in facioscapulohumeral muscular dystrophy, *Neurology* 66:1926–1928, 2006.
12. Hill M, Hughes T, Milford C: Treatment for swallowing difficulties (dysphagia) in chronic muscle disease, *Cochrane Database Syst Rev* (2) CD004303, 2004.
13. Jequier M, Todorov A: New aspects of Steinert's disease, *Rev Otoneuroophtalmol* 39:317–324, 1967.
14. Mueller LA, Camilleri M, Emslie-Smith AM: Mitochondrial neurogastrointestinal encephalomyopathy: manometric and diagnostic features, *Gastroenterology* 116:959–963, 1999.
15. Modolell I, Mearin F, Baudet JS, et al: Pharyngo-esophageal motility disturbances in patients with myotonic dystrophy, *Scand J Gastroenterol* 34:878–882, 1999.
16. Ludatscher RM, Kerner H, Amikam S, Gellei B: Myotonia dystrophica with heart involvement: an electron microscopic study of skeletal, cardiac, and smooth muscle, *J Clin Pathol* 31:1057–1064, 1978.
17. Ronnblom A, Forsberg H, Danielsson A: Gastrointestinal symptoms in myotonic dystrophy, *Scand J Gastroenterol* 31:654–657, 1996.
18. Lecointe-Besancon I, Leroy F, Devroede G, et al: A comparative study of esophageal and anorectal motility in myotonic dystrophy, *Dig Dis Sci* 44:1090–1099, 1999.
19. Nowak TV, Ionasescu V, Anuras S: Gastrointestinal manifestations of the muscular dystrophies, *Gastroenterology* 82:800–810, 1982.
20. de Swart BJ, van der Sluijs BM, Vos AM, et al: Ptosis aggravates dysphagia in oculopharyngeal muscular dystrophy, *J Neurol Neurosurg Psychiatry* 77:266–268, 2006.
21. Verma A, Bradley WG, Adesina AM, et al: Inclusion body myositis with cricopharyngeus muscle involvement and severe dysphagia, *Muscle Nerve* 14:470–473, 1991.
22. van der Meulen MF, Bronner IM, Hoogendijk JE, et al: Polymyositis: an overdiagnosed entity, *Neurology* 61:316–321, 2003.
23. Weston S, Thumshirn M, Wiste J, Camilleri M: Clinical and upper gastrointestinal motility features in systemic sclerosis and related disorders, *Am J Gastroenterol* 93:1085–1089, 1998.
24. Willig TN, Bach JR, Venance V, Navarro J: Nutritional rehabilitation in neuromuscular disorders, *Semin Neurol* 15:18–23, 1995.
25. Cameron A, Rosenfeld J: Nutritional issues and supplements in amyotrophic lateral sclerosis and other neurodegenerative disorders, *Curr Opin Clin Nutr Metab Care* 5:631–643, 2002.
26. Slowie LA, Paige MS, Antel JP: Nutritional considerations in the management of patients with amyotrophic lateral sclerosis (ALS), *J Am Diet Assoc* 83:44–47, 1983.
27. Worwood AM, Leigh PN: Indicators and prevalence of malnutrition in motor neurone disease, *Eur Neurol* 40:159–163, 1998.
28. Hardiman O: Symptomatic treatment of respiratory and nutritional failure in amyotrophic lateral sclerosis, *J Neurol* 247:245–251, 2000.
29. Heffernan C, Jenkinson C, Holmes T, et al: Nutritional management in MND/ALS patients: an evidence based review, *Amyotroph Lateral Scler Other Motor Neuron Disord* 5:72–83, 2004.
30. Kasarskis EJ, Berryman S, Vanderleest JG, et al: Nutritional status of patients with amyotrophic lateral sclerosis: relation to the proximity of death, *Am J Clin Nutr* 63:130–137, 1996.
31. Barbiera F, Condello S, De Palo A, et al: Role of videofluorography swallow study in management of dysphagia in neurologically compromised patients, *Radiol Med* 111:818–827, 2006.
32. Eckardt VF, Nix W, Kraus W, Bohl J: Esophageal motor function in patients with muscular dystrophy, *Gastroenterology* 90:628–635, 1986.
33. Hila A, Castell JA, Castell DO: Pharyngeal and upper esophageal sphincter manometry in the evaluation of dysphagia, *J Clin Gastroenterol* 33:355–361, 2001.
34. Swick HM, Werlin SL, Dodds WJ, Hogan WJ: Pharyngoesophageal motor function in patients with myotonic dystrophy, *Ann Neurol* 10:454–457, 1981.
35. Castell JA, Castell DO, Duranceau CA, Topart P: Manometric characteristics of the pharynx, upper esophageal sphincter, esophagus, and lower esophageal sphincter in patients with oculopharyngeal muscular dystrophy, *Dysphagia* 10:22–26, 1995.
36. Leigh PN, Abrahams S, Al-Chalabi A, et al: The management of motor neurone disease, *J Neurol Neurosurg Psychiatry* 74(Suppl 4):iv32–iv47, 2003.
37. Hillel AD, Miller R: Bulbar amyotrophic lateral sclerosis: patterns of progression and clinical management, *Head Neck* 11:51–59, 1989.
38. Andersen PM, Borasio GD, Dengler R, et al: EFNS task force on management of amyotrophic lateral sclerosis: guidelines for diagnosing and clinical care of patients and relatives, *Eur J Neurol* 12:921–938, 2005.

39. The role of percutaneous endoscopic gastrostomy in enteral feeding. Guidelines for clinical application, *Gastrointest Endosc* 34(3 Suppl):35S–36S, 1988.

40. Park RH, Allison MC, Lang J, et al: Randomised comparison of percutaneous endoscopic gastrostomy and nasogastric tube feeding in patients with persisting neurological dysphagia, *BMJ* 304:1406–1409, 1992.

41. Ramelli GP, Aloysius A, King C, et al: Gastrostomy placement in paediatric patients with neuromuscular disorders: indications and outcome, *Dev Med Child Neurol* 49:367–371, 2007.

42. Seguy D, Michaud L, Guimber D, et al: Efficacy and tolerance of gastrostomy feeding in pediatric forms of neuromuscular diseases, *JPEN J Parenter Enteral Nutr* 26:298–304, 2002.

43. Shimizu T, Hanaoka T, Hayashi H, et al: Percutaneous endoscopic gastrostomy in patients with intractable neurological diseases—retrospective study of the indication, complication and prognosis, *Rinsho Shinkeigaku* 47:565–570, 2007.

44. Mathus-Vliegen LM, Louwerse LS, et al: Percutaneous endoscopic gastrostomy in patients with amyotrophic lateral sclerosis and impaired pulmonary function, *Gastrointest Endosc* 40:463–469, 1994.

45. Mazzini L, Corrà T, Zaccala M, et al: Percutaneous endoscopic gastrostomy and enteral nutrition in amyotrophic lateral sclerosis, *J Neurol* 242:695–698, 1995.

46. Miller RG, Rosenberg JA, Gelinas DF, et al: Practice parameter: the care of the patient with amyotrophic lateral sclerosis (an evidence-based review): report of the Quality Standards Subcommittee of the American Academy of Neurology: ALS Practice Parameters Task Force, *Neurology* 52:1311–1323, 1999.

47. Miller RG, Jackson CE, Kasarskis EJ, et al: Practice parameter update: the care of the patient with amyotrophic lateral sclerosis: drug, nutritional, and respiratory therapies (an evidence-based review): report of the Quality Standards Subcommittee of the American Academy of Neurology, *Neurology* 73(15):1218–1226, 2009.

48. Akpunonu BE, Mutgi AB, Roberts C, et al: Modified barium swallow does not affect how often PEGs are placed after stroke, *J Clin Gastroenterol* 24:74–78, 1997.

49. Forbes RB, Colville S, Swingler RJ: Frequency, timing and outcome of gastrostomy tubes for amyotrophic lateral sclerosis/motor neurone disease—a record linkage study from the Scottish Motor Neurone Disease Register, *J Neurol* 251:813–817, 2004.

50. Kasarskis EJ, Scarlata D, Hill R, et al: A retrospective study of percutaneous endoscopic gastrostomy in ALS patients during the BDNF and CNTF trials, *J Neuro Sci* 169:118–125, 1999.

51. Boitano LJ, Jordan T, Benditt JO: Noninvasive ventilation allows gastrostomy tube placement in patients with advanced ALS, *Neurology* 56:413–414, 2001.

52. Birnkrant DJ, Pope JF, Martin JE, et al: Treatment of type I spinal muscular atrophy with noninvasive ventilation and gastrostomy feeding, *Pediatr Neurol* 18:407–410, 1998.

53. Pope JF, Birnkrant DJ, Martin JE, Repucci AH: Noninvasive ventilation during percutaneous gastrostomy placement in Duchenne muscular dystrophy, *Pediatr Pulmonol* 23:468–471, 1997.

54. Thornton FJ, Fotheringham T, Alexander M, et al: Amyotrophic lateral sclerosis: enteral nutrition provision—endoscopic or radiologic gastrostomy? *Radiology* 224:713–717, 2002.

55. Eisen GM, Baron TH, Dominitz JA, et al: Role of endoscopy in enteral feeding, *Gastrointest Endosc* 55:794–797, 2002.

56. Hassett JM, Sunby C, Flint LM: No elimination of aspiration pneumonia in neurologically disabled patients with feeding gastrostomy, *Surg Gynecol Obstet* 167:383–388, 1988.

57. Light VL, Slezak FA, Porter JA, et al: Predictive factors for early mortality after percutaneous endoscopic gastrostomy, *Gastrointest Endosc* 42:330–335, 1995.

58. Hull MA, Rawlings J, Murray FE, et al: Audit of outcome of long-term enteral nutrition by percutaneous endoscopic gastrostomy, *Lancet* 341:869–872, 1993.

59. Larson DE, Burton DD, Schroeder KW, DiMagno EP: Percutaneous endoscopic gastrostomy. Indications, success, complications, and mortality in 314 consecutive patients, *Gastroenterology* 93:48–52, 1987.

60. Mathus-Vliegen LM, Koning H: Percutaneous endoscopic gastrostomy and gastrojejunostomy: a critical reappraisal of patient selection, tube function and the feasibility of nutritional support during extended follow-up, *Gastrointest Endosc* 50:746–754, 1999.

61. Dormann AJ, Wigginghaus B, Risius H, et al: A single dose of ceftriaxone administered 30 minutes before percutaneous endoscopic gastrostomy significantly reduces local and systemic infective complications, *Am J Gastroenterol* 94:3220–3224, 1999.

62. Gossner L, Keymling J, Hahn EG, Ell C: Antibiotic prophylaxis in percutaneous endoscopic gastrostomy (PEG): a prospective randomized clinical trial, *Endoscopy* 31(2):119–124, 1999.

63. Jafri NS, Mahid SS, Minor KS, et al: Meta-analysis: antibiotic prophylaxis to prevent peristomal infection following percutaneous endoscopic gastrostomy, *Aliment Pharmacol Ther* 25:647–656, 2007.

64. Gottfried EB, Plumser AB, Clair MR: Pneumoperitoneum following percutaneous endoscopic gastrostomy. A prospective study, *Gastrointest Endosc* 32:397–399, 1986.

65. Gauderer MW, Ponsky JL, Izant RJ Jr, : Gastrostomy without laparotomy: a percutaneous endoscopic technique, *J Pediatr Surg* 15:872–875, 1980.

66. Brant CQ, Stanich P, Ferrari AP Jr, : Improvement of children's nutritional status after enteral feeding by PEG: an interim report, *Gastrointest Endosc* 50:183–188, 1999.

67. Mitsumoto H, Davidson M, Moore D, et al: Percutaneous endoscopic gastrostomy (PEG) in patients with ALS and bulbar dysfunction, *Amyotroph Lateral Scler Other Motor Neuron Disord* 4(3):177–185, 2003.

68. Langmore SE, Kasarskis EJ, Manca ML, Olney RK: Enteral tube feeding for amyotrophic lateral sclerosis/motor neuron disease, *Cochrane Database Syst Rev* (4) CD004030, 2006.

69. Brouillette D, Martel E, Chen LQ, Duranceau A: Pitfalls and complications of cricopharyngeal myotomy, *Chest Surg Clin N Am* 7:457–475, 1997, discussion 476.

70. Brigand C, Ferraro P, Martin J, Duranceau A: Risk factors in patients undergoing cricopharyngeal myotomy, *Br J Surg* 94:978–983, 2007.

71. Kuiper DH: Gastric bezoar in a patient with myotonic dystrophy. A review of the gastrointestinal complications of myotonic dystrophy, *Am J Dig Dis* 16:529–534, 1971.

72. Lewis TD, Daniel EE: Gastroduodenal motility in a case of dystrophia myotonica, *Gastroenterology* 81:145–149, 1981.

73. Rönnblom A, Andersson S, Hellström PM, Danielsson A: Gastric emptying in myotonic dystrophy, *Eur J Clin Invest* 32(8):570–574, 2002.

74. Hillemand B: Gastric emptying and amyotrophic lateral sclerosis (proceedings), *Lille Med* 24:13, 1979.

75. Toepfer M, Folwaczny C, Lochmüller H, et al: Noninvasive (13)C-octanoic acid breath test shows delayed gastric emptying in patients with amyotrophic lateral sclerosis, *Digestion* 60:567–571, 1999.

76. Abell TL, Camilleri M, Donohoe K, et al: Consensus recommendations for gastric emptying scintigraphy: a joint report of the American Neurogastroenterology and Motility Society and the Society of Nuclear Medicine, *Am J Gastroenterol* 103:753–763, 2008.

77. Borrelli O, Salvia G, Mancini V, et al: Evolution of gastric electrical features and gastric emptying in children with Duchenne and Becker muscular dystrophy, *Am J Gastroenterol* 100:695–702, 2005.

78. Rönnblom A, Hellström PM, Holst JJ, et al: Gastric myoelectrical activity and gut hormone secretion in myotonic dystrophy, *Eur J Gastroenterol Hepatol* 13:825–831, 2001.

79. Horowitz M, Maddox A, Maddern GJ, et al: Gastric and esophageal emptying in dystrophia myotonica. Effect of metoclopramide, *Gastroenterology* 92:570–577, 1987.

80. Horowitz M, Maddox A, Wishart J, et al: The effect of cisapride on gastric and oesophageal emptying in dystrophia myotonica, *J Gastroenterol Hepatol* 285–293, 1987.

81. Wysowski DK, Corken A, Gallo-Torres H, et al: Postmarketing reports of QT prolongation and ventricular arrhythmia in association with cisapride and Food and Drug Administration regulatory actions, *Am J Gastroenterol* 96:1698–1703, 2001.

82. Camilleri M: Diagnosis and treatment of enteric neuromuscular diseases, *Clin Auton Res* 13:10–15, 2003.

83. De Giorgio R, Camilleri M: Human enteric neuropathies: morphology and molecular pathology, *Neurogastroenterol Motil* 16:515–531, 2004.

84. Krishnamurthy S, Schuffler MD: Pathology of neuromuscular disorders of the small intestine and colon, *Gastroenterology* 93:610–639, 1987.

85. Antonucci A, Fronzoni L, Cogliandro L, et al: Chronic intestinal pseudo-obstruction, *World J Gastroenterol* 14:2953–2961, 2008.

86. De Giorgio R, Sarnelli G, Corinaldesi R, Stanghellini V: Advances in our understanding of the pathology of chronic intestinal pseudo-obstruction, *Gut* 53:1549–1552, 2004.

87. Sanders KM, Ordog T, Ward SM: Physiology and pathophysiology of the interstitial cells of Cajal: from bench to bedside. IV. Genetic and animal models of GI motility disorders caused by loss of interstitial cells of Cajal, *Am J Physiol Gastrointest Liver Physiol* 282:G747–G756, 2002.

88. Takakusaki S, Kudo T, Suzuki K, et al: Intestinal pseudo-obstruction associated with polymyositis successfully treated with somatostatin analog, *Nippon Naika Gakkai Zasshi* 97:398–400, 2008.

89. Anuras S, Mitros FA, Milano A, et al: A familial visceral myopathy with dilatation of the entire gastrointestinal tract, *Gastroenterology* 90:385–390, 1986.

90. Mansell PI, Tattersall RB, Balsitis M, et al: Megaduodenum due to hollow visceral myopathy successfully managed by duodenoplasty and feeding jejunostomy, *Gut* 32:334–337, 1991.

91. Ionasescu V, Christensen J, Hart M: Intestinal pseudo-obstruction in adult spinal muscular atrophy, *Muscle Nerve* 17:946–948, 1994.

92. Harvey JC, Sherbourne DH, Siegel CI: Smooth muscle involvement in myotonic dystrophy, *Am J Med* 39:81–90, 1965.

93. Pruzanski W, Huvos AG: Smooth muscle involvement in primary muscle disease. I. Myotonic dystrophy, *Arch Pathol* 83:229–233, 1967.

94. Faure C, Goulet O, Ategbo S, et al: Chronic intestinal pseudoobstruction syndrome: clinical analysis, outcome, and prognosis in 105 children. French-Speaking Group of Pediatric Gastroenterology, *Dig Dis Sci* 44:953–959, 1999.

95. Uncini A, Servidei S, Silvestri G, et al: Ophthalmoplegia, demyelinating neuropathy, leukoencephalopathy, myopathy, and gastrointestinal dysfunction with multiple deletions of mitochondrial DNA: a mitochondrial multisystem disorder in search of a name, *Muscle Nerve* 17:667–674, 1994.

96. Giordano C, Sebastiani M, Plazzi G, et al: Mitochondrial neurogastrointestinal encephalomyopathy: evidence of mitochondrial DNA depletion in the small intestine, *Gastroenterology* 130:893–901, 2006.

97. Gillis LA, Sokol RJ: Gastrointestinal manifestations of mitochondrial disease, *Gastroenterol Clin North Am* 32:789–817, v. 2003.

98. Munnich A, Rötig A, Chretien D, et al: Clinical presentations and laboratory investigations in respiratory chain deficiency, *Eur J Pediatr* 155:262–274, 1996.

99. Simon LT, Horoupian DS, Dorfman LJ, et al: Polyneuropathy, ophthalmoplegia, leukoencephalopathy, and intestinal pseudo-obstruction: POLIP syndrome, *Ann Neurol* 28:349–360, 1990.

100. Ravindra BS, Desai N, Deviprasad S, et al: Myotonic dystrophy in a patient of celiac disease: a new association? *Trop Gastroenterol* 29:114–115, 2008.

101. von der Ohe MR, Camilleri M: Measurement of small bowel and colonic transit: indications and methods, *Mayo Clin Proc* 67:1169–1179, 1992.

102. Stanghellini V, Camilleri M, Malagelada JR: Chronic idiopathic intestinal pseudo-obstruction: clinical and intestinal manometric findings, *Gut* 28:5–12, 1987.

103. Knowles CH, Silk DB, Darzi A, et al: Deranged smooth muscle alpha-actin as a biomarker of intestinal pseudo-obstruction: a controlled multinational case series, *Gut* 53:1583–1589, 2004.

104. De Giorgio R, Barbara G, Stanghellini V, et al: Review article: the pharmacological treatment of acute colonic pseudo-obstruction, *Aliment Pharmacol Ther* 15:1717–1727, 2001.

105. Abell TL, Camilleri M, DiMagno EP, et al: Long-term efficacy of oral cisapride in symptomatic upper gut dysmotility, *Dig Dis Sci* 36:616–620, 1991.

106. Attar A, Flourié B, Rambaud JC, et al: Antibiotic efficacy in small intestinal bacterial overgrowth-related chronic diarrhea: a crossover, randomized trial, *Gastroenterology* 117:794–797, 1999.

107. Soudah HC, Hasler WL, Owyang C: Effect of octreotide on intestinal motility and bacterial overgrowth in scleroderma, *N Engl J Med* 325:1461–1467, 1991.

108. Di Lorenzo C, Flores AF, Buie T, Hyman PE: Intestinal motility and jejunal feeding in children with chronic intestinal pseudo-obstruction, *Gastroenterology* 108:1379–1385, 1995.

109. Koretz RL, Lipman TO, Klein S: AGA technical review on parenteral nutrition, *Gastroenterology* 121:970–1001, 2001.

110. Kark AE, Greenstein AJ: Sigmoid volvulus in muscular dystrophy, *Am J Gastroenterol* 57:571–577, 1972.

111. Weiner MJ: Myotonic megacolon in myotonic dystrophy, *AJR Am J Roentgenol* 130:177–179, 1978.

112. Baltadzhieva R, Gurevich T, Korczyn AD: Autonomic impairment in amyotrophic lateral sclerosis, *Curr Opin Neurol* 18:487–493, 2005.

113. Toepfer M, Schroeder M, Klauser A, et al: Delayed colonic transit times in amyotrophic lateral sclerosis assessed with radio-opaque markers, *Eur J Med Res* 2:473–476, 1997.

114. Borasio GD, Miller RG: Clinical characteristics and management of ALS, *Semin Neurol* 21:155–166, 2001.

115. Johanson JF, Morton D, Geenen J, Ueno R: Multicenter, 4-week, double-blind, randomized, placebo-controlled trial of lubiprostone, a locally-acting type-2 chloride channel activator, in patients with chronic constipation, *Am J Gastroenterol* 103:170–177, 2008.

116. Camilleri M, Kerstens R, Rykx A, Vandeplassche L: A placebo-controlled trial of prucalopride for severe chronic constipation, *N Engl J Med* 358:2344–2354, 2008.

117. Herbaut AG, Nogueira MC, Panzer JM, et al: Anorectal incontinence in myotonic dystrophy: a myopathic involvement of pelvic floor muscles, *Muscle Nerve* 15:1210–1211, 1992.

118. Abercrombie JF, Rogers J, Swash M: Faecal incontinence in myotonic dystrophy, *J Neurol Neurosurg Psychiatry* 64:128–130, 1998.

119. Kiff ES, Swash M: Slowed conduction in the pudendal nerves in idiopathic (neurogenic) faecal incontinence, *Br J Surg* 71:614–616, 1984.

120. Eckardt VF, Nix W: The anal sphincter in patients with myotonic muscular dystrophy, *Gastroenterology* 100:424–430, 1991.

121. Holstege G, Tan J: Supraspinal control of motoneurons innervating the striated muscles of the pelvic floor including urethral and anal sphincters in the cat, *Brain* 110(Pt 5):1323–1344, 1987.

122. Pelliccioni G, Scarpino O, Piloni V: Procainamide for faecal incontinence in myotonic dystrophy, *J Neurol Neurosurg Psychiatry* 67:257–258, 1999.

123. Buntzen S, Rasmussen OO, Ryhammer AM, et al: Sacral nerve stimulation for treatment of fecal incontinence in a patient with muscular dystrophy: report of a case, *Dis Colon Rectum* 47:1409–1411, 2004.

124. Pucciani F, Iozzi L, Masi A, et al: Multimodal rehabilitation for faecal incontinence: experience of an Italian centre devoted to faecal disorder rehabilitation, *Tech Coloproctol* 7:139–147, 2003, discussion 147.

125. Coggrave M, Wiesel PH, Norton C: Management of faecal incontinence and constipation in adults with central neurological diseases, *Cochrane Database Syst Rev* (2) CD002115, 2006.

126. Bytzer P, Talley NJ, Leemon M, et al: Prevalence of gastrointestinal symptoms associated with diabetes mellitus: a population-based survey of 15,000 adults, *Arch Intern Med* 161:1989–1996, 2001.

127. Bytzer P, Talley NJ, Hammer J, et al: GI symptoms in diabetes mellitus are associated with both poor glycemic control and diabetic complications, *Am J Gastroenterol* 97:604–611, 2002.

128. Feldman M, Schiller LR: Disorders of gastrointestinal motility associated with diabetes mellitus, *Ann Intern Med* 98:378–384, 1983.

129. Dandona P, Fonseca V, Mier A, Beckett AG: Diarrhea and metformin in a diabetic clinic, *Diabetes Care* 6:472–474, 1983.

130. Walker JJ, Kaplan DS: Efficacy of the somatostatin analog octreotide in the treatment of two patients with refractory diabetic diarrhea, *Am J Gastroenterol* 88:765–767, 1993.

131. Mourad FH, Gorard D, Thillainayagam AV, et al: Effective treatment of diabetic diarrhoea with somatostatin analogue, octreotide, *Gut* 33:1578–1580, 1992.

Nicholas J. Silvestri, MD
Christopher H. Gibbons, MD, MMSc

Autonomic Dysfunction in Neuromuscular Disorders

5

Overview of the Autonomic Nervous System

The autonomic nervous system extends to every organ in the human body, creating a dizzying array of central and peripheral nerves, nuclei, ganglia, and neurotransmitters that often defy conventional attempts at learning through memorization. Although colloquial understanding of the autonomic nervous system is discovered in the medical students' mantra of "fight or flight," true comprehension of the system often occurs only after disease-specific disturbances of autonomic function are encountered in clinical practice. The autonomic nervous system modulates blood pressure, heart rate, thermoregulation, motility of the gastrointestinal system, micturition, pupillary function, and salivary gland secretion, among other things.[1] Dysfunction of one, or all, of these processes may occur in neuromuscular disorders that affect the autonomic nervous system. This chapter briefly reviews the anatomic structure and clinical implications of autonomic dysfunction, the evaluation of the autonomic nervous system, neuromuscular diseases that result in autonomic disturbances, and treatment options in patients with dysautonomia. A graphic overview of the autonomic nervous system is shown in Figure 5-1.

Sympathetic Nervous System

The sympathetic nervous system is composed of cells located in the lateral horn of the spinal cord (thoracic to lumbar levels), and for this reason, it has been referred to as the *thoracolumbar system*. The cell bodies of sympathetic preganglionic neurons are located from T1 to L3 in the intermediolateral columns.[1] The preganglionic neurons project ipsilaterally out the white rami to the paravertebral chain, where they synapse on postganglionic neurons in adjacent ganglia. There is a rough anatomic distribution to the ganglia, with the upper thoracic ganglia projecting to the head and the lumbar ganglia projecting to the lower extremities and lower trunk. The axons of the preganglionic sympathetic neurons are relatively short because of the close proximity of the paravertebral ganglia, and they use acetylcholine as their neurotransmitter. In contrast, the postganglionic neurons have longer axons that stimulate directly on their target end-organ through the neurotransmitter norepinephrine. One notable exception to this rule is the innervation to the postganglionic sudomotor (sweat) system, which also uses acetylcholine as the postganglionic neurotransmitter.[1]

Activation of the sympathetic nervous system can be considered an attempt to optimize energy expenditure in urgent situations. Bronchial dilation occurs to facilitate respiration. There is constriction of the arrector pili muscles, resulting in hairs standing on end. The piloerection response is seen prominently in households cohabitated by feline and canine species as the domesticated cat attempts to frighten the dog by appearing larger. Sphincters of the anus and bladder tighten (to prevent fluid release), with simultaneous relaxation of the detrusor muscle (to prevent fluid expulsion). Activation of the cardiovascular system results in increased heart rate and contractility, and vasodilation occurs in blood vessels to the lungs, heart, and striated muscle. Conversely, vasoconstriction occurs in the skin and gastrointestinal tract. During sympathetic activation, the pupil widens as a result of constriction of the dilator muscle, the tarsal muscle of the eyelid contracts, elevating the eyelid, and tightening of the orbital muscle results in protrusion of the eyeball. These ocular adjustments result in an increase in visual field size, but are well suited to stereotyping for cartoonists creating a caricature of a face with retracted eyelids and bulging eyes.

Parasympathetic Nervous System

The parasympathetic nervous system is composed of cells located in the brain stem and the sacral region of the spinal cord, and for this reason, it has been referred to as the craniosacral system. The cranial preganglionic neurons project to the cranial nerves with autonomic activity: III, VII, IX, and X. Unlike the sympathetic nervous system, the parasympathetic postganglionic neurons are located near to end-organ systems, resulting in long preganglionic axons and relatively short postganglionic axons.[1]

The brain stem nuclei involved in cranial nerve (CN) parasympathetic innervation include the following: (1) CN III: Preganglionic neurons from the Edinger-Westphal nucleus extend down the oculomotor nerve and synapse at the orbital ciliary ganglion, where postganglionic neurons extend to the ciliary muscles and iris, resulting in accommodation and pupillary constriction. (2) CN VII: Pontine preganglionic fibers from the superior salivatory nucleus extend down the facial nerve to the pterygopalatine ganglion, with postganglionic fibers extending to the lacrimal gland (tear production) and the cranial vasculature (resulting in vasodilation). Pontine preganglionic fibers also extend to the submandibular ganglion, with postganglionic fibers continuing on to the salivary glands (resulting in salivation).

61

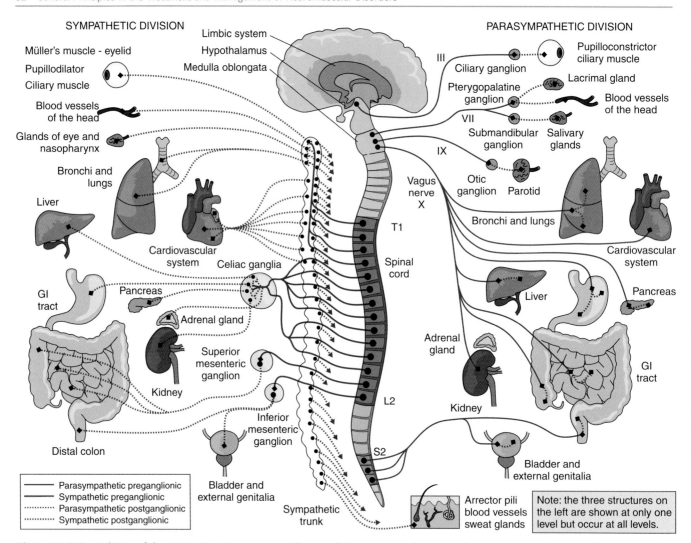

Figure 5-1 Major pathways of the autonomic nervous system, with sympathetic innervation shown in *red* and parasympathetic innervation shown in *blue*. Preganglionic fibers are shown as *solid lines*, and postganglionic fibers are represented by *dotted lines*. GI, gastrointestinal.

(3) CN IX: Medullary preganglionic fibers from the inferior salivatory nucleus extend down the glossopharyngeal nerve to the otic ganglion, where postganglionic fibers continue on to the parotid gland (resulting in salivation). (4) CN X: By far the largest parasympathetic output, the preganglionic fibers from the dorsal motor nucleus of the vagus and the ventrolateral portion of the nucleus ambiguus, extend down the vagus nerve to various ganglia. The fibers extending from the dorsal motor nucleus of the vagus provide input to the gastrointestinal tract (enteric system, described in more detail later), the respiratory tract, and some cardiac input, whereas fibers extending from the nucleus ambiguus extend primarily to the heart. The primary response to vagal activation is cardiac inhibition, visceromotor activation, and salivation.[1]

Sacral parasympathetic output begins in the lateral gray matter of segments S2–S3, with preganglionic fibers extending down the ventral roots to the splanchnic nerves. The parasympathetic fibers extend to the colon, bladder, and sexual organs. The Onuf nucleus innervates the rectal and urethral sphincters and the pelvic floor. Selective denervation of the Onuf nucleus in Parkinson disease enables differentiation (in some cases) from multiple system atrophy.[2]

The overall effect achieved with activation of the sacral parasympathetic system results is urination (relaxation of the bladder sphincter with simultaneous contraction of the detrusor muscle to facilitate micturition), defecation (relaxation of the rectal sphincter with increased peristalsis), and penile erection (ejaculation is mediated via sympathetic innervation). Unlike the sympathetic nervous system, the parasympathetic nervous system uses acetylcholine for both pre- and postganglionic neural transmission.

Enteric Nervous System

Although it was historically subsumed under the auspices of the parasympathetic nervous system, recent evidence suggests that the enteric nervous system is a discrete component of the autonomic nervous system. The enteric system is made up of two interconnected ganglia influenced by both sympathetic and parasympathetic pathways. The first ganglia are located between the longitudinal and circular muscle layers of the gastrointestinal tract, known as the myenteric or Auerbach plexus, and project to both external and internal muscle layers. The second ganglia are located in the submucosal layer, known as the submucosal or Meissner plexus, and project to the mucosal layer. Neurons from both the myenteric plexus and the submucosal plexus innervate nearby tissue as well as anteriorly and posteriorly along adjacent regions of the gastrointestinal tract. The enteric nervous system controls peristalsis, secretion, and absorption along the gastrointestinal tract.[1]

Evaluation of the Autonomic Nervous System

A number of testing techniques are available for clinical evaluation of the autonomic nervous system; far more are used for research investigation. This chapter describes the most commonly used clinical tests, but does not provide a comprehensive review. For additional details on evaluation of the autonomic nervous system, more comprehensive references are suggested.[3,4] The overall utility of autonomic testing has recently been reviewed and given a level B recommendation (probably effective) by an expert panel for the evaluation of autonomic neuropathy and a level C recommendation (possibly effective) in the evaluation of distal small fiber neuropathy.[5,6]

Indications for Autonomic Testing

Autonomic testing provides functional information on the parasympathetic, sympathetic adrenergic, and sympathetic cholinergic systems. Any patient presenting with suspected dysfunction of the autonomic nervous system resulting in orthostatic hypotension, syncope, postural tachycardia syndrome, peripheral neuropathy, or thermoregulatory abnormalities is a candidate for tests of autonomic function. Other common symptoms that suggest autonomic dysfunction include postural dizziness, visual graying in the upright position, impaired cognition, "coat hanger headache," lightheadedness, platypnea (shortness of breath in the upright position), weakness, and lethargy.[7]

Preparation for Autonomic Testing

Adequate preparation for autonomic testing is critical to obtain reliable and reproducible results. All medications that affect autonomic function should be discontinued for five half-lives before testing, if clinically appropriate, with guidance from the patient's treating physician as necessary. All patients referred for autonomic evaluation should avoid caffeine and nicotine on the day of testing. Food intake should be kept to a minimum, with no food 3 hours before testing.

Medications that commonly interfere with testing include anticholinergics (antihistamines, antidepressants, decongestants), antihypertensives, volume expanders (e.g., fludrocortisone), and volume contractors (e.g., diuretics), and should be discontinued for five half-lives, if possible. Analgesics (opioids or over-the-counter) and items that cause structural changes to blood flow (e.g., compression stockings or corsets) should be avoided the day of testing.[8]

Tests of Autonomic Function

A number of terms are frequently used when describing symptoms related to autonomic dysfunction, such as *orthostatic hypotension*, *orthostatic intolerance*, and *postural tachycardia*. A brief overview of these terms is provided in Table 5-1.

Hemodynamic Response to Standing

The transition from supine to standing causes hemodynamic stress on the cardiovascular system as approximately 500 to 1000 mL of blood moves from the central to the peripheral vasculature.[9] The immediate response to orthostatic stress occurs in the first 30 seconds, beginning with a rapid decrease in blood pressure and systemic resistance, followed by a rapid increase in peripheral vascular resistance, cardioacceleration, and blood pressure overshoot.[9] These dynamic changes allow two tests of autonomic function to be determined: (1) orthostatic vital signs and (2) the 30:15 ratio.

Table 5-1 Definitions of Frequently Used Terms

Term	Definition
Orthostatic intolerance	Symptoms that develop in the upright position and are relieved by recumbency; no physiologic measurements required
Orthostatic hypotension	Sustained drop in systolic blood pressure of ≥20 mm Hg or diastolic blood pressure of ≥10 mm Hg within 3 minutes of moving from the supine to the standing position or head-up tilt to ≥60 degrees
Postural tachycardia	Sustained increase in pulse of ≥30 beats/min within the first 10 minutes of moving from the supine to the standing position or head-up tilt to ≥60 degrees

To measure orthostatic vital signs, blood pressure and heart rate should be measured in the supine position after an adequate period of recumbency (typically, at least 5 minutes). Patients then move to the standing position, where blood pressure and heart rate are monitored again after 3 minutes. A diagnosis of orthostatic hypotension is made when a decrease in systolic blood pressure of 20 mm Hg or a decrease in diastolic blood pressure of 10 mm Hg occurs from the supine to the standing position.[10] There is a frequent misunderstanding among practitioners that an increase in pulse of 25 points or greater leads to a diagnosis of "orthostatic by pulse." In the appropriate clinical setting, this finding suggests that the patient may be hypovolemic, but there is appropriate tachycardia preventing orthostatic hypotension from occurring. However, in a normovolemic patient, a sustained increase in pulse of 30 points or greater (to a maximum of 120 bpm) from the supine to the standing position within 10 minutes results in a diagnosis of postural tachycardia syndrome.[11]

The 30:15 ratio is a measure of parasympathetic function that occurs when subjects move from the supine to the standing position. The immediate response to orthostatic stress is tachycardia, typically maximal at the 15th heartbeat after standing, followed by bradycardia, most pronounced at the 30th heartbeat after standing. The ratio of the RR interval at beat 30 to the RR interval at beat 15, called the 30:15 ratio, is an index of cardiovagal function (Fig. 5-2).[3]

Tilt-Table Testing

The tilt-table is an important tool in the evaluation of the autonomic nervous system. When a subject is tilted to an angle of 60 to 70 degrees, the orthostatic stress that occurs is similar to that of standing, but the muscles of the legs are relaxed. The "muscle pump" effect that occurs with the legs during standing is a powerful counter-maneuver to prevent orthostatic hypotension.[12]

Testing requires a period of recumbency, typically 20 minutes, followed by a gradual rise to a head-up tilt angle of 60 to 70 degrees. Testing for many laboratories extends to 45 minutes for adequate assessment of autonomic function.[8] Testing combines the use of oscillometric blood pressure recording at regular intervals and noninvasive beat-to-beat blood pressure recordings.[3] A diagnosis of orthostatic hypotension is made when a sustained decrease in systolic blood pressure of 20 mm Hg or a decrease in diastolic blood pressure of 10 mm Hg occurs from the supine to the upright position within the first 3 minutes of head-up tilt.[10] Decreases in blood pressure after 3 minutes have been described as delayed orthostatic hypotension.[13] A sustained increase in pulse of 30 points or greater (to a maximum of 120 bpm) from the supine to the standing position within 10 minutes, in a normovolemic patient, results in a diagnosis of postural tachycardia syndrome.[14]

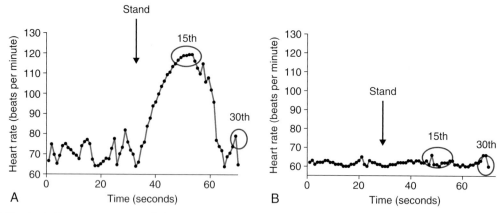

Figure 5-2 The 30:15 ratio. **A,** The patient moves rapidly from a supine to a standing position, causing initial tachycardia at approximately the 15th heartbeat, followed by bradycardia at approximately the 30th heartbeat. The RR interval at the 30th heartbeat is 0.89 seconds, and at the 15th beat it is 0.5 seconds, leading to a 30:15 ratio of 1.78. **B,** The same test is performed in a patient with severe diabetic autonomic neuropathy. There is no noticeable change in heart rate on standing, and the 30:15 ratio approaches 1.

Heart Rate Response to Deep Breathing

The heart rate varies during inspiration and expiration and has been described as the sinus arrhythmia. The maximal heart rate variation with respiration occurs at a breathing rate of 5 to 10 breaths/min. Patients are provided with a visual or auditory cue to regulate their breathing in combination with continuous electrocardiographic monitoring. Approximately 1 minute of respiration is recorded, and the average variation between the maximal and minimal heart rates is described (Fig. 5-3). This test provides a measure of parasympathetic function, and can be compared with age- and sex-matched normative values.[15]

Valsalva Maneuver

The Valsalva maneuver is a relatively simple test to perform, but it results in rapid and complex hemodynamic shifts that require continuous electrocardiographic and beat-to-beat blood pressure recordings to measure. The subject, in a supine position, blows into a tube with a pressure of approximately 40 mm Hg for 15 seconds.[3] The procedure is similar to blowing up a stiff balloon. The breathing tube should have an air leak to prevent glottic closure.

The Valsalva maneuver has four parts, as seen in Figure 5-4. Phase 1 occurs during the onset of exhalation with straining against resistance. The increase in intrathoracic pressure causes compression of the great vessels and an increase in blood pressure. Phase 2 of the Valsalva maneuver begins with decreased venous return (because of increased intrathoracic pressure) and decreased stroke volume, cardiac output, and blood pressure (phase 2 early), followed by sympathetically mediated peripheral vasoconstriction and an increase in blood pressure and heart rate (phase 2 late). Phase 3 occurs with cessation of forced exhalation, resulting in decreased intrathoracic pressure and a transient decrease in blood pressure. Phase 4 may extend for several minutes from the end of phase 3 and leads to an increase in blood pressure over baseline levels secondary to increases in stroke volume and cardiac output with peripheral vasoconstriction.[3]

Isometric Handgrip

The isometric handgrip is routinely used to measure the response to a "pressor" stimulus. Isometric handgrip is a relatively simple test to perform, but the result is a complex compilation of multiple factors,

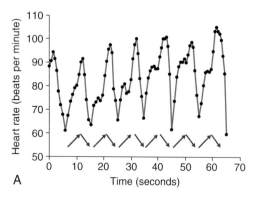

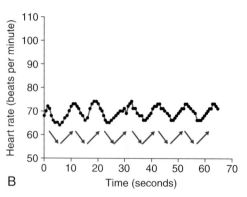

Figure 5-3 Heart rate response to deep breathing. **A,** A healthy subject takes slow, deep breaths (*up arrows* denote inspiration; *down arrows* denote expiration) with auditory or visual cues while the heart rate is monitored. The average variation in heart rate is calculated and can be expressed as the mean difference in heart rate (in this example, an average of 29), or the RR interval ratio between mean minimum and maximum heart rates (in this example, 1.52). This is a normal response. **B,** The heart rate response to deep breathing is seen in a patient with diabetic autonomic neuropathy. The average variation in heart rate is substantially reduced compared with the healthy individual shown in **A.** In this example, the average variation in heart rate is eight beats, with an RR interval ratio of 1.1.

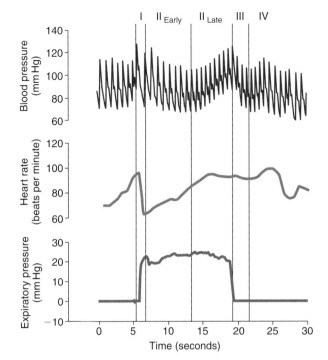

Figure 5-4 Valsalva maneuver. The patient exhales forcefully for 15 seconds. Expiratory pressure is shown at the bottom of the graph. The heart rate response is shown in the middle of the graph, whereas the beat-to-beat blood pressure response is shown at the top of the figure. The four phases of the Valsalva maneuver are as follows. Phase 1 occurs during the onset of exhalation with straining against resistance. The increase in intrathoracic pressure causes compression of the great vessels (with a transient increase in venous flow to the heart) and an increase in blood pressure. Phase 2 begins with decreased venous return (because of increased intrathoracic pressure compressing the great vessels and reducing venous flow) and decreased stroke volume, cardiac output, and blood pressure (phase 2 early), followed by sympathetically mediated peripheral vasoconstriction and an increase in blood pressure and heart rate (phase 2 late). Phase 3 occurs with cessation of forced exhalation, resulting in decreased intrathoracic pressure and a transient decrease in blood pressure. Phase 4 may extend for several minutes from the end of phase 3 and leads to an increase in blood pressure over baseline levels secondary to increases in stroke volume and cardiac output with peripheral vasoconstriction.

including sympathetic and parasympathetic output, baroreceptor function, norepinephrine reuptake, and central command. The subject is asked to provide a maximal voluntary contraction on a hand-grip dynamometer as a baseline. The test itself is conducted by monitoring blood pressure continuously in the nontested arm while the subject contracts to 30% of the maximal effort for 3 minutes. The blood pressure and heart rate responses have a moderate level of agreement with the findings of tilt-table testing.[16]

Tests of Sympathetic Cholinergic Function

Sympathetic Skin Response

The sympathetic skin response detects electrical potential changes between the dorsal and ventral surfaces of the hands and feet. A stimulus, such as an inspiratory gasp or electric shock, results in electrical potential changes to the palms of the hands and soles of the feet. This test can be easily performed with any electromyogram or evoked potential device. A typical example in a healthy individual and a patient with neuropathy is shown in Figure 5-5. The sympathetic skin response is a surrogate measure of sudomotor function, but does not actually measure sweat production. Attempts to correlate response amplitude and latency with disease severity have met with mixed results.[17] The absence of a sympathetic skin response is usually considered abnormal, although age-related changes occur in the lower extremities of individuals older than 50 years.[18]

Thermoregulatory Sweat Testing

The thermoregulatory sweat test detects the host's ability to generate sweat in response to an increase in core temperature. The subject is placed in a chamber, where the external temperature is increased to a degree sufficient to increase the core temperature by 1° to 1.5° C.[19] An indicator dye, typically alizarin red or iodinated corn starch, covers the individual and changes color in the presence of sweat. Photographic mapping of sweat patterns can determine patterns of abnormalities. A normal response is seen with symmetrical sweat production over the entire body (there is individual variation in maximal sweat production), as shown in Figure 5-6. Specific abnormalities can be seen in diseases of both the central nervous system and the peripheral nervous system because the thermoregulatory sweat test measures both the pre- and postganglionic response to an increase in core temperature. An abnormal response may suggest a specific diagnosis through a distribution of sweat loss, but cannot differentiate a preganglionic lesion from a postganglionic lesion.[19]

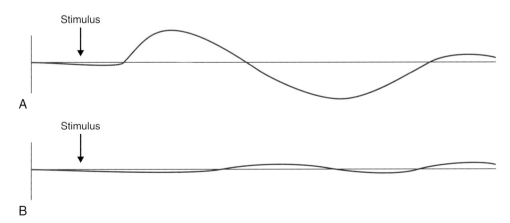

Figure 5-5 Sympathetic skin response. **A,** After a stimulus (a deep breath or an electric shock), a normal sympathetic skin response is shown, with negative and positive deflection noted. The onset latency and magnitude of response can be quantified. **B,** A patient with neuropathy has a much smaller magnitude of response and longer onset latency.

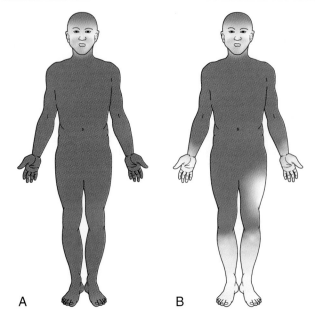

A   B

Figure 5-6 Thermoregulatory sweat testing. Two patients are shown after thermoregulatory sweat testing. The *dark areas* correspond to regions where sweating has occurred. **A,** Normal response. **B,** Loss of sweating in a stocking-glove distribution (length-dependent neuropathy, in this case, secondary to diabetes), with additional loss in the left lateral cutaneous nerve distribution.

Quantitative Sudomotor Axon Reflex Testing
Quantitative sudomotor axon reflex testing provides a measure of postganglionic sweat production. Activation of local sudomotor fibers through iontophoresis of a cholinergic agonist (typically, acetylcholine) results in the direct stimulation of local sweat glands. However, a local axon reflex occurs when an antidromic response is generated, travels to a more proximal nerve branch point, and then travels orthodromically to neighboring sweat glands that were not directly activated by the cholinergic agonist.[3] A small capsule over the skin is used to detect changes in humidity and provide a quantifiable measure of postganglionic sweat production. Well-established normative values have been published, and abnormalities can be seen early in distal small fiber neuropathies of many causes.[20]

Summary of Autonomic Testing

Tests of sympathetic adrenergic, sympathetic cholinergic, and parasympathetic function are shown in Table 5-2. Many tests fall under both sympathetic adrenergic and parasympathetic categories because of their effects on both heart rate and blood pressure. A large number of additional tests can be performed by other subspecialty groups in ophthalmology, gastroenterology, urology, cardiology, and others. For a complete review of available tests, the reader is referred to a number of excellent texts devoted entirely to these topics.[21,22]

One of the challenges inherent to autonomic testing is the differentiation of peripheral and central disorders of autonomic regulation, a problem compounded by the frequently overlapping test results. Most autonomic tests cannot differentiate between peripheral and central causes of autonomic disturbance in isolation; the results are usually combined with a detailed history and examination by a specialist to narrow the differential diagnosis. A few tests are more likely to differentiate central from peripheral autonomic disorders and are described in Table 5-3.

Table 5-2 Autonomic Testing

Sympathetic Adrenergic	Parasympathetic	Sympathetic Cholinergic
Blood pressure response to standing	Heart rate response to standing (30:15 ratio)	Sympathetic skin response
Blood pressure response to tilt-table testing	Heart rate response to tilt-table testing	Thermoregulatory sweat testing
Valsalva maneuver: phase 2 blood pressure recovery and phase 4 overshoot	Valsalva heart rate ratio	Quantitative sudomotor axon reflex testing
Isometric exercise: blood pressure response	Isometric exercise: heart rate response	Silicone impression testing*
Cold pressor test: blood pressure response*	Cold pressor test: heart rate response*	Quantitative direct and indirect axon reflex testing*
Plasma catecholamine levels*	Deep breathing: heart rate response	Acetylcholine sweat-spot testing*

*Tests not described in detail in this chapter. For further information, see Mathias and Bannister[21] and Low.[22]

Table 5-3 Findings Suggestive of Central or Peripheral Autonomic Dysfunction

Test	Central Autonomic Disorder	Peripheral Autonomic Disorder
Plasma catecholamines*	Normal or slightly elevated (150–300 pg/mL plasma norepinephrine)	Low (≤100 pg/mL plasma norepinephrine)
Thermoregulatory sweat test[†]	Abnormal	Abnormal
Quantitative sudomotor axon reflex test[†,‡]	Normal	Abnormal

*A minority (up to 20%) of patients will have plasma catecholamine levels that fall between the two ranges, resulting in diagnostic ambiguity.
[†]Thermoregulatory sweat testing and postganglionic tests of sudomotor function can be combined to identify central or peripheral disorders. If both test results are abnormal, it is a peripheral disorder; if only the result of the thermoregulatory sweat test is abnormal, it is central.
[‡]Any postganglionic test of sudomotor function can be used (quantitative sudomotor axon reflex testing, silicone impressions, acetylcholine sweat-spot testing, or quantitative direct and indirect reflex test of sudomotor function).

Types of Autonomic Neuropathy

Chronic Autonomic Neuropathies

Diabetic Autonomic Neuropathy
Diabetic autonomic neuropathy is the most common form of autonomic neuropathy in the developed world.[23] It is a system-wide disorder, affecting all parts of the autonomic nervous system.[24] The incidence of this form of neuropathy increases with age, with

duration of disease, and with chronic hyperglycemia, and it is almost universally accompanied by features of concomitant distal sensori-motor polyneuropathy.[23] The symptoms of autonomic neuropathy generally occur well after the onset of the endocrinologic manifestations of diabetes mellitus.[24] However, evidence of subclinical autonomic dysfunction may be seen as early as 1 year after initial diagnosis.[24] The prevalence of diabetic autonomic neuropathy is dependent on the criteria used for diagnosis and the population studied.[25] A population-based study in the United States found that symptomatic diabetic autonomic neuropathy affected 5.5% of patients with diabetes mellitus.[26] In a multicenter study in Europe involving nearly 1200 patients, there was evidence of abnormalities in the results of tests of autonomic function in 25.3% of patients with type 1 diabetes mellitus and in 34.3% of patients with type 2 diabetes mellitus.[27]

Autonomic neuropathy is associated with an increase in overall mortality and with a higher likelihood of sudden death, especially when cardiovascular autonomic neuropathy is present.[28] In a prospective study,[29] 56% of patients with diabetic cardiovascular autonomic neuropathy were dead at 5 years, and half of them died unexpectedly and possibly of causes related to underlying dysautonomia.

There are multiple hypotheses as to the pathogenesis of diabetic autonomic neuropathy, and the etiology is likely multifactorial. A metabolic injury to nerve fibers secondary to hyperglycemia, neurovascular insufficiency, autoimmune damage, and a neurohormonal growth factor deficiency are among the processes implicated.[24] As with most neuropathies, diabetic autonomic neuropathy is a length-dependent process and clinical manifestations are first seen in processes affecting longer nerves. Accordingly, the vagus nerve (the longest of the autonomic nerves) is affected early in the disease course. Because this nerve is responsible for approximately 75% of parasympathetic function, symptoms may occur from the beginning and may be widespread.[25] The clinical features of diabetic autonomic neuropathy are reflective of the multiple organ systems that it affects. Accordingly, these are discussed on a system-by-system basis.

Cardiovascular Autonomic Neuropathy in Diabetes

Cardiovascular autonomic neuropathy results from damage to autonomic nerves that innervate the heart and blood vessels, thereby leading to abnormalities in heart rate control and peripheral vascular dynamics.[24] The prevalence is estimated to be approximately 17% of patients with type 1 diabetes mellitus and 22% with type 2 diabetes mellitus.[30] The 5-year mortality rate among diabetic patients with symptomatic cardiovascular autonomic neuropathy is estimated to be five times higher than that of those without cardiovascular autonomic neuropathy.[30] The manifestations of cardiovascular autonomic neuropathy are multiple and reflect both parasympathetic and sympathetic dysfunction.

Exercise intolerance is frequently seen in patients with cardiovascular autonomic neuropathy. Early in the course of the disease, an increase in resting heart rate is often observed as a result of vagal neuropathy and unopposed sympathetic activity and may be the first sign of autonomic neuropathy. As the disease progresses, a fixed heart rate is observed.[29] Eventually, reduced response in heart rate and blood pressure during physical activity leads to decreased cardiac output, reflecting impairment of both parasympathetic and sympathetic responses that typically augment cardiac output during exercise.[24]

Orthostatic hypotension is also a typical feature of cardiovascular autonomic neuropathy and is defined as a decrease in blood pressure of greater than 20 mm Hg systolic or greater than 10 mm Hg diastolic in response to postural change. Orthostatic hypotension occurs secondary to damage to efferent sympathetic vasomotor fibers, predominantly in the splanchnic vasculature, reduced cardiac output, and a reduction in the normal increase in plasma norepinephrine.[31] Patients typically present with symptoms of lightheadedness or presyncope on change of position. Other symptoms may include nonspecific dizziness, weakness, fatigue, visual blurring, and neck pain.[7] Many patients may remain asymptomatic despite significant decreases in blood pressure on change of position.[24]

Other symptoms seen in cardiovascular autonomic neuropathy are intraoperative cardiovascular lability and sudden death, possibly as a result of malignant arrhythmogenesis.[24] In addition, silent myocardial infarction, likely as a result of cardiac denervation, is estimated to occur in approximately one third of patients with diabetes mellitus.[24]

Gastrointestinal Autonomic Neuropathy in Diabetes

Gastrointestinal symptoms are relatively common in patients with diabetes mellitus and are often caused by underlying autonomic neuropathy. The prevalence of gastrointestinal symptoms was reported to be as high as 76% in patients with type 2 diabetes mellitus in one series.[32] Symptoms are reflective of widespread disease and include esophageal dysfunction secondary to vagal neuropathy. This may manifest as heartburn or dysphagia for solids. Gastroparesis diabeticorum is seen in up to 50% of patients with diabetes mellitus. This can produce such symptoms as early satiety, anorexia, postprandial nausea and vomiting, and epigastric discomfort. In addition, delayed gastric emptying interferes with nutrient delivery to the small bowel and can have far-reaching implications.[33] Diarrhea, which is typically nocturnal, watery, and profuse, is frequently seen in those with diabetes. This may alternate with constipation as a result of gut dysmotility, and is estimated to occur in approximately 60% of patients with diabetes.[32] Fecal incontinence may also occur as a result of anal sphincter incompetence or reduced rectal sensation.

Genitourinary Autonomic Neuropathy in Diabetes

Neurogenic bladder is seen in approximately one third to one half of patients with diabetes mellitus. Early on, deafferentation leads to impaired bladder sensation and an increased threshold for initiating the micturition reflex. This leads to an increase in bladder capacity with urinary retention. Later, parasympathetic dysfunction results in reduced detrusor activity with urinary hesitancy and incomplete emptying. This causes further retention and overflow incontinence, as well as predisposing patients to urinary tract infections.[34]

Erectile dysfunction may actually be the earliest sign of diabetic autonomic neuropathy and is seen in 35% to 75% of men with diabetes mellitus.[23] The pathogenesis is likely multifactorial and due to neuropathy (leading to reduced cholinergic activation), vascular, metabolic, endocrinologic, pharmacologic, and psychological factors.[23] In addition to erectile dysfunction, ejaculatory failure and retrograde ejaculation may be seen.[23]

Sudomotor Dysfunction in Diabetes

Sudomotor dysfunction is a common feature of diabetic autonomic neuropathy. It typically manifests first as anhidrosis of the extremities in a stocking-glove distribution, conforming to the length dependency of the neuropathy. This progresses to involve the upper aspects of the limbs, the anterior abdomen, and the top of the head, and may ultimately result in global anhidrosis.[23] Hyperhidrosis of the trunk may be seen early in the disease as a compensatory phenomenon. Gustatory sweating (abnormal production of sweat over the face, head, neck, shoulders, and chest after eating) is also occasionally observed.[19] The gustatory pattern of sweating is believed to occur secondary to cervical sympathetic denervation and aberrant reinnervation.[35]

Other Manifestations of Diabetic Autonomic Neuropathy

Other manifestations of diabetic autonomic neuropathy include reduced or absent pupillary response to light and lacrimal gland dysfunction (resulting in dry eyes). Although impaired awareness of hypoglycemia as a result of blunting of the normal catecholamine surge has long believed to be secondary to autonomic neuropathy in patients with diabetes, the literature on this topic is controversial. Some studies found that peripheral neuropathy was a risk factor for episodes of severe hypoglycemia,[36,37] although others looking specifically at the presence of autonomic neuropathy found that neuropathy produced at best a modest increase in the risk of severe hypoglycemia because of a reduction in counter-regulatory catecholamine responses.[38,39]

Amyloid Autonomic Neuropathy

Overall, amyloidosis is a rare disease.[40] There are multiple forms of amyloidosis, including primary amyloidosis, secondary amyloidosis (caused by an underlying plasma cell dyscrasia or chronic inflammatory condition), and hereditary amyloidosis.[40] Of these, dysautonomia is seen in the primary and hereditary forms.[23] Neuropathy is present in 20% to 50% of patients with amyloidosis. The typical presentation is that of a distal painful small-fiber sensory neuropathy.[41] Autonomic neuropathy is also frequently observed and involves both sympathetic and parasympathetic nerve fibers.[35] Symptoms of autonomic dysfunction typically manifest early in the disease process and may be the presenting symptom in approximately 40% of cases.[40] These include orthostatic hypotension, heart block, anhidrosis, erectile dysfunction, gastroparesis, pupillary abnormalities, constipation, and diarrhea.[41]

The pathogenesis of the neuropathy in amyloidosis involves the deposition of insoluble beta-fibrillar proteins in the epi-, peri-, and endoneurium, as well as in the vasa nervorum, with resultant infiltrative, inflammatory, toxic, or ischemic damage to axons.[23]

Primary amyloidosis is most commonly of the amyloid light chain (AL) type and is a plasma cell dyscrasia whereby monoclonal immunoglobulin light chains are deposited as amyloid.[40] Patients typically present in the sixth or seventh decade. The survival is poor (median range, 13–35 months), despite treatment with prednisone and melphalan.[23]

There are many forms of hereditary amyloidosis, and the most common cause is mutant production of transthyretin protein.[40] Inheritance is autosomal dominant, and the disease usually presents in the third to fifth decade.[35] Autonomic symptoms are usually prominent. Survival is better than in the primary form of amyloidosis, but death generally occurs 5 to 15 years after diagnosis. There are reports of increased survival with orthotopic liver transplantation, although the autonomic symptoms typically do not improve.[23]

Autonomic Neuropathies in Association with Metabolic Disease

Renal Disease

Up to 60% of patients with chronic uremia show evidence of abnormalities on testing of autonomic function.[42] Parasympathetic dysfunction occurs more frequently than sympathetic dysfunction; the exact pathogenesis is unknown but presumably involves damage to axons of autonomic fibers by toxic compounds. Symptomatic autonomic neuropathy appears to be most severe in older patients with concomitant diabetes mellitus. Symptoms include gastrointestinal dysmotility, orthostatic hypotension, and anhidrosis.[42] It has also been hypothesized that dysautonomia contributes to instances of intradialytic hypotension.[41,42]

Hepatic Disease

In one study of patients with hepatic failure, 48% showed evidence of autonomic neuropathy, often subclinical. Most patients with symptoms reported gastrointestinal dysfunction and cardiovascular symptoms. The mechanism of the development of peripheral nerve damage is unclear.[43]

Porphyria

The porphyrias are autosomal dominant disorders of heme biosynthesis. The neuropathic syndrome has an acute to subacute onset, with a predominantly distal motor polyneuropathy. Autonomic symptoms are common in acute intermittent porphyria and reflect sympathetic overactivity as opposed to failure. Symptoms include tachycardia (which may go on to produce malignant cardiac arrhythmias), abdominal pain and cramping, nausea and vomiting, obstipation, bladder dysfunction, and anhidrosis.[44]

Nutritional Deficiencies

Finally, autonomic neuropathy is infrequently seen in patients with nutritional deficiencies, such as vitamin B_{12} deficiency. One study of 21 patients with documented vitamin B_{12} deficiency found abnormalities on testing of sympathetic and parasympathetic function, with patterns similar to those of patients with diabetic autonomic neuropathy.[45] It is unclear how frequently autonomic neuropathy is seen in conjunction with the more typical large-fiber deficits seen in patients with vitamin B_{12} deficiency.

Autonomic neuropathy has been described in two patients with concomitant sensory neuronopathy as a result of pyridoxine (vitamin B_6) intoxication. The autonomic symptoms were primarily of gastrointestinal and genitourinary dysfunction. Although changes in the autonomic ganglia have not been observed in animal models of pyridoxine excess, it has been posited that they are susceptible to damage by very high doses of pyridoxine because they lie outside the blood–brain barrier.[46]

Hereditary Sensory and Autonomic Neuropathies

A group of rare disorders known as hereditary sensory and autonomic neuropathies are characterized by prominent sensory loss and autonomic symptoms with minimal motor involvement. There are currently five types of hereditary sensory and autonomic neuropathy (HSAN), with several subtypes now recognized. HSAN I is the most common form (with subtypes 1A–1D) and has by far the most extensive list of historic names, including hereditary sensory radiculoneuropathy, Thévenard syndrome, familial trophoneurosis, familial syringomyelia, and ulceromutilating neuropathy. HSAN I presents in an autosomal dominant fashion during late childhood or early adolescence.[47] The primary deficit is in small unmyelinated fibers, leading to loss of pain sensitivity, although peroneal motor atrophy and auditory nerve deafness may be seen. HSAN II, or congenital sensory neuropathy, is autosomal recessive and presents in infancy or early childhood with loss of pain sensation. Multiple ulcerations and injuries to joints and extremities are common.[48] HSAN III, familial dysautonomia or Riley-Day syndrome, is an autosomal recessive disorder that presents at birth. In addition to impaired pain sensation, affected individuals have orthostatic hypotension, hypothermia, hypotonia, reduced tearing, and absent corneal reflexes.[48] HSAN IV, or congenital insensitivity to pain with anhidrosis, is an autosomal recessive condition presenting in infancy with hyperthermia, impaired pain sensation, and anhidrosis.[48] HSAN V, or congenital insensitivity to pain with partial anhidrosis, is autosomal recessive and presents in a similar fashion to

Table 5-4 Hereditary Sensory and Autonomic Neuropathies

HSAN Type	Nomenclature	Inheritance	Onset	Chromosomal Locus	Gene
IA	Hereditary sensory neuropathy	AD	Childhood, adolescence	9q22.1	SPTLC1
IB		AD	Childhood, adolescence	3p24–p22	Unknown
IC	CMT 2B, HMSN 2B	AD	Childhood, adolescence	3q21	RAB7A
ID		AD	Childhood, adolescence	Unknown	Unknown
II	Congenital sensory neuropathy	AR	Childhood	12p13.33	Unknown
III	Familial dysautonomia/Riley-Day syndrome	AR	Childhood	9q31	IKBKAP
IV	Congenital insensitivity to pain with anhidrosis	AR	Childhood	1q21–q22	NRTK1
V	Congenital insensitivity to pain with partial anhidrosis	AR	Childhood	1p13.1	NGFβ NTRK1

AD, autosomal dominant; AR, autosomal recessive; CMT, Charcot-Marie-Tooth disease; HMSN, hereditary motor/sensory neuropathy; HSAN, hereditary sensory and autonomic neuropathy.

HSAN IV, with the exception that anhidrosis is not complete.[47,48] A summary of HSAN I to V is shown in Table 5-4. Other inherited causes of autonomic neuropathy include Fabry disease, triple A syndrome, Navajo Indian neuropathy, Tangier disease, and the neuropathy seen in multiple endocrine neoplasia (MEN) type 2B.[23] Multiple endocrine neoplasia (MEN) type 2B consists of pheochromocytoma, medullary thyroid carcinoma, mucocutaneous neuroma, gastrointestinal symptoms (e.g., constipation and flatulence), and muscular hypotonia.

Subacute Autonomic Neuropathies

Paraneoplastic Autonomic Neuropathy

Autonomic neuropathy may occur in association with the development of anti-Hu antibodies in patients with malignancy, most commonly small cell lung cancer, but it is also seen with ovarian and breast cancer, lymphoma, and thymoma. Peripheral neuropathy eventually occurs in 60% to 95% of patients with anti-Hu antibodies.[49] As is the case with a majority of paraneoplastic phenomena, neurologic symptoms typically antedate the diagnosis of malignancy. Although the most common manifestation is subacute sensory neuronopathy with a progressive course,[50] autonomic neuropathy is present in 10% to 30% of patients and may be the presenting symptom in 4% to 9%.[49] The pathogenesis involves autoimmune targeting of postganglionic sympathetic and parasympathetic and myenteric neurons. Accordingly, symptoms include bowel dysmotility (which may be the sole autonomic symptom), orthostatic hypotension, and erectile, bladder, pupillomotor, and sudomotor dysfunction.[23]

Autonomic Neuropathies Associated with Rheumatologic Diseases

Autonomic neuropathy has been best illustrated in patients with Sjögren syndrome, but has also been described in association with rheumatoid arthritis, systemic lupus erythematosus, mixed connective tissue disease, and scleroderma.[41] Various forms of peripheral neuropathy have been seen in association with Sjögren syndrome, and the pathogenesis is unresolved. Autonomic symptoms were seen in a majority of patients with Sjögren syndrome in one study,[51] and a purely autonomic neuropathy was the predominant form in 3 of 92 patients who showed striking involvement of the sympathetic nervous system. In this series, symptoms of autonomic dysfunction included orthostatic hypotension, anhidrosis, evidence of cardiac

sympathetic dysfunction, pupillary abnormalities, diarrhea, constipation, and urinary dysfunction. In the one patient who went to autopsy, pathologic evaluation showed T cell invasion of the sympathetic ganglion cells.[51]

Toxic Autonomic Neuropathies

Autonomic neuropathies have been described with the use of a variety of prescription medications and industrial, organic, and environmental toxins. With regard to medications, chemotherapeutic agents are notable offenders. Cisplatin and other platinum-containing agents usually lead to large-fiber sensory neuropathy, but the development of autonomic neuropathy with prominent orthostatic hypotension and ileus has been described.[52] Vinca alkaloids (e.g., vincristine, vinblastine) characteristically cause motor neuropathy more than sensory neuropathy, but autonomic involvement has been reported.[53] The use of paclitaxel has also been associated with autonomic neuropathy.[54] Long-term use of the antiarrhythmic agent amiodarone may lead to a sensorimotor or motor neuropathy, but autonomic neuropathy has been reported.[55] Arsenic poisoning and thallium poisoning have been associated with autonomic neuropathy. Distal sudomotor dysfunction in combination with painful sensory neuropathy is the characteristic presentation of arsenic intoxication.[56] Hypertension and tachycardia, also in association with painful sensory neuropathy, have been described with thallium intoxication.[57] Exposure to organic solvents, vacor (a rat poison), hexacarbon compounds (inhaled when sniffing glue), acrylamide, and marine toxins (e.g., ciguatoxic fish) may lead to prominent autonomic symptoms, with or without evidence of distal sensory polyneuropathy.[23,58]

Infectious Autonomic Neuropathies

A number of infectious processes are associated with the development of autonomic neuropathy, including HIV/AIDS, leprosy, Chagas disease, and diphtheria.

The severity of autonomic symptoms seems to increase as HIV/AIDS progresses in severity, and these symptoms are usually seen in association with other signs of HIV-related neurologic disease, such as sensory polyneuropathy.[41] Patients with early HIV infection have abnormalities in autonomic testing, but symptoms are more severe in those with AIDS and low CD4 count.[59] The pathogenesis includes direct viral effects on small nerve fibers, but concomitant nutritional deficiencies and medications may have a role. Symptoms reflect both parasympathetic and sympathetic dysfunction and include resting tachycardia, orthostatic hypotension, bowel and bladder dysfunction, impotence, and sweating disturbances.[59]

Leprosy is caused by infection with *Mycobacterium leprae* and is a common cause of autonomic neuropathy in endemic regions. Focal anhidrosis in association with impaired pain and temperature perception is seen in cooler parts of the body and is usually the first sign of disease. This correlates with the loss of cutaneous innervation in these areas.[60] More widespread involvement of the autonomic nerves may occur and lead to orthostatic intolerance, impotence, and gustatory sweating.[61] Chagas disease is caused by infection with *Trypanosoma cruzi* and is found primarily in Central and South America. Autonomic (particularly parasympathetic) dysfunction may be seen in the chronic phase of the disease and manifests as cardiac conduction abnormalities and dysrhythmias, orthostatic intolerance, and bowel dysmotility.[62]

Diphtheria is caused by *Corynebacterium diphtheriae*. A toxin-mediated sensorimotor neuropathy characterized by multiple cranial neuropathies, a descending pattern of weakness, and absent reflexes is typically seen weeks after either pharyngeal or cutaneous diphtheria. Accommodation paralysis with preserved light reflex, cardiac vagal abnormalities, and bowel and bladder dysfunction may also be seen.[63]

Acute Autonomic Neuropathies

Dysautonomia Associated with Guillain-Barré Syndrome

Guillain-Barré syndrome, or acute inflammatory demyelinating polyradiculoneuropathy (AIDP), is an acute monophasic illness associated with sensorimotor neuropathy of variable severity. The sensorimotor symptoms are commonly accompanied by autonomic manifestations. As early as 1892, Osler observed that some patients with "acute febrile neuritis" died of "paralysis of the heart."[64] Some form of dysautonomia is seen in approximately two thirds of cases of AIDP.[65] Rarely, autonomic symptoms are the presenting feature of AIDP. Autonomic symptoms are more prominent in patients with respiratory failure, severe paresis, and the axonal variant of the disease.[66] With the availability of mechanical ventilation, autonomic symptoms are a major cause of mortality in AIDP,[67] which ranges from 3% to 7%.[65]

The clinical manifestations of dysautonomia in AIDP reflect both sympathetic and parasympathetic dysfunction. Cardiovascular abnormalities occur in as many as two thirds of patients with AIDP, although they are mild in most cases.[68] Blood pressure lability (hypertension alternating with hypotension), often in an unpredictable manner, may be observed and is believed to be primarily due to excessive sympathetic outflow.[69] Orthostatic hypotension as a result of sympathetic hypofunction may also be seen, occurring in 19% to 43% of patients.[70] Cardiac arrhythmias are frequently seen and are primarily caused by parasympathetic dysfunction. Vagal neuropathy may lead to the development of ectopic activity in the diseased nerve, manifesting as sudden bradyarrhythmias and even asystole.[67] These arrhythmias may be spontaneous or provoked by suctioning or Valsalva maneuvers. Tachyarrhythmias are also seen as a result of an overall reduction in vagal activity. Sinus tachycardia is the most frequently observed abnormality on cardiac telemetry. If brady- or tachyarrhythmias are problematic, temporary pacemaker insertion may be required.[67] A wide range of abnormalities may be observed on 12-lead electrocardiogram, including atrial fibrillation, atrial flutter, supraventricular tachycardia, ST segment depression, QT interval prolongation, and conduction block.[69]

In addition to cardiovascular abnormalities, other symptoms of dysautonomia are frequently seen in AIDP. Anhidrosis as a result of sympathetic hypofunction is often observed, and hyperhidrosis has been described. Gastrointestinal manifestations are relatively infrequent, but gastroparesis, ileus, and constipation may be seen in a minority of patients.[67,69] Urinary retention is seen in approximately one third of patients. Sexual dysfunction and pupillomotor abnormalities have also been observed.[67]

The management of patients with AIDP should include vigilance and awareness of the possibility of dysautonomia, especially in those with severe weakness. Routine cardiac telemetry and 12-lead electrocardiogram to evaluate for rhythm disturbances or conduction abnormalities should be performed. As discussed earlier, if malignant arrhythmias occur, temporary pacemaker insertion may be needed. In addition, attentive blood pressure monitoring should be performed with the knowledge that lability may occur. Patients with AIDP are usually very sensitive to most vasoactive drugs, and low doses of short-acting agents should be used only if absolutely necessary.[67]

The outcome of AIDP and associated autonomic symptoms is usually good. Typically, the autonomic neuropathy improves in concert with the motor and sensory nerve improvement, and long-term autonomic sequelae are uncommon.[35]

Dysautonomia in Chronic Demyelinating Polyradiculoneuropathy

Although much less common than in AIDP, autonomic dysfunction has also been described in patients with chronic inflammatory demyelinating polyradiculoneuropathy (CIDP). Dysautonomia in CIDP is rare because of the involvement of predominantly large myelinated nerve fibers, and has been attributed by some to concomitant involvement of postganglionic unmyelinated autonomic fibers, perhaps because of an immune-mediated attack on nonmyelin proteins.[71] Several studies have shown, however, that evidence of subclinical sympathetic or parasympathetic dysfunction exists in a minority of patients with CIDP.[72,73]

Dysautonomia in Autoimmune Autonomic Ganglionopathy

A syndrome affecting predominantly autonomic nerves has been referred to as *acute pandysautonomia*, or *autoimmune autonomic neuropathy*. An antecedent (usually viral) illness is followed by subacute onset of autonomic failure. A more chronic form is also seen and is more aptly referred to as autoimmune autonomic ganglionopathy.[74] The disease is secondary to antibodies to the nicotinic acetylcholine receptor of the autonomic ganglia, not the neuromuscular junction, as is seen in myasthenia gravis.[75] Sensory symptoms are reported in some patients, but not motor involvement.

Most commonly, patients present with profound orthostatic hypotension resulting in syncope, anhidrosis, fixed and dilated pupils, urinary retention, and severe constipation.[76] Purely cholinergic and adrenergic forms have been described.[76] In the acute form, some patients improve spontaneously but incompletely.[75] There is no proven treatment, although there are reports of a beneficial effect of intravenous immunoglobulin or plasmapheresis.[77] In the chronic form, these therapies have also been shown to be effective.[78]

Dysautonomia in Diseases of the Neuromuscular Junction

Lambert Eaton Myasthenic Syndrome

Lambert Eaton myasthenic syndrome (LEMS) is an acquired disorder of the neuromuscular junction as a result of antibody-mediated attack against the voltage-gated P/Q-type calcium channel. This syndrome is associated with an underlying malignancy (usually small cell lung cancer) in one half to two thirds of cases. Although proximal weakness, particularly in the lower extremities, is the most common presenting symptom, autonomic complaints are frequent. It has been estimated that 74% to 93% of patients with LEMS have some evidence of dysautonomia.[41,79] Although it is mild in most cases, autonomic dysfunction is severe in approximately 20% of cases, typically older patients with an underlying malignancy.[79] Autonomic symptoms reflect cholinergic dysfunction in LEMS. These include xerostomia (the most common symptom), blurred vision, pupillomotor dysfunction, impaired sweating, erectile dysfunction, constipation, and much less commonly, orthostatic hypotension.[41] The mechanism of autonomic dysfunction is believed to be secondary to a cross-reaction of the pathogenic antibody against N-type calcium channels in autonomic ganglia, which have approximately 60% homology with the P/Q type of channel.[79] As with all paraneoplastic diseases, treatment is directed against the underlying malignancy. There are reports, however, that treatment with 3,4-diaminopyridine leads to symptomatic improvement in the autonomic features of LEMS.[41]

Dysautonomia in Myasthenia Gravis

Autonomic dysfunction in association with myasthenia gravis is rare, with only 12 cases reported in the literature.[80] All patients were found to have thymomas and all were acetylcholine receptor antibody positive. These patients experienced subacute onset of symptoms ranging from isolated gastrointestinal dysmotility (the most commonly observed symptom) to severe panautonomic failure, including cardiovascular dysfunction.[80] Symptoms improved with acetylcholinesterase inhibitors in a majority of patients, supporting the concept of impaired cholinergic transmission as the underlying mechanism of dysautonomia.[80]

Botulism

Botulism is another important infectious cause of dysautonomia. Binding of the toxin released by *Clostridium botulinum* to the presynaptic nerve terminal prevents release of synaptic vesicles at the neuromuscular junction. This leads to the acute onset of ptosis, extraocular muscle weakness, and diplopia, dysphagia, and bulbar dysfunction, followed by progressive generalized limb weakness in a characteristically descending pattern. Autonomic symptoms reflect acute, severe cholinergic failure as a result of a similar mechanism of failed synaptic vesicle release in autonomic ganglia. This results in symptoms of blurred vision, xerophthalmia, xerostomia, anhidrosis, constipation, and urinary retention. Orthostatic intolerance has also been described.[81] Examination classically shows mydriasis with poor or absent reactivity to light or accommodation. Autonomic symptoms may rarely occur in the absence of evidence of concomitant neuromuscular disease.[81] In the more typical form of the disease, the autonomic symptoms generally improve in conjunction with other neuromuscular symptoms.

Symptomatic Treatment of Autonomic Disorders

Treatment of Orthostatic Hypotension

Nonpharmacologic Therapies

The mainstay of treatment of orthostatic hypotension is education. Patients need to develop the practical skills that will enable them to function independently in the face of dramatic decreases in blood pressure. Gradual transitions from the supine to the standing position will reduce symptoms of orthostatic intolerance. Maintaining adequate hydration, especially if subjected to unusual heat or humidity, is an absolute requirement. Individuals who enjoy vacationing in warmer climates often experience dramatic worsening of symptoms if intravascular volume is not maintained.

Physical countermaneuvers, such as leg crossing, fist clenching, or squatting can improve venous return and increase cerebral perfusion with a decrease in orthostatic intolerance.[82] The use of thigh-high or waist-high compression stockings, in combination with an abdominal binder, will reduce peripheral venous pooling.[83] Sleeping with the head of the bed elevated activates the renin-angiotensin-aldosterone system, reducing nocturia and improving hydration in the morning.

Additional nonpharmacologic therapies include sodium chloride ingestion. Adequate dietary intake in symptomatic individuals is typically 10 g/day or more, with sodium chloride tablets used as a supplement if necessary.[84] Adequate fluid intake is necessary for sodium chloride to result in an increase in plasma volume. In general, 2 L/day is appropriate for most individuals, although those with greater activity levels or living in warmer environments may require greater daily fluid intake. Caffeinated beverages may augment blood pressure transiently but tend to worsen orthostatic hypotension secondary to the diuretic effect of caffeine, so they should not be counted as part of the total volume of daily fluid intake.

Recent evidence has shown that rapid ingestion of pure water (approximately 500 mL) can result in a transient pressor effect in patients with dysautonomia. Water can increase systolic blood pressure by 30 mm Hg in the upright position for more than 1 hour and will work within 5 minutes.[85] This effect is unique to water, does not appear to work with other ingested liquids, and will not work in individuals without autonomic disturbance.[86] This "water effect" can be used by patients to counterbalance postprandial hypotension or to provide a brief pressor response for a short period of upright activity. A common scenario in which this might be used is while shopping. In this scenario, a patient experiences orthostatic hypotension and is forced to sit down. The patient does not have the necessary medications handy (or does not have time to wait for the medication to take effect) and is unable to walk back to the car. The ingestion of water will take effect quickly and will provide a brief period in which the patient can return to the car or can return home safely.

Finally, many patients with mild orthostatic intolerance have symptoms that worsen to a large degree after medication adjustments. Avoiding the use of the many iatrogenic causes of orthostatic hypotension, such as diuretics, antidepressants, antihypertensives, alpha blockers, and peripheral vasodilators, will frequently improve orthostatic tolerance.[87] The concomitant supine hypertension that is often seen in patients with orthostatic hypotension frequently results in overuse of long-acting antihypertensive medications. Short-acting antihypertensives dosed only at night may decrease supine hypertension without worsening orthostatic hypotension during the day.

Primary Therapy

An overview of pharmacologic therapies for the symptomatic treatment of orthostatic hypotension is shown in Table 5-5.

Fluodrocortisone

Fludrocortisone, a mineralocorticoid, results in modest volume expansion and improvements in orthostatic tolerance and is often considered first-line therapy for the treatment of orthostatic hypotension. Fludrocortisone has demonstrated effectiveness in several observational studies of patients with orthostatic hypotension and in patients with orthostatic intolerance.[88] Fludrocortisone may also enhance the sensitivity of blood vessels to circulating catecholamines.[89] Fludrocortisone is given at 0.1 to 0.5 mg daily;

Table 5-5 Pharmacologic Treatment of Orthostatic Hypotension

Drug	Dose	Side Effects	Monitoring/Special Considerations
Fludrocortisone	0.1–0.4 mg daily	Supine hypertension, peripheral edema, congestive heart failure, hypokalemia	Potassium levels, supine blood pressure
Midodrine hydrochloride	2.5–10 mg qd–tid	Severe supine hypertension, urinary retention, headache	Supine blood pressure
Ephedrine	25–50 mg tid	Supine hypertension, anxiety, restlessness, nervousness, tachycardia	Supine blood pressure
Pseudoephedrine	30–60 mg tid	Supine hypertension, anxiety, restlessness, nervousness, tachycardia	Supine blood pressure
Pyridostigmine	60 mg tid	Cramps, diarrhea, nausea, vomiting, miosis, salivation	Cholinergic overdose
Desmopressin acetate	Nasal spray (5–40 g) qhs Orally (0.1–0.8 mg qhs) Intramuscularly (2–4 g qhs)	Water intoxication, hyponatremia, supine hypertension	Sodium levels, supine blood pressure
Erythropoietin	25–75 units/kg tiw starting, 25 units/kg tiw maintenance	Edema, injection site reactions, headache, supine hypertension, constipation	Complete blood count with platelets and differential, supine blood pressure

however, with a half-life of 36 hours, a clinical effect typically is not seen for several days. Monotherapy is often inadequate for patients with more severe orthostatic hypotension. Supine hypertension is a common and dose-limiting side effect of treatment. Other side effects may include peripheral edema, congestive heart failure, and hypokalemia.[83]

Midodrine Hydrochloride

Midodrine is the only agent approved by the U.S. Food and Drug Administration for the treatment of orthostatic hypotension. Midodrine is an alpha-1 adrenoceptor agonist, resulting in both arterial and venous constriction and an increase in blood pressure. The efficacy of this agent was shown in double-blind placebo-controlled studies.[90,91] The minimum effective dose for symptomatic relief should be used, starting with 2.5 mg and titrating to clinical effect. The medication has a clinical effect within 30 minutes, and lasts for approximately 4 to 6 hours. The medication can be dosed three times daily, but is often written as TID, typically resulting in the last dose at bedtime. Doses should be administered only when patients are required to maintain the upright position. Midodrine given within 6 hours of sleep can result in severe supine hypertension, forced nocturnal diuresis, volume depletion, and more severe orthostatic hypotension in the morning. Doses are typically given at 8 AM, 12 noon, and 4 PM. The maximum recommended dose of 30 mg/day may be exceeded in rare patients with severe orthostatic hypotension. Supine hypertension is common and may require dose reductions in the latter part of the day and sleeping with the head of the bed elevated. Other side effects include piloerection, urinary retention, and headache. Concomitant use of digoxin can lead to bradycardia and atrioventricular block. Monoamine oxidase inhibitors can result in hypertensive crisis.

Ephedrine and Pseudoephedrine

Ephedrine and pseudoephedrine are mixed α-adrenoreceptor agonists that act through direct and indirect mechanisms to release norepinephrine from the postganglionic sympathetic neuron and increase blood pressure.[83,92] Both medications cross the blood–brain barrier, resulting in dose-dependent and dose-limiting side effects of anxiety, restlessness, nervousness, and tachycardia. Pseudoephedrine, a stereoisomer of ephedrine, may have less β-adrenoreceptor agonist activity than ephedrine and fewer central sympathomimetic

effects.[92,93] As with other sympathomimetic agents, these medications should not be given within several hours of bedtime to prevent severe supine hypertension. Typical doses of pseudoephedrine are 30 to 60 mg three times daily, and for ephedrine, 25 to 50 mg three times daily.

Secondary Therapy
Pyridostigmine

Pyridostigmine has improved orthostatic tolerance and blood pressure in patients with orthostatic hypotension in recent studies.[94] The mechanism of action is believed to be augmentation of autonomic ganglionic transmission. Theoretically, pyridostigmine has a lower risk of supine hypertension than sympathomimetic or volume-expanding agents by potentiating ganglionic transmission selectively during orthostatic stress. Typical doses are 60 mg up to three times daily. Cholinergic side effects are common (cramps, diarrhea, nausea, vomiting, increased salivation, and miosis) and may be dose-limiting.

Vasopressin Analogs

Desmopressin acetate is a synthetic analog of the natural pituitary hormone 8-arginine vasopressin, an antidiuretic hormone affecting renal water conservation. The postural release of arginine vasopressin is reduced in some patients with autonomic failure, in part, because of loss of vasopressin neurons in the suprachiasmatic nucleus of the hypothalamus.[95] Desmopressin acetate acts on the V2 receptors in the collecting ducts of the renal tubules, prevents nocturia and weight loss, and reduces the morning postural decrease in blood pressure in patients with autonomic failure when administered at bedtime.[92] Fluid and electrolyte status must be monitored because there is a risk of water intoxication and hyponatremia.[96] Desmopressin acetate can be administered as a nasal spray (5–40 µg), orally (0.1–0.8 mg), or intramuscularly (2–4 µg). A typical oral starting dose is 0.1 to 0.2 mg only at bedtime.

Erythropoietin

Erythropoietin increases standing blood pressure and improves orthostatic tolerance in patients with orthostatic hypotension.[97] This agent corrects the normochromic normocytic anemia that frequently accompanies autonomic failure and diabetic autonomic neuropathy.[97] The mechanism of action for the pressor effect of this agent is unresolved. Possibilities include an increase in red cell mass and central blood volume, alterations in blood viscosity, and direct or indirect neurohumoral effects on the vascular wall. There is also evidence that the effect of erythropoietin is related to vascular tone regulation mediated by the interaction between hemoglobin and the vasodilator nitric oxide.[98] Standard doses are 25 to 75 units/kg three times weekly until a normal hematocrit is achieved. Lower maintenance doses (approximately 25 units/kg three times weekly) should then be used. Iron supplementation is usually required, particularly during the period when the hematocrit is increasing.

Treatment of Genitourinary Disorders

Treatment of Urinary Retention
Although pharmacologic therapy for urinary retention is frequently used, many patients with complete urinary retention require clean intermittent catheterization or chronic indwelling catheterization as the primary treatment. Sacral nerve stimulation has been touted as an effective alternative to catheterization, although most patients must continue to catheterize, albeit at a lower frequency. The long-term safety, efficacy, and tolerability of these devices have not been completely established.[99,100]

Bethanechol
Bethanechol can augment urination in patients with residual bladder activity. For those with complete bladder atony, the medication is unlikely to be effective. Medication doses of 5 to 50 mg four times daily are used to induce urination on a scheduled basis.[101]

Common side effects are anticholinergic and include lightheadedness, diarrhea, abdominal cramps, salivation, and flushing.

Treatment of Erectile Dysfunction
An overview of pharmacologic therapies for the symptomatic treatment of erectile dysfunction is provided in Table 5-6.

Phosphodiesterase Type 5 Inhibitors
Over the last decade, phosphodiesterase type 5 inhibitors (i.e., sildenafil, tadalafil, vardenafil) have dramatically altered the treatment of erectile dysfunction. The mechanism of action is the relaxation of smooth muscle in the corpora cavernosa, resulting in increased penile arterial blood flow and erection. The phosphodiesterase type 5 inhibitors are effective in the treatment of erectile dysfunction as a result of diabetes, postradiation therapy for prostate cancer, spinal cord injury, and multiple sclerosis.[102–104] These medications are contraindicated in patients with active cardiovascular disease, those taking nitrates, and those with uncontrolled hypertension. Additionally, these medications should not be used in patients with autonomic dysfunction and orthostatic hypotension.[105] Doses per use

are as follows: sildenafil, 50 mg with a 4- to 5-hour half-life; tadalafil, 10 mg with a 17- to 18-hour half-life; and vardenafil, 5 to 10 mg with a 4- to 5-hour half-life.

Alprostadil
For those unresponsive to oral phosphodiesterase type 5 inhibitors, alprostadil is a naturally occurring form of prostaglandin E_1 used in an intracavernous injection for the treatment of erectile dysfunction. The mechanism of action is relaxation of smooth muscle in the corpora cavernosa and resulting erection. Although it is effective in up to 80% of patients, it is rarely used because of the route of administration.[106]

Treatment of Gastrointestinal Disorders

Patients with dysautonomia may experience gastrointestinal disorders that include esophageal dysmotility, delayed gastric emptying, gastroparesis, constipation, diarrhea, and incontinence.

Treatment of Gastroparesis
Nonpharmacologic therapies are used in the management of gastroparesis, including eating smaller, more frequent meals. In addition, diet modification may provide some relief. More invasive nonpharmacologic therapies have been suggested, and a number of small case reports have touted gastric pacemakers as effective treatments for gastroparesis. However, attempts to rigorously evaluate the value of these treatments have not been as successful.[107] Until controlled trials provide hard data, this treatment should be considered experimental. An overview of pharmacologic therapies for the symptomatic treatment of gastroparesis is provided in Table 5-7.

Metoclopramide
Metoclopramide improves the symptoms of gastroparesis through a number of different mechanisms. It reduces nausea by acting on serotonergic 5-HT3 receptors, increases gastrointestinal motility by facilitating acetylcholine release, and improves gastric emptying through an antidopaminergic effect on the fundus.[108] Typical doses are 5 to 10 mg one half hour before meals, with additional dosing at bedtime. Although it is highly effective, there are concerns about tardive dyskinesia, parkinsonism, myelosuppression, and cardiac arrhythmias with use.

Erythromycin
Erythromycin is a motilin receptor agonist (a G-protein-coupled receptor that stimulates contractions of smooth muscle in the gut) and has been used in the treatment of diabetic gastroparesis. The use of erythromycin immediately after meals leads to improved contraction and gastric emptying.[108] Typical doses are 250 to 500 mg

Table 5-6 Pharmacologic Treatment of Erectile Dysfunction

Drug	Dose	Side Effects	Monitoring/Special Considerations
Sildenafil	50 mg	Headache, flushing, dyspepsia, rhinitis	Contraindicated in patients with active cardiovascular disease or severe orthostatic hypotension
Tadalafil	10 mg	Headache, flushing, dyspepsia, rhinitis	Contraindicated in patients with active cardiovascular disease or severe orthostatic hypotension
Vardenafil	5–10 mg	Headache, flushing, dyspepsia, rhinitis	Contraindicated in patients with active cardiovascular disease or severe orthostatic hypotension
Alprostadil	2.5–40.0 μg injection	Pain, headache, hypotension	Contraindicated in patients with severe orthostatic hypotension

Table 5-7 Pharmacologic Treatment of Gastroparesis

Drug	Dose	Side Effects	Monitoring/Special Considerations
Metoclopramide	5–10 mg before meals and at bedtime	Tardive dyskinesia, parkinsonism, myelosuppression, cardiac arrhythmias, drowsiness, fatigue, anxiety, headache, depression	Extrapyramidal side effects, parkinsonism
Erythromycin	250–500 mg after meals	Nausea, vomiting, abdominal pain, diarrhea	Rare QTc prolongation
Domperidone	10 mg before meals	Menstrual irregularities, galactorrhea, breast engorgement	Not available in the United States
Clonidine	0.2–1.0 mg q12h	Confusion, hypotension, dry mouth, hallucinations, somnolence, dizziness	Sudden discontinuation can result in rebound hypertension

given immediately after meals. Side effects include nausea, vomiting, and diarrhea.

Domperidone

Domperidone is a selective antagonist of the dopamine (D2) receptor. It stimulates antral contractions and has promotility activity similar to that of metoclopramide. It does not cross the blood–brain barrier, so it is less likely to cause extrapyramidal side effects. Unfortunately, however, this medication is not available within the United States.[108] Domperidone is also dosed at 10 mg one half hour before meals and at bedtime.

Clonidine

Clonidine is an alpha-2 adrenergic agonist that reduces symptoms related to gastroparesis and dyspepsia by relaxing the fundus.[109] Typical doses of clonidine are 0.2 to 1.0 mg every 12 hours. Side effects may be dose-limiting and include confusion, hypotension, dry mouth, hallucinations, somnolence, and dizziness.

Treatment of Diarrhea

An overview of pharmacologic therapies for the symptomatic treatment of diarrhea is provided in Table 5-8.

Loperamide

Loperamide is U.S. Food and Drug Administration (FDA) approved for the treatment of diarrhea. Loperamide reduces watery stool by altering electrolyte and fluid absorption and inhibiting peristaltic activity.[110] The standard dose is 4 mg for the initial dose, followed by 2 mg after each loose stool (16 mg daily maximum).

Clonidine

Despite its use in gastroparesis, clonidine inhibits intestinal electrolyte secretion and may reduce diarrhea. Typical doses of clonidine are 0.2 to 1.0 mg every 12 hours. Side effects may be dose-limiting and include confusion, hypotension, dry mouth, hallucinations, somnolence, and dizziness.

Diphenoxylate

Diphenoxylate is FDA approved for the treatment of diarrhea. It is a synthetic opiate related to meperidine and is considered a controlled substance, category V.[111] The medication is dosed at 5 mg four times daily until diarrhea is controlled. Side effects include nausea, dizziness, sedation, euphoria, and miosis.

Treatment of Constipation

An overview of pharmacologic therapies for the symptomatic treatment of constipation is shown in Table 5-9.

Docusate Sodium

Docusate sodium is a stool softener often used as the initial treatment for chronic constipation, and it is FDA approved for this purpose. Although only useful as a single agent in mild to moderate constipation, it can be used in conjunction with other agents in cases of refractory constipation.[112] The medication is typically dosed at 100 mg twice daily.

Laxatives

Polyethylene glycol and lactulose are FDA-approved agents for the treatment of constipation. They are osmotic agents that increase

Table 5-8 Pharmacologic Treatment of Diarrhea

Drug	Dose	Side Effects	Monitoring/Special Points
Loperamide	4 mg initial dose, 2 mg after each loose stool (up to 16 mg/day)	Constipation, drowsiness, dizziness, fatigue	Rare reports of anaphylactic reactions
Clonidine	0.2–1.0 mg q12h	Confusion, hypotension, dry mouth, hallucinations, somnolence, dizziness	Sudden discontinuation can result in rebound hypertension; monitor orthostatic hypotension, mental status
Diphenoxylate	5 mg qid until diarrhea is controlled	Nausea, dizziness, sedation, euphoria, miosis	Controlled substance, category V

Table 5-9 Pharmacologic Treatment of Constipation

Drug	Dose	Side Effects	Monitoring/Special Considerations
Docusate sodium	50–200 mg bid	Abnormal taste, diarrhea, nausea, muscle cramps	Rare hepatotoxicity has been noted
Polyethylene glycol	17 g as needed (up to qid)	Diarrhea, flatulence, nausea, abdominal cramping, muscle cramping	Monitor electrolytes with long-term use
Lactulose	20–30 g as needed (up to qid)	Diarrhea, flatulence, nausea, abdominal cramping, muscle cramping	Contains galactose, which may alter blood glucose levels in patients with diabetes; bowel movements may not occur for 24–48 hours; monitor electrolytes with long-term use
Senna	15 mg daily	Nausea, vomiting, diarrhea, abdominal cramps	May discolor feces
Bisacodyl	5–15 mg daily	Electrolyte and fluid imbalance, nausea, rectal burning, vomiting, abdominal cramps	Should be taken with water on an empty stomach

the water content of stool.[113] The standard dose of polyethylene glycol is one heaping spoonful (17 g) and the standard dose of lactulose is two to three spoonfuls (20–30 g) administered as needed (up to four times daily). Osmotic laxatives that contain sodium or magnesium salts should be avoided in patients with chronic constipation because of the risk of electrolyte imbalance.[108]

Stimulant Laxatives

Stimulant laxatives are available both over the counter and by prescription. Many of the side effects and contraindications are similar. Two of the most commonly used are senna and bisacodyl.[113] Senna is an herbal supplement available in liquid or tablet form that causes mild colon-specific stimulation and changes in electrolyte absorption to produce bowel movements in 6 to 12 hours.[113] Bisacodyl is an FDA-approved treatment for chronic constipation. The mechanism of action is likely altered absorption and intestinal fluid accumulation, although it was initially assumed to be direct colonic stimulation.[113] There are concerns that long-term use of any stimulant laxative can result in physical dependence.

Pyridostigmine

In addition to use in orthostatic hypotension, there is limited evidence that pyridostigmine provides relief in patients with chronic constipation secondary to autonomic dysfunction.[114] A pilot study suggested doses of 60 mg three times daily or greater, but additional study is required before clinical conclusions on effectiveness can be made.

References

1. Benarroch EE: The autonomic nervous system: basic anatomy and physiology, *Continuum* 13:13–32, 2007.
2. Palace J, Chandiramani VA, Fowler CJ: Value of sphincter electromyography in the diagnosis of multiple system atrophy, *Muscle Nerve* 20:1396–1403, 1997.
3. Low PA: Testing the autonomic nervous system, *Semin Neurol* 23:407–421, 2003.
4. Low PA: Pitfalls in autonomic testing. In *Clinical Autonomic Disorders: Evaluation and Management*, Boston, 1993, Little, Brown, pp 355–365.
5. England JD, Gronseth GS, Franklin G, et al: Evaluation of distal symmetric polyneuropathy: the role of autonomic testing, nerve biopsy, and skin biopsy (an evidence-based review), *Muscle Nerve* 39:106–115, 2009.
6. England JD, Gronseth GS, Franklin G, et al: Practice parameter: evaluation of distal symmetric polyneuropathy: role of autonomic testing, nerve biopsy, and skin biopsy (an evidence-based review). Report of the American Academy of Neurology, American Association of Neuromuscular and Electrodiagnostic Medicine, and American Academy of Physical Medicine and Rehabilitation, *Neurology* 72:177–184, 2009.
7. Gibbons CH, Freeman R: Orthostatic dyspnea: a neglected symptom of orthostatic hypotension, *Clin Auton Res* 15:40–44, 2005.
8. Low PA: Laboratory evaluation of autonomic function. In *Clinical Autonomic Disorders: Evaluation and Management*, Philadelphia, 1997, Lippincott-Raven, pp 179–208.
9. Borst C, Van Brederode JF, Wieling W, et al: Mechanisms of initial blood pressure response to postural change, *Clin Sci (Colch)* 67:321–327, 1984.
10. Position paper: Orthostatic hypotension, multiple system atrophy (the Shy Drager syndrome) and pure autonomic failure, *J Auton Nerv Syst* 58:123–124, 1996.
11. Low PA, Schondorf R, Novak V, et al: Postural tachycardia syndrome. In Low PA, editor: *Clinical Autonomic Disorders*, Philadelphia, 1997, Lippincott-Raven, pp 681–697.
12. Gibbons C, Freeman R: The evaluation of small fiber function-autonomic and quantitative sensory testing, *Neuro Clin* 22:683–702, 2004 vii.
13. Gibbons CH, Freeman R: Delayed orthostatic hypotension: a frequent cause of orthostatic intolerance, *Neurology* 67:28–32, 2006.
14. Schondorf R, Low PA: Idiopathic postural orthostatic tachycardia syndrome: an attenuated form of acute pandysautonomia? *Neurology* 43:132–137, 1993.
15. Bennett T, Fentem PH, Fitton D, et al: Assessment of vagal control of the heart in diabetes. Measures of R-R interval variation under different conditions, *Br Heart J* 39:25–28, 1977.
16. Khurana RK, Setty A: The value of the isometric hand-grip test—studies in various autonomic disorders, *Clin Auton Res* 6:211–218, 1996.
17. Soliven B, Maselli R, Jaspan J, et al: Sympathetic skin response in diabetic neuropathy, *Muscle Nerve* 10:711–716, 1987.
18. Drory VE, Korczyn AD: Sympathetic skin response: age effect, *Neurology* 43:1818–1820, 1993.
19. Fealey RD, Low PA, Thomas JE: Thermoregulatory sweating abnormalities in diabetes mellitus, *Mayo Clinic Proc* 64:617–628, 1989.
20. Low PA, Caskey PE, Tuck RR, Fealey RD, Dyck PJ: Quantitative sudomotor axon reflex test in normal and neuropathic subjects, *Ann Neurol* 14:573–580, 1983.
21. Mathias CJ, Bannister R: *Autonomic Failure*, Oxford, 1999, Oxford University Press.
22. Low PA: *Clinical Autonomic Disorders: Evaluation and Management*, Philadelphia, 1997, Lippincott-Raven.
23. Freeman R: Autonomic peripheral neuropathy, *Lancet* 365:1259–1270, 2005.
24. Vinik AI, Maser RE, Mitchell BD, Freeman R: Diabetic autonomic neuropathy, *Diabetes Care* 26:1553–1579, 2003.
25. Vinik AI, Freeman R, Erbas T: Diabetic autonomic neuropathy, *Semin Neurol* 23:365–372, 2003.
26. Dyck PJ, Kratz KM, Karnes JL, et al: The prevalence by staged severity of various types of diabetic neuropathy, retinopathy, and nephropathy in a

population-based cohort: the Rochester Diabetic Neuropathy Study, [published erratum appears in *Neurology* 1993 Nov;43(11):2345]. *Neurology* 43:817–824, 1993.

27. Ziegler D, Gries FA, Spuler M, Lessmann F: The epidemiology of diabetic neuropathy. Diabetic Cardiovascular Autonomic Neuropathy Multicenter Study Group, *J Diabetes Complications* 6:49–57, 1992.

28. Maser RE, Mitchell BD, Vinik AI, Freeman R: The association between cardiovascular autonomic neuropathy and mortality in individuals with diabetes: a meta-analysis, *Diabetes Care* 26:1895–1901, 2003.

29. Ewing DJ, Campbell IW, Clarke BF: Heart rate changes in diabetes mellitus, *Lancet* 1:183–186, 1981.

30. Ziegler D, Gries FA, Muhlen H, et al: Prevalence and clinical correlates of cardiovascular autonomic and peripheral diabetic neuropathy in patients attending diabetes centers. The Diacan Multicenter Study Group, *Diabete Metab* 19(Pt 2):143–151, 1993.

31. Low PA, Walsh JC, Huang CY, McLeod JG: The sympathetic nervous system in diabetic neuropathy. A clinical and pathological study, *Brain* 98:341–356, 1975.

32. Maleki D, Locke GR III, Camilleri M, et al: Gastrointestinal tract symptoms among persons with diabetes mellitus in the community, *Arch Intern Med* 160:2808–2816, 2000.

33. Kong MF, Horowitz M, Jones KL, et al: Natural history of diabetic gastroparesis, *Diabetes Care* 22:503–507, 1999.

34. Ellenberg M: Development of urinary bladder dysfunction in diabetes mellitus, *Ann Intern Med* 92:321–323, 1980.

35. Low PA, Vernino S, Suarez G: Autonomic dysfunction in peripheral nerve disease, *Muscle Nerve* 27:646–661, 2003.

36. Akram K, Pedersen-Bjergaard U, Borch-Johnsen K, Thorsteinsson B: Frequency and risk factors of severe hypoglycemia in insulin-treated type 2 diabetes: a literature survey, *J Diabetes Complications* 20:402–408, 2006.

37. Pedersen-Bjergaard U, Pramming S, Heller SR, et al: Severe hypoglycaemia in 1076 adult patients with type 1 diabetes: influence of risk markers and selection, *Diabetes Metab Res Rev* 20:479–486, 2004.

38. Stephenson JM, Kempler P, Perin PC, Fuller JH: Is autonomic neuropathy a risk factor for severe hypoglycaemia? The EURODIAB IDDM Complications Study, *Diabetologia* 39:1372–1376, 1996.

39. Meyer C, Grossmann R, Mitrakou A, et al: Effects of autonomic neuropathy on counterregulation and awareness of hypoglycemia in type 1 diabetic patients, *Diabetes Care* 21:1960–1966, 1998.

40. Falk RH, Comenzo RL, Skinner M: The systemic amyloidoses, *N Engl J Med* 337:898–909, 1997.

41. Toth C, Zochodne DW: Other autonomic neuropathies, *Semin Neurol* 23:373–380, 2003.

42. Vita G, Messina C, Savica V, Bellinghieri G: Uraemic autonomic neuropathy, *J Auton Nerv Syst* 30(Suppl):S179–S184, 1990.

43. Chaudhry V, Corse AM, O'Brian R, et al: Autonomic and peripheral (sensorimotor) neuropathy in chronic liver disease: a clinical and electrophysiologic study, *Hepatology* 29:1698–1703, 1999.

44. Sack GH: Acute intermittent porphyria, *JAMA* 264:1290–1293, 1990.

45. Beitzke M, Pfister P, Fortin J, Skrabal F: Autonomic dysfunction and hemodynamics in vitamin B$_{12}$ deficiency, *Auton Neurosci* 97:45–54, 2002.

46. Albin RL, Albers JW, Greenberg HS, et al: Acute sensory neuropathy-neuronopathy from pyridoxine overdose, *Neurology* 37:1729–1732, 1987.

47. Axelrod FB, Chelimsky GG, Weese-Mayer DE: Pediatric autonomic disorders, *Pediatrics* 118:309–321, 2006.

48. Axelrod FB, Gold-von Simson G: Hereditary sensory and autonomic neuropathies: types II, III, and IV, *Orphanet J Rare Dis* 2:39, 2007.

49. Dalmau J, Graus F, Rosenblum MK, Posner JB: Anti-Hu–associated paraneoplastic encephalomyelitis/sensory neuronopathy. A clinical study of 71 patients, *Medicine* 71:59–72, 1992.

50. Lucchinetti CF, Kimmel DW, Lennon VA: Paraneoplastic and oncologic profiles of patients seropositive for type 1 antineuronal nuclear autoantibodies, *Neurology* 50:652–657, 1998.

51. Mori K, Iijima M, Koike H, et al: The wide spectrum of clinical manifestations in Sjögren's syndrome-associated neuropathy, *Brain* 128:2518–2534, 2005.

52. Rosenfeld CS, Broder LE: Cisplatin-induced autonomic neuropathy, *Cancer Treat Rep* 68:659–660, 1984.

53. Legha SS: Vincristine neurotoxicity. Pathophysiology and management, *Med Toxicol* 1:421–427, 1986.

54. Jerian SM, Sarosy GA, Link CJ Jr, et al: Incapacitating autonomic neuropathy precipitated by taxol, *Gynecol Oncol* 51:277–280, 1993.

55. Manolis AS, Tordjman T, Mack KD, Estes NA: A typical pulmonary and neurologic complications of amiodarone in the same patient. Report of a case and review of the literature, *Arch Intern Med* 147:1805–1809, 1987.

56. LeQuesne PM, McLeod JG: Peripheral neuropathy following a single exposure to arsenic, *J Neurol Sci* 32:437–451, 1977.

57. Bank WJ, Pleasure DE, Suzuki K, et al: Thallium poisoning, *Arch Neurol* 26:456–464, 1972.

58. Matikainen E, Juntunen J: Autonomic nervous system dysfunction in workers exposed to organic solvents, *J Neurol Neurosurg Psychiatry* 48:1021–1024, 1985.

59. Freeman R, Roberts MS, Friedman LS, Broadbridge C: Autonomic function and human immunodeficiency virus infection, *Neurology* 40:575–580, 1990.

60. Facer P, Mathur R, Pandya SS, et al: Correlation of quantitative tests of nerve and target organ dysfunction with skin immunohistology in leprosy, *Brain* 121(Pt 12):2239–2247, 1998.

61. Freeman R: Autonomic peripheral neuropathy, *Lancet* 365:1259–1270, 2005.

62. Iosa D, Dequattro V, De-Ping Lee D, et al: Pathogenesis of cardiac neuromyopathy in Chagas' disease and the role of the autonomic nervous system, *J Auton Nerv Syst* 30:S83–S87, 1990.

63. Idiaquez J: Autonomic dysfunction in diphtheritic neuropathy, *J Neurol Neurosurg Psychiatry* 55:159–161, 1992.

64. Osler W: *Principles and Practice of Medicine*, New York, 1892, Appleton.

65. Hughes RA, Cornblath DR: Guillain-Barré syndrome, *Lancet* 366: 1653–1666, 2005.

66. Winer JB, Hughes RAC: Identification of patients at risk of arrhythmia in the Guillain-Barré syndrome, *Q J Med* 257:735–739, 1988.

67. Zochodne DW: Autonomic involvement in Guillain-Barré syndrome: a review, *Muscle Nerve* 17:1145–1155, 1994.

68. Ropper AH, Wijdicks EFM, Truax BT: *Guillain Barré Syndrome*, Philadelphia, 1991, F.A. Davis.

69. Asahina M, Kuwabara S, Suzuki A, Hattori T: Autonomic function in demyelinating and axonal subtypes of Guillain-Barré syndrome, *Acta Neurol Scand* 105:44–50, 2002.

70. Singh NK, Jaiswal AK, Misra S, Srivastava PK: Assessment of autonomic dysfunction in Guillain-Barré syndrome and its prognostic implications, *Acta Neurol Scand* 75:101–105, 1987.

71. Yamamoto K, Watarai M, Hashimoto T, Ikeda S: Chronic inflammatory demyelinating polyradiculoneuropathy with autonomic involvement, *Muscle Nerve* 31:108–112, 2005.

72. Lyu RK, Tang LM, Wu YR, Chen ST: Cardiovascular autonomic function and sympathetic skin response in chronic inflammatory demyelinating polyradiculoneuropathy, *Muscle Nerve* 26:669–672, 2002.

73. Misra UK, Kalita J, Yadav RK: A comparison of clinically atypical with typical chronic inflammatory demyelinating polyradiculoneuropathy, *Eur Neurol* 58:100–105, 2007.

74. Klein CM, Vernino S, Lennon VA, et al: The spectrum of autoimmune autonomic neuropathies, *Ann Neurol* 53:752–758, 2003.

75. Vernino S, Low PA, Fealey RD, et al: Autoantibodies to ganglionic acetylcholine receptors in autoimmune autonomic neuropathies, *N Engl J Med* 343:847–855, 2000.

76. Sandroni P, Vernino S, Klein CM, et al: Idiopathic autonomic neuropathy: comparison of cases seropositive and seronegative for ganglionic acetylcholine receptor antibody, *Arch Neurol* 61:44–48, 2004.

77. Schroeder C, Vernino S, Birkenfeld AL, et al: Plasma exchange for primary autoimmune autonomic failure, *N Engl J Med* 353:1585–1590, 2005.

78. Gibbons CH, Vernino SA, Freeman R: Combined immunomodulatory therapy in autoimmune autonomic ganglionopathy, *Arch Neurol* 65: 213–217, 2008.

79. O'Suilleabhain P, Low PA, Lennon VA: Autonomic dysfunction in the Lambert-Eaton myasthenic syndrome: serologic and clinical correlates, *Neurology* 50:88–93, 1998.

80. Vernino S, Cheshire WP, Lennon VA: Myasthenia gravis with autoimmune autonomic neuropathy, *Auton Neurosci* 88:187–192, 2001.

81. Merz B, Bigalke H, Stoll G, Naumann M: Botulism type B presenting as pure autonomic dysfunction, *Clin Auton Res* 13:337–338, 2003.

82. Wieling W, van Lieshout JJ, van Leeuwen AM: Physical manoeuvres that reduce postural hypotension in autonomic failure, *Clin Auton Res* 3:57–65, 1993.

83. Gibbons CH, Freeman R: Treatment options for autonomic neuropathies, *Curr Treat Options Neurol* 8:119–132, 2006.

84. Freeman R: Current pharmacologic treatment for orthostatic hypotension, *Clin Auton Res* 18(Suppl 1):14–18, 2008.

85. Jordan J, Shannon JR, Black BK, et al: The pressor response to water drinking in humans: a sympathetic reflex? *Circulation* 101:504–509, 2000.

86. Raj SR, Biaggioni I, Black BK, et al: Sodium paradoxically reduces the gastropressor response in patients with orthostatic hypotension, *Hypertension* 48:329–334, 2006.

87. Meredith PA: Is postural hypotension a real problem with antihypertensive medication? *Cardiology* 96(Suppl 1):19–24, 2001.

88. van Lieshout JJ, ten Harkel AD, Wieling W: Fludrocortisone and sleeping in the head-up position limit the postural decrease in cardiac output in autonomic failure, *Clin Auton Res* 10:35–42, 2000.

89. Hickler RB, Thompson GR, Fox LM, Hamlin JT: Successful treatment of orthostatic hypotension with 9-alpha-fluorohydrocortisone, *N Engl J Med* 261:788–791, 1959.

90. Low PA, Gilden JL, Freeman R, et al: Efficacy of midodrine vs placebo in neurogenic orthostatic hypotension. A randomized, doubleblind multicenter study. Midodrine Study Group, *JAMA* 277:1046–1051, 1997.

91. Wright RA, Kaufmann HC, Perera R, et al: A double-blind, dose-response study of midodrine in neurogenic orthostatic hypotension, *Neurology* 51:120–124, 1998.

92. Freeman R: Treatment of orthostatic hypotension, *Semin Neurol* 23:435–442, 2003.

93. Jordan J, Shannon JR, Biaggioni I, et al: Contrasting actions of pressor agents in severe autonomic failure, *Am J Med* 105:116–124, 1998.

94. Singer W, Sandroni P, Opfer-Gehrking TL, et al: Pyridostigmine treatment trial in neurogenic orthostatic hypotension, *Arch Neurol* 63:513–518, 2006.

95. Ozawa T, Oyanagi K, Tanaka H, et al: Suprachiasmatic nucleus in a patient with multiple system atrophy with abnormal circadian rhythm of arginine-vasopressin secretion into plasma, *J Neurol Sci* 154:116–121, 1998.

96. Mathias CJ, Fosbraey P, da Costa DF, et al: The effect of desmopressin on nocturnal polyuria, overnight weight loss, and morning postural hypotension in patients with autonomic failure, *Br Med J Clin Res* 293:353–354, 1986.

97. Hoeldtke RD, Streeten DHP, Streeten DH: Treatment of orthostatic hypotension with erythropoietin, *N Engl J Med* 329:611–615, 1993.

98. Rao SV, Stamler JS: Erythropoietin, anemia, and orthostatic hypotension: the evidence mounts, *Clin Auton Res* 12:141–143, 2002.

99. White WM, Dobmeyer-Dittrich C, Klein FA, Wallace LS: Sacral nerve stimulation for treatment of refractory urinary retention: long-term efficacy and durability, *Urology* 71:71–74, 2008.

100. Datta SN, Chaliha C, Singh A, et al: Sacral neurostimulation for urinary retention: 10-year experience from one UK centre, *BJU Int* 101:192–196, 2008.

101. Apostolidis AN, Fowler CJ: Evaluation and treatment of autonomic disorders of the urogenital system, *Semin Neurol* 23:443–452, 2003.

102. Carson CC, Lue TF: Phosphodiesterase type 5 inhibitors for erectile dysfunction, *BJU Int* 96:257–280, 2005.

103. Boulton AJ, Selam JL, Sweeney M, Ziegler D: Sildenafil citrate for the treatment of erectile dysfunction in men with type II diabetes mellitus, *Diabetologia* 44:1296–1301, 2001.

104. Derry FA, Dinsmore WW, Fraser M, et al: Efficacy and safety of oral sildenafil (Viagra) in men with erectile dysfunction caused by spinal cord injury, *Neurology* 51:1629–1633, 1998.

105. Hussain IF, Brady CM, Swinn MJ, et al: Treatment of erectile dysfunction with sildenafil citrate (Viagra) in parkinsonism due to Parkinson's disease or multiple system atrophy with observations on orthostatic hypotension, *J Neurol Neurosurg Psychiatry* 71:371–374, 2001.

106. Linet OI, Ogrinc FG: Efficacy and safety of intracavernosal alprostadil in men with erectile dysfunction. The Alprostadil Study Group [see comments], *N Engl J Med* 334:873–877, 1996.

107. Frokjaer JB, Ejskjaer N, Rask P, et al: Central neuronal mechanisms of gastric electrical stimulation in diabetic gastroparesis, *Scand J Gastroenterol* 43:1066–1075, 2008.

108. Parkman HP, Hasler WL, Fisher RS: American Gastroenterological Association medical position statement: diagnosis and treatment of gastroparesis, *Gastroenterology* 127:1589–1591, 2004.

109. Thumshirn M, Camilleri M, Choi MG, Zinsmeister AR: Modulation of gastric sensory and motor functions by nitrergic and alpha2-adrenergic agents in humans, *Gastroenterology* 116:573–585, 1999.

110. Abrahamsson H: Gastrointestinal motility disorders in patients with diabetes mellitus. [Review] [33 refs], *J Intern Med* 237:403–409, 1995.

111. Harford WV, Krejs GJ, Santa Ana CA, Fordtran JS: Acute effect of diphenoxylate with atropine (Lomotil) in patients with chronic diarrhea and fecal incontinence, *Gastroenterology* 78:440–443, 1980.

112. Hurdon V, Viola R, Schroder C: How useful is docusate in patients at risk for constipation? A systematic review of the evidence in the chronically ill, *J Pain Symptom Manage* 19:130–136, 2000.

113. Rao SS: Constipation: evaluation and treatment, *Gastroenterol Clin North Am* 32:659–683, 2003.

114. Bharucha AE, Low PA, Camilleri M, et al: Pilot study of pyridostigmine in constipated patients with autonomic neuropathy, *Clin Auton Res* 18:194–202, 2008.

Daniel L. Menkes, MD

A Practical Approach to the Treatment of Painful Polyneuropathies

The prevalence of neuropathic pain in the U.S. population has not been firmly established. One conservative estimate predicts that between 1% and 2% of the population will eventually experience neuropathic pain (NP).[1] A higher estimate of 7% to 8% of the population, with 5% reporting severe pain, has been reported by other authors.[2,3] Even using the more conservative estimate, more people are afflicted with NP than with multiple sclerosis, myasthenia gravis, and amyotrophic lateral sclerosis combined. Given these statistics, every health care provider must have a working knowledge of the pathophysiology of NP as well as its treatment, supported by evidence-based medicine (EBM). NP and painful polyneuropathies (PPs) are not synonymous; pain management specialists consider NP to result from many types of dysfunction within the sensory nervous system or its central connections. Even if NP were restricted to conditions affecting the peripheral nervous system (PNS), numerous other entities other than polyneuropathy would be included, such as traumatic mononeuropathies, plexopathies, radiculopathies, and even cranial neuropathies, such as trigeminal neuralgia. Many studies that assess the treatment of NP combine one or more of these entities such that an "effective" NP treatment cannot necessarily be extrapolated to the treatment of PPs. Because there are numerous textbooks, book chapters, medical reviews, and editorials on the treatment of NP in general, this topic is not addressed in this chapter. Two related publications summarized the available evidence on topical and oral agents used in the treatment of NP.[4,5] Neither these articles nor this chapter discusses invasive methods to treat NP, such as spinal stimulators, intrathecal delivery systems, or radioablation techniques, because these methods are rarely used in a neuromuscular consultant's practice. Furthermore, this chapter addresses only the treatment of PP in adults, those 18 years and older. As such, these data cannot be used to guide treatment decisions in younger individuals. Medications used in the pediatric population should be adjusted for the patient's age, height, and weight and should be prescribed by pediatric neurologists who specialize in the treatment of PP in children.

This chapter provides a practical approach to the treatment of an adult patient presenting with a PP. It describes the available medical literature and clinical practice experience. Ideally, EBM should guide all treatment decisions, but EBM is only useful when the requisite studies have been conducted in an appropriate manner. Thus, EBM is limited when discussing the management of PP, for numerous reasons. One is that pain management experts tend to subdivide pain based on its presumed mechanism of action. Studies that evaluate "neuropathic pain" can assess a variety of conditions, such as post-herpetic neuralgia (PHN), diabetic peripheral neuropathic pain (DPNP), and even central nervous system (CNS) syndromes, such as post–spinal cord injury pain. Most studies of PP tend to focus on common disorders, such as DPNP, because a sufficient number of patients must be recruited to have an adequately powered study to detect a statistically significant difference. For this reason, there are far more studies on the treatment of DPNP and HIV-related neuropathy than there are of patients with unclassified small fiber neuropathies. Another issue is that older, more established medications, such as tricyclic antidepressants (TCAs) or opioids, were not studied to the same exacting standards as in modern-day trials. Furthermore, there are few head-to-head trials of generic medications versus brand name medications whose patents have not yet expired. Finally, there are few studies that allow for an accurate assessment of the use of combinations of agents versus monotherapy, especially with the newer proprietary drugs.

Previous publications tended to focus on the pharmacologic management of NP without specifically addressing commonly associated comorbid disorders, such as obstructive sleep apnea (OSA), major depression, and fibromyalgia (FM). These comorbid conditions have a significant negative effect on the patient's quality of life (QoL). Because one should always maximize the patient's QoL, it is important to identify and treat these comorbidities. The advantage of such an approach is that medication selection will be based on a "best for all conditions" approach rather than one that is simply focused on the PP. Although many practitioners disagree with this approach, it has proven to be consistent with EBM pain management guidelines and effective in clinical practice. It is important to provide some type of guidance on the treatment of PPs until more EBM is available to modify these recommendations. Finally, although the cranial nerves can be considered part of the PNS, this chapter only discusses the management of PP and does not address the mononeuropathy of trigeminal neuralgia. Those interested in this subject should review the recently published EBM guidelines for the treatment of trigeminal neuralgia.[6]

Table 6-1 Workup for Painful Polyneuropathy

Test	Comments
Routine Testing	
Complete blood count with differential	↑ White blood cell count may indicate infection Eosinophilia may indicate Churg-Strauss syndrome ↑ Mean corpuscular volume may reflect B_{12} deficiency
Electrolyte panel	Abnormalities may indicate renal disease Hyponatremia may also indicate SIADH
Hemoglobin A1C (known diabetic) Fasting blood sugar or glucose tolerance test (status unknown)	Ideal is < 7 in diabetics (<5% in normal subjects) Fasting blood sugar of 100–125 mg/dL = impaired glucose tolerance
Renal function studies (24-hour urine is preferred)	Consider urea clearance with impaired renal function (<50% of predicted)
Liver function studies	SGOT now AST/SGPT now ALT
Serum B_{12} and methylmalonic acid levels	↑ Methylmalonic acid levels may warrant B_{12} treatment even with normal B_{12} level
Folate levels	Rarely observed in isolation
Serum and urine immunoelectrophoresis	Immunoelectrophoresis is more sensitive
Thyroid-stimulating hormone	Complete thyroid panel rarely needed
Anti-nuclear antibody	Titers < 1:160 are nonspecific
Rheumatoid factor	May be first indication of HCV infection
Erythrocyte sedimentation rate ± C-reactive protein	Nonspecific indicators of inflammation
Workup for Painful Polyneuropathy (When Clinical History Warrants)[63,64]	
History of IV drug abuse, "needle-stick" blood transfusion, "unsafe sex"	HBV, HCV, HIV, serum cryoglobulins
Severe gastroenteritis preceding the neuropathy	24-hour urine test for heavy metals
Suspected rheumatologic condition	ACE level, ANCA, ENA, SS-A, SS-B
Suspected inherited neuropathy	DNA analysis
Dysautonomia	Autonomic testing Fat pad or skin biopsy for amyloidosis Transthyretin-related DNA testing in selected patients
Asymmetric polyneuropathy (suspected vasculitis)	Sural nerve ± muscle biopsy

ACE, angiotensin-converting enzyme; ALT, alanine aminotransferase; ANCA, anti-neutrophil cytoplasmic antibody; AST, aspartate aminotransferase; ENA, extractable nuclear antigen; HBV, hepatitis B virus; HCV, hepatitis C virus; SGOT, serum glutamic oxaloacetic transaminase; SGPT, serum glutamic pyruvic transaminase; SS-A, Sjögren syndrome (specific) antibody A (also known as anti-Ro); SS-B, Sjögren syndrome (specific) antibody B (also known as anti-La); SIADH, syndrome of inappropriate antidiuretic hormone.

This chapter reviews the definition of NP and the concept of EBM and discusses some of the potential mechanisms that may be responsible for the pain associated with PP. As with any disorder, the clinician should attempt to identify a potentially reversible cause for the PP (Table 6-1). If no specific etiology is identified, the treating practitioner should improve the patient's QoL by identifying and aggressively treating any comorbid conditions. This chapter discusses only oral and topical medications that have the highest level of EBM that supports their use for the treatment of at least one disease entity that manifests with a PP.

Definitions and Overview

Pain has been defined by the International Association for the Study of Pain as "an unpleasant sensory and emotional experience associated with actual or potential tissue damage, or described in terms of such damage."[7] Restated, pain can occur even in the absence of an actual injury. All that is required to experience pain is for the affected person to believe that such an injury is imminent or has occurred. The International Association for the Study of Pain also

recently updated its definition of NP as indicative of a direct consequence of diseases that affect the somatosensory system.[8] Many pain management experts further subdivide NP into noninflammatory and inflammatory subtypes. Examples of inflammatory NP include herpes zoster neuritis, cancer pain, and complex regional pain syndrome, whereas noninflammatory pain would include conditions, such as trigeminal neuralgia and phantom limb pain. PP cannot be as readily classified because the underlying etiology is not always identified. Even when the underlying cause is identified, pain may occur as a result of both inflammatory and noninflammatory mechanisms (e.g., inflammatory vasculitis with secondary axonal loss from ischemia). This is one of many reasons why the EBM recommendations regarding the treatment of NP in general do not necessarily apply to the treatment of PP.

Previously, acute pain was differentiated from chronic pain by stating that acute pain lasted less than 3 to 6 months.[9] However, this definition has fallen out of favor because of its arbitrary nature and because many patients with acute pain eventually have chronic pain. For these reasons, the American Pain Society revised this definition by stating, "Acute pain follows injury to the body and generally disappears when the bodily injury heals. It is often, but not always, associated with objective physical signs of autonomic nervous system activity. Chronic pain in contrast to acute pain is rarely accompanied by signs of sympathetic nervous system arousal."[10]

Turk and Okifuji proposed a different definition of pain that integrates its duration and perceived physical intensity.[11] They describe NP in terms of a "strength–duration curve" in which pain intensity is reported as severe over a relatively short period, whereas chronic pain tends to be reported as less severe but more persistent. From this perspective, they define acute pain as pain elicited by the injury of bodily tissues and activation of nociceptive transducers at the site of local tissue injury. They also opine that the nociceptive transmission may be altered through central processing and that coexistent autonomic phenomena are often observed. In contrast, chronic pain is usually elicited by an injury but may be augmented by other factors that are not necessarily related to the precipitating cause. Turk and Okifuji remarked, "Chronic pain extends for a long period of time, represents low levels of underlying pathology that does not explain the presence and extent of the pain, or both."[11] They also wrote that acute pain often responds to treatment, whereas chronic pain is "rarely effectively treated." Turk and Okifuji concluded that "cure" may be a reasonable goal for acute pain processes, whereas "management" would be more appropriate in patients with chronic pain.[11]

The division between acute and chronic pain should not lead to the misconception that one cannot transform into the other. One prospective study from New Zealand reported that acute NP accounted for 1% to 3% of consults on an acute pain service.[12] The same study reported that 78% of patients had persistent pain after 6 months and that 56% still had pain after 1 year. Thus, failure to treat acute NP may lead to chronic NP, implying that early intervention is the best course of action. Therefore, it is recommended that NP be treated as early and comprehensively as possible because a "wait and see" attitude is less likely to be effective than one in which the underlying disorder is treated in short order. Dworkin et al advised that moderate to severe pain must be treated quickly and aggressively in an attempt to reduce the probability that a chronic pain syndrome will result.[4] Although early and aggressive intervention in a patient with an acute pain process may not result in a "cure," it may mitigate the severity of the chronic pain syndrome. Patients with chronic pain syndromes rarely experience complete relief and may require long-term opioid medication, a course of action that should be viewed as a double-edged sword for reasons that are discussed later.

Nerve Anatomy

A simplified view of the peripheral nerve is to subdivide it into its three main structural components: Schwann cells with the myelin sheath that they produce, the vasa nervorum, and the axons. The axons are further classified as afferent or efferent fibers. The afferent, or sensory, fibers can be further subdivided into large, heavily myelinated fibers (Aβ), thinly myelinated fibers (Aδ), and unmyelinated fibers (C fibers). Most sensory fibers within a sensory nerve are the "small fibers" that are either thinly myelinated or unmyelinated. Further, these small fibers tend to be clustered toward the center of the nerve. The blood vessels to the nerves (vasa nervorum) do not penetrate the nerve itself, but stop at the epineurium so that the axons receive their nutrients and eliminate their wastes through diffusion. For this reason, the large, heavily myelinated axons at the edge of the nerve are at less risk from hypoxic-ischemic issues than are the small fibers that tend to be clustered in the center of the nerve.

The myelinated fibers have an additional advantage in that the myelin sheath acts as an electrical insulator such that the electrical impulse along these nerve fibers only needs to be boosted by firing an action potential at the nodes of Ranvier. In contrast, the unmyelinated fibers must fire an action potential at every contiguous membrane segment. After an action potential is generated, energy must be expended to reestablish the electrochemical gradient. The net result is that lesser myelinated and unmyelinated sensory axons are much more susceptible to toxic-metabolic pathologic processes than are the more heavily myelinated Aβ fibers. Because these "myelin-deficient" fibers must generate an action potential more frequently than their heavily myelinated counterparts, they are also more prone to ischemic processes. These smaller, less myelinated fibers require more energy per unit length than do the heavily myelinated fibers. Viewed from this perspective, the small fibers serve an important purpose as an early warning system indicative of an underlying ischemic or toxic-metabolic process. The smaller fibers thus serve a similar function to the "check engine" light on a car. Either the engine is fully functional or it is not. When nerve function is suboptimal, the "check engine" light is illuminated, advising the operator that there is a problem. In the same way that an illuminated "check engine" light cannot specify the severity of a problem, the severity of the patient's NP does not necessarily correlate with the severity of the underlying pathology. The presence of a PP usually indicates dysfunction of the smaller fibers or their central connections, often as a result of an ischemic or toxic-metabolic process. Contrast these disorders with those in which the small fibers are relatively spared, as in acquired demyelinating polyneuropathy. Although pain may be a feature of acquired demyelinating polyneuropathies, this is less common and often indicates collateral damage of small fibers secondary to inflammatory processes. The presence of a PP should initiate an investigation for potentially reversible causes, as suggested in Table 6-1.

Overview of Peripheral Neuropathic Pain Pathophysiology

The precise mechanisms by which NP occurs are incompletely understood. One early hypothesis advanced by Melzack and Wall was the "gate control theory."[13] They postulated both large and small fiber input onto a wide dynamic range (WDR) neuron remained quiescent until an imbalance in sensory input developed. This would result in the activation of a previously quiescent nociceptive WDR neuron. The WDR neuron would then engage in central NP transmission. This simplistic hypothesis has flaws because it does not predict what is observed in clinical practice. The activation of a WDR neuron as a result of small and large fiber imbalance predicts that loss of one or the other of these fiber types would result in NP. However, patients with hereditary sensory and autonomic neuropathies do not always experience pain. In fact, many have mutilated limbs because of an absence of small fiber function, the exact opposite of what the gate control theory would predict. Another example would be acquired demyelinating polyneuropathies, such as chronic inflammatory demyelinating polyradiculoneuropathy, wherein there is significant large fiber dysfunction, yet pain is not a common feature of this illness. For these reasons, the gate control hypothesis had to be modified.

No optimum theory can explain all of the mechanisms involved in NP, let alone the pain experienced in PP. As a first approximation, one can view this process as one in which there is a real or perceived injury to the sensory nervous system such that various mechanisms are activated. At every level of this process there will be events that favor nociceptive transmission and those that oppose it. From the periphery to the most rostral regions of the CNS, there will be a wider degree and an ever more complex series of inputs on this process. Even though the current understanding of this process is incomplete, some of these mechanisms have been elucidated, as summarized in Tables 6-2 to 6-4.

There is also some consensus that pain in polyneuropathy likely results from some change in the previous level of functioning of the sensory afferent pathways. Most NP conditions associated with PP develop after an injury to the PNS. Several potential mechanisms are responsible for peripheral NP, including phenotypic switch of nociceptors, ectopic activity in damaged axons, abnormal firing of dorsal root ganglion cells, unmaking of silent nociceptors, collateral sprouting, and invasion of dorsal root ganglia.[14] Each of these potential mechanisms provides a rationale for the use of the medications available for the treatment of pain in polyneuropathy.

Table 6-2 summarizes the various mechanisms by which NP can be generated in the PNS. These include direct pain impulse transduction by the transient receptor potential vanilloid channels and tyrosine kinase A (TrkA) receptors activated by nerve growth factor (NGF). In addition, they may induce previously dormant receptor subtypes that include purine receptors (P2X$_3$, P2X$_{2/3}$), the proteinase-activated receptor (PAR-2), and the bradykinin receptors B1 and B2.[15] Ion channels that regulate electrochemical transmission, such as voltage-gated sodium, potassium, and calcium channels, are also involved in the transmission of NP.[16–18] In most instances, activation of sodium and calcium channels tends to depolarize the

Table 6-2 Mechanisms Involved in Peripheral Neuropathic Pain

Channels/Receptors	Activated by	Function	Comments
TRPV channels (types 1, 2, and 3)	Noxious heat, low pH, capsaicin	Neuropeptide release	Proinflammatory
Neuropeptides*	TRPV channels	Nerve growth factor and cyokine release	Proinflammatory
TrkA receptors	Nerve growth factor	Upregulation of ion channels, receptors, and neuropeptides	Proinflammatory
	Creates NGF:TrkA complex		Channel activation
Sodium channels	Chronic inflammation	Linked to familial erythromelalgia and PEPD	Na$_v$1.7 has key role
TTX-R and TTX-S	Membrane voltage changes		Alters membrane potential
Calcium channel α2δ subunit	Membrane voltage changes	Calcium influx and cell damage	Gabapentinoids block calcium influx
Potassium channels	Membrane voltage changes	Membrane repolarization	Opening of K$_v$7 channels inhibits conduction
Purine receptors (P2X$_3$, P2X$_{2/3}$)	ATP	Neuropeptide release	Proinflammatory
Proteinase-activated receptor (PAR-2)	Tryptases/proteinases	Hyperalgesia	Proinflammatory?
Bradykinin receptor (B1 and B2)	Tissue injury	Inflammatory hyperalgesia	Proinflammatory

*Neuropeptides are neither receptors nor channels; they are proteins (e.g., substance P).

ATP, adenosine triphosphate; NGF, nerve growth factor; PEPD, paroxysmal extreme pain disorder; TrkA, tyrosine kinase A; TRPV, transient receptor potential vanilloid; TTX-R, tetrodotoxin resistant sodium channels; TTX-S, tetrodotoxin sensitive sodium channels.

Table 6-3 Mechanisms Involved in Peripheral Neuropathic Pain: Spinal Cord Level

Structures/Receptors	Activated by	Function	Comments
Small fiber afferents to dorsal horn of spinal cord	Ischemia/voltage changes	Release of neuropeptides and EAA	Activation of DHPTN
DHPTN		Pain transduction	Central sensitization
Neurokinin-1 receptors	Neuropeptides		
NMDA receptors	EAA		Mg-inactivated/Ca-activated
AMPA	EAA		
Kainate	EAA		
Metabotropic receptors*	EAA		
Microglia	Inflammation/trauma	Pain transduction	EAA, MAPK, prostaglandins, PIC release
		Inflammation	ATP, nitric oxide, reactive oxygen species production

*See text.

AMPA, α-amino-3-hydroxyl-5-methyl-4-isoxazole-propionate; ATP, adenosine triphosphate; Ca, calcium; DHPTN, dorsal horn pain–transmitting neurons; EAA, excitatory amino acids (e.g., glutamate, aspartate); MAPK, p38 mitogen-activated protein kinase; Mg, magnesium; NMDA, N-methyl-D-aspartate; PIC, proinflammatory cytokines (e.g., tumor necrosis factor-α, interleukin-1β, interleukin-6).

Table 6-4 Mechanisms Involved in Peripheral Neuropathic Pain: Pain Reducers/Inhibitors

Structure	Neurotransmitter	Other Functions	Comments
PNS and CNS	Opioid peptides	Sense of well-being	β-endorphin opposes bradykinin
NRM	Opioid peptides		Receives input from periaqueductal gray matter
Periaqueductal gray matter	5-HT, norepinephrine, glycine, GABA		Multiple inputs/outputs
Caudal DRN	5-HT	Satiety/initiates sleep	Projects to spinal cord and cerebellum
Rostral DRN	5-HT	Satiety/initiates sleep	Widespread
Locus coeruleus	Norepinephrine	Arousal and reward	Associated with 5-HT
CNS	GABA, glycine	Inhibit neurotransmission	Widespread

Dopamine and acetylcholine pathways in the CNS have effects on all of these pathways.
5-HT, 5-hydroxytryptamine or serotonin; CNS, central nervous system; DRN, dorsal raphe nucleus; GABA, gamma aminobutyric acid; NRM, nucleus raphe magnus; PNS, peripheral nervous system.

membrane and lead to electrical impulse propagation, whereas activation of potassium channels has the opposite effect. Several available medications modify ion conductance, and a more in-depth discussion of these channels is in order.

Sodium Channels

Sodium channels may be divided into tetrodotoxin-resistant and tetrodotoxin-sensitive subtypes, although chronic inflammation activates both. Primary nociceptive neurons express multiple voltage-gated sodium channels. There are nine alpha unit isoforms of the sodium channel, designated $Na_v1.1$ through $Na_v1.9$. Of these, pathologic mutations in $Na_v1.7$ have been shown to be responsible for certain specific disease states. Gain-of-function pathologic mutations in $Na_v1.7$ have been reported to result in the clinical syndromes of erythromelalgia and paroxysmal extreme pain disorder.[16] Conversely, an autosomal recessive "loss-of-function" mutation mapped to 2q24.3 in three northern Pakistani families resulted in a "'channelopathy-associated insensitivity to pain."[17] Affected persons experience painless injuries beginning in infancy, but have otherwise normal sensory function. Proprioception, joint vibratory sensation, tactile thresholds, and light touch perception are normal, as are reflexes and autonomic responses. The axonal flare response after an intradermal histamine injection is normal in these persons, a feature that distinguishes this condition from hereditary sensory and autonomic neuropathy.[18] Wada et al noted that mutations in the $Na_v1.7$ isoform of the sodium channel are not required because the aberrant upregulation/hyperactivity of even the native $Na_v1.7$ can produce pain associated with inflammation and nerve injury, as noted in rodents.[16]

Potassium Channels

Voltage-gated potassium channels may be viewed as the "brakes" on the sensory system in that they repolarize active neurons to the resting state.[19] Potassium channel, voltage-gated KQT-like subfamily (KCNQ) (K_v7) channels are responsible for the inhibitory M current in dorsal root ganglion (DRG) neurons.[20] The agent retigabine has been shown to facilitate the inhibitory M current through the opening of K_v7 channels in a dose-dependent manner.[21] Valeant Pharmaceuticals (Research Triangle Park, NC) recently filed an investigational new drug application to study the effects of this agent on PHN.[22] Retigabine is also being evaluated in phase 3 trials as an adjunctive anticonvulsant. The company's Web site also lists the most common side effects of retigabine as somnolence,

dizziness, abnormal vision, asthenia, headache, nausea, and diarrhea. There are also hyperpolarization-activated cyclic nucleotide-gated pacemaker cells that have structural similarities to potassium channels that are located in cardiac tissue and DRG neurons. These hyperpolarization-activated cyclic nucleotide-gated cells are permeable to both sodium and potassium ions and may subserve a role in Aδ-mediated mechanical allodynia.[19]

Calcium Channels

Calcium channels serve an important role with respect to nerve injury and pain transmission. Calcium influx is one of the final common pathways involved in cell injury and death. There are numerous calcium channel subtypes that can be divided into low-voltage, transient, or T-type and are associated with cardiac pacemaker rhythmicity and high-voltage calcium channels. The high-voltage calcium channels are further divided into subtypes L, N, P, Q, and R.[23] Of these subtypes, the one most germane to pain management is the N subtype, which has been shown to mediate persistent tactile allodynia after nerve injury in rats.[24] These N-type calcium channels are located in presynaptic terminals and mediate catecholamine release. At presynaptic nerve terminals, calcium entry is the initial trigger mediating the release of neurotransmitters via the calcium-dependent fusion of synaptic vesicles and involves interactions with the soluble N-ethylmaleimide-sensitive factor attachment protein receptor complex of synaptic release proteins.[25] Blockage of N-type calcium channel transmission is the postulated mechanism underlying the analgesic effect of the intrathecally administered medication ziconotide.[26] Because this medication is administered intravenously and only under specific circumstances, it is not discussed further. The gabapentinoids, gabapentin and pregabalin, exert their effects on the $\alpha_2\delta$ subunit of the Ca^{2+} channel at the N-, L- and P/Q-type channels.[27] Sutton et al further stated that the major effect of gabapentin, and by extension, pregabalin, is to affect N-type current.[27] The use of these medications may reduce calcium influx into the nerve fibers, reducing the degree of axonal injury and thus the degree of NP. The lack of their effect on T-type calcium channels may explain why these medications are not usually associated with cardiac arrhythmias.

Induction of nociceptive nerve fiber transmission may also occur. For example, the tyrosine kinase A receptor is expressed by nociceptors that bind NGF. NGF is produced by mast cells, several inflammatory cells, and endothelial cells. When the TrkA-NGF complex is formed, retrograde transport to the sensory neuron cell bodies located in the dorsal root ganglia occurs. This results in upregulation of numerous receptors and ion channels as well as the release of neuropeptides involved in pain transmission. Pappagallo and Werner cited evidence from other authors that sensory innervation of cortical and trabecular bone is mediated by this mechanism and that antibodies directed against NGF are effective in reducing pain in animal models of cancer-induced bone pain.[15,28,29]

Finally, the properties of the nociceptive fibers can be altered by inducing previously dormant receptor subtypes. The purine receptors ($P2X_3$, $P2X_{2/3}$) are activated by adenosine triphosphate, resulting in a release of neuropeptides.[15] $P2X_3$ receptors are located on peripheral sensory afferents, where their induction contributes to hyperalgesia and mechanical allodynia. Similar to the purine receptors, the proteinase-activated receptor (PAR-2) is activated by mast cell–derived tryptase and other proteinases that are believed to be involved in hyperalgesia. The bradykinin receptors B1 and B2 are also expressed on nociceptive neurons. The bradykinin receptor B1 is induced by tissue injury and contributes significantly to inflammatory hyperalgesia.

Regardless of the precise mechanisms involved, the nociceptive system can be viewed as an early warning system of actual or incipient tissue injury. Pain is a binary process; either tissue injury is perceived to be imminent or it is not. Pain alerts the organism to alter its behavior to minimize the amount of tissue damage, real or perceived. Failure to terminate the pain signal may result in permanent alteration of the sensory afferent system such that a chronic pain syndrome results. This is why PP should be treated as soon as possible.

Modification of Sensory and Nociceptive Afferents

Unlike the dorsal column/lemniscal system that conducts large fiber sensory pathway information to the cortex in a relatively direct manner, nociceptive afferents can be modified at various levels within the CNS. These often occur at synapses within the spinothalamic pathways, such as the dorsal horn of the spinal cord and the brain stem, as noted in Tables 6-2 and 6-3. With incoming nociceptive volleys to the dorsal horn, neuropeptides and excitatory amino acids are released and may result in the transient depolarization and central transmission of pain by the dorsal horn pain-transmitting neurons. These pain-inducing neuropeptides include substance P, calcitonin gene–related peptide, cholecystokinin, and neurokinin A.[15] The excitatory amino acids include glutamate and aspartate. N-methyl-D-aspartate receptors may subserve a role in pain modulation as well. These receptors are normally inactivated by the presence of magnesium.[15] However, intense or more frequent stimulation of nociceptive afferents by substance P and excitatory amino acids removes this protective "magnesium cap" such that intracellular calcium influx occurs. This calcium influx leads to a series of intracellular changes and prolonged sensitization of the pain-transmitting neurons in a phenomenon known as "wind-up."[30] Increased calcium influx has been implicated in both peripheral and central mechanisms of pain propagation. This is the presumed mechanism by which gabapentin and pregabalin produce their analgesic effects.

Wind-up may also occur through the activation of microglia, a process that can occur with peripheral nerve injury. This results in the expression of $P2X_4$ receptors on microglia in the spinal cord that leads to the release of brain-derived nerve growth factor. There is evidence that this results in activation of N-methyl-D-aspartate receptors in the dorsal horn of the spinal cord.[31] Ulmann et al also reported that $P2X_4$-deficient mice lacked mechanical hyperalgesia induced by peripheral nerve injury and showed impaired brain-derived neurotrophic factor (BDNF) signaling in the spinal cord.[31] Moreover, they noted that adenosine triphosphate stimulation did not stimulate BDNF release from $P2X_4$-deficient mice microglia in primary cultures. Another important mechanism involves the release of fractalkines, which are proteins in the chemokine family that are expressed by pain-transmitting neurons. In certain situations, fractalkines detach from neurons and activate nearby microglia.[32]

Pain can occur even in the absence of a peripheral nerve injury (e.g., thalamic syndrome of Dejerine-Roussy, complex regional pain syndrome type I). In these instances, pain may result from a change in the afferent traffic experienced by the CNS. Viewed from this perspective, either increased or decreased trafficking along the sensory pathways could give rise to pain perception. Restated, the CNS is constantly receiving sensory inputs, both somatic and visceral, from peripheral receptors that transmit reports back to the CNS for interpretation. Failure to transmit these signals might be interpreted as pain, as is observed in phantom limb pain. Interruption in normal transmission may also be responsible for the pain experienced contralateral to the lesion site in the thalamic syndrome of Dejerine-Roussy. Although these conditions are beyond the scope of this chapter, it is important to recognize that not all peripheral NP syndromes may be caused by alteration in nociceptive receptors or their central connections. Thus, compensating for the effects of a peripheral neuropathy with adaptive devices or physical therapy may actually reduce pain perception in addition to improving QoL.

Modification of sensory and nociceptive afferents may also occur in locations rostral to the dorsal horn of the spinal cord. Descending inhibitory pain pathways originate from various locations in the brain's cortical and subcortical areas. Three of the most important subcortical areas are the periaqueductal gray matter, locus ceruleus, and nucleus raphe magnus, as shown in Figures 6-1 and 6-2. The periaqueductal gray matter may be viewed as a hub that receives input from the cortex, thalamus, and hypothalamus. It expresses opioid receptors and stimulates the nucleus raphe magnus. The locus ceruleus inhibits the dorsal horn of the spinal cord through norepinephrine (NE)-mediated inhibitory pathways, whereas the nucleus raphe magnus inhibitory pathways project to the dorsolateral funiculus of the dorsal horn using serotonin or 5-hydroxytryptamine (5-HT) and enkephalins as their inhibitory neurotransmitters. Medications that increase transmission within these pathways should have a net effect of reducing perceived pain by increasing the effects of the neurotransmitters NE, 5-HT, and, to a lesser extent, dopamine (DA). Opioids, which have similarities to endorphins and enkephalins, most likely exert their effects by increasing transmission within the descending inhibitory pain pathways. Further modification of these ascending inputs occurs in more rostral CNS regions wherein the neurotransmitter gamma aminobutyric acid (GABA) and, to a lesser extent, acetylcholine subserve these functions. The GABA, 5-HT, and NE major pathways are shown in Figure 6-3. There is also significant influence of dopamine (DA)- and acetylcholine (Ach)-mediated pathways within the CNS on these afferent and efferent tracts.

These are the mechanisms that are believed to underlie the analgesic effects of the tricyclic antidepressants (TCAs), the selective serotonin and NE reuptake inhibitors (SSNRIs) such as duloxetine and venlafaxine, and opioid analgesics and their related compounds. Most of these data have been obtained in laboratory animals and have not necessarily been confirmed in humans. Nonetheless, Tables 6-5 to 6-7 summarize these agents' hypothesized mechanisms of action. Descending inhibitory pain pathways are believed to be mediated by 5-HT and NE such that increasing the availability of

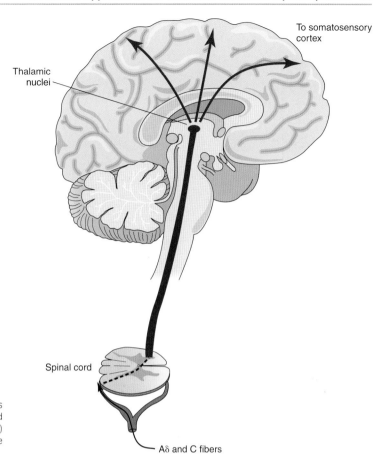

Figure 6-1 Thinly myelinated (A-delta) and unmyelinated (C) fibers cross within the spinal cord before ascending to the thalamus and somatosensory cortex. The large, heavily myelinated fibers (A-beta) that subserve vibration and position, not depicted here, cross at the cervicomedullary junction before ascending.

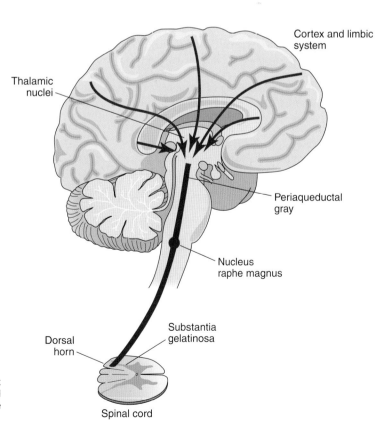

Figure 6-2 The descending pain pathways originate in the cortex and limbic system. They exert inhibitory effects on subcortical structures and the spinal cord. Serotonin and norepinephrine are important neurotransmitters in these pathways.

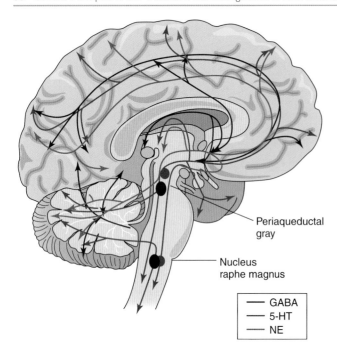

Figure 6-3 The major pathways that use these neurotransmitters within the central nervous system. Gamma aminobutyric acid (GABA) is an important inhibitory neurotransmitter, with numerous projections throughout the brain. 5-HT, serotonin; NE, norepinephrine.

these neurotransmitters within this pathway should reduce pain perception.[33] One such agent, duloxetine, is believed to have efficacy because of its relatively balanced inhibition of 5-HT and NE reuptake.[34] It has been approved by the FDA for the treatment of diabetic peripheral neuropathic pain (DPNP). Pregabalin is also approved for the same indication. The TCAs are believed to have a similar mechanism of action to duloxetine.[35,36] However, the TCAs are less specific than the SSNRIs because the TCAs have additional actions, such as anticholinergic and histamine blockade effects. Nonetheless, inhibition of 5-HT reuptake, alone or in combination with NE reuptake inhibition, has been invoked as the mechanism underlying the clinical effect of the older and newer antidepressants.[37] As discussed later, TCAs and SSNRIs have analgesic properties, whereas the selective serotonin reuptake inhibitors (SSRIs), such as fluoxetine and sertraline, have minimal, if any,

analgesic effects. With respect to the treatment of depression, a meta-analysis of 20 short-term comparative studies of 5 SSRIs, including citalopram, fluoxetine, fluvoxamine, paroxetine, and sertraline, showed no net difference in efficacy between individual compounds, but a slower onset of action for fluoxetine.[38] Thus, analgesic efficacy and antidepressant activity differ among these agents such that analgesic efficacy occurs when both NE reuptake and 5-HT reuptake are inhibited. Analogous to the SSRIs, no purely selective NE reuptake inhibitor has been conclusively shown to be an effective treatment for PP.

Narcotic analgesics can be subdivided into four main categories: natural alkaloids derived from opium (e.g., morphine and codeine), opium derivatives (e.g., heroin), synthetic agents that resemble the morphine molecule (e.g., methadone, meperidine), and opioid antagonists, such as naloxone. The precise mechanisms by which narcotic analgesics exert their effects remain to be firmly established. One important observation is that these substances resemble two endogenous pentapeptides known as enkephalins that differ in their last amino acid. It has been hypothesized that enkephalins prevent the release of acetylcholine, resulting in reduced nociceptive transmission. Other purported mechanisms include potentiation of the descending inhibitory pain pathways that originate from the cortex, limbic system, and periaqueductal gray matter. However, their use is limited by the effects of physical dependence, addiction, respiratory depression, and anticholinergic side effects, such as sedation and constipation. Regardless of the precise mechanisms involved, narcotic analgesics have been shown to be effective against many different types of NP. These substances interact with one or more of the four major subtypes of opioid receptors: δ (delta), κ (kappa), μ (mu), and the nociceptin receptor.[39] These receptors are widely distributed throughout the CNS. The nociceptin receptor subserves anxiety, depression, appetite, and the development of tolerance to μ agonists. The δ receptors, of which there are two subtypes, mediate analgesia, antidepressant effects, and physical dependence. The κ receptors, of which there are three subtypes, mediate spinal analgesia, sedation, miosis, and inhibition of antidiuretic hormone release. The μ receptors, of which there are also three subtypes, have the best characterized subtypes. Of these subtypes, the μ1 and μ2 receptors are the most important with respect to pain management. The μ1 receptors mediate supraspinal analgesia and physical dependence, whereas the μ2 receptors mediate respiratory depression, miosis, euphoria, reduced gastrointestinal motility, and respiratory

Table 6-5 Level A Recommendation Medications: Tricyclic Antidepressants[5,56]

Subtype	Generic Name	Mechanism of Action*	Number Needed to Treat (95% Confidence Interval)[†]	Additional Benefits
Secondary				
	Nortriptyline	NE	Similar to desipramine	
	Desipramine	NE	2.5 (1.9–3.6)	
	Amoxapine	5-HT ≈ NE/(-) DA/(-) HIS	ND	Useful in Huntington chorea
Tertiary				
	Amitriptyline	5-HT ≈ NE	2.1 (1.8–2.6)	
	Imipramine	5-HT ≈ NE	2.1 (1.8–2.6)	Panic disorder and generalized anxiety disorder
	Doxepin	NE/(-) HIS	ND	Used in fibromyalgia off-label
	Clomipramine	5-HT/(-) DA/some NE	ND	Useful in treating obsessive-compulsive disorder

*These mechanisms are based on preclinical data and have not been proven in humans.
[†]Based on an analysis of treatments for diabetic polyneuropathy.
5-HT, serotonin reuptake inhibitor; (-) DA, dopamine antagonist; (-) HIS, histamine antagonist; ND, no data available; NE, norepinephrine reuptake inhibitor.

Table 6-6 Level A Recommendation Medications: Selective Serotonin and Norepinephrine Reuptake Inhibitors, Gabapentinoids, and Topical Lidocaine[4,56]

Subtype	Generic Name	Mechanism of Action*	Number Needed to Treat (95% Confidence Interval)[†]	Other FDA Indications
Selective Serotonin and Norepinephrine Reuptake Inhibitors				
	Duloxetine	5-HT, NE	4 (3–9)	Depression, fibromyalgia
	Venlafaxine[‡]	5-HT; 5-HT/NE	5.5 (3.4–14.0)	Depression
Gabapentinoids				
	Gabapentin[‡,§]	Ca Ch α2δ antagonist	3.9 (3.2–5.1)	PS, PHN
	Pregabalin	Ca Ch α2δ antagonist	4.2 (3.4–5.4)	PS, PHN, fibromyalgia
Topicals				
	Lidocaine patch[‡]	Na Ch blocker	Unknown	PHN

*These mechanisms are based on preclinical data and have not been proven in humans.
[†]Based on an analysis of treatments in diabetic polyneuropathy.
[‡]Not U.S. Food and Drug Administration–approved for the treatment of pain in any type of polyneuropathy.
[§]For doses ≥ 2400 mg daily.
5-HT, serotonin reuptake inhibitor; Ca Ch α2δ antagonist, calcium channel α2δ antagonist; FDA, U.S. Food and Drug Administration; Na Ch blocker, sodium channel blocker; NE, norepinephrine reuptake inhibitor; PHN, post-herpetic neuralgia; PS, adjunctive therapy for partial seizures.

Table 6-7 Level A Recommendation Medications: Narcotics and Related Compounds[4,56,118,119]

Subtype	Generic Name	Mechanism of Action	Number Needed to Treat (95% Confidence Interval)
Derivative	Tramadol	μ receptor/weak 5-HT, NE	3.5 (2.4–6.4)
Opioids	See text	See text	

5-HT, 5-hydroxytryptamine or serotonin; NE, norepinephrine.

depression. From this brief description, one can see the advantage of developing an agent that only excited δ receptors or a combination of μ1 and δ receptors. Several such agents have been developed. Unfortunately, pure δ agonists are not as effective in producing analgesia as μ-receptor-mediated agents.[40] Furthermore, many δ agonists induce seizures at high doses, although not all δ agonists produce this effect.[41] One advantage of these δ opioid receptor agonists is that they have a novel antidepressant effect.[42] Antidepressant effects have also been noted with opioids that bind to μ and δ receptors.[43] Opioids have the advantages of providing pain control and antidepressant and antianxiety effects. Notwithstanding, opioids have numerous unwanted side effects that limit their use as first-line agents in the treatment of PP and should generally be used as second-line agents.[5]

Lastly, the mind is contained within the brain. A person's background, experiences, and psyche have an important effect on the perception of pain and its severity. The brain's cortex, in concert with the limbic system, interprets the noxious stimuli and makes assumptions about their meaning. Neurotransmitters involved in these processes include acetylcholine and DA. Although both are involved in the brain's "reward system," as well as in memory and cognition, DA plays a greater role than acetylcholine in the reward system, whereas the converse is true for memory and cognition. A person's emotional state and previous experiences play a significant role in the interpretation of incoming noxious stimuli. There are some experiences that few would interpret as pleasurable, such as voluntarily striking one's contralateral thumb with a hammer driven at full force. Nonetheless, the severity of the perceived noxious stimulus will vary between individuals and even within the same individual, depending on the circumstances. For example, stubbing one's toe after a sleep-deprived night on call will likely be perceived as more noxious than stubbing one's toe during a game of beach volleyball on vacation. The inciting stimulus is the same, but the

context is very different. Sunburn provides another example. Some persons are incapacitated for days after sunburn, whereas others view it as a minor inconvenience. Therefore, treating physicians should not base treatment decisions on their perception of what the patient should be experiencing, but rather on the basis of what the patient is actually reporting. Rating scales, such as the visual analog pain rating scale and the Wong-Baker faces model, have been used to classify a particular individual's perception of pain.[44,45] These provide reliable estimates that allow for a comparison between different points in time for the same individual in therapeutic trials. There are other, more comprehensive scales, such as the McGill Pain Questionnaire and the Walid-Robinson Pain Index (WRPI).[46,47] The McGill Pain Questionnaire gives a more specific indication of pain qualities, whereas the WRPI provides a description of both the intensity and duration of pain, measured in months. All of these rating scales have been validated, but they were not developed specifically for evaluating PP. Specifically, the WRPI was developed to measure low back pain in patients who were scheduled for spine surgery. Nonetheless, it is reasonable as a first approximation to use any of these pain rating scales when evaluating patients with a polyneuropathy so long as the same scale is used at every visit. The author prefers the simpler rating scales, such as the Wong-Baker faces model, because they are fairly quick and easy to perform. Their use allows for a longitudinal and reproducible assessment of the patient's perceived pain.

Evidence-Based Medicine

Evidence-based medicine is the conscientious, explicit, and judicious use of current best evidence in making decisions about the care of individual patients. The practice of EBM involves integrating one's individual clinical expertise with the best available external

Table 6-8 Evidence-Based Medicine Studies: U.S. Preventive Services Task Force[49]

Evidence Level	Source of Evidence		
Level I	At least one properly designed randomized controlled trial.		
Level II-1	Well-designed controlled trials without randomization.		
Level II-2	Well-designed cohort or case-control analytic studies, preferably from more than one site.		
Level II-3	Evidence obtained from multiple time series, with or without the intervention.		
Level III	Opinions of respected authorities, based on clinical experience, descriptive studies, or reports of expert committees.		
Quality of Evidence	**Summary**		
Good	Well-designed trials assessing health impact applicable to the population at large.		
Fair	Health impact assessable, but the evidence's strength has limitations.		
Poor	Unable to assess health impact let alone apply it to the population at large.		
Recommendation	**Recommendation to Provider**	**Benefit-to-Harm Ratio**	**Evidence Quality**
A	Strongly in favor	Very favorable	Good
B	In favor	Favorable	Fair or better
C	No position	Marginal	Fair
D*	Against	Equal or unfavorable	Fair or better
I	No position	Indeterminate	Poor

*D recommendations include asymptomatic patients as well.

clinical evidence from systematic research.[48] EBM reviews the available literature, assesses its quality, and makes a recommendation to guide clinical practice.

Unfortunately, EBM has limitations because there are some interventions in which it may be impractical, unethical, or inappropriate to subject patients to double-blind, placebo-controlled trials. For example, objections have been raised to the use of "sham surgery" in which a patient would be subjected to the risks of general anesthesia but would not benefit from receiving an actual surgical procedure. Prednisone treatment of myasthenia gravis provides another example. It is generally believed that it would be unethical to subject patients with myasthenia gravis to a trial of prednisone versus placebo to document the efficacy of prednisone therapy, a treatment that is widely believed to be beneficial based on historical controls. Finally, some interventions are so benign that it would not be practical to conduct a trial in which expert physical therapy would be compared against novice physical therapy to demonstrate an improvement in a patient's QoL. Assistive devices and other such modifications can be initiated and later discontinued at any time with no harm done to the patient. As such, some clinical questions may never be amenable to EBM analysis. Despite its limitations, EBM represents a great leap forward in patient treatment.

There are several different rating systems available, but the one most commonly used is derived from the U.S. Preventive Services Task Force (USPSTF), as noted in Table 6-8.[49] The American Academy of Neurology's Quality Standards' Subcommittee (AAN) modified this system, as noted in Tables 6-9 and 6-10.[6] These studies are ranked based on their level of evidence from I to III. The USPSTF's level I evidence reflects the "gold standard" of a well-designed, randomized clinical trial (equivalent to the AAN's Class I trial). On the opposite end of the spectrum, level III evidence reflects the opinions of authorities or descriptive studies (AAN Class IV). The USPSTF then ranks the quality of the evidence based on a rating of "good," "fair," or "poor," whereas the AAN methodology rates the evidence based on specific "levels." The AAN levels are subdivided into level A (established), level B

(probable), level C (possible), and level U (uncertain). Unlike the AAN system, the USPSTF's final assessment integrates these parameters to provide a level of recommendation for use in clinical practice, with grade A strongly supporting the clinical practice and grade D opposing this practice. In contrast, the AAN merely rates the quality and strength of the available evidence. Although these rating systems appear similar, an example demonstrates that they are very different. Consider three unethical randomized clinical trials

Table 6-9 Evidence-Based Medicine Studies: American Academy of Neurology[6]—Classification of Evidence Rating

Classification of Evidence Rating of a Therapeutic Trial	
Class I	Prospective, randomized, controlled clinical trial with masked outcome assessment in a representative population. The following are required: A. Concealed allocation. B. Primary outcome clearly defined. C. Inclusion/exclusion criteria clearly defined. D. Adequate accounting for a minimum number of dropouts and crossovers to minimize bias. E. Relevant baseline characteristics presented and substantially equivalent among treatment groups or appropriate statistical adjustment.
Class II	Prospective matched group cohort study in a representative population with masked outcome that meets criteria A–E above or a randomized controlled trial that lacks one criterion of A–D.
Class III	All other controlled trials (including well-defined natural history control subjects or patients serving as their own controls) in a representative population, where outcome is assessed independently or independently derived by an objective outcome measurement; a measure unlikely to be affected by an observer's expectation or bias.
Class IV	Evidence from uncontrolled studies, case series, case reports, or expert opinion.

Table 6-10 Evidence-Based Medicine Studies: American Academy of Neurology[6]—Level of Recommendation

Level of Recommendation	
Level A	Established as effective, ineffective, or harmful for the given condition in the specified population (requires two consistent Class I studies).*
Level B	Probably effective, ineffective, or harmful for the given condition in the specified population (requires at least one Class I study or two consistent Class II studies).
Level C	Possibly effective, ineffective, or harmful for the given condition in the specified population (requires at least one Class II study or two consistent Class III studies).
Level U	Inadequate or conflicting data. Treatment is unproven (studies not meeting Class I–III criteria).

*In exceptional cases, one convincing Class I study may suffice for a level A recommendation under the following conditions: all Class I criteria have been met; the magnitude of the effect is large; the relative rate of improved outcome exceeds 5; and the lower limit of the confidence interval is >2.

that assessed the use of hydrogen cyanide versus placebo for the treatment of PP wherein all of the patients who received cyanide died. Both the AAN and the USPSTF would concur that three Class I trials that obtained the same results would provide compelling clinical evidence against the use of cyanide for treating PP. The USPSTF would rate the quality of this evidence as "good," as would the AAN system, level A. The USPSTF would take one additional step and issue a grade D recommendation (harmful; not recommended). Restated, an AAN level A designation should not be interpreted as indicating that the data favor using this treatment, just that the data are conclusive. In fact, the AAN system does not actually make specific recommendations. Not all level I studies will result in a USPSTF grade A recommendation. As another example, assume that several level I studies found that a particular medication successfully treated hypertension in all African American men older than 50 years who served on active duty in the Vietnam War. This would likely lead to a USPSTF grade B recommendation at best because it is unclear whether these results could be generalized to the entire population. Finally, lack of evidence is not equivalent to "ineffective." As such, USPSTF grade I recommendations indicate "indeterminate" rather than "ineffective." Given these differences, the reader needs to be attuned to the rating system used.

Most practitioners are unlikely to follow this method for every clinical question that arises in the course of practice. Nonetheless, all clinicians should be aware of the clinical practice guidelines generated by these methods. Patients should be offered treatments with a USPSTF A or B grade recommendation and should not be advised to have treatments or interventions with a grade D recommendation. The AAN practice parameters must be read carefully to ascertain whether the treatment under consideration is helpful or harmful because this is not explicitly stated by the evidence class. Although EBM does not specifically advise against an intervention with an USPSTF grade of C, the practitioner should inform the patient that although the intervention may be helpful, the risk-to-benefit ratio is narrow. Furthermore, USPSTF grade I interventions may or may not be helpful. In such situations, the clinician needs to explain to the patient that there are no adequate data "for or against" this treatment and that "best judgment" should be used. For the remainder of this chapter, the USPSTF system will be the one employed because it incorporates all of the AAN criteria and then makes a specific recommendation.

Approved and "Off-Label" Medication Uses

Approval by the U.S. Food and Drug Administration (FDA) should not be equated with EBM. If a medication is approved by the FDA for a particular indication, then the agency has rendered an opinion that a particular medication is an effective treatment for that condition and that its benefits outweigh its risks. In general, FDA approval implies that this agency considers the medication or device to have efficacy for the approved indication as well as a favorable risk-to-benefit ratio. The FDA does not assign a grade to the level of evidence, but would be unlikely to approve a medication that was not at least grade B or better for the approved indication. However, the converse is not necessarily true in that a grade A recommendation may be warranted, even when the FDA has not given formal approval to that indication. For example, aspirin was shown to reduce the risk of myocardial infarction in patients with angina pectoris long before the FDA officially recognized this indication. Physicians can and should provide the best possible care to their patients, even if it means prescribing medications in an "off-label" manner.

According to the FDA's stated policy, "Neither the FDA nor the Federal government regulates the practice of medicine. Any approved product may be used by a licensed practitioner for uses other than those stated in the product label."[50] Once the medication has been approved for use, it may be prescribed "off-label" as seen fit by any licensed practitioner with the patient's informed consent.

Unfortunately, there is a paucity of data to guide clinicians as to the optimal drug to be used in specific conditions. A recent review of NP by Dworkin et al noted that only three broad classes of medications received a grade A recommendation for the first-line treatment of NP: antidepressants (TCAs and dual reuptake inhibitors of serotonin and NE), calcium channel $\alpha_2\delta$ ligands (gabapentin and pregabalin), and topical lidocaine.[4,5] Nonetheless, this publication addressed NP in general such that radiculopathy, PHN, and other conditions were included in this analysis. The review did not restrict its purview to the treatment of PP. The FDA has only approved two medications for the specific indication of DPNP: pregabalin and duloxetine. These agents have not received FDA approval for any other PP.

Although many patients are treated "off-label" with the other medications recommended by Dworkin et al, the FDA has not approved either the TCAs or gabapentin to be used as a treatment for pain associated with any type of painful peripheral neuropathy.[5] The two FDA-approved indications for gabapentin are as adjunctive therapy in the treatment of partial seizures with and without secondary generalization in patients older than 12 years with epilepsy and for the management of post-herpetic neuralgia (PHN) in adults.[51] A related compound, pregabalin, has been FDA approved only for use in adults as adjunctive therapy in the treatment of partial seizures and the management of PHN, DPNP, and FM.[52] Duloxetine is approved in adults for the treatment of major depressive disorder, generalized anxiety disorder, DPNP, and FM.[53] The only FDA-approved indication for the lidocaine patch is for the management of PHN in adults. Finally, although naturally occurring opioids, such as morphine, and synthetic opioids, such as tramadol, are FDA approved for the treatment of "pain," they have not been specifically FDA approved for the treatment of PP.

Previous Treatment Recommendations

Given the paucity of EBM guidance, many guidelines for the treatment of NP have been proposed.[4,5,54,55] Although these guidelines are all useful, most are based on meta-analyses and expert opinion because there are few double-blind placebo-controlled trials to provide guidance on each and every condition that results in NP. As previously discussed, the only PP that has been extensively evaluated in double-blind, multicenter, placebo-controlled trials is DPNP. Other authors have performed analyses regarding the treatment of DPNP, one of which analyzed the data to estimate the number needed to treat (NNT), the number of consecutive patients who would need to be treated for one person to report a 50% reduction in perceived pain.[56] Although this may have some utility, all analyses, including meta-analyses, are subject to numerous potential sources of bias, so their conclusions may not necessarily be accurate.[57] These biases may include such factors as not identifying negative trials because these are less likely to be published, ignoring publications in languages other than English, selection bias on the part of the reviewer, and overestimation of a drug's effect because a higher end of the dosage range was used. Even if a meta-analysis were bias-free and accurate, its findings cannot necessarily be generalized to the treatment of other painful neuropathic conditions. Therefore, there is a paucity of evidence to guide the treatment of pain in polyneuropathy other than DPNP. More importantly, there are few head-to-head trials wherein less expensive medications, such as the TCAs, are compared with newer agents. Given the paucity of EBM, a rational approach to the treatment of PP based on the available literature is in order.

There have been many publications on the treatment of DPNP, including an analysis by Huizinga and Peltier that summarized the relevant literature and made treatment recommendations.[56] Huizinga and Peltier reported that there were no head-to-head trials that allowed for an objective comparison of one recommended agent against another.[56] Therefore, they analyzed the available data to give a comparison based on the NNT. The mean NNT for these agents suggests that the TCAs and carbamazepine (which has a structure similar to that of the TCAs) have a better efficacy than the other medications listed. A closer evaluation notes a significant overlap in the 95% confidence intervals. As such, one cannot state with certainty that carbamazepine and the TCAs are truly superior to the other agents evaluated by this study. Furthermore, this analysis of DPNP cannot be extrapolated to the treatment of all PPs. Finally, these data report what the "average" patient with this condition would likely experience and not what an individual patient would experience. In the absence of clear treatment guidelines, a practitioner should discuss all of the potential treatment options with the patient so that the patient makes an informed decision.

Many physicians are tempted to combine two or more medications with different mechanisms of action, hoping that the combination will prove superior to either agent alone. Many pain management specialists combine pregabalin and duloxetine, assuming that their different mechanisms of action will be additive. However, physicians should recognize that such combination therapies have not been formally evaluated in prospective, double-blind, placebo-controlled trials. Nonetheless, trials combining opioids with nonopioid agents reported that a combination was superior to placebo, that a greater degree of pain reduction was achieved, and that fewer side effects were encountered.[58,59] Few, if any, level I studies compared a combination of an SSNRI with a gabapentinoid against these agents individually or against a placebo. Until such evidence is forthcoming, the treating physician should attempt to treat each patient individually, taking into consideration the patient's age, comorbid conditions, the patient's tolerance of side effects, medication cost, and evidence supporting the medication's efficacy.

General Approach to the Patient with Painful Neuropathy

The principles of neurology are applicable to PP as well. The treating physician needs to take a detailed history, perform a physical examination, and localize the lesion in the nervous system. The patient's symptoms, the distribution of physical examination abnormalities, and the findings of electrodiagnostic studies should narrow the range of diagnostic possibilities. Appropriate laboratory testing should then be used in an attempt to identify the underlying cause.

Pain should be considered the "fifth vital sign" such that its presence should prompt the physician to identify and treat the underlying cause.[60] Most practitioners would attempt to identify the underlying cause for a systolic blood pressure of 230 mm Hg, a pulse of 140 bpm, or a respiration rate of 36 breaths/min. The same sort of due diligence needs to be paid to a person who reports significant pain. A patient who presents with new onset of "10/10" pain demands a more emergent and extensive workup than someone with a 20-year history of "2/10" pain. Even if no specific cause for the pain is identified, the physician should not assume that there is no cause and should never tell the patient that it is "all in your head." This leads to significant and often irreparable damage to the physician–patient relationship. Physicians who are uncomfortable managing "idiopathic pain" should refer these patients to a colleague who specializes in pain management.

The best possible outcomes occur when the treating physician is able to identify and eliminate the underlying cause of the NP process. However, the precise etiology often remains undetected despite extensive evaluations. Thus, "cures" are rarely achieved because most processes causing NP are not identified or cannot be completely eliminated. Even when the underlying cause is identified, the underlying disease process may not be reversible. In such instances, treatments should be given that will retard or attenuate the disease process. If this is not possible, then the remaining course of action is to minimize the patient's symptoms and address any comorbid conditions. The patient should be informed that the goal is to maximize QoL and minimize the effect of the disease.

When PPs are observed, there is usually some degree of small fiber dysfunction. The etiologies can be subdivided into toxic-metabolic derangements, autoimmune disorders, and traumatic injury.[61,62] Nervous system tissue, both central and peripheral, is particularly susceptible to toxic-metabolic derangements. Restated, "Nervous tissues malfunction when other tissues malfunction." Examples would include pancreatic insufficiency (e.g., diabetes mellitus), liver disease, thyroid disorders, and kidney dysfunction. Toxic-metabolic derangements would include diverse etiologies such as hypoxic-ischemic disorders, vitamin deficiencies, and external toxins, including alcohol and heavy metal poisoning. Table 6-1 shows the author's recommended evaluation of a patient who presents with a PP, although recently published guidelines did not establish the highest level of evidence to warrant these recommendations, with the exception of DNA testing for suspected inherited neuropathy.[63,64] These PP-causing conditions, their means of diagnosis, and their treatment are discussed more extensively in other chapters and will not be repeated here. Diagnostic testing should only be performed if that diagnostic test will change the patient's management. For this reason, skin biopsies in patients with small fiber neuropathies should not be routinely performed because this test rarely establishes a specific diagnosis.

Moreira et al reported that patients with diabetes who have distal symmetrical diabetic polyneuropathy (DSDP) have an increased incidence of psychiatric disorders, especially anxiety and depression.[65] In this cohort of 65 diabetic patients, anxiety disorders were present in 81.8% of those with DSDP and 60.0 % of those without DSDP ($P = 0.01$). A current episode of major depression was present in 18.2% of patients with concomitant DSDP and 7.7% of those without DSDP ($P = 0.04$). Furthermore, the severity of the depressive symptoms correlated positively with the severity of DSDP symptoms ($r = 0.38$; $P = 0.006$), but not with the severity of diabetic symmetric peripheral neuropathy (DSPN) signs ($r = 0.07$; $P = 0.56$). The patient with PPs may have concomitant small myelinated and large fiber dysfunction as well, leading to comorbidities such as dysautonomia and gait impairment. Medications or assistive devices may improve the patient's QoL. For these reasons, the patient should be queried about any autonomic dysfunction. Questions regarding activities of daily living, such as ability to walk, bathe, and feed oneself, are also important. If a patient reports difficulties in these areas, then consultation with occupational and physical therapists is warranted.

Given the evidence that persons with PPs are at increased risk for comorbid conditions, the treating physician must screen for these disorders. Cormorbid conditions amenable to treatment include major depression, anxiety, sleep disorders, and FM. There are written screening tools for all of these disorders except for FM, which does require a physical examination. Although a psychiatric consultation would seem an obvious course of action, many patients are reluctant to consult a psychiatrist. Therefore, it is incumbent on the physician evaluating the patient with a PP to screen for depression. Few patients with PPs are not depressed after 6 months of constant pain. Uncomplicated, mild to moderate comorbid depression can and should be treated by a physician who is not a psychiatrist. Nonetheless, immediate psychiatric consultation would definitely be indicated for patients expressing suicidal or homicidal ideation as well as for patients who do not respond to routine antidepressant therapy. Numerous screening tools are available for assessing the probability and severity of coexisting depression. Two such scales that have no restrictions on their use are the Hamilton-D and Zung depression rating scales.[66–68] Both of these scales may be completed by the patient at home before the visit or in short order when arriving for a consultation. A physician can address these issues by asking patients whether the pain condition has altered their mood in any way. This allows the patient a chance to report changes in behavior that may have been unmasked by the PP. This may change the physician's opinion regarding the choice of drug. For example, a patient with depression may respond better to treatment with an antidepressant than to agents without antidepressant properties. There is still some controversy as to whether the use of antidepressants prescribed for the treatment of unipolar depression can precipitate mania in persons who actually may have bipolar disorder.[69] Until this issue is settled, prudence dictates that the physician counsel the patient to report any adverse symptoms with medication use, including symptoms of mania or hypomania. In such instances, referral to a psychiatrist for a definitive evaluation is recommended. The National Institute of Mental Health states that bipolar disorder has a prevalence of 2.6% of the population in the United States, whereas unipolar depression is found in 7% of men and 12% of women.[70–72] These data suggest that approximately 10% of the population will have unipolar depression, which is four times as many as those with bipolar illness. One review from the United Kingdom noted that persons who were depressed were twice as likely to have cardiovascular disease as nondepressed persons.[73] This report also noted that depressed persons were far less likely to be compliant with their medical regimen and more likely to refuse

rehabilitation services. Although there is some controversy as to whether depressed persons have a worse outcome when afflicted with cardiovascular disease, it has a significant negative effect on a patient's QoL and should be treated when present.

Anxiety disorder is more prevalent than depression because it affects approximately 18% of the adult population in a given year.[70] Anxiety disorders encompass a variety of disorders, including panic disorder, obsessive-compulsive disorder (OCD), post-traumatic stress disorder (PTSD), social anxiety disorder, phobias, and generalized anxiety disorder (GAD). These entities are discussed in greater detail in general psychiatry textbooks. Patients with PPs may report these symptoms for the first time because the PP may unmask these disorders. The reason that this chapter mentions these disorders is that specific medications are effective for these conditions. For example, the TCA imipramine is prescribed for panic disorder and GAD, whereas clomipramine is the only TCA noted to be useful for treating OCD. Persons who prefer to begin using a TCA for treatment of a PP should be asked about symptoms of anxiety disorders because this information may affect the selection of the TCA. In contrast, SSNRIs are effective for depression and anxiety disorders, although only duloxetine has the FDA indications for treatment of DPNP, depression, and GAD. Other agents, such as monoamine oxidase inhibitors and benzodiazepines, are also effective treatments for anxiety disorders.[74] Monoamine oxidase inhibitors and benzodiazepines have not been shown to be useful in the treatment of PP and should not be used for this indication. The treatment of PTSD remains controversial. Physicians should be aware that a patient who experienced a traumatic nerve injury may be experiencing PTSD. The patient should be questioned about the events surrounding this injury to ascertain whether PTSD might be present. Many patients, especially veterans, tend to underreport their PTSD symptoms. If PTSD cannot be excluded with confidence, then the patient should be referred to a psychiatrist specializing in PTSD.

Sleep disturbances are often reported by patients with polyneuropathies. Many patients with PPs have an inability to initiate or maintain sleep, which is a common symptom of anxiety and depression. Regardless of the underlying cause, lack of sleep usually worsens the underlying pain condition. Physicians should endeavor to improve the patients' sleep quality so that they feel rested on awakening in the morning. Although poor sleep may be a symptom of depression, other comorbid conditions may be responsible. Common causes encountered in patients include obstructive sleep apnea (OSA) and restless legs syndrome (RLS). The presence of a sleep disturbance can be assessed with the Epworth Sleepiness Scale.[75] This is an eight-item questionnaire in which patients rate their "likeliness of dozing" on a scale from 0 to 3 wherein the numbers indicate no chance (0), slight chance (1), moderate chance (2), and high chance (3) of dozing. These eight situations are sitting and reading, watching television, sitting inactive in a public place, riding as a passenger in a car for one hour, lying down to rest in the afternoon, sitting and talking, sitting quietly after a lunch without alcohol, and being stopped by traffic in a car for a few minutes. As with the previously mentioned scales, the patient can complete this before the visit or at the time of the visit. A total score of 9 or greater indicates a high probability that a sleep disturbance is present, but does not specify the cause. Additional history helps to narrow the differential diagnosis. Such questions should attempt to distinguish between OSA and RLS.

Population-based studies suggest that 2% of women and 4% of men older than 50 years have symptomatic OSA.[76] Both the incidence and the prevalence of this disorder are likely to increase over time as the average American's body mass index increases.

Patients with adult-onset diabetes mellitus, a common cause of PP, often have an elevated body mass index and are at greater risk for symptomatic OSA. A simple screening tool, neck circumference, has been shown to be highly sensitive for detecting OSA. A neck circumference of greater than 16 inches in a woman or greater than 17 inches in a man correlates with an increased risk of OSA.[77] In addition, increasing neck circumference has been shown to correlate with the severity of apnea.[78,79] Neck circumference should be assessed in all patients who report nonrefreshing sleep. Any woman with a neck circumference of greater than 16 inches ($\approx$40 cm) or a man with a neck circumference of greater than 17 inches ($\approx$43 cm) should be referred for a sleep study to evaluate for OSA. OSA is associated with an increased risk of hypertension and cardiovascular disease.[80]

An incompletely understood condition, RLS results in a compulsion to move one's legs, especially during or immediately before sleep.[81] Patients who report sleep disturbances should be asked about RLS because one potentially treatable cause is anemia. RLS is often associated with chronic diseases, such as renal insufficiency, diabetes mellitus, Parkinson disease, and polyneuropathy. Treating the underlying condition often provides relief from RLS symptoms.[82] DA agonists, such as ropinirole and benzodiazepines, are effective, whereas RLS is worsened by DA antagonists and phenytoin.

Fibromyalgia is a chronic pain disorder that is defined by the American College of Rheumatology as widespread pain lasting at least 3 months in combination with pain at 11 or more of 18 specific tender point sites on the body.[83] A different definition proposed by Pope and Hudson also considers FM to be present in the absence of trigger points if at least four of the following six comorbid conditions are present: headaches, generalized fatigue, sleep disturbance, neuropsychiatric complaints, numbness or tingling sensations, and irritable bowel symptoms.[84] This subject was recently reviewed in detail by Arnold.[85] FM tends to respond to the same types of medications that are useful for the treatment of NP.[86] Only two medications are FDA-approved for the treatment of FM: pregabalin and duloxetine. Although many practitioners consider FM a "dubious disease," it is unlikely that the FDA would have approved two medications for a "nonexistent" condition. Even if the treating physician does not "believe in" FM, this condition will have a significant negative effect on QoL. Given that FM is amenable to treatment, an assessment for myofascial trigger points should be part of every neuromuscular specialist's examination.

Certain medications may increase the risk of other cormorbid conditions. For example, some agents, such as the TCAs and pregabalin, have been associated with weight gain. As such, these agents may not be the drug of choice in a patient with adult-onset diabetes mellitus and a PP who has a large body mass index and sleep apnea. The FDA requires that all SSRIs and SSNRIs display a boxed warning that the risk of suicide may be increased in persons 18 to 24 years. As such, duloxetine may not be the drug of choice in an 18-year-old patient who reports a history of suicidal ideation. Anticonvulsant agents, such as the gabapentinoids, may not necessarily be a safer alternative because the FDA recently announced that it will require a warning label on all antiepileptic drugs (AEDs) because their use has been associated with increased suicidal ideation.[87] This article summarized an FDA review of 199 clinical trials of 11 antiepileptic drugs. The risk of suicidal behavior or thoughts was nearly doubled for patients receiving AEDs versus placebo (0.43% vs. 0.24%), leading to approximately one additional case of suicidality for every 500 patients treated with AEDs instead of placebo. However, there was no statistically significant difference in the number of actual or "completed" suicides when comparing AEDs (four cases) versus placebo (zero cases). Nonetheless, the FDA will

now require a warning label on all anticonvulsants, including the ones used for the treatment of NP: pregabalin, gabapentin, carbamazepine, oxcarbazepine, and phenytoin. This list also includes the benzodiazepines clonazepam and chlorazepate, which may be prescribed off-label for RLS and anxiety disorders. Furthermore, Dworkin et al reported that there were insufficient data to give the AEDs, other than the gabapentinoids, a grade A recommendation for the treatment of NP.[5] For these reasons, AEDs other than the gabapentinoids should not be used as first-line agents for the treatment of PP.

In summary, comorbid conditions have a significant negative effect on the patient's QoL. Certain conditions, such as OSA, may increase the patient's risk of hypertension and cardiovascular diseases. Also, there is a significant overlap in the symptoms of pain, psychiatric comorbidities, and FM. Given these associations, all neuromuscular consultants should be comfortable identifying and treating these conditions. This will allow the treating physician to select an agent that will treat the NP as well as any other comorbid conditions that may be present.

"First-Line" Neuropathic Pain Treatments

The available medical evidence and expert opinion support the use of the gabapentinoids, topical lidocaine, the TCAs, and SSNRIs as first-line agents for the treatment of the average person with NP. However, these medications differ in terms of their mechanism of action, additional benefits, side effects, and adverse effects. A summary of these data appears in Tables 6-5 to 6-7 and Tables 6-11 to 6-13. Because treatment must be individualized, the risks and benefits of each treatment should be discussed so that the patient makes the best informed decision. A brief discussion of each class of medication follows. Although the important data on these medications have been summarized, all practitioners should be completely familiar with all of the information regarding the risks and benefits for the medications that they are prescribing.

Tricyclic Antidepressants

A significant advantage of TCAs is that they are among the least expensive medications available for the treatment of pain in polyneuropathy. It is believed that these agents act by inhibiting the reuptake of NE and 5-HT. Their proposed mechanism of action is thought to be similar to that of the SSNRIs, such as duloxetine. Other authors consider these agents to have differing effects on 5-HT and NE inhibition that are reported according to "selectivity ratios."[88] Nonetheless, TCAs have numerous side effects that may limit their clinical utility. Of the TCAs, nortriptylene may be considered to have the most NE reuptake inhibition and the least 5-HT reuptake inhibition. Amitriptylene and imipramine would be classified as "balanced," and chlomipramine would have the most 5-HT reuptake inhibition and the least NE reuptake inhibition. TCAs may also be classified as secondary or tertiary amines. In general, the tertiary amines tend to affect both NE and 5-HT reuptake inhibition, whereas the secondary amines are less "balanced" and act primarily as NE reuptake inhibitors. However, the "balanced" tertiary amines are far more likely to produce anticholinergic side effects and orthostatic hypotension than are the secondary amines. Therefore, the tertiary amines are more likely to be effective, based on the current models of NP treatment, but they are more likely to produce side effects. Dworkin at al recommend that secondary amines should be used in preference to the tertiary amines.[4,5] However, younger persons who are more tolerant of side effects may

Table 6-11 Non-narcotic Medications and Dosing[4,5,56,118,119]

	Medication	First Dose (mg)*	Increase by (mg/wk)	Maximum Daily Dose (mg)	Adequate Trial Length
Tricyclic Antidepressants[†]	Nortriptyline[‡]	10–25 qhs	10–25 qhs	75–150	6–8 (2 wk at max dosage)
	Desipramine[‡]	10–25 qhs	10–25 qhs	75–150	6–8 (2 wk at max dosage)
	Amitriptyline[‡]	10–25 qhs	10–25 qhs	75–150	6–8 (2 wk at max dosage)
	Imipramine[‡]	10–25 qhs	10–25 qhs	75–150	6–8 (2 wk at max dosage)
Selective Serotonin and Norepinephrine Reuptake Inhibitors	Duloxetine[§]	20–30 qhs	20–30 qhs	60–120	4–6 wk
	Venlafaxine[‡]	37.5 qhs to bid	37.5–75	225	4–6 wk
Gamma Aminobutyric Acid Analogs	Gabapentin[‡]	100 qhs to bid	100–300[¶]	600 tid[#]	3–8 (2 wk at max dosage)
	Pregabalin	50–75 bid	150 mg q 3–7 days	600	4 wk
Other	Lidocaine patch[‡]	3 total q12h	NA		3–4 wk

*Starting dose and upward titration should be should be "lower and slower" in the elderly.
[†]Consider another agent if no response at 75 mg qhs for 2 weeks.
[‡]Not U.S. Food and Drug Administration–approved for the treatment of any specific painful polyneuropathy.
[§]Duloxetine showed no significant difference between 60 mg and 120 mg for diabetic peripheral neuropathic pain.
[¶]Some authors recommend a more rapid dose escalation (see reference 4).
[#]Some authors recommend a maximum dosage of 1200 mg po tid.
max, maximum; NA, not applicable.

Table 6-12 Oral Opioid "Around-the-Clock" Dosing in Opioid-Naïve Patients Weighing More than 55 kg[120,121]

Drug	Equipotent Dose (mg)	Starting Dose for Moderate to Severe Pain
Morphine	30 mg q3–4h	30 mg q3–4h
Morphine (controlled release)	90–120 mg q12h	90–120 mg q12h
Hydromorphone	7.5 mg q3–4h	6 mg q3–4h
Levorphanol	4 mg q6–8h	4 mg q6–8h
Methadone*	20 mg q6–8h	20 mg q6–8h
Codeine plus acetaminophen or aspirin	180 mg q3–4h	60 mg q3–4h
Hydrocodone	30 mg q3–4h	10 mg q3–4h
Oxycodone	30 mg q3–4h	10 mg q3–4h

*Methadone has unusual pharmacokinetics and side effects. It should be used with caution.

benefit from the tertiary amines, especially those with difficulty initiating and maintaining sleep. Otherwise, the secondary amines should be used preferentially because they have fewer adverse effects and can be tolerated more easily in older patients.

Because TCAs have been in use for nearly 50 years, their side effect profile and long-term effects are well known. They are also among the least expensive medications known to be effective for the treatment of NP. Their side effect profile limits their use, however. These side effects include anticholinergic symptoms, such as dry mouth, constipation, urinary retention, blurred vision, and confusion. Other significant side effects include weight gain, orthostatic hypotension, and arrhythmias. TCAs may cause unwanted side effects on the cardiac conduction system, such as lengthening of the PR interval and first-degree heart block.[89] Patients who have first-degree heart block while using TCAs can progress to more significant degrees of heart block.[90] Furthermore, a large, retrospective cohort analysis reported an increased risk of sudden cardiac death at doses of 100 mg daily or greater.[91] This led to a recommendation that TCAs should not be prescribed to persons with known ischemic cardiac disease. It has also become standard practice to order an electrocardiogram before initiating treatment and during TCA dose escalation in all patients older than 40 years.[92] A second electrocardiogram is prudent when the patient will be using a dose of 100 mg daily or greater. Given the previously cited association of depression and cardiovascular disease, it may not be prudent to prescribe a TCA to anyone who is depressed and has more than one risk factor for cardiovascular disease. In such instances, duloxetine may be preferable because it is FDA approved for the treatment of unipolar depression, as maintenance therapy for unipolar depression, and as a treatment for DPNP. TCAs should be used sparingly in the elderly because they may adversely affect cognition and gait, which puts the patient at increased risk for falling. TCAs should also be used only in persons who can tolerate their numerous side effects. The other issue with the TCAs is that they have a narrow therapeutic window. Patients who are depressed sometimes attempt to commit suicide by taking an overdose of TCAs. Therefore, it is advisable to prescribe less than 1 g in total of the agent when initiating therapy. The patient should also be warned about the risks inherent in a TCA overdose.

There are various recommended starting doses and dosing regimens for the TCAs. One should use the lowest dose that maximizes the degree of pain control while minimizing side effects. In patients who report being prone to side effects, treatment should be started at 10 mg by mouth at bedtime. In this manner, the patient will likely be asleep when the medication reaches its peak plasma level such that the side effects are minimized. Otherwise, the starting dose should be initiated in the range of 10 to 25 mg at bedtime. The dose can be titrated by 10 to 25 mg every 1 to 2 weeks until an effective dose is reached. Most patients who will respond to TCAs usually require a dose of 75 mg or less. If a patient reports no response after using a TCA at 75 mg for 2 weeks, then

Table 6-13 Medication Class, Side Effects, Precautions, and Safety[4,5,56,118,119]

Medication Class	Common Side Effects	Relative Contraindications	Benefit-to-Risk Ratio*
Tricyclic antidepressants	Anticholinergic effects,[†] weight gain	Cardiac disease, suicidal ideation Depression? Cognitive impairment	Second tier[‡]
Duloxetine	Nausea, headache, dry mouth	Renal or liver impairment	First tier
Pregabalin[§]	Lethargy/peripheral edema	Renal impairment	First tier
Lidocaine patch	Local irritation	Previous allergy	First tier
Tramadol[¶]	Similar to narcotics	History of substance abuse Cognitive impairment (initially) Suicidal ideation	Third tier
Opioids	Nausea, anticholinergic effects	Same as above	Third tier

*The author's assessment of which agents are likely to provide the best level of pain relief with the fewest side effects.

[†]Anticholinegic effects include dry mouth, dry eyes, cognitive impairment (especially in the elderly), constipation, urinary retention, and cardiac effects.

[‡]Tricyclic antidepressants have a narrow therapeutic window, but their long-term side effects are better established than with tramadol or opioids.

[§]These medicines have U.S. Food and Drug Administration approval for the treatment of pain associated with diabetic polyneuropathy. Others in their class do not have this approval and are not discussed here.

[¶]This medicine inhibits serotonin reuptake and should be used cautiously in combination with tricyclic antidepressants, selective serotonin reuptake inhibitors, selective serotonin and norepinephrine reuptake inhibitors, and triptans.

another medication should be considered. Those who do respond can have their dose increased slowly until a maximum dose of 150 mg daily is reached. Dworkin et al stated that the dose can be increased beyond this range as long as the serum level of the medication and its metabolite is less than 100 ng/mL.[4]

In summary, TCAs have the advantage of being inexpensive, with a well-established side effect profile and nearly 50 years of widespread use. However, they have a narrow therapeutic window and have numerous undesirable side effects. Unless cost is an issue, the newer agents may be preferable because of their wider therapeutic window and fewer side effects.

Selective Serotonin and Norepinephrine Reuptake Inhibitors

The SSNRIs represented a significant development in the treatment of NP. Unlike the TCAs, the SSNRIs have far fewer effects on neurotransmitters other than 5-HT and NE. SSNRIs have a higher therapeutic window and are less likely to cause side effects in case of an overdose. They also have the advantage of faster onset, more rapid titration, and a wider variety of FDA-approved indications. There are two main SSNRIs available on the market: venlafaxine and duloxetine. However, only duloxetine has received FDA approval to be marketed for the treatment of DPNP. The limiting side effects include nausea, dizziness, dry mouth, and erectile dysfunction. These side effects are not unique to SSNRIs because they occur with the SSRIs as well.

Venlafaxine tends to act more as an SSRI at the lower end of its dosage range and as an SSNRI at higher doses.[4] It also has weak DA reuptake inhibition at the higher end of the dosage range. Despite the fact that it does not have FDA approval for the treatment of pain in polyneuropathy, it does have FDA approval for the treatment of major depressive disorder, GAD, social anxiety disorder, and panic disorder in adult patients.[93] Because these are commonly encountered comorbid conditions, venlafaxine should remain a treatment option for patients with PP. Although duloxetine may have some advantages, venlafaxine should be considered for patients who have coexisting panic disorder or social anxiety disorder because duloxetine has not been FDA approved for these indications.

Duloxetine is a reasonable first choice for the treatment of PP as long as cost is not a factor. It has the advantages of once daily

dosing, a rapid titration schedule, and FDA approval for the treatment of DPNP. It is also FDA approved for the treatment of major depressive disorder and FM, two commonly encountered comorbid conditions associated with pain as a result of polyneuropathy. It also has the advantage of causing no statistically significant weight gain. Nonetheless, it does have limitations. It has been shown to cause a slight elevation in blood glucose and blood pressure. Given that it is metabolized both by the kidney and the liver, this agent should be given cautiously to persons with hepatic or renal impairment.

Gabapentinoids

The two medications in this class that are commonly used for the treatment of NP are gabapentin and pregabalin. Their use in NP has become widespread because these agents are generally well tolerated, are easily titrated, have few drug interactions, and do not require laboratory monitoring. However, cost may be a limiting factor for some patients. Although the basic GABA frame is the same in both compounds, they have somewhat different structures in that the beta carbon has a different side chain. Gabapentin has five additional carbons attached to form a ring structure, whereas pregabalin has a hydrogen atom and a propyl side chain. Unlike pregabalin, gabapentin has not received FDA approval for the treatment of DPNP. Although one well-designed clinical trial showed that gabapentin had a statistically significant benefit over placebo for the treatment of pain associated with diabetic polyneuropathy, the effects were modest in that there was a 1-point reduction on an 11-point rating scale at a daily dose of 1800 mg after 2 weeks.[94] Neither longer treatment durations nor higher doses showed any significant benefit. The main advantage of gabapentin over pregabalin is that gabapentin is not a controlled substance and it is available generically. Gabapentin's side effects include weight gain and cognitive impairment.[51] Although pregabalin and gabapentin are chemically related, they have different pharmacokinetic properties.[95] Preclinical studies with pregabalin and gabapentin showed similar anticonvulsant pharmacologic profiles, but pregabalin showed three- to sixfold greater potency as an anticonvulsant. Pregabalin, unlike gabapentin, exhibits linear absorption, with the observed maximum plasma drug concentration (C_{max}) and area under the plasma drug concentration–time profile increasing proportionally with dose.

In contrast, the extent of gabapentin absorption decreases with increasing dose. This may be one possible explanation as to why gabapentin was not more effective in higher doses in the trial previously referenced. The FDA approved pregabalin for the treatment of DPNP on the basis of two trials. One trial of 173 patients showed that pregabalin 100 mg three times daily by mouth for 8 weeks was both safe and effective in decreasing pain associated with DPN compared with placebo. Pregabalin also improved mood, sleep disturbance, and QoL, with minimal side effects.[96] A second, 8-week-long study of 338 patients stratified by creatinine clearance to receive pregabalin at a total of 75 mg, 300 mg, or 600 mg in three divided doses showed that the two higher doses were more effective than placebo.[97] Nevertheless, a recent report indicated that pregabalin was no more effective than placebo for the treatment of painful HIV neuropathy.[98]

No statistically significant difference in efficacy between the doses of 100 mg three times daily by mouth and 200 mg three times daily by mouth was detected, whereas adverse events were more common at the higher doses. Similar to what was observed in the duloxetine studies, pain relief was noted as early as 1 week after the initiation of treatment. A more recent publication analyzed seven separate trials using pregabalin for the treatment of DPNP and noted it to be effective.[99] Given these data, pregabalin should be preferred over gabapentin when treating PP. The most common side effects of pregabalin include dizziness, ataxia, and somnolence.[100] Unlike gabapentin, pregabalin is a Schedule V controlled substance because some patients with a history of alcohol or other substance abuse may be at increased risk for addiction to pregabalin. Despite these caveats, pregabalin may be considered a safe and effective treatment for DPNP with proper patient selection.

Topical Lidocaine

Topical lidocaine has FDA approval for the treatment of postherpetic neuralgia. However, Meier et al showed that this agent could be used effectively in persons with a variety of peripheral NP conditions and allodynia, including a subgroup without PHN.[101,102] When prescribed according to the package insert, the only side effects are the result of local skin irritation. Furthermore, the medication tends not to be absorbed systemically to any significant degree when the dose of three patches per day in a 12-hour-on/12-hour-off regimen is used or when four patches are used in an 18-hour period.[103] The main disadvantages of this therapy include cost, the inability to dose the medication continuously, and the issue that the patch must cover the area involved. As a practical matter, this medication should be reserved for patients with neuropathies that have not progressed much beyond the ankles bilaterally and who do not need around-the-clock analgesia.

"Second-Line" Neuropathic Pain Treatments

The other medications that have a grade A recommendation for the treatment of NP include the opioids and their related compounds. Opium and its derivatives have been used for the treatment of pain for millennia, although there is some controversy regarding the use of chronic opioids for the treatment of NP. Most authorities would agree that opioids have the advantage of being effective, relatively inexpensive, and potent analgesic medications. Few physicians would deny any patient narcotics for an acute pain syndrome, such as a broken bone or postoperative pain. In fact, narcotics are the treatment of choice in most acute pain conditions that are not responding to non-narcotic analgesics, such as nonsteroidal anti-inflammatory drugs. Common side effects include euphoria, drowsiness, nausea, vomiting, constipation, dilated pupils, and, in rare cases, respiratory depression.

The review by Dworkin et al makes several important points regarding opioid management.[4] The first is that multiple trials have shown that their efficacy is comparable to that of the other medications previously discussed, but they tend to produce more side effects. Moreover, these side effects may persist throughout the duration of treatment. As such, the benefit-to-risk ratio is not as favorable. Notably, the long-term safety of long-term opioid therapy has not been systematically evaluated. There is increasing evidence that long-term opioid use may result in clinically significant alteration of both the hypothalamopituitary-adrenal and the hypothalamopituitary-gonadal axes, resulting in suppression of luteinizing hormone, follicle-stimulating hormone, testosterone, estrogen, and cortisol.[104–109] There is also increasing evidence, both clinical and preclinical, that long-term opioid use may lead to immunosuppression.[110–112] For all of these reasons, patients with neuropathies as a result of autoimmune disorders should be counseled about this potential side effect. There is also some evidence to suggest that chronic opioid use can induce hyperalgesia.[113,114] One report stated that this phenomenon can occur during the initial treatment with a high-dose opioid.[115] Although this phenomenon has not been conclusively demonstrated in patients with chronic NP, its presence may make it difficult to distinguish from the phenomenon of tolerance or from an exacerbation of the underlying pain disorder. Given all of these potential adverse outcomes with long-term opioid use, patients who require this treatment should be referred to pain management experts.

It is unfortunate that the terms *dependence*, *addiction*, and *tolerance* are used interchangeably by patients as well as by some health care providers. Although these entities may be interrelated, they are not identical.[116] Dependence on a drug indicates that the body has come to rely on this agent for normal functioning such that lack of access to the drug will precipitate withdrawal symptoms. Opioid withdrawal symptoms may include sweating, tremor, vomiting, anxiety, insomnia, and muscle pain. All persons who are treated with opioids for a period will have dependence and withdrawal if they are denied access to the medication. As an example, a patient could be treated for tachycardia with a beta blocker because the patient is unable to have a normal heart rate without that medication. That person is, in effect, dependent on the beta blocker. If that person is admitted to a hospital without access to a beta blocker, withdrawal symptoms, such as tachycardia, are likely to recur. However, it would be inappropriate to state that this patient was "addicted" to the beta blocker.

Tolerance refers to the fact that escalating doses will be needed over time to achieve the same clinical effect. Some patients even have a cross-tolerance, in which prolonged use of one opioid results in a similar effect when using other opioids. Dose escalation is to be expected when prescribing opioids for the treatment of chronic pain. Dependence and tolerance should be anticipated by both the treating physician and the patient.

Addiction is an entirely different matter. Although exposure to a substance that induces tolerance and dependence is a prerequisite, addiction is not inevitable. Addiction appears to have a biochemical basis linked to the reward system in which DA is an important neurotransmitter. This system reinforces behaviors that are pleasurable because such behaviors tend to enhance survival. This is one explanation as to why humans tend to crave calorie-dense foods. Much as chronic NP can be viewed as a protective mechanism that has gone awry, there is increasing evidence of a genetic predisposition to addictive behavior. This is believed to result from pathologic alterations in this reward system. Addiction involves physical and psychological dependence separate from the need to avoid withdrawal symptoms. Addiction almost inevitably causes physiologic, chemical, and anatomic changes in the brain, along with behavioral changes. Addiction develops after an initial exposure to the addicting substance or activity. That initial exposure must occur for addiction to develop, but the exposure does not always lead to addiction. This is why some children of alcoholic parents avoid alcoholic beverages. Addictions lead to repeated behavioral problems, consume a lot of time and energy, and are marked by an increasing obsession with the drug. Furthermore, the cycle of quitting the addictive behavior, going through withdrawal, and relapsing may become self-reinforcing.[116] However, not all addictions are illegal or self-destructive. Many people are addicted to coffee and experience withdrawal symptoms if they are denied access to it. Despite this "caffeine dependence," there is no adverse effect on their professional or personal lives. Destructive addiction occurs when there is an adverse effect on the affected person's life. Addicted individuals may be willing to risk their family, their career, or their reputation to obtain the drug.

Despite these advances in the understanding of addiction, the laws that govern U.S. society often treat addiction as a crime rather than a disease entity. This has led to a hodgepodge of regulations that vary from state to state. There is a spirited debate in the medical community as to whether physicians are reluctant to prescribe opioid medications because they fear legal prosecution or enabling an addict. There seems to be a general consensus among the public that pain needs to be treated, but that addicts and those who enable them should be punished. In effect, the law is trying to minimize both type 1 and type 2 errors, a difficult, if not impossible, task. Although there are numerous guidelines and recommendations regarding how to distinguish addicts from nonaddicts, there is no perfect test. Further, the presence of an addiction should not prevent a person from receiving treatment. Addicts with chronic pain requiring opioids need to be followed very closely by a practitioner or a group of practitioners well versed in the use of opioids for pain management and well acquainted with the local and federal laws regarding prescribing opioids. As a practical matter, this usually involves a multidisciplinary pain clinic that can coordinate written agreements, perform drug testing where indicated, and arrange for the necessary and appropriate ancillary services. Few neuromuscular practitioners have the requisite time, expertise, and support staff to insure that these guidelines are followed. Nonetheless, clinicians should not be deterred from prescribing appropriate opioid therapy in accordance with the World Health Organization's "Pain Ladder."[117] This is a three-step tiered approach that begins with nonopioids and escalates to opioid use. Although this approach was developed for cancer pain, the basic principles may be used in any painful condition, as noted in Table 6-11. This table incorporates evidence-based neuropathic pain treatment guidelines,[118] the use of duloxetine,[119] opioid dosing guidelines,[120] and a comparison of opioid potency.[121] The only modification to the World Health Organization recommendation is that opioids are often required for moderate to severe acute pain. Practitioners should not withhold opioids from such patients because the goal of acute pain control is of paramount importance. Opioids are often required for the treatment of moderate to severe acute pain, but should be used with caution in other situations.

Ancillary Treatments

Little EBM literature supports the utility of occupational and physical therapy for patients with PP. Nonetheless, these allied health professionals have been of invaluable assistance in improving the QoL of patients with PP. Physical therapy, or physiotherapy, is an allied health profession that is dedicated to the development,

maintenance, and restoration of maximal movement and functional ability throughout the patient's life. There are many subspecialties within physical therapy, including cardiopulmonary, geriatric, neurologic, orthopedic, and pediatric. However, most neurologic and geriatric physical therapists tend to focus on CNS disorders rather than PNS disorders. Nonetheless, these subspecialties as well as nonsubspecialty physical therapists are skilled in gait and balance assessment. As such, a physical therapy consultation should be suggested to any patient with a gait disorder. Occupational therapists focus on maximizing a person's health and well-being in the activities of daily living by modifying the environment or adapting the activity. Occupational therapists are especially skilled at evaluating tasks that involve the use of the patient's hands and hand–eye coordination. Thus, the author recommends an occupational therapy consultation for all patients who have neurologic deficits affecting their hands, their activities of daily living, or their hand–eye coordination. Both of these allied health professions bring a valuable perspective to the management of a patient with PP. For these reasons, occupational therapy and physical therapy consultations are generally beneficial for all patients with polyneuropathies, painful or otherwise.

Conclusion

The treatment of PPs remains controversial and is an inexact science. Optimal outcomes are achieved when a physician–patient relationship based on mutual respect is established at the outset. The best outcomes occur when the underlying cause of pain is identified and removed. However, this is rarely achieved and therefore management of the condition is the norm. EBM has provided some guidelines regarding the medications that are most likely to have a beneficial outcome for the patient. The identification and treatment of all comorbid conditions will likely improve the patient's QoL. Some practitioners treating patients with PP underestimate the coincidence of depression, FM, and OSA. Acute pain syndromes that are moderate to severe often require the use of narcotic analgesics, and patients should receive them to reduce the likelihood that a chronic pain syndrome will develop. Once pain control is achieved, addition of a second, nonopioid agent, followed by a slow taper of the opioid, should be considered, although there is little EBM to support this recommendation. For mild acute pain syndromes, duloxetine and pregabalin have a relatively rapid onset of action and can be initiated without adjuvant therapy in most cases. The available evidence suggests that the agent of first choice to treat PP is duloxetine in depressed patients and pregabalin in nondepressed patients. In either case, the choice of medication should be left up to the patient after a discussion of the risks and benefits of all potential treatments. TCAs should be reserved for younger persons without cardiac risk factors who are able to tolerate their side effects and for whom cost is a factor. If an adequate trial of two medications from different classes is unsuccessful, the patient should be referred to a pain management specialist.

Conflict of Interest Statement

The author has previously served as a consultant for the Eli Lilly Company, manufacturer of duloxetine (Cymbalta). He has received honoraria in the past from this company for giving lectures on the diagnosis and treatment of diabetic peripheral neuropathic pain and FM. He is no longer a speaker for any pharmaceutical manufacturer.

References

1. Bennet GJ: Neuropathic pain: new insights, new interventions, *Hosp Pract (Minneap)* 33:95–98, 1998.

2. Torrance N, Smith BH, Bennett MI, Lee AJ: The epidemiology of chronic pain of predominantly neuropathic origin. Results from a general population survey, *J Pain* 7:281–289, 2006.

3. Bouhassira D, Lantéri-Minet M, Attal N, et al: Prevalence of chronic pain with neuropathic characteristics in the general population, *Pain* 136:380–387, 2008.

4. Dworkin RH, O'Connor AB, Backonja M, et al: Pharmacological management of neuropathic pain: evidence-based recommendations, *Pain* 132:237–251, 2007.

5. Dworkin RH, O'Connor AB, Audette J, et al: Recommendations for the pharmacological management of neuropathic pain: an overview and literature update, *Mayo Clin Proc* 85(Suppl 3):S3–S14, 2010.

6. Gronseth G, Cruccu G, Alksne J, et al: Practice parameter: the diagnostic evaluation and treatment of trigeminal neuralgia (an evidence-based review), *Neurology* 71:1183–1190, 2008.

7. Classification of chronic pain. Merskey H, Bogduk N, editors: *The International Association for the Study of Pain. Part III: Pain Terms. A Current List with Definitions and Notes on Usage*, ed 2, Seattle, 1994, IASP Press, pp 206–314.

8. Treede RD, Jensen TS, Campbell JN, et al: Neuropathic pain: redefinition and a grading system for clinical and research purposes, *Neurology* 70:1630–1635, 2008.

9. Acute pain, http://www.spine-health.com/glossary/a/acute-pain; Accessed 28.12.08.

10. Miaskowski CM, Bair M, Chou R, et al: *Principles of Analgesic Use in the Treatment of Acute Pain and Cancer Pain*, 6th ed. Glenview, IL, 2008, American Pain Society.

11. Turk DC, Okifuji A. Pain terms and taxonomies of pain. In Loeser JD, Bonica JJ, Butler SH, et al, editors: *Bonica's Management of Pain*, 3rd ed. New York, 2001, Lippincott Williams & Wilkins, pp 17–25.

12. Hayes C, Brown S, Lantry G, Burstal R: Neuropathic pain in the acute pain service: a prospective survey, *Acute Pain* 4:45–48, 2002.

13. Melzack R, Wall PD: Pain mechanisms: A new theory, *Science* 150:171–179, 1965.

14. Nurmikko TJ, Nash TP, Wiles JR: Recent advances: control of chronic pain, *BMJ* 317:1438–1441, 1998.

15. Pappagallo M, Werner M: *Chronic Pain: A Primer for Physicians*, Chicago, IL, 2007, Remedica.

16. Wada A, Wanke E, Gullo F, Sciavon E: Voltage-dependent Nav 1.7 sodium channels: multiple roles in adrenal chromaffin cells and peripheral nervous system, *Acta Physiologica* 192:221–231, 2008.

17. Cox JJ, Reimann F, Nicholas AK, et al: An SCN9A channelopathy causes congenital inability to experience pain, *Nature* 444:894–898, 2006.

18. Nagasako EM, Oaklander AL, Dworkin RH: Congenital insensitivity to pain: an update, *Pain* 101:213–219, 2003.

19. Bee LA, Dickenson AH: Neuropathic pain: multiple mechanisms at multiple sites, *Future Neurol* 2:661–671, 2007.

20. Passmore GM, Selyanko AA, Mistry M, et al: KCNQ/M currents in sensory neurons: significance for pain therapy, *J Neurosci* 23:7227–7236, 2003.

21. Rivera-Arconada I, Martinez-Gomez J, Lopez-Garcia JA: M-current modulators alter rat spinal nociceptive transmission: an electrophysiological study in vitro, *Neuropharmacology* 46:598–606, 2004.

22. Retigabine, http://www.valeant.com/researchAndDevelopment/pipeline/retigabine.jspf; Accessed 28.12.08.

23. Catterall WA, Perez-Reyes E, Snutch TP, Striessnig J: International Union of Pharmacology. XLVIII. Nomenclature and structure-function relationships of voltage-gated calcium channels, *Pharmacol Rev* 57:411–425, 2005.

24. Chaplan SR, Pogrel JW, Yaksh TL: Role of voltage-dependent calcium channel subtypes in experimental tactile allodynia, *Pharmacol Exp Ther* 269:1117–1123, 1994.

25. Snutch TP: Targeting chronic and neuropathic pain: the N-type calcium channel comes of age, *NeuroRx* 2:662–670, 2005.

26. Ziconotide, http://www.pdr.net/druginformation/FDAMonographsInfo.aspx?MonographID=2288; Accessed 26.11.08.

27. Sutton KG, Martin DJ, Pinnock RD, et al: Gabapentin inhibits high-threshold calcium channel currents in cultured rat dorsal root ganglion neurons, *Br J Pharmacol* 135:257–265, 2002.

28. Sevcik MA, Ghilardi JR, Peters CM, et al: Anti-NGF therapy profoundly reduces bone cancer pain and the accompanying increase in markers of peripheral and central sensitization, *Pain* 115:128–141, 2005.

29. Halvorson KG, Kubota K, Sevcik MA, et al: A blocking antibody to nerve growth factor attenuates skeletal pain induced by prostate tumor cells growing in bone, *Cancer Res* 65:9426–9435, 2005.

30. Staud R, Price DD, Robinso ME, et al: Maintenance of windup of second pain requires less frequent stimulation in fibromyalgia patients compared to normal controls, *Pain* 110:689–696, 2004.

31. Ulmann L, Hatcher JP, Hughes JP, et al: Up-regulation of P2X$_4$ receptors in spinal microglia after peripheral nerve injury mediates BDNF release and neuropathic pain, *J Neurosci* 28:11263–11268, 2008.

32. Harrison JK, Jiang Y, Chen S: Role for neuronally derived fractalkine in mediating interactions between neurons and CX3CR1-expressing microglia. http://www.pnas.org/content/95/18/10896.full; Accessed 19.11.08.

33. Bymaster FL, Dreshfield-Ahmad LJ, Threlkeld PG, et al: Comparative affinity of duloxetine and venlafaxine for serotonin and norepinephrine transporters in vitro and in vivo, human serotonin receptor subtypes and other neuronal receptors, *Neuropsychopharmacology* 25:871–880, 2001.

34. Iyengar S, Webster AA, Hemrick-Luecke SK, et al: Efficacy of duloxetine, a potent and balanced serotonin norepinephrine reuptake inhibitor in persistent pain models in rats, *J Pharmacol Exp Ther* 311:576–584, 2004.

35. Micó J, Ardid D, Berrocoso E, Eschalier A: Antidepressants and pain, *Trends Pharmacol Sci* 27:348–354, 2006.

36. McQuay H, Tramèr M, Nye B, et al: A systematic review of antidepressants in neuropathic pain, *Pain* 68:217–227, 1996.

37. Feighner JP: Mechanism of action of antidepressant medications, *J Clin Psychiatry* 60(Suppl 4):4–11, 1999. discussion 12–13.

38. Edwards JG, Anderson I: Systematic review and guide to selection of selective serotonin reuptake inhibitors, *Drugs* 57:507–533, 1999.

39. Corbett AD, Henderson G, McKnight AT, Paterson SJ: 75 years of opioid research: the exciting but vain quest for the Holy Grail, *Br J Pharmacol* 147 (Suppl 1):S153–S162, 2006.

40. Varga EV, Navratilova E, Stropova D, et al: Agonist-specific regulation of the delta-opioid receptor, *Life Sci* 76:599–612, 2004.

41. Jutkiewicz EM, Baladi MG, Folk JE, et al: The convulsive and electroencephalographic changes produced by nonpeptidic delta-opioid agonists in rats: comparison with pentylenetetrazol, *J Pharmacol Exp Ther* 317:1337–1348, 2006.

42. Broom DC, Jutkiewicz EM, Rice KC, et al: Behavioral effects of delta-opioid receptor agonists: potential antidepressants? *Jpn J Pharmacol* 90: 1–6, 2002.

43. Zhang H, Torregrossa MM, Jutkiewicz EM, et al: Endogenous opioids upregulate brain-derived neurotrophic factor mRNA through delta- and micro-opioid receptors independent of antidepressant-like effects, *Eur J Neurosci* 23:984–994, 2006.

44. Wong DL, Hockenberry-Eaton M, Wilson D, et al: *Wong's Essentials of Pediatric Nursing*, 6th ed. St. Louis, 2001, Mosby, p 1301.

45. Huskisson EC: Measurement of pain, *J Rheumatol* 9:768–769, 1982.

46. Melzack R: The McGill Pain Questionnaire: major properties and scoring methods, *Pain* 1:277–299, 1975.

47. Walid MS, Hyer L, Ajjan M, et al: Prevalence of opioid dependence in spine surgery patients and correlation with length of stay, *J Opioid Manag* 3:127–132, 2007.

48. Sackett DL, Rosenberg WMC, Gray JA: Evidence based medicine: what it is and what it isn't, *BMJ* 312:71–72, 1996.

49. U.S. Preventive Services Task Force Ratings: Grade Definitions: *Guide to Clinical Preventive Services, Third Edition: Periodic Updates*, Rockville, MD, 2000–2003, Agency for Healthcare Research and Quality. http://www.ahrq.gov/clinic/3rduspstf/ratings.htm; Accessed 31.12.08.

50. Center for Drug Evaluation and Research (CDER), U.S. Food and Drug Administration: *Oncology Tools: A Short Tour*, www.fda.gov; 2003; Accessed 15.06.04.

51. Neurontin, http://www.pfizer.com/files/products/uspi_neurontin.pdf; Accessed 26.11.08.

52. Lyrica, http://media.pfizer.com/files/products/uspi_lyrica.pdf; Accessed 28.11.08.

53. Cymbalta, http://pi.lilly.com/us/cymbalta-pi.pdf; Accessed 28.11.08.

54. Attal N, Cruccu G, Haanpää M, et al: EFNS guidelines on pharmacological treatment of neuropathic pain, *Eur J Neurol* 13:1153–1169, 2006.

55. Moulin DE, Clark AJ, Gilron I, et al: Pharmacological management of chronic neuropathic pain—consensus statement and guidelines from the Canadian Pain Society, *Pain Res Manag* 12:13–21, 2007.

56. Huizinga MM, Peltier A: Painful diabetic neuropathy: a management-centered review, *Clinical Diabetes* 25:6–15, 2007.

57. Egger M, Davey Smith G: Meta-analysis bias in location and selection of studies, *BMJ* 316:61–66, 1998.

58. Gilron I, Bailey JM, Tu D, et al: Morphine, gabapentin, or their combination for neuropathic pain, *N Engl J Med* 352:1324–1334, 2005.

59. Hanna M, O'Brien C, Wilson MC: Prolonged-release oxycodone enhances the effects of existing gabapentin therapy in painful diabetic neuropathy patients, *Eur J Pain* 6:804–813, 2008.

60. Walid MS, Donahue SN, Darmohray DM, et al: The fifth vital sign—what does it mean? *Pain Practice* 8:417–422, 2008.

61. Portenoy RK: Painful polyneuropathy, *Neurol Clin* 7:265–288, 1989.

62. Vaillancourt PD, Langevin HM: Painful peripheral neuropathies, *Med Clin North Am* 83:627–642, 1999.

63. England JD, Gronseth GS, Franklin G, et al: Evaluation of distal symmetric polyneuropathy: the role of autonomic testing, nerve biopsy and skin biopsy (an evidence-based review), *Muscle Nerve* 39:106–115, 2009.

64. England JD, Gronseth GS, Franklin G, et al: Evaluation of distal symmetric polyneuropathy: the role of laboratory and genetic testing (an evidence-based review), *Muscle Nerve* 39:116–125, 2009.

65. Moreira RO, Papelbaum M, Fontenelle LF, et al: Comorbidity of psychiatric disorders and symmetric distal polyneuropathy among type II diabetic outpatients, *Braz J Med Biol Res* 40:269–275, 2007.

66. Depression rating scales, http://neurotransmitter.net/depressionscales.html; Accessed 26.11.08.

67. Zung WW: A self-rating depression scale, *Arch Gen Psychiatry* 12:63–70, 1965.

68. Hamilton MA: Rating scale for depression, *J Neurol Neurosurg Psychiatry* 23:56–62, 1960.

69. Bhagwagar Z: Revisiting antidepressant-induced mania in bipolar disorder: Factor fiction? http://www.medscape.com/viewarticle/554129; Accessed 19.12.08.

70. Kessler RC, Chiu WT, Demler O, Walters EE: Prevalence, severity, and comorbidity of twelve-month DSM-IV disorders in the National Comorbidity Survey Replication (NCS-R), *Arch Gen Psychiatry* 62:617–627, 2005.

71. Weissman MM, Bland RC, Canino GJ, et al: Cross national epidemiology of major depression and bipolar disorder, *J Am Med Assoc* 276:293–299, 1996.

72. Narrow WE: One year prevalence of depressive disorders among adults 18 and over in the U.S.: NIMH ECA prospective data. Population estimates based on U.S. Census estimated residential population age 18 and over on July 1, 1998, Unpublished table. http://www.nimh.nih.gov/publicat/numbers.cfm#5; Accessed 26.11.08.

73. Tyrer F, Lawrenson RA, MacRae K, Farmer RDT: Prescribing of antidepressants in cardiovascular disease: a study using a computerised general practice data base, http://priory.com/fam/cardiodep.htm; Accessed 20.12. 2008.

74. Anxiety disorders, http://www.nimh.nih.gov/health/publications/anxiety-disorders/complete-publication.shtml#pub8; Accessed 26.11.08.

75. Epworth sleepiness scale, http://www.stanford.edu/~dement/epworth.html; Accessed 26.11.08.

76. Strollo PJ, Rogers RM: Obstructive sleep apnea, *N Engl J Med* 334:99–104, 1996.

77. Davies RJ, Stradling JR: The relationship between neck circumference, radiographic pharyngeal anatomy, and the obstructive sleep apnoea syndrome, *Eur Respir J* 3:509–514, 1990.

78. Flemons WW, Remmers JE, Whitelaw WA, Brant R: The clinical prediction of obstructive sleep apnea [abstract], *Am Rev Respir Dis* 145(4 pt 2):A722, 1992.

79. Katz I, Stradling J, Slutsky S, et al: Do patients with obstructive sleep apnea have thick necks? *Am Rev Respir Dis* 141(5 Pt 1):1228–1231, 1990.

80. Lanfranchi P, Somers VA: Obstructive sleep apnea and vascular disease, *Respir Res* 2:315–319, 2001.

81. Restless legs syndrome, http://www.irlssg.org/rlsinformation.html#a1; Accessed 26.11.08.

82. Restless legs syndrome, http://www.ninds.nih.gov/disorders/restless_legs/detail_restless_legs.htm; Accessed 26.11.08.

83. Wolfe F, Smythe HA, Yunus MB: The American College of Rheumatology 1990 criteria for the classification of fibromyalgia. Report of the Multicenter Criteria Committee, *Arthritis Rheum* 33:160–172, 1990.

84. Pope HG, Hudson JI: A supplemental interview for forms of "affective spectrum disorder". *Int J Psychiatry Med* 21:205–232, 1991.

85. Arnold LM: Management of fibromyalgia and comorbid psychiatric disorders, *J Clin Psychiatry* 69(Suppl 2):14–19, 2008.

86. Dworkin RH, Fields HL: Fibromyalgia from the perspective of neuropathic pain, *J Rheumatol* (Suppl 75):1–5, 2005.

87. Antiepileptic drug safety, http://www.fda.gov/medwatch/safety/2008/safety08.htm#Antiepileptic; Accessed 20.12.08.

88. Antidepressants and upper gastrointestinal bleeding, http://www.pubmedcentral.nih.gov/articlerender.fcgi?artid=1116881; Accessed 28.12.08.

89. Burckhardt D, Raeder E, Muller V, et al: Cardiovascular effects of tricyclic and tetracyclic antidepressants, *JAMA* 239:213–216, 1978.

90. Kantor ST, Bigger JT, Glassman AH, et al: Imipramine-induced heart block: a longitudinal case study, *JAMA* 231:1364–1366, 1975.

91. Ray WA, Meredith S, Thapa BP, et al: Cyclic antidepressants and the risk of sudden cardiac death, *Clin Pharmacol Therapeutics* 75:234–241, 2004.

92. Dworkin RH, Backonja M, Rowbotham MC, et al: Advances in neuropathic pain: diagnosis, mechanisms, and treatment recommendations, *Arch Neurol* 60:1524–1534, 2003.

93. Effexor (venlafaxine), http://www.effexorxr.com/medication-guide.aspx; Accessed 26.12.08.

94. Backonja M, Beydoun A, Edwards KR, et al: Gabapentin for the symptomatic treatment of painful neuropathy in patients with diabetes mellitus: a randomized controlled trial, *JAMA* 280:1831–1836, 1998.

95. Miller R, Bockbrader H, Chapel S: Comparison of pregabalin and gabapentin pharmacodynamics in patients with refractory partial seizures, Abstract of the Annual Meeting of the Population Approach Group in Europe, Brugge, Belgium, June 2006. http://www.page-meeting.org/?abstract=941; Accessed 26.11.08.

96. Rosenstock J, Tuchman M, LaMoreaux L, Shama U: Pregabalin for the treatment of painful diabetic peripheral neuropathy: a double-blind, placebo-controlled trial, *Pain* 110:628–638, 2004.

97. Lesser H, Sharma U, LaMoreaux L, Poole RM: Pregabalin relieves symptoms of painful diabetic neuropathy: a randomized controlled trial, *Neurology* 63:2104–2110, 2004.

98. Simpson DM, Schifitto G, Clifford DB, et al: Pregabalin for painful HIV neuropathy: a randomized, double-blind, placebo-controlled trial, *Neurology* 74(5):413–420, 2010.

99. Freeman RF, Durso-DeCruz E, Emir B: Efficacy, safety and tolerability of pregabalin treatment of painful diabetic peripheral neuropathy: findings from 7 randomized, controlled trials across a range of doses, *Diabetes Care* 31:1448–1454, 2008.

100. Block F: Gabapentin therapy for pain. *Nervenarzt* 72:69–77, 2001.

101. Meier T, Faust M, Huppe M, Schmucker P: Reduction of chronic pain for non-postherpetic peripheral neuropathies after topical treatment with a lidocaine patch, [Translated from German]*Schmerz* 118:172–178, 2004.

102. Meier T, Wasner G, Faust M, et al: Efficacy of lidocaine patch 5% in the treatment of focal peripheral neuropathic pain syndromes: a randomized, double-blind, placebo-controlled study, *Pain* 106:151–158, 2003.

103. Gammaitoni AR, Davis MW: Pharmacokinetics and tolerability of lidocaine patch 5% with extended dosing, *Ann Pharmacother* 36:236–240, 2002.

104. Mendelson JH, Meyer RE, Ellingboe J, et al: Effects of heroin and methadone on plasma cortisol and testosterone, *J Pharmacol Exp Ther* 195:296–302, 1975.

105. Daniell HW: Hypogonadism in men consuming sustained-action oral opioids, *J Pain* 3:377–384, 2002a.

106. Lee C, Ludwig S, Duerksen D: Low serum cortisol associated with opioid use: case report and review of the literature, *Endocrinologist* 12:5–8, 2002.

107. Paice JA, Penn RD, Shott S: Intraspinal morphine for chronic pain: a retrospective, multicenter study, *J Pain Symptom Manage* 11:71–80, 1996.

108. Finch PM, Roberts LJ, Price L, et al: Hypogonadism in patients treated with intrathecal morphine, *Clin J Pain* 16:251–254, 2000.

109. Abs R, Verhelst J, Maeyaert J, et al: Endocrine consequences of long-term intrathecal administration of opioids, *J Clin Endocrinol Metab* 85: 2215–2222, 2000.

110. Roy S, Loh HH: Effects of opioids on the immune system, *Neurochem Res* 21:1375–1386, 1996.

111. Risdahl JM, Khanna KV, Peterson PK, et al: Opiates and infection, *J Neuroimmunol* 83:4–18, 1998.

112. Peterson PK, Sharp BM, Gekker G, et al: Morphine promotes the growth of HIV-1 in human peripheral blood mononuclear cell cocultures, *AIDS* 4:869–873, 1990.

113. Angst MS, Clark DJ: Opioid-induced hyperalgesia: A qualitative systematic review, *Anesthesiology* 104:570–587, 2006.

114. Mao J: Opioid-induced abnormal pain sensitivity: Implications in clinical opioid therapy, *Pain* 100:213–217, 2002.

115. Celerier E, Laulin J-P, Corcuff J-B, et al: Progressive enhancement of delayed hyperalgesia induced by repeated heroin administration: a sensitization process, *J Neurosci* 21:4074–4080, 2001.

116. Nash MN: Addiction, http://www.emedicinehealth.com/addiction/article_em.htm; Accessed 20.12.08.

117. World Health Organization's Pain Ladder, http://www.who.int/cancer/palliative/painladder/en/; Accessed 20.12.08.

118. Finnerup NB, Otto M, McQuay HJ, et al: Algorithm for neuropathic pain treatment: an evidence-based proposal, *Pain* 118:289–305, 2005.

119. VHA Pharmacy Benefits Management Strategic Healthcare Group, and the Medical Advisory Panel. Duloxetine in painful diabetic neuropathy and fibromyalgia [article online]: http://www.pbm.va.gov/monograph/6upaeDuloxetine.pdf; Accessed 26.11.08.

120. Dosing threshold for selected opioids, http://www.agencymeddirectors.wa.gov/Files/OpioidGdline.pdf; Accessed 31.12.08.

121. Galvagno SM, Correll DJ, Narang S: Safe oral equianalgesic opioid dosing for patients with moderate-to-severe pain, http://www.residentandstaff.com/issues/articles/2007-04_06.asp; Accessed 31.12.08.

Christopher W. Mitchell, MD
Tulio E. Bertorini, MD

Principles and Guidelines of Immunotherapy in Neuromuscular Disorders

Among the variety of diseases seen by neuromuscular specialists, immune-mediated disorders generate tremendous interest. These disorders are relatively common and often respond favorably to treatment. The timely and accurate diagnosis and management of these entities can be a gratifying experience for both patient and physician. This chapter provides a general overview of the components and function of the immune system and discusses the use of individual therapies aimed at altering the immune response to treat these disorders. Lastly, the available evidence for the use of these drugs in the treatment of select neuromuscular disorders is summarized.

Basics of the Immune Response

The principal function of the immune system is the differentiation between self and non-self and resultant rejection of the latter. When infection with bacterial, viral, fungal, or parasitic organisms occurs, components of the pathogen are recognized by specialized immune cells. The first such cells to come into contact with the invading organism are macrophages and dendritic cells. These cells are able to recognize pathogens using a small number of constitutively expressed receptors called pattern-recognition receptors, such as the Toll-like receptors. Such receptors bind common elements of microorganisms that cause disease (e.g., endotoxin of gram-negative bacteria or lipoteichoic acid of group B *Streptococcus*) and help to provide a quick response to a threat but lack the exquisite specificity and plasticity of the adaptive immune system. The role of the innate immune response in human disease, particularly in the development of autoimmunity, is only beginning to be understood.[1,2]

Adaptive immunity refers to the ability of lymphocytes to respond to a specific threat, to amplify the response to that threat, and to retain memory of the threat to quickly respond when re-exposure occurs. Antigens, which are molecules that are capable of inducing an immune response, are presented to T lymphocytes via major histocompatibility complex (MHC) molecules. Class I MHC molecules present endogenous antigens, such as those present intracellularly during a viral infection. In contrast, class II MHC molecules are present on antigen-presenting cells, such as macrophages and dendritic cells, and present exogenous (i.e., extracellular) antigens to lymphocytes. In each case, recognition and response occurs by binding of the antigen with the

lymphocyte's T cell receptor (TCR) along with the interaction of appropriate costimulatory molecules (e.g., CD28 with CD80). The specificity of the adaptive immune response is due in large part to the vast repertoire of TCRs available. This enormous variety is generated through random rearrangement of the genes encoding for TCRs during lymphocyte development. The result is a unique TCR for each lymphocyte that binds with high affinity to a single antigen.

Once a pathogen is encountered and its antigens are presented to and recognized by a T lymphocyte, an intracellular signaling cascade is initiated that leads to an effective T cell response. The initial events in this signaling cascade consist of hydrolysis of components of the T cell's lipid bilayer to form inositol triphosphate and diacylglycerol. Diacylglycerol activates protein kinase C, and inositol triphosphate facilitates the entry of calcium into the cytosol. Calcium in turn activates numerous proteins, including calcineurin and several DNA-binding proteins. Calcineurin facilitates the release of interleukin-2 (IL-2), a powerful stimulator of T cell proliferation (discussed later), whereas DNA-binding proteins alter gene transcription. The end result of these changes is T cell proliferation and differentiation. Thus stimulated, T cells are ready to respond to the threat.

T lymphocytes bearing the cluster of differentiation marker 8 (i.e., CD8+ lymphocytes) respond by engaging in cell-mediated cytotoxicity and act most effectively against viruses by destroying host cells that have been invaded. The response of CD4+ T lymphocytes usually involves the secretion of substances, such as cytokines, that modify the cell-mediated or humoral immune response. T helper type 1 (Th1) cells are CD4+ lymphocytes that release cytokines that strengthen the cell-mediated, cytotoxic response to an antigen. T helper type 2 (Th2) cells, in contrast, release cytokines that may be anti-inflammatory or that favor the production of antibodies by B cells.

Immunoglobulins are also produced in a large variety and contribute to the specificity of the immune system. Like the TCRs, the genes for immunoglobulin heavy and light chains undergo random genetic rearrangement during B cell development, resulting in a complement of lymphocytes that each bear a unique receptor and respond to a particular antigen. In addition, mature B lymphocytes can alter immunoglobulin production from one immunoglobulin class to another when stimulated. Immunoglobulin A (IgA) is secreted at mucosal surfaces and is most useful in repelling pathogens in the gastrointestinal tract and respiratory tree.

IgE mediates the release of cytotoxic substances from eosinophils, mast cells, and basophils, and is most effective against parasitic organisms, but it also plays an important role in allergic reactions. IgM is the first subtype produced in response to a threat and is most effective at activating complement. IgG can also effectively activate complement and is able to coat, or *opsonize*, a pathogen for effective clearance by phagocytes. In addition to immunoglobulins, mature B lymphocytes are distinguished by their expression of cell markers CD19 and CD20.

Complement refers to a group of proteins that are produced in the liver and participate in humoral immune responses in association with antibodies, particularly IgM and most classes of IgG. Complement can be activated by immunoglobulin binding to an antigen or deposited through less specific mechanisms. The deposition of complement on a foreign substance, allowing for its recognition by other immune components and subsequent clearance, is called *opsonization*. In addition, serum complement proteins C5b, C6, C7, C8, and C9 associate to form a cytolytic structure called the *membrane attack complex*. Some products of complement activation (e.g., C5a) may also serve as chemotactic factors, drawing immune cells to the area for a more robust response.

A key feature of the immune system is the communication between cell types, allowing for the coordination of humoral and cellular responses. This communication is mediated in large part by proteins called *cytokines* that are secreted by many different types of cells, including antigen-presenting cells and lymphocytes. The interferons and interleukins are considered cytokines, as are tumor necrosis factor (TNF) and the chemokines, or chemotactic cytokines.

Interferons were first noted to be produced in the setting of viral infection, where they effectively interfered with viral replication. Interferons, which are generated by a wide variety of cell types, are also produced in response to other microorganisms as well as neoplasms. Once interferons bind to their receptors, they initiate a broad alteration of gene expression, ultimately leading to multiple antiviral and antioncogenic actions, including apoptosis.[3,4]

Interleukins are a large group of small polypeptide molecules that, in general, have pleiotropic effects on lymphocytes as well as many other cell types. This feature, combined with the baffling array of interactions among the different cytokines, makes the understanding of individual interleukins difficult. Still, some of these molecules have roles that are predictable enough to bear mentioning. IL-1 augments lymphocyte production of other cytokines, notably IL-2. It is also partly responsible for many of the symptoms of severe systemic illness, including fever, anorexia, myalgias, and decreased production of so-called housekeeping proteins, such as albumin. IL-2 primarily stimulates T lymphocyte proliferation. IL-10, in contrast, has a predominantly anti-inflammatory action and appears to help induce tolerance.[5]

Tumor necrosis factor is a pro-inflammatory cytokine that was initially named for its antioncogenic actions. Its effects are similar to those of IL-1, as discussed earlier. Both TNF and IL-1 can act on endothelium to increase intercellular and vascular adhesion molecules, facilitating egress of inflammatory cells into the tissues. In addition, TNF causes the cachexia seen in some patients with cancer.

Chemokines are named for their ability to draw inflammatory cells to an area along a chemical gradient, and like interleukins, have diverse functions. Chemokines can be subdivided based on the amino acid sequence on the N-terminal portion of the molecule. One group has two adjacent cysteine residues (i.e., the CC family of chemokines), whereas another has two cysteine residues separated by some other amino acid (i.e., the CXC family). It is believed that CC chemokines are more effective in attracting macrophages, eosinophils, and basophils, whereas CXC chemokines attract polymorphonuclear granulocytes.

Autoimmunity

The elements of the immune system described earlier usually work together in the differentiation of self from non-self with amazing fidelity. The importance of this system in fighting infection is highlighted by the various inherited immunodeficiency states as well as by the more recent HIV/AIDS epidemic. However, when the line between self and non-self becomes blurred in autoimmune disorders, these mechanisms, which are so effective in the destruction of invading pathogens, can be unleashed on the host, with devastating consequences.

Because of the random nature of recombination of genes involved in T and B cell receptor formation, there are always lymphocytes that have an affinity for self-antigens. Thankfully, many of these are eliminated during their development. In the bone marrow and thymus, primitive B and T lymphocytes are exposed to numerous self-proteins bound to MHC molecules. Those lymphocytes whose receptors have little or no affinity for the MHC molecule are unable to participate effectively in an appropriate immune response and are allowed to die. Lymphocytes with receptors that bind with very high affinity to the MHC molecule are likely to initiate autoimmunity and are actively targeted for destruction. Both groups undergo apoptosis, or programmed cell death. This process has been termed *clonal deletion*.[6]

Although many self-antigens are present in the bone marrow or thymus, not all are. Therefore, a peripheral mechanism for inducing tolerance must also be in operation. Some lymphocytes possess receptors that recognize antigens that are sequestered in immunologically privileged sites. Anatomic barriers, such as the blood–brain and blood–nerve barrier, prevent these lymphocytes from encountering their antigens under normal circumstances. Such T and B cells are said to be in a state of ignorance.[7] If there is a breakdown of the barrier or if the antigens are released through injury or infection, then an autoimmune response may occur.

Some autoreactive lymphocytes are held in check by regulatory T cells. These unique CD4+ T cells act through membrane-bound or soluble molecules, such as cytokines, to suppress immune responses. The absence of these cells promotes the development of numerous autoimmune diseases in mice.[8]

Even when an autoreactive T cell encounters its antigen, activation and an immune response do not always occur. In addition to TCR binding to the protein–MHC complex, costimulatory molecules such as CD28 must bind to their respective receptors on the antigen-presenting cell if activation is to take place. If such costimulatory molecules are not present, the lymphocyte undergoes apoptosis. The presence of Fas ligand, which is constitutively expressed in some tissues, and its interaction with its receptor CD95 can also directly trigger cell death of autoreactive T lymphocytes.[7] In addition, a proper balance of Th1 and Th2 cytokines (e.g., IL-2 and IL-10, respectively) helps to keep autoreactive lymphocytes in check.

To better explain how the cellular constituents and soluble factors of the immune system can damage the peripheral nervous system, following is a brief review of their role in the development and maintenance of chronic inflammatory demyelinating polyradiculoneuropathy (CIDP).

The initial trigger that leads to immune attack of peripheral nerves in CIDP remains obscure, as in most autoimmune disorders. The most popular notion, for which there is some existing evidence, is molecular mimicry. Approximately one third of patients with CIDP report a preceding illness or vaccination within 6 months before the development of symptoms.[9] In axonal forms of Guillain-Barré syndrome (GBS), certain infectious organisms, such as *Campylobacter jejuni*, are likely to cause a cross-reaction against nerve ganglioside antigens, such as GM1, and trigger the autoimmune cascade.[10] In rare cases, CIDP and malignant melanoma may coexist,[11] suggesting some molecular mimicry between epitopes on melanoma cells and Schwann cells, both of which develop from the neural crest.

Regardless of the inciting event, once autoreactive T cells or immunoglobulins against nerve antigens appear, the immune system's property of biologic amplification takes over (Fig. 7-1). Circulating immunoglobulins bind to their antigens and can be recognized by patrolling monocytes that then become activated to begin phagocytosis. Once nerve antigens are digested, they are presented via MHC II molecules to T cells. T cells that recognize these antigens become activated in the presence of appropriate costimulatory molecules. Th1 cells generate IL-2, which further activates these self-reactive T cells. In addition, both T cells and phagocytes produce TNF, which increases vascular permeability and increases endothelial intercellular and vascular adhesion molecules. These substances allow for adhesion to the vascular wall and transmigration of inflammatory cells into the area. Chemokines secreted by many different cell types in the immune response also ensure that lymphocytes and macrophages are drawn to the region. Th2 cells in the area are stimulated to release interleukins, such as IL-4 and IL-6, which promote immunoglobulin production by B cells. Immunoglobulins that recognize nerve antigens not only facilitate phagocytosis but also can activate complement, resulting in membrane attack complex formation and cell lysis as well as the production of chemotactic factors.[12] In addition, immunoglobulins against certain myelin proteins, such as P_0, may be partially responsible for the development of conduction block seen on nerve conduction studies.[13] A more comprehensive review of the proposed pathophysiology of CIDP is provided by Kieseier et al.[14]

Immunotherapy

After a review of the components of the immune system and the problem of autoimmunity, the next topic is the available medications and treatments that can alter the immune response for those affected by autoimmune neuromuscular conditions. As with all drugs, these medications have potential side effects, some modest and some considerable. The first agents discussed are those used most frequently. (For more details on immunotherapy in neuromuscular diseases, see Chapters 14, 18, and 21.)

Corticosteroids

All corticosteroids bind to the glucocorticoid receptor, which then enters the nucleus and binds to glucocorticoid-responsive elements within the chromosomal DNA. This results in alteration of the chromatin structure and subsequent up- or downregulation of gene transcription. As expected, the consequences of this shift in gene expression are varied. Corticosteroids are known to increase apoptosis, or programmed cell death, of autoreactive T cells as well as to inhibit T cell proliferation and shift cytokine profiles.[15]

Many corticosteroids are available, all with varying anti-inflammatory and mineralocorticoid actions. The most commonly used drug is prednisone. It is actually a prodrug and is converted by the liver to the active drug prednisolone. Although very low doses can be helpful for certain conditions, such as polymyalgia rheumatica,[16] most disorders require a more aggressive approach referred to as *slam and taper*. A high dose of 0.5 to 2.0 mg/kg is prescribed for daily use and after 1 month tapered to alternate-day dosing. The dose can then be further tapered to reach the lowest dose that controls symptoms. At alternate-day or daily doses of less than 20 mg, the rate of tapering may need to be very slow, perhaps no more than 10% per month, to avoid disease recurrence or adrenal insufficiency.

Corticosteroids are also used in focal neuropathies that are of autoimmune etiology, such as Bell palsy. In this disease, the combination of corticosteroids and antiviral agents was considered beneficial. However, in two new controlled studies, the addition of antivirals was not superior to prednisolone alone. Prednisolone was given in doses of 50[17] to 60 mg[18] daily. Deflazacort is another steroid preparation that has been used for the treatment of Duchenne muscular dystrophy and appears to cause less weight gain than prednisone.[19]

Other regimens for corticosteroids have been proposed. Some experts favor a gradual introduction of steroids with a 5- to 10-mg daily dose that is increased by 5 mg increments every few days until the 0.5- to 2.0-mg/kg dose is achieved. This is primarily used for patients with myasthenia gravis in whom there is a risk of disease exacerbation by sudden, high doses of steroids. Lopate et al[20] suggested a unique corticosteroid regimen for patients with CIDP. They performed a retrospective study of patients with CIDP who were treated with intravenous immunoglobulin (IVIg), oral corticosteroids or cyclosporine, or intermittent intravenous methylprednisolone. They found no difference in improvement in muscle strength between groups over an average of 4.5 years of follow-up; however, weight gain and cushingoid features were much less frequent in those treated with intermittent intravenous steroids.[20] Intravenous methylprednisolone is also sometimes used in the management of myasthenia gravis in crisis. A recent study also suggested that weekly pulses of oral methylprednisolone may be effective in the treatment of CIDP.[21]

The side effects of corticosteroids are well known (Box 7-1) and often limit treatment. Acutely, most patients tolerate steroids well, but some experience insomnia or depression. Rarely, acute psychosis may occur.[22] Hyperglycemia and hypertension can develop quickly as well. A low-calorie, low-carbohydrate, low-sodium diet may help to lessen these problems as well as later weight gain. Gastric ulceration is also a concern, and patients may need to take proton pump inhibitors prophylactically. Late effects of steroids include the development of type II muscle fiber atrophy, glaucoma, cataracts, acne, avascular necrosis, and osteoporosis.[23] Both calcium and vitamin D supplementation (with daily doses of 1000 mg and 800 IU, respectively) have been found to be effective in helping to prevent loss of bone mineral density in patients taking chronic glucocorticoids, and their use is strongly recommended.[24] More active forms of vitamin D, such as calcitriol, can also be used, but patients must be monitored for the development of hypercalcemia and hypercalciuria. Several randomized clinical trials have found bisphosphonates to be effective for the prevention and treatment of glucocorticoid-induced osteoporosis.[25-29] A recent study showed that human recombinant parathyroid hormone or teriparatide provided greater improvement in bone mineral density and fewer fractures than daily alendronate.[30] Bone densitometry is recommended at the initiation of corticosteroid therapy as well as yearly thereafter.[24]

In addition to the complications listed earlier, the development of infections while taking steroids is also feared. Patients may need to be evaluated even during the course of what appears to be a common upper respiratory illness. Patients undergoing long-term treatment with corticosteroids should be vaccinated yearly for influenza. Those taking glucocorticoids are also at risk for pneumococcal disease and should probably receive the multivalent vaccine that is available, especially if they are older than 65 years. Contrary to intuition, patients taking steroids appear to have intact immune responses to these vaccines.[31,32] Of course, these patients are susceptible to unusual infectious organisms as well. *Pneumocystis carinii*, in particular, is a concern, especially because effective prevention is available in the form of trimethoprim-sulfamethoxazole.[33] Because of the many side effects of corticosteroids, other immunosuppressive drugs are often used in an attempt to lower or eliminate the steroid dosage while keeping the disease in remission.

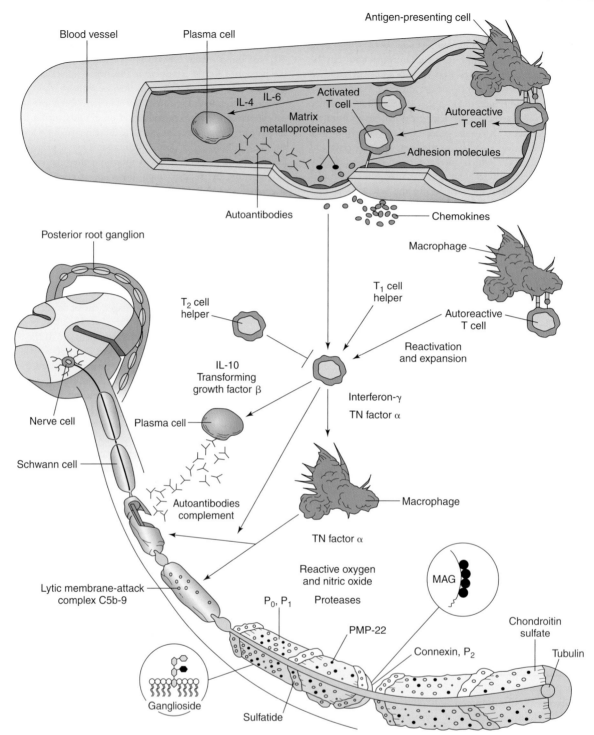

Figure 7-1 Immunopathogenesis of chronic inflammatory demyelinating neuropathy. A schematic illustration of the basic principles of the cellular and humoral immune responses shows that autoreactive T cells recognize a specific autoantigen in the context of major histocompatibility complex class II and costimulatory molecules on the surface of antigen-presenting cells (macrophages) in the systemic immune compartment. An infection might trigger this event through molecular mimicry, a cross-reaction toward epitopes shared between the microbial agent and nerve antigens. These activated T lymphocytes can cross the blood–nerve barrier in a process involving cellular adhesion molecules, matrix metalloproteinases, and chemokines. Within the peripheral nervous system, T cells activate macrophages that enhance phagocytic activity, the production of cytokines, and the release of toxic mediators, including nitric oxide reactive oxygen intermediates, matrix metalloproteinases, and proinflammatory cytokines, including tumor necrosis factor α and interferon γ. Autoantibodies crossing the blood–nerve barrier or locally produced by plasma cells contribute to demyelination and axonal damage. Autoantibodies can mediate demyelination by antibody-dependent cellular cytotoxicity, potentially block epitopes that are functionally relevant for nerve conduction, and activate the complement system by the classic pathway, yielding proinflammatory mediators and the lytic membrane-attack complex C5b-9. Termination of the inflammatory response occurs through the induction of T-cell apoptosis and the release of anti-inflammatory cytokines, including interleukin-10 and transforming growth factor β. The myelin sheath (*insets*) is composed of various proteins, such as myelin protein zero, that account for more than 50% of the total membrane protein in human peripheral nervous system myelin, myelin protein 22, myelin basic protein, myelin-associated glycoprotein, connexin 32, and gangliosides and related glycolipids. These molecules have been identified as target antigens for antibody responses with varying frequencies in patients with this disease. IL, interleukin; MAG, myelin-associated glycoprotein; PMP, peripheral myelin protein; TN, tumor necrosis. (Modified and reprinted with permission from Koller H, Keiseier BC, Jander S, Hartung HP. Chronic inflammatory demyelinating polyneuropathy. *N Engl J Med* 352:1343–1356, 2005.)

Box 7-1 Complications of Systemic Corticosteroids

Central Nervous System

Psychosis
Mania
Depression
Insomnia
Epidural lipomatosis

Ophthalmologic

Cataracts
Glaucoma
Corneal ulceration/perforation in those with HSV infections

Ear, Nose, and Throat

Epistaxis

Cardiovascular

Sodium and water retention
Peripheral edema
Worsening of congestive heart failure

Pulmonary

Reactivation of tuberculosis

Gastrointestinal

Gastric ulceration
Perforation (in the setting of infection)

Infectious

Increased susceptibility to infection
Poor wound healing

Genitourinary

Decreased spermatozoa number and motility

Endocrinologic/Musculoskeletal

Induction or worsening of diabetes mellitus
Adrenal insufficiency (on withdrawal or when stressed)
Osteoporosis
Central obesity
Avascular necrosis

Neuromuscular

Type II muscle fiber atrophy
Worsening of myasthenia gravis on initiation

Intravenous Immunoglobulin

Intravenous immunoglobulin is a unique therapy. This blood product is prepared from a large number of donors, on average, 5000 to 10,000 for each dosage. Although the main component of IVIg is IgG, many other molecules are present. Some of these include IgA, IgM, soluble anti-TCR, and various cytokines. There is unlikely to be a single mechanism of action for IVIg, but certain ones may be important for particular diseases. Some proposed mechanisms of action include promotion of T cell apoptosis, impaired migration of T cells, restoration of the balance between pro- and anti-inflammatory cytokines, suppression of autoreactive B cells, and enhanced clearance of IgG in the circulation.[34] As with many other medications, the role of genetic factors in predicting responsiveness to this form of therapy is just beginning to be realized.[35]

The standard dose of IVIg is 2 g/kg. At the initiation of therapy, the dose may be divided equally over 2 to 5 days. For young patients with normal cardiovascular and renal function, infusion over 2 days

may be preferred. Although there is some evidence that more rapid infusion over 2 days is superior to longer courses,[36] the data from trials in GBS show no such benefit.[37] For long-term use, a dose of 1 to 2 g/kg over 1 to 2 days is given. Infusions can be repeated every month to 6 weeks or as the patient's symptoms dictate.

Infusions of IVIg are well tolerated by most patients. The most common side effect is a mild headache. Rarely, a more severe headache from aseptic meningitis occurs. It is not uncommon for patients to have chills or myalgias during the initial infusion. These symptoms typically improve with acetaminophen and a slower rate of infusion. Patients may feel fatigued or mildly nauseated after treatment. Rash is not uncommon. Because of the risk of renal insufficiency as a result of acute tubular necrosis, patients should be well hydrated and electrolytes and serum creatinine should be monitored. This complication may be more common in preparations containing sucrose. Older patients and those with congestive heart failure could experience fluid overload, and more concentrated preparations may be preferred in this setting. Other serious side effects include thrombosis as a result of serum hyperviscosity. These thrombotic events include deep venous thrombosis and pulmonary embolism as well as stroke or myocardial infarction.[38] The use of aspirin or subcutaneous or low-molecular-weight heparin should be considered in patients who are at risk for these events. In addition, a less concentrated formula may reduce this risk. Anaphylaxis is a rare complication and may occur in individuals who have anti-IgA antibodies, such as those with IgA deficiency. Because all IVIg preparations contain some level of IgA and IgA deficiency is relatively common, IgA levels should be obtained before the administration of IVIg. If such a deficiency is identified, a preparation with a very low IgA level, such as immune globulin (Gammagard, Baxter, Westlake Village, CA), or an alternate therapy should be considered. Because IVIg is a blood product that is purified from thousands of donors, patients may be concerned about the risk of infection. They should be reassured that blood donors are screened for known transmissible infections, such as HIV and hepatitis viruses, but it is possible that currently unknown pathogens may be transmitted. Finally, some spurious laboratory test results may occur after IVIg infusion, namely, an elevated erythrocyte sedimentation rate and pseudohyponatremia.[36]

Although IVIg is safe and effective for several neuromuscular disorders, cost remains a major drawback to this mode of therapy. Additionally, shortages of individual preparations occur not infrequently and may limit its usage.

The need for intravenous access can become an issue for some patients, especially those needing treatment over several years. Subcutaneous administration of immunoglobulins via a small pump may be a viable option and could reduce the cost of treatment by 50%.[39] Further study of this mode of immunoglobulin administration is needed. An expert consensus on IVIg use in neuromuscular disorders was recently published.[40]

Therapeutic Plasma Exchange

Therapeutic plasma exchange has been used primarily for patients with GBS, although it can be beneficial in other disorders as well. This procedure is similar to IVIg in that its effects are usually believed to be on the humoral immune system or other soluble factors, such as cytokines. As with IVIg, its effects are transient, and repeated treatments or other immunosuppressives must be used for chronic disorders.

The procedure of therapeutic plasma exchange consists of removal of whole blood from the patient followed by separation of cellular and plasma components by one of several mechanisms. The cellular components and some plasma plus a replacement solution are then returned to the patient. When a centrifugation technique is used, whole blood is spun until the components separate. The plasma component is removed, along with immunoglobulins and other soluble large molecules. In a filtration technique, such large molecules are able to pass across the filter but the cellular elements are not. Centrifugation often uses a lower blood flow rate, and peripheral venous access may be used. Filtration devices, on the other hand, have higher flow rates and usually require central venous access. Regardless of which technique is used, a replacement solution consisting of fresh-frozen plasma, albumin, saline, or other volume expanders must be used to maintain euvolemia.[41] Immunoadsorption is a related technique that does not require the use of a replacement solution. The plasma component is exposed to an absorptive material of variable selectivity, and thus, only certain proteins, rather than a specific volume of plasma, are removed. Absorption columns can be designed for specific disease states, such as the acetylcholine receptor antibody–selective column used in a clinical trial for the treatment of myasthenia gravis.[42]

The main consideration when using therapeutic plasma exchange is venous access and the need for a central venous catheter, with its attendant risks of vascular or nerve injury, line infection, and pneumo- or hemothorax. The depletion of clotting factors during pheresis and the use of heparin if needed may predispose the patient to bleeding. Many devices use citrate as an anticoagulant, and this may lead to hypocalcemia or metabolic acidosis.[41]

Azathioprine

Azathioprine is commonly used as a steroid-sparing agent in the treatment of neuromuscular disorders, especially myasthenia gravis. Azathioprine is a prodrug and is converted to 6-mercaptopurine by the enzyme xanthine oxidase. The active compound interferes with the formation of purines and thus DNA synthesis. This broad antiproliferative action suppresses clonal expansion of lymphocytes but can also lead to bone marrow suppression.[43]

The usual effective dosage of azathioprine is 1 to 3 mg/kg. It can be given once daily or in twice-daily divided doses, which may be better tolerated. An important consideration when initiating azathioprine treatment is the activity of thiopurine methyltransferase (TPMT). Approximately 10% of individuals are deficient in this enzyme involved in azathioprine metabolism. When such deficiency exists, azathioprine toxicity can easily occur. Deficiency of TPMT has been recognized as a major risk factor for the development of severe myelotoxicity, and many recommend assay of enzyme activity before initiating therapy.[44] The level of activity can then be used to guide drug dosing to better prevent side effects.[45] Patients with very low or absent TPMT activity should probably not receive azathioprine. In situations in which the TPMT assay is not available, starting at a low dose, such as 50 mg daily, is recommended, with weekly monitoring of the complete blood count (CBC) during the first 2 months .

In addition to causing myelotoxicity, azathioprine may predispose patients to infection, particularly when combined with steroids or other agents. Mild nausea and vomiting are common side effects and may be alleviated by reducing or dividing the drug dose. Pancreatitis may rarely occur. An idiosyncratic reaction that is characterized by rash, fever, nausea, vomiting, and diarrhea may develop within the first month of treatment. Some patients can become quite ill and develop hypotension, tachycardia, and oliguria. The symptoms remit with discontinuation of therapy but recur, often immediately, on rechallenge with the drug.[46] There is some evidence that long-term use of azathioprine may increase the risk of cancer, particularly skin cancer[47] and lymphoma.[48] The overall risk appears low, but patients should be reminded to limit sun exposure and use sunscreen, especially if they are light-skinned. Liver enzyme elevations may also occur when using azathioprine but appear to be less common than with methotrexate.

Appropriate monitoring is key to preventing complications related to azathioprine therapy. CBC and liver enzymes should be assessed weekly for at least the first month, and then every 3 months thereafter. An effective dose of the drug often results in mild leukopenia. Additionally, mean corpuscular volume is often elevated when an effective dose has been reached. If the white blood cell count drops below 4000/mm^3, the dose should be reduced, whereas leukopenia of 2500/mm^3 or an absolute neutrophil count of less than 1000/mm^3 should prompt discontinuation of the drug and possible consultation with a hematologist.[44]

Azathioprine has numerous drug interactions. The most significant is the toxicity that can occur with concomitant administration of allopurinol for gout. This inhibitor of xanthine oxidase can significantly increase drug levels, and the dose of azathioprine should be reduced in these patients.[48] Angiotensin-converting enzyme inhibitors may also promote toxicity.[44] The anticoagulant warfarin is less effective when given with azathioprine.[49]

Despite these cautions, azathioprine is often well tolerated. It does not have a rapid onset of action, however, and response can be delayed by up to 6 months.

Methotrexate

Methotrexate is sometimes used in the treatment of inflammatory myopathies or the vasculitides as well as in some neuromuscular complications of rheumatologic disorders, such as overlap syndrome. Methotrexate, like azathioprine, inhibits DNA synthesis by interfering with purine nucleotide synthesis, but it acts through a different mechanism; methotrexate inhibits the enzyme dihydrofolate reductase. It is administered in weekly oral or parenteral doses, usually starting with 5 to 10 mg/wk and increasing the amount over several weeks to reach a maximum of 20 mg/wk. Doses higher than 20 mg/wk can be used, but the side effects are more troublesome. Additionally, oral bioavailability is variable and is further reduced at higher doses. For this reason, some practitioners may switch to weekly intravenous or intramuscular administration if patients do not respond to oral dosing.[50]

Methotrexate is usually well tolerated when given in small weekly doses, but several side effects merit mentioning. Complications such as oral ulcers, nausea and vomiting, myelosuppression, and flu-like symptoms are at least partially related to folate deficiency and improve with supplemental folic acid (e.g., 1 mg daily). The use of folic acid does not appear to significantly reduce the effectiveness of methotrexate.[51] Liver toxicity is a recognized complication but also appears to be reduced with folic acid supplementation.[52] Screening for hepatitis and counseling patients to avoid alcohol is recommended. Pulmonary fibrosis is also a concern. A baseline chest radiograph is recommended and may be repeated yearly. Measurement of complete blood count and liver enzymes every 4 to 8 weeks is also recommended.[53]

Cyclophosphamide

Cyclophosphamide is a prototypical alkylating agent and a descendant of the more toxic nitrogen mustard. This compound is sometimes used for the treatment of steroid-resistant or -dependent cases of the inflammatory myopathies, CIDP, and myasthenia gravis. In addition, it is a valuable therapy in the management of the vasculitides. As an alkylating agent, cyclophosphamide results in abnormal cross-linkage of DNA and RNA and consequent reduction of transcription and translation. It thus inhibits the proliferation of lymphocytes.

Cyclophosphamide appears to have a preferential effect on B cells[53-55] and actively reduces their number by promoting apoptosis.[56]

The drug is typically administered by monthly infusions at a dose of 0.5 to 1.0 g/m^2. Oral dosing is 1 to 2 mg/kg daily but is less commonly used because of increased side effects. Once it is administered, the parent drug is converted to active and inactive metabolites that are subsequently eliminated by the kidneys.

The potential complications of cyclophosphamide are well known and feared. Hemorrhagic cystitis is a classic side effect and may manifest as microscopic or gross hematuria. Mesna or 2-mercaptoethane sulfate is used to bind the metabolites of cyclophosphamide and inactivate them. It is usually administered to those receiving pulse doses of cyclophosphamide and is given before infusion as well as 4 and 8 hours after the treatment. Each dose of mesna is 60% of the dose of cyclophosphamide used.[56,57] Bladder toxicity may also be minimalized by adequate hydration and frequent voiding to prevent extended contact of the bladder mucosa with the drug's active metabolites.[58] Long-term exposure to cyclophosphamide can also result in bladder cancer. This, too, may be prevented by appropriate use of mesna.[58]

Infections are a common complication of cyclophosphamide therapy. In patients treated for Wegener granulomatosis, serious infections occurred in 70% of those receiving daily oral cyclophosphamide and in 41% of those receiving pulse doses of cyclophosphamide. A major contributor to this number is the rate of infection with *P. carinii*.[59,60] Appropriate prevention with trimethoprim-sulfamethoxazole or an equivalent drug in those with sulfa allergies is recommended.

Malignancy is a concern when using cyclophosphamide. One study of patients with rheumatoid arthritis who were treated with the drug showed a fourfold increase in the overall risk of cancer.[61] A lifetime cumulative dose of 80 g or greater may also increase the risk of myelofibrosis. In addition to these side effects, cyclophosphamide has been associated with cardiomyopathy,[62] infertility,[63] and pulmonary fibrosis.[64]

When using cyclophosphamide, the dose should be adjusted to avoid severe leukopenia below 2000 to 3000/mm^3. CBC should be obtained weekly for a month and then every 1 to 3 months.

Mycophenolate Mofetil

Mycophenolate mofetil (MMF) is a newer immunosuppressant that has been used most successfully—typically in combination with other drugs—for the prevention of renal transplant rejection.[65] Because of its enhanced safety profile compared with many of the medications listed earlier, it has been adopted for use in the treatment of neuromuscular disorders rather quickly. It has been used most often in the management of myasthenia gravis, but the recent results of two large randomized trials may curb enthusiasm for its use. Both trials found no steroid-sparing effect of mycophenolate over a period of 12 weeks[66] or 36 weeks.[67] It is still possible, however, that mycophenolate is effective in the treatment of myasthenia gravis but requires a longer duration of therapy, similar to azathioprine.

The parent drug is metabolized in the liver to the active metabolite mycophenolic acid. The latter inhibits inositol monophosphate dehydrogenase, which is the key enzyme in the de novo pathway for purine synthesis. Although most cells of the body acquire purines from both the de novo and salvage pathways, lymphocytes only use the former.[68] Therefore, MMF has a selective effect on both B and T lymphocytes and less toxicity than many of the drugs mentioned previously.

The typical dosage is 2 g daily in two divided doses. Higher doses, up to 4 or 5 g daily, may be used provided severe leukopenia does not occur. Monitoring of the CBC should be done weekly for the first month of therapy, then monthly for several months. Obtaining the blood count every 3 months beyond that is reasonable. Hepatic or renal toxicity is rare and did not occur in the largest trials in patients with myasthenia gravis.[66,67]

The most common side effects are headache, paresthesias, and abdominal cramping or diarrhea. Peripheral edema may also occur. As expected, serious infections are more common in those taking MMF with steroids.[67] Although believed to be an uncommon complication, a risk of progressive multifocal leukoencephalopathy or the development of malignancy, such as central nervous system lymphoma, has been reported.[69]

Cyclosporine

Cyclosporine is a potent T cell inhibitor that is commonly used to prevent rejection of transplanted organs. The drug interferes with calcineurin, a calcium-dependent phosphatase. This enzyme becomes activated when the TCR binds to MHC-presented antigen in the presence of appropriate costimulatory molecules. Calcineurin dephosphorylates a nuclear transcription factor that enters the nucleus and facilitates IL-2 gene transcription. Cyclosporine thus deprives T cells of a key cytokine needed for their activation and proliferation.[70] Cyclosporine has been used frequently for myasthenia gravis, and there is anecdotal evidence for its use in other neuromuscular disorders.

Cyclosporine is usually administered at 3 to 5 mg/kg in divided doses. The dose can be increased, but side effects become problematic. Proper attention to drug levels and renal function are needed. Trough drug levels should be drawn 12 hours after the last dose and are optimal at 100 to 200 mg/mL. Once a benefit is seen, the dose can be reduced gradually to find the lowest effective dose. In the hands of experienced physicians, a dose of 150 mg twice daily is tolerated with few serious side effects.[71]

The presence of some of these side effects has prevented cyclosporine from gaining widespread popularity in the neurology community. The most concerning of these is renal dysfunction. This is often insidious in onset and progressive unless the dose is reduced or the drug discontinued, but acute renal insufficiency can also occur, especially with high doses of cyclosporine. The concomitant use of nonsteroidal anti-inflammatory drugs and other nephrotoxic medications is dangerous and should be avoided. Using the lowest possible dose of cyclosporine helps to prevent nephrotoxicity.

In addition to nephrotoxicity, cyclosporine use can lead to hypertension, hyperlipidemia, diabetes mellitus, hypertrichosis, gingival hyperplasia, headache, and tremor. The incidence of serious infection is increased, as expected, especially when combined with steroids or other immunosuppressants.[72] Central nervous system toxicity also occurs. Although known variably as reversible posterior leukoencephalopathy or posterior reversible leukoencephalopathy syndrome, the manifestations are protean and the disorder can leave permanent deficits.[73]

Tacrolimus

Tacrolimus (FK506) is a macrolide drug and differs considerably in structure from cyclosporine, yet its mechanism of action is identical. There have been anecdotal reports and uncontrolled studies of its use in myasthenia gravis. Some investigators have used larger daily doses of 0.1 mg/kg with monitoring of trough levels,[74] whereas others have used a low, fixed daily dose of 3 to 4 mg that usually does not result in detectable trough blood levels.[75] All have reported benefit, but controlled trials are needed.

The advantage of tacrolimus is that, like cyclosporine, it appears to act quickly; some patients show improvement within a month, but the best response occurs after months of therapy.[76] In addition, tacrolimus, especially when used at a very low dosage, has fewer side effects in general than cyclosporine. Drug-induced diabetes mellitus, though, remains a concern.

Rapamycin

Rapamycin, or sirolimus, is similar to cyclosporine and tacrolimus in that it inhibits IL-2 production from T cells and antigen-presenting cells; however, it does so through a unique mechanism. Rapamycin inhibits the protein known, conveniently enough, as mammalian target of rapamycin. This results in decreased translation of messenger RNA and reduced IL-2 production. Although cyclosporine has been associated with the eventual development of malignancy, especially skin cancer,[77] rapamycin appears to have antioncogenic properties.[78] Rapamycin can cause hyperlipidemia, diarrhea, thrombocytopenia, anemia, and poor wound healing.[70] Successful treatment of a single patient with dermatomyositis has been reported.[79]

Rituximab

Rituximab is one of a host of monoclonal antibodies that are changing the approach to the treatment of autoimmune disorders. Unlike IVIg, in which a multitude of antibodies having different specificities are used, these new preparations contain a highly purified antibody that works against a single target. There is great hope that these more selective therapies will result in disease control with far fewer side effects than traditional immunosuppressive medications.

Monoclonal antibodies are derived from immortalized B cells that secrete antibodies of selected specificity. The amount of foreign immunoglobulin content in these drugs varies. Chimeric monoclonal antibodies are secreted from murine–human or other hybrid cell lines. Some monoclonal antibodies are further humanized by grafting only the portion required for antigen recognition (the complementarity-determining regions) onto a human IgG molecule. The newest antibodies are fully humanized by the use of transgenic animals that carry human immunoglobulin genes. The greater the nonhuman content of an antibody, the greater the risk of allergic reaction in patients. However, because of the presence of anti-idiotypic antibodies in patients, the use of even fully humanized antibodies is not without this risk.

Rituximab is the monoclonal antibody best known to neuromuscular physicians. It has been used anecdotally or in uncontrolled studies in anti-MAG neuropathy,[80-83] multifocal motor neuropathy,[81,84] CIDP,[85-87] inflammatory myopathies,[88,89] myasthenia gravis,[90-92] and the neuropathies associated with Sjögren syndrome[93] and Waldenstrom macroglobulinemia.[94]

Rituximab is a chimeric monoclonal antibody against CD20, a molecule found on the surface of developing and mature B cells. It may be expressed on plasma cells as well. The drug was initially used in the management of B cell lymphoma. A single course of rituximab is capable of depleting B cells within several weeks and maintaining depletion for months or years. IgM levels often decline after a single treatment, but IgG levels may be unaffected, presumably because of the survival of at least some plasma cells. Although the drug's effect on B cells and IgM levels is believed to play a significant role in its mechanism of action, the importance of other effects, such as the inhibition of cell migration, are still being considered.[95]

Rituximab is given as an intravenous infusion of 375 mg/m^2 weekly for 1 month or as two infusions of 1 g every other week. Because the drug's effects are long-lasting, repeat infusions may not be needed until several months or even years have passed; however, when necessary, the cycle can be repeated after 6 months. Rituximab is believed to be most helpful in IgM-mediated diseases, such as anti-MAG neuropathy and multifocal motor neuropathy. When used for other disorders, it is theoretically advantageous to administer rituximab along with another immunosuppressant, although this likely increases the risk of infection.

Rituximab infusions are typically well tolerated, with only cough and mild hypotension being common side effects. More severe reactions, such as bronchospasm, fever, and rigors, are more common when the drug is administered to those with high B cell counts (i.e., patients with lymphoma). Progressive multifocal leukoencephalopathy has been reported in patients treated with rituximab for lymphoma, rheumatoid arthritis, systemic lupus erythematosus, and inflammatory myopathies[96] and other neuromuscular disorders. This disease, which is caused by reactivation of latent JC virus, is usually fatal unless the immune system can be reconstituted.

Other Monoclonal Antibodies

Alemtuzumab is a humanized monoclonal antibody that targets CD52, a cell marker found on leukocytes and monocytes. The drug has been used in the management of leukemia and lymphoma and more recently showed promising results in the treatment of multiple sclerosis.[97] A single patient with CIDP who was successfully treated with alemtuzumab has been reported.[98] Side effects include the expected occurrence of transfusion reactions as well as the unusual development of thyroid disease and idiopathic thrombocytopenic purpura.[97]

Natalizumab has specificity for α4β1 integrin and inhibits adhesion and transmigration of leukocytes. The drug is approved for use in multiple sclerosis and, like rituximab, has been associated with the rare development of progressive multifocal leukoencephalopathy. No clinical trials or anecdotal reports of experience in neuromuscular disorders have been described, but these are almost certain to follow. Daclizumab is a monoclonal protein against CD25, the cell surface receptor for IL-2, that has been reported to be beneficial in ocular myositis. However, there have been no reports of its use in patients with polymyositis or dermatomyositis.[99]

Anti–Tumor Necrosis Factor-α Agents

Tumor necrosis factor-α is a potent proinflammatory cytokine that is likely involved in the pathogenesis of several autoimmune conditions, particularly rheumatoid arthritis and the inflammatory myopathies. Anti-TNF-α agents have been used with varied results in several neuromuscular disorders.

Infliximab is a chimeric monoclonal antibody against TNF-α. The drug has been reported to be of benefit to some patients with refractory inflammatory myopathies,[100,101] but a recent open-label trial found no improvement in muscle strength.[102] Etanercept is not a monoclonal antibody but rather a TNF-α receptor fusion protein that can bind and inactivate the cytokine. Although anecdotal reports of successful treatment of polymyositis with this agent exist,[103] other reports document a uniform worsening of disease status during treatment.[104] A pilot trial of etanercept in inclusion body myositis (IBM) found that the drug was well tolerated and a small improvement in hand grip at 1 year was noted.[105] Several phase II trials of anti-TNF-α agents in IBM are under way. Etanercept has also been used in a small open-label trial for the treatment of steroid-dependent myasthenia gravis. Although 5 of 11 patients improved significantly, 3 patients dropped out of the study, 1 because of a significant exacerbation of disease associated with upregulation of TNF-α levels.[106] A series of 10 patients with CIDP treated with etanercept showed definite improvement in 3 cases.[107]

Side effects of anti-TNF-α agents are usually mild, but several are of specific concern. Because TNF-α plays an important proinflammatory role in the immune system, the incidence of infection, particularly by intracellular organisms such as *Mycobacterium tuberculosis*, is increased.

The use of these agents has also been associated with the development or clinical worsening of leukocytoclastic vasculitis, a lupus-like syndrome, and interstitial lung disease.[108] Of particular interest to neuromuscular physicians, these drugs have also been associated with a wide variety of nerve and muscle disorders, including GBS, CIDP, mononeuritis multiplex, axonal sensorimotor polyneuropathy, and inflammatory myopathies.[108,109] Central demyelination during anti-TNF-α treatment has also been observed.[110]

Miscellaneous Agents

Anakinra, an IL-1 receptor antagonist, has been reported to be effective in a single patient with the antisynthetase syndrome.[111] Interferon-β-1a has been used successfully and safely for multiple sclerosis for more than a decade. Vallat et al explored its use for CIDP in a multicenter, open-label trial. They found that the drug was well tolerated, with no serious side effects, and only the typical asthenia and flu-like symptoms. There was a significant improvement in a measure of disability and in conduction velocities, although clinical muscle strength testing was not significantly altered.[112] As such, interferon-β-1a may be considered for patients with CIDP that does not respond to other therapies. Antithymocyte globulin (ATG) is a preparation of polyclonal antihuman T lymphocyte antibodies that results in apoptosis or complement-mediated cytolysis of T cells.[71] It has been used in a small open-label trial for the treatment of IBM, and methotrexate was given after induction with ATG to prevent repletion of autoimmune T cells. Patients treated with this combination stabilized muscle strength or had modest gains compared with the patients who were given methotrexate alone, who all showed deterioration. Because ATG is produced in animals (e.g., horses), serum sickness is an expected complication, although it did not occur in the pilot study by Lindberg et al.[113]

Evidence-Based Medicine and Treatment of Autoimmune Neuromuscular Disorders

Evidence-based medicine (EBM) simply refers to the incorporation of the best available clinical evidence or data when making medical decisions. The term was coined by epidemiology faculty at McMaster University in the 1990s, but the concept, although not as concisely articulated, has existed for much longer.[114] EBM emphasizes empiricism in medical decision making and elevates the randomized, controlled clinical trial to be the gold standard by which EBM decisions are made. That is not to say that EBM denies the importance of other aspects of medical management, such as personal experience, patient preferences, and the recognition that all patients are unique. At its best, EBM provides a stable foundation on which to make medical decisions by recognizing what is most likely to be beneficial for a patient. At the least, it should help us avoid interventions that are likely to cause serious harm.

The application of EBM to neuromuscular disorders can be challenging. Some disorders are sufficiently rare (e.g., congenital myasthenic syndromes) that large controlled trials may never be feasible. This lack of evidence should not prohibit the use of drugs that have a reasonable mechanism of action appropriate to the pathophysiology of the condition. Other disorders are so heterogenous (e.g., myotonia congenita) that a large randomized controlled trial may obscure the benefit of an intervention in a select subpopulation of those affected. Some interventions are universally agreed to be of benefit, and a randomized, controlled trial would be unnecessary and unethical (e.g., mechanical ventilation in severe acute inflammatory demyelinating polyradiculoneuropathy).

The evidence base for interventions in autoimmune neuromuscular disorders were evaluated according to the guidelines of the American Academy of Neurology (Table 7-1). Unfortunately, most of the

Table 7-1 Types of Immunotherapy

Drug	Dosage	Side Effects	Drug Monitoring	Indications	Evidence Level*
Corticosteroids					
Prednisone	0.5–2.0 mg/kg PO daily, then taper	See Box 7-1	Weight, blood pressure, glucose, bone density, eye examination	CIDP Myasthenia gravis Vasculitic neuropathy Dermatomyositis Duchenne muscular dystrophy	C U U U A
Methylprednisolone	1 g IV q day × 3–5 days as initial treatment then 1 g IV weekly for 1 month before tapering or 500 mg PO q week	See Box 7-1	As above	Discussed earlier	
IV Immunoglobulin	1–2 g/kg IV over 1–5 days; may be repeated monthly	Headache, chills, myalgia, renal insufficiency, thrombosis, rash, anaphylaxis	Blood pressure Serum creatinine during daily infusions Pseudohyponatremia and falsely elevated erythrocyte sedimentation rate may be seen	AIDP CIDP Myasthenia gravis Dermatomyositis	B B B C

Continued

Table 7-1 Types of Immunotherapy—Cont'd

Drug	Dosage	Side Effects	Drug Monitoring	Indications	Evidence Level*
Therapeutic Plasma Exchange	500–5000 mL plasma volume per exchange × 4 exchanges	Pneumo-/hemothorax, hypocalcemia, easy bruising or bleeding, hypertension	Blood pressure Calcium fibrinogen Serum calcium	AIDP CIDP Myasthenia gravis	B C C
Inhibitors of Purine Synthesis					
Azathioprine	1–3 mg/kg PO q day or divided bid Initiate with a small dose (i.e., 50 mg) if TPMT assay not available Reduce dose in those taking allopurinol or angiotensin-converting enzyme inhibitors	Myelotoxicity, nausea, idiosyncratic "flu-like" reaction, pancreatitis, malignancy, infections	Advise assessing TPMT activity before initiating treatment CBC weekly for 1 month, then q 3 months Liver function studies Amylase, lipase if pancreatitis is suspected	Myasthenia gravis CIDP Inflammatory myopathies	C U U
Methotrexate	5 mg/wk to 20 mg/wk PO or IV/IM	Nausea, oral ulcers, hepatotoxicity, pulmonary fibrosis, infections	Screen for hepatitis, interstitial lung disease on initiation CBC and liver function tests q 4–12 weeks Yearly chest X-ray Folic acid daily	Inflammatory myopathies Neuromuscular complications of 10 rheumatologic disorders	U
Mycophenolate mofetil	2–4 or 5 g daily, divided bid	Gastrointestinal upset, paresthesias/headache	CBC weekly to monthly initially, then trimonthly	Myasthenia gravis, CIDP	B U
Cyclophosphamide	0.5–1.0 g/m² IV q month	Myelosuppression, myelofibrosis, hemorrhagic cystitis, malignancy (especially bladder)	CBC weekly Liver function tests weekly for a month and then every 1 to 3 months Urinalysis every 1 to 3 months	Vasculitis CIDP Myasthenia gravis Inflammatory myopathies	U
Calcineurin Inhibitors					
Cyclosporin	3–5 mg/kg PO q day, divided bid	Hypertension, renal insufficiency, CNS toxicity, hirsutism	Trough drug levels weekly at first BMP weekly at first Avoid nonsteroidal anti-inflammatory drugs	Myasthenia gravis CIDP	C U
Tacrolimus	3–4 mg up to 1 mg/kg PO q day, divided bid	Same as discussed earlier, but less common Diabetes mellitus	Trough drug levels CMP monthly	Myasthenia gravis Dermatomyositis	U
Rapamycin	2–5 mg PO q day	Hyperlipidemia, diarrhea, thrombocytopenia	Periodic CMP Lipid levels	Dermatomyositis	U
Monoclonal Antibodies					
Rituximab	0.375 g/m² IV weekly × 4 or 1 g IV q other week × 2	Progressive multifocal leukoencephalopathy Infusion reactions	Brain magnetic resonance image, if indicated CBC CD20 and B cells monthly	Multifocal motor neuropathy CIDP Anti-MAG neuropathy Myasthenia gravis Inflammatory myopathies	U
Alemtuzumab	Varies	Infusion reactions idiopathic thrombocytopenic purpura	CBC CMP	CIDP	U

Continued

Table 7-1 Types of Immunotherapy—Cont'd

Drug	Dosage	Side Effects	Drug Monitoring	Indications	Evidence Level*
Anti–Tumor Necrosis Factor-α Agents					
Infliximab	3–6 mg/kg IV periodically	Infections Inflammatory neuropathy, vasculitis	CBC, CMP monthly	Dermatomyositis Polymyositis	U
Etanercept	25 mg sq biweekly	As above Infections, autoimmune disorders	CBC, CMP monthly	Polymyositis Inclusion body myositis Myasthenia gravis CIDP	U
Anakinra	100 mg sq q day	Injection site reactions, diarrhea Infections, autoimmune disorders	CBC, CMP monthly	Inflammatory myopathies	U
Interferon-β-1a	30 μg IM q week	Injection site reactions, flu-like symptoms Mild leukopenia, abnormal liver function tests, abnormal thyroid function tests	CMP, thyroid-stimulating hormone periodically	CIDP	U
Antithymocyte globulin	Varies	Serum sickness		Inclusion body myositis	U

*Evidence level: A, established as effective; B, probably effective; C, possibly effective; U, uncertain effectiveness.
AIDP, acute inflammatory demyelinating polyradiculoneuropathy; CBC, complete blood count; BMP, basic metabolic panel; CIDP, chronic inflammatory demyelinating polyradiculoneuropathy; CMP, complete metabolic panel; CNS, central nervous system; TPMT, thiopurine methyltransferase.

treatments discussed earlier, even clinically well-accepted interventions such as corticosteroids for myasthenia gravis, earned only a "U" recommendation. This does not imply that these treatments are not valuable but should spur additional and higher-quality (i.e., controlled) trials.

References

1. Akira S, Uematsu S, Takeuchi O: Pathogen recognition and innate immunity, *Cell* 124:783–801, 2006.
2. Cook DN, Pisetsky DS, Schwartz DA: Toll-like receptors in the pathogenesis of human disease, *Nat Immunol* 5(10):975–979, 2004.
3. Stetson DB, Medzhitov R: Type I interferons in host defense, *Immunity* 25(3):373–381, 2006.
4. Borden EC, Sen GC, Uze G, et al. Interferons at age 50: past, current and future impact on biomedicine. *Nat Rev Drug Discov.* 6(12):975–990.
5. Adkinson NF: *Middleton's Allergy: Principles and Practice*, 7th ed. Elsevier, Philadelphia, 2009.
6. Nossal GJ: A purgative mastery, *Nature* 412:685–686, 2001.
7. Kamradt T, Mitchison MA: Tolerance and autoimmunity, *N Engl J Med* 344(9):655–664, 2001.
8. Jonuleit H, Schmitt E: The regulatory T cell family: distinct subsets and their interrelations, *J Immunol* 171(12):323–327, 2003.
9. McCombe PA, Pollard JD, McCleod JG: Chronic inflammatory demyelinating polyradiculoneruopathy. A clinical and electrophysiological study of 92 cases, *Brain* 110:1617–1630, 1987.
10. Hughes RA, Cornblath DR: Guillain-Barré syndrome, *Lancet* 366(9497):1653–1666, 2005.
11. Bird SJ, Brown MJ, Shy ME, Sherer SS: Chronic inflammatory demyelinating polyneuropathy associated with malignant melanoma, *Neurology* 46(3):822–824, 1996.
12. Toyka KV, Gold R: The pathogenesis of CIDP: rationale for treatment with immunomodulatory agents, *Neurology* 60(Suppl 3):S2–S7, 2003.
13. Yan WX, Archelos JJ, Hartung H-P, Pollard JD: P0 protein is a target antigen in chronic inflammatory demyelinating polyradiculoneuropathy, *Ann Neurol* 50:286–292, 2001.
14. Kieseier BC, Dalakas MC, Hartung H-P: Immune mechanisms in chronic inflammatory demyelinating neuropathy, *Neurology* 59(Suppl 6):S7–S12, 2002.
15. Rhen T, Cidlowski JA: Antiinflammatory action of glucocorticoids—new mechanisms for old drugs, *N Engl J Med* 353(16):1711–1723, 2005.
16. Salvarani C, Cantini F, Hunder GG: Polymyalgia rheumatica and giant-cell arteritis, *Lancet* 372(9364):234–245, 2008.
17. Sullivan Frank M, Swan Iain RC, et al: Early treatment with prednisolone or acyclovir in Bell's palsy, *N Engl J Med* 357:1598–1607, 2007.
18. Engström M, Berg T, Stjernquist-Desatnik A, et al: Prednisolone and valaciclovir in Bell's palsy: a randomised, double-blind, placebo-controlled, multicentre trial, *Lancet Neurol* 7:993–1000, 2008.
19. Bonifati MD, Ruzza G, Bononetto P, et al: A multicenter, double-blind, randomized trial of deflazacort versus prednisone in Duchenne muscular dystrophy, *Muscle Nerve* 23:1344–1347, 2000.
20. Lopate G, Pestronk A, Al-Lozi M: Treatment of chronic inflammatory demyelinating polyneuropathy with high-dose intermittent intravenous methylprednisolone, *Arch Neurol* 62(2):249–254, 2005.
21. Muley SA, Kelkar P, Parry G: Treatment of chronic inflammatory demyelinating polyneuropathy with pulsed oral steroids, *Arch Neurol* 65:1460–1464, 2008.
22. Hong SI, Cho DH, Kang HC, et al: Acute onset of steroid psychosis with very low dose of prednisolone in Sheehan's syndrome, *Endocr J* 53(2):255–258, 2006.
23. Min DI, Monaco AP: Complications associated with immunosuppressive therapy and their management, *Pharmacotherapy* 11(5):119S–125S, 1991.
24. American College of Rheumatology Ad Hoc Committee on Glucocorticoid-Induced Osteoporosis: Recommendations for the prevention and treatment of glucocorticoid-induced osteoporosis: 2001 update, *Arthritis Rheum* 44(7):1496–1501, 2001.
25. Adachi JD, Bensen WG, Brown J, et al: Intermittent etidronate therapy to prevent corticosteroid-induced osteoporosis, *N Engl J Med* 337:382–387, 1997.
26. Saag KG, Emkey R, Schnitzer TJ, et al: Alendronate for the treatment and prevention of glucocorticoid-induced osteoporosis, *N Engl J Med* 339:292–299, 1998.
27. Roux C, Oriente P, Laan R, et al: Randomized trial of effect of cyclical etidronate in the prevention of corticosteroid-induced bone loss, *J Clin Endocrinol Metab* 83:1128–1133, 1998.
28. Cohen S, Levy RM, Keller M, et al: Risedronate therapy prevents corticosteroid-induced bone loss: a twelve-month, multicenter, randomized,

double-blind, placebo-controlled, parallel-group study, *Arthritis Rheum* 42:2309–2318, 1999.

29. Reid DM, Hughes RA, Laan RF, et al: Efficacy and safety of daily risedronate in the treatment of corticosteroid-induced osteoporosis in men and women: a randomized trial, *J Bone Miner Res* 15:1006–1020, 2000.

30. Saag KG, Shane E, Boonen S, et al: Teriparatide or alendronate in glucocorticoid-induced osteoporosis, *N Engl J Med* 357:2028–2039, 2007.

31. deRoux A, Marx A, Burkhardt O, et al: Impact of corticosteroids on the immune response to a MF59-adjuvanted influenza vaccine in elderly COPD-patients, *Vaccine* 24(10):1537–1542, 2006.

32. Kapetanovic MC, Saxne T, Sjoholm A, et al: Influence of methotrexate, TNF blockers and prednisolone on antibody responses to pneumococcal polysaccharide vaccine in patients with rheumatoid arthritis, *Rheumatology* 45(1):106–111, 2006.

33. Russian DA, Levine SJ: Pneumocystis carinii pneumonia in patients without HIV infection, *Am J Med Sci* 321(1):56–65, 2001.

34. Hartung H-P: Advances in the understanding of the mechanism of action of IVIg, *J Neurol* 255(Suppl 3):3–6, 2008.

35. Iijima M, Tomita M, Morozumi S, et al: Single nucleotide polymorphism of TAG-1 influences IVIg responsiveness of Japanese patients with CIDP, *Neurology* 73:1348–1352, 2009.

36. Dalakas MC: The use of intravenous immunoglobulin in the treatment of autoimmune neuromuscular diseases: evidence-based indications and safety profile, *Pharmacol Ther* 102(3):177–193, 2004.

37. Hughes RA, Swan AV, Raphael JC, et al: Immunotherapy for Guillain-Barré syndrome: a systemic review, *Brain* 130(Pt 9):2245–2257, 2007.

38. Bertorini TE, Nance AM, Horner LH, et al: Complications of intravenous gammaglobulin in neuromuscular and other diseases, *Muscle Nerve* 19 (3):388–391, 1996.

39. Lee D-H, Linker RA, Paulus W, et al: Subcutaneous immunoglobulin infusion: a new therapeutic option in chronic inflammatory demyelinating polyneuropathy, *Muscle Nerve* 37:406–409, 2008.

40. Donofrio PD, Berger A, Brannagan TH III, et al: Consensus statement: the use of intravenous immunoglobulin in the treatment of neuromuscular conditions: report of the AANEM ad hoc committee, *Muscle Nerve* 40(5): 890–900, 2009.

41. Lehmann HC, Hartung H-P, Hetzel GR, et al: Plasma exchange in neuroimmunological disorders. Part 1: rationale and treatment of inflammatory central nervous system disorders, *Arch Neurol* 63:930–935, 2006.

42. Yeh JH, Chiu HC: Comparison between double-filtration plasmapharesis and immunoadsorption plasmapharesis in the treatment of patients with myasthenia gravis, *J Neurol* 247(7):510–513, 2000.

43. Anstey A, Lear JT: Azathioprine: clinical pharmacology and current indications in autoimmune disorders, *BioDrugs* 9(1):33–47, 1998.

44. Goldsmith P, Lennox G, Bhalla N: Azathioprine prescribing in neurology, *J Neurol* 255(6):791–795, 2008.

45. Meggitt SJ, Gray JC, Reynolds NJ: Azathioprine dosed by thiopurine methyltransferase activity for moderate-to-severe eczema: a double-blind randomised controlled trial, *Lancet* 367(9513):839–846, 2006.

46. Knowles SR, Gupta AK, Shear NH, Sauder D: Azathioprine hypersensitivity-like reactions—a case report and a review of the literature, *Clin Exp Dermatol* 20(4):353–356, 1995.

47. O'Donovan P, Perrett CM, Zhang X, et al: Azathioprine and UVA light generate mutagenic oxidative DNA damage, *Science* 309:1871–1874, 2005.

48. Silman AJ, Petrie J, Hazleman B, Evans SJ: Lymphoproliferative cancer and other malignancy in patients with rheumatoid arthritis treated with azathioprine: a 20 year follow up study, *Ann Rheum Dis* 47:988–992, 1988.

49. GlaxoSmithKline: *Azathioprine data sheet.*

50. Cannella AC, O'Dell JR: Methotrexate, leflunomide, sulfasalasine, hydroxychloroquine and combination therapies. In Harris ED, editor: *Kelley's Textbook of Rheumatology*, ed 8, Philadelphia, 2008, Elsevier.

51. Morgan SL, Baggott JE, Vaughn WH, et al: Supplementation with folic acid during methotrexate therapy for rheumatoid arthritis. A double-blind, placebo-controlled trial, *Ann Intern Med* 121(11):833–841, 1994.

52. van Ede AE, Laan RF, Rood MJ, et al: Effect of folic or folinic acid supplementation on the toxicity and efficacy of methotrexate in rheumatoid arthritis: a forty-eight week, multicenter, randomized, double-blind, placebo-controlled study, *Arthritis Rheum* 44(7):1515–1524, 2001.

53. American College of Rheumatology Ad Hoc Committee on Clinical Guidelines: Guidelines for monitoring drug therapy in rheumatoid arthritis, *Arthritis Rheum* 39:723–731, 1996.

54. Zhu LP, Cupps TR, Whalen G, Fauci AS: Selective effects of cyclophosphamide therapy on activation, proliferation, and differentiation of human B cells, *J Clin Invest* 79(4):1082–1090, 1987.

55. Cupps TR, Edgar LC, Fauci AS: Suppression of human B lymphocyte function by cyclophosphamide, *J Immunol* 128(6):2453–2457, 1982.

56. Hemendinger RA, Bloom SE: Selective mitomycin C and cyclophosphamide induction of apoptosis in differentiating B lymphocytes compared to T lymphocytes in vivo, *Immunopharmacology* 35(1):71–82, 1996.

57. Freter CE, Perry MC: Systemic therapy. In Abeloff MD, Armitage J, Niederhuber J, et al, editors: *Abeloff's Clinical Oncology*, ed 4, Philadelphia, 2008, Elsevier.

58. Reingold-Keller E, Beuge N, Latza U, et al: An interdisciplinary approach to the care of patients with Wegener's granulomatosis: long-term outcome in 155 patients, *Arthritis Rheum* 43(5):1021–1032, 2000.

59. Stein CM, Taylor HG: Immunoregulatory drugs. In Firestein GS, editor: *Kelley's Textbook of Rheumatology*, ed 8, Philadelphia, 2008, Elsevier.

60. Guillevin L, Cordier JF, Lhote F, et al: A prospective, multicenter, randomized trial comparing steroids and pulse cyclophosphamide versus steroids and oral cyclophosphamide in the treatment of generalized Wegener's granulomatosis, *Arthritis Rheum* 40(12):2187–2198, 1997.

61. Baltus JA, Boersma JW, Hartman AP, Vandenbroucke JP: The occurrence of malignancies in patients with rheumatoid arthritis treated with cyclophosphamide: a controlled retrospective follow-up, *Ann Rheum Dis* 42(4): 368–373, 1983.

62. Kamezaki K, Fukuda T, Makino S, Harada M: Cyclophosphamide-induced cardiomyopathy in a patient with seminoma and a history of mediastinal irradiation, *Intern Med* 44(2):89–90, 2005.

63. Nicholson HS, Byrne J: Fertility and pregnancy after treatment for cancer during childhood or adolescence, *Cancer* 71(Suppl 10):3392–3399, 1993.

64. Fraiser LH, Kanekal S, Kehrer JP: Cyclophosphamide toxicity: characterising and avoiding the problem, *Drugs* 42:781–795, 1991.

65. Behrend M, Lueck R, Pichlmayr R: Long-term experience with mycophenolate mofetil in the prevention of renal allograft rejection, *Transplant Proc* 29:2927–2929, 1997.

66. The Muscle Study Group: A trial of mycophenolate mofetil with prednisone as initial immunotherapy in myasthenia gravis, *Neurology* 71:394–399, 2008.

67. Sanders DB, Hart IK, Mantegazza R, et al: An international, phase III, randomized trial of mycophenolate mofetil in myasthenia gravis, *Neurology* 71:400–406, 2008.

68. Chaudhry V, Cornblath DR, Griffin JW, et al: Mycophenolate mofetil: a safe and promising immunosuppressant in neuromuscular diseases, *Neruology* 56:94–96, 2001.

69. Vernino S, Salomao DR, Habermann TM, O'Neill BP: Primary CNS lymphoma complicating treatment of myasthenia gravis with mycophenolate mofetil, *Neurology* 65:639–641, 2005.

70. Magee CC, Ansari MJ, Milford EL: Renal transplantation: clinical management. In Brenner BM, editor: *Brenner and Rector's The Kidney*, ed 8, Philadelphia, 2008, Saunders Elsevier.

71. Dalakas MC: Therapeutic targets in patients with inflammatory myopathies: present approaches and a look to the future, *Neuromuscul Disord* 16:223–236, 2006.

72. Wolfe GI, Gross B: Treatment review and update for myasthenia gravis, *J Clin Neuromuscul Dis* 6:54–68, 2004.

73. Stott VL, Hurrell MA, Anderson TJ: Reversible posterior leukoencephalopathy syndrome: a misnomer reviewed, *Intern Med J* 35(2): 388–395, 2005.

74. Ponseti JM, Azem J, Fort JM, et al: Benefits of FK506 (tacrolimus) for residual, cyclosporine- and prednisone-resistant myasthenia gravis: one-year follow-up of an open-label study, *Clin Neurol Neurosurg* 107(3):187–190, 2005.

75. Nagaishi A, Yukitake M, Kuroda Y: Long-term treatment of steroid-dependent myasthenia gravis patients with low-dose tacrolimus, *Intern Med* 47(8):731–736, 2008.

76. Konishi T, Yoshiyama Y, Takamori M, Saida T: Long-term treatment of generalised myasthenia gravis with FK506 (tacrolimus), *J Neurol Neurosurg Psychiatry* 76(3):448–450, 2005.

77. Euvrard S, Kanitakis J, Claudy A: Skin cancers after organ transplantation, *N Engl J Med* 348:1681–1691, 2003.

78. Rowinsky EK: Signal events: cell signal transduction and its inhibition in cancer, *Oncologist* 8(Suppl 3):5–17, 2003.

79. Nadiminti U, Arbiser JL: Rapamycin (siroliumus) as a steroid-sparing agent in dermatomyositis, *J Am Acad Dermatol* 52(suppl 1):17–19, 2005.

80. Levine TD, Pestronk A: IgM antibody-related polyneuropathies: B-cell depletion chemotherapy using rituximab, *Neurology* 52:1701–1704, 1999.

81. Pestronk A, Florence J, Miller T, et al: Treatment of IgM antibody associated polyneuropathies using rituximab, *J Neurol Neurosurg Psychiatry* 74:485–489, 2003.

82. Renaud S, Gregor M, Fuhr P, et al: Rituximab in the treatment of polyneuropathy associated with anti-MAG antibodies, *Muscle Nerve* 27:611–615, 2003.

83. Renaud S, Fuhr P, Gregor M, et al: High-dose rituximab and anti-MAG-associated polyneuropathy, *Neurology* 66:742–744, 2006.

84. Ruegg SJ, Fuhr P, Steck AJ: Rituximab stabilizes multifocal neuropathy increasingly less responsive to IVIg, *Neurology* 63:2178–2179, 2004.

85. Briani C, Zara G, Zambello R, et al: Rituximab-responsive CIDP, *Eur J Neurol* 11:788, 2004.

86. Kilidireas C, Anagnostopoulos A, Karandreas N, et al: Rituximab therapy in monoclonal IgM-related neuropathies, *Leuk Lymphoma* 47:859–864, 2006.

87. Gorson KC, Natarajan N, Ropper AH, Weinstein R: Rituximab treatment in patients with IVIg-dependent immune polyneuropathy: a prospective pilot study, *Muscle Nerve* 35:66–69, 2007.

88. Levine TD: Rituximab in the treatment of dermatomyositis: an open-label pilot study, *Arthritis Rheum* 52:601–607, 2005.

89. Mok CC, Ho LY, To CH: Rituximab for refractory polymyositis: an open-label prospective study, *J Rheumatol* 34:1864–1868, 2007.

90. Hain B, Jordan K, Deschauer M, Zierz S: Successful treatment of MuSK antibody-positive myasthenia gravis with rituximab, *Muscle Nerve* 33:575–580, 2006.

91. Kerkeni S, Marotte H, Miossec P: Improvement with rituximab in a patient with both rheumatoid arthritis and myasthenia gravis, *Muscle Nerve* 38:1343–1345, 2008.

92. Zebardaost N, Patwa HS, Novella SP, Goldstein JM: Rituximab in the management of refractory myasthenia gravis, *Muscle Nerve* 41:375–378, 2010.

93. Seror R, Sordet C, Guillevin L, et al: Tolerance and efficacy of rituximab and changes in serum B cell biomarkers in patients with systemic complications of primary Sjögren's syndrome, *Ann Rheum Dis* 66:351–357, 2007.

94. Dimopoulos MA, Zervas C, Zomas A, et al: Treatment of Waldenstrom's macroglobulinemia with rituximab, *J Clin Oncol* 20:2327–2333, 2002.

95. Stubgen J-P: B cell-targeted therapy with rituximab and autoimmune neuromuscular disorders, *J Neuroimmunol* 204:1–12, 2008.

96. Molloy ES, Calabrese LH: Progressive multifocal leukoencephalopathy in patients with rheumatic diseases: are patients with systemic lupus erythematosus at particular risk? *Autoimmun Rev* 8:144–146, 2008.

97. CAMMS223 Trial Investigators, Coles AJ, Compston DA, et al: Alemtuzumab vs interferon beta-1a in early multiple sclerosis, *N Engl J Med* 359:1786–1801, 2008.

98. Hirst C, Raasch S, Llewelyn G, Robertson N: Remission of chronic inflammatory demyelinating polyneuropathy after alemtuzumab (Campath 1H), *J Neurol Neurosurg Psychiatry* 77:800–802, 2006.

99. Garcia-Pous M, Hernandez-Garfella ML, Diaz-Llopis M: Treatment of chronic orbital myositis with daclizumab, *Can J Ophthamol* 42:156–157, 2007.

100. Hengstman GJ, van den Hoogen FH, Barrera P, et al: Successful treatment of dermatomyositis and polymyositis with anti-tumor-necrosis-factor-alpha: preliminary observations, *Eur Neurol* 50:10–15, 2003.

101. Riley P, McCann LJ, Maillard SM, et al: Effectiveness of inliximab in the treatment of refractory juvenile dermatomyositis with calcinosis, *Rheumatology (Oxford)* 47:877–880, 2008.

102. Dastmalchi M, Grundtman C, Alexanderson H, et al: A high incidence of disease flares in an open pilot study of infliximab in patients with refractory inflammatory mopathies, *Ann Rheum Dis* 67:1670–1677, 2008.

103. Sprott H, Glatzel M, Michel BA: Treatment of myositis with etanercept (Enbrel), a recombinant human soluble fusion protein of TNF-alpha type II receptor and IgG1, *Rheumatology (Oxford)* 43:524–526, 2004.

104. Iannone F, Scioscia C, Falappone PC, et al: Use of etanercept in the treatment of dermatomyositis: a case series, *J Rheumatol* 33:1802–1804, 2006.

105. Barohn RJ, Herbelin L, Kissel JT, et al: Pilot trial of etanercept in the treatment of inclusion-body myositis, *Neurology* 66(2 Suppl 1):S123–S124, 2006.

106. Rowin J, Meriggioli MN, Tuzun E, et al: Etanercept treatment in corticosteroid-dependent myasthenia gravis, *Neurology* 63:2390–2392, 2004.

107. Chin RL, Sherman WH, Sander HW, et al: Etanercept (Enbrel) therapy for chronic inflammatory demyelinating polyneuropathy, *J Neurol Sci* 210:19–21, 2003.

108. Ramos-Casals M, Brito-Zeron P, Munoz S, et al: Autoimmune diseases induced by TNF-targeted therapies: analysis of 233 cases, *Medicine* 86:242–251, 2007.

109. Stubben J-P: Tumor necrosis factor-α antagonists and neuropathy, *Muscle Nerve* 281–292, 2008.

110. Robinson WH, Genovese MC, Moreland LW: Demyelinating and neurologic events reported in association with tumor necrosis factor alpha antagonism: by what mechanisms could tumor necrosis factor alpha antagonists improve rheumatoid arthritis but exacerbate multiple sclerosis? *Arthritis Rheum* 44:1977–1983, 2001.

111. Furlan A, Botsios C, Ruffatti A, et al: Antisynthetase syndrome with refractory polyarthritis and fever successfully treated with the IL-1 receptor antagonist, anakinra: a case report, *Joint Bone Spine* 75:366–367, 2008.

112. Vallat J-M, Hahn AF, Leger J-M, et al: Interferon beta-1a as an investigational treatment for CIDP, *Neurology* 60(Suppl 3):S23–S28, 2003.

113. Lindberg C, Trysberg E, Tarkowski A, Oldfors A: Anti-T-lymphocyte globulin treatment in inclusion body myositis: a randomized pilot study, *Neurology* 61:260–262, 2003.

114. Guyatt G: Evidence-based medicine, *ACP J Club* A-16:114, 1991.

Dorothy Weiss, MD, EdM
Lisa S. Krivickas, MD

Rehabilitation in Neuromuscular Disorders

8

Despite the explosion of research interest in the genetics of hereditary neuromuscular disorders (NMDs) and the numerous clinical trials that have been conducted over the past decade, clinicians treating many NMDs (e.g., amyotrophic lateral sclerosis [ALS], the muscular dystrophies, the hereditary neuropathies) are left without medications that significantly slow disease progression. Aggressive rehabilitation and symptom management can prolong life and improve quality of life for patients with these disorders to a greater extent than any currently available pharmacologic interventions. As researchers develop additional drugs that slow the progression of these diseases, life expectancy and quality of life will increase and rehabilitation will become even more important.

> Rehabilitation is the process of helping a person to reach the fullest physical, psychological, social, vocational, avocational, and educational potential consistent with his or her physiological or anatomic impairment, environmental limitations, and desires and life plans. Realistic goals are determined by the person and those concerned with his care. Thus, one is working to obtain optimal function despite residual disability, even if the impairment is caused by a pathological process that cannot be reversed.[1]

The pathologic processes underlying NMDs are often progressive and irreversible. Comprehensive care should include rehabilitation that restores patients to a level of optimal functioning in their normal societal environments and achieves the optimal quality of life possible throughout the course of the disease. Rehabilitation includes management of musculoskeletal dysfunction, respiratory failure, dysarthria, dysphagia, pain, mood, and cognition, and is attentive to the patient's environment, quality of life, and family and caregivers.

The nature of rehabilitation for individuals with NMDs can vary over time with changes in health and social supports. Thus, rehabilitation can be more challenging for these patients than for patients with static functional deficits caused by single events, such as spinal cord injury. One of the most difficult tasks for the rehabilitation team is to predict how quickly the patient's disease will progress so that the team can "stay ahead" of the disease process and can recommend interventions at appropriate times. This is most difficult with more rapidly progressing disease processes.

Rehabilitation and symptom management in NMDs may be approached in a problem-oriented manner. Rehabilitation topics addressed in this chapter include the role of exercise in patients with NMDs and management of impairments resulting in difficulties with mobility, activities of daily living (ADLs), communication, and the maintenance of oxygenation and nutrition. Musculoskeletal pain syndromes are discussed because of their direct effect on the ability to exercise, maintain mobility, and perform ADLs. Mood disorders and cognitive dysfunction are discussed because they are easily overlooked in the context of multiple rehabilitation needs and impaired communication; optimal management can allow patients to maintain social contacts, improve patient quality of life, and lessen caregiver and family stress. Palliative care falls at the end of the rehabilitation continuum and can become necessary for patients with some NMDs. Rehabilitation needs are best addressed by a multidisciplinary team, which can consist of some or all of the following individuals: physiatrist, neurologist, psychologist, physical therapist, occupational therapist, speech therapist, recreational therapist, nutritionist, respiratory therapist, orthotist, social worker, chaplain, peer visitor, palliative care specialist, and nurse. At the center of every team is the patient and family. Studies from the Netherlands, Ireland, and Italy have shown that patients with ALS who are cared for in a multidisciplinary clinic have a better quality of life, longer survival, and fewer emergency hospitalizations, and are more likely to use riluzole and noninvasive positive-pressure ventilation (NIPPV).[2–4] They are also more likely to have the appropriate equipment and assistive devices to meet their needs. The same findings hold true for those with other NMDs.

Rehabilitation is necessary during all stages of NMDs. As a disease progresses, however, rehabilitation strategies and needs change. Rehabilitation services are beneficial throughout the course of a person's life with an NMD, although services are frequently discontinuous for insurance coverage reasons. For example, a patient with early ALS may be referred to a physical therapist for help with designing an appropriate aerobic exercise and strengthening program. As increasing spasticity develops, the patient and family may return to physical therapy for a few sessions of education about stretching and range-of-motion exercises. If foot drop develops and the patient is prescribed an ankle-foot orthosis (AFO), he may return for a few sessions of gait training with the new brace. As weakness increases, additional sessions of physical therapy may be necessary to teach a caregiver how to transfer the patient between surfaces effectively.

Insurance carriers typically deny coverage for continuous physical, occupational, or speech therapy to patients with NMDs because they consider them "maintenance" therapies, with "no improvements" expected. This is faulty reasoning about which healthcare providers need to educate insurers. Most NMDs are not static; as function declines, patients develop needs for new treatment interventions to improve outcomes, and additional therapy is required. Frequently, therapy is also required to slow decline in function.

Management of Muscle Weakness

Exercise

Exercise is an important part of the rehabilitation process for individuals with NMDs of all severities. Early in the course of progressive disease, an exercise program can maximize strength and prolong independence. For those with disease states that respond to pharmacologic treatment (e.g., multifocal motor neuropathy), exercise can reverse acquired muscle weakness and cardiovascular deconditioning. For any patient for whom exercise is an important part of lifestyle, continuing to exercise improves mood, psychological well-being, and social engagement.

For many years, patients with progressive NMDs were advised not to exercise because of the fear that too much exercise might hasten the progression of their weakness by producing "overuse weakness." A critical review of the literature reveals only isolated case reports suggesting that overuse weakness occurs.[5,6] No controlled studies have demonstrated that this phenomenon actually exists. In fact, most studies of exercise in patients with a variety of NMDs, despite methodologic limitations, suggest that strength gains can occur as a result of exercise training in patients with slowly progressive disorders. Whether these strength gains translate into a functional benefit is less clear. Four forms of exercise training are relevant to patients with NMDs: *flexibility, strengthening, aerobic,* and *balance exercises*. The general benefits of these four forms of exercise are summarized in Table 8-1.

Several factors must be considered when assessing the ability of patients with NMDs to participate in and benefit from an exercise program. The specific diagnosis and rate of disease progression will affect the response to exercise. One might expect patients with neuropathic disorders to respond differently than those with myopathic disorders. In rapidly and relatively rapidly progressive diseases, slowing the rate of functional impairment is a positive outcome. In more slowly progressive diseases, a positive outcome might be actual gain of strength or aerobic exercise capacity. Response to an exercise program can be affected by patient age, baseline strength, baseline physical activity, cardiopulmonary health, and medication regimen. For example, the cardiomyopathy associated with some muscular dystrophies and the restrictive lung disease associated with both dystrophies and anterior horn cell disorders may limit aerobic capacity. Medications such as beta blockers can limit aerobic exercise capacity. Each of these factors must be considered when designing exercise programs as well as studies to investigate the role of exercise in patients with NMDs.

Flexibility Training

Flexibility training involves stretching and range-of-motion (ROM) exercises. Although there is little scientific literature on the role of flexibility training in patients with NMDs, it is widely accepted that this form of exercise helps prevent the development of contractures. Contractures may place weak muscles at biomechanical disadvantage, impairing their function. For example, a patient with a hip flexion contracture and weak quadriceps may be able to reduce the load on his quadriceps and improve his gait by decreasing the hip flexion contracture. Contractures may also produce pain and interfere with positioning and the performance of ADLs. Contractures typically develop in the shoulder when patients are too weak to raise their arms overhead and in the hips, knees, and ankles when patients

Table 8-1 Exercise Training Relevant to Patients with Neuromuscular Disorders

Type of Exercise	Description	General Benefits
Flexibility	Stretching and range of motion	Prevent contractures Prevent pain Reduce spasticity Increase joint blood flow and lubrication
Resistance	Strengthening Static (no joint movement) Isometric (constant length) Dynamic (involving joint movement) Isotonic (constant force) Isokinetic (constant velocity) Concentric (shortening contraction) Eccentric (lengthening contraction)	Reverse disuse weakness Strengthen minimally weak muscles Delay onset of impairment Muscle fiber hypertrophy Fiber type conversion Increase protein synthesis Increase capillary density Reduce mitochondrial density Reduce lipid storage Neural adaptations
Aerobic	Low-resistance dynamic activity using large muscle groups that has a cardiopulmonary training effect	Improve functional exercise capacity Decrease psychological stress Improve quality of life Improve sleep Prevent secondary diseases Help maintain bone density Greater independence with activities of daily living in the frail elderly
Balance	Improving unipedal stance and functional reach	Reduce risk of falls

spend most of their days in wheelchairs. Loss of range of motion can result in painful joints, including "frozen shoulder syndrome" and even complex regional pain syndrome.[7] In addition to preventing contractures, ROM exercises stimulate joint and cartilage blood flow, enhancing the health and lubrication of joints in both healthy individuals and those with NMDs.

Strengthening Exercises

Among the several forms of strengthening exercises, some may be safer than others for patients with NMDs. Strengthening exercises can be classified as static or dynamic. Static (also called *isometric*) exercises are those performed at a constant muscle length, such as "quadriceps setting," or straight-leg raises using ankle weights to strengthen the quadriceps. Dynamic exercise involves joint movement. Dynamic muscle actions can be described as *isotonic*, *isokinetic*, *concentric*, and *eccentric*. Isotonic muscle actions supply constant force throughout a muscle movement, which rarely or never occurs in real-life settings. Isokinetic muscle actions are those performed at a constant velocity and require the use of specially designed exercise machines. Concentric actions are those in which the muscle shortens as it produces force, and eccentric actions are those in which the muscle lengthens as it produces force. Elbow flexion using a dumbbell (a "curl") is a concentric action of the biceps muscle; if the weight is then slowly lowered by extending the elbow, an eccentric muscle action of the biceps occurs.

Eccentric muscle actions are more efficient than concentric actions and generate more force at a given level of exertion. In healthy individuals, a heavy bout of eccentric exercise can produce a long-lasting decrease in muscle twitch tension and elevated serum creatine kinase (CK). Muscle fiber necrosis and mononuclear cell infiltration may be seen on muscle biopsy specimens for up to 20 days after such a bout of exercise. In healthy individuals, this muscle damage may serve as a stimulus for hypertrophy. However, in patients with muscle diseases affecting the cell membrane, such as the dystrophinopathies and sarcoglycanopathies, there is concern that the damage may not be repairable. Although there is no human datum addressing this issue, animal studies suggest that this concern is valid. In one study, *mdx* mice (the mdx mouse is an animal model for Duchenne muscular dystrophy) suffered an irreversible loss of force-generating capacity after eccentric exercise.[8]

Both muscular and neural adaptations occur in response to strength training. Muscular adaptations take at least 6 to 8 weeks to develop. They include muscle fiber hypertrophy, conversion from type IIa to type IIx fibers, increased protein synthesis, decreased protein degradation, increased capillary density, reduced mitochondrial density, and decreased lipid storage. Neural adaptations may occur in as little as 2 weeks and account for early strength gains when a training program is initiated. Neural adaptations occur without muscle hypertrophy and may be due to increased motor unit activation and synchronization. Cross-transference is a neural adaptation in which a single limb is trained, but strength increases also occur in the contralateral untrained limb. This is an important consideration in reviewing the literature on strength training in NMDs because some studies have been designed such that a single limb is exercised, with the contralateral limb used as a control.

The strength training studies involving patients with NMDs can be divided into those with heterogeneous patient populations (a mixture of neuropathic and myopathic disorders), those with strictly myopathic subjects, and those with strictly neuropathic subjects (primarily those with post-polio syndrome [PPS]). Although the prescription of exercise for patients with neuromuscular junction disorders, such as myasthenia gravis, is particularly challenging, no studies have been performed with this population.

The largest number of strength training studies has been performed using patients with a mix of disorders.[9–15] Only one of these studies, enrolling 62 patients, was a randomized, controlled trial.[12] The studies cannot be directly compared with one another because they utilize different methodologies. The nonrandomized studies tend to involve unilateral exercise using the contralateral arm as a control.[9,10,13,14] Strength gains were documented in all studies. Strength gains in the nonexercised limb, a cross-transference training effect, were also demonstrated.[9] Muscle activation, assessed using the twitch interpolation technique, improved in one study, suggesting that some of the strength gain was due to neural adaptations.[13] Functional improvement, in the form of increased walking speed, was documented in one study.[12] Patients reported subjective benefit and did not report muscle weakness or soreness, even in one high resistance study in which the biceps muscle lost eccentric strength[10]; the disparity between the subjective and objective responses to this training regimen suggests that overuse weakness can occur without apparent muscle fatigue or soreness. However, no muscle damage as a result of exercise has been detected using a variety of techniques, including measurement of serum myoglobin and CK, muscle biopsy and histology, and computed tomography scan.[12,13]

A few studies have explored the effect of resistance training in specific myopathic disorders, including DMD, facioscapulohumeral dystrophy (FSHD), limb-girdle muscular dystrophy (LGMD), inclusion body myositis (IBM), and mitochondrial myopathy.[16–19] In general, the findings are similar to those described in patients with mixed diagnoses. Although the strength changes in boys with DMD as a result of training are not statistically significant, they may be clinically significant; a nonexercising control group of age-matched DMD subjects actually might be expected to lose strength over a similar 9- to 12-month study period.[16,19] In a 12-month study of adults with FSHD and LGMD, significant strength gains were achieved during the first 4 months, and strength then plateaued, suggesting that the initial positive response may have been due to reversal of disuse muscle atrophy or neural adaptation. In a study of patients with IBM, magnetic resonance imaging measurements of whole muscle cross-sectional area did not change despite a significant improvement in strength, supporting the idea that much of the strength gain may be neurally mediated.[17] In general, muscles with the greatest initial strength improved the most with training, but some improvement was seen in weaker muscles.[17,19]

An interesting case report of heavy resistance training in a patient with a mitochondrial myopathy demonstrates a possible "gene shifting" benefit induced by exercise.[18] When heavy resistance exercise damages muscle, satellite cells are incorporated into the muscle as part of the repair process. In mitochondrial disorders, satellite cells contain much lower levels of mutant mitochondrial DNA than do muscle cells. By incorporating satellite cells into muscle, the proportion of mitochondria carrying mutant DNA can be reduced. In a patient with Kearns-Sayre syndrome, wild-type mitochondrial DNA in the biceps increased by 33% with an 18-day training program. Interestingly, concentric exercise appears to cause greater gene shifting than eccentric exercise.

With regard to purely neuropathic disorders, there is a single randomized, controlled trial of strengthening exercise in patients with ALS,[20] and several studies have addressed the role of resistance training in PPS.[21–24] The ALS study involved 6 months of training three times per week following an individualized program for muscles with greater than grade 3/5 strength on the Medical Research Council (MRC) muscle strength scale. Those in the training group had higher ALS Functional Rating Scale (ALS FRS) and Short Form-36 (SF-36) Health Survey scores at the end of the training period, suggesting that resistance training may improve function and quality of life. There were no significant adverse events related to the exercise program.

Studies in PPS have all involved training of the quadriceps muscle group, and none enrolled control subjects. These studies, varying in length from 6 weeks to 2 years, all demonstrated increases in static or dynamic strength without evidence of histologic muscle damage, changes in serum CK, or changes in motor unit physiology, as assessed using single-fiber and macro electromyography techniques. Several of these studies utilized relatively high-resistance training protocols.[22–24] The fact that large strength gains occurred without an increase in muscle cross-sectional area once again suggests neurally mediated strength gains.[24] Thus, studies in patients with PPS suggest that strength can improve with resistance training in patients with progressive neuropathic disorders without adversely affecting muscle histology or producing overuse weakness.

Although most studies of strength training have focused on major muscle groups in the extremities that are important for mobility and ADLs, the impact of strength training on ventilatory muscle function is also important in patients with NMDs. A 3-month uncontrolled study of an inspiratory muscle training program in 24 adults with motor neuron disease, neuromuscular junction disorders (mainly myasthenia gravis), and myopathies demonstrated increases in forced vital capacity (FVC), maximum voluntary ventilation (MVV, a measure of ventilatory muscle endurance), and maximum inspiratory pressure (MIP) in all groups.[25] Interestingly, the patients with motor neuron disease were the weakest initially and made the greatest gains. Several studies have addressed the role of inspiratory muscle training in boys with DMD.[26–29] One study found an increase in MIP in those with an FVC greater than 25% of predicted[29]; another study documented an increase in MVV with no change in MIP.[26] FVC did not improve in any of these studies, but there was no evidence of overuse weakness. Inspiratory muscle training in patients with myasthenia gravis has also improved respiratory muscle strength and endurance.[30] The clinical impact of small increases in MIP and MVV is unknown.

Aerobic Exercise

Aerobic exercise refers to prolonged low-resistance dynamic activity utilizing large muscle groups; it has a cardiopulmonary training effect. The American College of Sports Medicine (ACSM) recommends that the minimum quantity and quality of training to maintain cardiorespiratory fitness in healthy adults is at least 30 minutes of aerobic activity at 55% to 90% of maximum heart rate (HR) or 40% to 85% of maximum oxygen uptake (VO_2max) reserve most days of the week; activity may be accumulated in 10-minute bouts. Maximum HR can be estimated using the formula: HR = 220 − age. In healthy individuals, aerobic exercise improves functional exercise capacity, decreases psychological stress, improves quality of life, helps prevent secondary diseases (i.e., heart disease, diabetes, cancer), improves sleep, helps maintain bone density if performed in a weight-bearing manner, and produces greater independence with ADLs in the frail elderly. Although one would expect the benefits to be similar for patients with NMDs, little research has been done in this area. The studies that have been performed have focused primarily on whether the response to aerobic training in patients with NMDs is similar to that of healthy controls and whether aerobic fitness can be improved by training in this population. Quality of life, psychological impact, and secondary disease prevention have not been primary outcome measures.

In general, the cardiovascular response to aerobic training in patients with NMDs appears to be the same as that in healthy adults. A study comparing the response of patients with a variety of myopathic disorders to control subjects during a cycle ergometer exercise test found that, in general, the patients had normal resting oxygen consumption and a normal oxygen cost of exercise.[31] Their VO_2max was reduced, reflecting their deconditioned status. Of the 24 patients in the study, 5 had an increased oxygen cost of exercise; their diagnoses were Becker muscular dystrophy, carnitine palmitoyltransferase deficiency, and mitochondrial myopathy. Training studies utilizing home-based cycle ergometry have been performed in patients with FSHD, myotonic dystrophy, LGMD type 2I, Guillain-Barré syndrome, and chronic inflammatory demyelinating polyradiculoneuropathy (CIDP). In all of these studies, VO_2max increased, with some self-reported improvement in strength, endurance, ability to perform ADLs, and mood.[32–35] Patients with McArdle disease (myophosphorylase deficiency) have also shown a positive response to a carefully controlled walking and cycling aerobic exercise program.[36]

Taivassalo et al have studied adaptations to aerobic training in patients with mitochondrial myopathy. In an initial study, 10 patients with varied mitochondrial disorders (chronic progressive external ophthalmoplegia, Kearns-Sayre syndrome, and myopathy) trained for 8 weeks on a treadmill at 60% to 80% of HR three to four times per week for 20 to 30 minutes.[37] Aerobic capacity and exercise duration improved by 30%. Serum lactate concentrations at rest and after exercise decreased by 30%, and magnetic resonance spectroscopy measurements of adenosine diphosphate recovery after exercise improved by 60%. In a follow-up study utilizing a similar protocol, patients with mitochondrial disorders, patients with other myopathies, and sedentary control subjects were trained.[38] Aerobic capacity improved in all three groups, but the gain was greatest in the group with mitochondrial disorders. There has been some concern that endurance training might shift the proportion of mutant to wild-type mitochondrial DNA in a deleterious manner. However, recent studies have demonstrated an increase in the overall mitochondrial DNA content without a change in the ratio of mutant to wild-type DNA.[39,40]

Several studies have documented aerobic training benefits in patients with PPS.[41–43] These studies have utilized both cycle ergometry and treadmill training and have demonstrated increases in VO_2max, endurance, and oxygen consumption at a given exercise intensity without any loss of strength or other adverse events.

A single study has addressed the response to aerobic exercise in patients with ALS.[44] Overall, the oxygen cost of exercise was increased, possibly because of spasticity. Ventilation and HR increases were proportional to those in oxygen consumption, as would be expected in healthy individuals. Interestingly, the expected increases in plasma free fatty acids, beta-hydroxybutyrate, and carnitine were blunted in patients with ALS, suggesting a possible defect in lipid metabolism.

A single study has documented the beneficial effects of a simple, moderate home exercise program in patients with ALS.[45] Patients with ALS were randomized to receive a moderate daily exercise program consisting of gentle aerobic activity, such as walking, stationary bicycling, or swimming, for 30 minutes or less or not to perform any physical activity beyond their usual daily requirements. At 3 months, patients who performed regular exercise showed less deterioration on the ALS FRS and Ashworth Scale of muscle tone. At 6 months, there was no significant difference between groups, although a trend toward less deterioration was observed in the exercise group. This study demonstrates that a regular moderate physical exercise program is safe and has a short-lived positive effect on disability in patients with ALS. A small study of patients with ALS and respiratory insufficiency who exercised on a treadmill while using bilevel positive airway pressure ventilation has suggested that the progression of respiratory failure may be slowed by aerobic exercise.[46]

Balance Exercises and Training

Balance often is impaired in patients with NMDs due to a combination of sensory neuropathy, proximal muscle weakness, and/or spasticity. Impaired balance, which may be defined as a unipedal stance time of less than 30 seconds, is a risk factor for falling among healthy older individuals.[47] One would presume that this is also true among patients with NMDs. Among patients referred to a university electromyography laboratory for lower extremity complaints, an abnormal unipedal stance time (<45 sec) had a sensitivity of 83% and specificity of 71% for predicting peripheral neuropathy.[48] The question of whether or not balance can be improved by a specific balance training exercise program and whether this can improve function in patients with NMDs is in the exploratory stages.

Richardson et al enrolled patients with diabetic neuropathy in a 3-week exercise program designed to improve balance.[49] The exercises included bipedal and unipedal toe raises, heel raises, and ankle inversion and eversion exercises as well as unipedal balance challenges. Patients improved their unipedal and tandem stance time as well as their functional reach. These results suggest that balance exercises may be a promising therapy for patients with NMDs if the improvements translate into a decreased incidence of falling.

Future Research in Exercise

Much additional research needs to be done regarding the safety and potential benefits of exercise for patients with NMDs. A key question that has not been entirely answered is whether overuse weakness develops. Other questions that require definitive answers are whether exercise training can improve strength, aerobic fitness, function in ADLs, quality of life, and mood in patients with NMDs. The impact of respiratory muscle training on the incidence of pneumonia and time to respiratory failure also remains to be shown.

When evaluating studies of exercise in patients with NMDs, particular attention must be given to the specific exercise prescription; the measurement methods used to determine strength, aerobic capacity, flexibility, and balance; and the specificity of the exercise and outcome measurement methods. A quantitative, reproducible method for measuring strength must be used in any strength training study, and the method for measuring strength should be as close to the training method as possible. For instance, if a study involves primarily dynamic exercise (such as lifting dumbbells), dynamic rather than static strength should be used as an outcome measure. Ideally, studies should be randomized and have a nonexercising control group with the same disease and baseline characteristics. Unfortunately, few randomized studies have been performed; one of the research challenges is convincing patients with NMDs to agree to be randomized to a nonexercising control group.

Exercise Recommendations

Existing research regarding exercise in patients with NMD is limited in scope, but some recommendations for exercise prescription can be formulated. An exercise prescription should include the form of exercise, as well as the intensity, duration, and frequency of training sessions. Research thus far has focused on the safety and efficacy of exercise with little work on the impact of exercise programs on performance of ADLs or less directly related factors such as mood, psychological well-being, sleep, and appetite. It may be that exercise has a minimal impact on function but a greater impact on quality-of-life parameters such as those mentioned here.

Flexibility and ROM exercises are certainly safe and should be prescribed to all patients with muscle tightness due to either limited mobility (i.e., contractures) or spasticity.

Strength training appears to be safe when performed with proper supervision. It can reverse disuse weakness and may improve absolute muscle strength in those with more slowly progressive NMDs or acquired NMDs that have responded to pharmacologic treatment (e.g., myasthenia gravis or dermatomyositis). Overuse weakness has not been documented with any moderate-resistance strengthening program, and moderate-resistance strength training can increase strength in muscles with an initial MRC grade of 3/5 or better. Strength gain appears to be proportional to the initial strength of the muscle, with the strongest muscles making the greatest gains. Thus, it is logical to institute a strengthening program as early in the course of a progressive disease as possible. The goal of a resistance training program should be to maximize the strength of unaffected or minimally affected muscles to delay the onset of impairment. To ensure safety, patients should be advised to avoid high-resistance eccentric exercise. A practical recommendation is to find a weight a patient can lift 15 to 20 times comfortably, and then ask him to perform several sets of 10 lifts each. Patients also should be counseled to reduce their training load if they experience persistent muscle soreness or fatigue after exercise sessions.

In general, patients with NMDs have a normal cardiovascular response to aerobic training. Unless they have significant cardiac or respiratory disease, there are no apparent contraindications to aerobic exercise. The benefits of aerobic training are similar to those in healthy individuals. Patients should select a mode of exercise with minimal risk of injury from falling; for example, in patients with poor balance, a cycle ergometer may be safer than a treadmill. ACSM guidelines regarding intensity, duration, and frequency of exercise should be followed.

Balance training is a promising form of exercise for patients with a variety of NMDs. In patients with neuropathy, training has been demonstrated to improve balance, and it is hoped that this will in turn reduce the risk of falling.

Orthoses and Mobility Aids

Over time, individuals with NMDs may require orthoses and mobility aids to maximize function and independence. Particularly in rapidly progressive disease, the rehabilitation focus may shift quickly from using exercise to optimize strength and physical fitness to utilizing assistive devices to maximize function and independence.

Orthoses

Orthoses are devices applied externally to the body to provide support, protection, and improved function. They support weak muscles, decrease stress on compensatory muscles, minimize fatigue, prevent deformity, and conserve energy. Orthoses can be prefabricated or individually fashioned. Orthoses are one component of a comprehensive rehabilitation program; orthosis needs must be frequently reassessed, as fit and needs change over time.

Spinal Orthoses

Weakness of neck extensor muscles, as can occur in inflammatory myopathies, neuromuscular junction disorders, and motor neuron diseases, can result in head drop. Head drop is associated with pain and

Table 8-2 Cervical Orthoses/Collars

Collar Type	Examples	Indication	Benefits	Disadvantages
Soft	Foam	Mild neck extensor weakness	Comfortable Well-tolerated	Minimal limitation of neck movement
Semirigid or hard	Aspen* Malibu* Miami-J* Philadelphia	Moderate to severe neck weakness	Limitation of neck flexion and extension	Discomfort Skin breakdown
Open air	Headmaster Executive Canadian		Often the most acceptable balance between stability and comfort	Limited lateral support
Baseball cap[50]	Can be individually fabricated by a therapist	Good neck extensor strength and adequate cervical spine range of motion	Cosmesis Comfort	

*These collars provide increased sagittal and lateral support, as well as anterior neck access.

fatigue, as well as impaired speech, swallowing, and interpersonal communication. In severe neck extensor muscle weakness, the cervical spine can become completely flexed, resulting in particularly significant pain. Cervical orthoses (collars) can be utilized to mitigate head drop. See Table 8-2 for types of cervical orthoses and their indications. Figure 8-1 depicts the Headmaster collar, which is commonly used for treatment of head drop.

In preadolescent children with neuromuscular scoliosis, including those with spinal muscular atrophy (SMA), the muscular dystrophies, and peripheral neuropathies, including the hereditary motor and sensory neuropathies/Charcot-Marie-Tooth disease, thoracolumbosacral orthoses can be used to provide support to the spinal column during growth.[51] Molded seating supports can be used adjunctively for spine support as well. Orthosis use cannot prevent curve progression; if the curve has progressed significantly or seating positioning is compromised, surgery is typically performed at the onset of puberty in those who qualify as surgical candidates. In many individuals, surgery is performed prophylactically in anticipation of curve progression. In those who are not surgical candidates, thoracolumbosacral orthoses and wheelchair modifications addressing seating and arm height can provide stability and comfort.

Upper Extremity Orthoses

Upper extremity orthoses compensate for weakness, position an extremity for comfort and function, and enforce directional control in the treatment and prevention of contractures. Orthoses can be static (to prevent deformity, reduce tone), serial static (to provide stretch), static progressive (to provide stretch), dynamic (to allow restricted motion), or adaptive/functional (to compensate for absent upper extremity function).

Considerations in selecting and fitting upper extremity orthoses include cosmesis, skin protection, extremity positioning, tolerability, and individual functional goals. Tolerability includes comfort and lack of interference with desired hand functions. Grasp is most effective with the wrist in extension and slight radial deviation. Most right-handed individuals write with the wrist slightly extended, whereas left-handed individuals write with the wrist slightly flexed. For maintenance of muscle stretch, it is desirable for joints to be held at the end range of motion for the maximal tolerated duration.

Weakness of proximal upper extremity muscles, as can be seen, for example, in FSHD, Emery-Dreifuss muscular dystrophy, proximal myopathies, and motor neuron disorders, can result in glenohumeral joint subluxation, contractures, pain, and diminished function. Although slings cannot always prevent subluxation, they can be used for support and pain relief. Slings can be used in conjunction with appropriate seating and arm rests for individuals who use wheelchairs. Types of slings include the humeral cuff and pouch/single strap. The humeral cuff sling consists of an arm cuff on the distal humerus secured by a figure-of-eight harness. The pouch sling supports the elbow and wrist; however, because this sling holds the upper extremity in adduction, internal rotation, and elbow flexion, it may promote the development of contractures over time.

For individuals with intrinsic hand muscle weakness, wrist-hand and hand-finger orthoses can be utilized. The resting hand splint (wrist-hand orthosis) can be used during the days or nights to maintain muscle length and reduce contracture risk. This orthosis promotes wrist and metacarpophalangeal extension and interphalangeal flexion.

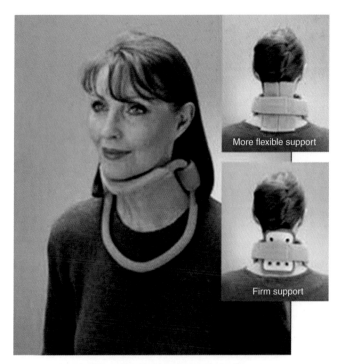

More flexible support

Firm support

Figure 8-1 Headmaster cervical collar.

An anti–claw hand splint can reduce claw-hand deformity and improve grasp by limiting metacarpophalangeal extension of digits four and five.

Individuals with finger flexor (notably IBM) or extensor weakness can use a variety of wrist-hand-finger orthoses to improve grasp and reduce contracture risk. These include the dynamic finger-extension splint for individuals with finger extensor weakness and adequate flexor strength; the volar cock-up splint for those with wrist and finger extensor weakness; and the opponens splint for those with abductor pollicis brevis, extensor pollicis longus, and extensor pollicis brevis weakness. The tenodesis orthosis (wrist-driven prehension orthosis) allows an individual with finger flexor and extensor weakness to create a three-jaw chuck handgrip using wrist extension. Figure 8-2 depicts several of the orthoses discussed here.

Functional upper extremity orthoses can afford individuals with upper extremity weakness increased independence in performing specific daily activities. These orthoses include the universal cuff to compensate for limited hand function and the balanced forearm orthosis to compensate for shoulder abduction weakness. The universal cuff is secured to the hand by an elastic strap and has a pocket that can hold utensils, hygiene tools, and writing implements. The balanced forearm orthosis (also known as a ball bearing feeder) supports the weight of the forearm and arm against gravity and utilizes ball bearings to allow for independent horizontal movement. These movements facilitate manipulation of desktop items and independent grooming and feeding. Balanced forearm orthoses can include adjustable resistance and ROM settings, as well as flexible mounting options. In the future, powered robotics, both externally and individually controlled, will likely become an increasingly utilized means of prolonging functional upper extremity independence as well.

Lower Extremity Orthoses

In NMDs, ankle dorsiflexion, knee extension, and hip flexion weakness can be quite marked. Similar to upper extremity orthoses, lower extremity orthoses are used to compensate for weakness, position an extremity for comfort and function, and enforce directional control. Orthoses should be as lightweight as possible. Cognitive status and upper body strength must be taken into account in optimizing ease of use of lower extremity orthoses. The physiatrist, orthotist, and physical therapist collaborate in assessing gait and orthosis needs and in training individuals in the use of the orthoses. Often, a nurse also participates in the care of individuals using orthoses by teaching about and screening for effects on the skin.

AFOs are the most commonly prescribed lower extremity orthoses in adults with NMDs. AFOs are prescribed for individuals with ankle dorsiflexion weakness to optimize safe, efficient ambulation (promote clearing of the toe during swing phase) and prevent ankle plantar flexion contractures. When prescribed for poorly selected candidates, however, AFOs can limit both gait and function. For example, solid-ankle AFOs reduce equinus, yet in children with DMD, for example, equinus gait may be compensatory for weak quadriceps muscles. Particularly in children, impaired gait may be more functional than braced gait. Generally, AFOs can be solid or hinged, static or dynamic, and can be modified to accommodate

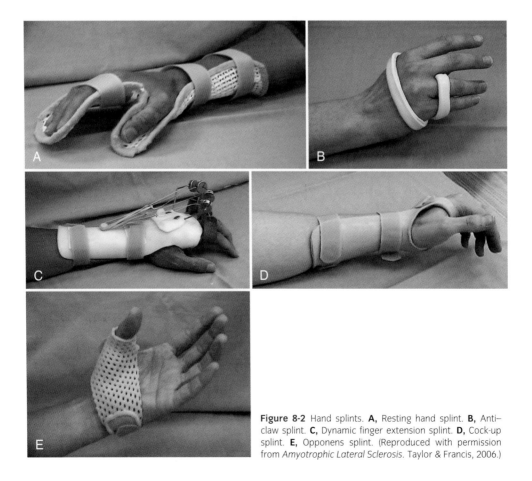

Figure 8-2 Hand splints. **A,** Resting hand splint. **B,** Anti–claw splint. **C,** Dynamic finger extension splint. **D,** Cock-up splint. **E,** Opponens splint. (Reproduced with permission from *Amyotrophic Lateral Sclerosis.* Taylor & Francis, 2006.)

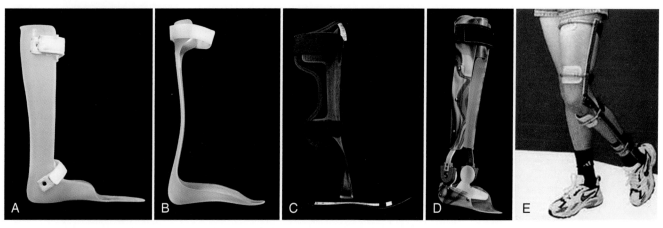

Figure 8-3 Lower extremity orthoses. **A,** Solid-ankle ankle-foot orthosis (AFO). **B,** Standard posterior leaf spring orthosis. **C,** Floor-reaction AFO. **D,** Hinged AFO with anterior shell. **E,** Stance control knee-ankle-foot orthosis. (**A–D,** Courtesy of Mitch Weiss, www.mitchweiss.com; **E,** with permission from Becker Orthopedic, www.beckerortho.com.)

quadriceps weakness, spasticity, and desired function. Often, new or modified shoes may be required to accommodate an AFO's bulk and shape. Figure 8-3 depicts examples of commonly used AFOs.

Solid (nonhinged) AFOs include the solid-ankle, semi-solid ankle, and posterior leaf spring AFOs. The standard solid-ankle AFO is made of thermoplastic material and provides maximal static stability in all planes of ankle-foot movement. This AFO encapsulates the posterior calf, with the proximal border 1 to 2 inches below the fibular head. Anterior and posterior trimlines are at the midlines of the malleoli. Because it is a static AFO, it does not allow for any ankle movement in the sagittal plane. This restriction of movement can limit sit-to-stand transfers and stair climbing. As needed, an AFO can be set in a few degrees of plantar flexion to help prevent buckling at the knee or a few degrees of dorsiflexion to limit hyperextension at the knee. If the AFO is set in dorsiflexion, an individual must have sufficient quadriceps control to compensate for rapid knee flexion during the loading phase of gait. Semi-solid ankle AFOs have trimlines posterior to the malleoli, and although they do not provide as complete ankle support as solid-ankle AFOs, semi-solid ankle AFOs may be better tolerated than solid-ankle AFOs when used bilaterally.

The posterior leaf spring AFO (PLS AFO) is a dynamic AFO, allowing for some flexibility of the anatomic ankle joint in the sagittal plane. The PLS AFO has trimlines posterior to the malleoli and has a narrow posterior calf component. It allows for tibial advancement over the forefoot during the stance phase of gait and for adequate clearance of the foot during the swing phase. However, it does not provide complete ankle stability in other planes of motion or provide firm equinus support. The PLS AFO is indicated for individuals with mild ankle dorsiflexion weakness but limited tone. Hypertonicity and spasticity can diminish the functionality of the PLS AFO by overcoming its flexibility.

Floor-reaction AFOs are solid-ankle AFOs that incorporate pretibial shells that limit tibial advancement during the stance phase of gait, thus reinforcing knee extension and overall gait stability. These AFOs are indicated when quadriceps strength is ≤3+/5 on the MRC scale and knee range of motion is good. Floor-reaction AFOs are not indicated for individuals with structural knee abnormalities. Individuals with poor postural control may need to use canes or other assistive devices along with the floor-reaction AFOs.

As compared with solid AFOs, hinged (or articulating) AFOs allow for easier sit-to-stand transfers and stair climbing. The

articulation across the ankle allows for improved anterior displacement of the tibia over the foot during the stance phase of gait. Hinged AFOs tend to be most appropriate for individuals with mild ankle dorsiflexion weakness and fairly preserved quadriceps strength. A 90-degree plantar flexion stop can be added to a hinged AFO to limit ankle plantar flexion in the setting of increased tone. A disadvantage of the hinged AFO is slightly increased weight and greater bulk around the ankle, making it more difficult to find shoes to accommodate it. Adductor spasticity and bilateral hinged AFO use can result in the medial aspects of the orthosis componentry catching, leading to falls.

In individuals with progressive quadriceps weakness, such as those with IBM, even a floor-reaction AFO may provide insufficient support over time. The relatively new stance-control knee-ankle-foot orthosis (KAFO) can lock and unlock without user manipulation, thus optimizing gait mechanics. The weight of this orthosis and the training required for its use may prohibit individuals with excessive weakness, fatigue, or cognitive impairment from successfully utilizing the device. Older KAFO designs include those with ratchet locks, drop locks, ball locks (for individuals with poor hand control), and dial locks (adjustable for knee flexion contractures). These older designs are often used by patients with a history of polio and some boys with DMD but are not practical for those with most other NMDs. They are relatively heavy and require walking with a locked knee, which is not possible in the setting of significant proximal weakness.

Antispasticity features that can be incorporated into AFOs and KAFOs include full foot plates, metatarsal head supports, built-up medial longitudinal arches, plantar flexion stops, and peroneal ridges.

If upper body strength allows, AFO and KAFO use can be accompanied by the use of crutches, canes, and walkers as needed for support and balance.

Canes, Crutches, and Walkers

Canes, crutches, and walkers can be used with or without orthoses to normalize gait pattern, reduce energy expenditure, and enhance balance, safety, and mobility. These aids can be considered extensions of the upper limbs; therefore, the maintenance of upper limb strength and range of motion can prolong their use. Device selection is based on strength, tone, and range of motion in the trunk and upper and lower extremities, degree of body weight

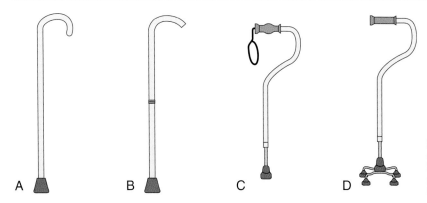

Figure 8-4 Canes. **A,** Standard wooden cane. **B,** Adjustable aluminum cane. **C,** Adjustable aluminum cane with offset handle. **D,** Four-point quad cane. (Reproduced with permission from *Amyotrophic Lateral Sclerosis.* Taylor and Francis, 2006.)

support needed, degree of fatigue present, rate of disease progression, individual desires and goals, and economic capabilities. Training by a physical therapist on any aid prescribed is recommended.

In general, canes provide the least support for gait stability and can be recommended for individuals with mild lower extremity weakness or balance impairments. Canes can be wooden or aluminum, solid or adjustable height, with one or four points of contact with the ground, and with narrow or wide bases. Grips on handles can be enlarged to accommodate handgrip weakness. A cane should be held in the arm opposite the weakest side and should be fitted for 20 degrees of elbow flexion. One should lead with the stronger limb on flat ground and in ascending stairs and with the weaker limb when descending stairs. Quad canes, which provide four points of contact with the ground, can be of standard or wide base, and provide additional stability as compared with standard canes. Different types of canes are shown in Figure 8-4.

Crutches provide support from the axilla to the floor. They are indicated for individuals with lower extremity weakness but preserved upper extremity and trunk strength. Lofstrand crutches are typically recommended over standard axillary crutches because they provide a forearm cuff that can free hands for use during standing. Platform forearm orthoses are useful for individuals with elbow flexion contractures or severe hand weakness. Crutch tips and handgrips must be routinely evaluated to ensure integrity and safety. Three types of crutches are depicted in Figure 8-5.

Walkers provide greater support for ambulation than canes and crutches, but their use may be limited by their weight and size. Options for walkers include folding, wheeled, and with brakes. Seating surfaces, baskets, and trays can also be added. When brakes are

selected, push-down brakes (engage when body weight is placed over the walker) are preferable to squeeze brakes for individuals with hand weakness. Although expensive, specialized wheeled walkers that can traverse multiple terrains are also available. Three walkers are depicted in Figure 8-6.

Seated Mobility Options

When independent or assisted ambulation is not feasible, seated mobility options can be used to maximize functional independence. These include power scooters, manual wheelchairs, and power wheelchairs. Power scooters should be recommended with caution for individuals with neuromuscular disorders. Power scooters require good upper extremity and trunk strength, cannot be modified for disease progression, and when covered by insurance, can preclude insurance coverage of power wheelchairs within a several-year time period. However, for those who can afford them, they may be good intermediate options before purchasing a power wheelchair. They are relatively lightweight and can be disassembled and transported in the trunk of a car.

A manual wheelchair can be used when an individual cannot ambulate long distances independently. Frequently, individuals with NMDs will not be able to self-propel a manual wheelchair due to easy fatigability and the need to conserve energy. For ease of transport, wheelchairs prescribed should be lightweight (<36 pounds) or ultra lightweight (<30 pounds) and with folding frames rather than rigid frames. Of note, a standard manual wheelchair, such as that used in hospitals, should not be prescribed, because it is heavier than these chairs and comes in a more restricted set of seat width, seat depth, and back height options. Standing capability for a manual wheelchair, which can provide weight-bearing and pressure relief, confers limited stability and flexibility for wheelchair modifications and is not typically prescribed for individuals with NMDs. Particularly for individuals with rapidly progressive diseases, such as ALS, a manual wheelchair should be rented or borrowed through organizations such as the Amyotrophic Lateral Sclerosis Association or Muscular Dystrophy

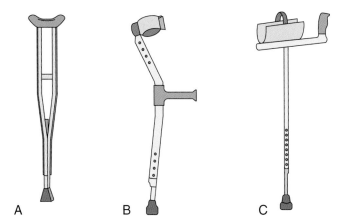

Figure 8-5 Crutches. **A,** Axillary crutch. **B,** Lofstrand or Canadian crutch. **C,** Platform crutch. (Reproduced with permission from *Amyotrophic Lateral Sclerosis.* Taylor and Francis, 2006.)

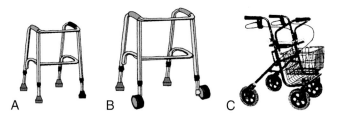

Figure 8-6 Walkers. **A,** Standard walker. **B,** Wheeled walker. **C,** Specialized walker. (Reproduced with permission from *Amyotrophic Lateral Sclerosis,* Taylor and Francis, 2006.)

Association, because most insurance companies will only reimburse for one wheelchair purchase over the course of several years. Insurance coverage for an eventual power wheelchair should be the priority.

Power-assist wheelchairs provide powered assistance to manually controlled use. They are heavier than manual wheelchairs and do not provide the flexibility of modifications available for fully powered wheelchairs. For these reasons, as well as the considerations described above, power-assist wheelchairs are typically not recommended for individuals with progressive NMDs.

When manual wheelchair use is no longer feasible due to weakness or the need for the use of ventilator or other equipment, full power wheelchairs are used. The transition from manual to power wheelchair use can be psychologically, physically, and logistically challenging. These challenges include psychological adjustment to disease progression, the need to modify previously used methods for performing ADLs and transfers, the need to modify home and work environments, and the need to modify vehicles and typical means of transportation.

Power wheelchairs are divided into three classifications by the Centers for Medicare and Medicaid Services. Class A wheelchairs are the conventional nonprogrammable power wheelchairs with basic seating. Class B wheelchairs can be modified based on an individual's needs in the realms of speed, acceleration, and braking. Class C wheelchairs, the most durable and modifiable, allow for seating, pressure relief, and ventilator modifications. Class C wheelchairs allow for the most flexibility and accommodation for long-term needs.

Specialty wheelchair and seating clinics, often coordinated by physical therapists, can provide expert recommendations to a rehabilitation team regarding optimal individualized wheelchair systems. Seat width, depth, and height, as well as back height and leg rest length, are based generally on the height and size of the user. Componentry for head and neck support (e.g., head rests), trunk support (e.g., lateral supports), seating/cushioning (e.g., molded cushioning to accommodate orthopedic abnormalities), pain and pressure relief (e.g., tilt-in-space or recline functionalities), upper and lower extremity support, and seatbelts can be individualized based on patient needs. Flexibility for adding items such as trays, ventilators, and communication or other equipment must also be specified.

Final factors that must be specified are type of drive and user-wheelchair interfaces. Wheelchairs can be rear-, front-, or mid-wheel drive. Mid-wheel drive chairs have the smallest turning radius and can negotiate some outdoor terrain. Rear-wheel drive chairs have the most consistent straight tracking but have a large turning radius and are most appropriate for patients who are heavy outdoor users.

The user-wheelchair interface refers to the means by which a user controls his wheelchair. Interfaces include the joystick, sip-and-puff mechanism, head array switch, and voice control. Joystick selection includes several features: proportional versus switched control, mounting site (joysticks can be operated by nearly any body part), and shape. The sensitivity of the input device must be programmed to match the user's capabilities. The sip-and-puff mechanism is particularly useful for individuals with SMA, who retain strong respiratory systems while losing significant extremity strength. Integrated controls are also available—for these, a single input device, such as a joystick, can be toggled between controlling the wheelchair and controlling other electronic devices in the home.

Wheelchair features can be designed to accommodate weakness, spasticity, contractures, and anticipated medical and functional needs. Allowing an individual to personalize a wheelchair through choice of aesthetic design features such as color is also recommended.

Stair-climbing wheelchairs have limited stability and require upper extremity strength and trunk balance. As a result, these wheelchairs are typically not prescribed for individuals with NMDs. In addition, they are extremely expensive and usually are not covered by insurance.

Orthoses and Mobility Devices in Pediatrics

The landscape of orthotics and mobility devices for children with NMDs can be somewhat different than that for adults. Orthotic options more often include KAFOs, hip-knee-ankle-foot orthoses, and reciprocating gait orthoses. Children tend to tolerate bulky orthoses better than adults do. In adults, other considerations, including rapidity of disease course, energy cost of using complicated, heavy orthoses, and psychological barriers, often restrict the range of orthoses used.

Upright environmental exploration promotes cognitive, motor, and social development, and so is encouraged to the greatest extent possible. Standing frames, caster carts, and reverse walkers can be used to optimize standing.

For children, wheelchair design considerations include flexibility to accommodate growth and the incorporation of educational technologies, capabilities for facilitating interactions with peers, and manageability and transportability by families. Options include seats that can lower to the floor to allow for play with peers.

Assistive Devices for Activities of Daily Living

Basic ADLs include self-care tasks such as eating and feeding, grooming and bathing, dressing and undressing, toileting, initiating functional mobility, caring for personal devices, sleeping and resting, and engaging in sexual activity. Instrumental ADLs (IADLs) are not required for daily functioning, but allow individuals to function within their homes and communities. IADLs include work outside the home, housework, meal preparation, childcare, shopping, driving, participation in safety and emergency procedures, and home, health, and financial management.

Several types of modifications can facilitate independence with ADLs and IADLs. A task can be modified, the tools needed to complete the task can be modified, or the environments in which the task is performed can be modified. Most often, a combination of these modifications is required. An introduction to assistive devices for ADLs and IADLs is provided below. Assistive devices for self-feeding and manipulating food; for grooming, bathing, and toileting; and for dressing and undressing can be found in Tables 8-3 to 8-5. To optimize their use, these devices must be appropriately placed near the individual using them and should be used when the individual is appropriately awake and attentive. Occupational therapists can provide additional recommendations as well as assistance with creating appropriate individualized aids.

Assistive Devices for Functional Mobility

Assisted ambulation and wheelchair mobility permit significant independence for individuals with NMDs. Daily functional mobility also includes bed mobility, transfers, and long-distance transportation. Bed mobility—getting into and out of bed, and repositioning while in bed—can be facilitated by overhead trapezes, step stools, and powered hospital beds. Transfers—transitioning between surfaces—can be facilitated by using ability-appropriate techniques

Table 8-3 Assistive Devices for Self-Feeding and Manipulating Food

Device	Use
Universal cuff	To hold utensils; compensate for intrinsic hand weakness
Balanced forearm orthosis	To bring food to mouth; compensate for upper extremity weakness
Built-up utensil and cup handles, rocker knives, swivel utensils, weighted utensils and cups, extended straws, straw holders	To manipulate utensils, cups, straws; compensate for intrinsic hand weakness
Scoop dishes, plate guards, food bumpers	To manipulate food, reduce spilling
Spork	To allow for multiple functions with one utensil
Nonslip matting, bowls and plates with suction bottoms	To prevent slipping
Sippy cups, cut-out cups, spouted cups, modified shapes for bottles	To consume liquids; compensate for upper extremity weakness and oromotor dysfunction

Table 8-4 Assistive Devices for Grooming, Bathing, and Toileting

Device	Use
Shower benches, bathtub seats, shower commode chairs, grab bars,* raised toilet seats	To accommodate weakness, conserve energy, promote safe transfers
Handheld shower heads, long-handled sponges, bath mitts, electric toothbrushes and shavers, long-handled combs, strap-fitted hairbrushes, swiveling back scrubbers, clamp-on adjustable mirrors, nail brushes with suction cup bases	To accommodate weakness and diminished range of motion, promote complete hygiene
Shoulder-mounted shampoo rinse trays	To facilitate hair-washing from a wheelchair over a sink
Toenail clippers with long handles	To accommodate spine flexion weakness

*It is important to educate patients and families that grab bars must be specifically and appropriately installed; typical towel racks are insufficient to support body weight.

Table 8-5 Assistive Devices for Dressing and Undressing

Device	Use
Mechanical button loopers, modified button and snap hooks, modified zipper pulls and hooks, hook-and-loop clothing closures, elastic shoelaces	To compensate for intrinsic hand weakness and impaired dexterity
Long-handled sock and shoe horns	To reduce the need for lumbar flexion for donning and doffing socks
Dressing sticks with mechanical graspers	To compensate for upper extremity weakness and allow an individual to pull the side of a sweater or shirt across the front of the body

as taught by a rehabilitation team, use of a slideboard, and use of wheelchair features such as adjustable seat height. Long-distance transportation can be facilitated by driving modifications such as hand controls and built-up knobs and handles, as well as transportation modifications such as wheelchair tie-down systems, power lifts and ramps, and custom car seats for children.

Public transportation systems are required by law to accommodate individuals with mobility and other impairments; often, these public transportation systems will provide both accessible areas of buses and trains and specialized paratransport systems. To enroll in the latter, patients require a physician's documentation of justification.

Assistive Devices for Environmental Control and Communication

Environmental controls and communication aids allow individuals to manipulate their surroundings and interact with others. Generally, inputs for environmental control and communication systems include switches, remote controls, and computers.

Environmental controls include key extenders to provide larger key grip surface areas, doorknob adapters that convert doorknobs to lever mechanisms, electric door openers, and lamp switch extenders. Higher-technology adaptations include integrated control systems, which allow an individual control over various aspects of the environment, including room temperature, sound, and light.

Communication devices include voice-activated inputs for electronic devices, remote control speaker phones with automatic dialing, and telecommunication devices for the deaf that allow for typewritten inputs over telephone lines. The latter can be particularly important for individuals with bulbar-predominant disorders that limit voiced communication. Call bells that connect to caregivers or emergency response systems can be accessed in a variety of ways, ranging from voice activation to hand control to respiratory (sip and puff) control. These should be carefully selected and tested, and should be evaluated frequently for ease of use.

Adjustable table angles, foam tubing to build up grips for devices, and carefully selected input devices (e.g., mouthstick, headstick) can facilitate the use of environmental control and communication devices. It is important to remember that even in individuals with some hand strength, mouth-operated controls might be faster and easier to engage, and these should be offered as options in care planning.

Other Activities of Daily Living/Independent Activities of Daily Living/Community Participation Aids

Additional equipment can be prescribed or created to optimize participation in the classroom, work environment, and leisure and athletic activities. Devices prescribed and created to meet individual needs are as numerous as the number of individuals who use them. Individual needs and desires can be optimized via evaluation by a rehabilitation team that includes a physical therapist, occupational therapist, recreational therapist, technology specialist, educational specialist, and physiatrist. Often, individuals and families create their own solutions to daily ADL and IADL challenges, and professional care teams can learn important tricks and tips from them that can be shared with other patients and families.

Environmental Evaluations and Modifications

Physical and occupational therapists can provide home evaluations and make recommendations for improved accessibility and safety. Home modifications and renovations typically are not reimbursable by Medicare or most private insurance companies but may be covered by Medicaid in some instances. The range of possible home modifications is vast; basic adaptations to accommodate wheelchair use are discussed here.

To access a home, portable ramps, vertical platform lifts, or permanent ramps can be installed. A ramp cannot exceed 1 foot of height per 12 feet of length. Doorframe widths of 32 inches will allow most wheelchairs and walkers to clear. If a wheelchair must enter a door from an angle, a doorframe width of 36 inches is usually required. Doors to small rooms can be made more accessible by reversing them to swing open instead of inward, replacing them with folding doors, or removing them entirely. Offset hinges can increase doorway width by 2 inches. These modifications can allow for sufficient space for room entry and maneuvering within the room. A minimum of 60 inches for a wheelchair turning radius and 30 to 36 inches to approach a surface for transfer are recommended as well. Door handles, light switches, soap dishes, and other reachable items should be between 30 and 36 inches from the floor to allow for accessibility from a seated position.

Home modifications for hygiene and toileting include eliminating rims from shower stalls and creating a space for commode use outside of bathrooms if there is inadequate bathroom space. Kitchen modifications include removing cabinets from under sinks to accommodate wheelchairs. Staircases can be fit with custom-made chair glides and stair lifts, but their use may be limited by cost, home infrastructure, and limited space to allow for transfers at the tops and bottoms of the staircases. Often, individuals who have upper floor bedrooms transform lower floor rooms, such as dens, into bedrooms.

School and Workplace Modifications

The Americans with Disabilities Act and the Individuals with Disabilities Education Act require modifications for the school and workplace, as well as other community venues, to accommodate individual needs generated by NMDs. Local and national support and advocacy organizations can provide specific information and recommendations for communicating with schools and workplaces and obtaining appropriate accommodations.

Orthopedic Considerations

Skeletal deformities most commonly encountered in the context of NMDs include scoliosis, joint contractures, and abnormalities of the feet. Despite conservative efforts at the prevention of these deformities, surgical orthopedic intervention is often required. The goals of both rehabilitation and orthopedic intervention include optimizing functional independence, comfort, pulmonary function, and personal hygiene.

Neuromuscular Scoliosis

Neuromuscular scoliosis—sagittal deformity of the spine in individuals with neuropathic or myopathic disease—is particularly common in rapidly progressive NMDs that begin in childhood. Although the precise mechanisms generating the scoliosis have not been fully elucidated, muscle strength imbalances, immobility, and possibly dominant handedness likely contribute. In DMD, the development of scoliosis seems to co-occur with the onset of wheelchair use, but no causal relationship between wheelchair use and curve progression has been established. Both scoliosis and the onset of wheelchair use occur during the pubertal growth spurt, around ages 13 to 15 years.

Scoliosis, particularly with curves greater than 40 degrees, creates significant difficulty with seating and positioning, use of the upper extremities, and comfort, as well as respiratory compromise.[52] Bracing does not prevent curve progression in neuromuscular scoliosis. Seating modification, optimizing muscle strength and use, and patient and family education have similarly not been shown to affect the progression of scoliosis.[53] Surgical spine fusion with instrumentation and early postoperative mobilization is the treatment of choice for individuals with progressive neuromuscular scoliosis. Current data suggest postoperative improvements in quality of life, sitting posture, and ease of care. There is insufficient data at this time regarding the impact of surgery on respiratory function or life expectancy.[54]

Joint Contractures

Joint contractures—limitations in full range of motion of joints—are a major consequence of immobility, diminished weight bearing, and muscle imbalance in NMDs. In particular, increased wheelchair use is associated with flexion contractures at the hip, knee, ankle, and elbow, especially in muscles with less than antigravity strength.[55] Because contractures can limit mobility, positioning, hygiene, and comfort, prevention of contractures remains a key component of rehabilitation management.

The cornerstone of contracture prevention is the use of physical modalities. These include daily upright weight bearing with uniform weight distribution, active and passive stretching, and the use of bracing and splinting to promote muscle stretch. For those who cannot perform active stretching of multijoint muscle groups, passive (performed by another person) stretching is especially important, because typical daily positions do not place key muscles—the gastrocnemius, hamstring, rectus femoris, tensor fascia lata, and iliopsoas muscles—at maximal stretch. Heat and ultrasound may augment the effects of stretching and positioning.[56] Individuals with sensory impairment who are using contracture prevention programs must be monitored for fractures and skin breakdown.

An individually tailored contracture prevention program should be initiated as early as possible. The program can be developed by a physical or occupational therapist and can be taught to family members or other caregivers to perform on at least a daily basis. In addition, the program should focus on muscle groups particularly affected in a given condition. For example, a program for an individual with DMD might include the gastrocnemius, soleus, hamstring muscles, the iliotibial band, and the wrist flexors. In Emery-Dreifuss muscular dystrophy, elbow flexors must be addressed early. In SMA type 2, the hip, knee, and wrist must be addressed.

Particularly in individuals who use wheelchairs as a primary means of mobility, contractures may develop despite stretching, positioning, and splinting. Surgical intervention for fixed deformities can promote ease of positioning and prolonged capacity for upright weight bearing and, in some cases, braced ambulation. Because loss of ambulation is associated with weakness more than with contractures, however, surgical intervention for contractures will typically not permit resumption of independent ambulation that was previously lost.

Abnormalities of the Feet

Bony and soft-tissue abnormalities of the feet, including cavus (high-arched) feet, equinus (excess plantar flexion), and hammer toes (fixed flexion of the proximal interphalangeal joints of the small toes with hyperextension of the metatarsophalangeal and distal interphalangeal joints), are associated with peripheral neuropathies and weakness of the intrinsic foot muscles, as in Charcot-Marie-Tooth disease. These deformities can result in pain, calluses, skin breakdown, gait instability, and ankle instability. Stretching, orthoses, and serial casting in children may delay progression to fixed deformities. However, surgical intervention is often required to promote stability.[55] Shoe medications such as a widened toebox can improve comfort and protect skin.

Chapter 9 provides further detail on these and other related topics.

Respiratory Failure

Progressive respiratory failure impairs quality of life and limits life expectancy in many neuromuscular disorders, including the anterior horn cell diseases (ALS, PPS, SMA), severe forms of neuropathy (Guillain-Barré syndrome), myasthenia gravis, and several forms of muscular dystrophies and myopathies. The rehabilitation team must be aware of the patient's respiratory status because it will affect the ability to participate in exercise programs and rehabilitation therapies.

Some physiatrists have specialized expertise in pulmonary rehabilitation and the management of patients with restrictive lung disease.[57,58] In particular, they are skilled in the management of patients using noninvasive ventilatory techniques and equipment, including noninvasive positive-pressure ventilation, the pneumobelt, and negative pressure devices such as a cuirass or poncho ventilator. The insufflator-exsufflator (Cough Assist) and manually assisted coughing are indicated to help clear secretions in patients with expiratory muscle weakness. Respiratory monitoring, respiratory therapy services, and care by a pulmonologist are integral to the rehabilitation program for many patients with NMDs. Pulmonary assessment, monitoring, management, and rehabilitation are discussed in greater detail in Chapter 2.

Dysarthria

Dysarthria is a motor speech disorder resulting in impaired articulation and speech intelligibility. It interferes with verbal communication when receptive language and other means of communication may be fully intact and can diminish social interaction and quality of life. In NMDs, dysarthria can result from dysfunction of upper motor neurons, lower motor neurons, both upper and lower motor neurons, the neuromuscular junction, and muscle itself. The rehabilitation team focuses on maximizing independent communication with attention to the type of dysarthria present, the rate of progression, and patient and family goals.

Identification

In upper motor neuron (also called *spastic* or *pseudobulbar*) dysarthria, speech can be slurred, strained, and harsh, with slowness of movements and occasional bursts of loudness and unanticipated stops. There can be associated brisk gag and jaw reflexes, and notable absence of tongue atrophy and fasciculations. In contrast, lower motor neuron (also called *flaccid* or *bulbar*) dysarthria features a weak voice and associated wasting and weakness of tongue, palatal, and facial muscles; diminished reflexes; and nasal phonation. Dysarthria resulting from neuromuscular junction or muscle pathology typically presents with lower motor neuron features. In motor neuron disease with lower motor neuron features, fasciculations of the tongue can also be seen. In mixed dysarthria, the degrees of flaccidity and spasticity in any single individual can vary.[59]

Dysarthria in Motor Neuron Diseases

Motor neuron diseases often feature dysarthria of the upper and/or lower motor neuron varieties.[60] Dysarthria in ALS, for example, is of the mixed type, typically with prominent lower motor neuron features. Early signs of this pattern of dysarthria include slow speech rate, altered voice quality, difficulty singing, difficulty enunciating, and diminished intelligibility, resulting in decreased communication effectiveness. Speech may also sound hoarse and hypophonic, related to vocal cord and respiratory muscle weakness.

The cornerstone of rehabilitation management in progressive dysarthria is the utilization of verbal and nonverbal strategies to optimize communication throughout the course of disease progression. Speech-language pathology, neurology, physiatry, and, occasionally, otolaryngology assessments can yield comprehensive rehabilitation management strategies with these goals in mind. Of note, aggressive speech therapy per se typically does not have lasting long-term benefits in motor neuron diseases and may worsen speech impairment by causing fatigue.

In mild dysarthria, the rehabilitation team focuses on training patients and social contacts in compensatory techniques to prolong verbal communication. These can include slowing speech rate, using alternative words, spelling, repeating and overarticulating consonants, speaking face to face, using monosyllabic speech, and conserving energy by minimizing environmental noise and the distance between the patient and listeners. Importantly, developing personalized communication strategies between patient and listener can also prolong effective communication; these can include shared strategies for understanding gestures, facial expressions, and eye contact, as well as a system for confirming understanding.

Palatal lifts and palatal augmentation prostheses can be utilized to address hypernasality/hypophonia and consonant articulation, respectively, although little data exists regarding their efficacy. A retrospective review of the use of lifts and prostheses suggests that patients experience improved ease of speaking with their use.[61]

As dysarthria progresses, the rehabilitation team can provide augmentative and alternative communication systems. Higher-technology devices are not necessarily better for patients; device recommendations must consider patient and caregiver physical capability, education level, cognitive functional status, socioeconomic means, and general preferences. Optimally, training begins before acute need for the technology. Equipment can often be rented or acquired from charitable organizations. See Table 8-6 for a listing of augmentative communication devices.

Asynchronous communication, including the use of e-mail, message boards, and online social networks, can promote maintenance of social contacts without hindrance by slowness of speech/impaired direct in-person communication, and should also be encouraged as appropriate.

Finally, brain-computer interfaces (BCIs) are an active area of current study with much promise for use in severe dysarthria/anarthria that prevents verbal communication and co-occurs with severe motor impairment preventing other means of communication. BCIs output information from the brain directly to a computer. The use of both noninvasive (scalp recordings of electroencephalographic changes) and invasive (direct recordings from the motor cortex) devices are being investigated in ALS and other conditions resulting in severe dysarthria/anarthria.[62,63]

Assessment and training by occupational and adaptive technology specialists can provide technology users with individually designed accessible communication systems, mounting systems, and switches. Importantly, any technologies selected should be flexible to accommodate changes in user capabilities over time.

Table 8-6 Common Augmentative Devices to Enhance Communication

Type of Technology	Examples
Low	Communication boards, with manual writing
	Letter/word/picture boards, with eye gaze selection
	Alarm systems, such as buzzers, with accessible triggers
Higher	Portable voice amplifiers
	Voice record/playback devices (a patient can record phrases while still intelligible and play them back when no longer able to produce them physiologically)
	Computerized voice synthesizers on personal computers or dedicated devices (selection of information can be manual, by eye gaze, or by infrared signal)
	Word prediction technology for spelling words
	Specialized telephone equipment: hands-free, voice-free, or both

Dysarthria in Neuromuscular Junction Disorders

Neuromuscular junction disorders, including myasthenia gravis and the Lambert-Eaton myasthenic syndrome (LEMS), can also produce dysarthria, typically with lower motor neuron–type features and a nasal tone. In myasthenia gravis, impairment severity can fluctuate over the course of the day and with medications that alter neuromuscular junction transmission. Bulbar symptoms are presenting symptoms in 15% of individuals with myasthenia gravis and approximately 5% of individuals with LEMS. The latter statistic may be higher in practice, because the recognition of bulbar symptoms as part of LEMS is only beginning to emerge.[64,65]

Treatment of the underlying disorders produces resolution or improvement of dysarthria. A study of intravenous immunoglobulin in the treatment of LEMS specifically addressed bulbar function by measuring drinking times before and after therapy; there was improvement in this outcome measure after treatment.[66]

When dysarthria persists despite attempts at disease treatment, rehabilitation management can be employed to optimize speech quality and communication. The rehabilitation program includes patient and family education, speech therapy, and adaptive equipment as needed. Patients and families should be educated about symptoms and triggers, medication compliance, and energy conservation. Speech therapists can offer training in the control of speech rate, articulation, and interpersonal communication strategies. Augmentative communication devices and environmental modifications can also be employed. Finally, there may be a role for respiratory muscle and breathing training in enhancing intelligibility of speech in the setting of dysarthria in neuromuscular junction disorders. Such training has shown positive effects on respiratory muscle strength and endurance[30]; in turn, improved breath support may enhance speech volume and intelligibility.

Dysarthria in Myopathies/Muscular Dystrophies/Peripheral Neuropathies

Myopathic (congenital myopathies, mitochondrial myopathies), muscular dystrophic (myotonic dystrophy, oculopharyngeal muscular dystrophy), and peripheral neuropathic (including the hereditary peroneal muscular atrophy syndromes) conditions can also feature lower motor neuron–type or flaccid dysarthria. The general management approach to these conditions is similar to that outlined above: optimizing native verbal communication as long as feasible and facilitating continued communication via augmentative and alternative technologies, with early training.

In notable distinction to many other NMDs, however, in which activity can worsen speech production, the opposite is true in myotonic dystrophy. In myotonic dystrophy, both muscle weakness and myotonia contribute to impaired articulation, and speaking loudly may provoke myotonia. Warm-up exercises with prolonged sound production may improve repetition rate and fluency of speech and decrease the myotonic component of dysarthria without producing fatigue.[67] This suggests that more aggressive speech therapy with practice exercises may be of benefit in the treatment of dysarthria in myotonic dystrophy, whereas there is no evidence of beneficial effects of aggressive speech therapy in the dysarthria of most other NMDs.

Dysphagia

Oropharyngeal dysphagia, resulting from weakness and discoordination of facial, oral, and pharyngeal musculature, is common in many NMDs. Dysphagia can result in aspiration of oral contents, leading to pulmonary infection, social embarrassment, inadequate oral intake, malnutrition, and weight loss. In fact, many patients with myotonic dystrophy, for example, report dysphagia as the most disabling symptom of their disease.[68]

Identification

Indicators of dysphagia include changes in the quality of speech (wet-sounding voice), drooling and leaking of liquids from the mouth, coughing, nasal regurgitation, and choking while eating. Patients may also develop pneumonia after an episode of choking, multiple episodes of pneumonia in 1 year, and increasingly prolonged eating time. Unintentional weight loss, dehydration, and malnutrition may develop over time. Patients and family members should be educated early about the signs and dangers of dysphagia. At the first sign of dysphagia, evaluation by a speech-language specialist and, in some cases, a dietitian, will allow prompt diagnosis and intervention.

Compensatory Strategies and Interventions

When oropharyngeal dysphagia is identified, the rehabilitation team can design a program of interventions and compensatory strategies to facilitate safe oral intake to the greatest extent possible. These include positional, behavioral, and dietary modifications. Positional changes include posterior head tilt with swallow initiation, chin tuck, and head turning to the side of greater weakness if there is asymmetry. Behavioral interventions include scheduling meals during times of maximal arousal and minimal distraction. Dietary changes include altering food consistency (e.g., thickening liquids) and increasing caloric density of foods. Finally, in cases in which dysphagia is exacerbated by preoral challenges (i.e., weakness in the extremities limiting ability to bring food and fluid to the mouth), balanced forearm orthoses, universal cuffs, and modified utensils can be used.

If oral intake remains inadequate despite conservative interventions, gastrostomy tubes can be used for supplemental nutrition, weight stabilizations, and possible prolongation of survival. The use of gastrostomy tubes has not been shown to reduce the risk of aspiration. The American Academy of Neurology recommends the placement of gastrostomy tubes for individuals with ALS while they can still tolerate oral intake and before the FVC falls below 50% of predicted because morbidity and mortality associated with the procedure are lower when individuals do not have severe respiratory insufficiency.[69] However, more recent studies have demonstrated that feeding tubes can be safely placed in individuals with lower FVCs if bilevel positive airway pressure assistance is used during the procedure or if radiologic insertion techniques are used.[70,71]

Additional surgical management in select cases of oropharyngeal dysphagia related to impaired relaxation of the cricopharyngeus muscle in neuromuscular disease—particularly IBM—include botulinum toxin injection, physical dilatation of the muscle, and cricopharyngeal myotomy.[72–74] Chapter 4 provides further detail on these and other related topics.

Pain

Among individuals with NMDs, pain is a common experience and can contribute significantly to decreased health-related quality of life. Pain may be acute or chronic, with less chronic pain experienced among individuals with SMA as compared with other neuromuscular conditions.[75]

With the exception of some peripheral neuropathic syndromes, pain is not typically a feature of the primary disease itself, but rather is secondary to the effects of the disease on the musculoskeletal system. Of a sample of 811 patients with a range of NMDs, 83% reported ongoing pain, most commonly in the back.[75] In PPS, shoulder pain is also quite common.[76] Pain can arise from weakness, abnormal posture and gait, immobility, loss of range of motion, contractures, spasticity, and cramps, as well as from joint instability, nerve impingement from muscle atrophy, and overuse injury. Pain is then potentiated by deconditioning, depression, and comorbid health conditions. It is associated with increased fatigue, diminished coping ability, and altered sleep patterns.[75] Pain can limit participation in daily activities and social interactions and can be a source of anxiety for family members and caregivers.[77,78] Pain in individuals with NMDs has also been shown to persist for many years,[77] suggesting that current practices in pain assessment and management are insufficient.

Assessment of Pain

The assessment of physical pain must begin with open-ended questions and sensitivity to the contributions of biologic, psychological, and social factors to both the experience of and description of pain. Recently, through surveys and structured interviews of patients with physical disability from non-neuromuscular causes who use adapted mobility equipment, a set of common pain descriptors in sensory, affective, and temporal dimensions was created. These descriptors may be helpful prompts for patients with NMDs who need assistance in describing their pain, and can be used over time to assess efficacy of treatments. Pain sensation descriptors include aching, jumping, sore, cool/cold, numbing, shooting, cramping, pulling, throbbing, heavy/dull, radiating, tight, hot/burning, sharp/stabbing, and tingling. Pain affect descriptors include tiring/exhausting, nagging/bothersome, frustrating, emotional/psychological, and worrisome/afraid. Temporal descriptors include steady/constant, momentary/brief, and comes and goes.[79] In NMDs, additional descriptors of discomfort include soreness and local discomfort from prolonged positioning or equipment. Increased rates of impaired glucose tolerance in patients with myotonic

dystrophy may predispose individuals with that condition to peripheral neuropathies and the typical symptoms associated with them. Of course, pain can have a host of non-NMD etiologies, and these must remain in the differential diagnosis of pain in NMDs.

The Functional Independence Measure (FIM) self-report instrument has been validated for use in patients with NMDs and chronic pain, and can be used to assess an individual's perception of independence in the settings of neuromuscular disease and pain.[80]

Prevention of Pain

In rapidly progressive NMDs, weakness and immobility cannot be prevented. However, musculoskeletal pain complications from weakness and immobility can often be prevented. Prevention includes optimizing cardiopulmonary fitness to maintain stable pain threshold and mood, stretching to preserve range of motion, and using appropriately fitted equipment to optimize positioning and skin care. The nature and role of exercise is described earlier in this chapter.

Management of Pain

Despite the best efforts at prevention, musculoskeletal pain syndromes do develop in individuals with NMDs. Pain and pain interference with daily life activities and social satisfaction can cause significant disability and diminished quality of life. Individuals with ALS and myotonic dystrophy seem to be particularly sensitive to the effects of pain on daily life activities.[81]

A rehabilitation team, including a physiatrist, physical therapist, occupational therapist, adaptive technology specialist, psychologist, and primary caregivers, is well-suited to provide comprehensive pain management.

Back pain resulting from weakness and immobility, often associated with the use of adaptive mobility equipment, is common in individuals with NMDs. In a recent retrospective survey, 66% of individuals with myotonic dystrophy and 74% of individuals with FSHD reported pain in the back—the most frequently cited region of pain in those conditions.[77] Back pain can be minimized by wheelchair seating that includes lumbar support, firm compressible cushions (gel), and foam wedges for proper positioning. Weight shifting/pressure relief, required as frequently as every 15 minutes for as long a duration as possible, can reduce pressure on the bony structures of the lower back and the skin over the ischial spines. Patients must be taught to perform appropriate weight shifts. If a patient cannot perform weight shifts independently, a power tilt-in-space wheelchair control can provide pressure relief and skin protection. Sleeping surfaces must also be optimized for pressure relief.

Neck pain resulting from neck weakness and head drop occurs in a range of neuromuscular disorders, including ALS, myasthenia gravis, and the inflammatory myopathies. Cervical orthoses, as well as wheelchair head supports and reclining capabilities, can mitigate neck pain. ROM exercises can prevent pain associated with the development of contractures.

Shoulder pain from subluxation, adhesive capsulitis, and complex regional pain syndrome can be a consequence of loss of range of motion associated with weakness and immobility.[7,82,83] Shoulder pain can also arise from, or be complicated by, fractures, calcification, and musculotendinous damage. Prevention of these painful conditions includes maintenance of range of motion, optimization of positioning, and prompt treatment of comorbid pain-generating conditions. A figure-of-eight humeral cuff sling can minimize pain in those with shoulder subluxation when forced to have the arm in a dependent position, such as during ambulation.

Spinal deformities, including scoliosis and kyphosis, are particularly common in muscular dystrophies and SMA. Hyperlordosis, with or without scoliosis, is frequently seen in many forms of muscular dystrophy[77] as well. Although in a large series individuals with SMA reported less overall chronic pain than counterparts with other NMDs, bony spinal deformities in that condition and others can result in pain due to both altered positioning and secondary limitations in movement and ambulation. There is no proven means of preventing the development of these major spinal deformities in patients with NMDs. However, pain resulting from these deformities can be minimized with proper seating and positioning.

A source of pain for which prophylaxis may exist is fractures related to disuse osteoporosis. Among individuals with DMD attending a sample of neuromuscular clinics, 21% were reported to have experienced a fracture, with a peak age of 8 to 11 years at the time of fracture.[84] Upper limb fractures were most common in individuals using KAFOs, and lower limb fractures were most common in individuals with independent mobility or wheelchair use. Fracture prevalence did not appear to be affected by steroid use. McDonald et al[84] were unable to ascertain whether this number is significantly different from fracture prevalence in an average pediatric population, but they do note that fracture site and peak age do differ from those of children without DMD. In children with DMD and fractures, early aggressive mobilization after the fracture may decrease limitations in ambulation, which in turn may reduce pain and contractures.

Low bone mass has been reported in individuals with DMD, and alendronate may prevent loss of bone mass in DMD. Further study is required to delineate the impact of preserved bone mass on fracture rate.[85] In adults with limited mobility, screening bone density scans can be used to identify diminished bone mass, and primary care physicians or endocrinologists can assist in determining appropriate candidates for treatments including bisphosphonates.

In NMDs with upper motor neuron features, spasticity can both directly cause pain and indirectly result in pain due to limitation of extremity movement. A recent Cochrane Neuromuscular Disease Group topic review revealed only one randomized, controlled trial in the treatment of spasticity in ALS; this showed that individualized, moderate-intensity walking, swimming, or cycling may help to reduce spasticity.[86] Additional treatment modalities that can be effective in spasticity management in NMDs include oral medications, sustained muscle stretching, positional splinting (with good skin care), modalities including heat and cold, botulinum toxin injections, nerve blocks, and intrathecal baclofen pumps. With respect to medications, one must be cautious with dantrolene because it can cause excessive weakness by acting directly on muscle. In motor neuron disease with a combination of upper and lower motor neuron signs, caution must be taken that spasticity treatment does not diminish function and comfort by excessively exacerbating weakness. Contracture prevention and management are described elsewhere in this chapter; when done effectively, this can prevent the development of significant pain as well.

Finally, cramping is a common symptom in neuromuscular conditions, including ALS, myotonic dystrophy, and Charcot-Marie-Tooth disease.[77,87] Drinking tonic water may alleviate cramping-related discomfort. There are no proven pharmacologic interventions for the management of cramps in NMDs; of specific note, quinine-containing agents are discouraged due to significant side effects.

Additional Pain Management Strategies

No single treatment has been shown to provide lasting relief of pain in NMDs. Often, treatments are initiated but soon discontinued due to lack of benefit.[76,81] Although the sample size of individuals using chiropractic treatment and nerve blocks was small, these modalities were shown in one study to provide the greatest pain relief as compared with physical therapy, massage, acupuncture, magnets, biofeedback/relaxation training, counseling, hypnosis, and medications. Of note, individuals with weakness of the cervical or trunk musculature should avoid high-velocity spine manipulation because they are at increased risk for neurologic or bony injury. Additional research is warranted in the use of complementary and alternative medicine approaches for pain control in NMDs.

Some pain relief can be obtained from oral medications, which include scheduled acetaminophen with or without nonsteroidal anti-inflammatories, tricyclic antidepressants, sodium channel–blocking anticonvulsants, and antiepileptics (especially if there is a neuropathic component to pain), opioids (morphine can also relieve "air hunger"), hydroxyzine (synergistic with opioids), dextromethorphan, and cannabinoids (can also promote saliva reduction, appetite stimulation, sleep induction, and bronchodilation). Muscle atrophy can limit the effectiveness of intramuscular injections, and excessive diaphoresis can limit the effectiveness of transdermal medications. Patient-controlled analgesia can be limited by an individual's capacity to control the unit, so it is rarely an option for individuals with NMDs. Medications should be titrated to patient comfort, and risks and benefits discussed thoroughly with patients before initiation.

More invasive interventions, including steroid injections to treat joint discomfort and manipulation under anesthesia to treat adhesive capsulitis, are available for selected patients. Manipulation under anesthesia should be attempted with great caution, because it can be associated with both anesthesia-related risks and significant joint damage.

When adhesive capsulitis and contractures develop, consideration of goals of care is important. For example, an individual with adhesive capsulitis with rapidly progressive NMD might prefer to be treated with conservative pain control rather than manipulation under anesthesia.

Mood Disorders

Psychological challenges for individuals with NMDs include grief, fear, coping, and adjustment. Although features of depressed mood and anxiety often manifest, these are not necessarily correlated with the degree of neuromuscular impairment.[88–90] In individuals with end-stage ALS, for example, major depression is relatively rare and does not increase as death approaches, even though health-related quality of life may decline.[91,92]

Symptoms of depression, such as fatigue, inanition, limited social interactions, decreased enjoyment of daily activities, and even tearfulness, may overlap with features of primary NMD. It is therefore important to routinely screen for symptoms of depression in individuals with NMDs and elicit information from caregivers and families regarding changes in patients' behaviors and moods. Recent studies of depressed mood in ALS suggest that hopelessness and concerns about end of life are not uncommon. Pseudobulbar affect can be treated with a combination of dextromethorphan and quinidine, although combination therapy has not yet been approved in the United States and side effects of dizziness, nausea, and somnolence frequently limit its use.[69] Pseudobulbar affect and its management are discussed in further detail in Chapter 11.

Family, social, religious, spiritual, and formal support networks can provide sources of hope and forums for both sharing feelings and acquiring strategies to address them. Consistent support by health-care professionals of both the patient and caregivers can also mitigate fears and promote acceptance of one's disease and life changes.

A variety of standard pharmacologic interventions to treat depression can be trialed in patients with neuromuscular disease.

Frequently, these agents can simultaneously address primary disease symptoms. For example, agents with anticholinergic properties can both improve mood and treat pseudohypersalivation and non–respiratory-based insomnia. See Chapter 11 for a more detailed discussion of sialorrhea/pseudohypersalivation and insomnia). A psychiatrist or clinical psychologist can provide cognitive behavioral and other interventions that facilitate coping and engagement in pleasurable activities. A spiritual advisor can also assist patients in drawing on personal sources of strength.

As with symptoms of depression, symptoms of anxiety can also overlap with features of primary NMDs. For example, breathlessness can occur with acute episodes of anxiety or result from respiratory failure, which simultaneously incites feelings of anxiety. After addressing medical causes of anxiety to the greatest extent possible, anxiety itself can be addressed with social, pharmacologic, and counseling interventions. Pharmacologic management includes benzodiazepines and buspirone. Benzodiazepines must be used with caution, because they can exacerbate respiratory depression and fatigue. They should not be used in individuals with severe respiratory insufficiency or with myasthenic syndromes. Buspirone does not suppress respiration, but it may take several weeks before anxiolysis is achieved; it is also contraindicated for individuals with myasthenia.

Cognitive Dysfunction

Cognitive dysfunction is a clinically important feature in many NMDs, distinct from motor, mood, and behavioral changes associated with the disorders. Cognitive dysfunction has implications for decision making, interactions with family and caregivers, and interactions with professional care providers. For the professional care team, cognitive dysfunction also affects the design of individualized rehabilitation programs and clinical trials. Particularly as rehabilitation technology options become more complex, providers must carefully select appropriate candidates for their use. It is important to educate patients and families about possible cognitive changes associated with their neuromuscular conditions and for family members and care providers to monitor for and address cognitive changes over time. Lack of familiarity with cognitive manifestations of these conditions may prevent providers from discussing them upfront with patients and from recommending early educational and technological interventions.

Muscular Dystrophies

Cognitive impairment is common in individuals with Duchenne, Becker, myotonic, and the set of congenital muscular dystrophies and has recently been reported in facioscapulohumeral dystrophy (FSHD) as well. The impairments in Duchenne and Becker muscular dystrophy are believed to be nonprogressive, although weakness, medications, and respiratory status can affect alertness, communication, and global functioning. In myotonic dystrophy type 1, cognitive function may decline with age.[94] Cognitive impairments are not frequently reported in Emery-Dreifuss, limb-girdle, and oculopharyngeal muscular dystrophies.

Among individuals with DMD, the population mean full-scale IQ score is one standard deviation below the population mean for unaffected individuals, with impairments demonstrated in both the verbal and performance subscores.[95] It is also believed that one third of males with DMD demonstrate learning disabilities, including dyslexia.[96] Individuals with Becker muscular dystrophy are believed to have a more heterogeneous cognitive profile than those with DMD, possibly correlated with the more heterogeneous dystrophin protein expression profile in brain tissue. In a recent small study,

the mean full-scale IQ score among individuals with Becker muscular dystrophy was found to be comparable to that of the nonaffected population, although individuals with Becker muscular dystrophy showed particular difficulty with verbal working memory and visual-motor integration.[97]

Cognitive profiles for the myotonic dystrophies (congenital and juvenile/adult onset types 1 and 2) have been described. The degree of cognitive impairment is not consistently directly linked to the extent of genetic abnormality present in an individual. In congenital myotonic dystrophy, the degree of cognitive impairment seems to be out of proportion to the degree of motor impairment; up to 90% of individuals have global impairment, with IQ scores between 40 and 80.[98] Individuals with myotonic dystrophy type 1 have more significant cognitive impairments than those with type 2; impairments are in the areas of linguistic, visuospatial, and executive function, with relative preservation of memory, praxis, and global IQ scores (these are still below mean scores for the unaffected population).[94,98] Cognitive impairments may worsen with increasing age, and a subset of patients may develop focal dementias.

A personality profile in myotonic dystrophy that includes avoidance and passive-aggressive tendencies has been reported, as have patterns including health care–related obsessive behaviors.[98] Although cognitive impairment in individuals with myotonic dystrophy type 2 is more mild overall than in those with type 1, it includes similar cognitive testing and personality profiles. In otherwise mild cases of myotonic dystrophy, cognitive impairment may be the most prominent clinical feature.[99]

The congenital muscular dystrophies are associated with central nervous system involvement, which often includes mental retardation. This is particularly notable in Fukuyama, muscle-eye-brain disease, and Walker-Warburg syndrome variants. Intellectual function is typically within normal range in individuals with Ullrich and congenital muscular dystrophy associated with rigid spine syndrome. Learning disabilities along with normal intelligence have been associated with merosin-deficient congenital muscular dystrophy. Routine vision and hearing examinations are recommended to address any possible treatable causes of cognitive impairment, particularly if an acute change in cognitive function is observed.

Children with learning challenges can benefit from individually designed educational programs in the least restrictive environments. Assessment and treatment must begin early to optimize preschool and in-school interventions and educational outcomes. Often, associated behavioral challenges, including attention deficit hyperactivity disorder in individuals with Duchenne and Becker muscular dystrophies, can complicate the design of educational programming. Despite this, many can ultimately participate in typical mainstream classrooms with appropriate supports. Rehabilitation teams for children with muscular dystrophies and learning impairments include early intervention teams, social workers, speech-language therapists, and special educators, in addition to physicians, psychologists, physical therapists, occupational therapists, and technology specialists.

FHSD has historically been regarded as a condition that spares the central nervous system. However, in congenital myopathies, mental retardation and seizures can be present. Recently, Zouvelou et al[100] reported a case of adult-onset FSHD in which the patient had impairments in attention, memory, verbal, visuospatial, and reasoning capacity, along with cerebellar atrophy. These findings suggest central nervous system involvement in FSHD; further research in this area is indicated. More than half of individuals with FSHD have high-frequency hearing loss; this tends to be fairly asymptomatic in adults, but more severe in infants. If untreated during childhood, hearing loss can significantly impair cognitive development.[101]

Myopathies

Mitochondrial myopathies are often associated with seizures, strokes, and lactic acid accumulation, all of which can impair cognitive function and communication. Vision and hearing impairments can also have an impact on learning and communication. Controlling seizures, minimizing lactic acid buildup (i.e., treating infections, maintaining good nutrition, optimizing respiratory function), and addressing vision and hearing function can optimize cognitive function in individuals with mitochondrial disorders.

To date, several myopathic conditions, including the inflammatory and distal myopathies, have not been associated with major cognitive impairments, although studies continue to emerge.

Neuromuscular Junction and Motor Neuron Diseases

Historically less well-defined, but emerging in contemporary literature, are cognitive changes/impairments in individuals with disorders of the neuromuscular junction and those of the motor neuron. In neuromuscular junction disorders, an abnormality of acetylcholine-mediated neurotransmission is present. There is debate regarding whether primary acetylcholine-mediated neurotransmission defects in the cortex may account for mild memory and learning impairments, or whether cognitive changes may have a secondary etiology.[102]

Cognitive impairment has been documented in motor neuron diseases, including ALS and primary lateral sclerosis. No specific profile of cognitive impairment has been described in SMA; in fact, these children are often extremely bright. Cognitive impairment in primary lateral sclerosis tends to be mild, whereas cognitive impairment in ALS occasionally can be quite pronounced and may be associated with precentral gyrus atrophy. From 20% to 50% of individuals with ALS develop subtle cognitive changes. In sporadic ALS, cognitive changes may be more common in bulbar-onset disease patients; in familial ALS, cognitive changes may be more associated with advancing age.[103,104] These changes may be difficult to detect in the context of changes in motor control over speech and communication. Currently, cognitive changes are not included in the El Escorial ALS diagnostic criteria.

Cognitive impairment in both sporadic and familial ALS typically consists of alterations in executive function and language. Impairments may include decreased attention, diminished working memory, apathy, and lack of insight. In addition, altered verbal fluency and word-finding difficulty with reliance on stereotypical phrases can be seen. Associated behavioral changes, seen with or without other cognitive changes, include irritability and inflexibility. At least 5% of all patients with ALS meet criteria for the frontal variant of frontotemporal lobar dementia (FTLD); it also seems that patients with FTLD may develop ALS at a higher rate than the general population. The clinical presentation of FTLD associated with ALS includes apathy, perseveration, and loss of insight. As a result of these latter findings, cognitive changes are not often reported by patients, but may be observed by families and caregivers. There is no standardized tool for clinical cognitive assessment in ALS; however, word-generation tasks seem to be highly sensitive for identifying patients who could benefit from additional neuropsychological testing.[105,106]

The possibility for loss of decision-making capacity due to cognitive impairment underscores the importance of facilitating early conversations and documentation regarding ultimate goals of care over the course of the disease. Because executive dysfunction can affect compliance with treatment and quality of life for patients and caregivers, it may decrease survival.[107]

There are currently no medications approved for the treatment of FTLD. Rehabilitation management includes optimizing participation in therapies, optimizing quality of life for both patients and families, and screening and treating reversible contributors to impaired cognition. These include medications (e.g., tricyclic antidepressants), sleep disturbance (e.g., nocturnal hypoventilation), depression, and nutritional deficiencies. Services offered should include speech-language, psychology for both patient and family/caregivers, and others as indicated clinically. Ultimately, education and long-term planning by the rehabilitation team can play an important role in easing the transition and adjustment to a family member's cognitive impairment.

Quality of Life

It is well-documented that degree of physical impairment does not directly correlate with satisfaction with life circumstances among individuals with NMDs.[108–113] Rather, decision-making capability, social interactions, setting of care provision, spirituality, feelings of hope, the nature of coping strategies, and amelioration of manageable disease-related conditions may more directly affect overall life satisfaction.[109,110,114] Both primary caregivers and professional care providers tend to underestimate patients' experienced quality of life. Therefore, the rehabilitation team—in fact, the entire care provision team—must be well-educated about and comfortable discussing features of disease processes and their implications for daily life and relationships, setting realistic expectations, and offering management options. If a patient makes extreme or uncharacteristic requests regarding his life or care, care providers must ensure that all efforts have been made to optimize quality of life before attributing the requests to nonmodifiable disease-related distress.

Measurement

Several tools to measure quality of life are used in clinical research, yet designing instruments to determine quality of life in the setting of NMD remains a challenge. Excess focus on measures of physical capability must be avoided, because so many additional parameters affect the experience of living. In any assessment, the patient's voice should be paramount. For example, in the oft-studied realm of the role of mechanical ventilation in NMD, it has been shown that most patients with ALS who opt for mechanical ventilation would choose the same option again if given the choice, whereas only half of their care providers would choose that option for themselves.[115]

Role of the Professional Care Team

Throughout the course of an NMD, the rehabilitation/care provision team is uniquely poised to positively affect patient quality of life. For example, at initial diagnosis with ALS, the most rapidly progressive of the NMDs, patients tend to have low expectations of future quality of life. Over time, however, experienced quality of life is higher than initially expected and typically remains stable despite health-related changes.[109] Opportunities to affect quality of life for both patient and family/caregivers are at diagnosis (framing expectations and long-term vision of comfort and support), throughout the course of the disease (addressing disease manifestations that diminish health-related quality of life), near and at death (facilitating education and appropriate services, respecting patient autonomy), and after death (providing continued support for family and other caregivers). The first three of these opportunities are discussed below; the lattermost is discussed in the next section, entitled Roles of the Caregiver and Family. It is important that care for the caregiver be provided simultaneously with care for the patient, because caregiver quality of life can significantly affect patient quality of life.

From the very beginning of the course of a disease, the care team can frame patient expectations and long-term visions of comfort and support, thereby influencing the quality-of-life experience around receiving the diagnosis and planning for the future. The American Academy of Neurology ALS Practice Parameter guidelines recommend the physician deliver the diagnosis in person, discuss implications at that time, respect patient wishes regarding the ways information is transmitted (e.g., to patient versus via family members), provide materials about support and advocacy organizations, and provide documentation that summarizes the discussion.[69]

Throughout the course of the disease, the professional care team can educate patients and caregivers so that they can make informed treatment decisions and establish meaningful, appropriate short- and long-term goals. The professional care team can also foster open, reliable relationships with patients and families, another component of support for quality of life.[78] It is important for care providers to discuss sexual activity with patients and partners. Although ability and interest in sexual activity can be affected by mobility impairments and pain, individuals can maintain fulfilling sex lives and intimate personal relationships. The care team must also treat disease manifestations that diminish health-related quality of life. Such conditions include dysarthria, dysphagia, respiratory failure, spasticity, sialorrhea, pain, mood changes, and weakness/fatigue-related decreases in capacity to perform ADLs. Advice regarding exercise regimens, as described earlier in this chapter, can promote physical activity, which can be followed by increases in overall psychological well-being.

Individuals cared for in multidisciplinary clinics are more likely to receive timely and appropriate treatment and equipment. In addition, independent of adaptive equipment and the number of visits to care providers, individuals who partake in multidisciplinary clinics report increased quality of life on the SF-36 measurement, particularly in social functioning and mental health scores.[3]

Near and at death, consideration of quality of death is an important component of the consideration of quality of life. Maintaining individual choice about circumstances and location of death, comfort as death nears, and respect for personal autonomy are important components of comprehensive quality-of-life care. Death in the home with comfort and dignity is the preferred option for many patients. Hospice services for patients with NMDs, as discussed in the section of this chapter entitled Palliative Care, tend to be underused yet have the potential to significantly increase quality-of-life and death.

Despite best efforts by professional and family care providers, not all individuals with NMDs maintain stable or positive experiences of satisfaction and meaning in their lives over time. Reasons for this are many, including loss of decision-making capacity, requirement for care provision outside of the home, loss of ability to communicate and perform other personally valued functions, and incomplete response shifts (incomplete reorganizations of internal values and standards, which allow individuals to derive equal pleasure from life activities performed in new, modified ways).

Notable differences in perceived quality of life are present across cultures as well, affecting major patient and family decisions, including preferences for mechanical ventilation and, in some countries, euthanasia. Cultural perspectives must be discussed with patients and families and taken into account in consideration of individual circumstances.

Roles of the Caregiver and Family

Primary caregivers for adults with NMDs are typically spouses and, for children with NMDs, parents. The roles of these primary caregivers extend beyond direct provision of medical care and physical accommodations. Caregivers hold responsibilities for emotional care, financial support, decision making, and advocacy.

The caregiver is also challenged to adapt to major life changes, manage anxieties about uncertainties for the future, cope with losses, find ways to find joy amid sadness and anxiety, and maintain personal health and hygiene. In multi-member families, care for an individual with a NMD can divert attention from other family members; this is a particularly difficult challenge. Family functioning predicts adjustment to these challenges better than degree of disability or illness in the individual requiring care.

Williams and Donnelly[116] describe a range of caregiver and family needs throughout the course of a loved one's illness. After initial adjustment to a diagnosis, caregivers state needs such as "I have a need to not fight with him/her because I feel guilty"; "I have a need to accommodate the intrusion of medical helpers into my family"; "I have to be careful that I don't say too much or express too many negative feelings because then my loved one gets too depressed." Some state, "I need reassurance from professionals (e.g., hospice) that I am caring for my husband in the best possible way"; "I need not to be alone when my loved one dies"; and "I have a need to have people be aware of my loved one's physical needs, especially in the hospital, when he can't speak and I can't be with him."

Financial expenses for care of an individual with a NMD, especially if mechanical ventilation is required, can exceed hundreds of thousands of dollars per year. In-home care for a patient who uses mechanical ventilation can be less expensive than care in a skilled nursing facility, and this fact typically must be actively presented to insurance companies when service coverage is being determined. A skilled case manager or social worker, along with medical clinicians, can assist in this process.

Costs of care can be defrayed somewhat by hiring private aides instead of hiring through agencies, selecting modifiable durable medical equipment, renting or borrowing equipment from charitable organizations, and using hospice services when appropriate. The federal Family and Medical Leave Act allows primary caregivers time off from work to care for loved ones, but this leave is unpaid.

Unfortunately, the challenges that beset caregivers and families—even the most committed, well-connected, and financially capable ones—often result in adverse outcomes for those caregivers and families. Social isolation, demands on time and financial resources, limitations on personal and family opportunities, and constant readjustment of routines and expectations can lead caregivers to feel burdened. In turn, feeling burdened leads to increased stress, guilt, anxiety, and depression.

Addressing caregiver burden is part of comprehensive rehabilitation care for an individual with a NMD. Increased home care services, support groups, and counseling interventions can reduce stress. Caregivers and families should be encouraged to draw on sources of strength, including spiritual and cultural community groups. Professional care providers can also mitigate stress through validation of caregiver concerns, reassurance of the positive impact of their care, reinforcement of the importance of their own self-care, and acknowledgment of caregiver and family as experts in the care of their loved one. Importantly, professional care providers can elicit, address, and allay sources of guilt in caregivers and family members as well.

Despite the many challenges in providing care for a loved one with a NMD, caregivers and family members can derive great satisfaction and life enrichment in caring for their loved ones. In a recent qualitative study of parents' experiences caring for children with NMDs requiring mechanical ventilation, one parent encapsulated a common sentiment, that the child's "lifeline is us." Similarly, the parents' lifeline is the child. The mutual dependence between parents and child defined each of their lives. These families would choose mechanical ventilation if given the decision to make again.[117]

For caregivers, families, and clinicians, appropriate closure at the end of a patient's life can set the stage for healthy grieving and recovery. Hospice services for families can smooth this transition. Both clinicians and families can find additional closure and support when clinicians attend funeral and memorial services.

Palliative Care

The focus of palliative care, in many ways like that of rehabilitation care, is on patient comfort and quality of life. Hospice care is the delivery of palliative care at the end of life. In the United States, individuals with a life expectancy of 6 months or less and the desire to limit invasive intervention can be eligible for hospice services. Hospice services include comprehensive symptom management, psychosocial and spiritual support for patients and families, respite care, supplies, planning for death and dying, and bereavement services. Care can be in one's home or in a hospital or other facility.

Individuals with progressive life-limiting illnesses, such as ALS, DMD, or myotonic muscular dystrophy, can often benefit from earlier hospice referrals than they receive in practice. Early hospice referrals are limited by clinician lack of awareness and difficulty prognosticating remaining length of life. Individuals with NMDs can qualify for hospice services even when prognosis is difficult to specify—some individuals with NMDs receive hospice services for several years. Although documentation of a life expectancy of 6 months or less is required for hospice eligibility, additional criteria for hospice services for individuals with ALS and, by extrapolation, other NMDs, are as follows: There must be an overall rapid progression of disease within the past 12 months and the patient and family must desire no further aggressive treatment or cardiopulmonary resuscitation. One of the following must also be present: increased respiratory distress, severely impaired nutrition, or life-threatening complications. Additional details can be found in the National Hospice and Palliative Care Organization's "Expanding Access to Hospice Care for People with ALS" document.[118] Patients can receive tube feeding and use noninvasive positive-pressure ventilation while receiving hospice services because these can be considered comfort measures. Although the goal of hospice services is to provide comfort and specifically not to focus on cure, on some occasions, treatment medications, such as riluzole, can be approved.

A clinician must discuss several topics with patients and families when he or she suspects that hospice services might be of benefit. First, hospice services have the connotations of hopelessness, imminent death, and the relinquishing of control and treatment. Clinicians must educate families about the reasons for their recommendations of hospice (e.g., increased home services, grief counseling, provision of medical supplies) and the continued hope and care that will be maintained. They can also provide reassurance that patients can go off hospice services at any time and that they can receive services for longer than 6 months. Clinicians must explain that although the hospice application requires a life expectancy of 6 months or less, the prognosis is not definite. It may be difficult for patients and families

to accept hospice services after a single conversation with a clinician, and the conversation may need to be held many times. Some visiting nurse associations offer a bridge to hospice program so that patients can keep some of the same home health aides and other care professionals when making the switch to hospice. Hospice services do not cover durable medical equipment, such as wheelchairs and bilevel positive airway pressure ventilation machines; such equipment must be obtained before the initiation of hospice services.

The provision of end-of-life care is significantly eased by the early assignment of a durable power of attorney and statement of advance directives. These considerations should be discussed with a patient early in the course of illness and throughout the course, because goals, wishes, and relationships with family members can change over time.

References

1. DeLisa JA: *Rehabilitation Medicine*, Hagerstown, MD, 1993, Lippincott-Raven.
2. Traynor B, Alexander M, Corr B, et al: Effect of a multidisciplinary amyotrophic lateral sclerosis clinic on ALS survival: a population based study, 1996–2000, *J Neurol Neurosurg Psychiatry* 74:1258–1261, 2003.
3. vandenBerg J, Kalmijn S, Lindeman E, et al: Multidisciplinary ALS care improves quality of life in patients with ALS, *Neurology* 65:1264–1267, 2005.
4. Chio A, Bottacchi E, Buffa C, et al: Positive effects of tertiary centres for amyotrophic lateral sclerosis on outcome and use of hospital facilities, *J Neurol Neurosurg Psychiatry* 77(8):948–950, 2006.
5. Bennett R, Knowlton G: Overwork weakness in partially denervated skeletal muscle, *Clin Orthop Relat Res* 12:22–29, 1958.
6. Johnson EW, Braddom R: Over-work weakness in facioscapulohumeral muscular dystrophy, *Arch Phys Med Rehabil* 52:333–336, 1971.
7. deCarvalho M, Nogueira A, Pinto A, et al: Reflex sympathetic dystrophy associated with amyotrophic lateral sclerosis, *J Neurol Sci* 169:80–83, 1999.
8. Moens P, Baatsen P, Marechal G: Increased susceptibility of EDL muscles from *mdx* mice to damage induced by contractions with stretch, *J Muscle Res Cell Motil* 14:446–451, 1993.
9. Aitkens SG, McCrory MA, Kilmer DD, et al: Moderate resistance exercise program: its effect in slowly progressive neuromuscular disease, *Arch Phys Med Rehabil* 74(7):711–715, 1993.
10. Kilmer DD, McCrory MA, Wright NC, et al: The effect of a high resistance exercise program in slowly progressive neuromuscular disease, *Arch Phys Med Rehabil* 75:560–563, 1994.
11. Lenman J: A clinical and experimental study of the effects of exercise on motor weakness in neurologic disease, *J Neurol Neurosurg Psychiatry* 22:182–194, 1959.
12. Lindeman E, Leffers P, Spaans F, et al: Strength training in patients with myotonic dystrophy and hereditary motor and sensory neuropathy: a randomized clinical trial, *Arch Phys Med Rehabil* 76(7):612–620, 1995.
13. McCartney N, Moroz D, Garner SH, et al: The effects of strength training in patients with selected neuromuscular disorders, *Med Sci Sports Exer* 20(4):362–368, 1988.
14. Milner-Brown H, Miller RG: Muscle strengthening through high resistance weight training in patients with neuromuscular disorders, *Arch Phys Med Rehabil* 69:14–19, 1988.
15. Milner-Brown H, Miller RG: Muscle strengthening through electric stimulation combined with low resistance weights in patients with neuromuscular disorders, *Arch Phys Med Rehabil* 69:20–24, 1988.
16. DeLateur BJ, Giacomi R: Effect on maximal strength of submaximal exercise in Duchenne muscular dystrophy, *Am J Phys Med Rehabil* 58:26–36, 1979.
17. Spector S, Lemmer J, Koffman B, et al: Safety and efficacy of strength training in patients with sporadic inclusion body myositis, *Muscle Nerve* 20:1242–1248, 1997.
18. Taivassalo T, Fu K, Jones T, et al: Gene shifting: a novel therapy for mitochondrial myopathy, *Hum Mol Genet* 8:1047–1052, 1999.

19. Vignos P, Watkins M: Effect of exercise in muscular dystrophy, *JAMA* 197:843–848, 1966.

20. DalBello-Haas V, Florence J, Kloos A, et al: A randomized controlled trial of resistance exercise in individuals with ALS, *Neurology* 68(23):2003–2007, 2007.

21. Agre JC, Rodriquez AA, Franke TM: Strength, endurance, and work capacity after muscle strengthening exercise in postpolio subjects, *Arch Phys Med Rehabil* 78:681–686, 1997.

22. Einarsson G: Muscle conditioning in late poliomyelitis, *Arch Phys Med Rehabil* 72:11–14, 1991.

23. Fillyaw M, Badger G, Goodwin G, et al: The effects of longterm non-fatiguing resistance exercise in subjects with postpolio syndrome, *Orthopedics* 14:1253–1256, 1991.

24. Spector S, Gordon P, Feuerstein I, et al: Strength gains without muscle injury after strength training in patients with postpolio muscular atrophy, *Muscle Nerve* 19:1282–1290, 1996.

25. Gross D, Meiner Z: The effect of ventilatory muscle training on respiratory function and capacity in ambulatory and bed-ridden patients with neuromuscular disease, *Monaldi Arch of Chest Dis* 48(4):322–326, 1993.

26. DiMarco AF, Kelling JS, DiMarco MS, et al: The effects of inspiratory resistive training on respiratory muscle function in patients with muscular dystrophy, *Muscle Nerve* 8:284–290, 1985.

27. Smith P, Coakley J, Edwards R: Respiratory muscle training in Duchenne muscular dystrophy, *Muscle Nerve* 11:784–785, 1988.

28. Stern L, Martin A, Jones N, et al: Training inspiratory resistance in Duchenne dystrophy using adapted computer games, *Dev Med Child Neurol* 31:494–500, 1989.

29. Wanke T, Toifl K, Merkle M, et al: Inspiratory muscle training in patients with Duchenne muscular dystrophy, *Chest* 105(2):475–482, 1994.

30. Fregonezi G, Resqueti V, Guell R, et al: Effects of 8-week, interval-based inspiratory muscle training and breathing retraining in patients with generalized myasthenia gravis, *Chest* 128(3):1524–1530, 2005.

31. Carroll J, Hagberg J, Brooke M, et al: Bicycle ergometry and gas exchange measurements in neuromuscular diseases, *Arch Neurol* 36:457–461, 1979.

32. Garssen M, Bussmann J, Schmitz P, et al: Physical training and fatigue, fitness, and quality of life in Guillain-Barré syndrome and CIDP, *Neurology* 63:2393–2395, 2004.

33. Olsen D, Orngreen M, Vissing J: Aerobic training improves exercise performance in facioscapulohumeral muscular dystrophy, *Neurology* 64:1064–1066, 2005.

34. Orngreen M, Olsen D, Vissing J: Aerobic training in patients with myotonic dystrophy type 1, *Ann Neurol* 57:754–757, 2005.

35. Sveen M, Jeppesen T, Hauerslev S, et al: Endurance training: an effective and safe treatment for patients with LGMD2I, *Neurology* 68:59–61, 2007.

36. Mate-Munoz J, Moran M, Perez M, et al: Favorable responses to acute and chronic exercise in McArdle patients, *Clin J Sport Med* 17:297–303, 2007.

37. Taivassalo T, DeStefano N, Argov Z, et al: Effects of aerobic training in patients with mitochondrial myopathies, *Neurology* 50:1055–1060, 1998.

38. Taivassalo T, DeStefano N, Chen J, et al: Short-term aerobic training response in chronic myopathies, *Muscle Nerve* 22:1239–1243, 1999.

39. Jeppesen T, Schwartz M, Olsen D, et al: Aerobic training is safe and improves exercise capacity in patients with mitochondrial myopathy, *Brain* 129:3402–3412, 2006.

40. Taivassalo T, Gardner J, Taylof R, et al: Endurance training and detraining in mitochondrial myopathies due to single large-scale mtDNA deletions, *Brain* 129:3391–3401, 2006.

41. Dean E, Ross J: Effect of modified aerobic training on movement energetics in polio survivors, *Orthopedics* 14:1243–1246, 1991.

42. Jones D, Speir J, Canine K, et al: Cardiorespiratory responses to aerobic training by patients with post poliomyelitis sequelae, *JAMA* 261:3255–3258, 1989.

43. Kriz J, Jones D, Speier J, et al: Cardiorespiratory responses to upper extremity aerobic training by post-polio subjects, *Arch Phys Med Rehabil* 73:49–54, 1992.

44. Sanjak M, Paulson D, Sufit R, et al: Physiologic and metabolic response to progressive and prolonged exercise in amyotrophic lateral sclerosis, *Neurology* 37:1217–1220, 1987.

45. Drory V, Goltsman E, Reznik J, et al: The value of muscle exercise in patients with amyotrophic lateral sclerosis, *J Neurol Sci* 191:133–137, 2002.

46. Pinto A, Alves M, Nogueira A, et al: Can amyotrophic lateral sclerosis patients with respiratory insufficiency exercise? *J Neurol Sci* 169:69–75, 1999.

47. Hurvitz E, Richardson J, Werner R, et al: Unipedal stance testing as an indicator of fall risk among older outpatients, *Arch Phys Med Rehabil* 81:587–591, 2000.

48. Hurvitz E, Richardson J, Werner R: Unipedal stance testing in the assessment of peripheral neuropathy, *Arch Phys Med Rehabil* 82:198–204, 2001.

49. Richardson J, Sandman D, Vela S: A focused exercise regimen improves clinical measures of balance in patients with peripheral neuropathy, *Arch Phys Med Rehabil* 82:205–209, 2001.

50. Fast A, Thomas M: The "baseball cap orthosis": a simple solution for dropped head syndrome, *Am J Phys Med Rehabil* 87(1):71–73, 2008.

51. Karol LA, Elerson E: Scoliosis in patients with Charcot-Marie-Tooth disease, *J Bone Joint Surg Am* 89:1504–1510, 2007.

52. Hsu JD: The natural history of spine curvature progression in the non-ambulatory Duchenne muscular dystrophy patient, *Spine* 8:771–775, 1983.

53. Werner BC, Skalsky AJ, McDonald CM, et al: Convexity of scoliosis related to handedness in identical twin boys with Duchenne's muscular dystrophy: a case report, *Arch Phys Med Rehabil* 89:2021–2024, 2008.

54. Cheuk DK, Wong V, Wraige E, et al: Surgery for scoliosis in Duchenne muscular dystrophy, *Cochrane Database Syst Rev* (1): CD005375, 2007.

55. McDonald CM: Limb contractures in progressive neuromuscular disease and the role of stretching, orthotics, and surgery, *Phys Med Rehabil Clin N Am* 9:187–211, 1998.

56. Hornyak JE 4th, Pangilinan PH Jr: Rehabilitation of children and adults-who have neuromuscular diseases, *Phys Med Rehabil Clin N Am* 18(4): 883–897, 2007.

57. Bach J: *Noninvasive Mechanical Ventilation*, Philadelphia, 2002, Hanley and Belfus.

58. Bach J, Bach J: *Management of Patients with Neuromuscular Disease*, Philadelphia, 2003, Hanley and Belfus.

59. Tomik B, Guiloff RJ: Dysarthria in amyotrophic lateral sclerosis: A review, *Amyotroph Lateral Scler* 14:1–12, 2008.

60. Traynor BJ, Codd MB, Corr B, et al: Clinical features of amyotrophic lateral sclerosis according to the El Escorial and Airlie House diagnostic criteria: a population-based study, *Arch Neurol* 57:1171–1176, 2000.

61. Esposito S, Mitsumoto H, Shanks M: Use of palatal lift and palatal augmentation prostheses to improve dysarthria in patients with amyotrophic lateral sclerosis: a case series, *J Prosthet Dent* 83:90–98, 2000.

62. Nijboer F, Sellers EW, Mellinger J, et al: A P300-based brain-computer interface for people with amyotrophic lateral sclerosis, *Clin Neurophysiol* 119:1909–1916, 2008.

63. Hochberg LR: Turning thought into action, *N Engl J Med* 359:1175–1177, 2008.

64. Burns TM, Russell JA, LaChance DH, et al: Oculobulbar involvement is typical with Lambert-Eaton myasthenic syndrome, *Ann Neurol* 53:270–273, 2003.

65. Wirtz PW, Sotodeh M, Nijnuis M, et al: Difference in distribution of muscle weakness between myasthenia gravis and the Lambert-Eaton myasthenic syndrome, *J Neurol Neurosurg Psychiatry* 73:766–768, 2002.

66. Bain PG, Motomura M, Newsom-Davis J, et al: Effects of intravenous immunoglobulin on muscle weakness and calcium-channel autoantibodies in the Lambert-Eaton myasthenic syndrome, *Neurology* 47(3):678–683, 1996.

67. de Swart BJ, van Engelen BG, van de Kerkhof JP, Maassen BA: Myotonia and flaccid dysarthria in patients with adult onset myotonic dystrophy, *J Neurol Neurosurg Psychiatry* 75:1480–1482, 2004.

68. Ronnblom A, Forsberg H, Danielsson A: Gastrointestinal symptoms in myotonic dystrophy, *Scand J Gastroenterol* 31:654–657, 1996.

69. Miller RG, Jackson CE, Kasarskis EJ, et al: Practice parameter update: the care of the patient with amyotrophic lateral sclerosis: drug, nutritional, and respiratory therapies (an evidence-based review), *Neurology* 73:1218–1226, 2009.

70. Thornton F, Fotheringham T, Alexander M, et al: Amyotrophic lateral sclerosis: enteral nutrition provision—endoscopic or radiologic gastrostomy? *Radiology* 224:713–717, 2002.

71. Rosenfeld J, Ellis A: Nutrition and dietary supplements in motor neuron disease, *Phys Med Rehabil Clin N Am* 19:573–589, 2008.

72. Jaradeh S: Muscle disorders affecting oral and pharyngeal swallowing, *GI Motility Online*. doi:10.1038/gimo35 (Published 16 May 2006).

73. Oh TH, Brumfield KA, Hoskin TL, et al: Dysphagia in inclusion body myositis: clinical features, management, and clinical outcome, *Am J Phys Med Rehabil* 87:883–889, 2008.

74. Urtizberea JA: Oculopharyngeal muscular dystrophy, *Orphanet Encyclopedia* 1–4, 2004. http://www.orpha.net/data/patho/GB/uk-OPMD.pdf.

75. Abresch R, Carter G, Jensen M, et al: Assessment of pain and health-related quality of life in slowly progressive neuromuscular disease, *Am J Hosp Palliat Care* 19(1):39–48, 2002.

76. Stoelb BL, Carter GT, Abresch RT, et al: Pain in persons with postpolio syndrome: frequency, intensity, and impact, *Arch Phys Med Rehabil* 89:1933–1940, 2008.

77. Jensen M, Hoffman A, Stoelb B, et al: Chronic pain in persons with myotonic dystrophy and facioscapulohumeral dystrophy, *Arch Phys Med Rehabil* 89:320–328, 2008.

78. Mah JK, Thannhauser JE, McNeil DA, et al: Being the lifeline: the parent experience of caring for a child with neuromuscular disease on home mechanical ventilation, *Neuromuscul Disord* 18:983–988, 2008.

79. Dudgeon BJ, Ehde DM, Cardenas DD, et al: Describing pain with physical disability: narrative interviews and the McGill Pain Questionnaire, *Arch Phys Med Rehabil* 86:109–115, 2005.

80. Jensen MP, Abresch RT, Carter GT: The reliability and validity of a self-report version of the FIM instrument in persons with neuromuscular disease and chronic pain, *Arch Phys Med Rehabil* 86:116–122, 2005.

81. Jensen MP, Abresch RT, Carter GT, et al: Chronic pain in persons with neuromuscular disease, *Arch Phys Med Rehabil* 86:1155–1163, 2005.

82. Johnson EWF Jr, Lieberman J: Contractures in neuromuscular disease, *Arch Phys Med Rehabil* 73:807–810, 1992.

83. Shibata M, Abe K, Jimbo A, et al: Complex regional pain syndrome type I associated with amyotrophic lateral sclerosis, *Clin J Pain* 19(1):69–70, 2003.

84. McDonald DG, Kinali M, Gallagher AC, et al: Fracture prevalence in Duchenne muscular dystrophy, *Dev Med Child Neurol* 44:695–698, 2002.

85. Hawker GA, Ridout R, Harris VA, et al: Alendronate in the treatment of low bone mass in steroid-treated boys with Duchennes muscular dystrophy, *Arch Phys Med Rehabil* 86(2):284–288, 2005.

86. Ashworth N, Satkunam L, Deforge D: Treatment for spasticity in amyotrophic lateral sclerosis/motor neuron disease, *Cochrane Database Syst Rev* (1): CD004156, 2004.

87. Redmond AC, Burns J, Ouvrier RA: Factors that influence health-related quality of life in Australian adults with Charcot-Marie-Tooth disease, *Neuromuscul Disord* 18:619–625, 2008.

88. Fisher J, Parkinson K, Kothari MJ: Self-reported depressive symptoms in myasthenia gravis, *J Clin Neuromuscul Dis* 4:105–108, 2003.

89. Hunter M, Robinson I, Neilson S: The functional and psychological status of patients with amyotrophic lateral sclerosis: some implications for rehabilitation, *Disabil Rehabil* 15(3):119–126, 1993.

90. Kalkman JS, Schillings ML, Zwarts MJ, et al: Psychiatric disorders appear equally in patients with myotonic dystrophy, facioscapulohumeral dystrophy, and hereditary motor and sensory neuropathy type I, *Acta Neurol Scand* 115:265–270, 2007.

91. Kiebert G, Green C, Murphy C, et al: Patients' health-related quality of life and utilities associated with different stages of amyotrophic lateral sclerosis, *J Neurol Sci* 191:87–93, 2001.

92. Rabkin JG, Albert SM, Del Bene ML, et al: Prevalence of depressive disorders and change over time in late-stage ALS, *Neurology* 65(1):62–67, 2005.

93. Averill AJ, Kasarskis EJ, Segerstrom SC: Psychological health in patients with amyotrophic lateral sclerosis, *Amyotroph Lateral Scler* 8:243–254, 2007.

94. Modoni A, Silvestri G, Vita MG, et al: Cognitive impairment in myotonic dystrophy type 1 (DM1): a longitudinal follow-up study, *J Neurol* 255:1737–1742, 2008.

95. Cotton S, Voudouris NJ, Greenwood KM: Intelligence and Duchenne muscular dystrophy: full-scale, verbal, and performance intelligence quotients, *Dev Med Child Neurol* 43:497–501, 2001.

96. Hendriksen JG, Vles JS: Are males with Duchenne muscular dystrophy at risk for reading disabilities? *Pediatr Neurol* 34:296–300, 2006.

97. Young HK, Barton BA, Waisbren S, et al: Cognitive and psychological profile of males with Becker muscular dystrophy, *J Child Neurol* 23:155–162, 2008.

98. Meola G, Sansone V: Cerebral involvement in myotonic dystrophies, *Muscle Nerve* 36(3):294–306, 2007.

99. Modoni A, Silvestri G, Pomponi MG, et al: Characterization of the pattern of cognitive impairment in myotonic dystrophy type 1, *Arch Neurol* 61 (12):1943–1947, 2004.

100. Zouvelou V, Rentzos M, Zalonis I, et al: Cognitive impairment and cerebellar atrophy in typical onset 4Q35 facioscapulohumeral dystrophy, *Muscle Nerve* 38:1523–1524, 2008.

101. Tawil R, Van Der Maarel SM: Facioscapulohumeral muscular dystrophy, *Muscle Nerve* 34(1):1–15, 2006.

102. Glennerster A, Palace J, Warburton D, et al: Memory in myasthenia gravis: neuropsychological tests of central cholinergic function before and after effective immunologic treatment, *Neurology* 46:1138–1142, 1996.

103. Phukan J, Pender NP, Hardiman O: Cognitive impairment in amyotrophic lateral sclerosis, *Lancet Neurology* 6:994–1003, 2007.

104. Wheaton MW, Salamone AR, Mosnik DM, et al: Cognitive impairment in familial ALS, *Neurology* 69:1411–1417, 2007.

105. Lomen-Hoerth C, Murphy J, Langmore S, et al: Are amyotrophic lateral sclerosis patients cognitively normal? *Neurology* 60:1094–1097, 2003.

106. Strong MJ, Lomen-Hoerth C, Caselli RJ, et al: Cognitive impairment, frontotemporal dementia, and the motor neuron diseases, *Ann Neurol* 54 (Suppl 5):S20–S23, 2003.

107. Olney RK, Murphy J, Forshew D, et al: The effects of executive and behavioral dysfunction on the course of ALS, *Neurology* 65:1774–1777, 2005.

108. Bach J, Campagnolo D, Hoeman S: Life satisfaction of individuals with Duchenne muscular dystrophy using long-term mechanical ventilatory support, *Am J Phys Med Rehabil* 70:129–135, 1991.

109. Bromberg MB: Quality of life in amyotrophic lateral sclerosis, *Phys Med Rehabil Clin N Am* 19:591–605, 2008.

110. Lee JN, Rigby SA, Burchardt F, et al: Quality of life issues in motor neurone disease: the development and validation of a coping strategies questionnaire, the MND Coping Scale, *J Neurol Sci* 191:79–85, 2001.

111. Natterlund B, Ahlstrom G: Activities of daily living and quality of life in persons with muscular dystrophy, *J Rehabil Med* 33:206–211, 2001.

112. Paul RH, Nash JM: Quality of life in patients with myasthenia gravis (Letter to the Editor), Reply to Padua L, Evoli A, et al. *Muscle Nerve* 25:466–467, 2002.

113. Robbins RA, Simmons Z, Bremer BA, et al: Quality of life in ALS is maintained as physical function declines, *Neurology* 56:442–444, 2001.

114. Moss A, Oppenheimer E, Casey P, et al: Patients with amyotrophic lateral sclerosis receiving long-term mechanical ventilation. Advance care planning and outcomes, *Chest* 110:249–255, 1996.

115. Oppenheimer E, Baldwin-Meyers A, Fuller, JA, et al: Ventilator use by patients with amyotrophic lateral sclerosis, 1985–1992, in the Kaiser Permanente home care program in California. Paper presented at 4th International Conference on Home Mechanical Ventilation, Lyon, France, March 3–5, 1993.

116. Williams M, Donnelly J: ALS: family caregiver needs and quality of life, *Amyotroph Lateral Scler* 9:279–286, 2008.

117. Mah J, Thannhauser J, McNeil DA, et al: Being the lifeline: the parent experience of caring for a child with neuromuscular disease on home mechanical ventilation, *Neuromuscul Disord* 18:983–988, 2008.

118. National Hospice and Palliative Care Organization: *Expanding Access to Hospice Care for People with ALS*, http://www.nhpco.org/i4a/pages/Index.cfm?pageID=5335. Accessed December 2009.

William C. Warner, Jr., MD

Orthopedic Surgery in Neuromuscular Disorders

9

Neuromuscular disorders (NMDs) in children include conditions that affect the spinal cord, peripheral nerves, neuromuscular junction, and muscles. Orthopedic treatment of children with NMD has been aimed at preventing worsening of deformities and providing stability to the skeletal system to improve the quality of life for these children. Patients with severe NMDs have listed their priorities as the ability to communicate with others, the ability to perform many of the activities of daily living, mobility, and ambulation.[1] The role of the orthopedic surgeon in achieving these goals includes prescribing orthoses for lower extremity control to facilitate transfer to and from wheelchairs, preventing or correcting joint contractures, and maintaining appropriate standing and sitting posture. Treatment must be individualized for each patient according to the particular disorder, the severity of involvement, and the ambulation status of the patient.

Fractures are common in children with NMDs because of disuse osteoporosis and frequent falls.[2] Fracture treatment with splinting, cast-bracing, or surgery emphasizes a quick return to walking if the patient is ambulatory. Spinal bracing may be necessary to assist with sitting balance, a knee-ankle-foot orthosis can provide stability for patients with proximal muscle weakness, and an ankle-foot orthosis (AFO) can help position the ankle and foot plantigrade to help prevent progressive deformities. Most children with NMD will eventually require the use of a wheelchair, and these chairs must be carefully contoured to accommodate the spinal deformities and pelvic obliquity that usually are present.

Muscular Dystrophy

The muscular dystrophies are a group of hereditary disorders of skeletal muscle that produce progressive muscle degeneration and associated weakness. The disorders differ in the distribution and severity of muscle weakness, the age of onset, the rate of progression, and the pattern of inheritance (Fig. 9-1).

Duchenne Muscular Dystrophy

Duchenne muscular dystrophy, a sex-linked recessive inherited trait, occurs in males and in females with Turner syndrome; carriers are female. It is reported to occur in 1 in 3500 live births.[3–5] There is a family history in 70% of patients, and the condition occurs as a spontaneous mutation in approximately 30% of patients.[6] In contrast, Becker muscular dystrophy, the second most common form, occurs in 1 in 30,000 live male births; other types of muscular dystrophy are rare. Children with Duchenne muscular dystrophy usually reach early motor milestones at appropriate times, but independent ambulation may be delayed; many are initially toe-walkers. The disease will usually become evident between ages 3 and 6 years. The ability to ambulate typically is lost by about age 10 years.

Clinical features include large, firm calf muscles; the tendency to toe-walk; a widely based, lordotic stance; a waddling Trendelenburg gait; and a positive Gowers test indicative of proximal muscle weakness (Fig. 9-2). The diagnosis usually is obvious by the time the child is 5 or 6 years old. Diagnosis is confirmed by a dramatically elevated level of creatine kinase (50 to 100 times normal) and DNA analysis of blood samples.[5,7] Muscle biopsy demonstrates variations in fiber size in internal nuclei, split fibers, degenerating or regenerating fibers, and fibrofatty tissue deposition. Dystrophin testing of the muscle biopsy will confirm the type of muscular dystrophy.

Orthopedic Physical Examination

The degree of muscular weakness depends on the age of the patient and the type of dystrophy. Because the proximal musculature weakens before the distal muscles, examination of the lower extremities demonstrates an early weakness of gluteal muscle strength. The weakness in the proximal muscles of the lower extremity can be demonstrated by a decrease in the ability to rise from the floor without assistance of the upper extremities (Gowers sign). The calf

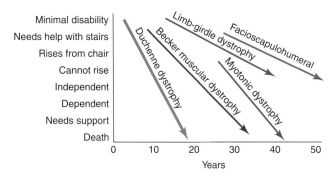

Figure 9-1 Natural history of muscular dystrophies. The *arrows* show the average clinical course with level of disability and age. (Adapted from Staheli LT: *Practice of Pediatric Orthopedics*, Philadelphia, 2001, Lippincott Williams & Wilkins, p 338.)

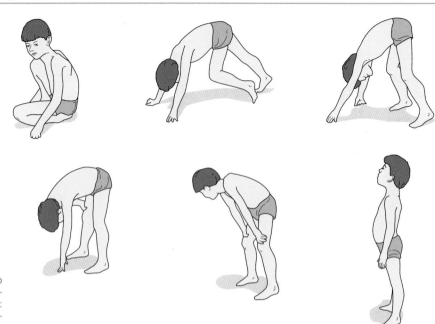

Figure 9-2 Gowers sign. Child must use hands to rise from a sitting position. (From Warner WC Jr: Neuromuscular disorders. In Canale ST, Beaty JH, editors: *Campbell's Operative Orthopaedics*, 11th ed. Philadelphia, 2008, Elsevier, p 1505.)

pseudohypertrophy is caused by infiltration of the muscle by fat and fibrosis, giving the calves the feel of hard rubber (Fig. 9-3). The extrinsic muscles of the foot and ankle retain their strength longer than the proximal muscles of the hip and knee. The posterior tibial muscle retains its strength for the longest time. This pattern of weakness causes an equinovarus deformity of the foot. Weakness

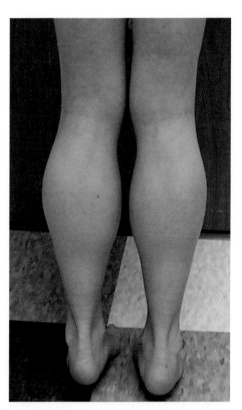

Figure 9-3 Pseudohypertrophy of the calf in a patient with muscular dystrophy. (From Warner WC Jr: Neuromuscular disorders. In Canale ST, Beaty JH, editors: *Campbell's Operative Orthopaedics*, 11th ed. Philadelphia, 2008, Elsevier, p 1505.)

of the shoulder girdle musculature can be demonstrated by the Meryon sign, which is elicited by lifting the child with one arm encircling the child's chest. Most children contract the muscles about the shoulder to increase shoulder stability and facilitate lifting. In children with muscular dystrophy, however, the arms abduct because of the severe shoulder abductor muscle weakness, until they eventually slide through the examiner's arms unless the chest is tightly encircled. Later in the disease process, the Thomas test demonstrates hip flexion contracture, and the Ober test demonstrates an abduction contracture of the hip.

Orthopedic Treatment

The major goal of early treatment is to maintain functional ambulation as long as possible. Between ages 8 and 14 years (with a median of 10 years), children with Duchenne muscular dystrophy typically have a sensation of locking of the joints. Contractures of the lower extremity may require early treatment to prolong the child's ability to ambulate, if even for 1 to 2 years. This requires prevention or retardation of the development of contractures of the lower extremity, which would eventually prohibit ambulation. It is easier to keep patients walking than to induce them to resume walking once they have stopped. When children with Duchenne muscular dystrophy stop walking, they also become more susceptible to the development of scoliosis and severe contractures of the lower extremities. Scoliosis will develop in nearly all children with Duchenne muscular dystrophy, usually when they require aided mobility or shortly after becoming wheelchair bound. Recently, the use of steroids has been suggested to possibly decrease the occurrence of scoliosis in these patients.

Correction of Lower Extremity Contractures

Three approaches have been used for surgical correction of lower extremity contractures:

1. Ambulatory approach. The goal of surgery during the ambulatory period is to correct any contractures in the lower extremity while the patient is still ambulatory. Early aggressive surgery may be indicated for the first appearance of contractures in the lower extremities; a plateau in muscle strength, usually around age 5 to 6 years; and difficulty maintaining an upright posture

with the feet together. Some surgeons suggest that surgery should be performed before deterioration of the Gowers maneuver time or time to rise from the floor[8-11]; others have recommended surgery later in the ambulatory phase, just before the cessation of ambulation.[12,13]

2. Rehabilitative approach. Surgery is done after the patient has lost the ability to walk but with the intention that walking will resume.[14] Surgery during this stage usually only allows for minimal ambulation with braces.

3. Palliative approach. The palliative approach treats only contractures that interfere with shoe wear and comfortable positioning in a wheelchair.

A comparison of ambulation and foot position in three groups of patients with Duchenne muscular dystrophy (those who had surgery to maintain ambulation, those who had surgery to correct and maintain foot position, and those who had no surgery) found that the mean age at cessation of ambulation for those who had surgery was 11.2 years, compared to 10.3 years in those who did not have surgery.[15] Foot position was neutral in 94% of those who had surgery, and none had toe flexion deformities; 96% of those who had surgery reported being able to wear any type of shoes, compared to only 60% of those who had no surgery. In contrast, another study of full-time wheelchair users with Duchenne muscular dystrophy found no significant differences between patients who did and did not have foot surgery with respect to shoe wear, hypersensitivity, or cosmesis.[16] Hindfoot motion was significantly better but equinus contracture was significantly worse in those who had not had surgery.

Currently the most common approach is to correct contractures just before the patient has a significant decline in ambulation and before the patient has to use a wheelchair (i.e., the ambulatory approach) (Fig. 9-4).

Mild equinus contractures of the feet can help force the knee into extension, which in turn helps prevent the knee buckling caused by severe weakness of the quadriceps. Stretching exercises and nightly bracing can be used to prevent the contractures from becoming severe. Flexion and abduction contractures of the hip, however, impede ambulation and should be minimized. Exercises to stretch the hip muscles and lower extremity braces worn at night to prevent the child's sleeping in a frog position are helpful initially. If surgery is indicated, the foot and hip contractures should be released simultaneously, usually through small incisions. Ambulation should be resumed immediately after surgery if possible. Polypropylene braces are preferred to long-term casting. Prolonged immobilization must be avoided to prevent or limit the progressive muscle weakness caused by disuse.

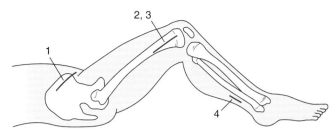

Figure 9-5 Tenotomy sites for release of hip flexors (1), tensor fasciae latae and fascia lata (2, 3), and Achilles tendon (4). (Redrawn from Siegel IM: Maintenance of ambulation in Duchenne muscular dystrophy: the role of the orthopaedic surgeon, *Clin Podiatr* 19:383–388, 1980.)

Percutaneous Release of Hip Flexion and Abduction Contractures and Achilles Tendon Contractures

A small (No. 15) blade is inserted percutaneously just medial and distal to the anterior superior iliac spine (Fig. 9-5) to release first the sartorius muscle, then the tensor fasciae femoris muscle, taking care to avoid the neurovascular structures of the anterior thigh. Then, through another small incision approximately 3 to 4 cm proximal to the upper pole of the patella, the fascia lata is released, as is the deeper lateral intermuscular septum. The Achilles tendon is released through a small posterolateral incision.

Open Lengthening of the Achilles Tendon

A posteromedial incision (Fig. 9-6A) is used to expose the Achilles tendon from its insertion to approximately 10 cm proximally, preserving the tendon sheath. The posteromedial two thirds of the tendon is divided near its insertion. With moderate dorsiflexion force applied to the foot, the medial two thirds of the tendon is divided approximately 5 to 8 cm proximal to the site of the distal division. The foot is then dorsiflexed so that the tendon lengthens to the desired length (Fig. 9-6B). The tendon can be sutured in a side-to-side fashion with absorbable suture, but this generally is unnecessary

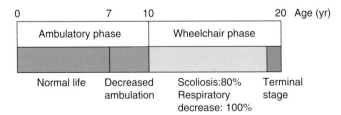

Figure 9-4 Natural course of Duchenne muscular dystrophy: age-related stages. Correction of contractures generally is done during the ambulatory phase. (From Rideau Y, Duport C, Delaubier A, et al: Early treatment to preserve locomotion for children with Duchenne muscular dystrophy, *Semin Neurol* 15:9–17, 1995.)

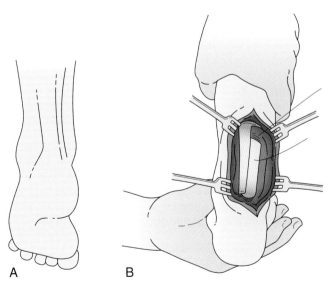

Figure 9-6 Sliding lengthening of the Achilles tendon. **A,** Posteromedial incision. **B,** Two cuts are made through one half of the tendon in opposite directions. Rotation of the fibers must be followed accurately. Placing the foot in dorsiflexion causes the tendon fibers to separate. (Redrawn from Green NE: Cerebral palsy. In Canale ST, Beaty JH, editors: *Operative Pediatric Orthopaedics*, 2nd ed. St. Louis, MO, 1995, Mosby.)

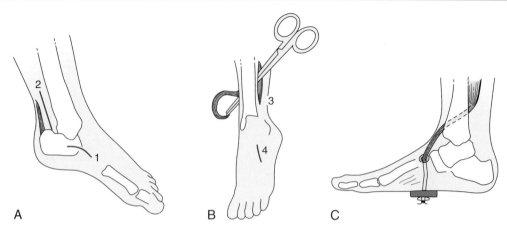

Figure 9-7 Posterior tibial tendon transfer. **A,** First (1) and second (2) incisions. **B,** Third (3) and fourth (4) incisions and clamp placement for pulling posterior tibial tendon from posterior to anterior compartment of the leg. **C,** Position of the transplanted tendon and suture tied over a felt pad and button the plantar aspect of the foot. (From Greene WB: Transfer versus lengthening of the posterior tibial tendon in Duchenne's muscular dystrophy, *Foot Ankle* 13:526–531, 1992.)

because this is a sliding technique; however, we prefer to suture the tendon. The tendon sheath and subcutaneous tissues are carefully closed to prevent adherence of the tendon to the overlying skin, and a short-leg cast is applied with the ankle in maximal dorsiflexion.

Transfer of Posterior Tibial Tendon to Dorsum of Foot

In patients with marked overpull of the posterior tibial muscle, transfer of the posterior tibial tendon to the dorsum of the foot (Fig. 9-7) combined with other tenotomies or tendon lengthening has been found to give better results than posterior tibial tendon lengthening alone. Although transfer of the posterior tibial tendon is technically more demanding and has a higher perioperative complication rate, most patients retain the plantigrade posture of their feet, even after walking ceases. Despite the more extensive surgical procedure, early ambulation of the patient usually is not impeded.

Transfer of Posterior Tibial Tendon to Dorsum of Base of Second Metatarsal

Transfer of the posterior tibial tendon to the dorsum of the base of the second metatarsal rather than the dorsum of the foot has as a cited advantage the more distal placement of the posterior tibial tendon, which increases the lever arm in dorsiflexion of the ankle. This technique also allows easier plantar flexion and dorsiflexion balancing of the ankle at the time of surgery. Lengthening of the posterior tibial tendon is required to have sufficient length for the tendon to be transferred to the second metatarsal with this technique.

Equinus contractures can be corrected by either a percutaneous or open Achilles tendon lengthening. If an open procedure is needed because of severe contractures, lengthening or release of the posterior tibial, flexor digitorum, and flexor hallicus longus tendons also may be needed. Once these lengthening procedures or releases are done, the child will need an AFO to continue to stand or ambulate.

Correction of Spinal Deformities

Approximately 75% to 90% of boys with Duchenne muscular dystrophy develop scoliosis.[5,17] The age of onset of scoliosis is generally about the same as the age at which they lose the ability to walk, between 10 and 14 years.[18] A significant association has been shown between prolonged ambulation and a reduced risk of scoliosis development,[19] and the use of steroids has been shown to slow the progression of scoliosis and perhaps delay the need for surgery.[20]

Weakness in the trunk and paraspinal muscles leads to collapse of the developing spine into what is usually a long C-shaped curve with the apex in the thoracolumbar region. Over time, the curve progresses and involves the entire thoracic and lumbar spine, resulting in pelvic obliquity (Fig. 9-8). This scoliosis does not respond to nonoperative treatment such as bracing and adaptive seating, and it is almost inevitably progressive, often increasing by 8 to 12 degrees per year.[21] Surgery generally is recommended when the scoliotic curve measures 20 to 30 degrees,[22–24] although some recommend spinal fusion at the onset of the deformity in patients who use a wheelchair full-time even when the curve is less than 20 degrees.[4,25,26] A delay in surgery allows the curve to progress further and pulmonary and cardiac function to worsen, adding to the risks of spinal surgery in these patients.

The patient's pulmonary function probably is more important than the size of the curve in decision making. Ideally, vital capacity should be 40% to 50% of normal. Patients who have a forced vital capacity of less than 35% are at high risk for pulmonary complications, whereas those with a forced vital capacity of greater than 50% are likely to have few postoperative pulmonary problems and usually can be weaned from the ventilator the night of surgery or the day after.[27,28] A few small studies have indicated that spinal surgery can be safely done on patients with a vital capacity of less than 30%.[29–31]

The goals of spinal surgery in patients with Duchenne muscular dystrophy are to obtain and maintain sitting balance and to correct pelvic obliquity so that the patient is able to use a wheelchair for the remainder of his life. The effect of spinal fusion on pulmonary function remains a matter of debate, with some studies finding no effect on the rate of pulmonary decline[19,28,32,33] and others finding reduced rates of decline.[25,27,34] Most authors agree that pulmonary function does not improve after surgical fusion of scoliosis[28,32,33]; however, patients who have spinal stabilization do have a substantially enhanced quality of life compared with patients who do not.[35,36] Suggested benefits of spinal fusion in patients with Duchenne muscular dystrophy include preservation of sitting balance, prevention of back pain, improvement in spinal decompensation, freeing the arms of the necessity of trunk support, improvement in body image, and possible slowing of the deterioration of pulmonary function.[37]

Segmental spinal instrumentation is recommended in patients with Duchenne muscular dystrophy because of the neuromuscular etiology and because the bone is relatively osteopenic due to nonambulation. Instrumentation with sublaminar wires and cross-link rods (Fig. 9-9) or a unit rod (Fig. 9-10) has been a useful technique

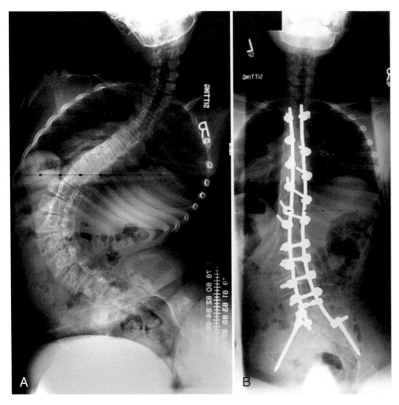

Figure 9-8 A, Spinal deformity in a 13-year-old boy with Duchenne muscular dystrophy; his forced vital capacity was 34%. **B,** After posterior spinal fusion with pedicle screw construct and iliac screws for pelvic fixation. (From Karol LA: Scoliosis in patients with Duchenne muscular dystrophy, *J Bone Joint Surg Am* 89 [Suppl 1]:159, 2007.)

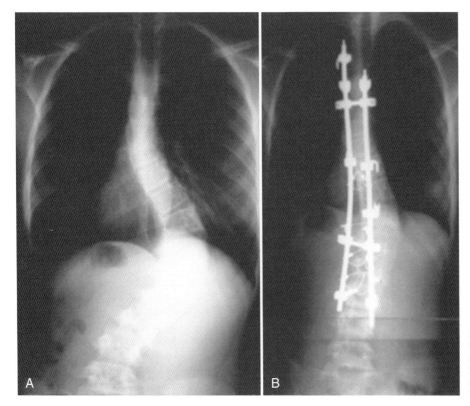

Figure 9-9 A, Thoracolumbar curve of 77 degrees. **B,** After correction with hooks and sublaminar cables, curve is 22 degrees. (From Freeman BL III: Scoliosis and kyphosis. In Canale ST, Beaty JH, editors: *Campbell's Operative Orthopaedics,* 11th ed. Philadelphia, 2008, Elsevier, 38:1960.)

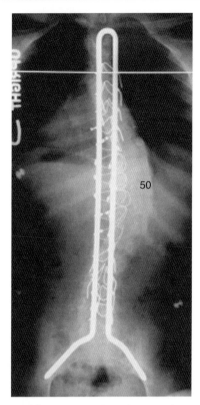

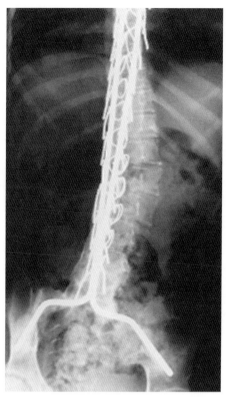

Figure 9-10 Unit rod for neuromuscular scoliosis. Single, continuous ¼-inch stainless steel rod has a U bend at the top and bullet-shaped ends for insertion into the pelvis. (From Freeman BL III: Scoliosis and kyphosis. In Canale ST, Beaty JH, editors: *Campbell's Operative Orthopaedics*, 11th ed. Philadelphia, 2008, Elsevier, 38:1960.)

Figure 9-11 Stabilization of the pelvis with the Galveston technique. Segment of rod is driven into each ilium. (From Freeman BL III: Scoliosis and kyphosis. In Canale ST, Beaty JH, editors: *Campbell's Operative Orthopaedics*, 11th ed. Philadelphia, 2008, Elsevier, 38:1960.)

for these patients. In patients with smaller curves and fixed pelvic obliquity, the fusion and instrumentation can end at L5. If fixed pelvic obliquity is more than 15 degrees, fusion to the pelvis with iliac screws, Galveston technique (Fig. 9-11), or S-rod pelvic fixation is recommended. The fusion should extend to the upper thoracic spine, to T2 or T3. The sagittal contours of the spine, especially lumbar lordosis, should be maintained for sitting balance and pressure distribution.

Because of the pulmonary compromise in these patients, rapid postoperative mobilization is important. We generally use no orthoses after surgery, although some recommend a bivalved plastic orthosis when the patient is sitting to minimize discomfort for 6 weeks postoperatively.[4]

Becker Muscular Dystrophy

Becker muscular dystrophy has a later onset and slower rate of muscle deterioration than Duchenne muscular dystrophy.[38] Orthopedic treatment of patients with Becker muscular dystrophy depends on the severity of the disease. In patients with large amounts of functional dystrophin, orthopedic procedures frequently are not needed until after childhood, and in patients with more severe forms of the disease, treatment considerations are the same as for patients with Duchenne muscular dystrophy. Contractures of the foot and overpull of the posterior tibial muscle can be treated effectively with Achilles tendon lengthening and posterior tibial tendon transfers with good long-term results. Patients rarely need soft-tissue releases around the hips. Because scoliosis is not as common in patients with Becker muscular dystrophy as in those with Duchenne muscular dystrophy, guidelines

for surgical correction of the scoliosis are not clearly defined and treatment must be individualized for each patient.

Emery-Dreifuss Muscular Dystrophy

During the first few years of life, patients with Emery-Dreifuss muscular dystrophy have muscle weakness, an awkward gait, and a tendency for toe-walking. The full syndrome, usually occurring in the teens, is characterized by fixed equinus deformities of the ankles, flexion contractures of the elbows, extension contracture of the neck, and tightness of the lumbar paravertebral muscles.[39,40] It is important to recognize Emery-Dreifuss muscular dystrophy because of the associated cardiac abnormalities that usually are asymptomatic but can lead to sudden cardiac death.[41–43]

Orthopedic treatment of patients with Emery-Dreifuss muscular dystrophy involves release of the heel cord contractures and other muscles around the foot, usually by Achilles tendon lengthening and posterior ankle capsulotomy.[44] Anterior transfer of the posterior tibial tendon also may be needed. Elbow flexion contractures usually do not exceed 35 degrees, but contractures of 90 degrees have been reported; these contractures generally do not require surgical release.[44] Full flexion and normal pronation and supination are maintained. Contractures around the neck and back should be treated conservatively with range-of-motion exercises, although full range of motion should not be expected. Scoliosis may occur in patients with this form of muscular dystrophy, but progression is less frequent and less severe than in those with Duchenne muscular dystrophy, and spinal fusion is infrequently necessary.

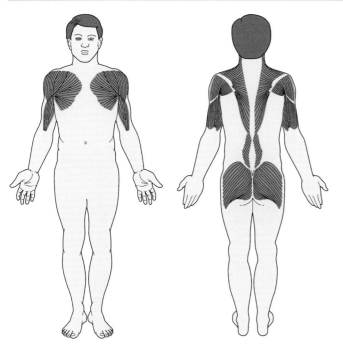

Figure 9-12 Pattern of weakness in limb-girdle muscular dystrophy. (From Warner WC Jr: Neuromuscular disorders. In Canale ST, Beaty JH, editors: *Campbell's Operative Orthopaedics*, 11th ed. Philadelphia, 2008, Elsevier, 38:1511.)

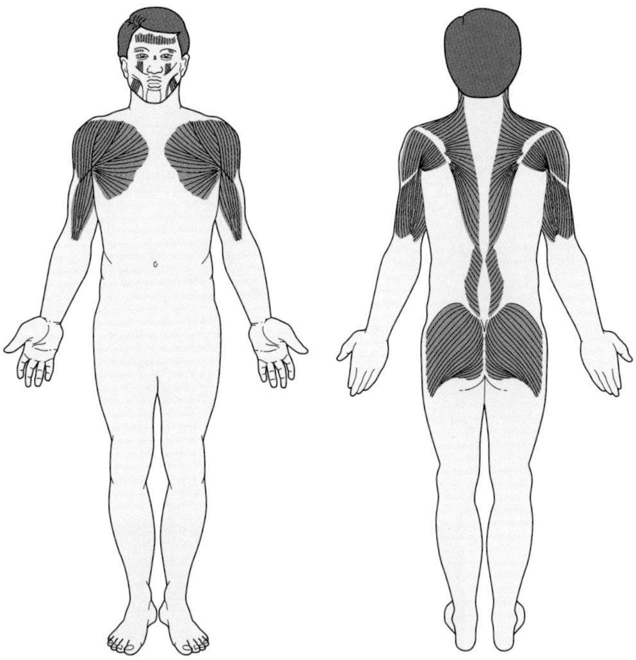

Figure 9-13 Pattern of weakness of facioscapulohumeral muscular dystrophy. (From Warner WC Jr: Neuromuscular disorders. In Canale ST, Beaty JH, editors: *Campbell's Operative Orthopaedics*, 11th ed. Philadelphia, 2008, Elsevier, 38:1512.)

Limb-Girdle Dystrophy

The clinical characteristics of limb-girdle dystrophy sometimes are indistinguishable from those of Becker and Duchenne muscular dystrophy, but normal dystrophin is noted on laboratory studies.[45–47] Limb-girdle dystrophy usually occurs in the first to fourth decades of life.[48] There are two major forms: the more common pelvic girdle type and a scapulohumeral type.[49] Initial muscle weakness involves the pelvic or shoulder girdle (Fig. 9-12). Lower extremity weakness usually involves the gluteus maximus, the iliopsoas, and the quadriceps muscles. Upper extremity weakness may involve the trapezius, the serratus anterior, the rhomboids, the latissimus dorsi, and the pectoralis major muscles. Some weakness also may develop in the prime movers of the fingers and wrists. Orthopedic surgery is seldom required for patients with limb-girdle dystrophy. Stabilization of the scapula to the ribs may be required for winging of the scapula; rarely muscle transfers around the wrist may be needed.

Facioscapulohumeral Muscular Dystrophy

The onset of facioscapulohumeral muscular dystrophy (FSHD) may be in early childhood, in which case the disease runs a rapid, progressive course, confining most children to a wheelchair by age 8 or 9 years; alternatively, onset may occur in patients age 15 to 35 years, in which case the disease progresses more slowly.

The most striking clinical manifestation is facial weakness with an inability to whistle, purse the lips, wrinkle the brow, or blow out the cheeks (Fig. 9-13). The greatest functional impairments are the inability to abduct and flex the arms at the glenohumeral joints and winging of the scapula, both caused by progressive weakness of the muscles that fix the scapula to the thoracic wall, while the muscles that abduct the glenohumeral joint remain strong. As the disease progresses, weakness of the lower extremities, especially in the peroneal and the anterior tibial muscles, results in a foot drop that requires the use of an AFO. Sometimes the quadriceps muscle is involved, requiring

expansion of the orthosis to a knee-ankle-foot orthosis. Scoliosis is rare, although extreme lumbar lordosis is common.

The inability to functionally flex and abduct the shoulder is usually treated by stabilization of the scapula with scapulothoracic arthrodesis.[49] Scapulothoracic fusion with strut grafts or with plates and screws provides a satisfactory fusion of the medial border of the scapula to the posterior thoracic ribs; however, it is associated with significant complications, including pneumothorax, pleural effusion, atelectasis, and pseudarthrosis.[50,51] A loss of pulses and motor and sensory function also has been reported after scapulothoracic arthrodesis.[52] The pulses and neurologic function returned when the scapula was repositioned to relieve compression of the neurovascular structures. A simplified technique (Fig. 9-14A) has produced good results after scapulocostal fusion in patients with FSHD[53] (Fig. 9-14B and C).

An early-onset form of FSHD has been described in which weakness is rapidly progressive and the lower extremities also are affected.[4,54,55] Patients become wheelchair bound by the second decade of life. Facial weakness is seen in infancy; this is followed by sensorineural hearing loss at an average age of 5 years. A progressive lumbar hyperlordosis develops and is almost pathognomonic for infantile FSHD. The hyperlordosis leads to fixed hip flexion contractures. Treatment consists of accommodation of the lordosis in the wheelchair. Spinal bracing has not been successful. Spinal fusion may be indicated to assist with sitting balance. Scapulothoracic fusion is not indicated in these patients because of the advanced weakness associated with this form of FSHD.

Congenital Muscular Dystrophies

Congenital muscular dystrophies are defined by the histologic appearance of the muscle biopsy rather than by specific clinical or molecular criteria.[56,57] Weakness and contractures at birth can cause hip dislocation, clubfeet, or other deformities. Respiratory weakness

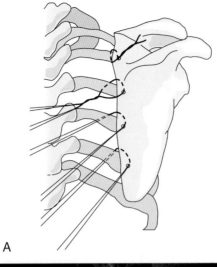

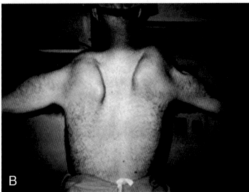

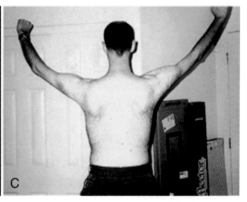

Figure 9-14 **A**, Technique for scapulocostal fusion in patients with facioscapulohumeral muscular dystrophy. **B**, Winging of the scapula in a patient with facioscapulohumeral dystrophy. **C**, After scapulocostal fusion. (**A**, From Jakab E, Gledhill RB: Simplified technique for scapulocostal fusion in the facioscapulohumeral dystrophy, *J Pediatr Orthop* 13:750, 1993.)

and difficulty with feeding and swallowing are common. The clinical appearance is one of dysmorphism, with kyphoscoliosis, chest deformities, a long face, and a high palate. Muscle tissue gradually is replaced with fibrous tissue, and contractures can become severe. Treatment is aimed at keeping the patient ambulatory and preventing contractures by exercises and orthotic splinting. Equinus and varus deformities of the feet may require releases if they interfere with ambulation. Congenital dislocation of the hip and clubfoot are treated conventionally, but recurrence is frequent.

Myotonic Dystrophy

Myotonic dystrophy is characterized by an inability of the muscles to relax after contraction. It is progressive and usually is present at birth, although it may develop in childhood. In addition to the inability of the muscles to relax, muscle weakness causes the most functional impairment. Other defects include hyperostosis of the skull, frontal and temporal baldness, gonadal atrophy, dysphasia, dysarthria, electrocardiographic abnormalities, and mental retardation.[58,59] The characteristic clinical appearance is a tent-shaped mouth, facial diplegia, and dull expression. About half of the children with myotonic dystrophy have clubfoot, and hip dysplasia and scoliosis may exist.[59,60] The hip dysplasia is treated conventionally but, because of capsular laxity, may not respond as readily as in other children. Serial casting can correct equinovarus deformity early on, but recurrence is likely and extensile release usually is required; triple arthrodesis may be required at skeletal maturity because of recurrence despite extensile releases. In patients with marked clubfoot deformity, extensive posteromedial release may not be sufficient to correct the deformity, and a talectomy may be needed. An AFO,

which frequently is needed for weakness in dorsiflexion, usually can maintain postoperative correction. In some adolescent patients, scoliosis develops and should be treated with the same principles as for the treatment of idiopathic scoliosis.[61] The high incidence of cardiac abnormalities and decreased pulmonary function will increase the risk of surgery and may prohibit surgery in these patients.

Hereditary Motor and Sensory Neuropathies

Hereditary motor and sensory neuropathies (HMSN) are a large group of inherited neuropathic disorders. The most common disorder among these neuropathies is Charcot-Marie-Tooth disease (CMT).

Charcot-Marie-Tooth Disease (Peroneal Muscular Atrophy)

Charcot-Marie-Tooth disease is an inherited degenerative disorder of the peripheral nervous system that causes muscle atrophy and loss of proprioception. It usually is an autosomal dominant trait but can be X-linked recessive or autosomal recessive. The incidence of the various forms of CMT ranges from 20 per 100,000 to 1 per 2,500.[62,63] Muscle atrophy is steadily progressive in most patients with the autosomal dominant form; less often, the disease arrests completely or manifests intermittently. The recessive forms have an early onset (first or second decade) and are more rapidly progressive. Initial complaints usually are general weakness of the foot and an unsteady gait. Foot problems include pain under the metatarsal heads, claw toes, foot fatigue, and difficulty in wearing regular shoes. Distal loss of proprioception and spinal ataxia are common. CMT should be suspected in patients with claw toes, high arches, thin legs, poor balance, and an unsteady gait. In addition to physical examination and family history, electromyograms showing an increased amplitude in duration of response and slow nerve conduction velocity typically confirm the diagnosis in the demyelinating types, but DNA testing also may be necessary.

Cavovarus Foot Deformity

The most common neuromuscular cause of cavovarus foot deformity in both adults and children is CMT.[64–66] This is a complex deformity of the forefoot and hindfoot. Surgery often is required to stabilize the foot.

Although muscle imbalance is known to cause the cavovarus deformity, theories explaining which muscles are involved and how the imbalances produce the rigid cavovarus deformity do not completely account for the clinical deformity. The most widely accepted explanation for the neuropathic cavovarus deformity of CMT is that it is caused by a combination of intrinsic and extrinsic muscle weakness, beginning with weakness of the intrinsic foot muscles and the anterior tibial muscle, with normal strength in the posterior tibial and peroneus longus muscles.[67–71] The triceps surae also is weak and may be contracted. The forefoot is pulled into equinus relative to the hindfoot, and the first ray becomes plantar-flexed. The long toe extensors attempt to assist the weak anterior tibial tendon in dorsiflexion but contribute to metatarsal plantar flexion. As the long toe extensors try to dorsiflex the foot, the toes are extended at the metatarsophalangeal joints (Fig. 9-15). This extension or clawing of the toes forces the heads of the metatarsals into a plantar-flexed position and increases the cavus deformity. The forefoot also is forced into a pronated position, with mild adduction of the metatarsals. Initially the foot is supple and plantigrade with weight-bearing, but as the forefoot becomes more rigidly pronated, the hindfoot will assume a varus position (Fig. 9-16). Weight-bearing becomes a "tripod" mechanism, with weight borne on the heel and the first and fifth metatarsal heads[72] (Fig. 9-17).

Clinical and Radiographic Evaluation

Although CMT is the most common neurologic cause of cavus foot deformity, it is essential to confirm the diagnosis. In one study, nearly 80% of pediatric patients with bilateral cavus foot deformities

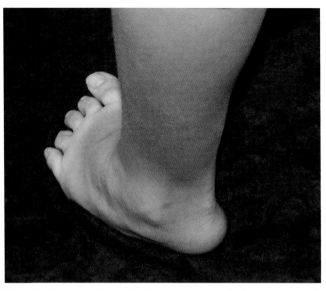

Figure 9-16 Varus position of hindfoot in a patient with Charcot-Marie-Tooth disease.

were diagnosed with CMT; among those with a family history, 91% had CMT.[73] Many adult patients with cavus feet have no clear etiology for the deformity. Other possible neurologic causes for the cavus foot should be considered (Box 9-1).

Physical Examination

Physical examination should include observation of the patient standing and walking to evaluate the degree of difficulty with balance and to assess for other associated deformities of the spine or hips. Patients often seek treatment because of frequent ankle sprains as a result of the cavovarus foot and underlying muscle weakness. In a patient with a cavus foot, the "peek-a-boo" sign is obvious when the foot is viewed from the front. Normally the heel is hidden behind the foot, but with a cavus foot its medial side is readily visible[74] (Fig. 9-18). The plantar fascia feels like a tight band in the sole of the foot as the forefoot is dorsiflexed. Calluses often are present on the soles of the feet, usually along the lateral border of the foot, especially in the area of the base of the fifth metatarsal.

Motor examination should focus on the relative balance of the agonist-antagonist pairs that generate the foot deformities. Active dorsiflexion against resistance can evaluate the anterior tibial muscle and help detect the use of the extensor hallucis longus as an accessory dorsiflexor, resulting in a claw toe deformity of the hallux. Resisted eversion of the foot directly tests the peroneus brevis, and the longus can be partially isolated by asking the patient to depress the first ray. A handheld dynamometry unit has been reported to provide reliable and objective measures of muscle strength in CMT patients.[75]

The rigidity of the deformity also must be determined because this indicates to what degree tendon transfers or bony procedures can be used for correction. The Coleman block test (Fig. 9-19) is used to help determine the rigidity of the hindfoot varus.[76] The patient stands on a block of wood with the heel and lateral forefoot supported by the block, allowing the plantar-flexed first ray to drop. If dropping the first ray over the edge of the block allows the hindfoot to correct to a valgus position, the hindfoot is flexible; if correction of the varus does not occur, the hindfoot is rigid. The hindfoot also can be examined for flexibility with the patient lying prone with the knee flexed.

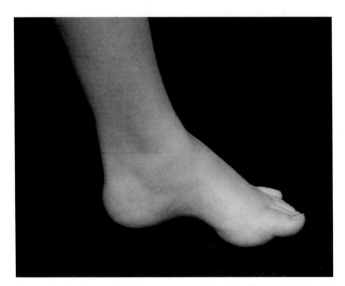

Figure 9-15 Clawing of left toe in a patient with Charcot-Marie-Tooth disease.

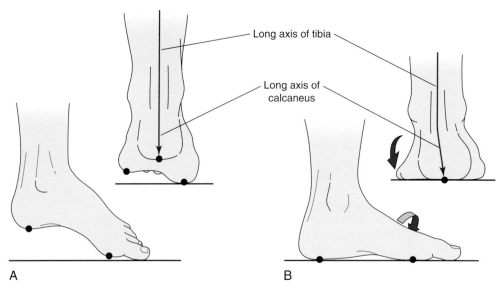

Long axis of tibia

Long axis of calcaneus

A   B

Figure 9-17 A, Posterior and lateral views of a cavus foot in a nonweight-bearing position. The long axes of the tibia and the calcaneus are parallel and the first metatarsal is pronated. *Dots* indicate the three major weight-bearing plantar areas (heel and first and fifth metatarsals). **B,** Posterior and lateral views of a cavus foot in weight-bearing position. The long axes of the tibia and the calcaneus are not parallel. With weight-bearing, a rigid equinus forefoot deformity forces the flexible hindfoot into varus, producing the tripod effect. (Adapted from Paulos L, Coleman SS, Samuelson KM: Pes cavovarus: review of a surgical approach using selective soft-tissue procedures, *J Bone Joint Surg Am* 62:942–953, 1980.)

Box 9-1 Potential Neurologic Causes of Cavus Foot Deformity Other Than Charcot-Marie-Tooth Disease
Infectious
Poliomyelitis
Degenerative
Friedreich ataxia
Hereditary cerebellar ataxia
Roussy-Lévy syndrome
Spinal muscular atrophy
Structural
Spinal cord tumor
Syringomyelia
Diastematomyelia
Spinal dysraphism
Central
Cerebral palsy

From Guyton GP: Current concepts review: orthopaedic aspects of Charcot-Marie-Tooth disease, *Foot Ankle Int* 27:1003–1010, 2006.

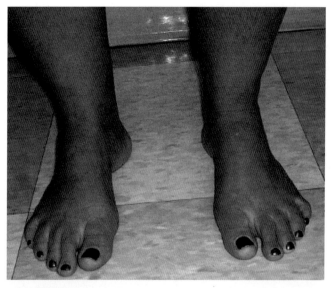

Figure 9-18 Peek-a-boo sign in a cavus foot. When viewed from the front, the heel is normally hidden behind the foot *(left)*, but with a cavus foot the medial side of the heel is readily visible *(right)*. (From Raikin SM, Slenker N, Ratigan B: The association of a varus hindfoot and fracture of the fifth metatarsal metaphyseal-diaphyseal junction. The Jones fracture, *Am J Sports Med* 36:1367–1373, 2008.)

Careful examination of the peripheral and central nervous systems is required, including electromyography and nerve conduction velocity studies. In demyelinating forms of CMT, electrophysiologic testing reveals slowing of the motor nerve conduction velocities due to loss of myelin. The hip and spine should be closely examined; hip dysplasia has been reported in 6% to 8% of children with CMT and scoliosis in as many as a third of children and half of adults with CMT.[77–81]

Radiographic Examination

Standard anteroposterior, lateral, and oblique radiographs are the most useful methods for evaluating the foot; however, to determine any significant relationships between the bones, it is essential that the anteroposterior and lateral views be made with the foot in a weight-bearing or simulated weight-bearing position. Anteroposterior views document the degree of forefoot adduction. The degree of cavus can be estimated on the lateral view by determining the talus-first metatarsal (Meary) angle, the angle between the long axis of the first metatarsal and long axis of the talus; the normal angle is 0 degrees; in the cavus foot, it usually measures greater than 5 degrees.[64] Other measurements include the Hibbs angle, defined as the angle between a line drawn along the longitudinal axis of the calcaneus and one drawn down the shaft of the first metatarsal (normally less than 45 degrees,

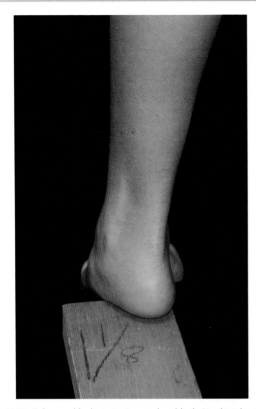

Figure 9-19 Coleman block test. A wooden block is placed under the hindfoot and lateral forefoot, with the first metatarsal head off the block. With a flexible deformity, the hindfoot everts into valgus when the plantar-flexed first metatarsal is not bearing weight. With a fixed deformity, the heel position does not change.

often near 90 degrees in the cavus foot), and the calcaneal pitch angle, which differentiates between calcaneocavus (more than 30 degrees) and forefoot cavus (less than 30 degrees)[4] (Fig. 9-20). Radiographs using the Coleman block test demonstrate the correction of the varus deformity if the hindfoot is flexible. Equinus can be measured by the lateral tibial calcaneal angle. If this angle exceeds 30 degrees, the ankle is dorsiflexed, and the tendency for patients to walk on their toes is specifically not due to ankle equinus. Cross-sectional imaging modalities have little role in the evaluation of CMT. Magnetic resonance imaging will show fatty infiltration in the peroneus brevis or anterior tibialis muscle, but muscle function is better determined clinically.

Orthopedic Treatment

Treatment is determined by the age of the patient and the severity of the deformity.

Nonoperative Treatment

Nonoperative treatment of the cavovarus foot generally has been unsuccessful, although a brace may help manage symptoms of drop foot and ankle instability.[65] In active patients with mild lateral ankle ligament laxity, a simple figure-of-eight Velcro-strap ankle brace often is sufficient.[65,82] For more severe foot drop, a posterior spring-leaf AFO provides dorsiflexion assistance and is lightweight and easy to transfer between shoes. A custom-molded leather boot brace or a conventional double-metal upright shoe-based AFO may be needed for more support, especially in obese patients. However, poor compliance with brace-wear has been found in patients with severe bilateral foot drop caused by CMT.[83] Reasons given for discarding the AFO were that it highlighted patients' disabilities, was not essential for limited daily walking, and was uncomfortable.

Some studies have suggested that neurotrophin-3 (NT-3) may augment nerve regeneration in animal models of CMT, and a small clinical study (eight patients) showed possible minor benefits, but currently there is no clear evidence that NT-3 is an effective treatment for CMT.[84] Small trials of exercise, creatine monohydrate,

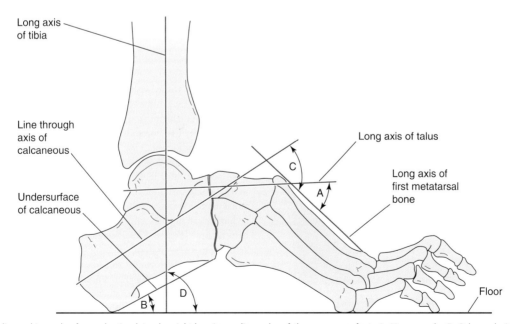

Figure 9-20 Radiographic angles for evaluating lateral weight-bearing radiographs of the cavovarus foot. A, Meary angle. B, Calcaneal pitch angle. C, Hibbs angle. D, Weight-bearing tibioplantar angle. (Adapted from Alexander IJ, Johnson KA: Assessment and management of pes cavus in Charcot-Marie-Tooth disease, *Clin Orthop Rel Res* 246:273–281, 1989.)

and purified bovine brain gangliosides have been done, but none showed significant benefit. Identification of the genes causing CMT may allow development of feasible gene therapy options.

Operative Treatment of Foot Deformities

Surgical procedures are of three types: soft-tissue (plantar fascia release, tendon release, or tendon transfer), osteotomy (metatarsal, midfoot, calcaneal), and joint-stabilizing (triple arthrodesis). The goals of operative treatment are correction of the deformity and rebalancing of the deforming muscle forces.

Experience in the treatment of foot deformities in CMT has demonstrated that early, aggressive treatment when the hindfoot is flexible and early soft-tissue releases can delay the need for more extensive reconstructive procedures. Even in a young patient with a fixed hindfoot deformity, limited soft-tissue release combined with osteotomies of the first metatarsal, midfoot, or calcaneus can provide a satisfactory functional outcome without the loss of hindfoot and midfoot joint motion that occurs with triple arthrodesis.

Initial treatment of a flexible cavus foot consists of plantar fascia release or plantar fascia and medial soft-tissue release (Fig. 9-21). This can be combined with appropriate tendon transfers to rebalance the foot.

Flexible claw toe deformity usually is corrected without additional surgery when the midfoot deformity is corrected. For clawing in a young child without severe weakness of the anterior tibial muscle, the extensor hallucis longus tendon can be transferred to the first metatarsal neck with tenodesis or fusion of the interphalangeal joint of the great toe (Fig. 9-22). This converts the extensor hallucis longus into an active dorsiflexor of the plantar-flexed first metatarsal. For adolescents or children with severe weakness of the anterior tibial muscle, the second through fifth long toe extensors can be transferred to the middle cuneiform, with fusion or tenodesis of the interphalangeal joint. For severe deformity, the posterior tibial tendon can be transferred anteriorly to the middle cuneiform instead of the long toe extensors. Anterior transfer of the posterior tibial tendon removes a deforming force and allows the posterior tibial muscle to assist with ankle dorsiflexion. The peroneus longus functions as a plantar flexor of the first metatarsal. Transfer of this muscle to the peroneous brevis changes its function from plantar flexion of the first metatarsal to eversion of the forefoot.

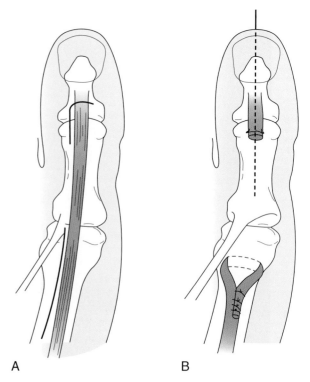

Figure 9-22 Transfer of extensor hallucis longus tendon for claw toe deformity (Jones procedure). **A,** Incisions. **B,** Completed transfer. (From Warner WC: Neuromuscular disorders. In Canale ST, Beaty JH, editors: *Campbell's Operative Orthopaedics,* 11th ed. Philadelphia, 2008, Elsevier, p 1518.)

Children younger than age 8 years with supple hindfeet usually respond to plantar releases and appropriate tendon transfers. A more extensive plantar-medial release and osteotomy of the first metatarsal can be used for rigid forefoot deformity. In children younger than age 12 years with rigid hindfoot deformities, radical plantar-medial release, first metatarsal dorsiflexion osteotomy or midfoot osteotomy, and a calcaneal osteotomy usually correct the deformity. For a fixed hindfoot varus deformity with a prominent calcaneus, a lateral closing wedge osteotomy may be preferred to shorten the heel. If the heel is not prominent, a sliding calcaneal osteotomy gives satisfactory results.

Many patients with CMT do not require triple arthrodesis; soft-tissue procedures and osteotomies are sufficient in skeletally immature feet and those with less severe deformity. Appropriate wedge resections correct both the hindfoot varus and midfoot component of the cavus deformity; soft-tissue release and muscle balancing are required for the forefoot deformity. Some authors recommend restoring hindfoot stability with a triple arthrodesis and transferring the posterior tibial tendon anteriorly to eliminate the need for a postoperative drop-foot brace. Because of early degenerative changes in the ankle, forefoot, and midfoot, triple arthrodesis generally is considered a salvage procedure for patients in whom other procedures were unsuccessful or in patients with untreated severe fixed deformities (Fig. 9-23); however, some surgeons prefer triple arthrodesis over midfoot osteotomy, because of a more reliable correction of the deformity and the possibility of arthritic changes caused by an osteotomy that crosses multiple joints.[85-87]

Surgical procedures usually are staged[88] (Fig. 9-24). The initial procedure is a radical plantar or plantar-medial release, with a dorsal closing wedge osteotomy of the first metatarsal base if necessary. Achilles tendon lengthening usually is not needed because ankle equinus usually is not present. If Achilles tendon lengthening is

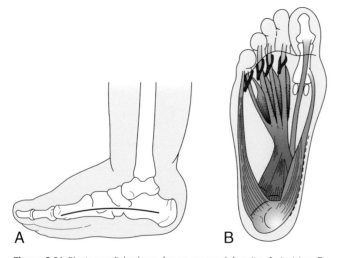

Figure 9-21 Plantar-medial release for cavovarus deformity. **A,** Incision. **B,** Release of musculotendinous mass. (Redrawn from Coleman SS: *Complex Foot Deformities in Children,* Philadelphia, 1983, Lea & Febiger.)

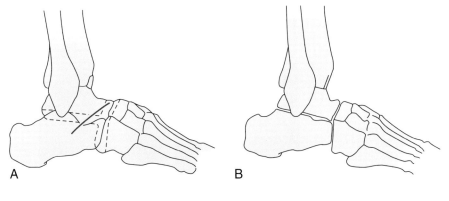

Figure 9-23 Triple arthrodesis. **A,** Oblique incision to expose subtalar, talonavicular, and calcaneocuboid joints. **B,** Cartilage and cortical bone are removed from all joint surfaces; appropriate bony wedges are removed if necessary for deformity correction. (From Warner WC: Paralytic disorders. In Canale ST, Beaty JH, editors: *Campbell's Operative Orthopaedics*, 11th ed. Philadelphia, 2008, Elsevier, p 1412.)

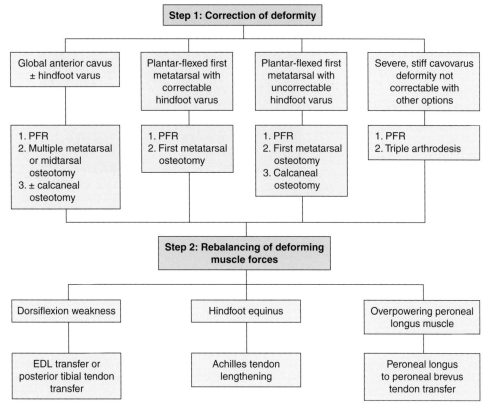

Figure 9-24 Treatment algorithm for correction of cavovalgus foot in pediatric patients with Charcot-Marie-Tooth disease. EDL, extensor digitorum longus; PFR, plantar fascia release. (From Olney B: Treatment of the cavus foot. Deformity in the pediatric patient with Charcot-Marie-Tooth disease, *Foot Ankle Clin* 5:305–315, 2000.)

needed for ankle equinus, it should not be done as part of the initial procedure because the force used to dorsiflex the forefoot would not allow for adequate correction of the equinus deformity. If the hindfoot is flexible and a posterior release is not necessary, posterior tibial tendon transfer can be done as part of the initial procedure for severe anterior tibial weakness.

Hip Dysplasia

Hip dysplasia has been reported in approximately 6% to 8% of patients with CMT.[77–79,89,90] Dysplasia is more likely to occur in HMSN type I than in HMSN type II. The treating physician should be aware of this association. If hip dysplasia is present, it should be corrected.

Spinal Deformities

Scoliosis is uncommon in association with CMT, usually reported to occur in approximately 10% of patients,[81] although Walker[79] reported frequencies of 37% in children and 50% in adults. In a review of 175 patients with HMSN, Horacek et al[80] found spinal deformity in 26%. The curve usually is mild to moderate and often does not require any treatment. In patients with CMT, Hensinger and MacEwen[91] reported associated kyphosis in half their patients with scoliosis. They reported that nonoperative treatment with a brace was well tolerated and successfully controlled the curve in many patients. Generally, spinal deformities in children with CMT can be managed by the same techniques used for idiopathic scoliosis. Because of the demyelinization of the peripheral nerves and degeneration of the dorsal root ganglion and dorsal column of the spinal cord, somatosensory-evoked potentials may be absent.

Charcot-Marie-Tooth Variants

Roussy-Lévy syndrome (hereditary areflexic dystaxia) is an autosomal dominant disease with the clinical characteristics of classic CMT plus a static tremor in the hands. The disease usually begins in infancy but may not have symptoms until adolescence. It is characterized by severe alterations in nerve conduction and sensory dysfunction.[68]

Dejerine-Sottas syndrome (familial interstitial hypertrophic neuritis) usually is an autosomal recessive disease but may show an autosomal dominant inheritance with variable penetrance. The disease usually begins in infancy but may not appear until adolescence. Along with the classic pes cavus deformity, marked sensory loss occurs in all four extremities, and patients also may have clubfoot or kyphoscoliosis.[68,92,93]

Refsum disease is an autosomal recessive disorder beginning in childhood or puberty in which the spinal fluid protein is increased. The gene responsible for Refsum disease is on chromosome 10. The condition is caused by a defect in phytanoyl-CoA hydroxylase, which is responsible for the degradation of phytanic acid. It is accompanied by retinitis pigmentosa and is characterized by a hypertrophic neuropathy with ataxia and areflexia. Distal sensory and motor loss occurs in the hands and feet. The course is unpredictable, with repeated reactivations and remissions, but the prognosis is poor.[94]

Neuronal-type CMT is an autosomal dominant disease with a usually late onset (middle age or later). The small muscles of the hands are not as weak as in other forms of the disease, but the ankle muscles and plantar muscles of the feet are much weaker and more atrophic.

Friedreich Ataxia

Friedreich ataxia is an autosomal recessive condition characterized by spinocerebellar degeneration. The prevalence of Friedreich ataxia is approximately 1 in 50,000.[95] An ataxic gait usually is the presenting symptom, with onset routinely between ages 7 and 15 years. The diagnosis is suggested by the clinical triad of ataxia, areflexia, and a positive Babinski reflex.[96] Definitive diagnosis can be made with DNA testing. The disease is progressive, and almost all patients are wheelchair bound by the first or second decade of life. Patients typically demonstrate progressive dysarthria or weakness, decreased vibratory sense in the lower extremities, cardiomyopathy, pes cavus, and scoliosis. Knee jerk and ankle jerk reflexes are lost quite early. Patients usually die in the fourth or fifth decade of life as a result of progressive cardiomyopathy, pneumonia, or aspiration.

The primary concern of the orthopedist is the correction of foot and spinal deformities (Fig. 9-25). In patients with Friedreich ataxia, the plantar reflex sometimes is so great that when standing is attempted, the feet and toes immediately plantar-flex and the posterior tibial tendon pulls the forefoot into equinovarus. If general anesthesia is contraindicated because of myocardial involvement or other medical conditions, tenotomies of the Achilles tendon, the posterior tibial tendon at the ankle, and the toe flexors at the plantar side of the metatarsophalangeal joints can be done with the patient under local anesthesia. Surgery should be delayed in patients who are able to walk and who have deformities that are either supple or can be controlled in braces; however, the cavovarus deformities tend to worsen and become rigid. In patients with rigid cavovarus deformity, primary triple arthrodesis provides a solid base of support with a fixed plantigrade foot. Because most patients become wheelchair bound, later development of ankle and midfoot degenerative changes seldom is clinically significant. Posterior tibial tenotomy, lengthening, or transfer should be combined with the triple arthrodesis. Bracing is routinely required after surgery.[97]

Scoliosis is frequent in patients with Friedreich ataxia, occurring in 60% to 100%.[98–100] Curve patterns are variable and may or may not resemble idiopathic curves.[99,101] Stabilization of the spine should be performed when the curve is greater than 40 to 50 degrees and the patient is no longer ambulatory. A single-stage posterior arthrodesis with segmental instrumentation is the treatment of

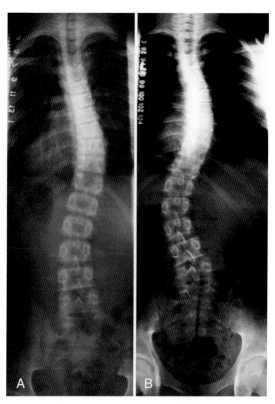

Figure 9-25 Scoliosis in a patient with Friedreich ataxia. **A,** At age 14, she had a 26-degree thoracic curve and a 25-degree lumbar curve; brace treatment was begun. **B,** At age 16.5 years, after 1 year of bracing and 1 year of follow-up, the residual thoracic curve is 30 degrees and the lumbar curve is 39 degrees. (From Milbrandt TA, Kunes JR, Karol LA: Friedreich's ataxia and scoliosis: the experience at two institutions, *J Pediatr Orthop* 28:236, 2008.)

choice. The fusion should extend from the upper thoracic spine to the lower region of the lumbar spine, as in patients with Duchenne muscular dystrophy.

Spinal Muscular Atrophy

Spinal muscular atrophy (SMA) is an inherited degenerative disease of the anterior horn cells of the spinal cord that occurs in 1 in 20,000 births.[102–104] It is generally transmitted by an autosomal recessive gene, but other hereditary patterns have been described. SMA has been classified into four types. In the acute infantile type (type I), severe generalized weakness manifests in patients younger than age 6 months, and terminal respiratory failure occurs early. A chronic infantile type (type II) occurs during the middle of the first year and, after initial progression of weakness, may remain static for long periods. The juvenile type (type III) develops later, with gradual onset of weakness and a slowly progressive course.[102–104] The fourth type is a rare adult form.

Orthopedic treatment generally is required for hip and spine problems.[105–109] Children with type I SMA are markedly hypotonic and generally succumb to the disease early in life. In these patients, orthopedic reconstruction is not warranted; however, patients with type I SMA may develop fractures that heal quickly with appropriate splinting. Many children with infantile SMA (Werdnig-Hoffmann disease) are never able to walk even with braces, but most patients with the juvenile form (Kugelberg-Welander disease) are able to walk for many years. Gentle passive range-of-motion exercises and positioning instructions can be beneficial initially. Surgical release of contractures rarely is required. Because of the absence of movement and

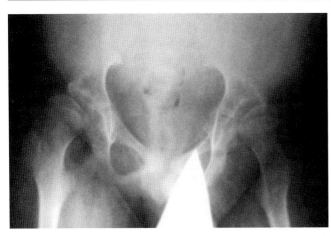

Figure 9-26 Coxa valga deformity and subluxation in a 12-year-old child with spinal muscular atrophy. (From Warner WC Jr: Neuromuscular disorders. In Canale ST, Beaty JH, editors: *Campbell's Operative Orthopaedics*, 11th ed. Philadelphia, 2008, Elsevier, 38:1521.)

weight-bearing, coxa valga deformity of the hip is frequent, and unilateral or bilateral hip subluxation may occur (Fig. 9-26). Because many of these children are sitters, a stable and comfortable sitting position is essential. Traditionally, proximal femoral varus derotational osteotomy has been used in nonambulatory patients to produce a more stable sitting base. Efforts to maintain the reduction of the hips for good sitting balance may prevent pain and pelvic obliquity. However, Sporer and Smith[107] recommended observation instead of surgical intervention because of the small number of patients who had symptoms or seating problems in their series.

Among children with SMA who survive childhood, scoliosis becomes the greatest threat during adolescence. Scoliosis is seen in nearly 100% of children with type II SMA and in children with type III SMA who become nonambulatory. It usually is progressive and severe and can limit daily function and cause cardiopulmonary problems. Bracing may be indicated during the growing years to slow curve progression, but spinal stabilization is ultimately required in almost all adolescent patients. Several authors have emphasized the importance of early surgery before the curve becomes severe and rigid. The treatment of choice is a long posterior fusion, using segmental instrumentation. This fusion and instrumentation usually should extend to the pelvis in nonambulatory patients to prevent pelvic obliquity. Intraoperative and postoperative complications are frequent in these patients, and thorough preoperative evaluation is mandatory.

References

1. Bleck EE: *Orthopaedic Management of Cerebral Palsy*, Philadelphia, 1979, WB Saunders.
2. Larson CM, Henderson RC: Bone mineral density and fractures in boys with Duchenne muscular dystrophy, *J Pediatr Orthop* 20:71–74, 2000.
3. Emery AE: Population frequencies of inherited neuromuscular diseases—a world survey, *Neuromuscul Disord* 1:19–29, 1991.
4. Shapiro F, Specht L: The diagnosis and treatment of inherited muscular diseases of childhood, *J Bone Joint Surg Am* 75:439–454, 1993.
5. Sussman M: Duchenne muscular dystrophy, *J Am Acad Orthop Surg* 10:138–151, 2002.
6. Hoffman EP, Pegoraro E, Scacheri P, et al: Genetic counseling of isolated carriers of Duchenne muscular dystrophy, *Am J Med Genet* 63:573–580, 1996.
7. Pasternak C, Wong S, Elson EL: Mechanical function of dystrophin in muscle cells, *J Cell Biol* 128:355–361, 1995.
8. Bach JR, McKeon J: Orthopaedic surgery and rehabilitation for the prolongation of brace-free ambulation of patients with Duchenne muscular dystrophy, *Am J Phys Med Rehabil* 70:323–331, 1991.
9. Forst J, Forst R: Lower-limb surgery in Duchenne muscular dystrophy, *Neuromuscul Disord* 9:176–181, 1999.
10. Goertzen M, Baltzer A, Voit T: Clinical results of early orthopaedic management in Duchenne muscular dystrophy, *Neuropediatrics* 257–259, 1995.
11. Rideau Y, Duport G, Delaubier A, et al: Early treatment to preserve quality of locomotion for children with Duchenne muscular dystrophy, *Semin Neurol* 5:9–17, 1995.
12. Manzur AY, Hyde SA, Rodillo E, et al: A randomized controlled trial of early surgery in Duchenne muscular dystrophy, *Neuromuscul Disord* 2:379–387, 1992.
13. Smith SE, Green NE, Cole RJ, et al: Prolongation of ambulation in children with Duchenne muscular dystrophy by subcutaneous lower limb tenotomy, *J Pediatr Orthop* 13:336–340, 1993.
14. Vignos PJ Jr, Wagner MB, Kaplan JS, et al: Predicting the success of re-ambulation in patients with Duchenne muscular dystrophy, *J Bone Joint Surg Am* 65:719–728, 1983.
15. Scher DM, Mubarak SJ: Surgical prevention of foot deformity in patients with Duchenne muscular dystrophy, *J Pediatr Orthop* 22:384–391, 2002.
16. Leitch KK, Raza N, Biggar D, et al: Should foot surgery be performed for children with Duchenne muscular dystrophy? *J Pediatr Orthop* 25:95–97, 2005.
17. Wilkins KE, Gibson DA: The patterns of spinal deformity in Duchenne muscular dystrophy, *J Bone Joint Surg Am* 58:24–32, 1976.
18. Karol LA: Scoliosis in patients with Duchenne muscular dystrophy, *J Bone Joint Surg Am* 89:155–162, 2007.
19. Kinali M, Messina S, Mercuri E, et al: Management of scoliosis in Duchenne muscular dystrophy: a large 10-year retrospective study, *Dev Med Child Neurol* 48:513–518, 2006.
20. Alman BA, Raza SN, Biggar WC: Steroid treatment and the development of scoliosis in males with Duchenne muscular dystrophy, *J Bone Joint Surg Am* 86:519–524, 2004.
21. Colbert AP, Craig C: Scoliosis management in Duchenne muscular dystrophy: prospective study of modified Jewett hyperextension brace, *Arch Phys Med Rehabil* 68:302–304, 1987.
22. Heller KD, Wirtz DC, Siebert CH, et al: Spinal stabilization in Duchenne muscular dystrophy: principles of treatment and record of 31 operative treated cases, *J Pediatr Orthop Br* 10:18–24, 2001.
23. Mubarak SJ, Morin WD, Leach J: Spinal fusion in Duchenne muscular dystrophy—fixation and fusion to the sacropelvis? *J Pediatr Orthop* 13:752–757, 1993.
24. Sussman MD: Advantage of early spinal stabilization and fusion in patients with Duchenne muscular dystrophy, *J Pediatr Orthop* 4:532–537, 1984.
25. Galasko CS, Delaney C, Morris P: Spinal stabilisation in Duchenne muscular dystrophy, *J Bone Joint Surg Br* 74:210–214, 1992.
26. Smith AD, Koreska J, Moseley CF: Progression of scoliosis in Duchenne muscular dystrophy, *J Bone Joint Surg Am* 71:1066–11064, 1989.
27. Jenkins JG, Bohn D, Edmonds JF, et al: Evaluation of pulmonary function in muscular dystrophy patients requiring spinal surgery, *Crit Care Med* 10:645–649, 1982.
28. Miller F, Moseley CF, Koreska J, et al: Pulmonary function and scoliosis in Duchenne dystrophy, *J Pediatr Orthop* 8:133–137, 1988.
29. Gill I, Eagle M, Mehta JS, et al: Correction of neuromuscular scoliosis in patients with preexisting respiratory failure, *Spine* 31:2478–2483, 2006.
30. Harper CM, Ambler G, Edge G: The prognostic value of preoperative predicted forced vital capacity in corrective spinal surgery for Duchenne's muscular dystrophy, *Anaesthesia* 59:1160–1162, 2004.
31. Marsh A, Edge G, Lehovsky J: Spinal fusion in patients with Duchenne's muscular dystrophy and a low forced vital capacity, *Eur Spine J* 12:507–512, 2003.
32. Kennedy JD, Staples AJ, Brook PD, et al: Effect of spinal surgery on lung function in Duchenne muscular dystrophy, *Thorax* 50:1173–1178, 1995.
33. Miller RG, Chalmers AC, Dao H, et al: The effect of spine fusion on respiratory function in Duchenne muscular dystrophy, *Neurology* 41:38–40, 1991.
34. Velasco MV, Colin AA, Zurakowski D, et al: Posterior spinal fusion for scoliosis in Duchenne muscular dystrophy diminishes the rate of respiratory decline, *Spine* 32:459–465, 2007.

35. Bridwell KH, Baldus C, Iffrig JM, et al: Process measures and patient/parent evaluation of surgery management of spinal deformity in patients with progressive flaccid neuromuscular scoliosis (Duchenne's muscular dystrophy and spinal muscular atrophy), *Spine* 24:1300–1309, 1999.

36. Granata C, Merlini L, Cervellati S, et al: Long-term results of spine surgery in Duchenne muscular dystrophy, *Neuromuscul Disord* 6:61–68, 1996.

37. Lonstein JE, Renshaw TS: Neuromuscular spine deformities, *Instr Course Lect* 36:285–304, 1987.

38. Herring JA, editor: *Tachdjian's Pediatric Orthopaedics* ed 4, vol. 29, Philadelphia, 2008, Elsevier, pp 1637–1638.

39. Emery AE: Emery-Dreifuss syndrome, *J Med Genet* 26:637–641, 1989.

40. Goncu K, Guzel R, Guler-Uysal F: Emery-Dreifuss muscular dystrophy in the evaluation of decreased spinal mobility and joint contracture, *Clin Rheumatol* 22:456–460, 2003.

41. Bialer MG, McDaniel NL, Kelly TE: Progression of cardiac disease in Emery-Dreifuss muscular dystrophy, *Clin Cardiol* 14:411–416, 1991.

42. Muntoni F: Journey into muscular dystrophies caused by abnormal glycosylation, *Acta Myol* 23:79–84, 2004.

43. Rakovec P, Zidar J, Sinkovec M, et al: Cardiac involvement in Emery-Dreifuss muscular dystrophy: role of a diagnostic pacemaker, *Pacing Clin Electrophysiol* 18(9 Pt 1):1721–1724, 1995.

44. Shapiro F, Specht L: Orthopedic deformities in Emery-Dreifuss muscular dystrophy, *J Pediatr Orthop* 11:336–340, 1991.

45. Guglieri M, Bushby K: How to go about diagnosing and managing the limb-girdle muscular dystrophies, *Neurol India* 56:271–280, 2008.

46. Pogue R, Anderson LV, Pyle A, et al: Strategies for mutation analysis in the autosomal recessive limb-girdle muscular dystrophies, *Neuromuscul Disord* 11:80–87, 2001.

47. Straub V, Bushby K: Therapeutic possibilities in the autosomal recessive limb-girdle muscular dystrophies, *Neurotherapeutics* 5:619–626, 2008.

48. Yamanouchi Y, Arikawa E, Arahata K, et al: Limb-girdle muscular dystrophy: clinical and pathological reevaluation, *J Neurol Sci* 129:15–20, 1995.

49. Letournel E, Fardeau M, Lytle JO, et al: Scapulothoracic arthrodesis for patients who have facioscapulohumeral muscular dystrophy, *J Bone Joint Surg Am* 72:78–84, 1990.

50. Berne D, Laude F, Laporte C, et al: Scapulothoracic arthrodesis in facioscapulohumeral muscular dystrophy, *Clin Orthop Relat Res* 409:106–113, 2003.

51. Krishnan SG, Hawkins RJ, Michelotti JD, et al: Scapulothoracic arthrodesis: indications, technique, and results, *Clin Orthop Relat Res* 435:126–133, 2005.

52. Mackenzie WG, Riddle EC, Earley JL, et al: A neurovascular complication after scapulothoracic arthrodesis, *Clin Orthop Relat Res* 408:157–161, 2003.

53. Jakab E, Gledhill RB: Simplified technique for scapulocostal fusion in facioscapulohumeral dystrophy, *J Pediatr Orthop* 13:749–751, 1993.

54. Klinge L, Eagle M, Haggerty ID, et al: Severe phenotype in infantile facioscapulohumeral muscular dystrophy, *Neuromuscul Disord* 16:553–558, 2006.

55. Korf BR, Bresnan MJ, Shapiro F, et al: Facioscapulohumeral dystrophy presenting in infancy with facial diplegia and sensorineural deafness, *Ann Neurol* 17:513–516, 1985.

56. Cardamone M, Darras BT, Ryan MM: Inherited myopathies and muscular dystrophies, *Semin Neurol* 28:250–259, 2008.

57. Sewry CA, Philpot J, Sorokin LM, et al: Diagnosis of merosin (laminin-2) deficient congenital muscular dystrophy by skin biopsy, *Lancet* 347:582–584, 1996.

58. Groh WJ, Groh MR, Saha C, et al: Electrocardiographic abnormalities and sudden death in myotonic dystrophy type 1, *N Engl J Med* 358:2688–2697, 2008.

59. Schara U, Schoser BG: Myotonic dystrophies type 1 and 2: a summary on current aspects, *Semin Pediatr Neurol* 13:71–79, 2006.

60. Ricker K: Myotonic dystrophy and proximal myotonic myopathy, *J Neurol* 246:334–338, 1999.

61. Themistocleous GS, Sapkas GS, Papagelopoulos PJ, et al: Scoliosis in Steinert syndrome: a case report, *Spine J* 5:212–216, 2005.

62. Holmberg BH: Charcot-Marie-Tooth disease in northern Sweden: an epidemiological and clinical study, *Acta Neurol Scand* 87:416–422, 1993.

63. Mendell JR: Charcot-Marie-Tooth neuropathies and related disorders, *Semin Neurol* 18:41–47, 1998.

64. Alexander IJ, Johnson KA: Assessment and management of pes cavus in Charcot-Marie-Tooth disease, *Clin Orthop Relat Res* 246:273–281, 1989.

65. Guyton GP: Current concepts review: orthopaedic aspects of Charcot-Marie-Tooth disease, *Foot Ankle Int* 27:1003–1010, 2006.

66. Schwend RM, Drennan JC: Cavus foot deformity in children, *J Am Acad Orthop Surg* 11:201–211, 2003.

67. Beals TC, Nickisch F: Charcot-Marie-Tooth disease and the cavovarus foot, *Foot Ankle Clin* 13:259–274, 2008.

68. Berciano J, Combarros O: Hereditary neuropathies, *Curr Opin Neurol* 16:613–622, 2003.

69. Mann RA, Missirian J: Pathophysiology of Charcot-Marie-Tooth disease, *Clin Orthop Relat Res* 234:221–228, 1988.

70. Sabir M, Lyttle D: Pathogenesis of pes cavus in Charcot-Marie-Tooth disease, *Clin Orthop Relat Res* 175:173–178, 1983.

71. Tynan MC, Klenerman L, Helliwell R, et al: Investigation of muscle imbalance in the leg in symptomatic forefoot pes cavus: a multidisciplinary study, *Foot Ankle* 13:489–501, 1992.

72. Paulos L, Coleman SS, Samuelson KM: Pes cavovarus: review of a surgical approach using selective soft-tissue procedures, *J Bone Joint Surg Am* 62:942–953, 1980.

73. Nagai MK, Chan G, Guille JT, et al: Prevalence of Charcot-Marie-Tooth disease in patients who have bilateral cavovarus feet, *J Pediatr Orthop* 26:438–443, 2006.

74. Beals TC, Manoli AII: The peek-a-boo heel sign in the evaluation of hindfoot varus, *Foot* 6:205–206, 1996.

75. Burns J, Redmond A, Ouvrier R, et al: Quantification of muscle strength in neurogenic pes cavus, compared to health controls, using hand-held dynamometry, *Foot Ankle Int* 26:540–544, 2005.

76. Coleman SS, Chesnut WJ: A simple test for hindfoot flexibility in the cavovarus foot, *Clin Orthop Relat Res* 123:60–62, 1997.

77. Chan G, Gowen JR, Kumar SJ: Evaluation and treatment of hip dysplasia in Charcot-Marie-Tooth disease, *Orthop Clin North Am* 37:203–209, 2006.

78. McGann R, Gurd A: The association between Charcot-Marie-Tooth disease and developmental dysplasia of the hip, *Orthopedics* 25:337–339, 2002.

79. Walker JL, Nelson KR, Heavilon JA, et al: Hip abnormalities in children with Charcot-Marie-Tooth disease, *J Pediatr Orthop* 14:54–59, 1994.

80. Horacek O, Mazanec R, Morris CE, et al: Spinal deformities in hereditary motor and sensory neuropathy: a retrospective qualitative, quantitative, genotypical, and familial analysis of 175 families, *Spine* 32:2502–2508, 2007.

81. Karol LA, Elerson E: Scoliosis in patients with Charcot-Marie-Tooth disease, *J Bone Joint Surg Am* 89:1504–1510, 2007.

82. Refshauge KM, Raymond J, Nicholson G, et al: Night splinting does not increase ankle range of motion in people with Charcot-Marie-Tooth disease: a randomised, cross-over trial, *Aust J Physiother* 52:193–199, 2006.

83. Vinci P, Gargiulo P: Poor compliance with ankle-foot-orthoses in Charcot-Marie-Tooth disease, *Eur J Phys Rehabil Med* 44:27–31, 2008.

84. Young P, De Jonghe P, Stögbauer F, et al: Treatment for Charcot-Marie-Tooth disease, *Cochrane Database Syst Rev* (1): CD006052, 2008.

85. Mann DC, Hsu JD: Triple arthrodesis in the treatment of fixed cavovarus deformity in adolescent patients with Charcot-Marie-Tooth disease, *Foot Ankle* 13:1–6, 1992.

86. Wetmore RS, Drennan JC: Long-term results of triple arthrodesis in Charcot-Marie-Tooth disease, *J Bone Joint Surg Am* 71:417–422, 1989.

87. Wukich DK, Bowen JR: A long-term study of triple arthrodesis for correction of pes cavovarus in Charcot-Marie-Tooth disease, *J Pediatr Orthop* 9:433–437, 1989.

88. Olney B: Treatment of the cavus foot. Deformity in the pediatric patient with Charcot-Marie-Tooth, *Foot Ankle Clin* 5:305–315, 2000.

89. Fuller JE, DeLuca PA: Acetabular dysplasia and Charcot-Marie-Tooth disease in a family: a report of four cases, *J Bone Joint Surg Am* 77:1087–1091, 1995.

90. Kumar SJ, Marks HG, Bowen JR, et al: Hip dysplasia associated with Charcot-Marie-Tooth disease in the older child and adolescent, *J Pediatr Orthop* 5:511–514, 1985.

91. Hensinger RN, MacEwen GD: Spinal deformity associated with heritable neurological conditions: spinal muscular atrophy, Friedreich's ataxia, familial dysautonomia, and Charcot-Marie-Tooth disease, *J Bone Joint Surg Am* 58:13–24, 1976.

92. Jani-Acsadi A, Krajewski K, Shy ME: Charcot-Marie-Tooth neuropathies: diagnosis and management, *Semin Neurol* 28:185–194, 2008.

93. Payerson D: Differential diagnosis of Charcot-Marie-Tooth disease and related neuropathies, *Neurol Sci* 25:75–82, 2004.

94. Wills AJ, Manning NJ, Reilly MM: Refsum's disease, *Q J Med* 94:403–406, 2001.

95. Pandolfo M: Friedreich ataxia, *Arch Neurol* 65:1296–1303, 2008.

96. Wood NW: Diagnosing Friedreich's ataxia, *Arch Dis Child* 78:204–207, 1998.

97. Delatycki MB, Holian A, Corben L, et al: Surgery for equinovarus deformity in Friedreich's ataxia improves mobility and independence, *Clin Orthop Relat Res* 430:138–141, 2005.

98. Cady BB, Bobechko WP: Incidence, natural history, and treatment of scoliosis in Friedreich's ataxia, *J Pediatr Orthop* 4:673–676, 1984.

99. Milbrandt TA, Kunes JR, Karol LA: Friedreich's ataxia and scoliosis: the experience at two institutions, *J Pediatr Orthop* 28:234–238, 2008.

100. Shapiro F, Specht L: The diagnosis and orthopaedic treatment of childhood spinal muscular atrophy, peripheral neuropathy, Friedreich ataxia, and arthrogryposis, *J Bone Joint Surg Am* 75:1699–1714, 1993.

101. Labelle H, Tohmé S, Duhaime M, et al: Natural history of scoliosis in Friedreich's ataxia, *J Bone Joint Surg Am* 68:564–572, 1986.

102. Han JJ, McDonald CM: Diagnosis and clinical management of spinal muscular atrophy, *Phys Med Rehabil Clin N Am* 19:661–680, 2008.

103. Lunn MR, Wang CH: Spinal muscular atrophy, *Lancet* 371 (9630):2120–2133, 2008.

104. Oskoui M, Kaufmann P: Spinal muscular atrophy, *Neurotherapeutics* 5:449–506, 2008.

105. Granata C, Cervellati S, Ballestrazzi A, et al: Spine surgery in spinal muscular atrophy: long-term results, *Neuromuscul Disord* 3:207–215, 1993.

106. Riddick MF, Winter RB, Lutter LD: Spinal deformities in patients with spinal muscle atrophy: a review of 36 patients, *Spine* 7:476–483, 1982.

107. Sporer SM, Smith BG: Hip dislocation in patients with spinal muscular atrophy, *J Pediatr Orthop* 23:10–14, 2003.

108. Thompson CE, Larsen LJ: Recurrent hip dislocation in intermediate spinal atrophy, *J Pediatr Orthop* 10:638–641, 1990.

109. Zenios M, Sampath J, Cole C, et al: Operative treatment for hip subluxation in spinal muscular atrophy, *J Bone Joint Surg Br* 87:1541–1544, 2005.

Tulio E. Bertorini, MD, Yingjun David Li, MD,
Bassam A. Bassam, MD, and Christopher W. Mitchell, MD

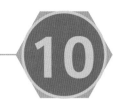

Perioperative Management of Patients with Neuromuscular Disorders

Patients with neuromuscular disorders (NMDs) are at increased risk for complications during or immediately after surgery. Some have significant weakness that can predispose them to respiratory failure and difficulty weaning from the ventilator, others may suffer cardiovascular complications, and still others are at risk of developing malignant hyperthermia.

Physicians should take measures to prevent such complications and should be able to recognize and manage them when they arise. Due to the variety of issues involved, a team approach (including a neuromuscular specialist, anesthesiologist, pulmonologist, and possibly a cardiologist) is ideal in providing perioperative care to patients with NMDs. In this chapter, we discuss some specific concerns that are pertinent to individual disorders as well as some more general issues that may occur in this clinical setting.

Perioperative Management in Specific Neuromuscular Disorders

Motor Neuron Diseases

Adults with motor neuron diseases, particularly amyotrophic lateral sclerosis, may undergo percutaneous endoscopic gastrostomy (PEG) tube placement and tracheostomy for management of the disorder. They also may undergo general surgical procedures common in those in late adulthood, and these should be performed under careful monitoring.

Dysphagia is a common symptom in patients with ALS, usually developing at about the same time as respiratory insufficiency; for this reason, pulmonary function should be assessed and oxygen saturation carefully monitored during PEG tube placement,[1–3] which requires sedation. The procedure is recommended to be done early and in patients whose vital capacity is more than 50% of predicted,[4] although there are insufficient data to suggest specific timing.[5] The use of noninvasive ventilation in those who are at risk and do not have a tracheotomy appears safe and reduces complications.[6] PEG tube placement does not prevent aspiration pneumonia, but it does

improve the patient's quality of life and nutritional state. In our center, we perform the procedure in the inpatient setting, followed by at least 24 hours of intravenous (IV) fluids until bowel sounds are present and tube feeding can be started.

Tracheostomy should be discussed early and performed in patients who do not tolerate noninvasive respiratory assistance or have inadequate ventilation. The procedure helps to reduce dead space and improves suctioning. Tracheostomy also should be done in the hospital setting after proper discussion with the patient and family concerning long-term care and complications, which include infections, excessive bleeding, and mucus plugs. Patients should be observed for at least 24 hours after the initiation of respiratory assistance[7] (see also Chapters 2 and 11).

Spinal Muscular Atrophy

Patients with type 1 spinal muscular atrophy (SMA) develop respiratory failure early, and tracheostomy and PEG tube placement are done in those whose parents opt for aggressive management. These procedures and their complications should be discussed as soon as the diagnosis is made.

Patients with types 2 and 3 SMA may develop respiratory failure later, but tracheostomy and PEG tube placement should be discussed early and performed as soon as they appear necessary.[8] This approach has been shown to prolong survival.[9]

Scoliosis surgery is done in patients with types 2 and 3 SMA, but those with type 1 SMA usually die before the procedure is necessary. The surgery should be performed before the curvature has become severe. Those with vital capacity below 35% usually have a poorer prognosis and might require permanent tracheotomy.[10] Surgical risks are increased for those with frequent respiratory infections.[11] Other orthopedic procedures that may be required by patients with SMA, such as correction of hip deformities, are discussed in Chapters 9 and 12. These procedures require careful preoperative and postoperative monitoring and management with respiratory therapy, including the use of incentive spirometry, with monitoring of pulse oximetry and arterial blood gases when necessary. Prompt mobilization is recommended.

Friedreich Ataxia

Individuals with Friedreich ataxia may undergo surgery to correct the orthopedic deformities that accompany the disease, such as surgical correction of foot abnormalities to improve ambulation.[11] Scoliosis may cause respiratory complications, and scoliosis surgery is the most important invasive procedure performed in this disorder. It is usually done on individuals who are wheelchair-bound, have vital capacities at least 40% of normal, and have a curvature of more than 60% of normal.[12]

Perioperative care of those with Friedreich ataxia is further complicated by the diabetes mellitus and hypertrophic cardiomyopathy that frequently accompany the neuromuscular symptoms. Thus, preoperative care of these patients requires not only oximetry but also cardiac assessment and monitoring as well as frequent electrolyte and glucose measurements. Other, more generalized complications are not uncommon in this population; these include aspiration pneumonia and pulmonary embolism.[13]

Peripheral Neuropathies

Patients with peripheral neuropathy, particularly those with Charcot-Marie-Tooth disease, might need orthopedic surgery for foot deformities,[14] but they usually do not require special monitoring. Spinal deformities are rare, but occur in some with the early childhood forms, and these should be managed similarly to those in patients with Friedreich ataxia, although careful cardiac monitoring is not necessary. Those with more severe forms, such as Dejerine-Sottas syndrome, might require a tracheostomy and even PEG tube placement.

Individuals with acute neuropathies, such as Guillain-Barré syndrome, may require tracheostomy and PEG tube placement, but these procedures usually are done when the patient is intubated and in the intensive care unit (ICU). Nonetheless, these patients require proper cardiac monitoring because of the possibility of dysautonomia and cardiac arrhythmias.

Myasthenia Gravis

Myasthenia gravis is a disease in which respiratory failure could occur during surgical procedures requiring deep sedation or general anesthesia. Special care should be taken to avoid the use of paralyzing agents or drugs that might aggravate the disease and cause a myasthenic crisis (see Chapter 18). Adequate electrolyte balance must be maintained to prevent hypokalemia, which can worsen weakness.[7]

Those receiving corticosteroids should take their daily dosage either orally or parentally, with a booster dose of 100 mg of Solu-Cortef (Pfizer, New York) IV the day of surgery and another the following day.

Thymectomy may be done, particularly in younger patients with generalized myasthenia gravis. The procedure has not definitively proved beneficial in controlled studies, but it is considered the standard of care.[15,16] Although there is substantial variation in the actual procedure performed, the surgery of choice is total or complete thymectomy.[17] Those with anti-MuSK-positive myasthenia gravis do not seem to respond to thymectomy, and it is not recommended in these patients at this time.[18]

Thymectomy in children may be beneficial because it appears to induce remissions of disease in uncontrolled trials.[19,20] There is lingering concern, however, that removal of this organ at a young age may lead to lasting, and potentially harmful, alterations of T-cell populations.[21–23] Thus, the decision to choose the procedure in children should be made on an individual basis.

Thymectomy has low incidences of morbidity and mortality, and it should be done early in generalized myasthenia.[24] Some clinicians recommend that thymectomy be done before the initiation of corticosteroid therapy,[25] but most patients are already receiving steroids when they undergo thymectomy. The chance of infection is not higher than in those receiving immunotherapy, but the risk is increased in those with severe disease.[26]

Severe myasthenia gravis should first be stabilized with corticosteroids and, if necessary, plasmapheresis[27,28] or IgG infusions before thymectomy using standard protocols. Both procedures appear to produce similar benefits.[29] Either procedure should be done about 2 weeks before thymectomy if pulmonary function is adequate.

After surgery, patients should be extubated promptly and monitored with pulse oximetry and, if necessary, measurements of arterial blood gases in the ICU setting for 24 to 48 hours.

The common practice of withholding anticholinesterase drugs for 48 hours after surgery is of questionable value. We administer the oral medication or its parenteral equivalent starting with half of the preoperative dosage 12 hours after the procedure, increasing to the full dose over 2 days. This method is in agreement with the findings of a large study of complications of 324 thymectomies in which the incidence of complications was higher in patients requiring prolonged intubation, apparently from withholding medications.[30]

Tracheostomy is performed only in patients who require prolonged intubation and respiratory assistance.

Muscular Dystrophies

Patients with myopathies, particularly muscular dystrophies or congenital myopathies, might undergo a series of surgeries during their lifetime. The risks and benefits should be carefully assessed, and the procedure should be done under careful pulmonary and cardiac monitoring.

Scoliosis surgery is performed in patients with myopathies who have curvatures between 10% and 20% and rarely in those with curvatures up to 30% but should be done in those whose vital capacity is at least 50% of normal.[31] Tendon releases should be done with minimal anesthesia, and patients should be carefully observed and promptly extubated.

Those with Emery-Dreifuss, Duchenne, and limb-girdle dystrophies that affect the heart (i.e., LGMD2I) must be carefully monitored during surgery for cardiac arrhythmias (see Chapter 3) and for electrolyte disturbance, which require immediate treatment.

Tracheostomy and rarely gastrostomy are necessary in patients with late stages of the disorders. The use of noninvasive ventilation helps to prevent complications.[32]

Patients with muscular dystrophy who undergo any surgical procedure should be evaluated closely by a medical team that includes a neuromuscular specialist, pulmonologist, and cardiologist, and the procedure should be done with monitoring for cardiac arrhythmias and with oximetry.

A unique and important complication to be avoided is the development of malignant hyperthermia (MH) or rather malignant hyperthermia-like syndrome (MHLS) or hyperkalemia-induced rhabdomyolysis.[33,34] Although patients who develop MH do not have the calcium channel mutations or all the features of malignant hyperthermia syndrome (MHS), the presentation and management are otherwise similar to those in other patients.[35] Drugs that can precipitate malignant hyperthermia should be avoided, and dantrolene should be available to be used when necessary.

It also should be pointed out that patients with Becker muscular dystrophy and limb-girdle muscular dystrophies with cardiomyopathy might undergo cardiac transplantation, particularly those in whom the weakness is not severe, and proper measures should be taken perioperatively and postoperatively[36] to prevent complications such as electrolyte disturbances and MHLS.

Myotonic Dystrophy

Myotonic dystrophy (DM) is discussed separately because these patients may develop multiple medical problems that require surgical intervention, which can be associated with complications.[37] Respiratory dysfunction can occur not only in patients with DM type 1,[38] but also in those with DM type 2. The risk of complications can be increased in these patients because of diabetes, respiratory failure, and cardiomyopathy.

Patients with DM have increased sensitivity to anesthetics[39–41] and muscle relaxants[42] and could develop cardiac conduction delays, diabetes, and respiratory insufficiency caused by muscle weakness,[37–40] as well as poor respiratory drive, which could result in alveolar hypoventilation.[39] Exacerbation of myotonia occurs with lower body temperatures when depolarizing relaxants are used.[41,42] MH also has been reported in these patients.[37]

It is recommended that general anesthesia be avoided when possible; surgical procedures should be done with monitoring for cardiac arrhythmia and for MH. Postoperatively, those with DM should receive proper early physical therapy and incentive respirometry. Noninvasive ventilation temporarily after surgical procedures is useful. A unique complication of DM is intestinal pseudo-obstruction or megacolon, which could be managed with a rectal tube placement.

Surgical guidelines for the preoperative and perioperative management of these patients are listed in Box 10-1.

Channelopathies

Channelopathies, particularly myotonia congenita, do not require surgery for management, but patients with these conditions might undergo procedures similar to those done in the general population. Complications include MH and exacerbation of myotonia from the use of agents such as succinylcholine.[43,44] Hypokalemia might exacerbate myotonia and cause arrhythmias and weakness, particularly in those with hypokalemic paralysis, whereas hyperkalemia causes weakness in those with hyperkalemic periodic paralysis and could also cause arrhythmias. For this reason, proper electrolyte balance and maintenance of potassium levels around 4 µg/L are advised. Patients should be monitored for at least 24 hours after surgery.

Propofol is recommended for anesthesia in patients with channelopathies; this drug acts by enhancing gamma-aminobutyric acid mediated sympathetic inhibition and might block sodium influx through the channels in the heart and brain. Propofol stabilizes membranes, decreasing their excitability.[45,46]

Malignant Hyperthermia Syndrome

MHS, a condition described initially by Denborough and Lovell in 1960,[47] is characterized by severe muscle rigidity, fever, cardiac arrhythmia, and rhabdomyolysis. MH occurs particularly with exposure to general anesthetics such as halothane and depolarizing muscle relaxants. Other manifestations include acidosis, hypermetabolism, fever, hyperkalemia, cardiac arrhythmias, and initial hypocalcemia due to intracellular calcium accumulation.

The syndrome has an incidence of 1 in 15,000 children and 1 in 50,000 adults.[48–50] It is an autosomal dominant inherited disorder more frequently associated with mutations of the ryanodine calcium channel genes, and this is allelic to central core disease.[51] It also has been reported in patients with dihydropyridine voltage-gated sodium calcium

Box 10-1 Preoperative and Postoperative Care and Complications of Anesthesia in Myotonic Dystrophy

Preoperative Evaluation, Care

Perform electrocardiogram (ECG)
Perform pulmonary function testing (including supine and upright forced vital capacity) and arterial blood gas measurement
Obtain chest radiograph
Encourage incentive respirometry

Intraoperative Monitoring

Monitor electrocardiograms
Measure arterial blood pressure
Use a peripheral nerve stimulator to monitor blockage of peripheral muscle
Monitor temperature
Warm mattress
Warm intravenous fluids
Maintain humidification of anesthetic gases

Postoperative Care

Retain endotracheal tube in place and ventilate if necessary in an ICU
Monitor oxygen saturation and Pco_2 for at least 24 hours postoperatively to avoid overlooking delayed-onset apnea
Use controlled-flow oxygen therapy with close monitoring of ventilation in patients relying on hypoxic drive due to chronic respiratory insufficiency
Provide early physiotherapy
Monitor ECG
Keep patient warm
Monitor swallowing closely to check for signs of aspiration
Treat all infections vigorously
Encourage incentive respirometry
Administer subcutaneous heparin if intubation is prolonged

Anesthetic Agents

When possible, use local or regional anesthesia, such as an epidural block
Avoid succinylcholine and other depolarizing muscle relaxants
Avoid or use only minimal dose of thiopental; for muscle relaxation, use short-acting agents (e.g., atracurium or vecuronium)
Avoid or use only minimal doses of opiates or other analgesics to avoid respiratory depression
When possible, avoid general anesthesia; if necessary, use combination of nitrous oxide/oxygen mixture with an agent such as 0.8% enflurane or 1.0% isoflurane; also consider propofol
Use anticholinesterases (e.g., neostigmine) with care; may be preferable to ventilate the patient until residual curarization wears off

Modified from: Moxley RT III: Myotonic muscular dystrophy. In Rowland LP, DiMauro S, editors: *Handbook of Clinical Neurology. Myopathies*, 2nd edition, Amsterdam, 1992, Elsevier Science, pp 209-244 with permission.

channel disorders.[52] Both channels are involved in muscle calcium release, and attacks of MH are caused by excessive release of calcium by the sarcoplasmic reticulum (SR) under certain conditions.[50]

The genetic mutations associated with MHS appear to lower the threshold for calcium release by the SR altering excitation-contraction coupling and manifesting as massive muscle necrosis, similar to what occurs in porcine stress syndrome.[53]

During attacks, the increased intracellular calcium causes muscle contractures that lead to increased oxygen consumption, glycogenolysis, and depletion of high energy phosphate compounds with elevation of body temperature. There also is a limitation of calcium reuptake by the SR for muscle relaxation, increasing muscle contractures, which further increases intramuscular calcium accumulation and necrosis (Fig. 10-1). This results in leakage of phosphate and potassium into the bloodstream, which could cause cardiac

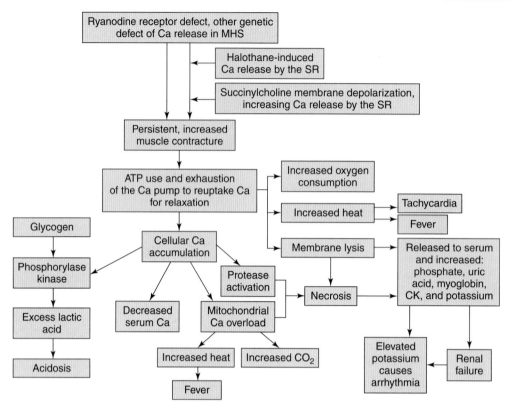

Figure 10-1 Possible mechanisms of clinical and laboratory abnormalities in malignant hyperthermia syndrome. ATP, adenosine 5′-triphosphate; Ca, calcium; CK, creatine kinase; CO_2, carbon dioxide; MHS, malignant hyperthermia syndrome; SR, sarcoplasmic reticulum. (Modified from Bertorini TE: Myoglobinuria, malignant hyperthermia, neuroleptic malignant syndrome and serotonin syndrome. *Neurol Clin* 15:658, 1997.)

arrhythmias. Serum uric and lactic acids, creatine kinase (CK), and myoglobin are increased, which could cause renal failure.[49,50]

Several mutations of the SR calcium receptor genes are associated with MHS.[51–55] MHS or MHLS also has been reported in a variety of muscle diseases, including channelopathies, muscular dystrophies, and congenital myopathies such as central core and mini-core disease.[50] Central core disease and mini-core disease are caused by mutations of the genes for calcium receptors that are associated with MHS.[55–57] A list of conditions in which MH or MHLS has been observed is given in Box 10-2. It also should be mentioned that, although halothane and depolarizing skeletal muscle relaxants are the drugs most often implicated in triggering the disorder, several other medications have been reported to induce attacks of MHS in subjects at risk (Box 10-3).

Box 10-2 Individuals at Risk for Malignant Hyperthermia or Malignant Hyperthermia-like Syndrome

Family history of malignant hyperthermia
King-Denborough syndrome
Evans myopathy
Central core disease
Multicore diseases
Muscular dystrophy (dystrophinopathy, myotonic dystrophy)
Periodic paralysis
Myotonia congenita
Carnitine palmitoyltransferase deficiency
Phosphorylase deficiency; possibly other glycogen storage myopathies
Brody's disease
Idiopathic hyperCKemia

Box 10-3 Medications and Their Relationship to Malignant Hyperthermia

Triggering Agents

Inhalation Anesthetics
Halothane
Enflurane
Isoflurane
Desflurane
Sevoflurane

Depolarizing Blockers
Succinylcholine
Decamethonium

Controversial Agents
Calcium, potassium salts
Ketamine
Catecholamines
Phenothiazines, monoamine oxidase inhibitors

Safe Agents

Nitrous oxide
Barbiturates
Local anesthetics
Narcotics
Nondepolarizing neuromuscular relaxants
Antibiotics
Propranolol
Propofol
Benzodiazepines

Modified from Kauss J, Rocko MA: Malignant hyperthermia, *Pediatr Clin North Am* 41:133, 1994.

Box 10-4 Clinical Events and Laboratory Findings during Malignant Hyperthermia

Clinical Events

Unexplained, sudden increase in end-tidal CO_2
Unexplained tachycardia, tachypnea, labile blood pressure, or arrhythmias
Masseter muscle rigidity or generalized muscle rigidity
Unanticipated respiratory or metabolic acidosis
Increasing patient temperature
Cola-colored urine (myoglobinuria)
Mottled, cyanotic, hot skin; sweating; decreased Spo$_2$

Laboratory Findings

Arterial blood gases; Paco$_2 \geq 60$ mm Hg, base excess more negative than -8 mEq/L, pH < 7.25
Potassium ion > 6 mEq/L
Creatine kinase $> 10,000$ IU/L after anesthetic without succinylcholine
Serum myoglobin > 170 g/L

Modified from Karlet MC: Malignant hyperthermia: considerations for ambulatory surgery, *J Perianesth Nurs* 13:306, 1998, with permission.

The diagnosis is based on the clinical presentation and should be suspected early in those who develop masseter contractures and then generalized muscle rigidity with a rapid rise in body temperature, tachycardia, acidosis, and hypermetabolism.[49,50]

Anesthesiologists should suspect MHS in patients who have early excessive masseter contractions and elevations of the end-tidal CO_2 during the induction of anesthesia, or if there are signs of acidosis with elevated body temperature and tachycardia (Box 10-4).

Recognition of individuals at risk before surgery is important. In patients considered to be at risk for MHS, particularly those with a strong family history, a muscle contracture test is recommended, but is not universally available.[58–61] DNA testing is of only limited usefulness because patients who do not have known mutations that are associated with MHS might still develop the syndrome.[50,51,62]

Patients with myopathies and elevated serum CK should undergo surgery with proper monitoring and should be considered as being at risk for this syndrome.

Treatment and Management

The treatment of MHS consists of correction of fluid and electrolyte imbalances, reduction of temperature, and especially the use of dantrolene, a muscle relaxant that decreases calcium release by the SR and thus inhibits muscle contractions. Preoperative use of dantrolene is recommended in patients at risk. Box 10-5 gives a detailed list of steps in the management of MHS, including proper dosing of dantrolene. Anesthetics that can contribute to an attack should be avoided in those at risk.[50,62]

Complications of Major Surgery and Organ Transplantation

Patients undergoing major surgery may manifest a variety of neurologic complications. Some could develop weakness or sensory symptoms from nerve or plexus injuries due to stretching or compression. Others may experience prolonged weakness and difficulty weaning from the ventilator due to neuromuscular blockade. For some patients, recovery from surgery will be difficult and the neuromuscular complications of critical illness and prolonged hospitalization become a concern. In addition to peripheral complications, certain subjects are

Box 10-5 Recommended Steps in Managing Patients with Suspected Malignant Hyperthermia

Discontinue the anesthetic and deliver 100% oxygen.
Administer dantrolene IV, 2 to 3 mg/kg every 5 minutes for a total of 10 mg/kg.
Get help; consult the malignant hyperthermia hotline for guidance.*
Administer sodium bicarbonate and ice in IV saline infusion, avoiding Ringer's lactate.
Cover the stomach, bladder, and rectum with iced saline and use cooling blankets while closely monitoring body temperature.
Treat arrhythmias by reducing hyperkalemia with antiarrhythmic drugs but not calcium channel blockers.
Monitor end-tidal CO_2 and blood gases; increase end-tidal CO_2.
Treat hyperkalemia with hyperventilation, bicarbonate, glucose, and insulin; in life-threatening cases, use calcium chloride.
Ensure urine output is greater than 2 mL/kg/hr by hydration, or by use of mannitol, furosemide, or both diuretics.
Treat unexpected cardiac arrests in children by treating hyperkalemia first.
Monitor blood gases, potassium, and calcium and check for the presence of myoglobulin in urine in the recovery room or ICU for a minimum of 24 hours. Monitor coagulation parameters; correct if necessary.
Administer dantrolene IV 1 mg/kg every 6 hours for 24 to 48 hours or up to 10 mg/kg/day followed by oral dantrolene for another day.
Observe patient in the ICU for at least 36 hours.
Refer patient and family to a malignant hyperthermia testing center; provide genetic counseling
Obtain information from: www.mhaus.org.
www.mhreg.org.
http://www.emhg.org1.

* www.mhous.org, U.S. and Canada: 1-800-644-9737, other countries: 011314647079.
Modified from Malignant Hyperthermia Association of the United States (MHAUS). *Emergency therapy for malignant hyperthermia.* New York: Malignant Hyperthermia Association of the United States, 1995.

at risk of central nervous system (CNS) injury (e.g., in the form of ischemia), particularly when undergoing cardiovascular procedures.

Those undergoing organ transplantation face additional risks from immunosuppression, including infections such as toxoplasmosis, herpes zoster, tuberculosis, and others.[63,64] The medications used for immunosuppression could cause other complications, as discussed in Chapter 7. Particularly, calcineurin inhibitors produce neurotoxicity, inducing tremors, posterior reversible leukoencephalopathy, seizures, mental status changes, paralysis, and speech abnormalities.[63–65] This section discusses some of the more common neuromuscular complications seen in association with surgery and transplantation.

Cardiothoracic Surgery and Transplantation

Most neurological complications of cardiac surgery and transplantation affect the CNS.[66,67] Cardiac surgery also might result in brachial plexopathies from retraction of the sternum, which causes weakness in muscles innervated by the lower trunk, with pain[68–71] and numbness that should be differentiated from ulnar compression, which can also occur in this setting.[72]

Another common presentation seen in those undergoing cardiovascular surgery is foot drop due to peroneal palsy. Recurrent laryngeal or phrenic nerve lesions causing hoarseness and difficulty breathing can also be seen. Phrenic nerve injury with resultant diaphragmatic paralysis may be particularly likely in those undergoing coronary revascularization with mobilization of the right internal mammary artery for bypass.[73] Catheterization procedures and pump placements could damage adjacent nerves in the limb (e.g., femoral or median nerves).

Mobilization or resection of a whole lung as in a transplantation procedure also carries a risk of nerve injury. Severe gastroesophageal reflux or even gastroparesis may result from damage to the vagus nerve.[74] Diaphragmatic paralysis and resultant ventilatory weakness could also develop from phrenic nerve injury.[75–78] Patients might also develop generalized weakness secondary to poor oxidative metabolism of muscle fibers.[79]

Evaluation and Diagnosis

A detailed neurologic examination should define if the weakness is generalized or focal, if it affects the upper motor neuron or lower motor neuron, and, in the latter, if this is caused by peripheral nerve or brachial plexus injuries. The evaluation should include the sniff test, nerve conduction studies, and needle electromyography (EMG).[79] Phrenic nerve studies and fluoroscopy are helpful for the diagnosis of phrenic neuropathy. Laryngoscopy is necessary in patients with recurrent laryngeal nerve paralysis.

Those with gastroparesis and gastroesophageal reflux disease require a proper gastrointestinal evaluation and esophageal motility studies; those with generalized weakness should have adequate electrolyte and CK measurements in addition to the electrophysiologic studies.

Treatment and Management

Measures to avoid complications include proper padding to avoid compressions, prompt mobilization, and physical therapy. Patients who develop phrenic nerve paralysis and dyspnea should be maintained in the upright position and receive intermittent noninvasive ventilation.

Patients with vagal nerve dysfunction with gastroparesis and gastroesophageal reflux disease may require metoclopramide and pump inhibitors as well as maintenance of the upright position.

The treatment of focal nerve paralysis is discussed in Chapter 16.

Abdominal Surgery and Transplantation

Abdominal surgery is associated with complications of anesthesia[79–81] and also with nerve compression or stretching from retractors. The lumbosacral plexus and lateral femoral cutaneous nerve may be injured, and compression may cause peroneal palsy.[82]

Intestinal surgery, particularly small-bowel resection, may cause malabsorption, with deficiencies of various vitamins manifesting as peripheral neuropathy or generalized weakness.[83] Encephalopathy may be seen in those undergoing liver transplantation.

In contrast to the encephalopathy commonly seen in liver failure, spastic paraparesis from so-called *hepatic myelopathy* is rare. Spinal cord compression from a structural lesion (e.g., hematoma or tumor) should be excluded radiographically. Orthotopic liver transplantation has been reported to improve the condition.[80,84] Another cause of myelopathy is spinal cord infarction, which is usually due to occlusion of the spinal artery of Adamkiewicz. This is a particular concern during procedures that involve cross-clamping of the aorta, such as surgical repair of an abdominal aortic aneurysm.

Steatorrhea from any cause may result in deficiencies of fat-soluble vitamins. Vitamin E deficiency might manifest with ataxia and peripheral neuropathy, whereas vitamin D deficiency could cause generalized weakness, and vitamin A deficiency could cause visual disturbances. Most vitamin B deficiencies are associated with peripheral neuropathies, but thiamine deficiency often presents with Wernicke's encephalopathy.

Evaluation and Diagnosis

Clinical evaluation is important, and this should be followed by EMG studies and measurement of electrolytes and serum CK.

Patients with generalized weakness require periodic measurements of electrolytes and of vitamin levels.

Treatment and Management

Avoidance of retractor injuries and the use of padding are very important. Patients require proper vitamin supplementation using periodic measurements of vitamins and nutrients, complete blood counts, and chemistry profiles. Pyridoxine and erythrocyte transketolase levels should be measured in those with symptomatic peripheral neuropathy; if reduced, replacement therapy should be initiated.

Ambulation, physical therapy, and respiratory assistance should be used when necessary.

Complications of Bariatric Surgery

Approximately 4.6% of patients who have bariatric surgery for weight reduction develop neurologic complications,[85] including encephalopathy,[86] vision loss,[87] ataxia, and neuromuscular manifestations such as radiculopathy, polyneuropathy, and myeloneuropathy.[88–91] Nerve entrapments such as carpal tunnel syndrome, ulnar neuropathy,[90] meralgia paresthetica,[91] and radiculoplexopathy also can occur.[90] Rarely, patients develop a myopathy, and rhabdomyolysis is not uncommon in these.[84–92]

Some complications occur during the procedure, such as retractor-induced nerve damage or compression such as peroneal palsy. Most other complications, however, are caused by malnourishment with deficiency of various micronutrients and vitamins.[90] Occasionally, a peripheral neuropathy is related to an autoimmune disorder.[90,92,93] A sensory neuropathy can be caused by copper,[94] pyridoxine, thiamine, and vitamin B_{12} deficiencies.[89,95]

Diagnosis and Evaluation

The evaluation includes obtaining measurements of electrolytes and serum CK immediately after surgery to document and prevent the development of severe rhabdomyolysis. Patients should then have measurements of nutrients and vitamin levels. The use of other tests depends on the clinical manifestations; for example, those with sensorimotor neuropathy or entrapment neuropathy should have electrophysiologic testing. The polyneuropathy in patients who have bariatric surgery is usually sensory or sensorimotor, and the electrodiagnosis documents the presence of axonal degeneration with some features of demyelination.[90] In those with prominent demyelination, an autoimmune etiology should be considered, especially if there is no evidence of vitamin deficiency or response to vitamin supplementation.[91]

Some patients may develop an acute paralysis similar to Guillain-Barré syndrome and should be properly diagnosed and treated. Although a nutritional polyneuropathy could present in this way, severe hypokalemia also should be considered.[87]

Myeloneuropathy manifests as long-tract findings presenting as combined degeneration, an ataxic neuropathy caused by vitamin B_{12} or copper deficiency, particularly in patients receiving zinc supplementation.[94] Neuroimaging to exclude a structural cause should be done, and somatosensory evoked potentials may also be useful.

Treatment and Management

Nerve compression during surgery should be prevented with adequate padding and avoidance of improper retraction and nerve stretching. After surgery, early mobilization and physical therapy are recommended.

Patients should be treated with good nourishment and vitamin supplementation. Clinical laboratory evaluation should be performed every 6 months, and this should include a complete blood count, chemistry profile, and measurements of iron, zinc, magnesium and selenium, vitamin B_{12}, and folate levels. In symptomatic patients, measurement of vitamin B_{12}, vitamin A, pyridoxine, copper, thiamine, zinc, and erythrocyte transketolase levels should be obtained.

Vitamin supplementation should include oral vitamin B_{12} in doses of 100 mcg and folate daily by mouth.[95,96] In patients with low levels of vitamin B_{12} who are symptomatic, parenteral administration of 1000 µg a week for 1 month and then 1000 µg monthly is needed. Thiamine deficiency is treated with intravenous administration of 50 to 100 mg of thiamine daily for up to 14 days, followed by 100 mg orally daily. Patients with frequent vomiting should receive vitamin C and calcium with vitamin D in doses of 1600 mg/day. Vitamin D deficiency should be treated with weekly vitamin D_2 in dosages of 50,000 units orally and multivitamin preparations.[96]

Those with copper deficiency should discontinue zinc supplementation and receive copper in dosages of 6 mg/day orally for 1 week, then 4 mg for an additional week, and then 2 mg permanently,[94] as discussed in Chapter 20.

Patients with severe demyelinating neuropathy who do not respond to vitamin therapy should be evaluated for an autoimmune etiology, which can be documented by a nerve biopsy, and then immunotherapy should be considered.[93]

Physical therapy and rehabilitation followed by an exercise program are very important in the care of these patients.

Neuromuscular Disorders Acquired in the Intensive Care Unit

Neuromuscular disorders acquired in the ICU are broadly categorized as critical illness polyneuropathy (CIP), critical illness myopathy (CIM), and prolonged neuromuscular junction blockade. After pulmonary and cardiac causes have been eliminated, an underlying neuromuscular condition should be suspected in patients in the ICU after surgery or for other causes who have limb weakness and difficulty weaning off the ventilator, who have sepsis or multi-organ failure, or who received neuromuscular blocking agents and steroids.

Singly or in combination, CIP and CIM are characterized by flaccid limbs and respiratory muscle weakness. These syndromes occur in critically ill patients during prolonged ICU hospitalization undergoing mechanical ventilation because of their critical illness or its treatment. Usually the weakness with, or less commonly without, failure to wean from the ventilator appears when the underlying critical illness improves, unmasking the NMD.

The diagnosis frequently is challenging, and a pre-existing NMD should be excluded. Electrodiagnostic studies are helpful to establish the diagnosis, in spite of the difficulty of performing such studies in the ICU environment.

Historical Note

In 1961, Mertens described *coma-polyneuropathies* in patients with severe metabolic crises and circulatory shock.[97] Bolton and colleagues (1983 and 1984) described patients in the ICU with severe limb weakness and difficulty weaning off the ventilator due to severe primary distal axonal motor sensory neuropathy.[98,99] Zochodne and colleagues in 1987 coined the term *critical illness neuropathy* to describe this event since it occurs in ICU patients with sepsis and multiple organ failure.[100]

Karpati and colleagues in 1972 described corticosteroid-induced myopathy, characterized by thick filament myopathy in animal models

after hind-limb nerve transection.[101] MacFarlane and colleagues in 1977 described acute quadriplegic myopathy in a young asthmatic patient who received high-dose corticosteroids.[102] Various other names for the primary myopathic disease in patients with critical illness were used in the 1990s; however, the term *critical illness myopathy*, coined by Latronico and colleagues in 1996, is now widely used.[103]

Critical Illness Polyneuropathy

As the length of time spent in the ICU increases, CIP occurs as a complication of sepsis and multi-organ failure. Despite improvements in medical and surgical care, the mortality rate in critically ill patients remains high—30% to 50%.[104] Sepsis, trauma, and burns can evoke a severe systemic response known as *systemic inflammatory response syndrome* (SIRS). As many as 70% of patients with a critical illness or SIRS may develop clinical, electrophysiologic, or histopathologic evidence of peripheral nerve dysfunction.[105] In SIRS, cellular and pro-inflammatory humoral responses are activated and interact with adhesion molecules to cause endothelial damage, local tissue edema, and subsequent disturbances of microcirculation. These disturbances may impair the delivery of oxygen and glucose to the peripheral and central nervous systems, causing septic encephalopathy and CIP.[106,107]

Critical illness polyneuropathy ranges from mild to severe and is usually recognized when a pre-existing encephalopathy associated with sepsis resolves. The severity of the neuropathy increases with time in the ICU, hyperglycemia, and hypoalbuminemia. This symmetric neuropathy is a sensorimotor axonal type that causes limb weakness and difficulty weaning from the ventilator. Tendon reflexes are attenuated or lost. Distal sensation is impaired, but this is difficult to assess in intubated ICU patients. Muscle atrophy in the distal muscles is common. Facial weakness is rare, and extraocular muscle movements are spared. Neuropathic pain is not characteristic of CIP, and autonomic dysfunction is uncommon. CIP may resemble axonal Guillain-Barré syndrome on the basis of clinical examination alone and may be difficult to differentiate from myopathic or neuromuscular junction disorders. CIP has been reported in children, but is less common in children than in adults.[108]

Evaluation and Diagnosis
Patient charts should be meticulously reviewed for documentation of sepsis and multi-organ failure. The use of IV corticosteroids, neuromuscular blocking agents, and drugs such as aminoglycosides or magnesium increases the incidence of CIP. The presence of significant facial or extraocular muscle weakness suggests prolonged neuromuscular junction blockade.

Nerve conduction studies typically show low amplitude of motor and sensory action potentials, with low normal or mildly slow conduction velocities, indicative of motor and sensory axonal loss. Compound muscle action potential (CMAP) amplitude decline predates clinical symptoms, whereas sensory nerve action potential (SNAP) decline occurs later. Because of the difficulty of performing nerve conduction studies in the ICU environment and the presence of tissue edema, sensory conduction studies can be difficult to assess, but needle EMG examination reveals predominant distal denervation and decreased recruitment of the motor unit action potentials (MUAP). Phrenic nerve conduction tests and needle EMG of the diaphragm help to establish the diagnosis in patients who have difficulty weaning from the ventilator. Laboratory testing and cerebrospinal fluid (CSF) studies usually are normal. Nerve biopsy is rarely indicated and shows varied degrees of primary axonal degeneration and lack of inflammatory cellular infiltrates or segmental demyelination.[109]

The differential diagnosis should include other axonal neuropathies, such as axonal Guillain-Barré syndrome, coexisting neuropathy, transient weakness secondary to prolonged neuromuscular junction blockade, and weakness secondary to CIM. Facial weakness, elevated CSF protein, and associated autonomic dysfunction are characteristic of Guillain-Barré syndrome, whereas an elevated serum CK level is more consistent with CIM. However, CIP may occur independently or in association with CIM.

Treatment and Management

Aside from the general principles of management, there are no known specific therapies for CIP. Early treatment of sepsis with appropriate antibiotics and avoidance of SIRS are critical. Adequate nutritional intake, correction of underlying metabolic abnormalities, maintenance of circulation, oxygenation, and management of airways and ventilator weaning are essential. Prophylaxis for deep venous thrombosis, physical therapy, rehabilitation, and basic care of paralyzed patients are warranted. Range-of-motion exercises and bracing are helpful to prevent contractures and disuse muscle atrophy; however, as patients improve, rehabilitation and assistive devices for ambulation may be required.

Treatment of CIP with IV immunoglobulins (IVIg) in a small group of patients produced no improvement.[110] A retrospective study of 33 patients showed that early treatment of sepsis or SIRS with IVIg may prevent the development of CIP.[111] Monoclonal and polyclonal antibodies against bacterial endotoxins, tumor necrosis factor-alpha, interleukin-1 receptor antagonists, and the oxygen radical scavenger N-acetylcysteine have been unsuccessful.[112,113] In one study, intensive insulin therapy in critically ill patients reduced the incidence of CIP, as well as the morbidity and mortality of critical illness.[114]

The mortality rate from sepsis and multi-organ failure in the ICU is high (30% to 50%). Recovery from CIP depends on the disease severity. Those with mild CIP usually recover within a matter of weeks, whereas recovery from severe CIP may take months. Recovery may not occur in patients with profound weakness, and nearly 22% may have severe residual deficits after 1 year.[115] Clinical and electrodiagnostic evidence of neuropathy may remain up to 5 years after the critical illness recovery.[116]

Critical Illness Myopathy

Critical illness myopathy is a rapidly evolving myopathy that affects critically ill patients; it can occur independent of or in association with CIP. Various names have been used to describe this entity, including acute quadriplegic myopathy, critical care myopathy, necrotizing myopathy of intensive care, thick filament myopathy, and others; however, the term critical illness myopathy is now widely accepted.

Critical illness myopathy usually afflicts patients exposed to high doses of IV corticosteroids, often in combination with nondepolarizing neuromuscular junction blocking agents.[117] It occurs in patients with asthma treated with high-dose IV corticosteroids and in 7% of organ transplant patients.[118,119] CIM also has been associated with propofol administration, high IV doses of corticosteroids in patients with myasthenia gravis, and rarely in patients with sepsis and multi-organ failure who were not exposed to corticosteroids.[120-122]

The main clinical feature of CIM is diffuse flaccid muscle weakness that occurs after the onset of critical illness. This usually is symmetric and proximal more than distal, although in some patients the weakness is more prominent distally. In most patients, all limb muscles, neck flexors, facial muscles, and diaphragm are involved. Respiratory failure is common, with subsequent difficulty weaning from mechanical ventilation. Tendon reflexes are often depressed,

but can be preserved or increased in some patients with concurrent encephalopathy. Variable muscle atrophy is common. Sensory perception usually is normal, when tested, in cooperative patients. Extraocular muscle weakness is rare in CIM and usually suggests prolonged neuromuscular junction blockade.

The pathogenesis of CIM is uncertain, although a number of triggering factors are recognized. Exposure to both corticosteroids and neuromuscular blocking agents suggests a potential pathogenic role; however, CIM also has been reported in patients who were not exposed to either of these classes of agents.[123,124] It appears that IV corticosteroids in conjunction with neuromuscular blocking agents, critical illness, protracted immobility, and a high-stress catabolic state trigger a proteolytic and apoptic mechanism that leads to myofibril atrophy, network disruption, and varying degrees of necrosis.[125-128] Animal models showed abnormalities in ion channels and inexcitability of myofibers due to increased sodium channel inactivation at their resting potential. Likewise, electrophysiologic studies in CIM demonstrated muscle membrane inexcitability to direct electrical stimulus, whereas denervated muscle maintained normal excitability.[129-132]

Evaluation and Diagnosis

Electrodiagnostic studies often show reduced CMAP amplitudes, normal nerve conduction velocities, and absence of CMAP amplitude changes on repetitive nerve stimulation. SNAP usually are normal, but may show mild abnormalities suggestive of concurrent neuropathy. Needle EMG examination reveals abnormal spontaneous activity, which indicates underlying muscle fiber necrosis and membrane irritability. Myopathic MUAPs are sparse initially, but prominent later in the course of the disease.[133]

Muscle biopsy shows myofiber atrophy, especially of type II fibers, and varied degrees of myofiber necrosis, degeneration, and regeneration. Selective loss of thick filament myosin is a characteristic finding in CIM, manifesting as a disrupted or patchy loss of myofiber visible with ATPase staining and best confirmed by immunohistochemical stains and electron microscopy[134] (Figs. 10-2 and 10-3). Widespread myofiber necrosis is seen in a more severe entity, known as acute necrotizing myopathy of intensive care.[133] Selective loss of thick filaments in human muscle is not specific to CIM and has been reported in other disorders, such as dermatomyositis, thrombocytopenic purpura, congenital myopathy, and myopathy associated with human immunodeficiency virus infection.[134,135] Laboratory studies in CIM show elevation of serum CK during the first 2 weeks, which can be missed if neuromuscular evaluation is delayed once medical complications obscure the weakness.[136]

Treatment and Management

There is no specific treatment for CIM. Avoidance of high-dose IV corticosteroids and cautious use of neuromuscular blocking agents, or limiting the duration of their use, reduces the risk of CIM occurrence. Treating the underlying illness, infection, and associated metabolic disorders should be initiated vigorously, along with adequate nutrition. Prophylaxis with subcutaneous heparin or enoxaparin (Lovenox) and pneumatic stockings are warranted to prevent deep venous thrombosis. Physical therapy and nursing care of paralyzed patients are necessary to prevent decubitus ulcers and joint contractures or superimposed disuse muscle atrophy. Monitoring of respiratory functions, mechanical ventilation, and early tracheostomy are indicated in patients with respiratory failure. In patients with an established or suspected diagnosis of CIM, corticosteroids and paralytic agents should be tapered off. Serial CK measurements during high-dose IV corticosteroid and paralytic agent administration in the ICU may allow an early diagnosis of CIM. In patients with

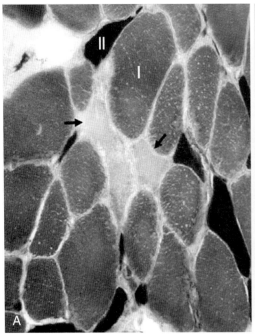
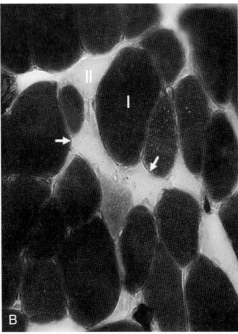

Figure 10-2 A, Muscle biopsy from a patient with critical illness myopathy stained with ATPase at pH 9.4. Notice the very pale fibers from loss of myosin *(arrows).* **B,** They also appear pale in the acid pH (4.3) *(arrows).* Magnification in both **A** and **B** is ×400.

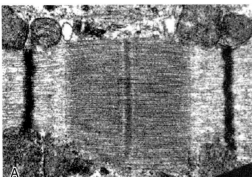
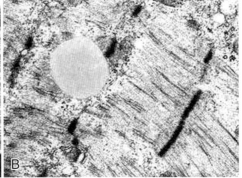

Figure 10-3 A, Normal biopsy specimen. **B,** Electron microscopy on the biopsy of the same patient as in Figure 10-2. There is a loss of the thick filaments, while thin filaments and Z lines are preserved. Magnification in both **A** and **B** is ×79,920.

rhabdomyolysis, IV hydration with alkaline diuresis is recommended. A rehabilitation program is highly recommended as patients improve.

In general, most patients with CIM who survive their critical illness recover fully within 2 to 3 months; however, CIM prolongs the ICU hospitalization and is associated with high medical costs.[136-138] Patients with more severe muscle necrosis may have a worse prognosis.

Prolonged Neuromuscular Junction Blockade

Neuromuscular blocking agents used to facilitate mechanical ventilation may cause a transient prolonged weakness. This usually occurs in patients with renal or liver failure treated with high doses of pancuronium or vecuronium.[139,140]

Neuromuscular blocking agents are metabolized by the liver and cleared by the kidneys; thus, the effect of these agents may last for several days or up to a week or two after their use has been discontinued. Concurrent use of corticosteroids and aminoglycosides may contribute to neuromuscular junction failure. Female gender, acidosis, and hypermagnesemia are risk factors.[141,142]

Like other ICU neuromuscular syndromes, prolonged neuromuscular junction blockade causes generalized flaccid muscle weakness; however, facial and extraocular muscle weakness and areflexia are characteristic of this syndrome. Some patients may have associated CIM, especially those who received concomitant corticosteroids in high doses.[137] Sensory disturbances usually are absent or minimal.

Evaluation and Diagnosis

Electrophysiologic studies demonstrate a decreased CMAP amplitude and area, which in some cases are further reduced during repetitive nerve stimulation.[143] Both presynaptic and postsynaptic defects in neuromuscular transmission have been suggested; abnormal responses to low and high stimulation rates have been described. Spontaneous activity and myopathic MUAP may be seen on needle

EMG examination in those with severe prolonged neuromuscular blockade.[144] Motor and sensory nerve conduction velocities and SNAP amplitude are normal.

Treatment and Management

Prevention of prolonged neuromuscular junction blockade by minimizing the use of paralytic agents or the use of a bolus instead of continuous administration is recommended. Administration of neostigmine may temporarily improve weakness. Hemodialysis is not an effective therapy and only partially reduces the paralytic agent's metabolites.[145] Hyperglycemia has a detrimental effect on nerve and muscle function, and glycemic control is warranted. In general, prolonged neuromuscular junction blockade is a self-limited syndrome that usually persists for a few days or a week until the paralytic agent metabolites are excreted. Patients who have persistent weakness lasting for more than 2 to 3 weeks are likely to have coexisting CIM or CIP.[144]

References

1. Mazzini L, Corra T, Zaccala M, et al: Percutaneous endoscopic gastrostomy and enteral nutrition in amyotrophic lateral sclerosis, *J Neurol* 242:695–698, 1995.
2. Kasarskis EJ, Neville HE: Management of ALS: nutritional care, *Neurology* 47(Suppl 2):S118–S120, 1996.
3. Albert SM, Murphy PL, Del Bene ML, et al: A prospective study of palliative care in ALS: choice, timing, outcomes, *J Neurol Sci* 169:108–113, 1999.
4. Miller RG, Rosenberg JA, Gelinas DF, et al: Practice parameter: the care of the patient with amyotrophic lateral sclerosis (an evidence-based review): report of the Quality Standards Subcommittee for the American Academy of Neurology. ALS Practice Parameters Task Force, *Muscle Nerve* 22:1311–1323, 1999.
5. Miller RG, Jackson CK, Kasarskis EJ, et al: Practice Parameter update: the care of the patient with amyotrophic lateral sclerosis: drug, nutritional and respiratory therapies (an evidence-based review), *Neurology* 73:1218–1226, 2009.
6. Boitano LJ, Jordan T, Benditt JO: Noninvasive ventilation allows gastrostomy tube placement in patients with advanced ALS, *Neurology* 56:413–414, 2001.
7. Bertorini TE: Perioperative management of neuromuscular diseases, *Neurol Clin North Am* 2:293–313, 2004.
8. Samaha FJ, Buncher CR, Russman BS, et al: Pulmonary function in spinal muscular atrophy, *J Child Neurol* 9:326–329, 1994.
9. Lyager S, Steffensen B, Juhl B: Indications of need for mechanical ventilation in Duchenne muscular dystrophy and spinal muscular atrophy, *J Child Neurol* 9:326–329, 1994.
10. Merlini L, Granata C, Bonfiglioli S, et al: Scoliosis in spinal muscular atrophy: natural history and management, *Dev Med Child Neurol* 31:501–508, 1989.
11. Hensinger RN, MacEwen GD: Spinal deformity associated with heritable neurological conditions: spinal muscular atrophy, Friedreich's ataxia, familial dysautonomia, and Charcot-Marie-Tooth disease, *J Bone Joint Surg Am* 58:13–24, 1976.
12. Labelle H, Tohme S, Duhaime M, et al: Natural history of scoliosis in Friedreich's ataxia, *J Bone Joint Surg* 68:564–572, 1986.
13. Delatychki MB, Holian A, Corben L, et al: Surgery for equinovarus deformity in Friedreich's ataxia improves mobility and independence, *Clin Orthop Relat Res* 430:138–141, 2005.
14. Alexander IJ, Johnson KA: Assessment and management of pes cavus in Charcot-Marie-Tooth disease, *Clin Orthop* (246):273–281, 1989.
15. Seybold M, Howard FM Jr, Duane DD, et al: Thymectomy in juvenile myasthenia gravis, *Arch Neurol* 25:385–392, 1971.
16. Olanow CW, Wechsler AS, Sirotkin-Roses M, et al: Thymectomy as primary therapy in myasthenia gravis, *Ann N Y Acad Sci* 505:595–606, 1987.
17. Jaretzki A III, Penn AS, Younger DS, et al: "Maximal" thymectomy for myasthenia gravis. Results, *J Thorac Cardiovas Surg* 95:747–757, 1988.
18. Sanders DB, El-Salem K, Massey JM, et al: Clinical aspects of MuSK antibody positive seronegative MG, *Neurology* 60:1978–1980, 2003.
19. Seybold ME: Thymectomy in childhood myasthenia gravis, *Ann N Y Acad Sci* 841:731–741, 1998.
20. Sarnat HB, McGarry JD, Lewis JE Jr: Effective treatment of infantile myasthenia gravis by combined prednisone and thymectomy, *Neurology* 27:550–553, 1977.
21. Brearly S, Gentle TA, Baynham MD, et al: Immunodeficiency following neonatal thymectomy in man, *Clin Exp Immunol* 70:322–327, 1987.
22. Mendell JR, Warmolts JR, Bass JC: Caution urged in childhood thymectomy for myasthenia gravis, *Neurology* 27:1182, 1977.
23. Halnon NJ, Jamieson P, Plunkett M, et al: Thymic function and impaired maintenance of peripheral T cell populations in children with congenital heart disease and surgical thymectomy, *Pediatr Res* 57:42–48, 2005.
24. Masaoka A, Monden Y: Comparison of the results of transsternal simple, transcervical simple, and extended thymectomy, *Ann N Y Acad Sci* 377:755–765, 1981.
25. Drachman DB: Myasthenia gravis, *N Engl J Med* 330:1797–1810, 1994.
26. Machens A, Emskotter T, Busch C, et al: Postoperative infection after transsternal thymectomy: a retrospective analysis of 125 cases, *Surg Today* 28:808–810, 1998.
27. d'Empaire G, Hoaglin DC, Perlo VP, et al: Effect of prethymectomy plasma exchange on postoperative respiratory function in myasthenia gravis, *J Thorac Cardiovasc Surg* 89:592–596, 1985.
28. Spence PA, Morin JE, Katz M: Role of plasmapheresis in preparing myasthenic patients for thymectomy: initial results, *Can J Surg* 27:303–305, 1984.
29. Jensen P, Bril V: A comparison of the effectiveness of intravenous immunoglobulin and plasma exchange as preoperative therapy of myasthenia gravis, *J Clin Neuromusc Dis* 9:352–355, 2008.
30. Kas J, Kiss D, Simon V, et al: Decade-long experience with surgical therapy of myasthenia gravis; early complications of 324 transsternal thymectomies, *Ann Thorac Surg* 72:1691–1697, 2001.
31. Shapiro F, Sethna N, Colan S, et al: Spinal fusion in Duchenne muscular dystrophy: a multidisciplinary approach, *Muscle Nerve* 15:604–614, 1992.
32. Pope JF, Birnkrant DJ, Martin JE, et al: Noninvasive ventilation during percutaneous gastrostomy placement in Duchenne muscular dystrophy, *Pediatr Pulmonol* 23:468–471, 1997.
33. Larach MG, Rosenberg H, Gronert GA, et al: Hyperkalemic cardiac arrest during anesthesia in infants and children with occult myopathies, *Clin Pediatr* 36:9–16, 1997.
34. Nathan A, Ganesh A, Godinez RI, et al: Hyperkalemic cardiac arrest after cardiopulmonary gastric bypass in a child with unsuspected Duchenne muscular dystrophy, *Anesth Ann* 100(3):672–674, 2005.
35. Hayes J, Veyckemans F, Bissonnette B: Duchenne muscular dystrophy: an old anesthesia problem revised, *Paediatr Anaesth* 18(2):100–106, 2008.
36. Komanapalli CB, Sera V, Slater MS, et al: Becker's muscular dystrophy and orthotopic heart transplantation: perioperative considerations, *Heart Surg Forum* 9(2):E604–E606, 2006.
37. Harper PS, Rudel R. Myotonic dystrophy. In Engel AG, Franzini-Armstrong C, editors: *Myology*, vol 2, New York, 1994, McGraw-Hill, pp 1192–1219.
38. Souayah N, Tick Chong PS, et al: Myotonic dystrophy type 1 presenting with ventilatory failure, *J Clin Neuromuscul Dis* 9(1):252–255, 2007.
39. Mathieu J, Allard P, Gobeil G, et al: Anesthetic and surgical complications in 219 cases of myotonic dystrophy, *Neurology* 49:1646–1650, 1997.
40. Kilburn KH, Eagon JT, Sieker HO, et al: Cardiopulmonary insufficiency in myotonic progressive muscular dystrophy, *N Engl J Med* 261:1089–1096, 1959.
41. Dundee J: Thiopentane in dystrophia myotonica, *Anesth Analg* 31:256–260, 1951.
42. Aldridge LM: Anaesthetic problems in myotonic dystrophy: a case report and review of the Aberdeen experience compromising 48 general anesthetics in a further 16 patients, *Br J Anaesth* 57:1119–1130, 1985.
43. Schwartz L, Rockoff MA, Koka BV: Masseter spasm with anesthesia: incidence and complications, *Anesthesiology* 61(6):772–775, 1984.
44. Russell SHE, Hirsch NP: Anasthesia and myotonia, *Br J Anaesth* 72:210–216, 1994.
45. England DE: Mutant sodium channels, myotonia and propofol, *Muscle Nerve* 24:713–715, 2001.

46. Haeseler G, Stormer M, Mohammadi B, et al: The anesthetic propofol modulates gating in paramyotonia congenita-mutant muscle sodium channels, *Muscle Nerve* 24:736–743, 2001.

47. Denborough MA, Lovell RRH: Anaesthetic deaths in a family, *Lancet* 2:45, 1960.

48. Jurkat-Rott K, McCarthy T, Lehmann-Horn F: Genetics and pathogenesis of malignant hyperthermia, *Muscle Nerve* 23:4–17, 2000.

49. Bertorini T: Malignant hyperthermia. In Kaminski HJ, editor: *Neuromuscular Disorders in Clinical Practice*, Boston, 2002, Butterworth-Heinemann, pp 1021–1027.

50. Gronert GA: Malignant hyperthermia. In Engel AG, Franzini-Armstrong C, editors: *Myology*, vol 2, New York, 1994, McGraw-Hill, pp 1661–1678.

51. Quane KA, Healy JM, Keating KE, et al: Mutations in the ryanodine receptor gene in central core disease and malignant hyperthermia, *Nat Genet* 5:51–55, 1993.

52. Monnier N, Procaccio V, Stieglitz P, et al: Malignant hyperthermia susceptibility is associated with a mutation of the A1 subunit of the human dihydropyridine-sensitive L-type voltage dependent calcium channel receptor in skeletal muscle, *Am J Hum Genet* 60:1316–1325, 1997.

53. Finsterer J: Current concepts in malignant hyperthermia, *J Clin Neuromusc Dis* 4:64–74, 2002.

54. Manning BM, Quane KA, Ording H, et al: Identification of novel mutations in the ryanodine receptor gene (ryanodine-receptor 1) in malignant hyperthermia: genotype phenotype, *Am J Hum Genet* 62:599–609, 1998.

55. Iles DE, Lehmann-Horn F, Scherer SW, et al: Localization of the gene encoding the alpha 2/delta-subunits of the L-type voltage-dependent calcium channel to chromosome 7q and analysis of the segregation of flanking markers in malignant hyperthermia susceptible families, *Hum Mol Genet* 3:969–975, 1994.

56. McCarthy TV, Healy JM, Heffron JJ, et al: Localization of the malignant hyperthermia susceptibility locus to human chromosome 19q12–13.2, *Nature* 343:562–564, 1990.

57. Loke J, MacLennan DH: Malignant hyperthermia and central core disease: disorders of Ca^{2+} release channels, *Am J Med* 104:470–486, 1998.

58. Heiman-Patterson TD, Rosenberg H, Fletcher JE, et al: Halothane-caffeine contracture testing in neuromuscular diseases, *Muscle Nerve* 11:453–457, 1988.

59. The European Malignant Hyperpyrexia Group: A protocol for the investigation of malignant hyperpyrexia (MH) susceptibility, *Br J Anaesth* 56:1267–1269, 1984.

60. Larach MG, North American Malignant Hyperthermia Group: Standardization of the caffeine halothane muscle contracture test, *Anesth Analg* 69:511–515, 1989.

61. Fletcher JE, Rosenberg H, Aggarwal M: Comparison of European and North American malignant hyperthermia diagnostic protocol outcomes for use in genetic studies, *Anesthesiology* 90:654–661, 1999.

62. Rosenberg H, Davis M, James D, et al: Malignant hyperthermia, *Orphanet J Rare Dis* 2:21–34, 2007.

63. Wijdicks EF: Neurotoxicity of immunosuppressive drugs, *Liver Transpl* 7 (11):937–942, 2001.

64. Walker RW, Brochstein JA: Neurologic complications of immunosuppressive agents, *Neurol Clin* 6:261–278, 1988.

65. Pless M, Zivkovic SA: Neurologic complications of transplantation, *Neurologist* 8:107–120, 2002.

66. Rush KB, Yip DS, Meschia JF: Neurologic sequelae of cardiac transplantation. In Biller J, editor: *Interface of Neurology and Internal Medicine*, Philadelphia, 2008, Lippincott Williams & Wilkins, pp 93–97.

67. Sila CA: Spectrum of neurologic events following cardiac transplantation, *Stroke* 20:1586–1589, 1989.

68. Dajczman E, Gordon A, Kreisman H, et al: Long-term postthoracotomy pain, *Chest* 99:270–274, 1991.

69. Lederman RJ, Breuer AC, Hanson MR, et al: Peripheral nervous system complications of coronary artery bypass graft surgery, *Ann Neurol* 12: 297–301, 1982.

70. Vahl CF, Carl I, Muller-Vahl H, et al: Brachial plexus injury after cardiac surgery. The role of internal mammary artery preparation: a prospective study on 1000 consecutive patients, *J Thorac Cardiovasc Surg* 102:724–729, 1991.

71. Wilbourn AJ: Plexopathies, *Neurol Clin* 25(1):139–171, 2007.

72. Watson BV, Merchant RN, Brown WF: Early postoperative ulnar neuropathies following coronary artery bypass surgery, *Muscle Nerve* 15:701–705, 1992.

73. Deng Y, Byth K, Paterson HS: Phrenic nerve injury associated with high free right internal mammary artery harvesting, *Ann Thorac Surg* 78:1517–1518, 2004.

74. Young LR, Hadjiliadis D, Davis RD, et al: Lung transplantation exacerbates gastroesophageal reflux disease, *Chest* 124:1689–1693, 2003.

75. Ferdinande P, Bruyninckx F, Van Raemdonck D, et al: Phrenic nerve dysfunction after heart-lung and lung transplantation, *J Heart Lung Transpl* 23:105–109, 2004.

76. Schweickert WD, Gruener G, Garrity ER Jr: Lung transplantation. In Biller J, editor: *Interface of Neurology and Internal Medicine*, Philadelphia, 2008, Lippincott Williams & Wilkins, pp 163–168.

77. Sheridan PH Jr, Cheriyan A, Doug J, et al: Incidence of phrenic neuropathy after isolated lung transplantation. The Loyola University Lung Transplant Group, *J Heart Lung Transpl* 14:684–691, 1995.

78. Maziak DE, Maurer JR, Kesten S: Diaphragmatic paralysis: a complication of lung transplantation, *Ann Thorac Surg* 61:170–173, 1996.

79. Zivkovic S, Linden PK: Liver transplantation. In Biller J, editor: *Interface of Neurology and Internal Medicine*, Philadelphia, 2008, Lippincott Williams & Wilkins, pp 290–294.

80. Kutcher JS: Askari. Gastrointestinal transplantation. In Biller J, editor: *Interface of Neurology and Internal Medicine*, Philadelphia, 2008, Lippincott Williams & Wilkins, pp 256–258.

81. Bronster DJ, Emre S, Boccagni P, et al: Central nervous system complications in liver transplant recipients—incidence, timing, and long-term follow-up, *Clin Transpl* 14(1):1–7, 2000.

82. Nonthasoot B, Sirichindakul B, Nivatvongs S, et al: Common peroneal nerve palsy: an unexpected complication of liver surgery, *Transpl Proc* 38:1396–1397, 2006.

83. Campellone JV, Lacomis D, Kramer DJ, et al: Acute myopathy after liver transplantation, *Neurology* 50(1):46–53, 1998.

84. Weissenborn K, Tietgu UJ, Bokemeyer M, et al: Liver transplantation improves hepatic myelopathy: evidence by three cases, *Gastroenterology* 124:346–351, 2003.

85. Abarbanel JM, Berginer VM, Osimani A, et al: Neurologic complications after gastric restriction surgery for morbid obesity, *Neurology* 37(2):196–200, 1987.

86. Salas-Salvado J, Garcia-Lorda P, Cuatrecasas G, et al: Wernicke's syndrome after bariatric surgery, *Clin Nutr* 19(5):371–373, 2000.

87. Banerji NK, Hurwitz LJ: Nervous system manifestations after gastric surgery, *Acta Neurol Scand* 47(4):485–513, 1971.

88. Pories WJ: Review: Bariatric surgery: risks and rewards, *J Clin Endocrin Metab* 93(11):S89–S96, 2008.

89. Koffman BM, Daboul I: Bariatric surgery. In: Biller J, editor: *Interface of Neurology and Internal Medicine*, Philadelphia, 2008, Lippincott Wilkins & Williams, pp 250–255.

90. Thaisetthawatkul P, Collazo-Clavell ML, Sarr MG, et al: A controlled study of peripheral neuropathy after bariatric surgery, *Neurology* 63 (8):1462–1470, 2004.

91. Macgregor AM, Thoburn EK: Meralgia paresthetica following bariatric surgery, *Obes Surg* 9(4):364–368, 1999.

92. Oliveira LD, Diniz MT, Diniz MD, et al: Rhabdomyolysis after bariatric surgery by Roux-en-Y gastric bypass: a prospective study, *Obes Surg* 1690:9780–9788, 2008.

93. Bertorini T: Case study #53. Inflammatory polyneuropathy after bariatric surgery. In Bertorini TE, editor: *Neuromuscular Case Studies*, Philadelphia, 2008, Butterworth-Heinemann, pp 352–356.

94. Kumar N: Copper deficiency myelopathy (human swayback), *Mayo Clin Proc* 81(10):1371–1384, 2006.

95. Schilling RF, Gohdes PN, Hardie GH: Vitamin B_{12} deficiency after gastric bypass surgery for obesity, *Ann Intern Med* 101(4):501–502, 1984.

96. MacLean LD, Rhode BM, Shizgal HM: Nutrition following gastric operations for morbid obesity, *Ann Surg* 198(3):347–355, 1983.

97. Mertens HG: Die disseminierte neuropathie nach koma, *Nervenarzt* 32:71–79, 1961.

98. Bolton CF, Brown JD, Sibbald WJ: The electrophysiologic investigation of respiratory paralysis in critically ill patients, *Abstr Neurol* 33:186, 1983.

99. Bolton CF, Gilbert JJ, Hahn AF, et al: Polyneuropathy in critically ill patients, *J Neurol Neurosurg Psychiatry* 47:1223–1231, 1984.

100. Zochodne DW, Bolton CF, Wells GA, et al: Critical illness polyneuropathy: a complication of sepsis and multiple organ failure, *Brain* 110:819–841, 1987.

101. Karpati G, Carpenter S, Eisen AA: Experimental core-like lesions and nemaline rods: a correlative morphological and physiological study, *Arch Neurol* 27:247–266, 1972.

102. MacFarlane IA, Rosenthal FD: Severe myopathy after status asthmaticus, *Lancet* 2:615, 1977.

103. Latronico N, Fenzi F, Recupero D, et al: Critical illness myopathy and neuropathy, *Lancet* 347:1579–1582, 1996.

104. Dellinger RP, Carlet JM, Masur H, et al: Surviving sepsis: campaign guidelines for management of severe sepsis and septic shock, *Crit Care Med* 32:858–873, 2004.

105. Bolton CF, Young GB, Zochodne DW: The neurological complications of sepsis, *Ann Neurol* 33:94–100, 1993.

106. Young GB, Bolton CF, Austin TW, et al: The encephalopathy associated with septic illness, *Clin Invest Med* 13:297–304, 1990.

107. Bolton CF: Critical illness polyneuropathy. In Thomas PK, Asbury A, editors: *Peripheral Nerve Disorders II*, Oxford, 1995, Butterworth-Heinemann, pp 262–270.

108. Dimachkie M, Austin SG, Slopis JM, et al: Critical illness polyneuropathy in childhood, *J Child Neurol* 9:207, 1994.

109. Zochodne DW, Bolton CF, Wells GA, et al: Critical illness polyneuropathy: a complication of sepsis and multiple organ failure, *Brain* 110:819–841, 1987.

110. Wijdicks EF, Fulgham JR: Failure of high dose intravenous immunoglobulins to alter the clinical course of critical illness polyneuropathy, *Muscle Nerve* 17:1494–1495, 1994.

111. Mohr M, Englisch L, Roth A, et al: Effects of early treatment with immunoglobulin on critical illness polyneuropathy following multiple organ failure and gram-negative sepsis, *Intensive Care Med* 23:1144–1149, 1997.

112. Dhainaut JF, Tenaillon A, Le Tulzo Y, et al: Platelet-activating factor receptor antagonist BN 52021 in the treatment of severe sepsis: a randomized, double-blind, placebo-controlled, multicenter clinical trial. BN 52021 Sepsis Study Group, *Crit Care Med* 22:1720–1728, 1994.

113. Spies CD, Reinhart K, Witt I, et al: Influence of *N*-acetylcysteine on indirect indicators of tissue oxygenation in septic shock patients: results from a prospective, randomized, double-blind study, *Crit Care Med* 22:1738–1746, 1994.

114. Mesotten D, Swinnen JV, Vanderhoydonc F, et al: Contribution of circulating lipids to the improved outcome of critical illness by glycemic control with intensive insulin therapy, *J Clin Endocrinol Metab* 89:219–226, 2004.

115. Witt NJ, Zochodne DW, Bolton CF, et al: Peripheral nerve function in sepsis and multiple organ failure, *Chest* 99:176–184, 1991.

116. Fletcher SN, Kennedy DD, Ghosh IR, et al: Persistent neuromuscular and neurophysiologic abnormalities in long-term survivors of prolonged critical illness, *Crit Care Med* 31:1012–1016, 2003.

117. Lacomis D, Giuliani MJ, Van Cott A, et al: Acute myopathy of intensive care: clinical, EMG, and pathologic aspects, *Ann Neurol* 40:645–654, 1996.

118. Douglass JA, Tuxen DV, Horne M, et al: Myopathy in severe asthma, *Am Rev Respir Dis* 146:517–519, 1992.

119. Perea M, Picon M, Miro O, et al: Acute quadriplegic myopathy with loss of thick (myosin) filaments following heart transplantation, *J Heart Lung Transpl* 20:1136–1141, 2001.

120. Hanson P, Dive A, Brucher J, et al: Acute corticosteroid myopathy in intensive care patients, *Muscle Nerve* 20:1371–1380, 1997.

121. Panegyres PK, Squier M, Mills KR, et al: Acute myopathy associated with large parenteral dose of corticosteroid in myasthenia gravis, *J Neurol Neurosurg Psychiatry* 56:702–704, 1993.

122. Deconinck N, Van Parijs V, Beckers-Bleukx G, et al: Critical illness myopathy unrelated to corticosteroids or neuromuscular blocking agents, *Neuromuscul Disord* 8:186–192, 1998.

123. Hirano M, Ott BR, Raps EC, et al: Acute quadriplegic myopathy: a complication of treatment with steroids, non-depolarizing blocking agents, or both, *Neurology* 42:2082–2087, 1992.

124. Deconinck N, Van Parijs V, Beckers-Bleukx G, et al: Critical illness myopathy unrelated to corticosteroids or neuromuscular blocking agents, *Neuromuscul Disord* 8:186–192, 1998.

125. Di Giovanni SD, Molon A, Broccolini A, et al: Constitutive activation of MAPK cascade in acute quadriplegic myopathy, *Ann Neurol* 55:195–206, 2004.

126. Lacomis D, Giuliani MJ, Van Cott A, et al: Acute myopathy of intensive care: clinical, electromyographic, and pathological aspects, *Ann Neurol* 40:645–654, 1996.

127. Danon MJ, Carpenter S: Myopathy with thick filament (myosin) loss following prolonged paralysis with vecuronium during steroid treatment, *Muscle Nerve* 14:1131–1139, 1991.

128. Danon MJ, Kumarasiri M, Etlinger J, et al: Steroid induced quadriplegic myopathy with selective thick filament loss: elevated proteasome content suggestive of increased proteolysis of myosin [abstract], *Neurology* 52(Suppl 2):S123, 1999.

129. Rich MM, Pinter MJ: Sodium channel inactivation in an animal model of acute quadriplegic myopathy, *Ann Neurol* 50:26–33, 2001.

130. Rich MM, Bird SJ, Raps EC, et al: Direct muscle stimulation in acute quadriplegic myopathy, *Muscle Nerve* 20:665–673, 1997.

131. Showalter CJ, Engel AG: Acute quadriplegic myopathy: analysis of myosin isoforms and evidence for calpain-mediated proteolysis, *Muscle Nerve* 20:316–322, 1997.

132. Danon MJ, Carpenter S: Myopathy with thick filament (myosin) loss following prolonged paralysis with vecuronium during steroid treatment, *Muscle Nerve* 14:1131–1139, 1991.

133. Zochodne DW, Ramsay DA, Saly V, et al: Acute necrotizing myopathy of intensive care: electrophysiological studies, *Muscle Nerve* 17:285–292, 1994.

134. Yarom R, Sphira Y: Myosin degeneration in a congenital myopathy, *Arch Neurol* 34:114–115, 1977.

135. Simpson DM, Bender AN: Human immunodeficiency virus-associated myopathy: analysis of 11 patients, *Ann Neurol* 24:79–84, 1988.

136. Hanson P, Dive A, Brucher JM, et al: Acute corticosteroid myopathy in intensive care patients, *Muscle Nerve* 20:1371–1380, 1997.

137. Gorson KC, Ropper AH: Generalized paralysis in the intensive care unit: emphasis on the complications of neuromuscular blocking agents and corticosteroids, *Intensive Care Med* 11:219–231, 1996.

138. Campellone JV, Lacomis D, Kramer DJ, et al: Acute myopathy after liver transplantation, *Neurology* 50:46–53, 1998.

139. Barohn RJ, Jackson CE, Rogers SJ, et al: Prolonged paralysis due to non-depolarizing neuromuscular blocking agents and corticosteroids, *Muscle Nerve* 17:647–654, 1994.

140. Gooch JL: Prolonged paralysis after neuromuscular blockade, *Muscle Nerve* 18:937–942, 1995.

141. Vanderheyden BA, Reynolds HN, Gerold KB, et al: Prolonged paralysis after long term vecuronium infusion, *Crit Care Med* 20:304–307, 1992.

142. Segredo V, Caldwell JE, Matthay MA, et al: Persistent paralysis in critically ill patients after long-term administration of vecuronium, *N Engl J Med* 327:524–528, 1992.

143. Gooch JL, Moore MH, Ryser DK: Prolonged paralysis after neuromuscular junction blockade: case reports and electrodiagnostic findings, *Arch Phys Med Rehabil* 74:1007–1011, 1993.

144. Barohn RJ, Jackson CE, Rogers SJ, et al: Prolonged paralysis due to non-depolarizing neuromuscular blocking agents and corticosteroids, *Muscle Nerve* 17:647–654, 1994.

145. Segredo V, Matthay MA, Sharma ML, et al: Prolonged neuromuscular blockade after long-term administration of vecuronium in two critically-ill patients, *Anesthesiology* 72:566–570, 1990.

Treatment and Management of Specific Neuromuscular Disorders

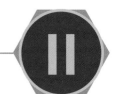

Catherine Lomen-Hoerth, MD, PhD

11

Treatment and Management of Adult Motor Neuron Diseases

Many diseases specifically affect the motor neurons, ranging from infectious processes such as polio and West Nile viruses to hereditary conditions such as spinal muscular atrophy (SMA) and Kennedy disease.[1] Radiation therapy can cause motor neuron degeneration many years later, mimicking the adult motor neuron disease amyotrophic lateral sclerosis (ALS).[2] Sometimes the motor neuron degeneration remains curiously restricted to just the cervical region, such as in Hirayama disease.[3] Central nervous system (CNS) lymphoma can directly infiltrate nerve roots, mimicking motor neuron disease. When motor neuron degeneration is accompanied by an adenocarcinoma, a paraneoplastic syndrome is suspected.[4]

Amyotrophic lateral sclerosis is a disease that is still little understood despite first being described in the late 1800s. It affects 1 in 100,000 people, with a slight male predominance and no ethnic or geographic preference. Typically, the disease is sporadic, but familial cases occur 10% of the time. Commercially available for testing in familial cases, the superoxide dismutase 1 gene (*SOD1*) present in approximately 10% to 20% of familial cases. Several other genes have been discovered, causing an even smaller proportion of familial cases; recently it was determined that the newly discovered gene *ALS6* accounts for another 5% of familial cases.[5,6]

In ALS, weakness starts in a limb or less frequently in the bulbar region and progressively spreads contiguously until ultimately respiratory depression and death occurs, approximately 3 to 5 years from symptom onset. The range of progression is variable, and death can occur within a couple of months from the first symptom or decades later. Diagnosis is difficult, particularly early in the disease course, because many conditions mimic ALS, and no definitive test is available for ALS.

No available treatments significantly alter the fatal outcome of the disease; however, tremendous strides have been made in the management of symptoms through technology and medications, leading to an improved quality of life. A new protein, TAR DNA-binding protein, or TDP-43, found in both ALS and frontotemporal dementia (FTD), may provide new clues to the pathogenesis of these diseases and hopefully lead to improved treatments in the future. Lastly, research into stem cell therapy keeps patients and physicians hopeful that we may have a meaningful therapy for ALS even before understanding its underlying mechanisms.[4]

Diagnosis and Evaluation

The evaluation of a potential motor neuron disease patient is primarily based on the clinical presentation (Figs. 11-1 to 11-3 and Table 11-1). Important features to determine what type of workup

is needed include the rate of progression of the weakness, the pattern of weakness, family history, associated symptoms such as parkinsonism or dementia, and the age of onset. The degree of upper versus lower motor neuron involvement is critical to identify; the symptoms of such involvement are shown in Figure 11-2. Once the degree of upper and lower motor neuron involvement is established and all ALS mimics are excluded, the revised El Escorial criteria can be used to establish the diagnosis (see Fig. 11-1). The different types of ALS presentations and the workup recommended in each case are described here and also diagrammed in Figure 11-3.

Family History

When there is a known family history of progressive weakness, it is important to determine the age of onset in family members, the disease duration, and the rate and pattern of the spread of weakness.

Symmetric proximal greater than distal lower motor neuron weakness in the limbs and bulbar involvement that is slowly progressive may indicate Kennedy disease. This is an X-linked, trinucleotide repeat, genetic disorder that occurs in 1 in 50,000 males and involves progressive degeneration of anterior motor neurons. Androgen receptor function is impaired, the severity of this impairment correlating with the length of the expansion of the CAG repeat within the receptor. There is also an inverse correlation between the number of CAG repeats and the age of onset of the disease. The key features include gynecomastia (in more than 50% of cases), areflexia, a subtle sensory neuropathy, and progressive, proximal greater than distal weakness in the limbs and bulbar muscles. Onset is usually in the third or fourth decade of life but may occur in the teenage years or later in life. Muscle cramps often occur years before the onset of weakness; fasciculations are common, particularly in the lower face and tongue. Creatine kinase (CK) measurements may be up to 5 times the upper limit of normal. Tremor of the limbs and chin is reported. Dysphagia and dysarthria usually occur later (10 to 20 years after symptoms start). Life expectancy in Kennedy disease is not particularly reduced unless complicated by aspiration pneumonia, so it is critical for the prognosis to distinguish this disorder from ALS. Testes may be small, and infertility is common. There can be associated diabetes.[7–9] Treatment is largely based on symptoms because treatment with testosterone makes the symptoms worse.[10]

If the weakness has an onset in childhood or late adulthood and the patient has a pure lower motor neuron presentation that is predominately proximal, SMA should be considered along with familial ALS. SMA is an autosomal recessive disorder with a defect in the survival motor neuron (*SMN1*) gene on chromosome 5.[11] It can also

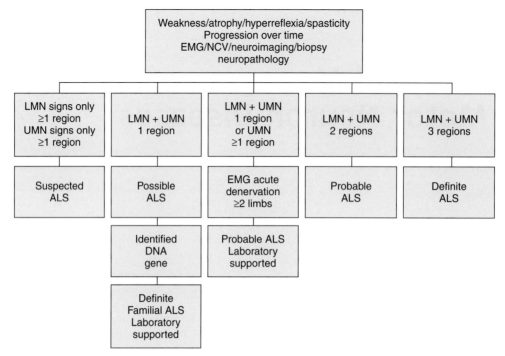

Figure 11-1 El Escorial revisited: revised criteria for the diagnosis of amyotrophic lateral sclerosis. ALS, amyotrophic lateral sclerosis; EMG, electromyography; LMN, lower motor neuron; NCV, nerve conduction velocity; UMN, upper motor neuron. (From Brooks BR, Miller RG, Swash M, et al, for the World Federation of Neurology Research Group on Motor Neuron Diseases: El Escorial revisited: revised criteria for the diagnosis of amyotrophic lateral sclerosis, *Amyotroph Lateral Scler Other Motor Neuron Disord* 1(5):293–299, 2000.)

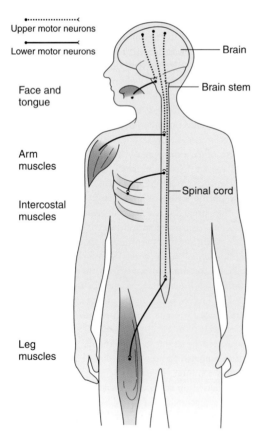

Figure 11-2 Upper motor neuron findings include slow speech; brisk gag and jaw jerk reflexes, brisk limb reflexes; spasticity; Hoffmann's or Babinski signs. Lower motor neuron findings include atrophy, fasciculations, and weakness.

occur in infants, in whom it is rapidly fatal. Due to the pattern of weakness and age of presentation, it can be difficult to distinguish from the limb-girdle muscular dystrophies without electromyographic (EMG) studies. There is no treatment for SMA; however, several trials are in progress examining hydroxyurea and valproic acid.[12,13]

Other inherited conditions that can be confused with ALS include adult-onset Tay-Sachs disease, Charcot-Marie-Tooth disease (CMT), and adult polyglucosan body disease. Adult-onset Tay-Sachs disease is caused by a mutation in the gene for hexosaminidase A and may cause lower more than upper motor neuron involvement. This disease tends to be slowly progressive; cerebellar atrophy on neuroimaging is a clue to this diagnosis. CMT can present with myriad clinical features that can be confused with those of ALS, including a mixture of upper and lower motor neuron involvement in rare cases and vocal cord paralysis. Adult polyglucosan body disease can also mimic ALS and should be included in the differential, particularly in patients of Ashkenazi Jewish background with associated dementia.[14] Commercially available genetic tests can exclude many of these possibilities. Muscular dystrophies may also be confused with ALS, particularly facioscapulohumeral muscular dystrophy (FSHD). FSHD is an autosomal dominant disorder affecting 1 in 20,000 persons. About 30% of patients are unaware of their condition, and new mutations can also occur, making it difficult to rely on family history to help with the diagnosis. FSHD is caused by a deletion of tandem 3.3kb repeats on chromosome 4q35. This results in the overexpression of upstream genes due to loss of binding of a transcriptional repressor protein. It is variable in severity and age of onset but is generally slowly progressive, with only about 20% of patients eventually needing a wheelchair. Typical onset is in the second or third decade with a nearly normal or normal life span. The facial muscles are involved, causing difficulty closing the

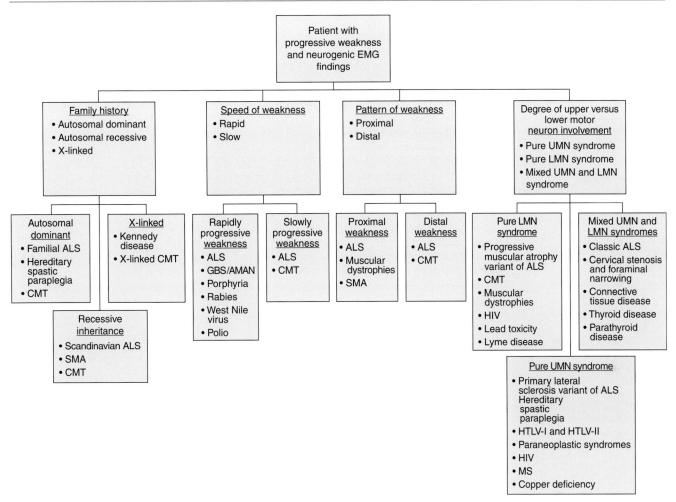

Figure 11-3 Critical questions for the workup of possible amyotrophic lateral sclerosis (ALS). AMAN, acute motor axonal neuropathy; CMT, Charcot-Marie-Tooth disease; EMG, electromyography; GBS, Guillain-Barré syndrome; HIV, human immunodeficiency virus; HTLV, human T-cell lymphotropic virus; MS, multiple sclerosis; SMA, spinal muscular atrophy; UMN, upper motor neuron.

eyes, smiling, and whistling. The face can appear to be pouting. The shoulder and upper arm muscles are affected, with relative sparing of the deltoid muscles and significant scapular winging. Foot drop occurs in the scapuloperoneal variety; interestingly, the extensor digitorum brevis muscle tends to be hypertrophied rather than atrophic as in neurogenic causes of foot drop. In the arms, the extensors are also affected more than the flexor muscles. The weakness can progress slowly with periods of arrests. Asymmetry of the weakness is not unusual. CK level may be normal or only mildly elevated, despite inflammation found on muscle biopsy.[15]

Once all mimics of familial ALS have been excluded, it is important to test for the presence of the *SOD1* gene, mutations of which are responsible for 10% to 20% of familial ALS cases. Establishing an *SOD1* case of ALS is helpful for other family members who desire testing and for researchers hoping to identify potential patients for upcoming clinical trials testing antisense mRNA for *SOD1* in familial ALS cases. The *SOD1* forms of ALS tend to be a pure lower motor neuron syndrome with a variable clinical course, from very rapidly progressive in the *A4V* variant to very slowly progressive with sensory involvement in the recessive Scandinavian type. Genetic counseling is critical both before and after testing, given the implications for other family members. Although it is frequently requested, asymptomatic genetic testing is not covered by insurance.

Because genetic testing only identifies a gene mutation in 10% to 20% of the familial cases, it is important to also screen for more common etiologies of weakness and not automatically assume that the weakness is from familial ALS rather than cervical radiculopathy, for example.

Pure Lower Motor Neuron Syndrome

When patients present with a pure lower motor neuron syndrome and no family history, it is important to still consider the differential discussed in this chapter for cases with a family history, because many patients with Kennedy disease and various muscular dystrophies are not aware of any family history until they are diagnosed themselves. This is not necessarily due to new sporadic mutations but rather to undiagnosed cases that may be too mild to seek clinical attention.

It is also important to consider the most common cause of lower motor neuron weakness—a polyradiculopathy. Neuroimaging of the affected areas is critical to look for this possibility. West Nile virus, Lyme disease, porphyria, diphtheria, Creutzfeldt-Jakob disease, acute motor axonal neuropathy (AMAN syndrome), and polio all cause a pure lower motor neuron syndrome, but the time from onset to deficit is much more rapid than in typical ALS and they are usually

Table 11-1 Workup for Adult Motor Neuron Disease

Symptom	Workup
Pure lower motor neuron syndrome	EMG and nerve conduction studies of at least one arm and one leg, tongue, and thoracic paraspinal muscles Neuroimaging of the affected body segments Routine blood work* Genetic testing for Kennedy's, ALS, and SMA if familial or if clinical presentation is classic in the absence of a family history HIV test if patient has risk factors Anti-GM1 antibodies Spinal tap with fluid sent for cytology, cell count, protein, glucose, and IgG index
Pure upper motor neuron syndrome	EMG and nerve conduction studies of at least one arm and one leg, thoracic paraspinal muscles, and tongue Neuroimaging of the affected body segments Routine blood work* Genetic testing for hereditary spastic paraplegia if familial Spinal tap with fluid sent for cytology, cell count, protein, glucose, IgG index, HTLV-I and -II, and VDRL Serum copper Paraneoplastic antibody tests HIV test if patient has risk factors
Progressive bulbar palsy	EMG and nerve conduction studies of at least one arm and one leg, thoracic paraspinal muscles, and tongue Neuroimaging of the brain Routine blood work* MuSK antibody if EMG not clearly neurogenic Spinal tap with fluid sent for cytology, cell count, protein, glucose, and IgG index
Upper and lower motor neuron syndrome	EMG and nerve conduction studies of at least one arm and one leg, thoracic paraspinal muscles, and tongue Neuroimaging of the affected body segments Routine blood work* Genetic testing for ALS if familial

*Routine blood work: complete blood count (CBC), electrolytes, calcium, thyroid-stimulating hormone (TSH), vitamin B_{12}, liver function tests (LFTs), serum protein electrophoresis, immunofixation, urine protein electrophoresis, glucose, blood urea nitrogen (BUN), creatinine (Cr), creatine kinase (CK), erythrocyte sedimentation rate (ESR), antinuclear antibody (ANA), and Lyme antibody (if in endemic area).

easily distinguishable from that disorder. Botulism also presents with rapidly progressive weakness but has characteristic findings on EMG and nerve conduction studies that distinguish this entity from motor neuron disease. Monoclonal gammopathies can be difficult to differentiate clinically, but can be screened by testing serum protein electrophoresis, immunofixation, and urine protein electrophoresis. Myasthenia gravis can easily be identified on nerve conduction studies with a decremental response on repetitive stimulation, and antibodies can be sent for the acetylcholine receptor. If an incremental response is seen on high-frequency repetitive stimulation suggesting a presynaptic disorder, then antibodies can be tested for the calcium channel. Eaton-Lambert syndrome presents with symmetric limb weakness and decreased reflexes, which can be confusing in the differential diagnosis of a pure lower motor neuron syndrome. Myopathies and muscular dystrophies can also be differentiated based on EMG studies and muscle biopsy. Blood should be tested for the presence of human immunodeficiency virus (HIV), particularly in patients with risk factors for HIV.[1]

When patients with a history of polio and residual weakness in a limb present later in life with new weakness, it is important to differentiate postpolio syndrome from other neurologic processes, including superimposed ALS. Postpolio syndrome occurs in a moderately severe or severely weak limb and usually involves small changes in the degree of strength that can sometimes lead to significant functional changes. It never occurs in a limb that is full strength, is not rapidly progressive, and does not occur in patients who have never had polio or had polio and recovered fully.[16]

One of the most important conditions to consider in the differential is multifocal motor neuropathy with conduction block; this is a highly treatable condition that mimics ALS. Patients have fasciculations; progressive weakness, typically in the distal upper limbs; preserved or brisk reflexes; and abnormalities on nerve conduction studies to support the diagnosis. Antibodies are produced to gangliosides, such as anti-GM1, which then, it is hypothesized, cause focal demyelination of motor neuron axons. When nerves are stimulated electrically at multiple points, a dropoff in the amplitude of the CMAP signifies conduction block. Anti-GM1 levels may be elevated or normal, making it difficult to achieve a definitive diagnosis with this test. To confound the issue more, patients with a classical clinical presentation but no conduction block identified on nerve conduction studies are sometimes responsive to intravenous immunoglobulin (IVIg), the treatment most typically given in this condition, with a 95% response rate. In contrast to chronic inflammatory demyelinating polyneuropathy, the spinal fluid protein in a patient with multifocal motor neuropathy with conduction block is typically normal. Sometimes a 3-month trial of IVIg at 2 g/kg/month is warranted to look for a treatment response in patients with a pure lower motor neuron syndrome.

After all the ALS mimics are excluded, patients with a pure lower motor neuron presentation of ALS are considered to have progressive muscular atrophy variant of ALS. This condition often starts with limb weakness; sometimes these patients progress more slowly than those with typical ALS, with progression more like that seen with SMA, but other times they progress just as rapidly as typical ALS patients. Over time, these patients may develop upper motor neuron signs and bulbar involvement, changing the diagnosis to classic ALS.[17,18] Development of these signs may change management of the disorder; for example, baclofen may be added to the treatment regimen to help with spasticity. In addition, the change in diagnosis may allow patients to be eligible for ALS clinical trials, because currently all such trials exclude patients with a pure lower or upper motor neuron presentation and require a diagnosis of probable or definite ALS (see Fig. 11-1).

Pure Upper Motor Neuron Syndrome

Patients with a pure upper motor neuron syndrome need a fairly aggressive workup to exclude mimics of *primary lateral sclerosis*, the term used for a pure upper motor neuron presentation of ALS. EMG studies should initially be performed in these patients to look for any subclinical motor neuron involvement, which might help to narrow the workup. If the EMG is normal or shows suprasegmental weakness (an interference pattern on EMG that is proportional to effort, consistent with an upper motor neuron pattern of weakness), extensive neuroimaging is critical to look for multiple sclerosis, tumor, or a compressive spinal cord lesion. Some conditions, such as spinal arteriovenous malformation or dural arteriovenous fistula, can be missed if the quality of the magnetic resonance study is poor or the neuroradiologist is inexperienced. These conditions may present with a more stepwise pattern of weakness. A lumbar puncture can help guide the workup, looking for elevated protein, IgG, and cells. The spinal fluid can also be tested for human T-cell lymphotropic virus 1 and 2 (HTLV-1 and HTLV-2) as well as syphilis with the VDRL. Serum can also be examined for presence of HTLV-1. Copper deficiency is a very rare cause of upper motor neuron syndrome, but it can be tested by examining serum copper levels. Paraneoplastic syndromes are also important to consider; measuring antineuronal antibodies is a typical part of the workup. It is also important to assess HIV status, as with pure lower motor neuron presentations.[1]

Hereditary spastic paraplegia can mimic an upper motor neuron presentation of ALS and can be difficult to distinguish from that disorder. Patients with spastic paraplegia usually have an earlier age of onset and a strong autosomal dominant family history, which is helpful in diagnosis. There can also be a superimposed neuropathy and cognitive deficits, and despite the name, arm involvement can occur. Vitamin B_{12} deficiency can cause a motor myelopathy, as can thyroid disease; these disorders can easily be ruled out with blood testing.[19]

As with the pure lower motor neuron presentation of ALS, patients with a pure upper motor neuron form can develop lower motor neuron involvement over time, even decades later. EMG studies at diagnosis and every 1 to 2 years can be useful to help identify subclinical lower motor neuron involvement. This can allow patients to be eligible for clinical trials if their diagnosis changes to ALS based on their EMG results (see Fig. 11-1).

Progressive Bulbar Palsy

Progressive bulbar palsy is a condition presenting with bulbar weakness. The differential is quite broad because patients can present with either pure lower motor neuron or pure upper motor neuron findings. Detailed neuroimaging is critical in a pure upper motor neuron presentation to look for any evidence of a structural lesion, such as stroke, tumor, or multiple sclerosis. In a pure lower motor neuron presentation, the Miller-Fisher variant of Guillain-Barré syndrome, myasthenia gravis, Lyme disease, and tumor infiltrating the nerve roots are part of the differential. MuSK-positive antibody myasthenia gravis is particularly difficult to distinguish from bulbar ALS because patients have proximal weakness, bulbar involvement, and sometimes significant muscle atrophy. Fasciculations, however, are not present in this condition.[20] A lumbar puncture, with a large

volume of cerebrospinal fluid sent for cytology, is important to aid in the diagnosis if neuroimaging is negative. When both upper and lower motor neuron findings are present and basic blood work, neuroimaging, and lumbar puncture results are negative, there is not much utility in further evaluations, because ALS is the most likely diagnosis. However, it may take years for the disease to involve the limbs. An EMG study can be useful to document the lower motor neuron involvement in the tongue and to establish any subclinical disease in the limbs.

Confounding Features

When patients have features in addition to those described in the revised El Escorial criteria shown in Figure 11-1, the term used is *ALS plus*.[21] This classification is unsatisfactory because it is not descriptive of the myriad associated findings patients can have in addition to the classic upper and lower motor neuron findings. A consensus paper recently published after the international ALS-FTD meeting in London, Ontario, Canada, suggested using the terms *Axis I* to describe the motor neuron disease variants and *Axis II* to describe the cognitive variants (Table 11-2).[22] The number of affected patients ranges from 3% to more than 50% of total patients with ALS, depending on the study published and the types of neuropsychological testing performed. The severity of frontotemporal deficits is on a continuum, with a significant proportion of ALS patients possessing a gradation of behavioral and cognitive changes.[23] Beyond being of interest for researchers, the associated cognitive and behavioral changes significantly affect survival due to their effects on compliance with treatment recommendations.[24] Obviously, before concluding that a patient has cognitive or behavioral problems due to ALS, a careful workup to exclude confounders, such as structural CNS causes, depression, nocturnal desaturations, sleep deprivation, and medication side effects, is critical. Although extensive progress has been made in developing screening studies to identify patients with cognitive and behavioral impairments in the clinic, the gold standard is still detailed neuropsychological testing and caregiver interviews. TDP-43 is a protein found in the neuronal inclusions of ALS, FTD, and ALS-FTD, and suggests a potentially common mechanism for these diseases.[25] TDP-43 may also be a way of distinguishing between *SOD1* and non-*SOD1* related cases of ALS, because it is not found in *SOD1* cases.[26]

Most drug development to date has been based on the *SOD1* murine model, which has identified just one treatment for ALS, riluzole. One proposed reason for the lack of effectiveness of this treatment is that the model of ALS on which it is based is present in only 10% of the population. Mutations have been found in the gene for TDP-43 (*TDPBP*), which can lead to the creation of new murine models for development of medications and offer treatments for ALS and FTD.

Electrodiagnostic Studies

Electrophysiology is the key to diagnosis in many cases. As demonstrated in Figure 11-1, the revised El Escorial criteria allow EMG findings to be included as identifying subclinical lower motor neuron involvement. Active and chronic denervation is required in at least two limbs. The denervation needs to be in at least two body segments innervated by different nerve roots in the limbs for a diagnosis of probable ALS (see Fig. 11-1). In the tongue and thoracic paraspinal muscles, this is not a requirement. Recently, EMG of the sternocleidomastoid and trapezius have been proposed to establish lower motor neuron cranial nerve involvement with greater sensitivity

Table 11-2 Axis II: Cognitive/Behavioral Characterization

Frontotemporal Lobar Degeneration with ALS			
ALS-FTD	ALS-bvFTD	ALS-dementia*, FTD-MND	ALS patient meeting either the Neary criteria (51) or Hodge's criteria (2) for FTD
	ALS-PNFA		ALS patient meeting Neary criteria for PNFA
	ALS-SD		ALS patient meeting Neary criteria for SD
ALSbi			ALS patient meeting at least two nonoverlapping supportive diagnostic features from either the Neary criteria (51) or Hodge's criteria (2) for FTD
ALSci			Evidence of cognitive impairment at or below the fifth percentile on at least two distinct tests of cognition that are sensitive to executive functioning
FTD-MND-like			A neuropathologic diagnosis in which FTLD is the primary diagnosis but in which there is neuropathologic evidence of motor neuron degeneration, but insufficient to be classified as ALS
ALS-dementia		ALS-dementia (ALS-D)*	ALS with dementia, not typical of FTLD
	ALS-AD		ALS in association with AD
	ALS-vascular dementia		ALS in association with vascular dementia
	ALS-mixed dementia		ALS in association with a mixed dementia (e.g., AD-vascular dementia)
ALS-parkinsonism-dementia complex		Western Pacific variant of ALS; Lytico- Bodig disease	ALS concurrent with dementia or parkinsonism occurring in hyperendemic foci of the Western Pacific

*Note that the term *ALS-dementia* has been used generically within the literature to imply the presence of any clinical or neuropathologic evidence of cognitive or behavioral impairment and thus appears in two synonymous categories. The participants recommend restriction of the use of *ALS-dementia* to refer to specific dementias.
AD, Alzheimer's disease; ALS, amyotrophic lateral sclerosis; ALSbi, amyotrophic lateral sclerosis with behavioral impairment; ALSci, amyotrophic lateral sclerosis with cognitive impairment; bvFTD, behavioral variant, frontotemporal dementia; FTD, frontotemporal dementia; FTLD, frontotemporal lobar dementia; MND, motor neuron disease; PNFA, progressive nonfluent aphasia; SD, semantic dementia.
From Strong MJ, Grace GM, Freedman M, et al: Consensus criteria for the diagnosis of frontotemporal cognitive and behavioural syndromes in amyotrophic lateral sclerosis. *Amyotroph Lateral Scler* 10:131–146, 2009; erratum in *Amyotroph Lateral Scler* 10:252, 2009.

than the tongue muscle.[27] In addition to establishing the degree of lower motor neuron involvement, the EMG and nerve conduction studies are required to exclude some of the mimics of ALS, such as myopathies, myasthenia gravis, muscular dystrophies, and neuropathies such as multifocal motor neuropathy. For some conditions such as polyradiculopathy, the EMG findings are indistinguishable from those of ALS, and detailed neuroimaging is critical.

Laboratory Evaluations

The laboratory evaluations are performed based on the clinical presentation and, in some cases, with serial testing to prevent costly workups (see Table 11-1). Basic blood work is important to test in most cases, including complete blood count, CK, erythrocyte sedimentation rate, glucose, liver function tests, electrolytes, kidney function tests, thyroid-stimulating hormone, and protein electrophoresis (serum and urine). Other specialized tests can be ordered on a case-by-case basis. For example, if Kennedy disease is highest in the differential diagnosis, then the androgen receptor DNA test would be performed before ordering other tests. Rapidly progressive weakness should prompt evaluations of various infectious causes. Remember: ALS is a clinical diagnosis based on the exclusion of other causes; there is currently no direct testing that can be done to confirm the diagnosis in non-*SOD1* ALS.

How to Deliver the Diagnosis

During the evaluation process, it is important to be careful about the delivery of information to the patient and family. When performing a workup of ALS mimics, the clinician should avoid mentioning that ALS is in the differential diagnosis, because this can cause significant

stress for the patient and family given the extensive amount of information about ALS available on the Internet. If the diagnosis of ALS is confirmed, it is critical for the clinician to allow plenty of time for the discussion, to pace the discussion appropriately based on the reactions of the patient and family, and to allow opportunity for questions to be asked. Specific guidelines for breaking the news are outlined in the American Academy of Neurology's practice parameters.[28] At the end of the discussion, it is important to provide hope with the offer of symptomatic and experimental therapies. Handouts are useful because patients may not absorb information well after hearing the word *ALS*. It is important to provide reassurance that the doctor and management team will be present throughout the disease course, that second opinion requests will be honored if desired, and that the disease will likely progress at the same rate without suddenly speeding up. Both the Muscular Dystrophy Association (MDA) and the ALS Association (ALSA) have many resources available for patients, including support groups, educational materials, and financial assistance for equipment needs (www.mda.org; www.alsa.org).

Treatment and Management

Drug Therapies

Treatments to slow disease progression include riluzole. This glutamate antagonist was shown in a large clinical trial with hundreds of ALS patients to slow disease progression by 10%.[29,30] The dose of riluzole is typically 50 mg BID; if the patient experiences side effects of somnolence, taking one tablet at night may be sufficient. A recent Italian study suggested benefit from combining low doses of lithium (which delays mitochondrial vacuolization) with riluzole when compared to treatment with riluzole alone. The dose used in the study ranged from 300 mg/day (divided BID) to 450 mg/day to keep the blood levels between 0.4 and 0.8 mEq/L. The benefit was much more dramatic than with riluzole; however, it was a very small study with a short follow-up time.[31,32] In a parallel study on a genetic ALS animal model, the G93A mouse, lithium delayed disease onset and duration and improved survival. Lithium caused activation of autophagy, increased the number of mitochondria in motor neurons, and suppressed reactive astrogliosis. Lithium reduced the slow necrosis characterized by mitochondrial vacuolization and increased the number of neurons counted in lamina VII that were severely affected in saline-treated G93A mice.[31] In response to this potentially intriguing use for this drug, two trials have been initiated in the United States to examine these findings. One of these trials was stopped early due to lack of efficacy.[33]

Experimental Trials

Experimental drug trials have been disappointing in ALS and in other motor neuron diseases (such as Kennedy disease and SMA). A large number of potentially beneficial therapies, such as several neurotrophic factors, antioxidant agents (such as coenzyme Q_{10}), anti-inflammatory agents (such as celecoxib [Celebrex]), topiramate (Topamax), and the caspase-1 inhibitor minocycline, have had negative results or have accelerated progression in ALS.[34] Current trials in progress include those of the antioxidant edaravone, the glutamate antagonists ceftriaxone and talampanel, lithium, a vascular endothelial growth factor activator, and R+pramipexole. Mecasermin (Iplex), a recombinant form of insulin-like growth factor-1, was recently released by the Food and Drug Administration for a limited number of patients who had an existing IND on file, and they are being tracked for any potential benefit or toxicity. Its potential benefit is controversial; there is some concern about inappropriate marketing of the drug to ALS patients.[35] The ALS, MDA, and National Institutes of Health (NIH) Web sites are excellent sources for information on ongoing clinical trials for ALS (www.alsa.org, www.mda.org, and www.nih.gov). Placebo-controlled trials have been important in ALS because previous trials have tested drugs that were safe in the general population, such as Topamax and minocycline, but these drugs caused decreased survival in ALS.[36,37]

Nonpharmaceutical trials in ALS are also occurring. Based on potentially exciting preliminary data on the ability of diaphragm-pacing electrodes to help with breathing, tests are being conducted on this device to determine if its use can delay patients with ALS being placed on a ventilator.[38] Exercise has been shown to be beneficial for improving both quantity and quality of life. A carefully constructed program is important to avoid overexercising weak muscles or underexercising strong muscles. Ideally, a physical therapist can work with the patient to help guide the exercise program at the beginning and throughout the disease process as weakness changes. Massage, water therapy, and use of recumbent bicycles are helpful adjuncts to physical therapy.

Stem cell trials are planned for ALS in addition to many other neuromuscular diseases and offer great hope for improvement of already weak muscles rather than strictly slowing down disease progression, which has been the sole focus of pharmaceutical trials in ALS.

Nutritional Management

One of the most important interventions to improve survival in ALS has been the improvement of nutritional function. Patients with bulbar onset ALS previously had a decreased survival rate compared to limb onset ALS, but with improved nutrition the differences in survival were eliminated. Advances in placement of percutaneous endoscopic gastrostomy (PEG) tubes have made it possible for even those patients with low forced vital capacity (FVC) to obtain PEG tubes safely. PEG tube placement is usually recommended before patients lose weight and should be considered when the FVC drops to 50% of predicted, when swallowing or bringing food to the mouth is burdensome due to weakness. Advances in nutritional supplements and equipment have made maintaining weight easier even without a PEG tube (see also Chapter 4).

Breathing Management

Supporting breathing with noninvasive breathing machines has prolonged survival in ALS by more than a year—a more significant improvement than seen with riluzole. Typically, these machines are recommended for patients once their breathing function declines to an FVC less than 50% or when their maximal inspiratory flow (MIF) is less than −60 cm H_2O. Most patients can acclimate to these machines over time if different interfaces are tried and saliva is well managed. If patients have fatigue, confusion, or shortness of breath, they may have diaphragm dysfunction, and further testing is indicated. The FVC can be tested in the supine position or patients can undergo nocturnal oximetry testing to see if they might qualify for noninvasive ventilation. At the point of the FVC declining to 30% of expected, patients are presented with the choice of pursuing invasive ventilation or enrolling in hospice. Artificial ventilation is discussed in detail in Chapter 2 and hospice is discussed in this chapter.

Symptomatic Management

Many ALS symptoms, including cramps, excessive saliva, spasticity, urinary urgency, pseudobulbar affect, constipation, pain, depression, and agitation, can be managed with medications (Table 11-3). Symptomatic therapies are also appropriate for any of the motor neuron diseases. Few direct comparison studies have been done to determine the most effective medications to treat these symptoms, but a small range of drugs are typically tried.[39,40]

Pseudobulbar affect is a condition of easy laughing and crying, which is common in ALS and is sometimes disabling. It responds well to tricyclic antidepressants such as amitriptyline and somewhat to the selective serotonin-reuptake inhibitors (SSRIs). A combination of dextromethorphan and quinidine being tested at two different doses in current clinical trials is hoped to be more effective than currently available therapy.[41]

Cramps, a very common symptom in ALS, were well controlled with quinine sulfate until it was pulled from the market in the United States due to safety concerns. Patients can continue to obtain this drug from Canada or in some cases are able to obtain insurance coverage for Qualaquin, the nongeneric form of quinine sulfate approved for malaria treatment. Tonic water contains small amounts of quinine and may be effective in patients with mild cramps. Carbamazepine and baclofen may also be effective in some cases.

Excessive saliva becomes a problem in ALS due to difficulty swallowing. It is usually treated with glycopyrrolate at first; atropine pills or drops are added when glycopyrrolate is no longer effective. A typical dose of glycopyrrolate is 1 to 2 mg every 4 hours as needed. Atropine is given in 0.04-mg pills or 1% drops every couple of hours as needed. It is safe to take both medications together, but constipation inevitably occurs with these drugs. These treatments

Table 11-3 Symptom Management in ALS

Symptom	Treatment
Sialorrhea	Amitriptyline (Elavil) 10–50 mg HS Atropine 1% solution 1–2 drops q4h Glycopyrrolate (Robinul) 10–20 mg q4h Scopolamine patch Radiation therapy to the salivary glands Botulinum toxin injection (Botox) to the parotid and submandibular salivary glands (2500 units)
Cramps	Tonic water containing quinine Quinine (Qualaquin) 324 mg HS or BID Carbamazepine 100–200 mg TID
Spasticity	Baclofen 10–30 mg TID Diazepam (Valium) 10–40 mg HS Tizanidine (Zanaflex) 4–12 mg TID Baclofen pump titrated to patient's spasticity
Urinary urgency	Oxybutynin (Ditropan) 5 mg BID Tolteridine (Detrol) 2 mg BID
Pseudobulbar affect	Amitriptyline (Elavil) 10–50 mg HS Dextromethorphan 30 mg and quinidine 10 mg (compounded)
Constipation	Stool softeners, fluids, fiber, and lactulose 20–40 g BID
Sleep	Bilevel positive airway pressure (BiPAP) at least 4 hours/day Mirtazapine (Remeron) 15–30 mg HS Trazodone 100–200 mg HS Zolpidem (Ambien) 5–10 mg HS Diazepam (Valium) 10–40 mg HS
Depression	Selective serotonin reuptake inhibitors (SSRIs) varying doses Mirtazapine (Remeron) 15–30 mg HS Trazodone 100–200 mg HS Bupropion (Wellbutrin) 100 mg TID
Anxiety	Lorazepam (Ativan) 0.5–1 mg q4h prn Buspirone 10–30 mg BID SSRIs varying doses

trial is performed with intrathecal injections of increasing doses of baclofen and careful monitoring of the patient's ability to walk. A bell-shaped curve is desired to best predict response to pump placement. Sometimes this treatment is so effective that patients can eliminate their oral medications, but typically less than 50% of patients referred demonstrate a good response to intrathecal baclofen.

Urinary difficulties in ALS typically manifest as increased urinary urgency, but it is unusual to have incontinence unless the patient cannot reach the bathroom in time due to mobility issues. Tolterodine (Detrol) and oxybutynin (Ditropan) may be prescribed for bladder control; a urinal or condom catheter may be useful for male patients. Prostate hypertrophy needs to be excluded as a cause for urinary urgency in men because treatment for that condition is very different. Frank incontinence or urine retention should be evaluated by a urologist because these are unusual for ALS.

Sleep disturbances are a major problem in ALS, with often multifactorial causes. Mobility issues prevent patients from being able to turn in bed, causing discomfort; difficulty breathing can cause disrupted sleep and fatigue. A hospital bed with an air mattress can be helpful; more sophisticated turning beds are also available, but sometimes the only solution is having caregivers turn the patient throughout the night. Breathing difficulties can be determined from FVC and MIF measurements along with the clinical history; a nocturnal oximetry study can be done at home during sleep to look for nocturnal desaturations. Noninvasive mechanical ventilation is an easy solution to the problem in these cases.

Sometimes even when breathing and mechanical problems are resolved, patients may still have trouble sleeping. In these cases, sedating medications such as zolpidem (Ambien), mirtazapine (Remeron), and trazodone may be effective. Although depression rarely occurs in ALS, when present, it is usually responsive to antidepressants.[43,44] Anxiety may be a sign of comorbid FTD or executive dysfunction. It is best managed with behavioral therapy and SSRIs but is often hard to fully control.[24,43] Fatigue can be managed by improving sleep, conserving energy, and taking modafinil.[45] Lastly, constipation should be managed well to avoid unnecessary discomfort. It frequently occurs in ALS due to decreased fluid intake, constipating medications, and mobility issues. Initially a high-fiber diet, hydration, and stool softeners work, but later in the disease course, stronger medications such as lactulose are needed to maintain a good bowel regimen.

Equipment Management

Advances in equipment for patients with ALS have been tremendous in the past 10 years. A myriad of options for power wheelchairs are available, including those that fold in the trunk, such as the At'm wheelchair. In addition, manual wheelchairs have become lighter and more compact. Ramps and lifts are now cheaper and more easily installed in the home for patients with stairs. Communication devices range from a simple laser pointer with an alphabet board to eye-gaze systems and even implanted brain chips. Home physical therapy and occupational therapy allow patients to receive professional guidance before remodeling their home or purchasing equipment.

Social Management

Social work involvement is critical for managing the financial, emotional, and physical impacts of the disease. The financial consequences of an ALS diagnosis can be severe. Patients may lose their jobs due to progressive weakness, and it is critical to connect

become less effective as swallowing worsens further; at that point, botulinum toxin injections into the parotid and submandibular glands are effective in drying up saliva.[42] When the saliva is dried with these medications, it often becomes thick; it can be thinned by using a humidifier, increasing fluids, and taking guiafenesin (Robitussin). Robitussin is available over the counter in liquid and pill forms and can be taken up to 400 mg every 4 hours.

For patients with significant upper motor neuron involvement, spasticity even more than weakness can limit mobility. It is important to caution patients that relieving their spasticity may cause the legs to become too limp if that spasticity is the main factor keeping them upright. It is a delicate balance between keeping patients from being too stiff or too loose to maximize function, and it is a continuously changing problem as the disease progresses. Baclofen, diazepam, and tizanidine are the main drugs used in the management of spasticity. Diazepam is usually started at 10 mg per night and increased as tolerated. Baclofen is usually started at 5 mg TID and gradually increased until maximum effectiveness. Tizanidine has more side effects than the other two drugs and is usually started at 4 mg TID. When patients have maximized medical therapy and still have refractory spasticity, a baclofen pump is considered. Usually a them with all the social services for which they are eligible, such as compensation from the Veterans Administration if they are veterans, Social Security disability, Medicare, long-term care insurance, and early payout of life insurance benefits. Patients with ALS are immediately eligible for Medicare, and veterans with ALS receive full-service connection. Counseling is often beneficial to help the patient and family cope with the stress at the time of diagnosis and as the disease progresses. The time of diagnosis has been determined to be the most stressful time of the disease process. It is important to provide patients and families as many resources as possible at this critical time.

Multidisciplinary Care

Several studies have shown the benefit of multidisciplinary care in affecting both the quality and quantity of life in ALS.[46,47] The typical multidisciplinary team includes a speech pathologist, communication specialist, dietitian, social worker, respiratory therapist, ALS nurse, neurologist, physical therapist, and occupational therapist. Other members of the team available as needed for consultation include a neuropsychologist, gastroenterologist, equipment specialist, and pulmonologist. Unfortunately, insurance reimbursement is not robust for coverage of these specialists, and few medical centers are able to offer comprehensive services for ALS patients. Both the MDA and the ALSA recognize those centers with comprehensive care, and details regarding the closest center can be obtained from either the ALSA or MDA Web sites.

End-of-Life Considerations

Once the patient's FVC is less than 30% of normal, he or she qualifies for hospice, because typically life expectancy will be less than 6 months at this point. Hospice is able to provide psychological support for the patient and family as well as other services to ensure comfort.

Many hospitals now have palliative care teams that can be employed for patients desiring to die in the hospital rather than at home or for those patients whose discomfort cannot be managed easily with home hospice. Inpatient hospice is available in some areas and is a good alternative for patients who may not have the social support or resources to be able to be maintained at home during the end stages of the disease. ALS patients rarely chose long-term ventilation, mostly due to the costs of the care, which can easily be as high as $250,000 per year. If they do chose long-term ventilation, most patients do so only for a limited time, perhaps to reach a significant milestone in their family life or until the disease progresses to the point that quality of life is not optimal (see also Chapter 8).

References

1. Shook SJ, Pioro EP: Racing against the clock: recognizing, differentiating, diagnosing, and referring the amyotrophic lateral sclerosis patient, *Ann Neurol* 65(Suppl 1):S10–S16, 2009.
2. Glenn SA, Ross MA: Delayed radiation-induced bulbar palsy mimicking ALS, *Muscle Nerve* 23(5):814–817, 2000.
3. Zhou B, Chen L, Fan D, Zhou D: Clinical features of Hirayama disease in mainland China, *Amyotroph Lateral Scler* 10:1–7, 2009.
4. Rowland LP, Shneider NA: Amyotrophic lateral sclerosis, *N Engl J Med* 344(22):1688–1700, 2001.
5. Vance C, Rogelj B, Hortobágyi T, et al: Mutations in FUS, an RNA processing protein, cause familial amyotrophic lateral sclerosis type 6, *Science* 323:1208–1211, 2009.
6. Kwiatkowski TJ Jr, Bosco DA, Leclerc AL, et al: Mutations in the FUS/TLS gene on chromosome 16 cause familial amyotrophic lateral sclerosis, *Science* 323:1205–1208, 2009.
7. Manganelli F, Iodice V, Provitera V, et al: Small-fiber involvement in spinobulbar muscular atrophy (Kennedy's disease), *Muscle Nerve* 36(6):816–820, 2007.
8. Lee JH, Shin JH, Park KP, et al: Phenotypic variability in Kennedy's disease: implication of the early diagnostic features, *Acta Neurol Scand* 112(1):57–63, 2005.
9. Sinnreich M, Klein CJ: Bulbospinal muscular atrophy: Kennedy's disease, *Arch Neurol* 61(8):1324–1326, 2004.
10. Kinirons P, Rouleau GA: Administration of testosterone results in reversible deterioration in Kennedy's disease, *J Neurol Neurosurg Psychiatry* 79(1):106–107, 2008.
11. Cuscó I, Barceló MJ, Rojas-García R, et al: SMN2 copy number predicts acute or chronic spinal muscular atrophy but does not account for intrafamilial variability in siblings, *J Neurol* 253(1):21–25, 2006.
12. Tsai LK, Yang CC, Hwu WL, Li H: Valproic acid treatment in six patients with spinal muscular atrophy, *Eur J Neurol* 14(12):e8–e9, 2007.
13. Liang WC, Yuo CY, Chang JG, et al: The effect of hydroxyurea in spinal muscular atrophy cells and patients, *J Neurol Sci* 268(1–2):87–94, 2008.
14. McDonald TD, Faust PL, Bruno C, et al: Polyglucosan body disease simulating amyotrophic lateral sclerosis, *Neurology* 43(4):785–790, 1993.
15. Dmitriev P, Lipinski M, Vassetzky YS: Pearls in the junk: dissecting the molecular pathogenesis of facioscapulohumeral muscular dystrophy, *Neuromuscul Disord* 19(1):17–20, 2009.
16. Halstead LS: Assessment and differential diagnosis for post-polio syndrome, *Orthopedics* 14(11):1209–1217, 1991.
17. Kim WK, Liu X, Sandner J, et al: Study of 962 patients indicates progressive muscular atrophy is a form of ALS, *Neurology* 73:1686–1692, 2009.
18. Van den Berg-Vos RM, Visser J, Kalmijn S, et al: A long-term prospective study of the natural course of sporadic adult-onset lower motor neuron syndromes, *Arch Neurol* 66:751–757, 2009.
19. Salinas S, Proukakis C, Crosby A, et al: Hereditary spastic paraplegia: clinical features and pathogenetic mechanisms, *Lancet Neurol* 7(12):1127–1138, 2008.
20. Sanders DB, El-Salem K, Massey JM, et al: Clinical aspects of MuSK antibody positive seronegative MG, *Neurology* 60(12):1978–1980, 2003.
21. Brooks BR, Miller RG, Swash M, et al, for the World Federation of Neurology Research Group on Motor Neuron Diseases: El Escorial revisited: revised criteria for the diagnosis of amyotrophic lateral sclerosis, *Amyotroph Lateral Scler Other Motor Neuron Disord* 1(5):293–299, 2000.
22. Strong MJ, Grace GM, Freedman M, et al: Consensus criteria for the diagnosis of frontotemporal cognitive and behavioural syndromes in amyotrophic lateral sclerosis. *Amyotroph Lateral Scler* 10:131–146, 2009; erratum in *Amyotroph Lateral Scler* 10:252, 2009.
23. Murphy J, Henry R, Lomen-Hoerth C: Establishing subtypes of the continuum of frontal lobe impairment in amyotrophic lateral sclerosis, *Arch Neurol* 64(3):330–334, 2007.
24. Olney RK, Murphy J, Forshew D, et al: The effects of executive and behavioral dysfunction on the course of ALS, *Neurology* 65(11):1774–1777, 2005.
25. Kwong LK, Neumann M, Sampathu DM, et al: TDP-43 proteinopathy: the neuropathology underlying major forms of sporadic and familial frontotemporal lobar degeneration and motor neuron disease, *Acta Neuropathol (Berl)* 114:63–70, 2007.
26. Mackenzie IR, Bigio EH, Ince PG, et al: Pathological TDP-43 distinguishes sporadic amyotrophic lateral sclerosis from amyotrophic lateral sclerosis with SOD1 mutations, *Ann Neurol* 61(5):427–434, 2007.
27. Sonoo M, Kuwabara S, Shimizu T, et al: Utility of trapezius EMG for diagnosis of amyotrophic lateral sclerosis, *Muscle Nerve* 39(1):63–70, 2009.
28. Miller RG, Rosenberg JA, Gelinas DF, et al: Practice parameter: the care of the patient with amyotrophic lateral sclerosis (an evidence-based review): report of the Quality Standards Subcommittee of the American Academy of Neurology: ALS Practice Parameters Task Force, *Neurology* 52(7):1311–1323, 1999.
29. Bensimon G, Lacomblez L, Meininger VA: controlled trial of riluzole in amyotrophic lateral sclerosis. ALS/Riluzole Study Group, *N Engl J Med* 330(9):585–591, 1994.
30. Rowland LP: Riluzole for the treatment of amyotrophic lateral sclerosis—too soon to tell? *N Engl J Med* 330(9):636–637, 1994.
31. Fornai F, Longone P, Cafaro L, et al: Lithium delays progression of amyotrophic lateral sclerosis, *Proc Natl Acad Sci U S A* 105(6):2052–2057, 2008.

32. Bedlack RS, Maragakis N, Heiman-Patterson T: Lithium may slow progression of amyotrophic lateral sclerosis, but further study is needed, *Proc Natl Acad Sci U S A* 105(16):E17, 2008.

33. Aggarwal S, Zinman L, Simpson E, et al: Clinical trial testing lithium in ALS terminates early for futility, *Lancet Neurology* 2010, in press.

34. Brooks BR: Managing amyotrophic lateral sclerosis: slowing disease progression and improving patient quality of life, *Ann Neurol* 65(Suppl 1):S17–S23, 2009.

35. Bedlack RS, Silani V, Ester Cudkowicz M: IPLEX and the Telephone Game: the difficulty in separating myth from reality on the Internet, *Amyotroph Lateral Scler* 10:1–3, 2008.

36. Gordon PH, Moore DH, Miller RG, et al: Efficacy of minocycline in patients with amyotrophic lateral sclerosis: a phase III randomised trial, *Lancet Neurol* 6(12):1045–1053, 2007.

37. Cudkowicz ME, Shefner JM, Schoenfeld DA, et al: A randomized, placebo-controlled trial of topiramate in amyotrophic lateral sclerosis, *Neurology* 61(4):456–464, 2003.

38. Onders RP, Carlin AM, Elmo M, et al: Amyotrophic lateral sclerosis: the Midwestern surgical experience with the diaphragm pacing stimulation system shows that general anesthesia can be safely performed, *Am J Surg* 197(3):386–390, 2009.

39. Forshew DA, Bromberg MB: A survey of clinicians' practice in the symptomatic treatment of ALS, *Amyotroph Lateral Scler Other Motor Neuron Disord* 4(4):258–263, 2003.

40. Lomen-Hoerth C: Amyotrophic lateral sclerosis from bench to bedside, *Semin Neurol* 28(2):205–211, 2008.

41. Brooks BR, Thisted RA, Appel SH, et al: Treatment of pseudobulbar affect in ALS with dextromethorphan/quinidine: a randomized trial, *Neurology* 63:1364–1370, 2004.

42. Jackson CE, Gronseth G, Rosenfeld J, et al: Randomized double-blind study of botulinum toxin type B for sialorrhea in ALS patients, *Muscle Nerve* 39(2):137–143, 2009.

43. Kurt A, Nijboer F, Matuz T, et al: Depression and anxiety in individuals with amyotrophic lateral sclerosis: epidemiology and management, *CNS Drugs* 21(4):279–291, 2007.

44. Rabkin JG, Albert SM, Del Bene ML, et al: Prevalence of depressive disorders and change over time in late-stage ALS, *Neurology* 65(1):62–67, 2005.

45. Rabkin JG, Gordon PH, McElhiney M, et al: Modafinil treatment of fatigue in patients with ALS: a placebo-controlled study, *Muscle Nerve* 39(3):297–303, 2009.

46. Mayadev AS, Weiss MD, Distad BJ, et al: The amyotrophic lateral sclerosis center: a model of multidisciplinary management, *Phys Med Rehabil Clin N Am* 19(3):619–631, 2008.

47. Zoccolella S, Beghi E, Palagano G, et al: LS multidisciplinary clinic and survival. Results from a population-based study in Southern Italy, *J Neurol* 254(8):1107–1112, 2007.

Cristian Ionita, MD
Susan T. Iannaccone, MD

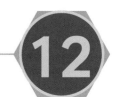

Treatment and Management of Spinal Muscular Atrophy and Congenital Myopathies

Although spinal muscular atrophy (SMA) and the congenital myopathies (CMs) have different etiologic features, they have similar clinical characteristics, and the decision to address them together is consistent with the similarities in the management of these two groups. This is not to say that there are no differences in both clinical presentations and management. When significant, these differences will be noted. Common clinical features include early onset, proximal symmetrical weakness, hypotonia, preserved mentation, and absence of extraocular involvement. Some of the severe, neonatal forms of CM resemble SMA type 1. Respiratory support is necessary frequently for both groups and there is high rate of morbidity and mortality related to restrictive lung disease (RLD). The prognosis of severe forms of CM is more favorable than that for SMA type 1. The natural history of SMA type 2 shares similarities with moderate forms of CM. RLD is the most common cause of morbidity and death in these patients. Type 3 SMA and late onset CM have a good prognosis and normal life expectancy. Both groups of disorders are genetic diseases. There is no cure for any of them.

Diagnosis and Evaluation

Spinal muscular atrophy (SMA) is an autosomal recessive neuromuscular disorder of infancy, childhood, and young adulthood. Its incidence is estimated to be 10 in 100,000 live births. First described at the end of the nineteenth century,[1,2] its causative gene, *SMN1*, was discovered in 1995.[3] Homozygous deletion or other mutations of the *SMN1* gene located on chromosome 5q causes degeneration of anterior horn motor neurons. 5q SMA represents 95% of all SMAs. The rest represent a heterogeneous group of disorders sharing the same involvement of anterior horn motor neurons, such as Kennedy disease, SMA with respiratory distress (SMARD), Hirayama disease, and juvenile amyotrophic lateral sclerosis. Clinical entities with established genetic linkage are included in Table 12-1. SMA is characterized by progressive, predominantly proximal symmetrical muscle weakness with normal sensation, depressed or absent reflexes, and preserved cognition. An acute phase of rapid decline in muscle strength is followed by a phase of relative stabilization, which extends over long periods of time. This course is especially evident in type 2 and 3 SMA. At the time of diagnosis, most patients are already in the chronic phase.

Since the initial classification in 1961,[4] multiple classification systems were described. A largely accepted classification includes types 1 to 3. Type 1 patients have symptom onset in the first 6 months, are able to sit supported, and die by age 2 years. Respiratory involvement is severe. Pectus excavatum and paradoxical breathing are common (Fig. 12-1). With aggressive respiratory intervention, life can be prolonged in some of these patients, this being a subject of intense ethical debate. Type 2 SMA is characterized by onset between 6 and 18 months; patients sit unsupported and survive into young adulthood or later. They have proximal symmetrical muscle weakness of the lower extremities more than upper. They often present with failure to walk. Type 3 patients have onset after 18 months of age, walk independently at some time, and can have normal life expectancy. Some lose ambulation by midadolescence and some develop RLD. A functional classification is based on the maximal motor milestone attained and consists of three groups.[5] The nonsitter group corresponds to type 1, sitter group with type 2, and walker group with type 3. This clinical heterogeneity was in great part explained with the discovery of the *SMN2* gene whose transcription produces a small amount of full length (fl-) SMN protein. In general, the more copies of *SMN2* gene, the less severe and the later the onset of the disease.[6] Classically, SMA diagnosis used to rely on electrodiagnostic studies (EDS) (denervation with normal motor and sensory nerve conductions) and muscle biopsy (grouped atrophy). Currently, targeted mutation analysis is used to detect deletion of exons 7 and 8 of the *SMN1* gene and it is the initial test in an infant or child with typical presentation. A homozygous *SMN1* deletion is diagnostic. Serum creatine kinase (CK) can be normal or mildly elevated in SMA. Serum CK values above 500 U/L should direct the diagnostic workup toward a myopathy. If targeted mutation analysis detects one copy of the *SMN1* gene in an otherwise typical patient, gene sequencing is necessary as a small proportion of SMA patients (2%–5%) may have an intragenic mutation of *SMN1*. Occasional patients with double heterozygote *SMN1* point mutations are seen. *SMN1* gene sequencing should be considered in typical patients with two *SMN1* copies and negative SMARD genetic testing. If SMA genetic testing is negative, then 5q SMA is not confirmed and further testing with EDS and with muscle and nerve biopsy should be pursued.

Congenital myopathies (CMs) are a genetically and pathologically heterogeneous group of muscle disorders that share a similar clinical picture dominated by neonatal or infantile weakness and hypotonia,

Table 12-1 Clinical Motor Neuron Entities with Established Genetic Linkage

Clinical Entity	Gene	Linkage	Inheritance	Age at Onset	Genetic Testing	Clinical Features
Distal SMA Syndromes						
Distal HMN type I	?	7q34–q36?	AD	2–20 years	N/A	Peroneal muscular atrophy and normal life expectancy
Distal HMN type II	HSPB8	12q24.3	AD	20–40 years	Clinical	Allelic with CMT2L
	HSPB	7q11.23	AD	Juvenile-adulthood	Clinical	Allelic with CMT2F; some with onset as early as age 4
Distal HMN type III	?	11q13	AR	Infancy to early adulthood	N/A	Distal weakness Diaphragm involvement possible
Distal HMN type IV	PLEKHG5	1p36	AR	Childhood	Research	Generalized weakness, progressive
Distal HMN type V	GARS	7p15	AD	Adolescent-young adult	Clinical	Upper limb weakness, slow progression; Allelic with CMT2D
Distal HMN type V (Silver phenotype)	BSCL2	11q12–q14	AD	Childhood-adulthood	Clinical	Upper limb weakness, lower limb spasticity
Distal HMN type VI (SMARD1)	IGHMBP2	11q13.2–13.4	AR	Infantile	Clinical	Severe form with early respiratory distress
Distal HMN type VII (with vocal cord paralysis)	?	2q14	AD	Childhood	N/A	Upper extremity distal weakness and atrophy, vocal cord paralysis,
	DCTN1	2p13	AD	Young adult	Clinical	Upper extremities weakness and atrophy, vocal cord paralysis, facial weakness
Distal HMNJ (Jerash type)	?	9p21.1–p12	AR	Childhood	N/A	Pyramidal signs
Distal HMN/ALS 4	SETX	9q34	AD	Childhood to young adult	Clinical	Pyramidal signs
Distal HMN X-linked (SMAX3)	?	Xq13–q21	X-L	Childhood	N/A	Feet deformities, slow progression
Distal SMA congenital	?	12q23–q24	AD	Congenital	N/A	Arthrogryposis, lower extremities weakness, nonprogressive
Proximal SMA Syndromes						
SMA type 1				<6 months		Severe, never sit, fatal before age of 2
SMA type 2	SMN1	5q12.2–q13.3	AR	6–18 months	Clinical	Chronic, sit independently, lower extremity predominance
SMA type 3				>18 months		Chronic, walk independently, milder
Kennedy disease (SMAX1)	Androgen receptor	Xq11–q12	X-L R	20–40 years	Clinical	Mostly adults, occasional teenager; gynecomastia, bulbar involvement, hyperlipoproteinemia
SMA infantile X-linked (SMAX2)	UBE1	Xp11.23	X-L R	Neonatal, early infantile	Research	Severe, fatal arthrogryposis, fractures
Scapuloperoneal SMA New England type	?	12q24.1–q24.31	AD	Young adult to adult	N/A	Scapuloperoneal weakness

AD, autosomal dominant; AR, autosomal recessive; BSCL2, seipin; DCTN1, dynactin; GARS, glycyl tRNA synthetase; HMN, hereditary motor neuropathy; HSPB1, heat shock 27-kD protein 1; HSPB8, heat shock 22-kD protein 8; IGHMBP2, immunoglobulin μ-binding protein 2; PLEKHG5, pleckstrin homology domain-containing family G member 5; SETX, senataxin; SMA, spinal muscular atrophy; SMN1, survival motor neuron 1; UBE1, ubiquitin-activating enzyme 1; X-L R, X-linked recessive (see also Table 13-1).

and characteristic morphologic changes on muscle biopsy (Table 12-2). Facial and bulbar weakness are common. Extraocular muscles are usually not involved but ptosis is nearly universal. Other common characteristics include early feeding problems, small muscle bulk, craniofacial deformities, and spine and limb deformities. CK level is normal or mildly elevated.

The incidence of CM is estimated to be 6 in 100,000.[7] More than 40 entities are described; many of them are still awaiting full recognition. The most common and better described are central core

disease (CCD), nemaline myopathy (NM), and centronuclear/myotubular myopathy (MM). Although many disease genes are now known, the genotype does not always predict phenotype. Genetic testing is available for some CMs (see Table 12-2). The spectrum of severity of CM extends from fatal neonatal forms to minimally symptomatic adult forms. Most CMs have a nonprogressive course.

CCD typically presents with infantile hypotonia and delayed motor milestones. Neonatal cases do occur and tend to be severe.[8]

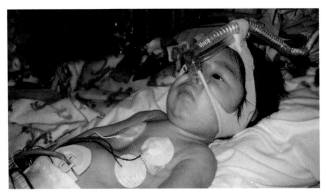

Figure 12-1 Paradoxical breathing in infant with type 1 spinal muscular atrophy on Infant Flow SiPAP by nasal mask.

Central cores lacking oxidative activity are seen usually in type 1 muscle fibers by light microscopy. Most cases are associated with *RYR1* gene mutations.

NM is a genetically heterogeneous entity. The congenital forms present with "floppy infant" syndrome, delayed motor milestones, or gait abnormalities. Respiratory involvement is severe in the neonatal onset group (severe and intermediate congenital forms); many patients succumb because of respiratory failure or aspiration pneumonia in the first year of life.

MM is characterized by centrally located nuclei that resemble fetal myotubules. The X-linked severe form has prenatal onset and high mortality and morbidity rates from pulmonary complications in the first year of life.[9] The disease gene was identified as *MTM1*.[10] MM is often associated with vertical gaze palsy that may progress to complete ophthalmoplegia.

Table 12-2 Identified Genes in Congenital Myopathies and Congenital Muscular Dystrophies

Congenital Myopathy	Genes	Chromosomal Locus	Inheritance	Testing
Nemaline myopathy	*ACTA1*	10q22–q24	AD/AR	Clinical
	TPM3	1q22–q23	AD/AR	Clinical
	NEB	2q22	AR	Clinical
	TPM2	9p13.2–p13.1	AD	Research
	TNNT1	19q13.4	AD?	Research
Central core disease	*RYR1*	19q13.1	AD/AR	Clinical
X-linked myotubular myopathy	*MTM1*	Xq28	X-linked recessive	Clinical
Centronuclear myopathy	*DNM2*	19q13.2	AD	Clinical
Multiminicore disease	*SEPN1*	1p36–p35	AR	Clinical
	RYR1	19q13.1	AR	Clinical
Congenital myopathy with fiber-type disproportion	*ACTA1*	10q22–q24	AD	Clinical
	SEPN1	1p36–p35	AR	Clinical
	TPM3	1q22–q23	AD	Clinical
Myofibrillar myopathy	*DES*	2q35	AD/AR?	Clinical
	CRYAB	11q22.3–q23.1	AD	Research
	MYOT	5q31	AD	Research
	LDB3	10q22.2–q23.3	AD	Clinical
	FLNC	7q32	AD	Research
Hyaline body myopathy	*MYH7*	14q12	AD	Clinical
Walker-Warburg syndrome	*POMT1*	9q34.1	AR	Clinical
	POMT2	14q24.3	AR	Clinical
Fukuyama CMD	*FCMD*	9q31	AR	Clinical
Muscle-eye-brain disease	*POMGnT1*	1p34–p33	AR	Clinical
CMD type 1D	*LARGE*	22q12.3–q13.1	AR	Clinical
CMD 1A	*LAMA2*	6q22–q23	AR	Clinical
CMD 1C	*FKRP*	19q13.3	AR	Clinical
CMD with integrin alpha-7 mutation	*ITGA7*	12q13	AR	Clinical
CMD with rigid spine	*SEPN1*	1p36–p35	AR	Clinical
Ullrich CMD	*COL6A1*	21q22.3	AR/AD	Clinical
	COL6A2	21q22.3	AR/AD	Clinical
	COL6A3	2q37	AR/AD	Clinical
Epidermolysis bullosa CMD	*Plectin1*	8q24.3	AR	Research

ACTA1, actin alpha skeletal muscle 1; AD, autosomal dominant; AR, autosomal recessive; CMD, congenital muscular dystrophy; COL6A1, COL6A2, COL6A3, collagen, type 6 subunit alpha-1, alpha-2, and alpha-3, respectively; CRYAB, alpha-beta crystalline; DES, desmin; DNM2, dynamin 2; FCMD, fukutin; FKRP, fuktin-related protein; FLNC, filamin C; ITGA7, integrin alpha7; LAMA2, laminin alpha-2 chain; LARGE, glycosyltransferase-like protein; LDB3, LIM domain-binding protein; MTM1, myotubularin; MYH7, myosin heavy chain 7; MYOT, myotilin; NEB, nebulin; POMT1, protein *O*-mannosyltransferase 1; POMT2, protein *O*-mannosyltransferase 2; POMGnT1, protein *O*-mannoside beta-1,2-*N*-acetylglucosaminyltransferase 1; RYR1, ryanodine receptor 1; SEPN1, selenoprotein N1; TNNT1, troponin T1; TPM2, tropomyosin beta-2 chain; TPM3, tropomyosin alpha-3 chain (see also Table 19-1).

Treatment and Management

Current management is focused on symptomatic treatment of the complications of weakness and hypotonia while maintaining quality of life.[11-14] Management is multidisciplinary and should take place in specialized neuromuscular clinics under direct supervision of a pediatric subspecialist (usually a pediatric neurologist) with expertise in SMA and CM. Specialties involved should, at minimum, include orthopedics, pulmonology, and gastroenterology as well as a physical therapist and speech therapist. The family physician should remain involved for emergency or triage care. Patient and parent education is paramount and should start at the time of diagnosis. Parents should be exposed to all available options of treatment/palliation and supported to make the best decisions in their particular circumstance. They should have a clinic contact number and clear guidelines for when to seek medical attention and fast access into the specialty hospital.

Developmental Delay

Muscle weakness leads to developmental delay. Gross motor milestones are predominantly affected with sparing of cognitive and social skills. Fine motor skills are variably affected. With few exceptions, CMs have a stable, nonprogressive course, while regression of motor milestones is the hallmark of SMA. Regression may not be obvious in infants with type 1 SMA as no significant milestones are achieved. SMA type 2 and 3 patients lose milestones (sitting/walking) after variable periods of time.

Children with SMA have normal intelligence, demonstrate good social skills, and often appear more mature than their peers. Their verbal intelligence quotient (IQ) is higher than average by adolescence, probably as a compensation to their physical disability.[15] With some exceptions, CM patients have normal intelligence.[16,17] Proper educational placement is important. Too often, their normal intelligence is overlooked and school placement is based on their motor handicaps. This leads to deficient education and psychological trauma in these children, who are already at high risk for low self-esteem. When in doubt, formal neuropsychological testing should be used to guide school placement. The level of education correlates with level of employment as adults.[18]

Failure to Thrive and Gastroenterologic Complications

Thirty-seven percent of patients with SMA type 2 have weight 2 SD below normal.[19] Most of the CM patients are underweight as well, some of them severely. The main causes for failure to thrive (FTT) are dysphagia, fatigue during feeding, chewing difficulties, and limitation in mouth opening (seen especially in older patients with SMA). Other factors, including depression, hypersalivation, and poor dentition, may have a role. In older patients, weakness of the arm may affect feeding. All these factors may lead to long feeding times and decreased caloric intake. Increased work of breathing induces increased energy expenditure. FTT exacerbates muscle weakness and increases susceptibility for infections.[20] Greater awareness of malnutrition (low basal metabolic index, BMI) and its deleterious effects justifies an aggressive approach with early percutaneous gastrostomy placement. Gastrostomy plays a role in increased survival in patients with SMA type 1.[21]

Assessment of feeding and swallowing by a speech therapist should be considered in every child with SMA and CM. Simple questioning about change in diet, feeding time, and choking or coughing during feeding, although very important, may fail to identify dysphagia. Observing the patient during feeding can be informative. A modified barium swallow test (video fluoroscopy) is necessary for suspected dysphagia and when there is recurrent or aspiration pneumonia. Barium swallow test not only proves swallowing dysfunction and microaspiration but also guides interventions. An upper gastrointestinal series is recommended before placement of the gastrostomy tube. Initial interventions include change in food consistency and caloric content, small frequent meals, and adjustment in positioning during and after feeding. In patients with severe swallowing difficulties, institution of an alternate feeding route is indicated.[20] There are currently no randomized clinical trials to evaluate the efficacy of different methods of treatment for dysphagia[22]; current recommendations are based on expert opinion.[23] When conservative measures fail and high risk of aspiration persists, gastrostomy placement remains the preferred alternative. Occasionally, the older patient may choose intermittent nasogastric tube placement instead of permanent gastrostomy. Temporary nasogastric tube can be used in patients awaiting gastrostomy placement.

There is disagreement between experts about the timing of gastrostomy placement in SMA.[23] Early placement of gastrostomy tube has the advantage of better respiratory status at the time of intervention. In addition, early gastrostomy placement may prevent episodes of pneumonia or aspiration. A minimally invasive procedure, such as percutaneous endoscopic gastrostomy, is preferred. When simultaneous Nissen fundoplication is necessary, laparoscopic approach is preferred to open surgical approach.

Delayed gastric emptying and gastroesophageal reflux (GER) are frequent in type 1 and severe type 2 SMA as well as severe CM. Frequent "spitting up" and vomiting, food regurgitation, and chest discomfort as well as frequent pulmonary infections are common presentations of GER. Fatal episodes of aspiration pneumonia are well recognized complications in these children.[13,24] Treatment of GER can be medical or surgical. Stable patients may benefit from a trial of antireflux medication (i.e., proton pump inhibitors or histamine blockers). However, a recent study reveals increased incidence of pneumonia in patients taking gastric acid inhibitors for GER disease.[25] Those with severe reflux and respiratory compromise will benefit from a combined laparoscopic gastrostomy and an antireflux procedure like Nissen fundoplication. Gastric emptying can be improved with erythromycin and metoclopramide.

As a consequence of abdominal muscle weakness, hypotonia, and immobility, constipation is common in type 1 and type 2 SMA and severe forms of CM. It is usually associated with abdominal distention and bloating that together may negatively affect respiratory status. In general, constipation in SMA responds to dietary changes: increase fiber intake and hydration. Ambulatory patients are less likely to develop constipation.

Often overlooked, xerostomia causes discomfort and predisposes to dental breakdown and can be treated with artificial saliva. Excessive salivation can be treated with glycopyrrolate and atropine.

Orthopedic Deformities

Although infrequent in young "nonsitters," scoliosis develops in a majority of type 2 and type 3 SMA patients as a consequence of weakness and immobility. The age of onset is around 4 and 9 years for "sitter" group and "walker" group, respectively. It remains mild while the patient is ambulatory and rapidly worsens once wheelchair bound.[26] Typically, scoliosis seen in SMA is a single, C-shaped curve that involves the predominantly thoracolumbar segments.[27] As it progresses, sacrum can be involved with consequent pelvic obliquity.[28] Often scoliosis has a progressive course despite the nonprogressive weakness of many forms of CM. Scoliosis worsens RLD, impedes sitting and mobility, causes ischial bursitis, leads to back and chest wall pain, and may cause functional loss of the arm. Although there is only weak evidence that spinal orthotics slow progression, orthotics are often recommended in young patients with curves larger than 40 degrees.[29] Scoliosis worsens at different rates despite bracing, progressing faster (8 degrees/year) in type 1 SMA and slower (3 degrees/year) in milder cases.[30] Spinal bracing in SMA patients with type 1 and type 2 may cause decreased tidal breathing. Initial fitting with a spinal brace and subsequent adjustments should be coordinated with the pulmonary team.[31,32] In order to minimize the effect on tidal breathing, spinal orthotics should have an abdominal cutout to allow free diaphragm movements.[23]

Surgical correction of scoliosis is generally recommended once the curvature worsens over 50 to 60 degrees[29] (see also Chapter 9). In patients with severe scoliosis, surgical intervention may have a palliative goal of relieving the pain secondary to impingements on the ribs. Preoperative evaluation should include respiratory, neurologic, and rehabilitation assessment in order to achieve the best possible functional status. Evidence exists for beneficial effects of surgical correction of scoliosis in this population. The benefits include improved sitting balance, improved endurance,[33] improved aesthetic appearance, and an increased sense of well-being.[34] A majority of studies report a correction of 40% to 60% of the preoperative angle of curvature.[34,35] Respiratory function continues to deteriorate after surgery but the rate of deterioration appears to be slower.[36] With advances in noninvasive ventilation and assisted cough devices, spine surgery is relatively safe even in type 1 SMA patients. More frequent complications of spine surgery include pseudarthrosis, failed correction, infectious complications, and respiratory failure. Frequently surgical intervention in flexible patients is preceded by traction to decrease the curve as much as possible prior to surgery. Traction has a positive effect on respiratory function as well.[35] Spine surgery should be undertaken under continuous somatosensory evoked potentials (SSEPs) monitoring to avoid permanent motor dysfunction. Posterior approach with fusion and segmental instrumentation is preferred for correction of neuromuscular scoliosis. An anterior approach may be necessary in the most severe cases but requires good respiratory function.[29] Harrington and Luque rod instrumentation is frequently used. Fusion to the pelvis is advocated in order to prevent further worsening of pelvic obliquity. Postoperative immobilization can be avoided if new techniques of posterior segmental fixation (pedicle screw fixation, sublaminar wires) instead of posterior fusion and instrumentation are used.[37] Young children with significant scoliosis may benefit from a dual growing rod technique that allows spinal growth while maintaining the initial correction. This approach may avoid subsequent lengthening procedures.[38]

Hip dislocation is common in nonambulatory children with both SMA and CM. Age of onset varies with severity of their weakness, ranging from 3 to 4 years in nonsitters to teenage years in sitters. It can be unilateral or bilateral. Mildly affected patients can develop hip subluxation.[28] A relationship of causality between pelvic obliquity and hip dislocation was not proved.[26] Surgical correction of hip dislocation is not recommended in patients with type 2 SMA.[39,40] There is a high rate of redislocation after surgical correction in patients with SMA.[40,41] Treatment of hip dislocation in various forms of CM is not well studied, with both conservative and surgical approaches being used. In general, a more aggressive stance is needed in patients with milder disease.

Congenital clubfoot occurs occasionally in patients with genetically proven SMA as well as some CMs.[42–44] A combination of serial casting and surgical repair may be effective.

Acquired equinovarus deformity is frequently seen in nonambulatory SMA patients. Type 3 SMA patients may develop equinovarus deformity that responds well to ankle-foot orthoses.[28] MM patients have a high incidence of equinovarus deformity, with

onset from birth to 6 years. The deformity responds well to treatment with ankle-foot orthoses but may require Achilles tendon lengthening.[45]

Large joint contractures are frequently seen in SMA and CM. The joints most frequently and severely involved are hips and knees and are directly related to the amount of time spent sitting. Upper extremity joint contractures tend to remain mild. A flexion contracture of more than 45 degrees is considered intractable. Stretching and passive range-of-motion exercises are the recommended initial intervention. However, night splints that apply tension to stretch tendons during sleep can be much more effective than passive stretch. Otherwise, surgical soft tissue release can be performed, keeping in mind that there is a significant risk of recurrence without postoperative bracing. The treatment goal should be adjusted to patient functional status and potential for ambulation. Because most patients are unlikely to ambulate independently, the goals should be improving seating, preventing hip subluxations, and reducing pain.

Congenital fractures have been reported in SMA type 1 and congenital NM.[24] Congenital fractures in SMA are secondary to intrauterine immobility, although recent studies suggest an intrinsic role of SMN1 in bone remodeling.[46] Patients with SMA may have the lowest bone mineral density of all neuromuscular patients.[47] As a consequence, SMA type 2 and 3 patients have significantly increased risk of bone fractures as compared to general population. Common locations for fractures include vertebrae, femur (with a relative risk [RR] of 15.1 when compared with the general population), lower leg, and arm. Approximately one fifth of fractures result in loss of function. The main predictor of fracture is the use of a wheelchair, consistent with the importance of ambulation for bone health.[48] Frequent fractures were noted in patients with MM,[45] NM,[24] and other forms of CM.

Dual-energy x-ray absorptiometry scans can be useful for assessment of bone mineral density and identification of patients at risk for fractures.[47] However, there are still issues to be resolved regarding the validity of this test in SMA patients. Maintaining ambulation is probably the most important factor in prevention of bone fractures, and monitoring dietary calcium and vitamin D intake is important.

Facial and Jaw Deformities

Craniofacial abnormalities are secondary to facial weakness. Frequently encountered deformities in CM include high, narrow palate; micrognathia; retrognathia; temporomandibular joint (TMJ) contracture; and open mouth. Although craniofacial abnormalities are prominent in CM, they occur in SMA as well.[49] The main consequences are malocclusion and jaw deformities. An open mouth and taking nothing by mouth (NPO) predispose patients to dental problems and occasionally create significant air leak that may interfere with proper mask ventilation.

Pulmonary Management

The past two decades have brought major technological advances for children with SMA and CM. Such advances include interfaces (masks) made of patient-friendly materials, in all sizes for all ages, as well as portable ventilators and bilevel positive airway pressure (BiPAP) and devices for airway clearance. Pathophysiology of respiratory failure in SMA is depicted in Figure 12-2.

Weak Cough

Weakness of inspiratory and expiratory muscles results in ineffective cough, which may lead to atelectasis and predispose the patient to pneumonia. Cough ability is further impaired during respiratory

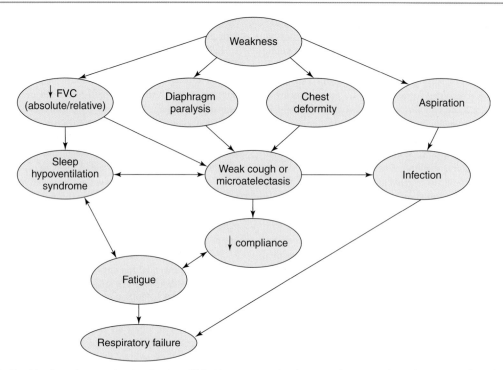

Figure 12-2 Algorithm for pulmonary deterioration in a child with neuromuscular disease and restrictive lung disease. FVC, forced vital capacity.

infections.[50] Weak cough is one of the initial manifestations of RLD in patients with SMA and CM. While a peak cough flow (PCF) of 160 to 200 L/min is considered sufficient for airway clearance, a PCF of 270 L/min may be necessary to overcome cough impairment during respiratory infections.[51]

Simple measures such as proper air humidity and good hydration decrease mucus viscosity.

Manual techniques for secretion mobilization include chest physiotherapy and postural drainage, often used together. The caregiver should be taught these techniques as well as the use of oximetry and PCF measurements to help guide therapy. Postural drainage and chest percussion remain useful, especially in young patients with SMA and CM who cannot actively participate in therapy.[52] Mechanical chest percussion devices are available, some of them designed for neonates and young infants (Neo-Cussor, General Physical Therapy, St. Louis, MO).

Different respiratory muscle training techniques (autogenic drainage, positive expiratory pressure therapy, and flutter valve) as well as devices that use oscillations of air column (Acapella, Smiths Medical Inc., Carlsbad, CA; and Quake, Thayer Medical, Tucson, AZ) rely on good respiratory muscle function and are unlikely to be useful in SMA and CM, except in mildly affected patients.

Augmentation of a patient's expiratory cough effort with few abdominal thrusts provided by a caregiver improves PCF in neuromuscular patients with RLD. If, in addition, an inspiratory assist is provided, the PCF is further increased. This can be accomplished by a number of modalities (glossopharyngeal breathing, air stacking, use of Ambu-bag, or intermittent positive pressure breathing [IPPB] device). IPPB devices are scarce but can be used at home as well as in hospital and are inexpensive. At home, IPPB therapy is usually performed two to four times a day, depending upon patient clinical status. Pressures used in one study in children varied between 22 and 40 mbar.[53] Higher pressures are not recommended because of risk of pneumothorax.

Out of the mechanically assisted cough devices, CoughAssist (mechanical insufflator-exsufflator [MI-E]) gained popularity within the SMA population and is helpful for all patients with RLD. This device provides a deep insufflation followed abruptly by application of a negative, expiratory pressure mimicking the rate and flow of air during natural cough. MI-E was proved beneficial for both adults[54] and children[55] with ineffective cough secondary to neuromuscular weakness. MI-E was well tolerated in children at pressures as high as 40 cm $H_2O/-40$ cm H_2O, with significant improvement in a number of respiratory parameters (sniff nasal inspiratory pressure [SNIP], PCF/peak expiratory flow [PEF]).[56] MI-E can be used prophylactically, but it is especially useful in the setting of infection and atelectasis. Early use can prevent hospitalizations and shorten recovery time. However, there is significant cost difference between the relatively inexpensive IPPB and MI-E. Appeals to insurance carriers are often successful in finding reimbursement for individual cases.

Other devices, such as The Vest (Hill-Rom, Batesville, IN) and Impulsator Percussionator Ventilator (IPV) (Percussionaire, Sandpoint, ID), loosen secretions in the small airways and may be helpful in preparation for assisted cough. IPV use reduced days of antibiotic requirement and hospitalization for respiratory infection in adolescents with neuromuscular disease.[57]

The use of different airway clearance techniques and devices should be individualized for each patient. They should be instituted as soon as the PCF drops. Patients with mild impairment may require airway clearance only during respiratory infection, while those more affected may benefit from daily use. In the hospital, these techniques must be used aggressively for treatment of any respiratory congestion. Use preoperatively, postoperatively, and at the time of extubation may be crucial.

Recurrent Infections

As a consequence of weak cough, children with SMA and CM develop respiratory infections more frequently than people in the general population. Most episodes of pneumonia and atelectasis follow upper respiratory infections when excessive secretions accumulate and become secondarily infected. Lower lobe pneumonia is frequent. Its clinical appearance is initially mild with only low-grade fever and tachypnea. Guidelines for treatment of acute respiratory infections in patients with neuromuscular weakness have been published.[51] Aggressive therapy should be initiated at home with use of assisted cough devices. This, by itself, may prevent hospitalization.[58] Treatment with broad-spectrum antibiotics should be initiated early, but oral antibiotics are generally ineffective. In the hospital, the patient will require frequent clinical evaluations and continuous monitoring of oxygen saturation and blood gases. Supplemental oxygen may be necessary in the face of hypoxemia secondary to pneumonia or atelectasis. However, supplemental oxygen without ventilation should not be used without a clear indication. Careful monitoring for hypercapnia and respiratory rate is mandatory. Aggressive airway clearance should be instituted under respiratory care coordination. With persistent hypoxemia, mechanical ventilation may be necessary. First consideration should be given to noninvasive positive pressure ventilation via mask. In the hospital, this is usually accomplished with a pressure-controlled ventilator with a backup rate and delivered through a face mask or nasal mask. Continuous noninvasive ventilation is initiated for patients with respiratory failure ($P_{CO_2} >$ 50 mm Hg). With improvement, over several days, a slow wean of noninvasive ventilation to the premorbid level is done. Only if this fails or there are clear contraindications to noninvasive ventilation should intubation follow. The relative contraindications for noninvasive ventilation include high risk of aspiration, mental status change, life-threatening hypoxemia, and cardiac instability. Nutritional support is important in critically ill patients. Since respiratory distress increases the risk of aspiration, patients should be NPO. A nasogastric tube (NGT) or nasojejunal tube should be placed.[58] Some patients may require total parenteral nutrition for a few days.

Aspiration

Aspiration secondary to dysphagia, weak cough, and GER is a significant cause of morbidity and death in these patients. It can take the form of the life-threatening event or a silent, repeated event. Fatal aspiration can occur in the setting of mild pulmonary disease.[24] Repeated microaspirations are often responsible for an increased incidence of chest infection. Early placement of gastrostomy tube (GT) and concomitant Nissen fundoplication is well tolerated even in children with type 1 SMA and may decrease the number of admissions and optimize quality of life.[59,60] IPV has been successfully used in treatment of refractory segmental atelectasis secondary to aspiration.[61]

Sleep-disordered Breathing

Sleep-disordered breathing (SDB) is an early and common complication of neuromuscular RLD. Early recognition and treatment of SDB improves quality of life and chance of survival.[62] SDB is a direct consequence of sleep-related changes: decreased muscle tone especially during the REM (rapid eye movement) stage, decrease of the respiratory drive, and increase in upper airway resistance. These changes pose a significant burden on the already limited respiratory reserve of these patients. Sleep-disordered breathing evolves over time from REM-associated hypopneas to REM hypopneas and hypoventilation and finally to non-REM nocturnal hypoventilation. Nocturnal hypoventilation will often progress to daytime hypoventilation and respiratory failure in SMA patients.[63] In SMA, the diaphragm is relatively spared; this is not the case in CMs, in particular NM. Involvement of the diaphragm puts patients at high risk for nocturnal hypoventilation, especially during REM sleep, when the diaphragm remains the main respiratory muscle. Occasional patients with

CM may have decreased respiratory drive of central origin, independent of muscle weakness.[64] Severe nocturnal hypoventilation with hypercapnia and cor pulmonale was described in NM with diaphragm paralysis despite relatively normal gross motor function. Patients responded well to nocturnal noninvasive ventilation.[65]

Until recently, SDB in children was frequently overlooked and intervention delayed until after onset of daytime hypoventilation.[66] New care guidelines for children with RLD include annual monitoring of forced vital capacity (FVC) and polysomnography. For young patients who cannot cooperate with spirometry, a history of frequent chest infections, early morning end tidal (ET) CO_2 measurement, and blood gases help in assessing the risk of SDB. FVC less than 65% predicted indicated a high risk of SDB in children with RLD. Nocturnal hypoventilation may be confirmed with polysomnography or overnight oxymetry.[51] If nocturnal noninvasive ventilation is started, regular, at least annual, reevaluation with overnight oximetry or polysomnography should be performed in order to assess effects and guide adjustments as the child grows. A number of CM and type 1 SMA patients will have a superimposed pattern of upper airway obstruction secondary to facial and cranial abnormalities or bulbar weakness. Fortunately, the treatment for nocturnal hypoventilation and obstructive apnea is similar. If untreated, nocturnal hypoventilation may progress to daytime hypoventilation and often causes daytime somnolence and poor school performance.[67] Nocturnal ventilation is initiated with BiPAP. Occasionally, as patients reach late adolescence, BiPAP may be replaced by a pressure-controlled ventilator using the same interface.[68]

Psychosocial Issues

Secondary to motor deficits, wheelchair use, and dependence on respiratory technology, children with SMA and CM cannot participate in many age-related physical and social activities. Their physical, social, and school functioning is reduced with a decreased quality of life when compared to healthy children. This not only creates a degree of isolation but also represents a challenge for their self-esteem. Owing to their normal intelligence, these children are able to adapt. Normal mother-infant bonding requires close contact, nursing, and intimacy; this is often compromised in SMA infants. Stress in families affected by SMA is high secondary to a number of factors (social isolation, conflicts within family, permanent commitment to the child in need, job-related problems, and financial factors), but it does not appear to be affected by use of home mechanical ventilation.[69] Interestingly, the healthy siblings of patients with SMA seem to suffer from more behavioral problems than SMA patients.[70] Somewhat unexpected, depression appears to be rare in children with SMA. However, when there is loss of mobility, adolescents express disappointment.[68] In general, children and adolescents with SMA have a low rate of psychiatric comorbidity, not different from control individuals.[71] The most common psychiatric comorbidity was separation anxiety disorder.[70] A number of studies revealed that the quality of life of children with neuromuscular disorders is higher than expected.[71–73]

Novel Therapies

In the absence of a specific cure, a number of pathways for therapeutic intervention in SMA have been considered. The main focus is on neuroprotection and compounds that increase *SMN2* expression. *SMN1* (telomeric) and *SMN2* (centromeric) genes have a single nucleotide difference, which causes production of a truncated protein that lacks exon 7 (delta 7-SMN) by *SMN2*.[74] The severity of SMA is ameliorated by *SMN2* copies. Milder cases have more *SMN2* copies.[74,75] The *SMN2* gene produces only a small amount of full-length SMN mRNA. Animal studies showed that increasing the amount of SMN2 protein, even the truncated form, may be a reasonable therapeutic option.[11,76,77] Physiologically, gene transcription is inhibited by a large group of proteins, histone deacetylases (HDACs). Inhibitors of HDACs (HDACIs) can increase transcription of certain genes, including the *SMN2* gene.[78] HDACIs include valproic acid, phenylbutyrate, and hydroxyurea. Current research effort is focused on a number of targets: the National Institute of Neurological Disorders and Stroke (NINDS), through the "SMA Project," is involved in identification and testing of candidate therapies and compounds at the preclinical level. Collaborative clinical trial groups are focused on testing candidate compounds already available in the marketplace. American SMA Randomized Trials (AmSMART), Project Cure SMA, and Pediatric Neuromuscular Clinical Research Network are the three North American collaborative groups. Similar groups exist in Europe (European Neuromuscular Center). Clinical trials in SMA face a number of challenges to enrollment: fragility of type 1 SMA patients, lack of standardized care, and lack of surrogate markers.[79] Outcome measures for muscle strength, gross motor function, pulmonary function, and quality of life were validated for a spectrum of ages in the last decade. Current research is directed at identification of surrogate markers for SMA that might eliminate the need for large numbers of subjects and long periods of observation. The low incidence of CMs and their great genetic heterogeneity explains the lack of trials in these disorders. One single trial in NM showed improvement in bulbar function with L-tyrosine.[80] A list of completed and ongoing drug trials in SMA is compiled in Table 12-3.

Table 12-3 Treatments for Spinal Muscular Atrophy

Study	Drug	Proposed Mechanism	Patients (number/ SMA type)	Type of Study	Status	Outcome
Weihl et al[81]	Valproic acid	Increases SMN2 expression	7/SMA type 3 and 4	Open label, pilot	Completed	Modest improvement in muscle strength and function
Brichta et al[82]	Valproic acid	Increases SMN2 expression	10 SMA carriers, 20 SMA patients (types 1, 2, 3)	Open label pilot	Completed	7/10 carriers and 7/20 patients with SMA showed increased SMN2 mRNA levels
Kinali et al[83]	Albuterol	Beta-2 agonist (has anabolic effect on muscle)	13/SMA types 2, 3	Open label pilot	Completed	Modest increase in muscle strength, forced vital capacity, and lean body mass
Miller et al[84]	Gabapentin	Neuroprotection	84/SMA types 2, 3	randomized, double-blind placebo control	Completed	No difference between the placebo and drug groups
Merlini et al[85]	Gabapentin	Neuroprotection	120/SMA types 2, 3	Randomized Gabapentin vs. no treatment	Completed	Modest improvement in strength
Mercuri et al[86]	Phenylbutyrate	Increases SMN2 expression	10/SMA type 2	Open label pilot	Completed	Modest improvement of function
Mercuri et al[87]	Phenylbutyrate	Increases SMN2 expression	107/SMA type 2	Randomized double blind placebo control	Completed	No functional improvement
Russman et al[88]	Riluzole	Glutamate inhibitor, neuroprotection	10/SMA type 1 (7/10 riluzole; 3/10 placebo)	Randomized Riluzole vs. placebo blinded	Completed	Possible benefit
Liang et al[89]	Hydroxyurea	Increases SMN2 expression	33/SMA types 2, 3	Open label pilot	Completed	Slight increase in muscle strength
NPTUNE02	Phenylbutyrate	Increases SMN2 expression	Est: 24 +6/SMA types 1, 2	Open label, phase 1/2	Recruiting	Obj: maximum tolerable dose; effect on SMN mRNA, protein Type 2 study closed for AEs
CARNI-VAL type 1	Valproic acid carnitine	Increases SMN2 expression	Est: 36/SMA type 1	Open label	Recruiting??	Obj: assessment of safety: nutritional status; various other
VALIANT SMA	Valproic acid	Increases SMN2 expression	Est: 36/SMA type 3, 4	Randomized, double-blind placebo control	Recruiting??	Obj: muscle strength
STOP SMA	Phenylbutyrate	Increases SMN2 expression	12/presymptomatic SMA types 1, 2	Open label	Recruiting	Obj: assess safety, tolerability and efficacy
A trial of hydroxyurea in SMA	Hydroxyurea	Increases SMN2 expression	60/SMA types 2, 3	Randomized, double-blind, placebo control	Recruiting	Obj: safety and efficacy

Est, estimated; Obj, objective; SMA, spinal muscular atrophy.

SMN2 alleles are not functionally equivalent and this could explain at least in part the variable phenotype in patients with the same number of SMN2 copies. SMN2 expression is dependent on DNA-methylation pattern, which differs from one patient to another and correlates with disease severity. HDACIs like valproic acid and phenylbutyrate are not able to bypass SMN2 gene silencing by DNA methylation. New agents such as vorinostat and romidepsin, which can do so, may represent future directions for clinical trials.[90] Correction of abnormal splicing of SMN2 exon 7 holds the promise for cure. A number of splicing enhancers and splicing silencers were identified at the level of exon 7 and flanking introns. Transient exon 7 incorporation was possible using antisense oligonucleotides targeting different regulatory motifs. Recently, a sustained correction of SMN2 splicing defect was achieved.[91,92] This strategy can potentially be applied to some of the CMs caused by abnormal splicing.[93] In addition to the SMN2 gene, other modifying genes are possibly involved in modulation of SMA severity. A recent study found overexpression of the Plastin 3 gene in asymptomatic patients with homozygous deletion of SMN1 while symptomatic siblings with a similar number of SMN2 copies had normal expression. The Plastin 3 gene is involved in axonogenesis by increasing F-actin levels. This may open a new avenue for possible therapeutic intervention.[94]

Post-translation control therapeutics promotes selective ribosomal read-through of premature stop codon but not a normal, terminal stop codon. This strategy is being currently investigated in patients with nonsense mutations of the dystrophin gene with encouraging results. This method has therapeutic potential for any genetic disorder caused by nonsense mutations, but whether it can be applied in SMA is not yet clear.

Progress in experimental therapies for CMs is hindered by the great genetic heterogeneity. Taking advantage of existence of different protein isoforms, one strategy involves increasing the expression of a structurally close isoform. For example, in CMs caused by mutations of skeletal muscle actin, increasing the expression of cardiac actin is currently under study.[95]

Conclusion

SMA and CM are incurable disorders that affect children more than adults. Recent advances in clinical management may improve quality of life and survival for many patients. Drug development and clinical trials in SMA hold great promise for the future.

References

1. Hoffmann J: Über chronische spinale Muskelatrophie im Kindesalter, auf familiärer Basis, *Dtsch Z Nervenheilk* 3, 1893.
2. Groger H: *Guido Werdnig in the Founders of Child Neurology*, San Francisco, 1990, Norman Publishing.
3. Lefebvre S, Bürglen L, Reboullet S, et al: Identification and characterization of a spinal muscular atrophy-determining gene, *Cell* 80(1):155–165, 1995.
4. Byers RK, Banker BQ: Infantile muscular atrophy, *Arch Neurol* 5:140–164, 1961.
5. Iannaccone ST, Russman BS, Browne RH, et al: Prospective analysis of strength in spinal muscular atrophy. DCN/Spinal Muscular Atrophy Group, *J Child Neurol* 15(2):97–101, 2000.
6. Mailman MD, Heinz JW, Papp AC, et al: Molecular analysis of spinal muscular atrophy and modification of the phenotype by SMN2, *Genet Med* 4(1):20–26, 2002.
7. Wallgren-Pettersson C: Congenital nemaline myopathy. A clinical follow-up of twelve patients, *J Neurol Sci* 89(1):1–14, 1989.
8. De Cauwer H, Heytens L, Martin JJ: Workshop report of the 89th ENMC International Workshop: Central Core Disease, 19–20 January 2001, Hilversum, The Netherlands, *Neuromusc Disord* 12(6):588–595, 2002.
9. Herman GE, Finegold M, Zhao W, et al: Medical complications in long-term survivors with X-linked myotubular myopathy, *J Pediatr* 134(2):206–214, 1999.
10. de Gouyon BM, Zhao W, Laporte J, et al: Characterization of mutations in the myotubularin gene in twenty-six patients with X-linked myotubular myopathy, *Hum Mol Genet* 6(9):1499–1504, 1997.
11. Iannaccone ST, Smith SA, Simard LR: Spinal muscular atrophy, *Curr Neurol Neurosci Rep* 4(1):74–80, 2004.
12. Bach JR, Baird JS, Plosky D, et al: Spinal muscular atrophy type 1: management and outcomes, *Pediatr Pulmonol* 34(1):16–22, 2002.
13. Birnkrant DJ, Pope JF, Martin JE, et al: Treatment of type I spinal muscular atrophy with noninvasive ventilation and gastrostomy feeding, *Pediatr Neurol* 18(5):407–410, 1998.
14. Simonds AK: Ethical aspects of home long term ventilation in children with neuromuscular disease, *Paediatr Respir Rev* 6(3):209–214, 2005.
15. von Gontard A, Zerres K, Backes M, et al: Intelligence and cognitive function in children and adolescents with spinal muscular atrophy, *Neuromuscul Disord* 12(2):130–136, 2002.
16. Kim JJ, Armstrong DD, Fishman MA: Multicore myopathy, microcephaly, aganglionosis, and short stature, *J Child Neurol* 9(3):275–277, 1994.
17. Chudley AE, Rozdilsky B, Houston CS, et al: Multicore disease in sibs with severe mental retardation, short stature, facial anomalies, hypoplasia of the pituitary fossa, and hypogonadotrophic hypogonadism, *Am J Med Genet* 20(1):145–158, 1985.
18. Fowler WM Jr, Abresch RT, Koch TR, et al: Employment profiles in neuromuscular diseases, *Am J Phys Med Rehabil* 76(1):26–37, 1997.
19. Messina S, Pane M, De Rose P, et al: Feeding problems and malnutrition in spinal muscular atrophy type II, *Neuromuscul Disord* 18(5):389–393, 2008.
20. Tilton AH, Miller MD, Khoshoo V: Nutrition and swallowing in pediatric neuromuscular patients, *Semin Pediatr Neurol* 5(2):106–115, 1998.
21. Oskoui M, Levy G, Garland CJ, et al: The changing natural history of spinal muscular atrophy type 1, *Neurology* 69(20):1931–1936, 2007.
22. Hill M, Hughes T, Milford C: Treatment for swallowing difficulties (dysphagia) in chronic muscle disease, *Cochrane Database Syst Rev* (2): CD004303, 2004.
23. Wang CH, Finkel RS, Bertini ES, et al: Consensus statement for standard of care in spinal muscular atrophy, *J Child Neurol* 22(8):1027–1049, 2007.
24. Ryan MM, Schnell C, Strickland CD, et al: Nemaline myopathy: a clinical study of 143 cases, *Ann Neurol* 50(3):312–320, 2001.
25. Canani RB, Cirillo P, Roggero P, et al: Therapy with gastric acidity inhibitors increases the risk of acute gastroenteritis and community-acquired pneumonia in children, *Pediatrics* 117(5):817–820, 2006.
26. Granata C, Merlini L, Magni E, et al: Spinal muscular atrophy: natural history and orthopaedic treatment of scoliosis, *Spine* 14(7):760–762, 1989.
27. Kouwenhoven JW, Van Ommeren PM, Pruijs HE, et al: Spinal decompensation in neuromuscular disease, *Spine* 31(7):E188–E191, 2006.
28. Evans GA, Drennan JC, Russman BS: Functional classification and orthopaedic management of spinal muscular atrophy, *J Bone Joint Surg Br* 63B(4):516–522, 1981.
29. Sucato DJ: Spine deformity in spinal muscular atrophy, *J Bone Joint Surg Am* 89(Suppl 1):148–154, 2007.
30. Merlini L, Granata C, Bonfiglioli S, et al: Scoliosis in spinal muscular atrophy: natural history and management, *Dev Med Child Neurol* 31(4):501–508, 1989.
31. Tangsrud SE, Carlsen KC, Lund-Petersen I, et al: Lung function measurements in young children with spinal muscle atrophy; a cross sectional survey on the effect of position and bracing, *Arch Dis Child* 84(6):521–524, 2001.
32. Morillon S, Thumerelle C, Cuisset JM, et al: Effect of thoracic bracing on lung function in children with neuromuscular disease, *Ann Readapt Med Phys* 50(8):645–650, 2007.
33. Phillips DP, Roye DP Jr, Farcy JP, et al: Surgical treatment of scoliosis in a spinal muscular atrophy population, *Spine* 15(9):942–945, 1990.
34. Granata C, Cervellati S, Ballestrazzi A, et al: Spine surgery in spinal muscular atrophy: long-term results, *Neuromuscul Disord* 3(3):207–215, 1993.
35. Aprin H, Bowen JR, MacEwen GD, et al: Spine fusion in patients with spinal muscular atrophy, *J Bone Joint Surg Am* 64(8):1179–1187, 1982.

36. Chng SY, et al: Pulmonary function and scoliosis in children with spinal muscular atrophy types II and III, *J Paediatr Child Health* 39(9):673–676, 2003.

37. Mullender M, Blom N, De Kleuver M, et al: A Dutch guideline for the treatment of scoliosis in neuromuscular disorders, *Scoliosis* 3:14, 2008.

38. Akbarnia BA, Marks DS, Boachie-Adjei O, et al: Dual growing rod technique for the treatment of progressive early-onset scoliosis: a multicenter study, *Spine* 30(Suppl 17):S46–S57, 2005.

39. Sporer SM, Smith BG: Hip dislocation in patients with spinal muscular atrophy, *J Pediatr Orthop* 23(1):10–14, 2003.

40. Zenios M, Sampath J, Cole C, et al: Operative treatment for hip subluxation in spinal muscular atrophy, *J Bone Joint Surg Br* 87(11):1541–1544, 2005.

41. Thompson CE, Larsen LJ: Recurrent hip dislocation in intermediate spinal atrophy, *J Pediatr Orthop* 10(5):638–641, 1990.

42. Echenne B, Rivier F, Roubertie A, et al: Congenital club foot with survival of motor neuron 1, telomeric (*SMN1*) gene deletion, *J Child Neurol* 19(3):212–213, 2004.

43. Zanette G, Robb N, Zadra N, et al: Undetected central core disease myopathy in an infant presenting for clubfoot surgery, *Paediatr Anaesth* 17(4):380–382, 2007.

44. Schwentker EP, Gibson DA: The orthopaedic aspects of spinal muscular atrophy, *J Bone Joint Surg Am* 58(1):32–38, 1976.

45. Cahill PJ, Rinella AS, Bielski RJ: Orthopaedic complications of myotubular myopathy, *J Pediatr Orthop* 27(1):98–103, 2007.

46. Shanmugarajan S, Swoboda KJ, Iannaccone ST, et al: Congenital bone fractures in spinal muscular atrophy: functional role for SMN protein in bone remodeling, *J Child Neurol* 22(8):967–973, 2007.

47. Khatri IA, Chaudhry US, Seikaly MG, et al: Low bone mineral density in spinal muscular atrophy, *J Clin Neuromusc Dis* 10(1):11–17, 2008.

48. Vestergaard P, Glerup H, Steffensen BF, et al: Fracture risk in patients with muscular dystrophy and spinal muscular atrophy, *J Rehabil Med* 33(4):150–155, 2001.

49. Houston K, Buschang PH, Iannaccone ST, et al: Craniofacial morphology of spinal muscular atrophy, *Pediatr Res* 36(2):265–269, 1994.

50. Mier-Jedrzejowicz A, Brophy C, Green M: Respiratory muscle weakness during upper respiratory tract infections, *Am Rev Respir Dis* 138(1):5–7, 1988.

51. Wallgren-Pettersson C, Bushby K, Mellies U, Simonds A; ENMC: 117th ENMC workshop: ventilatory support in congenital neuromuscular disorders—congenital myopathies, congenital muscular dystrophies, congenital myotonic dystrophy and SMA (II) 4–6 April 2003, Naarden, The Netherlands, *Neuromusc Disord* 14(1):56–69, 2004.

52. Langenderfer B: Alternatives to percussion and postural drainage. A review of mucus clearance therapies: percussion and postural drainage, autogenic drainage, positive expiratory pressure, flutter valve, intrapulmonary percussive ventilation, and high-frequency chest compression with the ThAIRapy Vest, *J Cardiopulm Rehabil* 18(4):283–289, 1998.

53. Dohna-Schwake C, Ragette R, Teschler H, et al: IPPB-assisted coughing in neuromuscular disorders, *Pediatr Pulmonol* 41(6):551–557, 2006.

54. Bach JR: Mechanical insufflation-exsufflation. Comparison of peak expiratory flows with manually assisted and unassisted coughing techniques, *Chest* 104(5):1553–1562, 1993.

55. Miske LJ, Hickey EM, Kolb SM, et al: Use of the mechanical in-exsufflator in pediatric patients with neuromuscular disease and impaired cough, *Chest* 125(4):1406–1412, 2004.

56. Fauroux B, Guillemot N, Aubertin G, et al: Physiologic benefits of mechanical insufflation-exsufflation in children with neuromuscular diseases, *Chest* 133(1):161–168, 2008.

57. Reardon CC, Christiansen D, Barnett ED, et al: Intrapulmonary percussive ventilation vs incentive spirometry for children with neuromuscular disease, *Arch Pediatr Adolesc Med* 159(6):526–531, 2005.

58. Birnkrant DJ, Pope JF, Eiben RM: Management of the respiratory complications of neuromuscular diseases in the pediatric intensive care unit, *J Child Neurol* 14(3):139–143, 1999.

59. Durkin ET, Schroth MK, Helin M, et al: Early laparoscopic fundoplication and gastrostomy in infants with spinal muscular atrophy type I, *J Pediatr Surg* 43(11):2031–2037, 2008.

60. Yuan N, Wang CH, Trela A, et al: Laparoscopic Nissen fundoplication during gastrostomy tube placement and noninvasive ventilation may improve survival in type I and severe type II spinal muscular atrophy, *J Child Neurol* 22(6):727–731, 2007.

61. Birnkrant DJ, Pope JF, Lewarski J, et al: Persistent pulmonary consolidation treated with intrapulmonary percussive ventilation: a preliminary report, *Pediatr Pulmonol* 21(4):246–249, 1996.

62. Mellies U, Dohna-Schwake C, Stehling F, et al: Sleep disordered breathing in spinal muscular atrophy, *Neuromusc Disord* 14(12):797–803, 2004.

63. Ragette R, Mellies U, Schwake C, et al: Patterns and predictors of sleep disordered breathing in primary myopathies, *Thorax* 57(8):724–728, 2002.

64. Wilson DO, Sanders MH, Dauber JH: Abnormal ventilatory chemosensitivity and congenital myopathy, *Arch Intern Med* 147(10):1773–1777, 1987.

65. Maayan C, Springer C, Armon Y, et al: Nemaline myopathy as a cause of sleep hypoventilation, *Pediatrics* 77(3):390–395, 1986.

66. Guilleminault C, Philip P, Robinson A: Sleep and neuromuscular disease: bilevel positive airway pressure by nasal mask as a treatment for sleep disordered breathing in patients with neuromuscular disease, *J Neurol Neurosurg Psychiatry* 65(2):225–232, 1998.

67. Ward S, Chatwin M, Heather S, et al: Randomised controlled trial of noninvasive ventilation (NIV) for nocturnal hypoventilation in neuromuscular and chest wall disease patients with daytime normocapnia, *Thorax* 60(12):1019–1024, 2005.

68. Iannaccone ST: Modern management of spinal muscular atrophy, *J Child Neurol* 22(8):974–978, 2007.

69. Mah JK, Thannhauser JE, Kolski H, et al: Parental stress and quality of life in children with neuromuscular disease, *Pediatr Neurol* 39(2):102–107, 2008.

70. Laufersweiler-Plass C, Rudnik-Schöneborn S, Zerres K, et al: A. Behavioural problems in children and adolescents with spinal muscular atrophy and their siblings, *Dev Med Child Neurol* 45(1):44–49, 2003.

71. von Gontard A, Backes M, Laufersweiler-Plass C, et al: Psychopathology and familial stress—comparison of boys with fragile X syndrome and spinal muscular atrophy, *J Child Psychol Psychiatry* 43(7):949–957, 2002.

72. Kohler M, Clarenbach CF, Böni L, et al: Quality of life, physical disability, and respiratory impairment in Duchenne muscular dystrophy, *Am J Respir Crit Care Med* 172(8):1032–1036, 2005.

73. Bach JR, Vega J, Majors J, et al: Spinal muscular atrophy type 1 quality of life, *Am J Phys Med Rehabil* 82(2):137–142, 2003.

74. Lorson CL, Hahnen E, Androphy EJ, et al: A single nucleotide in the *SMN* gene regulates splicing and is responsible for spinal muscular atrophy, *Proc Natl Acad Sci U S A* 96(11):6307–6311, 1999.

75. Campbell L, Potter A, Ignatius J, et al: Genomic variation and gene conversion in spinal muscular atrophy: implications for disease process and clinical phenotype, *Am J Hum Genet* 61(1):40–50, 1997.

76. Hsieh-Li HM, Chang JG, Jong YJ, et al: A mouse model for spinal muscular atrophy, *Nat Genet* 24(1):66–70, 2000.

77. Monani UR, Sendtner M, Coovert DD, et al: The human centromeric survival motor neuron gene (*SMN2*) rescues embryonic lethality in Smn$^{-/-}$ mice and results in a mouse with spinal muscular atrophy, *Hum Mol Genet* 9(3):333–339, 2000.

78. Jarecki J, Chen J, Whitney M, et al: Identification and profiling of compounds that increase full-length SMN2 nRNA levels, Chicago, IL, 2002, Sixth Annual International Spinal Muscular Atrophy Research Group Meeting.

79. Kaufmann P, Iannaccone ST: Clinical trials in spinal muscular atrophy, *Phys Med Rehabil Clin North Am* 19(3):653–660, 2008.

80. Ryan MM, Sy C, Rudge S, et al: Dietary L-tyrosine supplementation in nemaline myopathy, *J Child Neurol* 23(6):609–613, 2008.

81. Hauke J, Riessland M, Lunke S, et al: Survival motor neuron gene 2 silencing by DNA methylation correlates with spinal muscular atrophy disease severity and can be bypassed by histone deacetylase inhibition, *Hum Mol Genet* 18(2):304–317, 2008.

82. Singh NN, Shishimorova M, Cao LC, et al: A short antisense oligonucleotide masking a unique intronic motif prevents skipping of a critical exon in spinal muscular atrophy, *RNA Biol* 6(3):341–350, 2009.

83. Marquis J, Meyer K, Angehrn L, et al: Spinal muscular atrophy: SMN2 pre-mRNA splicing corrected by a U7 snRNA derivative carrying a splicing enhancer sequence, *Mol Ther* 15(8):1479–1486, 2007.

84. Laing NG, Wallgren-Pettersson C: 161st ENMC International Workshop on nemaline myopathy and related disorders, Newcastle upon Tyne, 2008, *Neuromusc Disord* 19(4):300–305, 2009.

85. Oprea GE, Kröber S, McWhorter ML, et al: Plastin 3 is a protective modifier of autosomal recessive spinal muscular atrophy, *Science* 320(5875):524–527, 2008.

86. Crawford K, Flick R, Close L, et al: Mice lacking skeletal muscle actin show reduced muscle strength and growth deficits and die during the neonatal period, *Mol Cell Biol* 22(16):5887–5896, 2002.

87. Weihl CC, Connolly AM, Pestronk A: Valproate may improve strength and function in patients with type III/IV spinal muscle atrophy, *Neurology* 67 (3):500–501, 2006.

88. Brichta L, Holker I, Haug K, et al: In vivo activation of SMN in spinal muscular atrophy carriers and patients treated with valproate, *Ann Neurol* 59 (6):970–975, 2006.

89. Kinali M, Mercuri E, Main M, et al: Pilot trial of albuterol in spinal muscular atrophy, *Neurology* 59(4):609–610, 2002.

90. Miller RG, Moore DH, Dronsky V, et al: A placebo-controlled trial of gabapentin in spinal muscular atrophy, *J Neurol Sci* 191(1–2):127–131, 2001.

91. Merlini L, Solari A, Vita G, et al: Role of gabapentin in spinal muscular atrophy: results of a multicenter, randomized Italian study, *J Child Neurol* 18 (8):537–541, 2003.

92. Mercuri E, Bertini E, Messina S, et al: Pilot trial of phenylbutyrate in spinal muscular atrophy, *Neuromusc Disord* 14(2):130–135, 2004.

93. Mercuri E, Bertini E, Messina S, et al: Randomized, double-blind, placebo-controlled trial of phenylbutyrate in spinal muscular atrophy, *Neurology* 68 (1):51–55, 2007.

94. Russman BS, Iannaccone ST, Samaha FJ: A phase 1 trial of riluzole in spinal muscular atrophy, *Arch Neurol* 60(11):1601–1603, 2003.

95. Liang WC, Yuo CY, Chang JG, et al: The effect of hydroxyurea in spinal muscular atrophy cells and patients, *J Neurol Sci* 268(1–2):87–94, 2008.

Thomas E. Lloyd, MD, PhD
Vinay Chaudhry, MD

13

Treatment and Management of Hereditary Neuropathies

The past decade has seen an explosion in our understanding of the molecular etiology of hereditary neuropathies. Nonetheless, hereditary neuropathy remains a major cause of undiagnosed neuropathy in patients referred to tertiary centers. The characterization of genetic mutations underlying these familial diseases has led to an understanding of disease pathogenesis and has heralded a new era of rational drug design. Identification of mutations has allowed the generation of animal models of these diseases in which new therapeutics can be tested. By identifying mechanisms and pathways important in these rare inherited neuropathies, this understanding holds promise for application to more common sporadic and acquired neuropathies. Some of these diseases now have specific therapies to offer patients, and most of these patients can benefit from symptomatic therapies.

Most chapters and reviews on inherited neuropathies focus on the underlying genetic mutations, the function of the mutated gene, and the pathogenesis of the disease. This chapter, on the other hand, takes a practical approach to caring for patients with familial neuropathy and discusses the clinical presentation, diagnosis, and treatment of these diseases. We cover both disorders specifically affecting peripheral nerves (referred to as *nonsyndromic inherited neuropathies*, listed in Table 13-1) and systemic genetic disorders in which peripheral neuropathy is a major clinical feature (referred to as *multiple system-inherited* or *syndromic neuropathies*, listed in Table 13-2). We first consider the hereditary motor and sensory neuropathies, also called Charcot-Marie-Tooth disease, and hereditary sensory and autonomic neuropathies summarized in Table 13-1. Because there is considerable overlap between hereditary motor neuropathies and motor neuron diseases, these disorders are briefly discussed here; specific management of motor neuron diseases is discussed in Chapters 11 and 12. As shown in Table 13-2, the list of syndromic neuropathies is long; we focus on inherited syndromes in which neuropathy is a primary feature and in which specific treatments are available: familial amyloid polyneuropathy, lysosomal storage diseases (Fabry disease, Krabbe disease, and metachromatic leukodystrophy), Friedreich ataxia, adrenomyeloneuropathy, and porphyria.

The list of genetic causes of neuropathy is continuously expanding, making them difficult to diagnose, even for the neuromuscular specialist (see Tables 13-1 and 13-2). The online database, OMIM (Online Mendelian Inheritance in Man, Johns Hopkins University School of Medicine; http://www.ncbi.nlm.nih.gov/Omim), is an extremely useful reference for clinicians; it is a publicly funded, up-to-date, searchable database in which a physician can

enter a patient's clinical findings and potential inherited diseases can be rapidly identified. Diagnosis relies on keeping inherited causes in the differential diagnosis and taking a careful family history. Rather than merely asking general questions as to whether family members have neuropathy or similar symptoms, patients should be asked if their parents or siblings had foot deformities, remained mobile or were confined to a wheelchair, or dragged their feet when they walked. When possible, family members should be interviewed and examined and, if appropriate, should have electrodiagnostic studies performed.

Once an inherited neuropathy is suspected, making the molecular diagnosis is often challenging. Genetic testing is usually best done along with a genetic counselor who can discuss costs and benefits of genetic testing with multiple family members. Patients need to be well educated regarding the implications of a molecular diagnosis, both for themselves and for family members. Genetic testing is of utmost relevance to family members of childbearing age, because for many disorders, genetic testing is available in utero and even pre-implantation. It is worth noting that the first genetic nondiscrimination law (GINA, Genetic Information Nondiscrimination Act; P.L. 110–233) was signed into law in 2008, giving patients protection from discrimination by employers and health insurance companies. In most cases, minors should not be offered genetic testing to determine future health or reproductive risks, unless screening provides a clear and timely medical benefit with minimal psychosocial risks. Although testing is expensive and often not covered by insurance, genetic diagnosis is extremely valuable to many patients and clinicians in part because it can potentially give a definitive diagnosis not available by any other means and can obviate invasive testing (e.g., nerve biopsy) and unnecessary treatment (e.g., intravenous gamma globulin). Knowing the cause of their symptoms can often empower patients to follow research progress and enroll in clinical trials. This chapter discusses the genetic tests that are commercially available in 2010, but others will certainly be available in the near future. The GeneTests Web site (www.ncbi.nlm.nih.gov/sites/GeneTests), funded by the National Institutes of Health, is a valuable resource for identifying gene tests, both those available clinically and those performed on a research basis, and includes online reviews of most diseases (GeneReviews).

Unfortunately, specific pharmacologic therapies are not yet available for most syndromic and all nonsyndromic inherited neuropathies. Given that the first genes causing Charcot-Marie-Tooth disease (CMT) were discovered less than 20 years ago, and given

Table 13-1 Nonsyndromic Inherited Neuropathies*

Disease	Inheritance Patterns	Gene or Locus[†]	Clinical Features
Hereditary Motor and Sensory Neuropathies (HMSN)[‡]			
Demyelinating			**Forearm NCV usually <38 m/sec**
CMT1	AD		Young adult onset, NCV 10–35 m/sec; most common (70% of all CMT1); mutations also cause CMT3
CMT1A		PMP22 (usually duplication)	Mutations also cause CMT2 and CMT3
CMT1B		MPZ (P$_0$)	
CMT1C		LITAF/SIMPLE	Broad clinical spectrum (also CMT3)
CMT1D		EGR2	DSS phenotype common
CMT1F		NEFL	
HNPP	AD	PMP22 (usually deletion)	Adult-onset episodic entrapment neuropathies, mild slowing (NCV 40–50 m/sec)
CMT3			Severe, early-onset demyelinating; onset before age 3 yr
DSS	AD/X	CMT1 genes PRX, MTMR2	
	AR		
CHN	AD	PMP22, MPZ	Congenital onset
	AR	EGR2	Also known as CMT4E
CMT4	AR		Childhood onset, usually severe
CMT4A		GDAP1	Both axonal and demyelinating types
CMT4B1		MTMR2	Biopsy shows focally folded myelin
CMT4B2		SBF2/MTMR13	Same as above ± early-onset glaucoma
CMT4C		SH3TC2	Scoliosis often severe, also axonal types
CMT4D		NDRG1	Dysmorphic features, deafness
CMT4F		PRX	DSS phenotype
CMT4H		FGD4	
CMT4J		FIG4	
Slow NCV only	AD	ARHGEF10	Asymptomatic NCV slowing without clinical manifestations
Intermediate			**NCV 25–45 m/sec**
CMTX	X		
CMTX1		GJB1/Cx32	Similar to CMT1, but males more severely affected; CNS involvement common
CMTX2		Xq24-q26	Cowchuck syndrome: mental retardation, deafness, axonal
CMTX5		PRPS1	Deafness, optic atrophy
DI-CMT	AD		
DI-CMTA		10q24	
DI-CMTB		DNM2	Neutropenia
DI-CMTC		YARS	
Axonal			**NCV >38 m/sec**
CMT2	AD		Young adult onset
CMT2A		MFN2 KIF1B (rare)	Most common; also HMSN V (optic atrophy), VI (spasticity), and early onset
CMT2B		RAB7	Severe sensory loss like HSAN1
CMT2C		TRPV4	Vocal cord/diaphragm weakness
CMT2D		GARS	Arm > leg, motor predominant, similar to dHMN caused by BSCL2 mutations
CMT2E		NEFL	Allelic with CMT1E; variable phenotype
CMT2F		HSP27 (HSPB1)	Motor predominant
CMT2G		12q12-13.3	Proximal > distal weakness
CMT2H, K		GDAP1	Allelic with CMT4A
CMT2I, J		MPZ (P0)	Cough, pain, autonomic/pupil, deafness
CMT2L		HSP22 (HSPB8)	Motor predominant, allelic with HMNIIa
HMSN-P		3p14-q13	Proximal > distal
AR-CMT2A	AR	LMNA	Also called CMT2B1 and CMT4C1

Table 13-1   Nonsyndromic Inherited Neuropathies*—Cont'd

Disease	Inheritance Patterns	Gene or Locus[†]	Clinical Features
Hereditary Sensory and Autonomic Neuropathies (HSAN)[¶] and Hereditary Motor Neuropathies (HMN)			
HS(A)N			**Sensory (± autonomic) neuropathy**
HSAN1A	AD	SPTLC1	Late onset, slowly progressive sensory axonal neuropathy ±SNHL, weakness Variant with cough, GERD, deafness
HSAN1B	AD	3p24-p22	Congenital sensory loss, acral mutilation
HSAN2	AR	HSN2	Severe dysautonomia, Ashkenazi Jews
HSAN3	AR	IKBKAP	
HSAN4	AR	TRKA	Anhidrosis, acral mutilation, ± CNS; congenital insensitivity to pain
HSAN5	AR	NGFB	
HMN/dSMA			**Distal wasting and weakness**
HMNIIa	AD	HSPB8 (HSP22)	Adult onset, allelic with CMT2L
HMNIIb	AD	HSP27 (HSPB1)	Allelic with CMT2F
HMNVa	AD	GARS	Upper limb predominant
HMNVb	AD	BSCL2	Allelic with SPG17/Silver syndrome
HMNVI	AR	IGHMBP2	Severe infantile respiratory distress/SMARD Adult onset, vocal cord paralysis
HMNVIIa	AD	2q14	Same as above
HMNVIIb	AD	DCTN1	
HMNX	X	Xq13.1-q21	Childhood-onset (Jerash type)
HMNJ	AR	9p21.1-p12	
SBMA	X	Androgen receptor (CAG repeat)	Adult onset bulbar signs, proximal weakness, sensory neuronopathy, gynecomastia

*The inherited neuropathies are generally considered to exclusively or predominantly affect peripheral nerve, though, as shown in the clinical features column, many of these diseases affect the CNS and other tissues.

[†]The affected gene(s) is listed if known; otherwise the chromosomal locus is listed. In cases where the mutation is not a missense mutation, the type of mutation is listed in parentheses (duplication, deletion, or CAG repeat).

[‡]The diseases are grouped according to phenotype: HMSN, hereditary motor and sensory neuropathy; HS(A)N, hereditary sensory and (± autonomic) neuropathy; HMN, hereditary motor neuropathy, also called dSMA (distal spinal muscular atrophy); SBMA, spinal bulbar and muscular atrophy. The HMSNs are further divided into demyelinating, axonal, and intermediate forms based on the usual range of nerve conduction velocity (NCV).

[¶]See also Table 5-4 and Table 12-1, where the chromosomal loci of these disorders are also listed.

AD, autosomal dominant; AR, autosomal recessive; CHN, congenital hypomyelinating neuropathy; CMT, Charcot-Marie-Tooth disease; CNS, central nervous system; DI-CMT, dominant intermediate CMT; DSS, Dejerine-Sottas syndrome; GERD, gastroesophageal reflux disease; HNPP, hereditary neuropathy with liability to form pressure palsies; SMARD, spinal muscular atrophy with respiratory distress; SNHL, sensorineural hearing loss; SPG, hereditary spastic paraplegia (see Table 13-2); X, X-linked.

Table 13-2 Syndromic Neuropathies*

Disease	Inheritance Pattern	Gene or Locus[†]	Clinical Features
HNA	AD	SEPT9	Recurrent brachial neuritis, dysmorphic features in some
Friedreich ataxia	AR	Frataxin (GAA repeats)	Ataxia, sensory large-fiber axonal neuropathy, positive Babinski sign, cardiomyopathy
AVED	AR	TTPA	Friedreich ataxia–like, vitamin E deficiency
SCAN1	AR	TDP1	Spinocerebellar ataxia, sensory neuropathy
Ataxia-telangiectasia	AR	ATM	Ataxia, telangiectasias, malignancy, infections
SCA			**Sensory neuropathy, variable in most**
SCA3/MJD	AD	ATXN3	Ataxia, spasticity, severe axonal neuropathy
SCA4	AD	PLEKHG4	Prominent axonal sensory neuropathy
SCA10	AD	ATXN10	±Sensorimotor neuropathy
SCA25	AD	2p21-p13	Prominent axonal sensory neuropathy
SCA27	AD	FGF14	Mild axonal sensory neuropathy

Continued

Table 13-2 Syndromic Neuropathies*—Cont'd

Disease	Inheritance Pattern	Gene or Locus[†]	Clinical Features
HSP			**"Complicated HSP" with neuropathy**
SPG2	X	*PLP*	CNS white matter disease ± neuropathy
SPG7	AR	Paraplegin	±Neuropathy, dysarthria, dysphagia
SPG9	AD	10q23.3-24.1	Amyotrophy, cataracts, GERD
SPG10	AD	*KIF5A*	±Distal atrophy
SPG11	AR	Spatacsin	Mental retardation, nystagmus, thin corpus callosum
SPG14	AR	3q27-q28	Distal motor neuropathy, mental retardation, visual agnosia
SPG15	AR	Spastizin	Pigmented maculopathy, mental retardation, dysarthria
SPG17	AD	*BSCL2*	Silver syndrome: hand atrophy prominent
SPG20	AR	Spartin	Troyer syndrome: distal atrophy, dysarthria
FAP			
Transthyretin	AD	*TTR*	Early adult onset, painful sensorimotor and autonomic neuropathy, entrapment neuropathy, cardiomyopathy, GI symptoms
(Iowa)		*APOAI*	Similar to transthyretin, but progressive renal failure
(Finnish)		Gelsolin	Cranial neuropathies, corneal dystrophy
Fabry	X	α-galactosidase-A	Child onset painful SFSN, renal failure, cardiac disease, strokes
Leukodystrophies			**Some associated with demyelinating neuropathy**
GLD/Krabbe's	AR	*GALC*	Progressive mental retardation, hyperreflexia, seizures, optic atrophy
MLD	AR	*ARSA*	Same as above, although CNS signs less severe
PCWH/ Wartenburg syndrome	AD	*SOX10*	CHN, central dysmyelination, Wartenburg syndrome, and Hirschprung disease
Adrenomyeloneuropathy	X	*ABCD1*	Spastic paraparesis, large-fiber sensory loss, bowel and bladder incontinence
Merosin def	AR	*LAMA2*	Neuropathy and muscular dystrophy
Refsum disease	AR	*PAHX* *PEX7*	Ataxia, retinitis pigmentosa, demyelinating neuropathy, cardiac, deafness, ichthyosis
Mitochondrial diseases			**Neuropathy common, axonal or demyelinating**
Leigh disease	AR mitochondrial	Multiple genes	Early-onset CPEO, ptosis, ataxia, mental retardation, pyramidal signs, demyelinating neuropathy
NARP	Mitochondrial	*MTATP6*	Sensory neuropathy, ataxia, retinitis pigmentosa
MNGIE	AR	*ECGF1 POLG*	Ptosis, CPEO, leukoencephalopathy, neuropathy, myopathy, GI dysmotility
Porphyria	**AD**		
AIP		*PBGD*	Acute neuropathy, abdominal pain, psychosis, seizures
Coproporphyria		*CPO*	Similar to AIP, but also skin photosensitivity
Variegate porphyria		*PPOX*	Similar to AIP, but also skin photosensitivity
Tangiers disease	AR	*ABC1*	Orange tonsils, organomegaly, low HDL, atherosclerosis
Abetalipoproteinemia	AR	*MTTP*	Ataxia, acanthocytosis, steatorrhea, low LDL
Hypobetalipoproteinemia	AD	Apo-B	Ataxia, sensory axonal polyneuropathy
GAN	AR	Gigaxonin	Mental retardation, kinky hair; biopsy shows giant axons
ACCPN	AR	*KCC3*	Agenesis of corpus callosum, French Canadian
CCFDN	AR	CTDP1	Congenital cataracts, facial dysmorphism

*These are the inherited neuropathies in which the neuropathy is part of a systemic disease.
[†]The affected gene(s) is listed if known; otherwise the chromosomal locus is listed. ACCPN, agenesis of the corpus callosum and peripheral neuropathy, also known as Anderman's syndrome; AD, autosomal dominant; AIP, acute intermittent porphyria; AR, autosomal recessive; AVED, ataxia with isolated vitamin E deficiency; CCFDN, congenital cataracts, facial dysmorphism, neuropathy; CNS, central nervous system; CPEO, chronic progressive external ophthalmoplegia; FAP, familial amyloidotic polyneuropathy; GAN, giant axonal neuropathy; GERD, gastroesophageal reflux disease; GI, gastrointestinal; GLD, globoid-cell dystrophy; HNA, hereditary neuralgic amyotrophy; HSP, hereditary spastic paraplegia; MJD, Machado-Joseph disease; MNGIE, mitochondrial neurogastrointestinal encephalopathy syndrome; SCA, spinocerebellar ataxia; MLD, metachromatic leukodystrophy; NARP, neuropathy, ataxia, and retinitis pigmentosa; PCWH, peripheral demyelinating neuropathy, central dysmyelination, Waardenburg syndrome, and Hirschprung disease; SCAN1, spinocerebellar ataxia with axonal neuropathy 1; SFSN, small-fiber sensory neuropathy; SPG, spastic gait; X, X-linked.

the magnitude of discoveries achieved since then, there is certainly reason to be optimistic that specific therapies will soon become available. Nonetheless, symptomatic therapies are available, mostly to treat the orthopedic complications that arise. These physiatric and surgical therapies are covered in detail in Chapters 8 and 9, respectively, and are only briefly discussed here as they relate to specific disorders. Neuropathic pain is uncommon in most inherited neuropathies and is treated in the same way as in acquired neuropathies; however, in a few inherited neuropathies, pain may be the presenting symptom, particularly in Fabry disease and familial amyloid polyneuropathy. Chapter 6 discusses treatment of painful neuropathy. Importantly, several patient support groups offer valuable services to patients and their families. The Muscular Dystrophy Association (MDA, www.mda.org) supports patients with CMT and Friedreich ataxia (FRDA), and this organization can be helpful to patients. Other patient resources include the Charcot-Marie-Tooth Association (www.charcot-marie-tooth.org), the Hereditary Neuropathy Foundation (www.hnf-cure.org), and the Neuropathy Association (www.neuropathy.org).

This chapter covers both available and experimental treatments, as it is expected that the principles of drug development will apply to new therapies for inherited neuropathies in the future. Figure 13-1 shows a schematic of the drug discovery process, beginning with identification of the mutated gene. Identification of the genetic mutations causing inherited neuropathies is the critical step in the development of disease-specific therapy. The next critical question is whether the mutations cause a loss of function (most autosomal recessive and some autosomal dominant mutations) or a gain of function (usually autosomal dominant). Loss-of-function mutations can be treated with gene or protein replacement strategies (e.g., Fabrazyme in Fabry disease), whereas gain-of-function mutations require a strategy to reduce the toxicity of the mutated gene product (e.g., ascorbic acid in CMT1A). As with all drug development, generation of animal models for testing compounds is paramount. The vast majority of genes known to cause neuropathy are highly conserved in mammals, and many are even conserved in simple genetic model systems such as yeast and fruit flies. Thus, studies of the basic biology and pathogenesis of inherited diseases in animal models has proven to be especially relevant to our understanding of inherited human diseases.

Once a mechanism of pathogenesis is proposed and animal models are developed, the drug development process can begin either using a rational drug design approach or using high-throughput screening (see Fig. 13-1). Rational drug design utilizes our understanding of the basic biology and of disease pathogenesis to test specific compounds for efficacy; for example, substrate inhibitors in lysosomal storage disorders are being developed to prevent the toxic storage products from being synthesized.[1] High-throughput screening, on the other hand, requires the generation of an assay in which a library of compounds can be tested for efficacy. For example, a high-throughput assay has recently been developed to screen compounds for modification of *PMP22* (peripheral myelin protein of 22 kD) gene expression. Importantly, candidate compounds with general neuroprotective or neuroregenerative properties may also be effective in acquired neuropathies as well.

After candidate drugs are identified and undergo rigorous toxicity, efficacy, and dosage testing in animal models, they can then be tested in clinical trials. Several factors have limited the success of clinical trials of treatments for inherited neuropathies. First, because these diseases individually are rare, most trials have been done on a small number of patients and thus have not been adequately powered to determine if the drug under investigation has efficacy. The development of large consortia that can enroll many patients from sites around the world is now allowing much larger and better-quality studies to be performed. Furthermore, the slowly progressive nature of many of these disorders with difficult-to-measure clinical parameters makes it difficult to quantitate the treatment effects. The development of quantitative scales to measure disease severity and the ability to assay biomarkers that are relevant to disease pathogenesis are improving the quality of clinical trials in these diseases. Thus, through continued advancements in our understanding of inherited neuropathies, progress in the development of new drugs, and improvements in the design and implementation of clinical trials, effective therapies for inherited neuropathies can be expected in the near future.

Hereditary Motor and Sensory Neuropathies

Hereditary motor and sensory neuropathies (HMSN), commonly referred to as Charcot-Marie-Tooth disease, are the most common inherited neurologic disease, affecting 1 in 2500 people, and thus encompasses the largest group of inherited neuropathies. These diseases are commonly classified based on clinical presentation

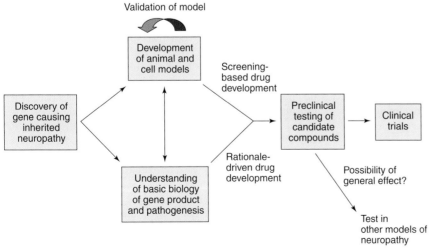

Figure 13-1 Drug development for inherited neuropathies. The initial step in drug development involves the identification and characterization of the gene that is mutated in a disease. By introducing these mutations into animals or cells, animal models can be developed and validated and can assist in understanding the basic biology of the disease. One can then identify therapeutic targets and design drugs based on a rationale-driven approach. Alternatively, animal or in vitro models can be screened with pharmaceutical and chemical libraries to identify novel potential therapeutics, which then undergo preclinical testing in animal models to show efficacy and safety. Once candidate compounds pass these tests, they can be tested in clinical trials. Some drugs developed for inherited neuropathies may have a general neuroprotective or regenerative effect and may be tested in other disease models.

(age of onset and inheritance pattern) and pathology/electrophysiology; for example, autosomal dominant neuropathies are classified as primarily demyelinating (CMT1) or axonal (CMT2). X-linked CMT is classified as CMTX, and autosomal recessive CMT is CMT4. The term CMT3 refers to severe, congenital or early childhood onset CMT, and is best considered a variant of CMT1, because the genes that are mutated are the same. Approximately 70% of cases of CMT are demyelinating, and approximately 70% of cases of demyelinating CMT are due to a duplication of the peripheral myelin protein (PMP22) gene (CMT1A). Thus, although more than 40 genetic loci have been described in CMT patients, almost half of patients with CMT have a single, well-characterized mutation. However, with the discovery of the genetic basis for most of these disorders, it is clear that different mutations in the same gene can cause multiple distinct phenotypes; similarly, the same phenotype is often caused by mutations in different genes (see Table 13-1 and the Inherited Peripheral Neuropathies Mutation Database; www.molgen.ua.ac.be/CMTMutations for a list of known HMSN genes). For example, mutations in the myelin protein zero (MPZ) gene have been found in all forms of CMT (axonal and demyelinating, dominant and recessive). Thus, classification based on the genetic mutation and molecular pathogenesis of the disease may be more relevant than the clinical presentation when discussing therapeutic options.

Clinical Presentation

Most patients with CMT develop slowly progressive weakness and atrophy in their feet beginning in childhood or early adulthood. Pain or sensory loss is variable but is usually not a chief complaint. Foot deformities (pes cavus, or high arches, and hammertoes) are common and may lead to disability (see Figs. 9-15 through 9-17). Mildly affected patients may only be limited in their ability to walk on their heels and play sports, whereas more severely affected patients will have foot drop and steppage gait (hence the initial description of this disease as peroneal muscular atrophy). However, due to the insidious nature of this disease, many patients do not complain of motor or sensory symptoms until late in the course of the disease, and most remain ambulatory. Thus, it is not uncommon to find asymptomatic family members with classical examination and electrophysiologic features of CMT.

On examination, patients typically have distal weakness and atrophy in the feet, areflexia, and length-dependent sensory loss of both large- and small-fiber sensory modalities. More severely affected patients will develop sensory ataxia or tremor (Roussy-Lévy syndrome), palpably enlarged nerves (demyelinating CMT), and weakness, atrophy, and sensory loss of the hands. Patients with motor findings only and without evidence of sensory involvement on examination or electrodiagnostic testing are classified as having hereditary motor neuropathy, whereas patients with sensory findings only and without evidence of motor involvement are classified as hereditary sensory or hereditary sensory and autonomic neuropathy (see Table 13-1 and below). Less commonly, patients can have a severe form of CMT (CMT3) that is congenital (congenital hypomyelinating neuropathy) or with onset before age 3 (Dejerine-Sottas syndrome). Some forms of CMT have unusual features, such as central nervous system (CNS) involvement in CMTX, vocal cord paralysis with CMT2C, and specific thenar involvement in CMT2D (see Table 13-1).

Whereas CMT1A is caused by a duplication of the PMP22 locus, hereditary neuropathy with liability to pressure palsies (HNPP) is caused by a deletion of the same locus.[2] As the name suggests, these patients often present with painless, recurrent entrapment neuropathies, often precipitated by minor trauma or compression. Furthermore, HNPP patients usually have a mild length-dependent demyelinating neuropathy. Another disorder occasionally confused with HNPP is hereditary neuralgic amyotrophy. These patients present essentially the same as those with idiopathic brachial neuritis (Parsonage-Turner syndrome) with episodic, painful weakness and numbness of one upper extremity, often triggered by an infection, exercise, or stress.

Diagnosis and Evaluation

Charcot-Marie-Tooth disease is usually suspected when there is a family history of peripheral neuropathy, because most forms of CMT are autosomal dominant. However, mutations causing CMT occur de novo in about a third of patients, so CMT should be considered in patients with slowly progressive peripheral neuropathy even in the absence of family history. Thus, CMT is underdiagnosed in sporadic cases and is a common diagnosis made in tertiary referral centers of patients with undiagnosed peripheral neuropathy.[3] Less commonly, CMT can be X-linked or autosomal recessive. Examination and electrodiagnostic testing of affected family members can often be extremely helpful in determining the inheritance pattern of neuropathy, if any.

The most useful tests to perform when CMT is clinically suspected are nerve conduction studies (NCS). Classification of the disease as axonal or demyelinating can usually limit the genetic testing required, because the common mutations causing CMT1 (demyelinating) are, in general, different from those causing CMT2 (axonal). History and clinical examination cannot reliably distinguish these distinct forms of CMT, although an early age of onset and palpable nerves would favor a diagnosis of demyelinating CMT. In addition to classifying the disease as primarily axonal or demyelinating, NCS may identify features suggestive of an acquired neuropathy such as chronic inflammatory demyelinating polyneuropathy (CIDP), including asymmetry and conduction block. For example, the most common form of CMT, CMT1A, typically shows severe, uniform reduction of motor and sensory conduction velocities (usually 15 to 30 m/sec). In congenital or early childhood cases (CMT3), the conduction velocity is usually less than 20 m/sec. HNPP shows only mild slowing of conduction velocities but frequently shows focal slowing or conduction block at common sites of entrapment.

When electrophysiology suggests a uniform, symmetric demyelinating polyneuropathy (forearm conduction velocities < 38 m/sec), the clinical diagnosis of CMT can be made and confirmed with genetic testing. When discussing the potential benefits of genetic testing, it is important that patients be educated that although there are currently no proven, specific therapies available for CMT, there are many ongoing clinical trials for patients with specific forms of CMT in which they may be eligible to participate. It is tempting for the clinician to order the entire "CMT gene test panel" to quickly rule in or rule out CMT as the diagnosis. Because insurance often does not cover the cost of genetic testing and ordering all the commercial tests is hardly cost-effective, a shotgun approach is not advisable. The diagnostic yield for a single genetic test (i.e., testing for the PMP22 duplication) for a patient with CMT1 is very high (approximately 70%), whereas the yield of complete sequencing of all known CMT2 genes in a family with CMT2 is low (<20% in one series).[4–6] Thus, the chance of making a definitive molecular diagnosis in a patient with CMT1 is quite high, whereas it remains low in CMT2, as additional genes remain to be discovered. For these reasons, it is generally advisable to first perform only the tests with

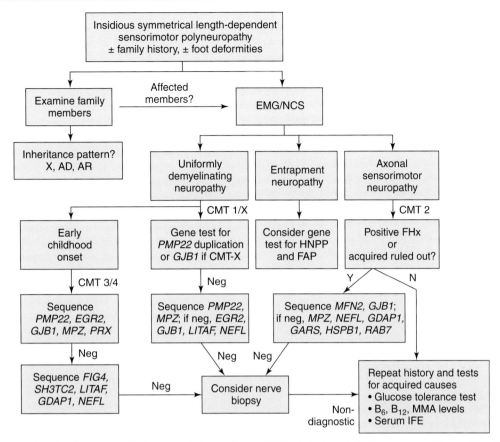

Figure 13-2 Diagnostic algorithm for suspected Charcot-Marie-Tooth disease (CMT). Patients and family members with possible CMT should undergo examination and neurometric testing (EMG/NCS) to evaluate for the presence and type of neuropathy. Depending on the age of onset, inheritance pattern, and physiologic characteristics, patients can be divided into different disease types (in bold). CMT3 and CMT4 (**CMT3/4**) are severe, early onset, AD (CMT3) or AR (CMT4) demyelinating neuropathies. CMT1 and CMTX (**CMT1/X**) are less severe, late childhood or adult onset demyelinating neuropathy with AD (CMT1) or X-linked (CMTX) inheritance. The presence of multiple entrapment neuropathies in a family suggests the possibility of HNPP or FAP. CMT2 is considered in axonal neuropathies in which acquired causes have been ruled out. Commercially available gene tests are listed; the most common genes mutated are listed first. Nerve biopsy is occasionally helpful in difficult cases. If genetic testing and biopsy do not confirm an inherited neuropathy, a repeat evaluation for acquired causes of neuropathy is warranted, particularly diabetes (glucose tolerance test), vitamin deficiency, and toxin exposure. AD, autosomal dominant; AR, autosomal recessive; CMT, Charcot-Marie-Tooth disease; EMG/NCS, electromyography/nerve conduction studies; FAP, familial amyloidotic polyneuropathy; FHx, family history; HNPP, hereditary neuropathy with liability to pressure palsies; IFE, immunofixation electrophoresis; MMA, methylmalonic acid; Neg, negative; X, X chromosome.

the highest likelihood of being positive and only search for rare mutations if the initial tests are negative.

A reasonable diagnostic algorithm for CMT is shown in Figure 13-2; an American Academy of Neurology practice parameter on diagnostic testing of distal symmetric polyneuropathy was recently published showing an algorithm for genetic testing similar to that one.[7] In patients with uniformly demyelinating neuropathy on NCS, a reasonable diagnostic approach is to first test for the *PMP22* duplication/deletion, because this will be positive in the majority of patients. The second most common genetic cause of demyelinating polyneuropathy is CMTX1, with mutations in the gap junction protein beta 1 (*GJB1*) gene (also called *connexin 32*), responsible for approximately 7% of cases. These mutations are X-linked dominant, and females are often affected, though often with milder phenotypes than males with the same mutation. Although usually clinically indistinguishable from other CMTs, CNS demyelination presenting with ataxia, dysarthria, aphasia, disorientation, weakness, and hearing loss, especially in males, has been described in a few families. Spontaneously resolving confluent white matter changes may be seen on brain magnetic resonance imaging (MRI). Furthermore, peripheral nerve demyelination is less

severe than in CMT1A with forearm nerve conduction velocities of 30 to 40 m/sec in males and 30 to 50 m/sec in females; nonuniform slowing and conduction block mimicking findings of CIDP may occur. If CMTX is suspected, it is reasonable to first sequence the *GJB1* gene. If this test is negative, one should consider performing genetic testing for the other genes associated with the CMT1 or CMTX phenotype (see Fig. 13-2 and Table 13-1). Less common mutations include dominantly inherited point mutations in *PMP22*, *MPZ*, early growth response 2 (*EGR2*), LITAF/SIMPLE genes, and recessively inherited mutations in ganglioside-induced differentiation-associated protein 1 (*GDAP1*), myotubularin related protein 2 (*MTMR2*), *SH3TC2*, *FIG4*, and periaxin (*PRX*) genes (see Table 13-1). The autosomal recessive demyelinating neuropathies usually have an earlier onset than autosomal dominant forms and may give an early childhood (Dejerine-Sottas syndrome) or congenital hypomyelinating neuropathy phenotype.

Interestingly, although CMT2 patients with axonal physiology usually have mutations in genes distinct from CMT1, mutations in several of the above genes mutated in CMT1 and expressed in Schwann cells can also cause CMT2. This finding highlights the dependence of Schwann cell–axon interactions on axonal health.

The most common form of CMT2, CMT2A, is caused by mutations in the mitofusin 2 gene (*MFN2*) and may be the second most common cause of CMT overall.[8] Mitofusin is a mitochondrial GTPase that regulates fusion of mitochondria and, in fact, most genes causative of axonal CMT are implicated in either mitochondrial function, axonal transport, or both.[9] Although genes causing CMT2 are ubiquitously expressed, the phenotype is believed to be selective to peripheral nerve due to profound energy demand along axons at long distances from the cell soma. Other genes that have been found mutated in CMT2 are listed in Table 13-1. Several genes have been described that cause dominant intermediate CMT, in which the conduction velocity is intermediate between CMT1 and CMT2, similar to that of CMTX. Many genes that cause CMT2 await discovery; thus, most patients will not be able to have molecular diagnosis. Because acquired causes of distal axonal sensorimotor polyneuropathy are much more common than inherited causes, the diagnosis of CMT2 is usually made by excluding other causes of axonal neuropathy, such as diabetes mellitus, alcoholism, heavy metal and drug toxicity, nutritional deficiency, monoclonal gammopathy, and renal disease.

When the available genetic tests are negative, nerve biopsy may be useful in determining etiology. For example, uniform onion bulb formations are the pathologic hallmark of demyelinating CMT (Fig. 13-3) and, if present, would strongly support the diagnosis of CMT. In patients with a severe early-onset neuropathy, CNS involvement, and tightly curled hair, biopsy findings of giant axonal swellings are diagnostic of giant axonal neuropathy. Furthermore, findings of amyloid deposition (see section on familial amyloid polyneuropathy) or inflammation would point to an alternative diagnosis. One should also reconsider acquired causes of neuropathy and repeat blood tests for vitamin B_1, B_6, B_{12}, and E levels; glucose tolerance test; and serum and urine immunofixation. In cases in which an exhaustive search is negative, one should consider toxins, such as alcohol. When a clear diagnosis cannot be made, referral to a tertiary center rather than a trial of immunotherapy is recommended for possible diagnosis of CIDP, because the expense and risks of intravenous immunoglobulins or steroids rarely justify empiric use of these drugs in slowly progressive cases.

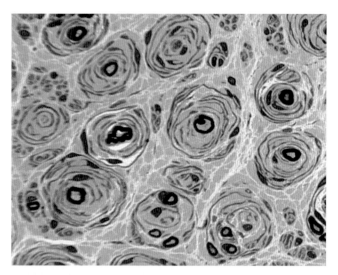

Figure 13-3 Osmicated and toluidine blue stained sural nerve biopsy section showing increased connective tissue and decreased number of myelinated axons; the most prominent finding is the presence of onion bulbs (400×).

Treatment and Management

There are no specific therapies for CMT currently available. Physical and occupational therapy should be offered to patients because orthotics, including ankle bracing and aids to improve dexterity (e.g., button and zipper holders), may improve quality of life. Orthopedic surgery for correction of foot deformities is often recommended, though surgery is often not necessary (see Chapter 9 for surgical management of neuropathies). Surgery such as tendon transfers may help prevent pressure ulcers or relieve pain caused by severe pes cavus, inverted feet, or other deformities. Well-made, specially fitted shoes and daily inspection of feet may be all that is required to prevent ulcers and pain over pressure points. Physical and occupational therapy are often helpful with regard to orthotics and exercises to maintain muscle bulk and coordination; however, evidence showing a benefit for most orthotics is lacking[10] (see Chapter 8 for more information). A 12-week controlled study showed that moderate exercise is beneficial for CMT patients, but overexercising can be detrimental.[11,12] Patients in whom pain is a significant complaint may benefit from medications used for neuropathic pain, such as antiepileptics and antidepressants (see Chapter 6). Although weak ankles and decreased sensation often affect balance, the majority of patients remain ambulatory and life expectancy is not shortened. A certified genetic counselor should be available to advise and help in the management of these patients and their families.

Physicians are often asked whether drugs prescribed for other purposes may potentially be harmful in CMT. Neurotoxic drugs, especially the chemotherapeutic agents paclitaxel, vincristine, and cisplatin, should be avoided if possible, but evidence demonstrating adverse effects of other drugs is limited. The CMT Association Web site (www.charcot-marie-tooth.org/med_alert.php) lists drugs that have been reported to exacerbate CMT, but this potential risk should be weighed against any benefit. Regardless of whether the underlying pathophysiology is primarily demyelinating or axonal, disability in CMT correlates with axonal loss. Thus, muscle atrophy and reduction in compound muscle action potential (CMAP) amplitude are much more important measures of functional status than conduction velocity on NCS or demyelination on biopsy. Chronic demyelination eventually leads to axonal degeneration through an unclear mechanism, though one that is an area of active investigation. Thus, therapies targeted at promoting neuronal survival and preventing axonal degeneration may be broadly applicable to all causes of inherited and acquired neuropathies.

There are reports of patients with CMT1 developing superimposed CIDP with acute or subacute progression, proximal involvement, or markedly elevated cerebrospinal fluid (CSF) protein, asymmetric NCS, and an inflammatory sural nerve biopsy. Whether there is an increased association of CIDP with CMT is unclear, but prednisone, immunoglobulin, or other immunotherapies should be considered in patients who develop rapid clinical deterioration.[13,14] There is evidence in mouse models that the immune system plays a role in the pathogenesis of CMT[15]; however, there is no evidence that immunosuppressive therapies are beneficial in typical CMT.

Because of the susceptibility of patients with HNPP and hereditary neuralgic amyotrophy to develop entrapment neuropathies, counseling these patients to avoid compression of the nerves at susceptible sites is of utmost importance in this disease (see Chapter 16 regarding specific therapies for compression neuropathies). As in noninherited entrapment neuropathies, the most common sites of compression are the wrist, elbow, knee, and shoulder. Patients should be advised to avoid repetitive and strenuous use of these joints and to avoid static or awkward positioning. Focal neuropathies usually recover spontaneously, although frequently the recovery is incomplete; surgical release of the entrapment is controversial[16] and generally not advisable because nerves are especially vulnerable to manipulation and minor trauma.

Experimental Therapies for CMT: Modifying PMP22 Expression and Neuroprotection

As the molecular basis of inherited neuropathies becomes better understood, specific therapies will likely become available. The best example of this rational therapeutic approach applied to CMT is development of modifiers of *PMP22* gene expression. The gene dosage of *PMP22* is critical for peripheral nerve myelination, as a duplication of the *PMP22* locus (increasing gene expression by only 50%) causes CMT1A, whereas a deletion of this locus (reducing expression by 50%) causes HNPP. The relatively high frequency of CMT1A can be explained by the genomic location of the *PMP22* gene, in a region of chromosome 17 that is flanked by two tandem duplications, thereby increasing the frequency of unequal crossing-over during meiosis.[17]

The most common inherited neuropathy, CMT1A is responsible for about half of all CMT cases and may be caused by both duplication of (most common) or point mutations in *PMP22*. Transgenic mice and rats overexpressing human *PMP22* replicate many of the pathologic features of CMT1A and thus have been used to model human CMT. Ascorbic acid (vitamin C) had previously been shown to be required for in vitro myelination of axons by Schwann cells in culture,[18] and vitamin C along with other antioxidant vitamins is believed to have neuroprotective properties.[19] Passage and colleagues showed in 2004 that administration of high-dose ascorbic acid to mice overexpressing *PMP22* led to marked improvement of locomotor deficits and reduced demyelination.[20] Interestingly, ascorbic acid, but not other antioxidants, specifically inhibits *PMP22* gene expression; thus, ascorbic acid may treat the underlying cause of CMT1A. However, ascorbic acid has not shown efficacy in recently completed phase II studies of patients with CMT1A.[21,22]

As with all slowly progressive neurodegenerative diseases, the primary limitation for determination of efficacy in these clinical trials is the need for sensitive biomarkers and clinical tests, because clinically significant functional measures require long-term follow-up of a large number of patients. A recently validated primary clinical outcome used in current studies is the CMT neuropathy score.[23] Skin biopsies may also be performed to evaluate *PMP22* expression. These large clinical trials demonstrate how identification of the underlying gene defect in CMT1A and development of animal models can rapidly translate to clinical trials for patients (see Fig. 13-1). A similar approach is currently being carried out with progesterone antagonists, shown to decrease *PMP22* expression in Schwann cell cultures and transgenic animals.[24] The available progesterone antagonist, onapristone, shows severe toxicity in humans[25]; thus, new progesterone antagonists are currently under development. Because HNPP is caused by reduced expression of *PMP22*, progesterone agonists may have efficacy in treatment of HNPP.

However, promising results in animal models do not always translate into effective human treatments, as has been shown too often in clinical trials for ALS[26]; thus, caution must be taken when counseling patients regarding taking these available, yet experimental, drugs outside of clinical trials. Furthermore, high-throughput screens for additional chemical modulators of *PMP22* expression are currently under development and funded by the CMT Association; for example, using Schwann cell lines expressing luciferase downstream of the *PMP22* promoter. Other potential treatments that may be available in the future for specifically inhibiting *PMP22* expression include gene therapy with RNA interference or antisense oligonucleotides to *PMP22*.

Although the above therapies address the cause of CMT1A, there is considerable evidence that the cause of disability in CMT is due to axonal loss rather than demyelination. This is believed to be due to disruption of interactions between Schwann cells and axons. Thus, therapies of neurotrophic factors devised to prevent axonal degeneration may also be efficacious in inherited demyelinating neuropathies.[27] One such trophic factor that has shown promise in CMT1A is neurotrophin-3 (NT-3). NT-3 is a small peptide produced by Schwann cells that autoregulates their proliferation and differentiation. Sahenk and colleagues performed a single-blinded pilot study of NT-3 in eight CMT1A patients.[28] They reported that subcutaneous administration of NT-3 (5 μg/kg three times weekly) led to a significant improvement of sensory symptoms and reflexes, but no change in motor outcome. Furthermore, NT-3 increased axonal regeneration in two CMT1A animal models.[28] A recent Cochrane Database review concluded that the NT-3 trial was the only randomized clinical trial for CMT in which the effect of treatment was able to be identified.[29] Although this therapy shows promise, larger studies are needed to determine the efficacy of NT-3.

Hereditary Motor Neuropathy

The term *hereditary motor neuropathy* (HMN) primarily refers to degenerative disorders of lower motor neurons that innervate *distal* muscles, whereas when proximal muscles are preferentially affected, the disorder is referred to as *spinal muscular atrophy* (SMA), which is discussed in Chapter 12. Because HMNs are about 10 times less common than SMA, these disorders are often referred to as distal SMA (dSMA) or occasionally as distal HMN (dHMN) to emphasize this distinction from typical SMA. Not surprisingly, there is significant overlap between HMN and CMT2, including several allelic disorders that differ in their classification depending on whether there is sensory involvement (e.g., *GARS* mutations cause both CMT2D and HMNVa). There is also overlap in clinical presentation of some hereditary forms of amyotrophic lateral sclerosis (ALS) with HMN; for example, ALS-4, a juvenile form of ALS, has very slowly progressive distal muscle weakness and atrophy (see Chapter 11). Genetic testing is not available for most of these disorders, and most are very rare (see Table 13-1). There are no specific therapies yet available, but patients' symptoms are treated similarly to those of patients with CMT.

Hereditary Sensory and Autonomic Neuropathies

The hereditary sensory and autonomic neuropathies (HSAN) comprise a group of rare disorders with the primary manifestation of peripheral sensory loss and autonomic dysfunction (also discussed in Chapter 5). These disorders must be distinguished from inherited neuropathies of large primary afferent sensory neurons with or without involvement of cerebellar or spinocerebellar neurons (spinocerebellar degeneration such as Friedreich ataxia or spinocerebellar ataxia). As shown in Table 13-1, HSAN is typically classified based on inheritance pattern into autosomal dominant (type 1) and autosomal recessive (types 2 through 5) forms.

Clinical Presentation

The autosomal dominant and recessive forms have very different clinical presentations. Autosomal dominant HSAN (HSAN type 1, also called HSN type 1 or HSN-1) presents as a slowly progressive, length-dependent sensory axonal neuropathy.[30] Onset is usually in the second or third decade of life. Motor and autonomic manifestations (usually loss of sweating) are variable, but are usually much less severe than the sensory symptoms. Examination also reveals distal loss of reflexes and sensation of all modalities, and foot ulcers are common. In addition, there are characteristic but variable findings seen in subtypes of HSAN type 1. Patients with a mutation in the serine palmitoyltransferase long-chain (*SPTLC1*) gene frequently develop hearing loss, peroneal weakness, and hyperhydrosis.[31] A second locus on chromosome 3 has been found in families with prominent cough and gastroesophageal reflux, variable sensorineural hearing loss, and lack of motor involvement.[32] Although the phenotypes often overlap, HSAN type 1 can often be distinguished from CMT2B, caused by *RAB7* mutations, because CMT2B patients usually have distal muscle weakness in addition to distal ulceromutilation and profound sensory loss.

In contrast, the autosomal recessive forms of HSAN (types 2 to 4) are usually congenital in onset with a generalized loss of sensory and autonomic fibers.[33] An insensitivity to pain frequently causes severe acral mutilation and arthropathy, frequently leading to more severe morbidity than seen in CMT patients. HSAN type 2 is a rare autosomal recessive disorder characterized by congenital sensory loss and severe acral mutilation. HSAN type 3, also known as *familial dysautonomia*, is probably the most common form of HSAN and is seen almost exclusively in the Ashkenazi Jewish population. Infants present with hypotonia and profound dysautonomia, causing poor feeding, high fevers, skin blotching, and cardiovascular instability. Pain and temperature sensation are less affected than in other forms of HSAN. HSAN type 4 is characterized by anhidrosis, causing recurrent high fevers and characteristic skin thickening, severe ulceromutilation and arthropathy due to pain insensitivity, and CNS involvement in more severely affected patients.

Diagnosis and Evaluation

Hereditary sensory and autonomic neuropathy type 1 (also called *HSN type 1*) can be difficult to distinguish from other causes of slowly progressive, length-dependent sensory neuropathy. This diagnosis should be considered in patients developing a sensory-predominant axonal neuropathy at a young age (often second or third decade of life) or with an autosomal dominant inheritance pattern. The chronicity and severity of the sensory loss leads to severe foot complications in some kindreds, including plantar ulcers, spontaneous fractures, and osteomyelitis. Electrodiagnostic testing is performed to confirm the presence of a sensory axonal neuropathy, and laboratory testing, including a glucose tolerance test, is helpful in excluding more common acquired sensory neuropathies. Distinguishing this disease from CMT2 may be difficult, but generally HSAN patients have more severe sensory symptoms and little or no motor involvement, whereas the reverse is usually true in CMT. Skin biopsy and sudomotor testing may be helpful in confirming small-fiber sensory and autonomic involvement, respectively. Nerve biopsy may be helpful in difficult cases to exclude amyloidosis and vasculitis. In HSAN types 2 to 5, diagnosis is usually based on the constellation of clinical signs.

As with other inherited neuropathies, genetic testing should be performed for definitive diagnosis if possible. HSAN type 1 is genetically heterogeneous, with additional genes yet to be discovered, but both *SPTCL1* and *RAB7* genetic testing are commercially available. In contrast, among the recessive HSANs, genetic testing is only available for familial dysautonomia/HSAN 3 (*IKBKAP*), allowing carrier status determination in the Ashkenazi Jewish population, a frequency estimated to be about 1 in 30.[34]

Treatment and Management

The mainstay of treatment in HSAN types 1 and 2 is in preventing ulcerations, the major cause of morbidity. Because sensory loss is length-dependent in HSAN type 1, the same general precautions and treatments for diabetic feet are recommended (see Chapters 8 and 20). In contrast, in HSAN types 2 and 4, prevention and treatment of self-mutilation is much more difficult given the infantile onset and generalized symptoms. Smoothing of teeth or tooth extractions may be required in children with severe ulceromutilation. A recent case study demonstrated a 98% reduction in self-injurious behavior in an 11-year-old boy using habit-reversal behavioral therapy.[35] Braces may be helpful to prevent osteoarthropathy of weight-bearing joints. Treatment of dysautonomia in patients with HSAN types 3 and 4 is particularly challenging and is discussed in detail in Chapter 5.

Familial Amyloidic Polyneuropathy

Like HSAN type 1, familial amyloid polyneuropathy (FAP) is also an autosomal dominant, adult-onset polyneuropathy, predominantly affecting small-caliber sensory and autonomic fibers.[36] Unlike HSAN, though, FAP is a systemic disease, and patients frequently develop restrictive cardiomyopathy, nephropathy, ocular symptoms, or involvement of other tissues. In addition to inherited amyloidoses, acquired forms of systemic amyloidosis also cause neuropathy.[37] Approximately 20% of patients with immunoglobulin light-chain amyloidosis develop neuropathy, and even more of these patients have symptoms of carpal tunnel syndrome or other entrapment neuropathies. Also, patients on chronic dialysis can develop amyloidosis and carpal tunnel syndrome from deposition of β_2-microglobulin. Here, we focus on the inherited amyloid neuropathies.

Familial amyloid polyneuropathy is most commonly caused by a missense mutation in the transthyretin gene (*TTR*), which encodes for an abundant plasma protein synthesized in the liver that binds and transports thyroid hormone and vitamin A.[38] More than 100 missense mutations in *TTR* that are believed to cause misfolding of the protein and a propensity to form amyloidogenic fibrils that are deposited extracellularly have been described. A V30M mutation is by far the most common, though there is little correlation between genotype and phenotype with a few exceptions. Two other genes have been shown to be mutated in a few families with FAP: apolipoprotein A-I (*APOAI*) and gelsolin, which both have distinctive clinical features discussed below (see Table 13-2). The mechanism whereby amyloid induces neuropathy is unclear, but is believed to be due to a direct toxic effect of amyloid oligomers on neurons.

Clinical Presentation

Patients with FAP from mutant *TTR* typically present in their second or third decade, with slowly progressive pain and allodynia in their limbs.[39] Patients may also develop autonomic symptoms, including impotence and orthostatic hypotension. As in diabetic neuropathy, this initial small-fiber neuropathy typically progresses to involve large myelinated sensory fibers, and later in the course of disease patients develop a length-dependent axonal sensorimotor polyneuropathy. Carpal tunnel syndrome is rarely a presenting complaint in families with the V30M mutation but is common in families with several other mutations. The course of the disease is usually slowly progressive, though rare cases of rapidly progressive disease have been reported. Patients typically become wheelchair-bound by an average of 10 years after onset and succumb to infection or cardiovascular collapse.

The involvement of other systems is variable and depends on the tissues in which the amyloid becomes deposited. Involvement of the cardiovascular system is common, and patients frequently develop progressive conduction abnormalities and restrictive cardiomyopathy, often leading to arrhythmias and heart failure, respectively. In addition to being produced in the liver, transthyretin is also produced at lower levels in the retina and choroid plexus, explaining the finding of amyloid deposits in the vitreous and leptomeninges, respectively. Some patients may develop CNS involvement due to leptomeningeal amyloid deposits and may have elevated CSF protein and meningeal enhancement on MRI. The gastrointestinal system may be affected both due to involvement of autonomic nerves supplying the gut and to amyloid deposition in the bowel wall causing a protein-losing enteropathy. Though other organs such as the kidneys frequently develop amyloid deposits in patients with *TTR* mutations, these deposits are usually asymptomatic.

Patients with mutations in *APOAI* develop a clinical presentation very similar to that of patients with *TTR* mutations; however, these patients also develop progressive renal failure.[40] Patients with gelsolin mutations have a very distinctive clinical presentation, initially presenting with a pathognomic lattice corneal dystrophy, often leading to diagnosis. These patients usually develop cranial neuropathies in their fourth or fifth decade and later develop a length-dependent polyneuropathy.[41]

Diagnosis and Evaluation

Early diagnosis of FAP depends on it being considered in all patients who present with an otherwise unexplained progressive sensorimotor axonal polyneuropathy, particularly in patients with autonomic or cardiovascular symptoms, early small-fiber involvement, or a family history of neuropathy. The primary differential diagnostic considerations are acquired amyloidosis, diabetes, human immunodeficiency virus infection, leprosy, and toxic neuropathies. In a cohort of 90 FAP patients who presented without family history, the most common misdiagnosis was CIDP, likely due to elevated CSF protein, slowed nerve conduction velocities, or negative biopsy.[42] Other inherited neuropathies that may mimic FAP are HSAN and Fabry disease, discussed later in this chapter.

If there is a family history of FAP, diagnosis is best made with genetic testing. However, in the majority of cases in which there is not a positive family history, usually the first step toward making the diagnosis is to perform a tissue biopsy, although a negative biopsy does not rule out FAP. Sural nerve biopsy has been reported to be insensitive for making the diagnosis of amyloidosis in one small case series,[43] but in several other studies, nerve biopsy has been shown to be at least as sensitive as biopsies from other sites, with a sensitivity of approximately 80%.[42] Biopsy of other tissues, such as rectum, labial salivary gland, and subcutaneous fat pad, has been reported to have a similar sensitivity and can also be examined. Skin biopsy is useful in evaluating small-fiber neuropathy but has not been shown to be sensitive or specific for diagnosing amyloidosis.[44] Biopsies stained with Congo Red reveal amorphous deposits of congophilic material that are apple-green birefringent under polarized light (Fig. 13-4).

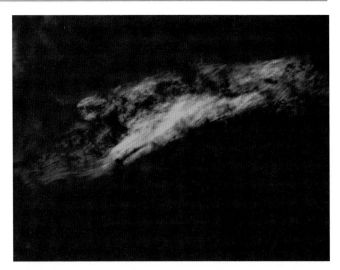

Figure 13-4 Amyloid deposits seen with polarized light, giving apple-green birefringence (400×).

However, due to the patchy nature of the deposits, multiple sections may be required to identify the amyloid.

Once the diagnosis of amyloidosis has been made by biopsy or, in the case of a negative biopsy in a patient in whom amyloidosis is considered, the next step is genetic testing. Specific mutations can be screened for in patients with a family history of a known mutation. Sequencing the entire *TTR* open reading frame is commercially available to identify unknown mutations. In patients with amyloid on biopsy and negative *TTR* sequencing, immunohistochemistry for light chains, transthyretin, and serum amyloid A protein are occasionally useful in determining the nature of the amyloid deposit. Serum and urine immunofixation electrophoresis should be performed to evaluate for a monoclonal plasma cell dyscrasia causing light-chain amyloid. Though sequencing for *APOAI* and gelsolin mutations is not commercially available, it can be performed by specialized laboratories. If the diagnosis of FAP is confirmed by DNA sequencing, further genetic counseling of the patient and family members should be performed. The presence of cardiac involvement should be determined with electrocardiogram and echocardiogram.

Treatment and Management

The only specific therapy proven to be effective in FAP is liver transplantation. Because transthyretin is predominantly produced in the liver, removal of the source of the amyloid often stops progression of the disease, but rarely does it lead to improvement in symptoms. In a recent, large series of 84 patients undergoing transplantation for FAP in Sweden over a 15-year period (1990–2005), less than 10% had improvement in symptoms, although in more than half, transplantation halted the progression of the disease.[45] Furthermore, orthotopic liver transplantation is a complicated procedure with significant perioperative mortality, particularly in patients with cardiac amyloidosis. In this same cohort of patients, there was a dramatic improvement in survival in patients transplanted over the last 10 years (92% at 5 years) compared with the first 5 years (67%). However, in this large group of patients, only a minority of patients' symptoms improved. The improvement in survival is believed to at least partially be due to transplanting patients earlier in their disease course; the factors that independently predicted survival included age less than 40 years, duration of disease of less than 7 years, and good nutritional status (mBMI > 600). Thus, it is generally recommended that patients be transplanted early in the course of their disease. Some mutations appear to benefit more from transplantation than others, with the greatest benefit seen in patients with the Val30Met mutation. In patients who do not respond to transplantation, the progression is thought to be due to continued deposition of wild-type transthyretin. Patients with *APOAI* mutations who also develop severe renal involvement may benefit from combined liver and kidney transplant,[46] and patients with gelsolin amyloidosis may be effectively treated with corneal transplantation.

Drugs in development for FAP include compounds that bind to amyloid and prevent its deposition.[47] The salicylate diflunisal has been shown to have such biochemical properties,[48,49] and because it is an FDA-approved drug, is currently in clinical trials despite not being tested in animal models. Because FAP is a systemic disease, many symptomatic treatments may be considered. As in acquired painful neuropathies, neuropathic pain may respond to antiepileptic and antidepressant medications (see Chapter 6). Vitrectomy is often effective for ocular amyloidosis. A pacemaker may be required for patients who develop arrhythmias or cardiomyopathy.

Friedreich Ataxia and Other Spinocerebellar Ataxias

Inherited diseases causing degeneration of the spinocerebellar tract have many genetic causes and are commonly associated with peripheral neuropathy. Large-fiber sensory neuropathy is a common clinical feature of Friedreich ataxia and spinocerebellar atrophy with axonal neuropathy and is a variable finding in most other spinocerebellar ataxias and ataxia-telangiectasia. Vitamin E deficiency (either acquired or rare inherited forms abetalipoproteinemia and ataxia with vitamin E deficiency [AVED]; see below and Table 13-2) can mimic the neurologic manifestations of Friedreich ataxia and should be considered in the differential diagnosis given that patients respond to high-dose vitamin E (100 mg/kg/day) and fat restriction. Here, we focus on Friedreich ataxia, the most common genetic ataxia in North America and Europe.

Clinical Presentation

Friedreich ataxia is an autosomal recessive neurodegenerative disease characterized by progressive ataxia, dysarthria, nystagmus, and sensory loss. Loss of sensory neurons in the dorsal root ganglion occurs early, followed by degeneration of the spinocerebellar tract, posterior columns, and pyramidal tracts. Although the clinical picture is usually dominated by ataxia, large-fiber neuropathy is a common cause of disability. Patients usually develop progressive proprioceptive loss, foot deformity, and kyphoscoliosis. On examination, they classically have absence of deep tendon reflexes with extensor plantar reflexes. Other common clinical findings include hypertrophic cardiomyopathy (a common cause of morbidity and mortality in Friedreich ataxia), diabetes, sensorineural hearing loss, and optic neuropathy.[50]

Diagnosis and Evaluation

Genetic testing of the frataxin (*FXN*) gene reveals an expansion of the GAA triplet-repeat in the first intron, causing a reduction in frataxin levels. Normally, there are less than 33 GAA repeats, whereas in patients with Friedreich ataxia, repeats range from 67 to more than 1,000 in length. Rarely (in approximately 3% of cases), one allele contains a point mutation elsewhere in the gene rather than an expanded triplet repeat.[51] Electrodiagnostic testing shows a sensory axonal neuropathy/neuronopathy (non–length-dependent decrease in sensory amplitudes), and sural nerve biopsy shows axonal atrophy with mild demyelination and remyelination.

Treatment and Management

As the molecular etiology of Friedreich's ataxia has been elucidated, targeted pharmacotherapies affecting specific pathogenic pathways have become increasingly promising (Fig. 13-5). Friedreich ataxia is often considered a nuclear-encoded mitochondrial disease, because the disorder is thought to be due to loss of frataxin function in neuronal mitochondria. Increasing evidence suggests that, as in fragile X syndrome, the triplet repeats in noncoding portions of the gene causes the DNA to form a "sticky" triple-helical structure, leading to decreased expression of frataxin.[52] To combat these structural changes, certain polyamides, small cell-permeable molecules able to specifically bind to GAA repeats and thereby disrupt aberrant DNA conformations, have been developed and shown to increase frataxin transcription in vitro.[53] Furthermore, these abnormal triple-helical structures are subject to deacetylation and hypermethylation of DNA, thereby condensing local chromatin and decreasing gene

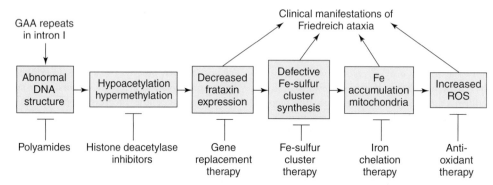

Figure 13-5 Pathogenesis and therapeutic development of Friedreich's ataxia. The *arrows* designate a hypothesized pathogenic cascade of Friedreich's ataxia in which the cause of disease is believed to be due to decreased frataxin expression. An expansion of the GAA triplet repeat causes DNA structural changes that cause the DNA to become hypoacetylated and hypermethylated, thereby reducing gene expression. Reduced frataxin protein leads to defective iron (Fe)-sulfur cluster synthesis, mitochondrial iron accumulation, and increased reactive oxygen species (ROS). Each of these abnormalities may contribute to the disease phenotype directly and indirectly (thus *multiple arrows* leading to clinical manifestations), and it is likely that an effective therapy will target multiple pathogenic steps. Therapies currently under development are listed below each pathogenic step and described in the text; ⊣ indicates therapy to ameliorate this pathogenic step.

expression. Thus, histone deacetylation (HDAC) inhibitors or DNA demethylation agents could potentially treat the underlying causes of these diseases, and small-molecule drugs are in various stages of preclinical development. Indeed, specific HDAC inhibitors have been shown to normalize frataxin expression in patient-derived lymphoid cell lines.[54] Friedreich ataxia mouse models have been generated that replicate many of the epigenetic and pathologic changes seen in human patients,[55,56] and HDAC inhibitors fed to a mouse model restore frataxin expression without signs of toxicity.[57] These and other studies have led to considerable excitement in the field and have paved the way for clinical trials of HDAC inhibitors in this disease.

In addition to rational drug design, high-throughput screening is being undertaken to develop new small molecules that increase frataxin expression. A previously FDA-approved drug, erythropoietin, was identified in a candidate-based screen for such agents and has been shown to increase frataxin expression in patient-derived cell lines through an as-yet unclear mechanism.[58] In a recent open-label "proof-of-principle" study of 12 patients, subcutaneous erythropoietin given three times a week to Friedreich ataxia patients for 6 months increased frataxin levels, decreased urinary oxidative stress markers, and improved a clinical ataxia score.[59] The short time frame at which clinical improvement was seen suggests that the improved ataxia score is unlikely to be due to an effect on degeneration and could be due to placebo effect. Furthermore, if the findings from this nonblinded pilot study are replicated in a well-controlled study, the frequent blood monitoring required and safety concerns of erythropoietin use would need to be weighed against any proven benefit.

Not only are therapies being designed to increase *FXN* gene expression, but they are also being developed to counteract the downstream consequences of frataxin loss. Frataxin functions in iron metabolism and is required for the mitochondrial generation of iron-sulfur clusters, cofactors essential to the function of several enzymes of the respiratory chain and Krebs cycle, such as aconitase. Decreased frataxin expression causes iron overload in mitochondria, and the abnormal iron chemistry generates increased reactive oxygen species and sensitivity to oxidative stress. As shown in Figure 13-5, all of these consequences of frataxin loss are investigational targets for Friedreich ataxia drug therapy. For example, compounds that increase iron-sulfur cluster synthesis are in development. Also, iron chelation therapy to reduce iron overload has been attempted; however, recent studies suggest that iron chelation may further reduce *FXN* expression via a feedback mechanism and impair aconitase activity.[60]

The most investigated therapy in Friedreich ataxia, initiated before the *FXN* gene was discovered, is antioxidant therapy.[61] One of the early rationales for this treatment was the similarity of symptoms between Friedreich ataxia and vitamin E–deficient ataxia. Once the increase in reactive oxygen species was identified in Friedreich ataxia and oxidative stress became a widely believed mechanism of neurodegeneration, antioxidant therapy became widely used in patients despite the lack of evidence of efficacy. Although a large number of studies have been performed with antioxidant agents in Friedreich ataxia, most of these have been uncontrolled, underpowered, and without clearly defined clinical endpoints, allowing few firm conclusions to be drawn. Recently, the use of standardized rating scales (e.g., the International Cooperative Ataxia Rating Scale [ICARS]) and the establishment of international consortia have significantly improved the quality of these studies.

The most promising candidate antioxidant therapy is idebenone, a synthetic coenzyme Q analog that has shown promise in phase I and II clinical trials. Several recent reviews have discussed the details of

these studies[61–63]; here, we summarize their conclusions. Although some of the studies are contradictory, likely due to problems with study design, generally a trend toward slowing of neurologic deterioration is observed in children treated with idebenone at high doses. The optimal dose is not at all clear, but clinical effects were generally not seen at low doses (5 mg/kg/day), and studies showing benefit used doses of 45 to 75 mg/kg/day. These higher doses are generally very well tolerated, although there are reports of neutropenia that is reversible on drug cessation.[64] Thus, patients taking high doses should have routine monitoring of blood counts. In addition, several studies have also shown a reduction in cardiac hypertrophy with idebenone, although this has not translated to improved cardiac function. In summary, idebenone has shown promise in Friedreich ataxia patients, but clearly further studies are needed; indeed, a pivotal phase III trial of 70 patients is currently under way in the United States and close to completion. Newer analogs of idebenone (e.g., Mito-Q) have been developed and are in clinical trials targeted to the mitochondria, theoretically increasing their efficacy.

Although antioxidant therapies and other therapies targeted toward the downstream effects of frataxin deficiency have shown promise, most experts believe that the goal of new investigational agents should be to restore frataxin levels and thereby target the underlying cause of the disease. The potential arises for treating two or more of these pathogenic steps shown in Figure 13-5 with a cocktail of drugs targeting different pathogenic events.

Despite the promise that these investigational agents have shown in early studies, there is, as yet, no proven pharmacotherapy for Friedreich ataxia. As in other inherited neuropathies, orthopedic procedures and devices are critical to the maintenance of mobility (see Chapters 8 and 9). This is particularly true in Friedreich ataxia, because foot deformities may compound the imbalance caused by the underlying ataxia. In one series of patients, although surgery to correct equinovarus foot deformity was effective in improving function (predominantly ability to transfer independently), three of seven patients had life-threatening complications (aspiration pneumonia or pulmonary embolus).[65] Thus, aggressive physiotherapy to prevent foot deformity is paramount. In a large series of patients undergoing treatment for scoliosis, surgical fusion was effective, whereas bracing was not.[66] Furthermore, the primary cause of death in these patients is related to cardiac complications; thus, prevention and treatment of hypertrophic cardiomyopathy is paramount. Finally, patients should be screened for glucose intolerance due to the risk of developing diabetes.

Inherited Dyslipidemic Neuropathies

Abetalipoproteinemia and Hypobetalipoproteinemia

Abetalipoproteinemia (also known as *Bassen-Kornzweig syndrome*) is a rare autosomal recessive disorder causing undetectable plasma apolipoprotein B (apoB) and low low-density lipoprotein (LDL) and total cholesterol (<50 mg/dL). The disease is caused by mutations in the microsomal triglyceride transfer protein (*MTTP*) gene, leading to an inability to transfer lipids to apoB and a severe defect in fat absorption. Fat malabsorption, hypocholesterolemia, and acanthocytosis are present in infancy; in adolescence, patients develop signs and symptoms of fat-soluble vitamin deficiency, particularly vitamin E. Disease features include cerebellar ataxia, spastic gait and neuropathy, myopathy, coagulopathy, retinitis pigmentosa and impaired night vision, nystagmus and ophthalmoplegia, anemia, and cardiac arrhythmia. Hypobetalipoproteinemia is a milder form of this disorder with autosomal dominant inheritance caused by truncation mutations in ApoB. These patients have a clinical presentation similar to Friedreich ataxia with progressive ataxia and peripheral neuropathy. Like Friedreich ataxia, the neuropathy of these diseases is predominantly a distal axonal sensory polyneuropathy. Importantly, the neuropathy and other features of these disorders have been reported to be treatable with high-dose vitamin E (100 mg/kg/day) and other fat-soluble vitamins.

Analphalipoproteinemia (Tangier Disease)

Tangier disease is a rare autosomal recessive disorder caused by mutations in the *ABCA1* gene, a member of the ABC transporter family similar to the *ABCD1* gene mutated in adrenoleukodystrophy. Loss of transporter activity leads to the inability of cells to secrete excess cholesterol in the form of high-density lipoprotein (HDL) and an accumulation of cholesterol esters in cells. This defect is manifest in patients as enlarged orange-yellow tonsils, corneal opacities, hepatosplenomegaly, a relapsing sensorimotor neuropathy, and premature coronary artery disease. Diagnosis is made by finding markedly reduced HDL levels and elevated triglyceride levels in plasma. Treatment aimed at elevating HDL has been generally ineffective, and no treatment is currently available for these patients.

Lysosomal Storage Diseases: Fabry Disease

Lysosomal storage diseases (LSDs) constitute a diverse group of more than 40 inherited disorders with multiorgan involvement that frequently affect the nervous system. Peripheral nerve manifestations are especially prominent in the sphingolipidoses, including Fabry disease, metachromatic leukodystrophy (MLD), and Krabbe's disease or globoid cell leukodystrophy (GLD), but has also been reported in many other LSDs. Many LSDs present with progressive neurodegeneration beginning in early childhood, but some have adult-onset forms. Although individually uncommon, as a group they make up a significant portion of inherited neuropathies, and many of these diseases are potentially treatable with enzyme replacement therapy (ERT) or hematopoietic stem cell therapy (HCT). Thus, LSDs should be considered in the differential diagnosis of unexplained neuropathy, especially in those with CNS or other organ involvement.

Fabry disease is one of the more common lysosomal storage disorders, and painful small-fiber neuropathy is the earliest and often the most disabling symptom of this multisystem disease. This disease is X-linked, and although symptoms occur earlier and are more severe in men, female carriers are variably affected, partially due to skewed X-inactivation. Fabry disease is caused by a deficiency of α-galactosidase A, leading to accumulation of globotriaosylceramide (Gb3) in vascular endothelium and other tissues. The lysosomal storage of Gb3 in blood vessels is believed to cause ischemic damage in multiple tissues.

Clinical Presentation

The symptoms of Fabry disease begin in childhood (usually about age 5 years in boys and late childhood or early adulthood in girls) with painful paresthesias in the hands and feet, decreased sweating, and gastrointestinal symptoms (nausea, abdominal pain, postprandial diarrhea), frequently leading to difficulty in school. Pain is typically chronic with episodic exacerbations or "crises," often triggered by environmental stimuli (e.g., heat, exercise, or stress). Untreated

patients develop progressive disease of the kidneys, heart, and brain, usually leading to premature death in the 40s or 50s. Renal disease starts with proteinuria and progresses to renal insufficiency and end-stage renal disease if untreated. Early cardiac manifestations include left ventricular hypertrophy and mitral insufficiency; these often progress to coronary artery disease, hypertrophic cardiomyopathy, and arrhythmias. Patients are at approximately a 10-fold increased risk for transient ischemic attacks and strokes, and brain MRI frequently shows evidence of microvascular ischemic disease. Boys usually have multiple angiokeratomas, punctate red telangiectasias commonly found on the skin of the lower trunk, buttocks, and scrotum. Other signs and symptoms include sensorineural hearing loss, corneal opacities, endocrine dysfunction, and mood disorders. As with other LSDs, there are rare late-onset variants of this disease, usually affecting only the heart or kidney. Recently, a family with adult-onset cramp-fasciculation syndrome was shown to have Fabry disease.[67]

Diagnosis and Evaluation

Diagnosis is frequently missed or delayed due to the nonspecific nature of the initial symptoms. In this regard, the neurologist or neuromuscular specialist is well suited to make the diagnosis when evaluating the patient for neuropathy. This disorder should be considered in children presenting with progressive length-dependent small-fiber neuropathy, particularly if there are associated angiokeratomas, gastrointestinal symptoms, sweating abnormalities, exercise intolerance or fatigue, and a family history of renal failure, cardiovascular disease, and stroke. NCS shows mildly reduced conduction velocity in approximately two thirds of patients, and sural nerve biopsies show a selective loss of small myelinated and unmyelinated fibers. In boys, diagnosis can reliably be made by testing α-galactosidase A activity in peripheral leukocytes or plasma; however, in girls, genetic testing is required to make the diagnosis.

Due to the multiorgan nature of the disease, patients are best served in a multidisciplinary clinic where they can be seen with cardiologists, nephrologists, and neurologists familiar with the disease. Cardiac monitoring with electrocardiogram and echocardiogram should be performed at least every 2 years, and renal function monitoring, including measurement of creatinine clearance and urine protein, should be performed on an annual basis. Brain MRI and magnetic resonance angiography is performed to evaluate for subclinical strokes and cerebrovascular disease, and unmyelinated fiber density may be followed with physical examination of pain and temperature sensation, sudomotor testing, and skin biopsy.

Treatment and Management

LSDs are uniquely amenable to ERT, because lysosomal enzymes can be secreted extracellularly and endocytosed into lysosomes by binding to the mannose-6-phosphate receptor on the surface of the cell (Fig. 13-6). As shown in Table 13-3, two recombinant α-galactosidase A preparations are available; agalsidase beta (Fabrazyme) made by Genzyme (Cambridge, MA) and agalsidase alfa (Replagal) made by Transkaryotic Therapies (Cambridge, MA). Both of these therapies have proven effective and are available in Europe, and no significant differences have been shown between them; nonetheless, only Fabrazyme has been approved in the United States; it gained orphan drug exclusivity status in 2003.

In a randomized, placebo-controlled, double-blind, multicenter trial of 58 adult patients, Fabrazyme given IV every 2 weeks for 20 weeks led to clearance of Gb3 deposits from the microvascular

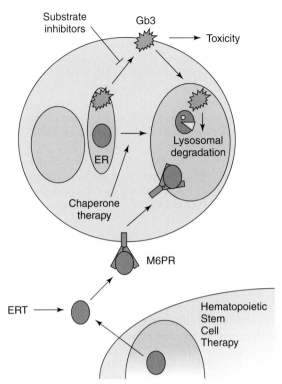

Figure 13-6 Therapeutic strategies for Fabry disease and other lysosomal storage diseases. Most lysosomal storage diseases are caused by deficiency of a lysosomal enzyme (*light green structure*) leading to an accumulation of the toxic enzyme substrate (*yellow blob*),which in the case of Fabry disease is Gb3). Enzyme replacement therapy (ERT) for Fabry disease and other lysosomal storage diseases is effective because when delivered intravenously, the enzyme is internalized by cells by binding to the mannose 6-phosphate receptor (M6PR) on the surface of the cell and is delivered to the lysosome, where it is activated. Hematopoietic stem cells and gene therapy are methods of having an endogenous source of enzyme. Because many enzyme mutations lead to misfolding and retention in the endoplasmic reticulum (ER), chaperone therapy aims to improve folding and thereby delivery of the mutant enzyme to the lysosome. Substrate inhibitor therapy aims to reduce the synthesis of the toxic enzyme substrate.

endothelium of kidneys, skin, and heart in 69% of patients, compared to 0% in the placebo group.[68] A 3-year phase IV open-label extension of this study showed sustained safety and efficacy of Fabrazyme with improvements in renal function and Gb3 clearance.[69] In a similarly designed placebo-controlled study of 26 adult patients, IV Replagal given every 2 weeks significantly reduced pain and renal pathology, increased creatinine clearance, and reduced plasma and urinary sediment Gb3 levels.[70] Subsequent studies have

substantiated a beneficial effect of ERT in Fabry disease, including a decrease in cardiac hypertrophy and decrease in the frequency of pain crises.[71,72] Furthermore, these studies have suggested that the earlier the initiation of therapy, the greater the treatment effect.

In addition to the reduction in pain described above, a few studies have specifically investigated the effects of ERT on neuropathy. Studies performing quantitative sensory and sudomotor testing on Fabry patients suggest a modest but significant improvement in thermal sensation and sweating with ERT.[73,74] However, an analysis of intraepidermal nerve fiber (IENF) density in the distal thigh did not show a treatment effect over the 6 months of the placebo-controlled trial[75]; there was no evidence of IENF regeneration with therapy, and in fact, patients had a significant reduction in IENF density after 18 months of treatment.

These medications are well tolerated, with the most concerning adverse effect being an allergic infusion reaction (see Table 13-3). These symptoms can often be prevented with pretreatment with antihistamines and hydrocortisone, and the incidence decreases with repeated infusions. Initially, Fabrazyme is infused slowly over 4 to 6 hours to ensure that the drug is tolerated, but with subsequent infusions, the rate can be significantly increased (see Table 13-3 and package insert for dosing information for Fabrazyme and Replagal). A significant number of patients (55% to 80%) generate IgG antibodies against the enzyme (as would be expected in patients who do not produce detectable levels of the enzyme); however, it is unclear whether antibody production reduces efficacy of the treatment, and antibody titers decrease over time, suggesting induction of immune tolerance.

Despite these encouraging results, many open questions remain. The optimal dosing of these drugs has not been determined, and no well-designed head-to-head trials have been performed to determine if one preparation has advantages over the other. Furthermore, although measurements of Gb3 levels from blood and urine have been used as a biomarker in clinical trials, there is significant variability in levels that do not allow it to be a reliable measurement to assess ERT response in individual patients. One critical question is when treatment should be initiated in females. There is considerable evidence in Fabry disease and other LSDs that much of the pathology is irreversible and that the earlier treatment is initiated the better. Because of this finding, most experts recommend ERT as early as possible in all patients with Fabry disease and in asymptomatic males. Indeed, ERT has been shown to be safe and effective in children as young as 8 years old.[76] However, the long-term efficacy and safety data are unknown for ERT in Fabry disease, and caution should be taken before recommending its use in asymptomatic women. Although asymptomatic female carriers are at increased risk for developing disease, it is unclear whether treatment reduces

Table 13-3 Enzyme Replacement Therapy for Fabry Disease*

Drug	Dose	Infusion Rate[†]	Side Effects[‡]
Agalsidase beta (Fabrazyme)	1.0 mg/kg IV q 2 weeks	0.25 mg/min initially, ↑ to 3–5 mg/min if tolerated	Infusion reaction; premedicate with antihistamines, acetaminophen, ± corticosteroids
Agalsidase alfa (Replagal)	0.2 mg/kg IV q 2 weeks	Over 40 min	Infusion reaction; premedicate with antihistamines, acetaminophen, ± corticosteroids

*See package inserts for more information for the two available forms of enzyme replacement therapy for Fabry disease. Only Agalsidase beta (Fabrazyme) is available in the United States. Both drugs are administered intravenously every 2 weeks, and the major potential adverse reaction is an infusion reaction (e.g., fever, chills, dyspnea, headache, nausea, pruritus, rash, tachycardia, dizziness, paresthesias).
[†]See package insert.
[‡]Patients should be premedicated with an antihistamine such as Benadryl and acetaminophen; and if a mild infusion reaction develops, corticosteroids such as hydrocortisone can be administered 30 minutes before subsequent infusions.

this risk and whether the cost and risks of treatment outweigh the potential benefit.

Although several studies have shown an improvement in pain with ERT, most patients still require pain medication. In fact, the neuropathic pain frequently gets worse with the initial ERT treatment before getting better. The chronic neuropathic pain typically appears to respond best to antiepileptic medications (see Chapter 6 for details). Pain crises in Fabry disease may be vascular rather than neuropathic in origin, and are best prevented by avoiding environmental triggers such as heat or stress if possible, but when severe, may require acute treatment with narcotics.

Other potential treatments for Fabry disease and other LSDs in preclinical trials include substrate reduction therapies, pharmacologic chaperone therapy, and gene therapy. As shown in Figure 13-6, the idea of substrate reduction therapy is that toxic levels of Gb3 can be reduced by inhibiting its synthesis. Chaperone therapy aims to increase the lysosomal delivery of the mutant enzyme, because most of the more than 200 mutations in α-galactosidase A are missense mutations that produce a misfolded but enzymatically active protein that is retained in the endoplasmic reticulum and degraded. Although both classes of therapies have shown efficacy in animal models and in preclinical trials, these compounds are not yet clinically available.[77] Furthermore, continuous delivery of enzyme replacement would likely be more efficacious and physiologic than a bolus infusion every other week. Such a delivery would be possible via gene therapy; indeed, because much of the breakdown of Gb3 normally occurs in the reticuloendothelial system, gene replacement via hematopoietic stem cells is a promising therapy currently under development. In the future, it is possible that a combination of ERT and the above therapies may prove most efficacious in treating Fabry disease.

Lysosomal Leukodystrophies: Metachromatic Leukodystrophy and Krabbe Disease

Lysosomal leukodystrophies are autosomal recessive LSDs with a specific defect in the breakdown of both CNS and peripheral nervous system myelin, and include MLD and GLD, also called *Krabbe disease*. The most common, infantile-onset forms of these diseases present with progressive walking difficulty beginning in infancy, followed by progressive mental retardation, pyramidal signs, seizures, and blindness due to optic atrophy. However, LSDs have variable presentations, including juvenile and adult-onset forms. Rarely, patients may initially present with progressive neuropathic symptoms, including pain in the extremities, areflexia, and weakness in the absence of other symptoms.[78,79] Patients with GLD have a similar presentation as in MLD, although the CNS involvement usually begins earlier and is more severe. The peripheral nervous system involvement was classically thought to be less profound in GLD, although a recent electrophysiologic study has shown that demyelinating peripheral neuropathy occurs early, is profound, and correlates in severity with that of CNS involvement.[80]

Diagnosis and Evaluation

Diagnosis is usually suspected based on clinical history and brain MRI showing nonspecific periventricular demyelination. Occasionally, these patients may be misdiagnosed with an inflammatory demyelinating polyneuropathy, because lumbar puncture reveals markedly elevated CSF protein and NCS shows evidence of demyelination (however, nerve conduction velocities are usually severely and uniformly reduced to 10 to 20 m/sec). MLD is caused by a deficiency of arylsulfatase A, leading to progressive central and peripheral demyelination. A blood test is available for diagnosing arylsulfatase A deficiency in leukocytes, and can be confirmed by genetic testing to identify mutations in the arylsulfatase A gene or in the activator protein, saposin B. Diagnosis of GLD can be made by testing galactosylceramide-β-galactosidase activity in leukocytes or with genetic testing. Although nerve biopsy is not necessary for diagnosis, toluidine blue staining shows demyelination and remyelination, and in MLD will show metachromatic (brown) lysosomal granules due to the accumulation of sulfatide in Schwann cell perikarya. Electron microscopy performed on thin sections of nerve or skin biopsies shows characteristic lysosomal inclusions in both MLD and GLD.

Treatment and Management

One important limitation of ERT (see Fabry disease discussion) is that intravenously delivered enzymes generally do not cross the blood–brain barrier. To circumvent this problem, patients can undergo hematopoietic stem cell transplantation (HSCT), because bone marrow–derived microglia can enter the CNS and secrete lysosomal enzymes that can enter affected cells. However, these therapies have significant risks, are extremely expensive, rely on the ability of stable enzyme to be secreted extracellularly, and are usually only effective if patients are treated early in the course of the disease, preferably presymptomatically.

HSCT was first shown to have efficacy in treating Hurler syndrome (mucopolysaccharidosis type 1) in 1981, long before the molecular defect causing that disorder was understood.[81] Since that time, HSCT has shown variable efficacy in treating several LSDs, including GLD and MLD.[82] The safety and efficacy of HSCT has improved over the past decade, and banking of umbilical cord blood allows the possibility of rapidly identifying a suitable donor. Furthermore, in the future autologous hematopoietic stem cells can potentially be modified with gene therapy to correct the lysosomal deficiency in one's own cells (critical when a suitable donor cannot be found).

In principle, both GLD and MLD can be treated with allogeneic HSCT. However, in practice, HSCT has been much less effective in MLD even when treated presymptomatically. The reasons for this difference are not known, but may be due to low amounts of stable arylsulfatase secreted by microglia. Supporting this hypothesis, bone marrow–derived hematopoietic stem cells from an arylsulfatase A–deficient mouse genetically engineered to produce high levels of the enzyme dramatically improved the neurologic outcome of these mice treated with HSCT.[83] In contrast, patients with the infantile, juvenile, and late-onset forms of GLD have shown improved neurologic outcomes when compared with patients receiving no therapy.[84,85] In a study of infantile GLD patients treated with umbilical-cord blood stem cells, asymptomatic newborns had a marked response to HSCT with only a few having delays in expressive language and motor function. However, the long-term outcome of transplantation is unclear. Important to our focus on neuropathy, an electrodiagnostic study showed a significant improvement in the neuropathy in Krabbe disease patients treated with HSCT, demonstrating an ability for these patients to regrow and myelinate axons with treatment.[86] In comparison, infants treated after the onset of symptoms had minimal neurologic improvement. Because of this marked effect on outcome if treated presymptomatically, newborn screening tests for GLD have been developed, but have thus far only been implemented in New York State in 2006.

Other promising therapies in development include small-molecule drugs and gene therapy. Chemicals that can cross the blood–brain barrier are being developed to increase expression of the deficient enzyme or to reduce synthesis of the toxic storage product. In summary, because LSDs associated with neuropathy are potentially treatable if identified early, these diagnoses should be considered and tested for, particularly in children with unexplained demyelinating neuropathy.

Peroxisomal Disorders: Adrenomyeloneuropathy and Refsum Disease

Adrenoleukodystrophy (ALD) and adrenomyeloneuropathy (AMN) are different clinical presentations of the same X-linked genetic disease characterized biochemically by accumulation of saturated very long chain fatty acids (VLCFA) (reviewed in Pillion et al[87]). The mutated protein, known as ABCD1, is a member of the ABC transporter family and is believed to function by transporting VLCFAs into the peroxisome where they undergo beta-oxidation. However, the mechanism of disease pathogenesis is unclear. Refsum disease (also known as *heredopathia atactica polyneuritiformis* and previously designated HMSN IV) is also a leukodystrophy characterized by an accumulation of specific long-chain fatty acids called *phytanic acids*. Phytanic acids are exclusively derived from the diet and normally undergo alpha-oxidation in the peroxisome. Refsum disease is a rare autosomal recessive disorder usually caused by a deficiency in phytanoyl-CoA hydroxylase.

Adrenoleukodystrophy/Adrenomyeloneuropathy: Clinical Presentation

The classic childhood-onset ALD phenotype affects boys age 4 to 8 years with an initial onset of attention deficit hyperactivity disorder and other behavioral symptoms, followed by rapidly progressive cortical blindness, spastic paraparesis, deafness, seizures, and adrenal insufficiency. Pathologically, brains of these patients show intense inflammatory demyelination beginning in the occipital lobes and progressing anteriorly. The intense CD8+ T-cell infiltrate and cytolytic death of oligodendrocytes has led to the hypothesis that immune recognition of abnormal VLCFAs causes an autoimmune response; however, myeloablation does not slow progression of the disease.[88] These children do not develop neuropathy.

In contrast, AMN develops in adults with a slowly progressive spastic paraparesis, large-fiber sensory loss, and bowel and bladder incontinence. The pathologic characteristics are very different in this disease, with evidence of a noninflammatory distal axonopathy affecting the corticospinal tract, dorsal columns, and peripheral nerve. AMN frequently affects males in their 20s and 30s and, surprisingly, also affects about 50% of carrier females in their 30s and 40s. Most patients do not develop cerebral manifestations, although approximately 20% to 40% of patients will develop cerebral inflammatory demyelination later in the course of their disease. Recent magnetic resonance spectroscopy imaging studies have shown that even patients with "pure AMN" have metabolic changes evident in the corticospinal tract and parieto-occipital white matter.[89,90] Almost 500 mutations in the *ABCD1* gene have been described (see www.x-ald.nl for an updated list), and there is almost no correlation between mutation and phenotype, suggesting that additional modifier genes or environmental factors determine whether a given

patient develops ALD, AMN, or remains asymptomatic. The majority of patients with ALD or AMN (approximately 70%) develop adrenal insufficiency, usually preceding neurologic symptoms. Symptoms include nausea, vomiting, fatigue, hyperpigmentation, and hyponatremia.

Diagnosis and Evaluation

Childhood cerebral ALD is difficult to diagnose in its early stages, because it must be distinguished from attention deficit hyperactivity disorder, autism spectrum disorders, and other neuropsychiatric disorders. However, with its inexorable progression, once brain MRI is performed, revealing the posterior demyelination, the diagnosis is quickly suspected. Adult-onset AMN must be distinguished from other causes of myelopathy and myeloneuropathy, and is frequently misdiagnosed as multiple sclerosis, particularly if abnormalities are seen on brain MRI. The differential diagnosis also includes vitamin deficiencies such as vitamin B_{12} and copper, primary lateral sclerosis and amyotrophic lateral sclerosis, HTLV1 infection, and hereditary spastic paraparesis.

Diagnosis is made using a plasma VLCFA assay. Both affected and asymptomatic males have a markedly elevated C26:0 level and an increased ratio of C24:0 and C26:0 to C22:0. Female carriers also have elevated VLCFAs, but false-negative tests do occur in approximately 20% of heterozygous females, so DNA sequencing is recommended. Once a mutation is identified, other family members can be rapidly tested for the presence of that mutation. VLCFAs are elevated in chorionic villus cells and cultured amniocytes, allowing prenatal diagnosis with chorionic villus sampling and amniocentesis. Neonatal screening assays have been recently developed that, if validated and implemented, could potentially prevent much of the morbidity and mortality of this devastating disease.[91]

The neuropathy of AMN is mild relative to the myelopathy and is frequently overlooked given the brisk reflexes. However, careful examination identifies evidence of a length-dependent peripheral neuropathy in most AMN patients. NCS shows mixed multifocal demyelination and axonal loss,[92] consistent with the AMN pathology initially described by Griffin and colleagues.[93] Interestingly, NCS abnormalities correlate with disability status and plasma VLCFA levels. In this regard, peroneal motor NCS were most useful in screening for neuropathy in these patients and for longitudinal follow-up.

Once the diagnosis of AMN is made, patients should be evaluated and regularly monitored for adrenal insufficiency. Testing is done by measuring serum corticotropin level and, if equivocal, performing a corticotropin-stimulation test. Serum cortisol levels are not sufficiently sensitive for detecting adrenal insufficiency in these patients. Furthermore, MRI of the brain should be performed on a regular basis to evaluate for cerebral inflammation. Newer imaging modalities, including magnetization transfer imaging and diffusion tensor imaging, show promise in quantifying and following axonal pathology in the brain and spinal cord.

Treatment and Management

Because about 70% of males with X-ALD develop adrenal insufficiency, which is potentially fatal if untreated, the most critical treatment of these patients is corticosteroid replacement if needed. This treatment is usually in the form of glucocorticoids (e.g., hydrocortisone 10 to 40 mg/day in divided doses) without mineralocorticoids (Table 13-4). Testosterone treatment may also be effective in patients with hypogonadism, although steroid treatment has no effect on the neurologic manifestations. Other symptomatic

Table 13-4 X-ALD/AMN Phenotypes and Treatment

Phenotype	Symptoms	Treatment
Boys		
Asymptomatic	None (elevated VLCFAs)	Lorenzo's oil Adrenal HRT
Early cerebral involvement*	Behavioral changes, dementia, white matter changes on MRI	HSCT Adrenal HRT
Adults (Men or Women)		
Pure AMN	Spastic paraparesis, large-fiber sensory loss, bowel/bladder symptoms	Possibly Lorenzo's oil† Adrenal HRT
Cerebral AMN*	AMN (above) + cognitive changes or white matter changes on MRI	Possibly HSCT Adrenal HRT

*Benefit of HSCT has only been reported early in the course of X-ALD or cerebral AMN.

†Studies have shown conflicting results as to benefit of Lorenzo's oil (see text).
AMN, adrenomyeloneuropathy; HRT, hormone replacement therapy; HSCT, hematopoietic stem cell transplantation; VLCFA, very long chain fatty acids; X-ALD, X-linked adrenoleukodystrophy.

treatments include treatment of spasticity (e.g., baclofen) and bowel and bladder symptoms.

Regarding specific therapy, Lorenzo's oil has recently proven effective in preventing or delaying onset in asymptomatic boys with X-ALD and may be of benefit in patients with AMN.[94] Lorenzo's oil, popularized by the 1992 movie of the same name, is a 4:1 mixture of two long-chain fatty acids, glyceryl trioleate and glyceryl trierucate. This combination competitively inhibits endogenous VLCFA synthesis, and Lorenzo's oil taken orally (1 mL/kg/day) along with a low-fat diet results in normalized VLCFA levels in most patients.[95] VLCFA levels are monitored regularly, and the Lorenzo's oil dose is adjusted accordingly in consultation with a nutritionist. This treatment initially was thought to be a potential cure for this devastating disease; however, despite anecdotal reports of cure, numerous controlled trials have shown that Lorenzo's oil is not effective in slowing progression in symptomatic boys. Recently, however, a prospective study performed on 89 asymptomatic boys (identified through relationship to a carrier) found that reduction of VLCFAs by Lorenzo's oil was associated with a decrease in developing MRI abnormalities, suggesting the need to treat asymptomatic boys before onset of cerebral manifestations.[94]

Whether Lorenzo's oil therapy is effective in patients with AMN is unknown. In a recent study by Koehler and Sokolowski,[96] 84% of patients taking Lorenzo's oil stabilized or progressed at a slower rate than they had before treatment; however, this was an open-label study. In contrast, several earlier studies did not show a benefit of Lorenzo's oil in AMN.[97,98] A large double-blinded study of Lorenzo's oil in AMN is currently being performed at the Kennedy Krieger Institute. Lorenzo's oil is expensive and is not available to patients outside of research studies in the United States.

The only therapy proven to have benefit in early symptomatic X-ALD is HSCT.[99] In approximately 50% of X-ALD boys treated with HSCT, disease progression is halted, and this effect is long-term. The earlier transplantation is performed, the greater the likelihood of clinical effect. However, as discussed earlier, HSCT is a risky procedure with a mortality rate of 10% to 20%; therefore, the risk-to-benefit ratio is considered unfavorable in patients with pure AMN. Nonetheless, HSCT should be considered as an option for AMN patients who develop cerebral inflammation if discovered early (e.g., subclinically with MRI). Other drugs in development for ALD and AMN include phenylbutyrate, lovastatin, and compounds that up-regulate the expression of *ABCD2*, which could potentially compensate for loss of *ABCD1*.

Refsum Disease: Clinical Presentation, Diagnosis, and Treatment

Refsum disease typically presents in late childhood with worsening night vision, although age of onset is variable, ranging from infancy to late adulthood. Constant and early disease features include pigmentary retinopathy and anosmia. Although symptoms of neuropathy are usually not present initially, a distal, demyelinating sensorimotor and autonomic polyneuropathy invariably develops as the disease progresses in untreated patients, often occurring subacutely. Other common findings include optic atrophy, cataracts, deafness, skin changes (ichthyosis), shortened bones in hands and feet, cardiac conduction defects, and cardiomyopathy.

Although Refsum disease is rare, this diagnosis should be considered in patients with retinitis pigmentosa because this disease is treatable. Elevated plasma phytanic acid over 200 µmoL/L (normal is < 30 µmoL/L) is pathognomonic for this disease. Because phytanic acid is solely derived from the diet, plasma levels can be markedly lowered and the disease treated by reducing dietary intake. Patients are advised to take less than 10 mg/day (normal is about 100 mg/day) by avoiding foods with high levels of phytanic acid, including dairy products, beef and lamb, and certain fatty fish. Abrupt weight loss or fasting should be avoided because mobilization of fat releases phytanic acid into the blood. In patients who develop subacute worsening of symptoms, plasmapheresis reduces phytanic acid levels and reportedly has led to a dramatic improvement in symptoms in a small case series. Patients should be counseled that they can prevent progression of the disease by strictly adhering to the diet.

Porphyric Neuropathy

Hepatic porphyrias are autosomal dominant disorders of heme metabolism that typically present with the triad of acute neuropathy, psychiatric symptoms, and abdominal involvement.[100] Variegate porphyria and hereditary coproporphyria are distinguished by the presence of skin blisters and bullae in approximately 50% of patients, whereas patients with the more common acute intermittent porphyria do not develop skin manifestations. Patients are usually asymptomatic between attacks, and episodes can occur spontaneously or be precipitated by factors that increase heme synthesis (and thereby increase the toxic porphyrin metabolites). Exacerbating factors include stress, hormonal factors, reduced caloric intake, and certain drugs. The active site of cytochrome P450 contains heme; therefore, drugs that induce hepatic synthesis of cytochrome P450 such as barbiturates are potent triggers of attacks. The earliest signs of an episode are usually abdominal pain, constipation, vomiting, and mental changes. Peripheral neuropathy has an acute onset and may be preceded or accompanied by autonomic manifestations such as tachycardia, hypertension, and postural hypotension. The neuropathy usually progresses over 2 to 4 weeks to cause diffuse weakness (often proximal > distal and upper > lower extremities) and areflexia. Sensory loss is generally mild and may be more prominent proximally in a "bathing trunk" distribution.

Table 13-5 Diagnosis of Porphyric Neuropathies*

	Acute Intermittent Porphyria	Hereditary Coproporphyria	Variegate Porphyria	ALA Dehydratase Deficiency
Inheritance	AD	AD	AD	AR
Enzyme deficiency	PBG deaminase	Copro oxidase	Proto oxidase	ALA dehydratase
Photosensitivity	None	Present	Present	None
Porphyrin excretion				
Urine	ALA, PBG, Uro	ALA, PBG, Uro, Copro	ALA, PBG, Uro, Copro	ALA, Copro
Feces	Normal	Copro > Proto	Proto > Copro	Normal

*Porphyrias can be diagnosed by urinary and fecal porphyrin excretion. As shown in the chart, hereditary coproporphyria and variegate porphyria are distinguished by the fecal porphyrin measurement.
AD, autosomal dominant; ALA, α-aminolevulinic acid; AR, autosomal recessive; Copro, coproporphyrinogen; PBG, porphobilinogen; Proto, protoporphyrin; Uro, uroporphyrin.

Diagnosis and Evaluation

The disease is named after the Greek word *porphuros* for purple, and indeed, urine of patients with hepatic porphyria turns purple/red when exposed to air and light due to oxidation of excess porphyrin precursors. Spinal fluid is similar to that seen in Guillain-Barré syndrome, with an albuminocytologic dissociation; in fact, some experts recommend screening all patients with Guillain-Barré clinical syndrome for porphyria. Acute attacks are invariably associated with increased urinary excretion of aminolevulinic acid or porphobilinogen, and a random urine test for porphobilinogen is a useful screen for acute porphyria. Although this test is sensitive, it lacks specificity, and porphyrins can be elevated secondary to many drugs and alcohol and to chronic diseases, such as diabetes mellitus, liver disease, and iron-deficiency anemia. Measuring 24-hour urinary excretion of porphobilinogen and aminolevulinic acid and 24-hour fecal excretion of protoporphyrin and coproporphyrin during a symptomatic period is the definitive test for porphyria. It can distinguish between variegate porphyria and hereditary coproporphyria (Table 13-5). Because porphyrins are light sensitive, specimens must be stored in the dark

and tested as soon as possible. In difficult diagnostic cases or to diagnose latent porphyria in an asymptomatic patient, enzyme activity can be measured in erythrocytes, and genetic testing is available.

Treatment and Management

Treatment of acute porphyria involves a three-pronged approach of removing the disease trigger, providing specific therapy aimed at decreasing hepatic porphyrin synthesis, and offering supportive care. The most important treatment during the acute crisis is supportive care, including fluid management, ventilatory support, management of heart rate and blood pressure (autonomic dysfunction), and avoidance of medications that are known to precipitate or worsen an acute attack (Table 13-6). As shown in Table 13-6, identifying safe drugs can be difficult, because most anticonvulsants and many analgesics and hypnotics may exacerbate porphyria. The offending agent should be identified, which is usually a drug known to induce cytochrome P450 synthesis. Other triggers include menstruation, fasting, and alcohol. Pharmacologic therapy including oral or intravenous

Table 13-6 Drugs That Are Potentially Safe or Harmful in Porphyria*

Drug Class	Reported to be Safe	Uncertain	Reported to Trigger Attacks
Analgesics	Acetaminophen, aspirin, narcotics	Ibuprofen, naproxen	Diclofenac, ergots
Anesthetics	Propofol	Lidocaine	Ketamine
Sedatives	Chloral hydrate, benzodiazepines[†]	Baclofen, benzodiazepines[†]	Barbiturates, alcohol
Antidepressants	Selective serotonin reuptake inhibitors	Nortryptyline	Amitriptyline
Antipsychotics	Phenothiazines	Olanzepine	
Antiepileptics	Gabapentin, vigabatrin	Benzodiazepines[†], levetiracetam	Phenytoin, carbamazepine, valproic acid
Cardiovascular	Beta blockers, digoxin, atropine, epinephrine	Amiodarone, angiotensin-converting enzyme inhibitors, thiazides	Calcium channel blockers, hydralazine
Gastrointestinal	Cimetidine, ranitidine	Promethazine, erythromycin	Metoclopramide
Endocrine	Insulin, glucocorticoids, estrogen	Danazol	Glipizide, tamoxifen, progestins
Antibiotics	Penicillin, acyclovir, vancomycin, zidovudine	Ketoconazole, isoniazid, chloroquine, trimethoprim	Sulfonamides, rifampin, pyrazinamide, nitrofurantoin

*This is an incomplete list, and is meant to serve as a general guide. The classification is based on information from clinical case reports and drug ability to induce cytochrome P450 synthesis. Individual patient responses to these drugs will vary.
[†]Benzodiazepines are reported to be safe at low doses (e.g., lorazepam for acute seizure), but are potentially harmful at high doses. Additional information on specific drugs can be obtained at http://www.drugs-porphyria.org/.

Table 13-7 Childhood or Adult Onset Inherited Neuropathies: Genetics, Common Clinical Presentation, Diagnosis, and Treatment of Selected Hereditary Neuropathies

	CMT/HMN/ HSN	Familial Amyloid Polyneuropathy	Friedreich Ataxia	Fabry Disease	Adrenomyeloneuropathy	Porphyria
Inheritance	AD, AR, X, sporadic	AD	AR	X-linked	X-linked	AD (rare AR)
Genetic defect	Many (see Table 13-1); CMT1: *PMP22*; CMT2: *MFN2*	TTR most common	Frataxin	α-Gal-A	*ABCD1*	PBG deaminase
Age at onset	Childhood to adult	Second or third decade	Childhood	Childhood (boys earlier than girls)	Adult (men earlier than women)	Adult
Early features of neuropathy	Motor, sensory, or autonomic. Demyelinating (two thirds) or axonal (one third)	Painful axonal small > large-fiber, sensory and autonomic > motor	Large-fiber sensory axonal, often foot deformities and kyphoscoliosis	Painful axonal small > large-fiber, sensory and autonomic > motor	Mixed axonal and demyelinating sensorimotor	Acute axonal motor and autonomic > sensory. Proximal > distal Upper > lower
Additional clinical features	None, except occasional CNS symptoms in CMTX	Entrapment neuropathy, cardiomyopathy, GI symptoms	Ataxia, nystagmus, positive Babinski, cardiomyopathy, SNHL	Renal failure, cardiac disease, stroke, GI symptoms, angiokeratomas	Spastic paraparesis, bowel and bladder incontinence, adrenal insufficiency	Abdominal pain, psychosis, seizures, skin rash in some forms
Diagnosis	Genetic testing (e.g., *PMP22* in CMT1)	Genetic testing or biopsy (nerve, fat pad, rectum, or lip)	Genetic testing (frataxin)	Boys: α-Gal A activity in blood; Girls: genetic testing	Plasma VLCFA levels or genetic testing	Screen: Urine porphobilinogen; Diagnosis: 24 hr urine/fecal porphyrins
Specific Treatment	Symptomatic only: PT/OT, orthotics	Liver transplant	Idebenone?	Agalsidase ERT	Adrenal HRT Lorenzo's oil? HSCT?	Hematin and glucose for acute attacks, avoid certain drugs

AD, autosomal dominant; AR, autosomal recessive; CMT, Charcot-Marie-Tooth disease; CNS, central nervous system; ERT, enzyme replacement therapy; α-Gal-A, alpha-galactosidase A; GI, gastrointestinal symptoms such as abdominal pain, nausea, vomiting; HRT, hormone replacement therapy; HSCT, hematopoietic stem cell transplantation; HMN, hereditary motor neuropathy; HSN, hereditary sensory neuropathy; PBG, porphobilinogen; PT/OT, physical/occupational therapy; SNHL, sensorineural hearing loss; TTR, transthyretin; VLCFA, very long chain fatty acids; X, X-linked. (?) indicate therapies of questionable benefit; see text.

glucose (300 to 500 g/day) and heme arginate (hematin) should be instituted as soon as possible. Hematin is administered in daily infusions of 4 mg/kg over a period of 3 to 5 days. Only one placebo-controlled study has been performed, which showed a modest benefit of hematin that was greatest if started early.[101] Recovery from an acute attack may take several months. Patients need to be educated to avoid triggers of acute attacks, and patients whose attacks correspond with the menstrual cycle can be treated with low-dose estrogen or gonadotropin-releasing hormone agonist therapy.

Conclusion

Every year, additional genetic causes of peripheral neuropathy are being discovered and we are learning more about the pathophysiology of inherited neuropathies. As shown in Table 13-7, the clinical presentation of hereditary neuropathies is quite variable, and inherited disease should always be considered in the differential diagnosis of unexplained neuropathy, even in the absence of family history. Both genetic and biochemical testing is available to diagnose many hereditary neuropathies, and specific therapies are available for many of the more common inherited neuropathies. With improved cell and animal models and increased understanding of these diseases, there is optimism that new therapeutic agents being developed to target these uncommon hereditary neuropathies will have efficacy in acquired neuropathies as well.

Acknowledgments

The authors thank Charlotte Sumner, Gerald Raymond, and Kathryn Wagner for their helpful feedback on this chapter.

References

1. Abe A, Gregory S, Lee L, et al: Reduction of globotriaosylceramide in Fabry disease mice by substrate deprivation, J Clin Invest 105:1563–1571, 2000.

2. Chance PF: Inherited focal, episodic neuropathies: hereditary neuropathy with liability to pressure palsies and hereditary neuralgic amyotrophy, Neuromolecular Med 8:159–174, 2006.

3. Pareyson D: Diagnosis of hereditary neuropathies in adult patients, J Neurol 250:148–160, 2003.

4. Bienfait HM, Baas F, Koelman JH, et al: Phenotype of Charcot-Marie-Tooth disease type 2, Neurology 68:1658–1667, 2007.

5. Szigeti K, Nelis E, Lupski JR: Molecular diagnostics of Charcot-Marie-Tooth disease and related peripheral neuropathies, Neuromolecular Med 8:243–254, 2006.

6. Klein CJ, Dyck PJ: Genetic testing in inherited peripheral neuropathies, J Peripher Nerv Syst 10:77–84, 2005.

7. England JD, Gronseth GS, Franklin G, et al: Practice parameter: evaluation of distal symmetric polyneuropathy: role of laboratory and genetic testing (an evidence-based review), Report of the American Academy of Neurology, American Association of Neuromuscular and Electrodiagnostic Medicine, and American Academy of Physical Medicine and Rehabilitation. Neurology 72:185–192, 2009.

8. Verhoeven K, Claeys KG, Zuchner S, et al: MFN2 mutation distribution and genotype/phenotype correlation in Charcot-Marie-Tooth type 2, Brain 129:2093–2102, 2006.

9. Zuchner S, Vance JM: Emerging pathways for hereditary axonopathies, J Mol Med 83:935–943, 2005.

10. Sackley C, Disler PB, Turner-Stokes L, et al: Rehabilitation interventions for foot drop in neuromuscular disease, Cochrane Database Syst Rev CD003908, 2007.

11. Aitkens SG, McCrory MA, Kilmer DD, et al: Moderate resistance exercise program: its effect in slowly progressive neuromuscular disease, Arch Phys Med Rehabil 74:711–715, 1993.

12. Kilmer DD, McCrory MA, Wright NC, et al: The effect of a high resistance exercise program in slowly progressive neuromuscular disease, Arch Phys Med Rehabil 75:560–563, 1994.

13. Dyck PJ, Swanson CJ, Low PA, et al: Prednisone-responsive hereditary motor and sensory neuropathy, Mayo Clin Proc 57:239–246, 1982.

14. Ginsberg L, Malik O, Kenton AR, et al: Coexistent hereditary and inflammatory neuropathy, Brain 127:193–202, 2004.

15. Gabriel CM, Gregson NA, Wood NW, et al: Immunological study of hereditary motor and sensory neuropathy type 1a (HMSN1a), J Neurol Neurosurg Psychiatry 72:230–235, 2002.

16. Grossman MJ, Feinberg J, Dicarlo EF, et al: Hereditary neuropathy with liability to pressure palsies: case report and discussion, HSS J 3:208–212, 2007.

17. Saifi GM, Szigeti K, Snipes GJ, et al: Molecular mechanisms, diagnosis, and rational approaches to management of and therapy for Charcot-Marie-Tooth disease and related peripheral neuropathies, J Invest Med 51:261–283, 2003.

18. Carey DJ, Todd MS: Schwann cell myelination in a chemically defined medium: demonstration of a requirement for additives that promote Schwann cell extracellular matrix formation, Brain Res 429:95–102, 1987.

19. Grandis M, Shy ME: Current therapy for Charcot-Marie-Tooth disease, Curr Treat Options Neurol 7:23–31, 2005.

20. Passage E, Norreel JC, Noack-Fraissignes P, et al: Ascorbic acid treatment corrects the phenotype of a mouse model of Charcot-Marie-Tooth disease, Nat Med 10:396–401, 2004.

21. Micallef J, Attarian S, Dubourg O, et al: Effect of ascorbic acid in patients with Charcot-Marie-Tooth disease type 1A: a multicentre, randomised, double-blind, placebo-controlled trial, Lancet Neurol 8(12):1103–1110, 2009.

22. Burns J, Ouvrier RA, Yiu EM, et al: Ascorbic acid for Charcot-Marie-Tooth disease type 1A in children: a randomised, double-blind, placebo-controlled, safety and efficacy trial, Lancet Neurol 8(6):537–544, 2009.

23. Shy ME, Blake J, Krajewski K, et al: Reliability and validity of the CMT neuropathy score as a measure of disability, Neurology 64:1209–1214, 2005.

24. Sereda MW, Meyer zu Horste G, Suter U, et al: Therapeutic administration of progesterone antagonist in a model of Charcot-Marie-Tooth disease (CMT-1A), Nat Med 9:1533–1537, 2003.

25. Klijn JG, Setyono-Han B, Foekens JA: Progesterone antagonists and progesterone receptor modulators in the treatment of breast cancer, Steroids 65:825–830, 2000.

26. Lanka V, Cudkowicz M: Therapy development for ALS: lessons learned and path forward, Amyotroph Lateral Scler 9:131–140, 2008.

27. Chao MV, Rajagopal R, Lee FS: Neurotrophin signalling in health and disease, Clin Sci (Lond) 110:167–173, 2006.

28. Sahenk Z, Nagaraja HN, McCracken BS, et al: NT-3 promotes nerve regeneration and sensory improvement in CMT1A mouse models and in patients, Neurology 65:681–689, 2005.

29. Young P, De Jonghe P, Stogbauer F, et al: Treatment for Charcot-Marie-Tooth disease, Cochrane Database Syst Rev CD006052, 2008.

30. Auer-Grumbach M: Hereditary sensory neuropathy type I, Orphanet J Rare Dis 3:7, 2008.

31. Klein CJ, Wu Y, Kruckeberg KE, et al: SPTLC1 and RAB7 mutation analysis in dominantly inherited and idiopathic sensory neuropathies, J Neurol Neurosurg Psychiatry 76:1022–1024, 2005.

32. Spring PJ, Kok C, Nicholson GA, et al: Autosomal dominant hereditary sensory neuropathy with chronic cough and gastro-oesophageal reflux: clinical features in two families linked to chromosome 3p22–p24, Brain 128:2797–2810, 2005.

33. Axelrod FB, Gold-von Simson G: Hereditary sensory and autonomic neuropathies: types II, III, and IV, Orphanet J Rare Dis 2:39, 2007.

34. Rubin BY, Anderson SL: The molecular basis of familial dysautonomia: overview, new discoveries and implications for directed therapies, Neuromolecular Med 10:148–156, 2008.

35. Kuhn D, Hagopian L, Terlonge C: Treatment of life-threatening self-injurious behavior secondary to hereditary sensory and autonomic neuropathy type II: a controlled case study, J Child Neurol 23:381–388, 2008.

36. Benson MD, Kincaid JC: The molecular biology and clinical features of amyloid neuropathy, *Muscle Nerve* 36:411–423, 2007.

37. Adams D: Hereditary and acquired amyloid neuropathies, *J Neurol* 248:647–657, 2001.

38. Plante-Bordeneuve V, Said G: Transthyretin related familial amyloid polyneuropathy, *Curr Opin Neurol* 13:569–573, 2000.

39. Andrade C: A peculiar form of peripheral neuropathy: familiar atypical generalized amyloidosis with special involvement of the peripheral nerves, *Brain* 75:408–427, 1952.

40. Van Allen MW, Frohlich JA, Davis JR: Inherited predisposition to generalized amyloidosis. Clinical and pathological study of a family with neuropathy, nephropathy, and peptic ulcer, *Neurology* 19:10–25, 1969.

41. Hornigold R, Patel AV, Ward VM, et al: Familial systemic amyloidosis associated with bilateral sensorineural hearing loss and bilateral facial palsies, *J Laryngol Otol* 120:778–780, 2006.

42. Plante-Bordeneuve V, Ferreira A, Lalu T, et al: Diagnostic pitfalls in sporadic transthyretin familial amyloid polyneuropathy (TTR-FAP), *Neurology* 69:693–698, 2007.

43. Simmons Z, Blaivas M, Aguilera AJ, et al: Low diagnostic yield of sural nerve biopsy in patients with peripheral neuropathy and primary amyloidosis, *J Neurol Sci* 120:60–63, 1993.

44. Kennedy WR, Nolano M, Wendelschafer-Crabb G, et al: A skin blister method to study epidermal nerves in peripheral nerve disease, *Muscle Nerve* 22:360–371, 1999.

45. Yamamoto S, Wilczek HE, Nowak G, et al: Liver transplantation for familial amyloidotic polyneuropathy (FAP): a single-center experience over 16 years, *Am J Transplant* 7:2597–2604, 2007.

46. Gillmore JD, Stangou AJ, Tennent GA, et al: Clinical and biochemical outcome of hepatorenal transplantation for hereditary systemic amyloidosis associated with apolipoprotein AI Gly26Arg, *Transplantation* 71:986–992, 2001.

47. Ando Y: Liver transplantation and new therapeutic approaches for familial amyloidotic polyneuropathy (FAP), *Med Mol Morphol* 38:142–154, 2005.

48. Sekijima Y, Hammarstrom P, Matsumura M, et al: Energetic characteristics of the new transthyretin variant A25T may explain its atypical central nervous system pathology, *Lab Invest* 83:409–417, 2003.

49. Tojo K, Sekijima Y, Kelly JW, et al: Diflunisal stabilizes familial amyloid polyneuropathy-associated transthyretin variant tetramers in serum against dissociation required for amyloidogenesis, *Neurosci Res* 56:441–449, 2006.

50. Pandolfo M: Friedreich ataxia, *Arch Neurol* 65:1296–1303, 2008.

51. Lynch DR JM, Balcer LJ, et al: Friedreich ataxia: effects of genetic understanding on clinical evaluation and therapy, *Arch Neurol* 59:743–747, 2002.

52. Wells RD: DNA triplexes and Friedreich ataxia, *FASEB J* 22:1625–1634, 2008.

53. Burnett R, Melander C, Puckett JW, et al: DNA sequence-specific polyamides alleviate transcription inhibition associated with long GAA.TTC repeats in Friedreich's ataxia, *Proc Natl Acad Sci USA* 103:11497–11502, 2006.

54. Herman D, Jenssen K, Burnett R, et al: Histone deacetylase inhibitors reverse gene silencing in Friedreich's ataxia, *Nat Chem Biol* 2:551–558, 2006.

55. Puccio H, Simon D, Cossee M, et al: Mouse models for Friedreich ataxia exhibit cardiomyopathy, sensory nerve defect and Fe-S enzyme deficiency followed by intramitochondrial iron deposits, *Nat Genet* 27:181–186, 2001.

56. Al-Mahdawi S, Pinto RM, Ismail O, et al: The Friedreich ataxia GAA repeat expansion mutation induces comparable epigenetic changes in human and transgenic mouse brain and heart tissues, *Hum Mol Genet* 17:735–746, 2008.

57. Rai M, Soragni E, Jenssen K, et al: HDAC inhibitors correct frataxin deficiency in a Friedreich ataxia mouse model, *PLoS One* 3:e1958, 2008.

58. Sturm B, Stupphann D, Kaun C, et al: Recombinant human erythropoietin: effects on frataxin expression in vitro, *Eur J Clin Invest* 35:711–717, 2005.

59. Boesch S, Sturm B, Hering S, et al: Friedreich's ataxia: clinical pilot trial with recombinant human erythropoietin, *Ann Neurol* 62:521–524, 2007.

60. Li K, Besse EK, Ha D, et al: Iron-dependent regulation of frataxin expression: implications for treatment of Friedreich ataxia, *Hum Mol Genet* 17:2265–2273, 2008.

61. Pandolfo M: Drug Insight: antioxidant therapy in inherited ataxias, *Nat Clin Pract Neurol* 4:86–96, 2008.

62. Tonon C, Lodi R: Idebenone in Friedreich's ataxia, *Expert Opin Pharmacother* 9:2327–2337, 2008.

63. Cooper JM, Schapira AH: Friedreich's ataxia: coenzyme Q_{10} and vitamin E therapy, *Mitochondrion* 7(Suppl):S127–S135, 2007.

64. Di Prospero NA, Baker A, Jeffries N, et al: Neurological effects of high-dose idebenone in patients with Friedreich's ataxia: a randomised, placebo-controlled trial, *Lancet Neurol* 6:878–886, 2007.

65. Delatycki MB, Holian A, Corben L, et al: Surgery for equinovarus deformity in Friedreich's ataxia improves mobility and independence, *Clin Orthop Relat Res* 430:138–141, 2005.

66. Milbrandt TA, Kunes JR, Karol LA: Friedreich's ataxia and scoliosis: the experience at two institutions, *J Pediatr Orthop* 28:234–238, 2008.

67. Nance CS, Klein CJ, Banikazemi M, et al: Later-onset Fabry disease: an adult variant presenting with the cramp-fasciculation syndrome, *Arch Neurol* 63:453–457, 2006.

68. Eng CM, Guffon N, Wilcox WR, et al: Safety and efficacy of recombinant human alpha-galactosidase A—replacement therapy in Fabry's disease, *N Engl J Med* 345:9–16, 2001.

69. Wilcox WR, Banikazemi M, Guffon N, et al: Long-term safety and efficacy of enzyme replacement therapy for Fabry disease, *Am J Hum Genet* 75:65–74, 2004.

70. Acierno JS Jr, Kennedy JC, Falardeau JL, et al: A physical and transcript map of the *MCOLN1* gene region on human chromosome 19p13.3–p13.2, *Genomics* 73:203–210, 2001.

71. Beck M, Ricci R, Widmer U, et al: Fabry disease: overall effects of agalsidase alfa treatment, *Eur J Clin Invest* 34:838–844, 2004.

72. Banikazemi M, Bultas J, Waldek S, et al: Agalsidase-beta therapy for advanced Fabry disease: a randomized trial, *Ann Intern Med* 146:77–86, 2007.

73. Schiffmann R, Floeter MK, Dambrosia JM, et al: Enzyme replacement therapy improves peripheral nerve and sweat function in Fabry disease, *Muscle Nerve* 28:703–710, 2003.

74. Hilz MJ, Brys M, Marthol H, et al: Enzyme replacement therapy improves function of C-, AH-, and A-nerve fibers in Fabry neuropathy, *Neurology* 62:1066–1072, 2004.

75. Schiffmann R, Hauer P, Freeman B, et al: Enzyme replacement therapy and intraepidermal innervation density in Fabry disease, *Muscle Nerve* 34:53–56, 2006.

76. Wraith JE, Tylki-Szymanska A, Guffon N, et al: Safety and efficacy of enzyme replacement therapy with agalsidase beta: an international, open-label study in pediatric patients with Fabry disease, *J Pediatr* 152:563–570, e561, 2008.

77. Hollak CE, Vedder AC, Linthorst GE, et al: Novel therapeutic targets for the treatment of Fabry disease, *Expert Opin Ther Targets* 11:821–833, 2007.

78. Comabella M, Waye JS, Raguer N, et al: Late-onset metachromatic leukodystrophy clinically presenting as isolated peripheral neuropathy: compound heterozygosity for the IVS2+1GCA mutation and a newly identified missense mutation (Thr408Ile) in a Spanish family, *Ann Neurol* 50:108–112, 2001.

79. Haberlandt E, Scholl-Burgi S, Neuberger J, et al: Peripheral neuropathy as the sole initial finding in three children with infantile metachromatic leukodystrophy, *Eur J Paediatr Neurol* 13:257–260, 2009.

80. Siddiqi ZA, Sanders DB, Massey JM: Peripheral neuropathy in Krabbe disease: electrodiagnostic findings, *Neurology* 67:263–267, 2006.

81. Hobbs JR, Hugh-Jones K, Barrett AJ, et al: Reversal of clinical features of Hurler's disease and biochemical improvement after treatment by bone-marrow transplantation, *Lancet* 2:709–712, 1981.

82. Cartier N, Aubourg P: Hematopoietic stem cell gene therapy in Hurler syndrome, globoid cell leukodystrophy, metachromatic leukodystrophy and X-adrenoleukodystrophy, *Curr Opin Mol Ther* 10:471–478, 2008.

83. Biffi A, De Palma M, Quattrini A, et al: Correction of metachromatic leukodystrophy in the mouse model by transplantation of genetically modified hematopoietic stem cells, *J Clin Invest* 113:1118–1129, 2004.

84. Krivit W, Shapiro EG, Peters C, et al: Hematopoietic stem-cell transplantation in globoid-cell leukodystrophy, *N Engl J Med* 338:1119–1126, 1998.

85. Escolar ML, Poe MD, Provenzale JM, et al: Transplantation of umbilical-cord blood in babies with infantile Krabbe's disease, *N Engl J Med* 352:2069–2081, 2005.

86. Siddiqi ZA, Sanders DB, Massey JM: Peripheral neuropathy in Krabbe disease: effect of hematopoietic stem cell transplantation, *Neurology* 67:268–272, 2006.

87. Pillion JP, Moser HW, Raymond GV: Auditory function in adrenomyeloneuropathy, *J Neurol Sci* 269:24–29, 2008.

88. Nowaczyk MJ, Saunders EF, Tein I, et al: Immunoablation does not delay the neurologic progression of X-linked adrenoleukodystrophy, *J Pediatr* 131:453–455, 1997.

89. Dubey P, Fatemi A, Barker PB, et al: Spectroscopic evidence of cerebral axonopathy in patients with "pure" adrenomyeloneuropathy, *Neurology* 64:304–310, 2005.

90. Fatemi A, Smith SA, Dubey P, et al: Magnetization transfer MRI demonstrates spinal cord abnormalities in adrenomyeloneuropathy, *Neurology* 64:1739–1745, 2005.

91. Raymond GV, Jones RO, Moser AB: Newborn screening for adrenoleukodystrophy: implications for therapy, *Mol Diagn Ther* 11:381–384, 2007.

92. Chaudhry V, Moser HW, Cornblath DR: Nerve conduction studies in adrenomyeloneuropathy, *J Neurol Neurosurg Psychiatry* 61:181–185, 1996.

93. Griffin JW, Goren E, Schaumburg H, et al: Adrenomyeloneuropathy: a probable variant of adrenoleukodystrophy, I. Clinical and endocrinologic aspects. *Neurology* 27:1107–1113, 1977.

94. Moser HW, Raymond GV, Lu SE, et al: Follow-up of 89 asymptomatic patients with adrenoleukodystrophy treated with Lorenzo's oil, *Arch Neurol* 62:1073–1080, 2005.

95. Moser HW, Moser AB, Hollandsworth K, et al: "Lorenzo's oil" therapy for X-linked adrenoleukodystrophy: rationale and current assessment of efficacy, *J Mol Neurosci* 33:105–113, 2007.

96. Koehler S, Sokolowski P: *Clinical Phenotypes, Diagnosis and Treatment of Adulthood X-linked Adrenoleukodystrophy*, Heilbronn, 2005, SPS Verlagsgesellschaft.

97. Aubourg P, Adamsbaum C, Lavallard-Rousseau MC, et al: A 2-year trial of oleic and erucic acids ("Lorenzo's oil") as treatment for adrenomyeloneuropathy, *N Engl J Med* 329:745–752, 1993.

98. van Geel BM, Assies J, Haverkort EB, et al: Progression of abnormalities in adrenomyeloneuropathy and neurologically asymptomatic X-linked adrenoleukodystrophy despite treatment with "Lorenzo's oil," *J Neurol Neurosurg Psychiatry* 67:290–299, 1999.

99. Moser HW, Raymond GV, Dubey P: Adrenoleukodystrophy: new approaches to a neurodegenerative disease, *JAMA* 294:3131–3134, 2005.

100. Albers JW, Fink JK: Porphyric neuropathy, *Muscle Nerve* 30:410–422, 2004.

101. Herrick AL, McColl KE, Moore MR, et al: Controlled trial of haem arginate in acute hepatic porphyria, *Lancet* 1:1295–1297, 1989.

Zachary Simmons, MD

Treatment and Management of Autoimmune Neuropathies

14

Autoimmune neuropathies constitute a broad, heterogeneous group of disorders, spanning the spectrum from acute to chronic, from sensory to sensorimotor to motor, and from focal to multifocal to generalized. They may occur as isolated entities or in association with systemic autoimmune disorders. Because they represent such a varied group of disorders, virtually all neurologists will encounter some of these relatively frequently in the course of their practice. The agents used for treatment are common to many of these conditions, but the evidence for their use varies widely. This chapter is meant not as an exhaustive reference, but as a clinically oriented guide to evaluation and immunologic management. References are provided primarily for treatment-related literature.

Guillain-Barré Syndrome

Guillain-Barré syndrome (GBS) is an acute, immune-mediated disorder of the peripheral nervous system in which an inflammatory response is directed against peripheral nerve myelin or axons. In contrast to the older concept of GBS as an acute, acquired, demyelinating polyneuropathy (acute inflammatory demyelinating polyradiculoneuropathy, or AIDP) characterized by an ascending paralysis, it is now clear that GBS is a heterogeneous syndrome clinically, electrodiagnostically, and histopathologically. The differential diagnosis is broad (Box 14-1). Approximately two thirds of patients have an infection 6 weeks or less before the onset of GBS symptoms, most commonly a flulike illness, followed in frequency by gastroenteritis.[1,2] Surgery and trauma as antecedent events have been reported anecdotally. The relationship between vaccinations and GBS has been the subject of much study since the identification of an increased incidence of GBS after swine flu vaccinations in 1976. Overall, the incidence of GBS after vaccination is low, and occurs most commonly with influenza vaccine.[3]

GBS usually presents as progressive, symmetric weakness of more than one limb, associated with depressed or absent reflexes. Cranial nerve involvement is not uncommon, particularly facial weakness (50% of patients at some point during the illness), ophthalmoplegia (15%), and oropharyngeal weakness (40%). Classic ascending paralysis is seen only about half the time, and the clinical presentation may vary widely.[4] Sensory signs usually are mild, although paresthesias are common. Autonomic dysfunction may be present, including tachycardia and other arrhythmias, postural

hypotension, and hypertension. The condition may progress for up to 4 weeks.

Diagnosis and Evaluation

The diagnosis often is challenging initially because weakness may be mild, the pattern of weakness may be atypical, and reflexes may be preserved. Diagnostic criteria for GBS have been published and include clinical, cerebrospinal fluid (CSF), and electrodiagnostic components.[5–7] The variants of GBS include pharyngeal-cervical-brachial, paraparetic, and pure motor, sensory, and autonomic presentations.[8–12] Fisher's variant is characterized by ophthalmoplegia, ataxia, and areflexia and usually is associated with IgG antibodies to GQ1b.[13–15]

Blood and imaging studies should be tailored to the clinical presentation, taking into account the diagnostic possibilities in Box 14-1. In the demyelinating form of GBS, the CSF commonly shows an elevated protein level without pleocytosis—the classic albuminocytologic dissociation.[4] CSF protein may be normal, particularly during the first few days of symptoms. A CSF pleocytosis, particularly more than 2 weeks after onset of symptoms, should raise suspicion of Lyme disease or of human immunodeficiency virus (HIV) infection.[6,7] Electrodiagnostic findings in the most common variant of GBS are those of an acquired demyelinating polyneuropathy, including prolonged distal latencies, slowed conduction velocities, prolonged F-wave latencies, and partial conduction block or abnormal temporal dispersion (Fig. 14-1).[7,16] The earliest abnormalities usually are prolonged distal latencies and prolonged F-wave latencies. Sensory studies often demonstrate the phenomenon of sural sparing, characterized by a pattern of normal sural and abnormal median sensory nerves.[17,18] Needle examination usually demonstrates only reduced recruitment initially. At a later time, it can be used to help assess secondary axon loss. Electrodiagnostic findings in Fisher's variant include low-amplitude or absent sensory responses and few or no motor nerve abnormalities.[19,20] Not all patients with GBS will meet electrodiagnostic criteria, particularly early in the course. Because treatment appears to be most effective when given early, it should be initiated even when electrodiagnostic criteria are not met if the clinical findings are consistent with GBS and other disorders have been excluded.

Axonal variants of GBS include acute motor axonal neuropathy (AMAN) and acute motor and sensory axonal neuropathy (AMSAN). AMAN was first clearly described in northern China, where it most commonly affects children and young adults in rural

Box 14-1 Differential Diagnosis of Guillain-Barré Syndrome

Brain or Brain Stem Disorders

Stroke
Bleed
Tumor
Encephalitis

Spinal Cord Disorders

Myelopathy
Myelitis

Other Peripheral Nervous System Causes of Acute Flaccid Paralysis

Diphtheria
Porphyria
Vasculitis
Tick paralysis
Toxic neuropathy
Neuropathy of critical illness
Lyme disease
West Nile virus
Poliovirus
Other enteroviruses

Disorders of Neuromuscular Transmission

Botulism
Myasthenia gravis

Disorders of Muscle

Rhabdomyolysis
Inflammatory
Hypophosphatemia
Periodic paralysis

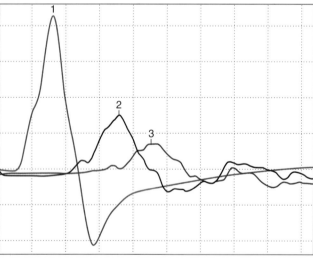

Figure 14-1 Abnormal temporal dispersion. Nerve conduction study of the ulnar motor nerve, with stimulation at the wrist (1), below the elbow (2), and above the elbow (3) in a patient with an acquired demyelinating polyneuropathy demonstrates an increasingly dispersed waveform with proximal stimulation.

areas during the summer months.[21,22] It has now been documented worldwide. The presentation usually is similar to that of typical AIDP, with a rapidly progressive quadriparesis that may be associated with respiratory failure. Patients often have elevated antiganglioside antibody titers, specifically IgG antibodies against GM_1,

GM_{1b}, GD_{1a}, and GalNac-GD_{1a}.[23–25] Within the first week, CSF usually is normal, but later in the illness albuminocytologic dissociation commonly occurs. Electrodiagnostic studies usually demonstrate an axonal neuropathy with normal sensory responses, although some patients have a rapidly reversible conduction block and so may initially mimic AIDP electrodiagnostically. Diarrhea often precedes the onset of weakness, and serologic evidence of a recent infection with *Campylobacter jejuni* is present in 67% to 92% of patients.[26–28] *AMSAN* is the term used for axonal GBS in which sensory as well as motor fibers are involved. AMSAN, often more severe than AMAN, is characterized by rapid progression and inexcitable nerves with severe axonal degeneration.[29,30] The CSF usually shows albuminocytologic dissociation. Electrodiagnostic studies demonstrate markedly decreased compound muscle action potential (CMAP) and sensory nerve action potential (SNAP) amplitudes, or absent CMAPs and SNAPs, within 7 to 10 days of onset.

Treatment and Management

Supportive Care

Evidence-based guidelines for supportive care for patients with GBS were recently published.[31] Unfortunately, the authors found that evidence is lacking for many management recommendations, leaving the clinician with uncontrolled clinical data and expert opinion (Class IV evidence) as the basis for best management practices. The following general management guidelines, also summarized in Table 14-1, are an overview and are followed by specific guidelines for immunotherapy. The reader is referred to other sources for details regarding the management of respiratory, bulbar, and cardiovascular issues in the intensive care unit (ICU).[4]

Most patients with GBS are admitted to an ICU, or at least to an intermediate care (step-down) unit, because this permits close neurologic and cardiovascular/hemodynamic observation and allows the treating physician to determine how rapidly the patient's

Table 14-1 Guillain-Barré Syndrome: Supportive Care and Symptomatic Management

Area of Management	Guidelines
Admit to intensive or intermediate care unit	**Procedures** Continuous cardiac monitoring Forced vital capacity and maximum inspiratory pressure every 2–4 hours, then less frequently Close monitoring of bulbar function Intubation if indicated
Monitoring and treatment of autonomic dysfunction	**Monitor for These Autonomic Manifestations:** Hypertension Hypotension (including orthostatic) Arrhythmias Urine retention Gastrointestinal (see text, next page)
Pain	**Medications** Acetaminophen Nonsteroidal anti-inflammatory medications Gabapentin Carbamazepine Tricyclic antidepressants Tramadol Mexiletine

respiratory and bulbar functions are changing. Frequent and accurate respiratory and bulbar assessments are essential to determining if and when to intubate a patient with GBS. In general, a vital capacity of less than 20 mL/kg or a maximum inspiratory pressure of less than 30 cm H_2O raises concerns of imminent respiratory failure.[4,32–34] Just as important as the absolute value of a respiratory measure, however, is the rate of change. That is, a patient who has had slow progression of symptoms for 5 days and now has a vital capacity or maximum inspiratory pressure at the levels specified above represents a much different management issue than one whose respiratory status has reached this level 12 hours after the development of the initial symptoms of GBS, and thus is at much higher risk of rapid respiratory failure. It is always best practice to admit a GBS patient to the ICU if there is any concern at all about respiratory status and certainly prudent to do so if changes in neurologic function overall are rapid. Similarly, any bulbar dysfunction places the patient at risk for aspiration and is an indication to admit to the ICU for observation to determine trends. Once in the ICU, respiratory measures, consisting of at least a forced vital capacity and maximum inspiratory pressure, should be performed frequently enough to catch worrisome trends in time to perform intubation electively. Often, these are measured every 2 to 4 hours initially. Intubation should be considered under several circumstances: impending respiratory failure, bulbar dysfunction with inability to handle secretions, and ineffective cough. It is almost always better to err on the side of intubating early and electively if respiratory and bulbar status are borderline, because most patients with GBS will become weaker after they are first evaluated. Guidelines have been offered as to when to perform a tracheostomy on an intubated patient with GBS: "The decision to place a tracheostomy may be postponed for 2 weeks. If after 2 weeks the pulmonary function tests do not show any significant improvement from baseline, tracheostomy should be performed. If the pulmonary function test tends to improve above baseline, tracheostomy could be deferred for an additional week, allowing the patient to attempt to be weaned from the ventilator."[31]

Other key reasons for an ICU admission are cardiovascular and other autonomic dysfunction, found in 65% of cases of typical GBS in one hospital series.[4] This can take many forms, including hypertension, hypotension, orthostatic hypotension, sinus tachycardia (very common), other arrhythmias (much less common), urine retention, and gastrointestinal autonomic dysfunction (constipation, ileus or gastric distention, diarrhea, fecal incontinence). Patients may be sensitive to medications used to treat cardiovascular dysautonomia or may react in an atypical manner to them, so caution is advised.

Pain control is an important category of symptom management. Retrospective series indicate that pain occurs in 33% to 71% of patients with GBS.[31] A prospective series found pain in 89%, severe in 47.3%.[35] The major types of pain and frequencies of occurrence were deep aching or throbbing pain in the low back with radiation into the buttocks, thighs, calves (61.8%); dysesthetic extremity pain (burning, tingling, shocklike; 49.1%); myalgic-rheumatic extremity pain (34.5%); and visceral pain (20%). In many patients, pain does not respond adequately to acetaminophen or nonsteroidal anti-inflammatory medications. In such patients, both gabapentin and carbamazepine have been shown to be superior to placebo for controlling pain in GBS.[36,37] For refractory pain, published guidelines suggest adjuvant therapy with tricyclic antidepressants, tramadol, carbamazepine, or mexiletine.[31] Some patients may require narcotic analgesics.

Immunotherapy

Immunotherapy for the treatment of GBS is summarized in Table 14-2. Two major randomized, controlled studies documented the benefits of plasma exchange (PE) when performed within about 2 weeks of onset of symptoms, with the greatest benefit when treatment was initiated within 7 days.[38,39] On completion of these studies, PE became a part of the standard of care for treatment of patients with GBS. A subsequent French study clarified three other aspects of PE[40]: (1) PE can be useful when given within 1 month of onset of symptoms, not just within 2 weeks, (2) a short course of PE (two exchanges) can be beneficial for patients with mild disease, and (3) the number of exchanges should not be reduced to two for those with moderate disease.

Two randomized, controlled studies have compared the efficacy of intravenous immunoglobulin (IVIg) 2 g/kg divided over 4 to 5 days in treating GBS to that of PE, and found them to be equal.[41,42] A randomized, controlled trial found that 6 days of IVIg 0.4 g/kg/day may be better than 3 days, but the study was small.[43] Most neurologists use 2 g/kg divided over 2 to 5 days. IVIg is used as first-line treatment at most centers because the efficacy of IVIg and PE is equal and because PE is available at a limited number of centers, often requires a central line, and may be difficult to arrange as an emergency procedure at night or on weekends. A large randomized study found no added benefit from combining PE with IVIg.[44] At least eight studies of corticosteroids have shown them to be uniformly unsuccessful in treating GBS.[45] There have been no controlled treatment trials limited to Fisher's variant, AMAN, or AMSAN, but patients usually are treated with IVIg or PE.

Table 14-2 Therapy for Guillain-Barré Syndrome

Therapy	Dose	Effective?	Evidence	Recommendation
Intravenous immunoglobulin (IVIg)	2 g/kg divided over 2–5 days	Yes	Randomized, controlled trials	First-line therapy, equal to plasma exchange
Plasma exchange	5 exchanges of 1 plasma volume each every other day	Yes	Randomized, controlled trials	First-line therapy, equal to IVIg
Plasma exchange followed by IVIg	Same as above	Same as IVIg or PE alone	Randomized, controlled trial	Not recommended
Corticosteroids	Various oral and intravenous	No	Various: double-blind, single and multiple centers, parallel groups	Not recommended

Outcome

The death rate in GBS has been reported to vary from 2.4% to 6.3%.[45,46] The rate of death or disability (unable to walk 5 meters without support after 1 year) ranges from 10.9% to 16.8%.[45] Factors found to be associated with a poorer prognosis are preceding diarrhea, older age, more severe disease, more rapid onset of disease, axonal involvement by electromyography (EMG), need for mechanical ventilation, and some specific preceding infections.[41,44,47,48] Persistent fatigue is common.[49,50] Outcome in patients with AMAN is similar to that in AIDP. The rapid recovery is thought to be due to reversible paranodal demyelination with conduction block or to axonal degeneration, primarily at the nerve terminals.[24] In those patients in whom axonal loss occurs more proximally, such as those with AMSAN, recovery takes longer and is more likely to be incomplete.[23] Fisher's variant usually is associated with a good recovery. Relapse rate in GBS patients treated with PE or IVIg is 4% to 7%.[45]

Chronic Inflammatory Demyelinating Polyradiculoneuropathy

Chronic inflammatory demyelinating polyradiculoneuropathy (CIDP) is a chronic acquired autoimmune demyelinating disorder of the peripheral nervous system with a relapsing, monophasic, or progressive course of 2 months duration or greater.[51] Since 1975, descriptions of a number of large series of patients with CIDP have provided insight into the clinical presentation, electrodiagnostic findings, clinical course, and prognosis. Antecedent events occur in about 30% of patients, most commonly upper respiratory infections, gastroenteritis, other infections, vaccinations, surgery, and trauma.[52–56] Some patients present acutely, and the disorder resembles GBS before a relapsing course typical of CIDP develops, whereas others present after months of progressive symptoms. The major symptom in more than 90% of patients at presentation is weakness. Numbness and paresthesias, usually distal, occur at onset in 64% to 82%. Pain is the presenting feature only 14% to 20% of the time.[57] Cranial nerve symptoms and dysautonomia are uncommon.[53–55,58]

Diagnosis and Evaluation

On examination, both proximal and distal weakness are common, usually in a symmetric manner. Reflexes are decreased or absent in most patients. Sensory deficits are present in more than 80%, with vibratory impairment more common than deficits to pinprick. Cranial nerve dysfunction occurs in up to 16% and may include ophthalmoplegia, facial weakness, and bulbar weakness. Papilledema may occur.[53–55,59] A pure sensory variant has been described.[60,61] Published criteria categorize CIDP as being definite, probable, or possible, based on clinical, electrodiagnostic, pathologic, and CSF findings.[51] However, as with GBS, many patients who do not meet criteria for definite CIDP are (and should be) diagnosed with and treated for CIDP.

When CIDP is suspected on clinical grounds, electrodiagnostic studies are performed (see next paragraph). Findings of an acquired demyelinating polyneuropathy should lead to some laboratory studies. Sedimentation rate, a good screen for underlying systemic inflammatory and infectious disorders, is commonly normal in CIDP. Autoimmune serology will help to screen for systemic lupus erythematosus (SLE). A fasting blood glucose level should be obtained, and a 2-hour glucose tolerance test should be considered if diabetic neuropathy is a serious consideration. HIV titers should be drawn in those patients suspected to be at risk for HIV infection. Screening tests for other causes of polyneuropathy are helpful, including thyroid function tests, vitamin B_{12} level, VDRL, and (in some geographic regions) Lyme titers, in an attempt to determine whether these factors are contributing to the abnormalities of nerve conduction, although they would not account for all of the electrodiagnostic abnormalities found in CIDP. Serum and urine immunofixation or immunoelectrophoresis should be performed looking for a monoclonal gammopathy in the serum and Bence-Jones proteins in the urine. If the IgM level is elevated, antibody titers to myelin-associated glycoprotein (MAG) should be assessed. If the immunofixation studies are abnormal, an evaluation by a hematology/oncology specialist is warranted because of the association of polyneuropathy with paraproteinemias. CIDP may coexist with other diseases, including SLE, HIV infection, CNS demyelination, and malignancies. In patients with CIDP who have atypical clinical findings, particularly those patients in whom the response to standard therapies is poor, a broader search for associated diseases should be performed.[62–68] The association with diabetes mellitus poses particularly challenging diagnostic and management issues. It is important to recognize CIDP in diabetic patients, because CIDP is treatable. Patients with diabetes who develop a progressive, painless, relatively symmetric polyneuropathy over several weeks to months, characterized by proximal and distal involvement of motor more than sensory modalities should be suspected of having CIDP and may fulfill published CIDP diagnostic criteria.[69–71]

On electrodiagnostic testing, motor nerve conduction abnormalities generally demonstrate multifocal demyelination, characterized by prolonged distal latencies, slowed conduction velocities, prolonged F-wave latencies, and partial conduction block or abnormal temporal dispersion (see Fig. 14-1), as has been described in the AIDP form of GBS.[18,52–55,59,72] However, not all patients who are ultimately diagnosed with CIDP will fulfill electrodiagnostic criteria.[73] A review of the electrodiagnostic studies of 70 patients who carried the diagnosis of CIDP found that only 48% to 64% of those in whom a sufficient number of nerves were tested fulfilled electrodiagnostic criteria for CIDP, depending on which criteria were used.[74] Motor nerve studies are particularly helpful in distinguishing patients with hereditary demyelinating polyneuropathies (most commonly type 1 Charcot-Marie-Tooth disease) from those with CIDP. Those with CIDP generally demonstrate differences in the degree of slowing of conduction velocity between different segments of a given nerve, and between similar segments of different nerves, whereas those with hereditary neuropathies are more likely to demonstrate uniform slowing of conduction velocity both within and between nerves. In addition, temporal dispersion and conduction block on proximal stimulation generally are characteristics of acquired but not hereditary demyelinating polyneuropathies.[75] Sensory responses usually are absent or of low amplitude.[52,53,55,72] The findings on needle examination reflect the amount of secondary axonal degeneration that has occurred. CSF analysis usually demonstrates an elevated protein level without a pleocytosis (albuminocytologic dissociation), although the CSF protein level may be normal.[53–55,59] A radiologic bone survey should be done for the possibility of osteosclerotic myeloma. If abnormal, an evaluation by a hematology/oncology specialist is warranted. Other radiologic studies usually are not necessary in CIDP. Magnetic resonance imaging (MRI) of the cord, if done, may reveal hypertrophy and gadolinium enhancement of nerve roots.[76–79]

Treatment and Management

A variety of immunomodulating agents have been used. In most series, the overall response rate has been good, with 65% to 95% of patients responding to these therapies, either alone or in combination.[53–56] However, the response to any single therapy is probably not that good, and failure to respond to one modality should lead to treatment with another. In one series, only 39% of CIDP patients improved with corticosteroids, whereas in another 39% responded to their first treatment with either steroids, IVIg, or PE.[56,59] The three cornerstones of CIDP treatment are corticosteroids, PE, and IVIg. Rigorous randomized, controlled trials exist only for PE and IVIg.

The earliest reports of effective treatment described the use of steroids.[80–83] A prospective, randomized, but nonblinded trial of prednisone demonstrated a small but significant improvement in patients with CIDP who were treated with prednisone compared to those with no treatment.[84] A recent Cochrane Review of the use of steroids for the treatment of CIDP noted that this trial was small (35 subjects) and the weight of evidence was weak.[85] There are no other controlled trials of corticosteroids. Despite the dearth of controlled trials, steroids have been observed for years to be effective treatment for CIDP and are one of the most commonly used therapies. The effects of prednisone are not immediate. The mean time for initial improvement was 1.9 months, and the mean time to reach a clinical plateau was 6.6 months in one series.[54] Oral dosage regimens vary, but generally begin at 60 to 100 mg/day for 2 to 4 weeks or longer, followed by a gradual taper.[86] Intermittent pulse oral or intravenous methylprednisolone at a dose of 500 or 1000 mg/week demonstrated efficacy and was better tolerated than oral steroids in uncontrolled studies.[87,88] Prospective, double-blind, sham-controlled studies of PE have demonstrated its efficacy in CIDP.[89,90] A Cochrane Review recently confirmed these findings, noting that short-term improvement occurred in about two thirds of patients, but that rapid worsening may occur afterward.[91] The time to improvement is generally short, with one series finding improvement beginning 2 days to 3 weeks after beginning PE.[92] Although patients may demonstrate a monophasic course and not relapse after PE treatment, most responders relapse after about 7 to 14 days.[89,90] A recent Cochrane Review noted that there are seven randomized, controlled studies of IVIg for the treatment of CIDP: five comparing IVIg with placebo, one with corticosteroids, and one with PE.[93] The usual dose is 2 g/kg divided over 2 to 5 consecutive days. Like PE, IVIg produces a rapid improvement in responders, but this is often transient, beginning in 3 to 8 days (mean, 5 days), and usually lasting 3 to 22 weeks (mean and median, about 6 weeks).[94–96] Patients with relapsing courses have continued to respond to intermittent infusions of IVIg for years.[95,96–100] Small open-label series and case reports have demonstrated that patients with CIDP and concomitant diabetes also respond to IVIg,[101] as do those with CIDP and concomitant multiple sclerosis.[68]

A recent Cochrane Review concluded that there is not sufficient evidence to determine whether any immunomodulating treatment other than corticosteroids, IVIg, and PE is beneficial in the treatment of CIDP.[102] This has not deterred physicians from trying a variety of agents, often in an attempt to reduce dependence on steroids and thus lessen steroid-associated side effects. There is one small randomized, controlled study in which the addition of azathioprine to prednisone resulted in no better an outcome than prednisone alone, but the study is considered to have sufficient methodologic flaws to render a definitive conclusion unreliable.[102] Uncontrolled series and case reports of patients refractory to IVIg,

Box 14-2 Principles of Treatment of Chronic Inflammatory Demyelinating Polyradiculoneuropathy

Some patients with mild sensory deficits and no weakness at presentation can be observed without treatment for a period of days to weeks, because spontaneous improvement may occur. In those patients who do not improve, continue to worsen, or have motor as well as sensory deficits at presentation, treatment should be initiated.

Begin with intravenous immunoglobulin (IVIg) if available and if there are no contraindications. Plasma exchange (PE) and prednisone represent alternatives if circumstances warrant.

Be persistent, and try other agents if the initial medications are not effective.

Once control is achieved, minimize the dosage of medication needed to maintain the patient in remission, and periodically attempt to taper the patient off immunosuppressant medication.

If a patient initially responds but then becomes refractory to a particular treatment, repeat portions of the diagnostic evaluation to determine whether an underlying disorder may be responsible.

PE, and corticosteroids point to the utility, in some but not all patients, of cyclophosphamide, rituximab, cyclosporine, interferon, mycophenolate mofetil, methotrexate, alemtuzumab, etanercept, tacrolimus, and autologous stem cell transplantation.[103–125]

In view of the massive amount of literature, what is a reasonable therapeutic approach to the patient with CIDP? Overarching principles of CIDP treatment appear in Box 14-2, and a general outline of therapeutic choices appears in Table 14-3. Initial therapy should consist of IVIg, PE, or prednisone. Because all are beneficial in some patients with CIDP, the decision of which to use as initial therapy must be based on other factors, such as severity of the patient's disability, need for rapid onset of action, side effects, availability, convenience, and cost. For patients who are moderately to severely affected and in need of rapid improvement, IVIg or PE is the treatment of first choice. For those patients who are mildly affected, corticosteroids or IVIg is a reasonable initial treatment; IVIg often is preferred because some patients experience long-term, sustained improvement with IVIg, thus avoiding the adverse effects of long-term corticosteroid treatment. In general, the widespread availability of IVIg has made this the treatment of first choice for most neurologists.

Table 14-3 Therapy for Chronic Inflammatory Demyelinating Polyradiculoneuropathy

Therapeutic Hierarchy	Treatment
First-line therapy (randomized, controlled trials)	Intravenous immunoglobulin Plasma exchange Corticosteroids
Second-line therapy	Azathioprine Cyclophosphamide Cyclosporine Mycophenolate mofetil
Third-line therapy	Alemtuzumab Etanercept Interferon Methotrexate Rituximab Tacrolimus
Fourth-line therapy	Autologous stem cell transplantation

Intravenous immunoglobulin is given at 2 g/kg body weight over 2 to 3 consecutive days. In some patients, the effects of IVIg will be sustained and the course of the disease will be monophasic, thus eliminating the need for any additional treatment. If improvement occurs but is unsustained (the patient relapses), IVIg can be given again at the same dose, but prednisone 60 to 80 mg/day should be started concomitantly. The prednisone should be maintained at this dose for 2 to 3 months, then tapered to 60 mg every other day over 3 months, then to 20 mg every other day over the next 3 months, with further tapering as tolerated, aiming for an alternate-day regimen at the lowest dose that maintains the patient in remission. Azathioprine 2 to 3 mg/kg or another immunosuppressant agent can be added in an attempt to minimize the prednisone dose. For patients in whom prednisone is contraindicated or those who do not tolerate prednisone, the IVIg can be given at progressively decreasing doses and progressively longer intervals between doses, attempting to minimize the dose and maximize the interval between doses. Azathioprine or another immunosuppressant can be added to the IVIg regimen in an attempt to facilitate taper of the IVIg. Maintenance doses of IVIg may be low, and efficacy is often maintained for years. In some patients, treatment can be eventually discontinued, but most patients require lifelong maintenance therapy. PE is usually given as one plasma volume per exchange, five times over 2 weeks. If the effect is sustained, no further treatment is required. If improvement occurs but the patient relapses, PE may be repeated while prednisone is begun simultaneously, according to the guidelines above. As with IVIg, PE can be used alone and tapered to a less intensive regimen to control the disease in those patients who cannot be given prednisone. Azathioprine or other immunosuppressants can be added, as with IVIg. Prednisone can be given without IVIg or PE for patients with mild chronic deficits, or for those with moderate deficits for whom IVIg and PE are not available or are ineffective. Azathioprine or other immunosuppressants can be added as a steroid-sparing agent.

Patients who fail to respond to these therapies or who do not tolerate them require treatment with other immunosuppressant regimens (see Chapter 7). There is no single, accepted regimen. Cyclosporine, a commonly used medication, is given at 3 to 5 mg/kg body weight daily, divided into twice-daily dosing, with close monitoring of renal function. Mycophenolate mofetil 1000 to 1500 mg twice daily is another agent that is relatively commonly used. Cyclophosphamide may be the agent most likely to produce a relatively rapid response, either at 1 to 2 mg/kg daily orally or 1 g/m^2 monthly intravenously but eventually must be discontinued because of its toxicity. The other agents described above represent options for those patients who are unresponsive to or intolerant of these more commonly used agents. With immunosuppression, care should be taken to monitor hematologic parameters carefully and to minimize the total dose and duration of therapy so as to reduce the long-term risk for developing malignancies.

Outcome

In the older literature, the prognosis of patients with CIDP was not good. A Mayo Clinic series found that 11% died from CIDP, 28% were in a wheelchair or in bed at last follow-up, and only 34 (64%) were recovered or were ambulatory and working.[59] More recent series have generally documented a better outcome, with mild or no disability in 87%.[126] Good outcomes are still not universal, however. The death rate from CIDP is 3% to 6%, and even with treatment, some CIDP patients are either quadriplegic (2%) or at least unable to live independently (4%).[53,54,126,127] The major factor

influencing long-term outcome in CIDP is the degree of axon loss.[128] Often, treatment must be given long-term to treat or prevent relapses.[54,126]

Multifocal Motor Neuropathy

Multifocal motor neuropathy (MMN) with persistent conduction block is an autoimmune, acquired demyelinating polyneuropathy that was first clearly described in 1988.[129,130] The reason for the intense focus on this relatively uncommon condition is that it may mimic motor neuron disease, albeit without upper motor neuron manifestations, and that it is treatable. Onset of symptoms and progression over time are usually insidious, commonly over many years.

Diagnosis and Evaluation

MMN is characterized by asymmetric multifocal weakness in a peripheral nerve distribution. Predominant upper limb involvement is usually seen. Bulbar and respiratory involvement are absent. Reflexes may be preserved or asymmetrically lost. Sensation is characteristically normal. No upper motor neuron signs are present. Elevated titers of antibodies to GM_1 gangliosides are found in about half of the patients with MMN.[131] The electrodiagnostic hallmark of MMN is the presence of persistent multifocal motor conduction blocks at nerve sites not prone to compression. Sensory conduction through these regions is unaffected. The key to diagnosis is the clinical phenotype. Anti-GM_1 antibodies and foci of conduction block are important findings that can support the diagnosis of MMN, but their absence does not rule it out. A number of papers have clearly demonstrated that patients with clinical features of MMN who do not meet criteria for conduction block or who lack anti-GM_1 antibodies respond to treatment.[132–135]

Treatment and Management

IVIg is the treatment of choice, usually given as 2 g/kg body weight divided over 2 to 5 days. Its efficacy has been demonstrated in randomized, double-blind, placebo-controlled trials.[136–139] With one exception (see below), all other treatment recommendations for patients with MMN are class IV evidence. After initial therapy, maintenance IVIg usually is administered at the lowest dose needed to maintain remission. Commonly, this is 1 g/kg every 2 to 4 weeks or 2 g/kg every 4 to 8 weeks. We usually begin with 2 g/kg every 4 weeks and then gradually lower the dose of IVIg to the lowest dose needed to maintain good control.

Of course, not all patients with MMN respond to IVIg. Cyclophosphamide usually has been effective, although there is a report of a patient who worsened after treatment with cyclophosphamide and autologous blood stem cell transplantation.[130,140–142] Careful consideration of risks versus benefits must be made when using this toxic medication. Rituximab has produced conflicting results.[108,143] The only other randomized, placebo-controlled treatment trial in MMN has involved mycophenolate mofetil, which did not alter the disease course or permit a reduction in the IVIg dosage.[144] This is in agreement with a case report of one patient, but differs from a favorable effect found in an open-label series of four patients.[115,117] PE and corticosteroids have been unsuccessful, with steroids having been reported to cause worsening.[145] Treatment is summarized in Table 14-4. We recommend IVIg as first-line therapy and maintenance therapy, proceeding to rituximab or cyclophosphamide as second-line therapy if needed.

Table 14-4 Therapy for Multifocal Motor Neuropathy

Therapy	Dose	Effective?	Evidence	Recommendations
Intravenous immunoglobulin (IVIg): initial therapy	2 g/kg divided over 2–5 days	Yes	Randomized, controlled trials	Initial first-line therapy
IVIg: maintenance therapy	1 g/kg every 2–4 weeks or 2 g/kg every 4–8 weeks, then taper	Yes	Uncontrolled open-label series, case reports, expert opinion	Maintenance therapy
Rituximab	375 mg/m² weekly for 4 weeks	Conflicting results	Small, open-label series	Consider when IVIg ineffective or not tolerated
Cyclophosphamide	1–2 mg/kg orally or 1 gm/m² IV	Usually	Case reports, small open-label series	Consider as second- or third-line therapy, but weigh risks
Mycophenolate mofetil	500–1,000 mg twice a day, added to IVIG	Results vary	Randomized, controlled trial; open-label studies	Consider if therapies above are ineffective
Plasma exchange	Various	No	Uncontrolled open-label series, case reports	Not recommended
Corticosteroids	Various oral and IV	No	Uncontrolled open-label series, case reports	Not recommended

Outcome

Untreated, worsening is seen clinically and electrodiagnostically over time, characteristically at a very slow pace over many years.[146] A retrospective review found that most patients required ongoing periodic IVIg treatments, although a small number went into remission.[147] With treatment, some patients appear to stabilize, whereas others have a slow decline in strength, although likely at a slower rate than if untreated.[147,148]

Lewis-Sumner Syndrome

In 1982, Lewis and colleagues described five patients with a chronic, acquired, asymmetric sensorimotor demyelinating polyneuropathy that clinically resembled a mononeuritis multiplex.[149] Subsequently, many similar patients have been described.[150–154] The syndrome has been given various names, most commonly *Lewis-Sumner syndrome* and *multifocal acquired demyelinating sensory and motor (MADSAM) neuropathy*.

Diagnosis and Evaluation

Patients have a slowly progressive course, commonly over many years. The upper extremities are usually involved before the lower extremities. Both weakness and numbness may be present, and the pattern of involvement is asymmetric, usually in the distribution of discrete nerves such as one sees in a mononeuritis multiplex. Pain is more common than in MMN. Cranial neuropathies may occur but are rare. Reflexes are usually decreased in an asymmetric multifocal manner, but rarely are completely absent.

Blood and urine tests are usually the same as those performed in the evaluation of CIDP. In contrast to MMN, anti-GM₁ antibodies are rarely present.[150–153] Electrodiagnostic studies demonstrate features of multifocal demyelination as described for CIDP, but in an asymmetric manner. CSF protein is usually normal to mildly elevated, without pleocytosis. Many consider Lewis-Sumner syndrome to be a variant of CIDP, based on clinical findings, electrodiagnostic abnormalities, and response to treatment.[152,155]

Treatment and Management

No controlled trials of treatment have been conducted, although a number of small series have used open-label treatments, most commonly IVIg and steroids.[149,151–154,156] Reported response rates vary widely. More than half of those treated responded to IVIg. Steroid responsiveness varied from no responses to 11 of 14 patients treated. There are occasional reports of responses to azathioprine and cyclophosphamide. Based on the evidence available, it appears that IVIg is the treatment of choice and that steroids represent a reasonable alternative. PE appears to be less effective, so it should be performed in those patients unresponsive to IVIg and steroids, whereas immunosuppression with azathioprine, cyclophosphamide, and other agents should be reserved for those unresponsive or suboptimally responsive to other therapies. Recommendations are provided in Table 14-5. As with CIDP, immunosuppressant agents can be considered for use in lessening dependence on IVIg or steroids.

Paraproteinemic Neuropathies: Chronic Inflammatory Demyelinating Polyradiculoneuropathy Associated with Monoclonal Gammopathy of Undetermined Significance

Monoclonal gammopathy of undetermined significance (MGUS) is found in approximately 60% of patients with a monoclonal gammopathy.[157] The association of CIDP with MGUS has been of considerable interest because of the possible causal relationship between the neuropathy and the MGUS, particularly IgM monoclonal gammopathy.

Diagnosis and Evaluation

Patients with CIDP and MGUS (CIDP-MGUS) have been compared to those with CIDP but no MGUS (idiopathic CIDP, or CIDP-I).[55] CIDP-MGUS patients generally present with a more

Table 14-5 Treatment of Lewis-Sumner Syndrome

Therapy	Dose	Effective?	Evidence	Recommendations
Intravenous immunoglobulin (IVIg): initial therapy	2 g/kg divided over 2–5 days	Usually	Uncontrolled open-label series, case reports	Initial first-line therapy
IVIg: maintenance therapy	1 g/kg every 2–4 weeks or 2 g/kg every 4–8 weeks, then taper	Usually	Uncontrolled open-label series, case reports	Maintenance therapy
Corticosteroids	60 mg/day, then taper	Some cases	Uncontrolled open-label series, case reports	Second-line therapy
Plasma exchange	5 exchanges of 1 plasma volume each over 10–14 days, then taper	Probably less so than IVIG or steroids	Uncontrolled open-label series, case reports	Third-line therapy
Azathioprine	2–3 mg/kg/day	Some cases	Case reports	Consider when above treatments ineffective or not tolerated
Cyclophosphamide	1–2 mg/kg orally or 1 gm/m^2 IV	Some cases	Case reports	Consider after other treatments, but weigh risks

slowly developing disease. Other features of CIDP-MGUS compared to CIDP-I are less severe weakness and more sensory impairment.[55,158] Such comparisons are somewhat problematic because patients with CIDP-MGUS represent a heterogeneous group of patients with IgM, IgG, and IgA monoclonal gammopathies, and IgM appears to play a unique role. Some studies have found IgM MGUS patients with neuropathy to be different from those with IgG or IgA MGUS due to more frequent sensory loss, more frequent ataxia, more progression over time, and a higher frequency of nerve conduction abnormalities.[159–161] Patients with CIDP, IgM MGUS, and high titers of antibodies to MAG are particularly likely to constitute a relatively homogeneous group of predominantly male, middle-aged to elderly patients with chronic, slowly progressive polyneuropathies characterized by distal sensory loss, gait ataxia, normal strength or mild distal weakness, and some distinguishing features on their nerve conduction studies.[162–169] The term *distal acquired demyelinating symmetric neuropathy* has been applied to such patients.[170]

The laboratory evaluation of these patients is carried out as described for CIDP-I. When the presence of a monoclonal protein is confirmed, an evaluation by a hematology/oncology specialist is usually necessary to differentiate a MGUS from other paraproteinemias. A radiologic bone survey is needed to identify the presence of one or more bone lesions characteristic of sclerotic myeloma. For CIDP-MGUS patients as a group, electrodiagnostic findings in motor nerves are similar to those of patients with CIDP-I, whereas sensory nerve conduction studies are more abnormal.[55,56] However, patients with IgM monoclonal gammopathies and high titers of anti-MAG antibodies usually do not demonstrate conduction block and have disproportionately prolonged motor distal latencies.[162–169,171] CSF findings are similar to those in CIDP-I.

Treatment and Management

Treatment of patients with CIDP-MGUS, particularly those patients with IgM monoclonal gammopathy, has not generally been as successful as treatment of patients with CIDP-I. A recent Cochrane Review concluded that the evidence is inadequate to support any particular immunosuppressant therapy for anti-MAG

neuropathies.[172] This conclusion reflects the combination in the literature of some treatment studies of PE and IVIg that are relatively scientifically rigorous, and studies of other immunosuppressant agents that produce class IV evidence. However, one subsequently published double-blind, placebo-controlled study of patients with IgM monoclonal gammopathies of undetermined significance and elevated titers of anti-MAG antibodies found that rituximab 375 mg/m^2 weekly for 4 consecutive weeks led to improvement of neuropathy over 8 months in 4 of 13 patients, compared to improvement in none of the patients treated with placebo.[173]

PE, in a double-blind, sham-controlled trial and in an open-label study, has been shown to produce improvement in CIDP-MGUS patients, although less effectively in IgM than in IgG and IgA patients.[174,175] A regimen of monthly PE treatments on 2 consecutive days followed by intravenous cyclophosphamide resulted in clinical improvements in four patients with polyneuropathy associated with anti-MAG antibodies.[176] The effects of IVIg have been assessed via two double-blind, placebo-controlled studies of patients with neuropathies associated with IgM monoclonal gammopathy. Short-term benefit was found in about half of patients in one study, and 2 of 11 improved in another.[177,178] The evidence for other therapeutic modalities is largely class IV, is focused mostly on IgM MGUS, and includes studies using cyclosporine, chlorambucil, fludarabine, mycophenolate mofetil, and rituximab, all of which demonstrated benefit in some patients but none in others.[179–186] One patient with Waldenström macroglobulinemia, elevated titers of anti-MAG antibodies, and a demyelinating polyneuropathy improved after autologous bone marrow transplantation.[187]

In view of the large number of therapies that have been tried, what should be the approach to treating patients with CIDP-MGUS? Those patients with IgG or IgA MGUS should be treated using the same approach as used for those with CIDP-I. Although only PE has been evaluated in a controlled fashion, experience has shown that these patients often respond to therapy in a manner similar to patients with CIDP-I. For those patients with CIDP-IgM gammopathy, we have summarized our approach in Table 14-6. Ideally, in view of the recently published controlled study, treatment would be initiated with rituximab, 375 mg/m^2 weekly for 4 weeks, with close follow-up of serum IgM levels regularly. If the serum

Table 14-6 Therapy for Demyelinating Polyneuropathy Associated with IgM Monoclonal Gammopathy of Undetermined Significance

Therapy	Dose	Effective?	Evidence	Recommendations
Rituximab	375 mg/m^2 weekly ×4 weeks. Repeat single infusions every 3 months if needed	Sometimes	One randomized, controlled study; other open-label series, case reports	Consider as first-line therapy if available
Intravenous immunoglobulin	2 g/kg over 2–5 days monthly for at least 3 months	Sometimes	Randomized, controlled trials	First-line therapy
Plasma exchange	2 exchanges weekly for at least 3 months	Sometimes; better for IgG and IgA	Randomized, controlled trials	Second-line therapy
Plasma exchange plus cyclophosphamide	Monthly	Probably	Case reports	Third-line therapy
Cyclosporine Chlorambucil Fludarabine Mycophenolate mofetil	Various	Sometimes	Open-label series, case reports	Fourth-line therapy Comparative efficacy of choices has not been assessed
Corticosteroids	Various	No	Open-label series, case reports	Not recommended

IgM level does not decline as expected, then single infusions of 375 mg/m^2 may be given every 3 months to achieve lowering of the IgM level. Improvement, when it occurs, is gradual. The high cost of this medication, combined with the lack of FDA approval for this indication, often leads to insurers declining to pay for such treatment. In that case, we usually begin with a trial of IVIg. Due to the chronic nature of these neuropathies, we often treat monthly for 3 months and then assess the response to treatment. Unfortunately, many patients do not respond to IVIg. The goal of therapy should then be to lower the serum IgM level to less than 50% of baseline and maintain it there. One means to do this is with PE. We recommend a prolonged course, consisting of two exchanges per week for 3 months, then one or two exchanges per week for at least another 3 months, monitoring serum IgM levels. The other agents can then be tried if necessary, although the probability of a response to any one of them cannot be predicted. Corticosteroids have not been found to be beneficial in these patients.

Outcome

The course of the disease in patients with CIDP-IgM MGUS is more likely to be progressive than in patients with idiopathic CIDP-I and to evolve more slowly, with much of the functional impairment due to sensory impairment and with a poorer long-term outcome.[126,158] As with CIDP-I, most patients require continued immunosuppressant treatment to maintain remission.[126] Patients with IgG and IgA MGUS and polyneuropathy generally follow a clinical course similar to that seen in patients with CIDP-I.

Paraproteinemic Neuropathies: Primary Systemic Amyloidosis

Primary amyloidosis is characterized by deposition of immunoglobulin light chains in various tissues, resulting in dysfunction of those organs. It can occur without or in association with multiple myeloma. At the time of diagnosis, 17% of patients with primary amyloidosis have peripheral neuropathy.[188] The clinical presentation is usually that of a distal, symmetric, sensorimotor polyneuropathy that

is painful and is often characterized by autonomic involvement. Carpal tunnel syndrome is common. Systemic involvement of other organs, particularly kidneys, heart, liver, and gastrointestinal tract, is common.

Diagnosis and Evaluation

Examination initially reveals sensory more than motor involvement. Electrodiagnostic findings are those of an axonal sensorimotor polyneuropathy, often with superimposed carpal tunnel syndrome.[162] Laboratory studies may demonstrate thrombocytopenia. Approximately 90% of patients with primary systemic amyloidosis will have a paraprotein in their serum or urine on immunofixation or immunoelectrophoresis, most commonly IgG or IgAλ in the serum and free monoclonal light chains in the urine.[189] Definitive diagnosis is made by nerve biopsy, which demonstrates axonal loss and amyloid deposits on Congo red staining or metachromatic stains such as methyl violet. Immunohistochemical staining identifies the amyloid deposits as consisting of light chains. Often the deposition of amyloid is patchy and is easily missed on biopsy of peripheral nerve.[190] Biopsy of other tissue may be required for definitive diagnosis.

Treatment and Management

Unfortunately, there is little data, none of it controlled, on the response of peripheral neuropathy to treatment of amyloidosis, although the neuropathy generally has been observed to worsen despite treatment. Treatment of primary systemic amyloidosis traditionally has consisted of a combination of melphalan and prednisone, which was shown to be beneficial in a placebo-controlled, double-blind study.[191] An open-label study of melphalan and high-dose dexamethasone shows that this appears to be preferable.[192] A randomized trial of high-dose melphalan followed by autologous hematopoietic stem cell transplantation was found to be no more effective than melphalan plus dexamethasone.[193] Because of widespread multiorgan involvement, prognosis is poor. The search for more effective therapies has been well-summarized recently.[194] Symptomatic management of the peripheral neuropathy usually is aimed at pain and autonomic symptoms, including orthostatic hypotension.[195]

Paraproteinemic Neuropathies: POEMS Syndrome (Osteosclerotic Myeloma)

The POEMS (polyneuropathy, organomegaly, endocrinopathy, monoclonal protein, skin changes) syndrome is also known as *osteosclerotic myeloma*. The systemic features include hepatomegaly, splenomegaly, peripheral edema, ascites, thrombocytopenia, and skin hyperpigmentation.[196] Not all patients demonstrate all features, but all have polyneuropathy, osteosclerotic myeloma (a plasma cell dyscrasia and at least one bone lesion) or Castleman disease (angiofollicular lymph node hyperplasia), and at least one of the other features. Up to 50% of patients with osteosclerotic myeloma have peripheral neuropathy.[196] The peripheral neuropathy often is the initial clinical manifestation and begins with distal sensory symptoms, usually evolving into a motor-predominant pattern, often with prominent proximal weakness.[197]

Diagnosis and Evaluation

Electrodiagnostically, the features are those of a demyelinating polyneuropathy with axonal degeneration.[198] CSF analysis reveals an elevated protein level without pleocytosis. The neurologist's role, particularly when the initial manifestation is that of peripheral neuropathy, centers around evaluation for the other features of POEMS syndrome once a demyelinating polyneuropathy has been identified. Laboratory studies are performed as for CIDP, and other clinical features of POEMS syndrome are searched for. A bone survey will demonstrate single or multiple bone lesions, which are most commonly sclerotic or mixed sclerotic and lytic, but which on occasion may be lytic only. A biopsy of such a lesion usually is needed for diagnosis. Castleman disease and other features of POEMS are usually identified in consultation with a hematology/oncology consultant. Failure to identify such extra-neurologic manifestations may result in a misdiagnosis of CIDP and consequently to ineffective treatment.

Treatment and Management

All evidence of efficacy of treatment of neuropathy in patients with osteosclerotic myeloma or POEMS syndrome is uncontrolled class IV evidence. Radiation of a solitary plasmacytoma generally is recommended. For patients with multiple lesions or with Castleman disease, the usual treatment is chemotherapy, often with a combination of an alkylating agent and corticosteroids. PE alone and IVIg alone appear to be ineffective.[196,199] Two uncontrolled series found that a combined regimen of high-dose chemotherapy and autologous peripheral blood stem cell transplantation appears to be effective in improving nerve conduction studies and neurologic function.[200,201]

Vasculitis

Vasculitis is a term that is applied to a variety of conditions that result in inflammation and destruction of blood vessel walls. In systemic vasculitis, there is involvement of organs outside of the nervous system, commonly the skin, kidneys, joints, liver, GI tract, and lungs. Nonsystemic vasculitic neuropathy (NSVN) refers to a localized type of vasculitis, restricted to the peripheral nerves. Neuropathy is common in systemic vasculitis, occurring in 20% to 80% of patients with primary vasculitides.[202] Of all patients presenting with vasculitic neuropathy, more than one fourth will have NSVN; nearly as many will have polyarteritis nodosa or microscopic

---

Box 14-3 Vasculitides Associated with Neuropathy

Primary Systemic Vasculitides Most Likely to Cause Vasculitic Neuropathy

Polyarteritis nodosa
Microscopic polyangiitis (MPA)
Churg-Strauss syndrome
Wegener's granulomatosis

Secondary Systemic Vasculitides Most Likely to Cause Vasculitic Neuropathy

Connective tissue diseases
  Rheumatoid arthritis
  Systemic lupus erythematosus
  Sjögren's syndrome
  Mixed connective tissue disease
Infectious agents
  Usually viral, including human immunodeficiency virus, cytomegalovirus, hepatitis B, hepatitis C with mixed cryoglobulinemia
Drugs
  Including cocaine, amphetamines, heroin, and many legally prescribed medications
Paraneoplastic
  Solid malignancies and hematologic disorders

Nonsystemic Vasculitic Neuropathy

Limited to nerve and muscle

---

polyangiitis. Rheumatoid vasculitis, undifferentiated connective tissue disease, Churg-Strauss syndrome, SLE, Sjögren's syndrome, and Wegener's granulomatosis account for 14%, 10%, 7%, 4%, 2%, and 2%, respectively, of vasculitic neuropathies.[203] One simple classification scheme, identifying the most common causes of vasculitic neuropathy, is presented in Box 14-3.

Diagnosis and Evaluation

Mononeuritis multiplex is the classic presentation of vasculitic neuropathy. Affected individuals develop stepwise, acute, or subacute dysfunction of multiple peripheral nerves.[203] In some patients, the areas of peripheral nerve damage may coalesce to produce a polyneuropathy that most commonly is asymmetric but on rare occasions may be indistinguishable from a nonvasculitic distal sensorimotor polyneuropathy. The evolution of vasculitic neuropathy usually occurs over weeks to months but may be very rapid (days) or very indolent (years). Most patients have sensory and motor involvement, whereas isolated sensory involvement is present in a small number. The neuropathy is painful in most patients.[203-205] Laboratory studies usually are undertaken to identify markers of inflammation and autoantibodies that indicate a systemic vasculitis or underlying connective tissue disease, and to identify organ involvement outside of the peripheral nervous system. The erythrocyte sedimentation rate is elevated in approximately 60% of patients with NSVN, usually mildly so. In contrast, approximately 90% of patients with systemic vasculitis have an elevated sedimentation rate, usually markedly so. A variety of autoimmune serologic markers are commonly assayed for, including antinuclear antibodies, rheumatoid factor, anti-double-stranded-DNA, anti-Ro (SSA), anti-La (SSB), anti-Sm, and the antineutrophil cytoplasmic antibodies c-ANCA and p-ANCA. Serum complement levels may be low in various connective tissue diseases. Cryoglobulins, Lyme antibodies, hepatitis B and C testing, HIV serology, and angiotensin-converting enzyme levels should be checked. Renal and liver function tests, a urinalysis, and a chest radiograph are used to screen for other organ involvement. A more extensive evaluation for an underlying malignancy should be considered. A lumbar puncture usually is not necessary, because CSF generally is normal, although the protein level may be elevated. If a polyradiculopathy is present, CSF may be useful to assess for carcinomatous meningitis or Lyme disease. A contrast-enhanced MRI of the involved region of the spine may be useful in this situation as well.

Electrodiagnostic studies demonstrate an axonal sensorimotor polyneuropathy, which is often asymmetric. Electrodiagnostic features of conduction block may occur.[206,207] Thus, a multifocal process such as one due to vasculitis should be suspected when there is a significant difference in amplitudes between responses from the same nerves on opposite sides, or between different nerves in the same limb, or when the upper extremities are affected more than the lower extremities, all of which would be atypical for a length-dependent process such as a distal axonal sensorimotor polyneuropathy. However, some patient with a vasculitic neuropathy may have symmetric findings indistinguishable from those seen in nonvasculitic distal sensorimotor polyneuropathies.[203,208] Nerve biopsy is the definitive diagnostic procedure. The sural nerve or superficial peroneal nerve is usually biopsied. Ideally, one should biopsy a nerve that is abnormal clinically or electrodiagnostically. The diagnostic pathologic findings in vasculitis are inflammatory infiltrates within the blood vessel wall and fibrinoid necrosis, hemorrhage, or endothelial cell disruption. Findings suggestive of, but not diagnostic for, vasculitis include thickening of blood vessel walls, narrowing or obliteration of the vascular lumen, thrombosis, perivascular hemosiderin deposits, and nerve fiber loss that is asymmetric within and between nerve fascicles.[203,209] Because of the limited number of nerves available for biopsy and the patchy nature of vasculitis, the nerve biopsy may be nondiagnostic. The yield can be increased by simultaneously performing a muscle biopsy. Superficial peroneal nerve/peroneus brevis muscle biopsy or sural nerve/peroneus brevis muscle biopsy are common combinations.[209–211]

Treatment and Management

Treatment for vasculitic neuropathy associated with primary vasculitis is based on treatment regimens for systemic vasculitis. These depend on the underlying disease and usually are chosen and managed by a rheumatologist. Details are beyond the scope of this review, but have been summarized elsewhere.[203,212] The usual treatment regimen consists of corticosteroids in combination with an immunosuppressant agent, most commonly cyclophosphamide. The cyclophosphamide usually is changed to azathioprine or methotrexate after remission is achieved (commonly 3 to 12 months), and the patient is treated with one of these other immunosuppressant agents for a number of months. A recent open-label, prospective, randomized study of patients with Wegener's granulomatosis or microscopic polyangiitis found no difference in safety or efficacy when comparing methotrexate with azathioprine.[213] A variety of other oral and intravenous treatments, including cyclosporine, mycophenolate mofetil, IVIg, and PE, each of which may have utility depending on the specific clinical syndrome. For patients with secondary systemic vasculitis in which there is an underlying infection, drug, toxin, or malignancy, treatment regimens are directed toward removal of the underlying drug or toxin and treatment of the infection or malignancy. Immunosuppression is used for some of these patients.[203,212]

Treatment of NSVN more often falls within the scope of the neurologist's expertise. A recent Cochrane Review found no controlled trials of treatment of NSVN.[214] Thus, treatment has been based largely on class IV evidence. In NSVN, less aggressive therapy can be considered than in systemic vasculitis because the prognosis is better, although this must be weighed against what appears to be a higher rate of relapse in those treated initially with corticosteroids alone versus those treated with corticosteroids plus immunosuppression.[202,203,212,215–217] Nonetheless, we recommend corticosteroids alone initially, administered as prednisone 60 mg/day for 2 to 3 months or until clinical stabilization occurs, followed by a very slow taper to 60 mg every other day over 3 months, then to 20 mg/day over 3 additional months, then slowly down to zero. Cyclophosphamide 1 to 2 mg/kg is added for those who fail to respond or who relapse as the prednisone is tapered. Pain control should be attempted with agents usually used for neuropathic pain or with other analgesics. High-dose corticosteroids often bring about a rapid reduction in pain. Long-term treatment with gradual tapering of the steroids or immunosuppression over months is necessary for these diseases, and some patients require steroids or immunosuppression indefinitely. Improvement, if it occurs, will be slow, because of the axonal nature of these neuropathies.

Outcome

NSVN is a more benign disease than neuropathy associated with systemic vasculitis. Survival rates are considerably higher, and residual disability is lower (Table 14-7).[204,205,210,216] There is only about a 6% chance of NSVN spreading to involve other organs.[210]

Cryoglobulinemia

Cryoglobulinemia is characterized by serum proteins that precipitate in the cold but dissolve back into solution when warmed. The proteins may be monoclonal immunoglobulins (type I), mixed monoclonal and polyclonal immunoglobulins (type II), or polyclonal immunoglobulins (type III). Cryoglobulins are associated with many underlying systemic illnesses. When no underlying disease can be identified, the term *essential cryoglobulinemia* is used.[218–221] Types II and III usually are associated with chronic hepatitis C infection. Mixed cryoglobulins induce immune complex–mediated inflammation of small blood vessels, resulting in peripheral neuropathy 40% to 75% of the time.[203]

Diagnosis and Evaluation

A distal, symmetric sensory or sensorimotor polyneuropathy or a mononeuritis multiplex may occur, usually characterized by painful distal dysesthesias and sensory loss.[221,222] The detection of

Table 14-7 Long-Term Disability in Survivors with Nonsystemic Vasculitic Neuropathy and in Those with Systemic Vasculitis

Disability	Nonsystemic Vasculitic Neuropathy	Systemic Vasculitis
Asymptomatic	14%	9%
Mild to moderate disability	67%	56%
Walking with assistance	16%	22%
Unable to walk	3%	14%

cryoglobulins in the blood involves collecting blood into warm tubes, which are later cooled to allow precipitation of cryoglobulins. Types II and III generally produce concentrations of 1 to 5 mg/dL.[223] Electrodiagnostic studies demonstrate an axonal neuropathy.[219,221,222] Nerve biopsies demonstrate axon loss, with an epineurial vasculitis characterized by thickening of the walls and obliteration of the lumens of endoneurial microvessels.[218,222,224]

Treatment

Corticosteroids, PE, and cyclophosphamide have been used empirically in the treatment of cryoglobulinemic vasculitis (class IV evidence) with varying degrees of success.[221,225,226] Rituximab, alone or in combination with PE, has recently been found to be effective in a few refractory patients.[227–229] Interferon alfa, when used to treat underlying hepatitis, has been found at times to improve and at other times to worsen these neuropathies, and may be combined with ribavirin. The decision of which of these various agents to use depends on the severity of the disease.[224,230–233] For treatment of hepatitis C–associated cryoglobulinemic vasculitis, induction is achieved with corticosteroids, cyclophosphamide, and PE, followed by maintenance with interferon alfa and ribavirin.[203]

Nonvasculitic Neuropathies Associated with Connective Tissue Disease

Although some patients with connective tissue disease develop a vasculitic neuropathy, others develop focal neuropathies as a result of entrapment or develop nonvasculitic polyneuropathies. Because connective tissue diseases are relatively common, neuropathies associated with these disorders are seen frequently, and careful evaluation is needed to distinguish the vasculitic neuropathies from nonvasculitic neuropathies, so as to permit rational treatment decisions.

Rheumatoid arthritis, Sjögren syndrome, SLE, scleroderma, and mixed connective tissue disease all may be associated with a distally predominant, painful, sensory-more-than-motor polyneuropathy, with axonal features on electrodiagnostic testing and without features of vasculitis on nerve biopsy.[234–239] Cranial neuropathies, particularly trigeminal sensory neuropathies, occur in many of these disorders. Autonomic neuropathies, though rare, have been reported. Sjögren syndrome may also be associated with a sensory neuronopathy, also classified as an inflammatory sensory polyganglionopathy or dorsal root ganglionitis.[240] This neuronopathy is characterized by numbness and tingling of the limbs and possibly the face, often asymmetric at onset and multifocal. Onset is usually subacute but may be sudden and severe.[241]

Diagnosis and Evaluation

The identification of distal symmetric sensorimotor polyneuropathies, cranial neuropathies, and autonomic neuropathies is undertaken with the usual clinical and electrodiagnostic methods. For those patients with sensory neuronopathy associated with Sjögren's syndrome, examination demonstrates prominent sensory loss, especially to proprioception and vibration. Gait ataxia is common, as is pseudoathetosis of the limbs due to sensory loss. Autonomic dysfunction may be present as well. Reflexes are usually absent. Strength is normal although frequently difficult to assess adequately due to the difficulty coordinating the limbs for testing as a result of the prominent sensory loss. The patient often has dry eyes and dry mouth, a combination termed *sicca complex*.

Serologic evidence of Sjögren syndrome should be sought with testing for SSA (Ro) and SSB (La) antibodies. Schirmer test usually demonstrates decreased tear production. A salivary gland biopsy is a useful test. More than one focus of lymphocytes per 4 mm² is considered diagnostic.[242,243] Electrodiagnostic studies demonstrate low-amplitude or absent sensory responses, but normal motor nerve studies, often asymmetric. The needle EMG examination is usually normal. Sural nerve biopsy reveals axon loss affecting primarily large fibers and perivascular inflammation without vasculitis. Biopsy of a dorsal root ganglion demonstrates loss of neurons and mononuclear inflammatory infiltrates without vasculitis.[240,244] A painful small-fiber neuropathy also may occur in Sjögren syndrome in which nerve conduction studies are normal but intraepidermal nerve fiber studies are abnormal.[245] SLE may be associated with an acute or chronic demyelinating polyneuropathy (AIDP or CIDP).[246,247] Clinical findings and electrodiagnostic features are as described elsewhere.

Treatment

No controlled trials have been directed specifically toward the treatment of nonentrapment, nonvasculitic peripheral neuropathies associated with the various connective tissue disorders. Thus, all recommendations are based on class IV evidence. Generally, the response of these nonvasculitic axonal sensorimotor polyneuropathies to corticosteroids and immunotherapy is poor. Thus, one must carefully consider whether the severity of the neuropathy is sufficient to justify the toxicities associated with immunotherapy or whether limiting treatment to the symptomatic management of pain would be the more prudent course. Generally, we recommend symptomatic treatment. The same caution applies to the cranial, autonomic, and small-fiber neuropathies seen in these disorders. For the sensory neuronopathy associated with Sjögren syndrome, treatment is often ineffective, although responses to corticosteroids, IVIg, PE, D-penicillamine, and infliximab have all been reported.[240,248–252] Treatment or GBS and CIDP associated with lupus should follow the same guidelines as for the idiopathic forms of these disorders.

Autoimmune Lumbosacral Plexopathy

An autoimmune lumbosacral plexopathy has been most commonly described in patients with diabetes and has also been called *diabetic amyotrophy*, *proximal diabetic neuropathy*, *diabetic lumbosacral plexopathy*, and *Bruns-Garland syndrome*. Perhaps the best descriptive term is *lumbosacral radiculoplexus neuropathy*.[253,254] The same condition also has been well-described in nondiabetic patients.[255,256] The underlying mechanism is thought to be ischemic neuropathy due to microvasculitis. The onset of symptoms often is abrupt, usually beginning with asymmetric or unilateral pain affecting the proximal lower extremity, the lower thoracic dermatomes, or both. The pain often is severe, and the distal portion of the limb may be involved. Pain usually is followed by progressive weakness and atrophy of involved muscles, not confined to one segmental level or one peripheral nerve. Weight loss is common. The syndrome may progress to involve the contralateral side. Weakness is often severe; half of the patients in one series were wheelchair bound and most of the others required an aid to ambulate.[254] Although less common, the upper limbs may be clinically involved either before, after, or simultaneously with lower limbs.[257] Progression of symptoms over several months is common but at a rate that may vary greatly; peak deficits may occur as quickly as weeks or as long as a year or more after onset. The condition may plateau and begin to improve on one side, only to then develop on the other.

Diagnosis and Evaluation

Laboratory studies are performed to assess for an underlying autoimmune disorder or vasculitis, as may be present in a mononeuritis multiplex, and are described in the section in this chapter on vasculitic neuropathy. Some patients have an elevated sedimentation rate or abnormal autoimmune serology, but most do not. CSF studies are indicated if the clinical or electrodiagnostic features are suggestive of a polyradiculopathy, as may occur in carcinomatous or lymphomatous meningitis or in an infectious process. In the absence of such underlying causes, CSF protein levels usually are elevated, without pleocytosis.[254–256] MRI of the lumbar spine and pelvis is commonly performed to rule out structural abnormalities or to look for nerve root enhancement, as may occur in neoplastic or infectious cases. Electrodiagnostic studies usually indicate involvement of peripheral nerves, lumbosacral plexus, and roots, with changes of active and chronic denervation seen on needle EMG examination of muscles of the lower extremities and of the thoracic and lumbar paraspinal regions. There may be an associated peripheral neuropathy. Biopsies demonstrate microvasculitis affecting peripheral nerves, lumbosacral plexus, and the thoracic and lumbar nerve roots, but are generally not done as part of the evaluation.[254–256]

Treatment and Management

Pain is often severe and is treated with medications used for neuropathic pain or with narcotic analgesics. Immunotherapy has been used to treat the microvasculitis. All evidence to date is based on case reports or uncontrolled studies. Efficacy is challenging to evaluate because spontaneous improvement occurs. IVIg and corticosteroids have been used most frequently, often with reported improvement. PE, cyclophosphamide, and azathioprine also have been reported to be effective in those with diabetes.[69,258–263] Perhaps the clearest description of efficacy comes from a Mayo Clinic open-label trial of intravenous methylprednisolone infusions 1 g/weekly for 8 to 16 weeks in 11 patients. All had marked improvement of pain, and some demonstrated improvement of weakness. Before treatment, six patients were wheelchair bound and four used a walking aid. After treatment, one was in a wheelchair and six walked independently.[264] Controlled clinical trials are under way. Because this is a self-limited condition, symptomatic treatment of pain alone generally is the accepted mode of management for those patients who have mild weakness. In those patients with severe and progressive weakness, corticosteroids or IVIg may be considered.

Outcome

Outcome data are available for those not treated with immunotherapy. Recovery generally occurs but is slow and frequently incomplete. Most patients do not recover entirely and may require leg brace, cane, walker, or wheelchair at maximal recovery.[253,254,256,265]

Autoimmune Brachial Plexopathy

Idiopathic brachial plexopathy was first described in 1948[266] and is also known as *neuralgic amyotrophy*, *Parsonage-Turner syndrome*, and *idiopathic brachial plexus neuropathy*. The mechanism is thought to be that of microvasculitis, as described for lumbosacral plexopathy.[267,268] The most common antecedent event is a febrile illness (25% to 55% of cases), although this syndrome also has commonly been reported after vaccinations and surgery, and less commonly after exercise, medications, illicit drug use, neoplasms, pregnancy, and trauma.[268–272] The onset may occur within 24 hours of the antecedent event, or as long as 2 or more weeks after the event. In virtually all cases, pain is the initial symptom, usually severe and of abrupt onset. It most commonly appears in the shoulder and scapula, often with upper extremity radicular pain. A unilateral onset is most common, although bilateral, asymmetric symptoms may be seen at presentation. In most patients, the pain resolves in 2 or 3 weeks, although in some it persists much longer. Muscle weakness appears within 2 weeks of onset of pain, usually as the pain improves, and commonly occurs in a patchy, multifocal pattern. The shoulder girdle and proximal upper extremity are the most common sites of weakness, which may be limited to the distributions of peripheral nerves (most commonly long thoracic, suprascapular, axillary nerves), portions of the brachial plexus (including one or more trunks), or rarely to C5–6 roots.[268–272]

Diagnosis and Evaluation

Results of laboratory studies usually are normal; studies should be carried out as described for lumbosacral plexopathy. CSF analysis usually demonstrates a normal to mildly increased protein level without pleocytosis. MRI of the cervical spine and the brachial plexus is commonly performed to rule out structural abnormalities, including neoplastic infiltration. On electrodiagnostic testing, sensory nerve conduction studies may be abnormal, depending on the region of the plexus involved. Motor nerve studies reveal low to normal amplitudes. Needle EMG examination may reveal active denervation, depending on when in the course of the illness the study is performed. Overall, the distribution of the abnormalities is consistent with a multifocal process producing axonal damage within the brachial plexus and isolated peripheral nerves of the upper extremities.

Treatment and Management

As with lumbosacral plexopathy, no controlled treatment trials have been conducted. Even open-label studies are scarce, and there is little evidence to guide treatment. Corticosteroids may decrease the initial pain.[269] Retrospectively, those patients treated with corticosteroids had a shorter time to onset of recovery of strength, but no other differences in outcome were noted among multiple variables assessed.[271] Treatment with IVIg has been reported to hasten recovery.[273–275] Because this is a self-limited condition, symptomatic treatment of pain is generally the accepted mode of management. However, in those patients with severe and progressive weakness, corticosteroids or IVIg may be considered.

Outcome

Outcome data is available for those not treated with immunotherapy. A follow-up study of 84 cases found that recovery occurred in 36% within 1 year, 75% by the end of the second year, and 89% by the end of the third year.[269] The degree of recovery depends on the severity of denervation and weakness[270] but also is length-dependent, with recovery occurring more quickly and being more complete in muscles closer to the site of damage. A recent series with a follow-up period of 3 years or more emphasized the persistent nature of symptoms and signs. More than 60% of patients had persistent pain; residual weakness was mild in 69.4%, moderate in 13.9%, and severe in 2.8%.[271]

Celiac Disease

Gluten sensitivity is a broad term that encompasses gluten-sensitive enteropathy (celiac disease), dermatopathy (dermatitis herpetiformis), and neurologic disorders (gluten ataxia and neuropathy). The term *gluten sensitivity* often is used for those patients with antigliadin antibodies but normal small-bowel mucosa, whereas those with diagnostic abnormalities on small-bowel biopsy are classified as having *celiac disease*. Nutritional deficiency is unlikely to be the cause of the neuropathy, because most patients with gluten sensitivity and neuropathy do not have abnormalities on small-bowel biopsy and have normal nutritional status.[276] The etiology likely is immunologic and T cell–mediated.[277] Nongastroenterologic symptoms can occur in the absence of the enteropathy and may be the presenting features of gluten sensitivity. Several series have found that 6% to 10% of patients with celiac disease develop neurologic manifestations, most commonly ataxia or peripheral neuropathy.[276–278] One review found that fully 23% of patients with celiac disease had axonal peripheral neuropathy on electrodiagnostic testing.[279] Conversely, in one series of 140 patients with axonal peripheral neuropathy of unknown cause, 47 (34%) were found to have IgG or IgA antigliadin antibodies, compared to a 12% prevalence in controls.[276]

Diagnosis and Evaluation

Patients with gluten sensitivity and peripheral neuropathy demonstrate a mean age at onset of neuropathy of 55 years (range, 24 to 77). Symptoms usually are those of a symmetric, distally predominant sensorimotor polyneuropathy; electrodiagnostic testing in these patients demonstrates a length-dependent axonal polyneuropathy. Some patients present clinically and electrodiagnostically with a mononeuritis multiplex, pure motor neuropathy, or small-fiber sensory neuropathy. Antigliadin IgG antibodies alone occur in 57%, IgA alone in 16%, and both IgG and IgA in 27%. Not all patients with gluten sensitivity and peripheral neuropathy have symptomatic gluten-sensitive enteropathy. In one series, this was present in only 29%.[276] Sural nerve biopsies generally are not part of the standard evaluation but when performed show axonal loss, with or without inflammatory cell infiltration. Rare patients present with a rapidly progressive neuropathy associated with CNS involvement, most commonly an ataxia.[276,280,281] It is not clear why gluten sensitivity can result in different clinical manifestations.

Treatment and Management

One case-control study found a gluten-free diet to improve neurophysiologic measures and neuropathy symptoms in patients with gluten sensitivity and sensorimotor axonal peripheral neuropathy.[282] Based on this study, it has been suggested that all patients with idiopathic axonal neuropathy be screened for gluten sensitivity by assaying for antigliadin antibodies and that those with such antibodies be offered a gluten-free diet even in the absence of enteropathy. At the level of class IV evidence, the published literature provides conflicting results. Some case reports and small series have found that the ataxia and peripheral neuropathy may improve with a gluten-free diet, but some patients worsen despite such treatment.[279–281,283–285] Based on the presumed immunologic basis of gluten sensitivity and on success in treating gluten ataxia,[286,287] IVIg was used for treatment of the neuropathy. Specifically, three patients with biopsy-proven celiac disease are described who developed cerebellar ataxia and neuropathic pain despite a gluten-free diet. Two had small-fiber neuropathy by skin biopsy. IVIg improved the

ataxia and the neuropathy symptoms, which then recurred with discontinuation of the IVIg and improved with its resumption.[277] Based on this sparse literature, it is certainly reasonable to consider a gluten-free diet in patients with gluten neuropathy. If the neuropathy is severe, IVIg may be considered.

Paraneoplastic Sensory Neuronopathy

Paraneoplastic neurologic disorders occur in patients with cancer but are not due to the direct effects of metastases or direct invasion of neural structures. The most common syndromes are cerebellar degeneration, limbic encephalitis, sensory neuronopathy, and encephalomyelitis. The syndrome of paraneoplastic subacute sensory neuronopathy and encephalomyelitis (SSN) has also been called the *anti-Hu syndrome*. Most patients have an underlying small cell lung cancer, but large series have documented a variety of other underlying malignancies.[288,289] No cancer is found in some patients, even at autopsy.[288,289] Despite the presence of anti-Hu antibodies as useful markers, these antibodies are not thought to be the cause of the paraneoplastic syndrome. They are probably part of an immune response against Hu antigens to control tumor growth, with the immunologic response ultimately being misdirected against components of the nervous system. The pathogenic mechanism for SSN appears to be primarily a T-cell process involving cell-mediated immunity.[290,291]

Diagnosis and Evaluation

The neurologic symptoms may precede or follow the identification of the malignancy. Sensory symptoms predominate, but encephalitis, cerebellar dysfunction, motor weakness, brain stem dysfunction, and autonomic symptoms may be present. The clinical features usually develop subacutely over several weeks but may be explosive over days or even hours. The course is relentlessly progressive in most patients, although it may stabilize with fixed neurologic deficits in some.[288,289] Anti-Hu antibodies are found in the blood with a specificity of 99% and a sensitivity of 82%.[292] The antibodies are also present in CSF, which otherwise may be normal or may demonstrate a mildly to moderately elevated protein level (<300 mg/dL in most) or a mild pleocytosis.[287,292] Electrodiagnostic testing demonstrates low-amplitude or absent sensory responses. However, although the syndrome has been characterized as a sensory neuronopathy, motor nerve studies are often abnormal, demonstrating low-amplitude CMAPs, with minor slowing of conduction velocities and mild prolongation of distal latencies.[293,294] Sural nerve biopsies demonstrate axonal loss and may show epineurial, endoneurial, or perivascular inflammatory infiltrates.[288,293] Pathologic studies of dorsal root ganglia demonstrate mononuclear cell infiltrates surrounding sensory neurons undergoing degeneration.[295] Patients with anti-Hu antibodies and no identifiable malignancy develop clinical symptoms identical to those in patients with such antibodies and malignancies.[296]

Treatment and Management

No controlled studies of treatment of SSN have been conducted. Treatment of the underlying malignancy appears to be of paramount importance and was an independent predictor of at least stabilization of the paraneoplastic syndrome in one large retrospective series.[289] The utility of immunotherapy is less clear. One series of 17 patients who were treated aggressively with IVIg, cyclophosphamide, and methylprednisolone found that most did not respond, although 3 who were not yet severely disabled stabilized.[297] In a series of 22 patients with paraneoplastic disorders, most of whom had SSN, treatment with IVIg resulted in improvement in only 1 with SSN, whereas 8 patients with SSN, most of whom had stabilized before treatment, remained stable, and 8 deteriorated despite treatment.[298] Based on these studies, early initiation of treatment may be more effective. Careful lifelong follow-up for malignancy should be part of the care of those patients in whom a malignancy is not identified as part of the initial evaluation. In some, the malignancy is so small as to remain undetected for years; in others no malignancy is ever identified, and it is believed that the immune response may eliminate the underlying cancer.[299]

Outcome

Prognosis is poor for most patients. Median survival in one large series was 11.8 months, but with a wide range of 0.7 to 121.4 months. The probability of survival to 12, 36, and 60 months was 47%, 20%, and 12%, respectively.[289] In another series, the 3-month, 1-year, and 3-year survival rates were 64%, 40%, and 22%, respectively.[300]

References

1. Winer JB, Hughes RAC, Anderson MJ, et al: A prospective study of acute idiopathic neuropathy. I. Antecedent events, *J Neurol Neurosurg Psychiatry* 51:613–618, 1988.
2. Guillain-Barré Syndrome Study Group : Guillain-Barré syndrome: an Italian multicentre case-control study, *Neurol Sci* 21:229–234, 2000.
3. Souayah N, Nasar A, Fareed M, et al: Guillain-Barré syndrome after vaccination in United States: a report from the CDC/FDA Vaccine Adverse Event Reporting System, *Vaccine* 25:5253–5255, 2007.
4. Ropper AH, Wijdicks EFM, Truax BT: *Guillain-Barré Syndrome*, Philadelphia, 1991, FA Davis.
5. Asbury AK, Arnason BG, Karp HR, et al: Criteria for diagnosis of Guillain-Barré syndrome, *Ann Neurol* 3:565–566, 1978.
6. Asbury AK: Diagnostic considerations in Guillain-Barré syndrome, *Ann Neurol* 9(Suppl):1–6, 1981.
7. Asbury AK, Cornblath DR: Assessment of current diagnostic criteria for Guillain-Barré syndrome, *Ann Neurol* 27(Suppl):S21–S24, 1990.
8. Thomashefsky AF, Horowitz SF, Feingold MH: Acute autonomic neuropathy, *Neurology* 22:251–255, 1972.
9. Young RR, Asbury AK, Corbett JL, et al: Pure pan-dysautonomia with recovery: discussion and description of diagnostic criteria, *Brain* 98:613–636, 1975.
10. Ropper AH: Unusual clinical variants and signs in Guillain-Barré syndrome, *Arch Neurol* 43:1150–1152, 1986.
11. Sterman AB, Shaumburg HH, Asbury AK: The acute sensory neuronopathy syndrome: a distinct clinical entity, *Ann Neurol* 7:354–358, 1986.
12. Dawson DM, Samuels MA, Morris J: Sensory form of acute polyneuritis, *Neurology* 38:1728–1731, 1988.
13. Chiba A, Kusunoki S, Obata H, et al: Serum anti-GQ1b antibody is associated with ophthalmoplegia in Miller-Fisher syndrome and Guillain-Barré syndrome: clinical and immunohistochemical studies, *Neurology* 43:1911–1917, 1993.
14. Willison HJ, Veitch J, Patterson G, et al: Miller-Fisher syndrome is associated with serum antibodies to GQ1b ganglioside, *J Neurol Neurosurg Psychiatry* 56:204–206, 1993.
15. Yuki N, Sato S, Tsuji S, et al: Frequent presentation of anti-GQ1b antibody in Miller-Fisher's syndrome, *Neurology* 43:414–417, 1993.
16. Hadden RDM, Cornblath DR, Hughes RAC, et al: Electrophysiological classification of Guillain-Barré syndrome: clinical associations and outcome, *Ann Neurol* 44:780–788, 1998.
17. Albers JW, Donofrio PD, McGonagle TK: Sequential electrodiagnostic abnormalities in acute inflammatory demyelinating polyradiculoneuropathy, *Muscle Nerve* 6:504–509, 1985.
18. Albers JW, Kelly JJ: Acquired inflammatory demyelinating polyneuropathies: clinical and electrodiagnostic features, *Muscle Nerve* 12: 435–451, 1989.
19. Fross RD, Daube JR: Neuropathy in the Miller Fisher syndrome: clinical and electrophysiologic findings, *Neurology* 37:1493–1498, 1987.
20. Dumitru D, Amato AA, Zwarts MJ: *Electrodiagnostic Medicine*, 2nd ed, Philadelphia, 2002, Hanley & Belfus.
21. McKhann GM, Cornblath DR, Ho TW, et al: Clinical and electrophysiological aspects of acute paralytic disease of children and young adults in northern China, *Lancet* 338:593–597, 1991.
22. McKhann GM, Cornblath DR, Griffin JW, et al: Acute motor axonal neuropathy: a frequent cause of acute flaccid paralysis in China, *Ann Neurol* 33:333–342, 1993.
23. Ogawara K, Kuwabara S, Koga M, et al: Anti-GM1b IgG antibody is associated with acute motor axonal neuropathy and *Campylobacter jejuni* infection, *J Neurol Sci* 210:41–45, 2003.
24. Tamura N, Kuwabara S, Misawa S, et al: Time course of axonal regeneration in acute motor axonal neuropathy, *Muscle Nerve* 35:793–795, 2007.
25. Lopez PH, Zhang G, Bianchet MA, et al: Structural requirements of anti-GD1a antibodies determine their target specificity, *Brain* 131:1926–1939, 2008.
26. Ho TW, Mishu B, Li CY, et al: Guillain-Barré syndrome in northern China: relationship to *Campylobacter jejuni* infection and anti-glycolipid antibodies, *Brain* 118:597–605, 1995.
27. Visser LH, Schmitz PIM, Meulstee J, et al: Prognostic factors of Guillain-Barré syndrome after intravenous immunoglobulin or plasma exchange, *Neurology* 53:598–604, 1999.
28. Yuki N, Kuwabara S: Axonal Guillain-Barré syndrome: carbohydrate mimicry and pathophysiology, *J Peripher Nerv Syst* 12:238–249, 2007.
29. Feasby TE, Hahn AF, Brown WF, et al: Severe axonal degeneration in acute Guillain-Barré syndrome: evidence of two different mechanisms? *J Neurol Sci* 116:185–192, 1993.
30. Griffin JW, Li CY, Ho TW, et al: Pathology of the motor-sensory axonal Guillain-Barré syndrome, *Ann Neurol* 39:17–28, 1996.
31. Hughes RAC, Wijdicks EFM, Benson E, et al: Supportive care for Guillain-Barré syndrome, *Arch Neurol* 62:1194–1198, 2005.
32. Pontoppidan H, Geffin B, Lowenstein E: Acute respiratory failure in the adult, 2, *N Engl J Med* 287:743–752, 1972.
33. McKhann GM, Griffin JW, Cornblath DR, et al: Plasmapheresis and Guillain-Barré syndrome: analysis of prognostic factors and the effect of plasmapheresis, *Ann Neurol* 23:347–353, 1988.
34. Sunderrajan EV, Davenport J: The Guillain-Barré syndrome: pulmonary-neurologic correlations, *Medicine* 64:333–341, 1995.
35. Moulin DE, Hagen N, Feasby TE, et al: Pain in Guillain-Barré syndrome, *Neurology* 48:328–331, 1997.
36. Tripathi M, Kaushik S: Carbamazepine for pain management in Guillain-Barré syndrome patients in the intensive care unit, *Crit Care Med* 28:655–658, 2000.
37. Pandey CK, Bose N, Garg G, et al: Gabapentin for the treatment of pain in Guillain-Barré syndrome: a double-blinded, placebo-controlled, crossover study, *Anesth Analg* 95:1719–1723, 2002.
38. Guillain-Barré Syndrome Study Group : Plasmapheresis and acute Guillain-Barré syndrome, *Neurology* 35:1096–1104, 1985.
39. French Cooperative Group on PE in Guillain-Barré Syndrome : Efficiency of PE in Guillain-Barré syndrome: role of replacement fluids, *Ann Neurol* 22:753–761, 1987.
40. French Cooperative Group on PE in Guillain-Barré Syndrome : Appropriate number of PEs in Guillain-Barré syndrome, *Ann Neurol* 41:298–306, 1997.
41. Van der Meché FG, Schmitz PI, Dutch Guillain-Barré Study Group: A randomized trial comparing intravenous immune globulin and plasma exchange in Guillain-Barré syndrome, *N Engl J Med* 326:1123–1129, 1992.
42. Bril V, Ilse WK, Pearce R, et al: Pilot trial of immunoglobulin versus PE in patients with Guillain-Barré syndrome, *Neurology* 46:100–103, 1996.

43. Raphael J-C, Chevret S, Harboun M, et al: French Guillain-Barré Syndrome Cooperative Group: Intravenous immunoglobulins in patients with Guillain-Barré syndrome and contraindications to PE: 3 days versus 6 days, J Neurol Neurosurg Psychiatry 71:235–238, 2001.

44. Plasma Exchange/Sandoglobulin Guillain-Barré Syndrome Trial Group: Randomised trial of plasma exchange, intravenous immuoglobulin, and combined treatments in Guillain-Barré syndrome, Lancet 349:225–230, 1997.

45. Hughes RAC, Swan AV, Raphael JC, et al: Immunotherapy for Guillain-Barré syndrome: a systematic review, Brain 130:2245–2257, 2007.

46. Alshekhlee A, Hussain Z, Sultan B, et al: Guillain-Barré syndrome: incidence and mortality rates in US hospitals, Neurology 70:1608–1613, 2008.

47. Chiò A, Cocito D, Leone M, et al: Guillain-Barré syndrome: a prospective, population-based incidence and outcome survey, Neurology 60:1146–1150, 2003.

48. Dhar R, Stitt L, Hahn AF: The morbidity and outcome of patients with Guillain-Barré syndrome admitted to the intensive care unit, J Neurol Sci 264:121–128, 2008.

49. Merkies IS, Schmitz PI, Samijn JP, et al: European Inflammatory Neuropathy Cause and Treatment (INCAT) Group: Fatigue in immune-mediated polyneuropathies, Neurology 53:1648–1654, 1999.

50. Garssen MP, Bussmann JB, Schmitz PI, et al: Physical training and fatigue, fitness, and quality of life in Guillain-Barré syndrome and CIDP, Neurology 63:2393–2395, 2004.

51. Ad hoc subcommittee of the American Academy of Neurology AIDS task force: Criteria for diagnosis of chronic inflammatory demyelinating polyneuropathy (CIDP), Neurology 41:617–618, 1991.

52. Prineas JW, McLeod JG: Chronic relapsing polyneuritis, J Neurol Sci 27:427–458, 1976.

53. McCombe PA, Pollard JD, McLeod JG: Chronic inflammatory demyelinating polyradiculoneuropathy: a clinical and electrophysiological study of 92 cases, Brain 110:1617–1630, 1987.

54. Barohn RJ, Kissel JT, Warmolts JR, et al: Chronic inflammatory demyelinating polyradiculoneuropathy: clinical characteristics, course, and recommendations for diagnostic criteria, Arch Neurol 46:878–884, 1989.

55. Simmons Z, Albers JW, Bromberg MB, et al: Presentation and initial clinical course in patients with chronic inflammatory demyelinating polyradiculoneuropathy: comparison of patients without and with monoclonal gammopathy, Neurology 43:2202–2209, 1993.

56. Gorson KC, Allam G, Ropper AH: Chronic inflammatory demyelinating polyneuropathy: clinical features and response to treatment in 67 consecutive patients with and without a monoclonal gammopathy, Neurology 48:321–328, 1997.

57. Boukhris S, Magy L, Khalil M, et al: Pain as the presenting symptom of chronic inflammatory demyelinating polyradiculoneuropathy (CIDP), J Neurol Sci 254:33–38, 2007.

58. Sakakibara R, Hattori T, Kuwabara S, et al: Micturitional disturbance in patients with chronic inflammatory demyelinating polyneuropathy, Neurology 50:1179–1182, 1998.

59. Dyck PJ, Lais AC, Ohta M, et al: Chronic inflammatory polyradiculoneuropathy, Mayo Clin Proc 50:621–637, 1975.

60. Oh SJ, Joy JL, Kuruoglu R: "Chronic sensory demyelinating neuropathy:" chronic inflammatory demyelinating polyneuropathy presenting as a pure sensory neuropathy, J Neurol Neurosurg Psychiatry 55:677–680, 1992.

61. Simmons Z, Tivakaran S: Acquired demyelinating polyneuropathy presenting as a pure clinical sensory syndrome, Muscle Nerve 19:1174–1176, 1996.

62. Antoine JC, Mosnier JF, Lapras J, et al: Chronic inflammatory demyelinating polyneuropathy associated with carcinoma, J Neurol Neurosurg Psychiatry 60:188–190, 1996.

63. Bird SJ, Brown MJ, Shy ME, et al: Chronic inflammatory demyelinating polyneuropathy associated with malignant melanoma, Neurology 46:822–824, 1996.

64. Sugai F, Abe K, Fujimoto T, et al: Chronic inflammatory demyelinating polyneuropathy accompanied by hepatocellular carcinoma, Intern Med 36:53–55, 1997.

65. Abe K, Sugai F: Chronic inflammatory demyelinating polyneuropathy accompanied by carcinoma, J Neurol Neurosurg Psychiatry 65:403–404, 1998.

66. Greenspan BN, Felice KJ: Chronic inflammatory demyelinating polyneuropathy (CIDP) associated with seminoma, Eur Neurol 39:57–58, 1998.

67. Falcone M, Scalise A, Minisci C, et al: Spreading of autoimmunity from central to peripheral myelin: two cases of clinical association between multiple sclerosis and chronic inflammatory demyelinating polyneuropathy, Neurol Sci 27:58–62, 2006.

68. Sharma KR, Saadia D, Facca AG, et al: Chronic inflammatory demyelinating polyradiculoneuropathy associated with multiple sclerosis, J Clin Neuromusc Dis 9:385–396, 2008.

69. Krendel DA, Costigan DA, Hopkins LC: Successful treatment of neuropathies in patients with diabetes mellitus, Arch Neurol 52:1053–1061, 1995.

70. Stewart JD, McKelvey R, Durcan L, et al: Chronic inflammatory demyelinating polyneuropathy (CIDP) in diabetics, J Neurol Sci 142:59–64, 1996.

71. Uncini A, De Angelis MV, Di Muzio A, et al: Chronic inflammatory demyelinating polyneuropathy in diabetics: motor conductions are important in the differential diagnosis with diabetic polyneuropathy, Clin Neurophysiol 110:705–711, 1999.

72. Dalakas MC, Engel WK: Chronic relapsing (dysimmune) polyneuropathy: pathogenesis and treatment, Ann Neurol 9(Suppl):134–145, 1981.

73. Van den Bergh PYK, Pieret F: Electrodiagnostic criteria for acute and chronic inflammatory demyelinating polyradiculoneuropathy, Muscle Nerve 29:565–574, 2004.

74. Bromberg MB: Comparison of electrodiagnostic criteria for primary demyelination in chronic polyneuropathy, Muscle Nerve 14:968–976, 1991.

75. Lewis RA, Sumner AJ: The electrodiagnostic distinctions between chronic familial and acquired demyelinative neuropathies, Neurology 32:592–596, 1982.

76. De Silva RN, Willison HJ, Doyle D, et al: Nerve root hypertrophy in chronic inflammatory demyelinating polyneuropathy, Muscle Nerve 17:168–170, 1994.

77. Goldstein JM, Parks BJ, Mayer PL, et al: Nerve root hypertrophy as the cause of lumbar stenosis in chronic inflammatory demyelinating polyradiculoneuropathy, Muscle Nerve 19:892–896, 1996.

78. Schady W, Goulding PJ, Lecky BRF, et al: Massive nerve root enlargement in chronic inflammatory demyelinating polyneuropathy, J Neurol Neurosurg Psychiatry 61:636–640, 1996.

79. Mizuno K, Nagamatsu M, Hattori N, et al: Chronic inflammatory demyelinating polyradiculoneuropathy with diffuse and massive peripheral nerve hypertrophy: distinctive clinical and magnetic resonance imaging features, Muscle Nerve 21:805–808, 1998.

80. Austin JH: Recurrent polyneuropathies and their corticosteroid treatment, Brain 81:157–192, 1958.

81. Thomas PK, Lascelles RG, Hallpike JF, et al: Recurrent and chronic relapsing Guillain-Barré polyneuritis, Brain 92:589–606, 1969.

82. DeVivo DC, Engel WK: Remarkable recovery of a steroid-responsive recurrent polyneuropathy, J Neurol Neurosurg Psychiatry 33:62–69, 1970.

83. Matthews WB, Howell DA, Hughes RC: Relapsing corticosteroid-dependent polyneuritis, J Neurol Neurosurg Psychiatry 33:330–337, 1970.

84. Dyck PJ, O'Brien PC, Oviatt KF, et al: Prednisone improves chronic inflammatory demyelinating polyradiculoneuropathy more than no treatment, Ann Neurol 11:136–144, 1982.

85. Mehndiratta MM, Hughes RAC: Corticosteroids for chronic inflammatory demyelinating polyradiculoneuropathy, Cochrane Database Syst Rev CD002062, 2002.

86. Brannagan TH: Current treatments of chronic immune-mediated demyelinating polyneuropathies, Muscle Nerve 39:563–578, 2009.

87. Lopate G, Pestronk A, Al-Lozi M: Treatment of chronic inflammatory demyelinating polyneuropathy with high-dose intermittent intravenous methylprednisolone, Arch Neurol 62:249–254, 2005.

88. Muley SA, Kelkar P, Parry GJ: Treatment of chronic inflammatory demyelinating polyneuropathy with pulsed oral steroids, Arch Neurol 65:1460–1464, 2008.

89. Dyck PJ, Daube J, O'Brien P, et al: PE in chronic inflammating polyradiculoneuropathy, *N Engl J Med* 314:461–465, 1986.

90. Hahn AF, Bolton CF, Pillay N, et al: Plasma-exchange therapy in chronic inflammatory demyelinating polyneuropathy: a double-blind, sham-controlled, cross-over study, *Brain* 119:1055–1066, 1996.

91. Mehndiratta MM, Hughes RAC, Agarwal P: PE for chronic inflammatory demyelinating polyradiculoneuropathy, *Cochrane Database Syst Rev* CD003906, 2004.

92. Donofrio PD, Tandan R, Albers JW: PE in chronic inflammatory demyelinating polyradiculoneuropathy, *Muscle Nerve* 8:321–327, 1985.

93. Eftimov F, Winer JB, Vermeulen M, et al: Intravenous immunoglobulin for chronic inflammatory demyelinating polyradiculoneuropathy, *Cochrane Database Syst Rev* CD001797, 2009.

94. Van Doorn PA, Brand A, Strengers PFW, et al: High-dose intravenous immunoglobulin treatment in chronic inflammatory demyelinating polyneuropathy: a double-blind, placebo-controlled, crossover study, *Neurology* 40:209–212, 1990.

95. Van Doorn PA, Vermeulen M, Brand A, et al: Intravenous immunoglobulin treatment in patients with chronic inflammatory demyelinating polyneuropathy, *Arch Neurol* 48:217–220, 1991.

96. Hahn AF, Bolton CF, Zochodne D, et al: Intravenous immunoglobulin treatment in chronic inflammatory demyelinating polyneuropathy: a double-blind, placebo-controlled, cross-over study, *Brain* 119:1067–1077, 1996.

97. Choudhary PP, Hughes RAC: Long-term treatment of chronic inflammatory demyelinating polyradiculoneuropathy with PE or intravenous immunoglobulin, *Q J Med* 88:493–502, 1995.

98. Hughes RA, Donofrio P, Bril V, et al: Intravenous immunoglobulin (10% caprylatechromatography purified) for the treatment of chronic inflammatory demyelinating polyradiculoneuropathy (ICE Study): a randomized placebo-controlled trial, *Lancet Neurol* 7:136–144, 2008.

99. Dyck PJ, Litchy WJ, Kratz KM, et al: A PE versus immunoglobulin infusion trial in chronic inflammatory demyelinating polyradiculoneuropathy, *Ann Neurol* 36:838–845, 1994.

100. Rajabally YA, Seow H, Wilson P: Dose of intravenous immunoglobulins in chronic inflammatory demyelinating polyneuropathy, *J Periph Nerv Syst* 11:325–329, 2006.

101. Jann S, Bramerio MA, Facchetti D, et al: Intravenous immunoglobulin is effective in patients with diabetes and with chronic inflammatory demyelinating polyneuropathy: long term follow-up, *J Neurol Neurosurg Psychiatry* 80:70–73, 2009.

102. Hughes RAC, Swan AV, van Doorn PA: Cytotoxic drugs and interferons for chronic inflammatory demyelinating polyradiculoneuropathy, *Cochrane Database Syst Rev* CD003280, 2004.

103. Good JL, Chehrenama M, Mayer RF, et al: Pulse cyclophosphamide therapy in chronic inflammatory demyelinating polyradiculoneuropathy, *Neurology* 51:1735–1738, 1998.

104. Brannagan TH, Pradhan A, Heiman-Patterson T, et al: High-dose cyclophosphamide without stem-cell rescue for refractory CIDP, *Neurology* 58:1856–1858, 2002.

105. Gladstone DE, Prestrud AA, Brannagan TH: High-dose cyclophosphamide results in long-term disease remission with restoration of a normal quality of life in patients with severe refractory chronic inflammatory demyelinating polyneuropathy, *J Periph Nerv Syst* 10:11–16, 2005.

106. Bodley-Scott DD: Chronic inflammatory demyelinating polyradiculoneuropathy responding to rituximab, *Pract Neurol* 5:242–245, 2005.

107. Benedetti L, Franciotta D, Beronio A, et al: Rituximab efficacy in CIDP associated with idiopathic thrombocytopenic purpura, *Muscle Nerve* 38:1076–1077, 2008.

108. Gorson KC, Natarajan N, Ropper AH, et al: Rituximab treatment in patients with IVIg-dependent immune polyneuropathy: a prospective pilot trial, *Muscle Nerve* 35:66–69, 2007.

109. Matsuda M, Hoshi K, Gono T, et al: Cyclosporin A in treatment of refractory patients with chronic inflammatory demyelinating polyradiculoneuropathy, *J Neurol Sci* 224:29–35, 2004.

110. Sabatelli M, Mignogna T, Lippi G, et al: Interferon-alpha may benefit steroid unresponsive chronic inflammatory demyelinating polyneuropathy, *J Neurol Neurosurg Psychiatry* 58:638–639, 1995.

111. Gorson KC, Allam G, Simovic D, et al: Improvement following interferon-alpha 2a in chronic inflammatory demyelinating polyneuropathy, *Neurology* 48:777–780, 1997.

112. Gorson KC, Ropper AH, Clark BD, et al: Treatment of chronic inflammatory demyelinating polyneuropathy with interferon-alpha 2a, *Neurology* 50:84–87, 1998.

113. Kuntzer T, Radziwill AJ, Lettry-Trouillat R, et al: Interferon-T1a in chronic inflammatorydemyelinating polyneuropathy, *Neurology* 53:1364–1365, 1999.

114. Vallat JM, Hahn AF, Léger JM, et al: Interferon beta-1a as an investigational treatment for CIDP, *Neurology* 60:S23–S28, 2003.

115. Umapathi T, Hughes R: Mycophenolate in treatment-resistant inflammatory neuropathies, *Eur J Neurol* 9:683–685, 2002.

116. Gorson KC, Amato AA, Ropper AH: Efficacy of mycophenolate mofetil in patients with chronic immune demyelinating polyneuropathy, *Neurology* 63:715–717, 2004.

117. Benedetti L, Grandis M, Nobbio L: Mycophenylate mofetil in dysimmune neuropathies: a preliminary study, *Muscle Nerve* 29:748–749, 2004.

118. Radziwill AJ, Schweikert K, Kuntzer T, et al: Mycophenolate mofetil for chronic inflammatory demyelinating polyradiculoneuropathy: an open-label study, *Eur Neurol* 56:37–38, 2006.

119. Fialho D, Chan YC, Allen DC, et al: Treatment of chronic inflammatory demyelinating polyradiculoneuropathy with methotrexate, *J Neurol Neurosurg Psychiatry* 77:544–547, 2006.

120. Hirst C, Raasch S, LLewelyn G, et al: Remission of chronic inflammatory demyelinating polyneuropathy after alemtuzumab (Campath 1H), *J Neurol Neurosurg Psychiatry* 77:800–802, 2006.

121. Chin RL, Sherman WH, Sander HW, et al: Etanercept (EnbrelR) therapy for chronic inflammatory demyelinating polyneuropathy, *J Neurol Sci* 210:19–21, 2003.

122. Ahlmen J, Andersen O, Hallgren G, et al: Positive effects of tacrolimus in a case of CIDP, *Transplant Proc* 30:4194, 1998.

123. Vermeulen M, Van Oers MH: Successful autologous stem cell transplantation in a patient with chronic inflammatory demyelinating polyneuropathy, *J Neurol Neurosurg Psychiatry* 72:127–128, 2002.

124. Oyama Y, Sufit R, Loh Y, et al: Nonmyeloablative autologous hematopoietic stem cell transplantation for refractory CIDP, *Neurology* 69:1802–1803, 2007.

125. Axelson HW, Oberg G, Askmark H: Successful repeated treatment with high dose cyclophosphamide and autologous blood stem cell transplantation in CIDP, *J Neurol Neurosurg Psychiatry* 79:612–614, 2008.

126. Simmons Z, Albers JW, Bromberg MB, et al: Long-term follow-up of patients with chronic inflammatory demyelinating polyradiculoneuropathy, without and with monoclonal gammopathy, *Brain* 118:359–368, 1995.

127. Harvey GK, Pollard JD, Schindhelm K, et al: Chronic experimental allergic neuritis: an electrophysiological and histological study in the rabbit, *J Neurol Sci* 81:215–225, 1987.

128. Bouchard C, Lacroix C, Planté V, et al: Clinicopathologic findings and prognosis of chronic inflammatory demyelinating polyneuropathy, *Neurology* 52:498–503, 1999.

129. Parry GJ, Clarke S: Multifocal acquired demyelinating neuropathy masquerading as motor neuron disease, *Muscle Nerve* 11:103–107, 1988.

130. Pestronk A, Cornblath DR, Ilyas AA, et al: A treatable multifocal neuropathy with antibodies to GM$_1$ ganglioside, *Ann Neurol* 24:73–78, 1988.

131. Taylor BV, Willison HJ: Multifocal motor neuropathy and conduction block. In Dyck PJ, Thomas PK, editors: *Peripheral Neuropathy*, 4th ed, Philadelphia, 2005, Saunders, pp 2277–2298.

132. Pakiam A, Parry G: Multifocal motor neuropathy without overt conduction block, *Muscle Nerve* 21:243–245, 1998.

133. Nobile-Orazio E, Cappellari A, Meucci N, et al: Multifocal motor neuropathy: clinical and immunological features and response to IVIg in relation to the presence and degree of motor conduction block, *J Neurol Neurosurg Psychiatry* 72:761–766, 2002.

134. Delmont E, Azulay JP, Giorgi R, et al: Multifocal motor neuropathy with and without conduction block: a single entity? *Neurology* 67:592–596, 2006.

135. Slee M, Selvan A, Donaghy M: Multifocal motor neuropathy: the diagnostic spectrum and response to treatment, *Neurology* 69:1680–1687, 2007.

136. Federico P, Zochodne DW, Hahn AF, et al: Multifocal motor neuropathy improved by IVIg. Randomized double-blind, placebo-controlled study, *Neurology* 55:1256–1262, 2000.

137. Leger JM, Chassande B, Musset L, et al: Intravenous immunoglobulin therapy in multifocal motor neuropathy: a double-blind, placebo-controlled study, *Brain* 124:145–153, 2001.

138. Azulay JP, Blin O, Pouget J, et al: Intravenous immunoglobulin treatment in patients with motor neuron syndromes associated with anti-GM₁ antibodies: a double-blind, placebo-controlled study, *Neurology* 44: 429–432, 1994.

139. Van den Berg LH, Kerkhoff H, Oey PL, et al: Treatment of multifocal motor neuropathy with high dose intravenous immunoglobins: a double-blind, placebo controlled study, *J Neurol Neurosurg Psychiatry* 59:248–252, 1995.

140. Pestronk A, Lopate G, Kornberg AJ, et al: Distal lower motor neuron syndrome with high-titer serum IgM anti-GM1 antibodies: improvement following immunotherapy with monthly PE and intravenous cyclophosphamide, *Neurology* 44:2027–2031, 1994.

141. Brannagan TH, Alaedini A, Gladstone DE: High-dose cyclophosphamide without stem cell rescue for refractory multifocal motor neuropathy, *Muscle Nerve* 34:246–250, 2006.

142. Axelson HW, Oberg G, Askmark H: No benefit of treatment with cyclophosphamide and autologous blood stem cell transplantation in multifocal motor neuropathy, *Acta Neurol Scand* 117:432–434, 2008.

143. Pestronk A, Florence J, Miller T, et al: Treatment of IgM antibody associated polyneuropathies using rituximab, *J Neurol Neurosurg Psychiatry* 74:485–489, 2003.

144. Piepers S, Van den Berg-Vos R, Van der Pol WL, et al: Mycophenolate mofetil as adjunctive therapy for MMN patients: a randomized, controlled trial, *Brain* 130:2004–2010, 2007.

145. Donaghy M, Mills KR, Boniface SJ, et al: Pure motor demyelinating neuropathy—deterioration after steroid treatment and improvement with intravenous immunoglobulin, *J Neurol Neurosurg Psychiatry* 57:778–783, 1994.

146. Lang DJ, Weimer LH, Trojaborg W, et al: Multifocal motor neuropathy with conduction block: slow but not benign, *Arch Neurol* 63:1778–1781, 2006.

147. Leger JM, Viala K, Cancalon F, et al: Intravenous immunoglobulin as short- and long-term therapy of multifocal motor neuropathy: a retrospective study of response to IVIg and of its predictive criteria in 40 patients, *J Neurol Neurosurg Psychiatry* 79:93–96, 2008.

148. Taylor BV, Wright RA, Harper CM, et al: Natural history of 46 patients with multifocal motor neuropathy with conduction block, *Muscle Nerve* 23:900–908, 2000.

149. Lewis RA, Sumner AJ, Brown MJ, et al: Multifocal demyelinating neuropathy with persistent conduction block, *Neurology* 32:958–964, 1982.

150. Gibbels E, Behse F, Kentenich M, et al: Chronic multifocal neuropathy with persistent conduction block (Lewis-Sumner syndrome), *Clin Neuropathol* 12:343–352, 1993.

151. Oh SJ, Claussen GC, Kim DS: Motor and sensory demyelinating mononeuropathy multiplex (multifocal motor and sensory demyelinating neuropathy): a separate entity or a variant of chronic inflammatory demyelinating polyneuropathy? *J Peripher Nerv Syst* 2:362–369, 1997.

152. Saperstein DS, Amato AA, Wolfe GI, et al: Multifocal acquired demyelinating sensory and motor neuropathy: the Lewis-Sumner syndrome, *Muscle Nerve* 22:560–566, 1999.

153. Van den Berg-Vos RM, Van den Berg LH, Franssen H, et al: Multifocal inflammatory demyelinating neuropathy: a distinct clinical entity? *Neurology* 54:26–32, 2000.

154. Viala K, Renie L, Maisonobe T, et al: Follow-up study and response to treatment in 23 patients with Lewis-Sumner syndrome, *Brain* 127:2010–2017, 2004.

155. Lewis RA: Neuropathies associated with conduction block, *Curr Opin Neurol* 20:525–530, 2007.

156. Gorson KC, Ropper AH, Weinberg DH: Upper limb predominant, multifocal chronic inflammatory demyelinating polyneuropathy, *Muscle Nerve* 22:758–765, 1999.

157. Kyle RA, Rajkumar SV: Monoclonal gammopathies of undetermined significance, *Best Pract Res Clin Haematol* 18:689–707, 2005.

158. Notermans NC, Franssen H, Eurelings M, et al: Diagnostic criteria for demyelinating polyneuropathy associated with monoclonal gammopathy, *Muscle Nerve* 23:73–79, 2000.

159. Gosselin S, Kyle RA, Dyck PJ: Neuropathy associated with monoclonal gammopathies of undetermined significance, *Ann Neurol* 30:54–61, 1991.

160. Suarez GA, Kelly JJ Jr: Polyneuropathy associated with monoclonal gammopathy of undetermined significance: further evidence that IgM-MGUS neuropathies are different than IgG-MGUS, *Neurology* 43: 1304–1308, 1993.

161. Notermans NC, Wokke JHJ, Lokhorst HM, et al: Polyneuropathy associated with monoclonal gammopathy of undetermined significance: a prospective study of the prognostic value of clinical and laboratory abnormalities, *Brain* 117:1385–1393, 1994.

162. Kelly JJ: The electrodiagnostic findings in peripheral neuropathy associated with monoclonal gammopathy, *Muscle Nerve* 6:504–509, 1983.

163. Melmed C, Frail D, Duncan I, et al: Peripheral neuropathy with IgM kappa monoclonal immunoglobulin directed against myelin-associated glycoprotein, *Neurology* 33:1397–1405, 1983.

164. Hafler DA, Johnson D, Kelly JJ, et al: Monoclonal gammopathy and neuropathy: myelin-associated glycoprotein reactivity and clinical characteristics, *Neurology* 36:75–78, 1986.

165. Nobile-Orazio E, Marmiroli P, Baldini L, et al: Peripheral neuropathy in macroglobulinemia: incidence and antigen-specificity of M proteins, *Neurology* 37:1506–1514, 1987.

166. Kelly JJ, Adelman LS, Berkman E, et al: Polyneuropathies associated with IgM monoclonal gammopathies, *Arch Neurol* 45:1355–1359, 1988.

167. Kaku DA, England JD, Sumner AJ: Distal accentuation of conduction slowing in polyneuropathy associated with antibodies to myelin-associated glycoprotein and sulphated glucuronyl paragloboside, *Brain* 117:941–947, 1994.

168. Nobile-Orazio E, Manfredini E, Carpo M, et al: Frequency and clinical correlates of anti-neural IgM antibodies in neuropathy associated with IgM monoclonal gammopathy, *Ann Neurol* 36:416–424, 1994.

169. Chassande B, Leger JM, Younes-Chennoufi AB, et al: Peripheral neuropathy associated with IgM monoclonal gammopathy: correlations between M-protein antibody activity and clinical/electrophysiological features in 40 cases, *Muscle Nerve* 21:55–62, 1998.

170. Katz JS, Saperstein DS, Gronseth G, et al: Distal acquired demyelinating symmetric neuropathy, *Neurology* 54:615–620, 2000.

171. Cocito D, Isoardo G, Ciaramitaro P, et al: Terminal latency index in polyneuropathy with IgM paraproteinemia and anti-MAG antibody, *Muscle Nerve* 24:1278–1282, 2001.

172. Lunn MPT, Nobile-Orazio E: Immunotherapy for IgM anti-myelin-associated glycoprotein paraprotein-associated peripheral neuropathies, *Cochrane Database Syst Rev* CD002827, 2006.

173. Dalakas MC, Rakocevic G, Salajegheh M, et al: Placebo-controlled trial of rituximab in IgM anti-myelin-associated glycoprotein antibody demyelinating neuropathy, *Ann Neurol* 65:286–293, 2009.

174. Dyck PJ, Low PA, Windebank AJ, et al: PE in polyneuropathy associated with monoclonal gammopathy of undetermined significance, *N Engl J Med* 325:1482–1486, 1991.

175. Sherman WH, Olarte MR, McKiernan G, et al: PE treatment of peripheral neuropathy associated with plasma cell dyscrasia, *J Neurol Neurosurg Psychiatry* 47:813–819, 1984.

176. Blume G, Pestronk A, Goodnough LT: Anti-MAG antibody-associated polyneuropathies: improvement following immunotherapy with monthly PE and IV cyclophosphamide, *Neurology* 45:1577–1580, 1995.

177. Comi G, Roveri L, Swan A, et al: A randomised controlled trial of intravenous immunoglobulin in IgM paraprotein associated demyelinating neuropathy, *J Neurol* 249:1370–1377, 2002.

178. Dalakas MC, Quarles RH, Farrer RG, et al: A controlled study of intravenous immonoglobulin in demyelinating neuropathy with IgM gammopathy, *Ann Neurol* 40:792–795, 1996.

179. Mahattakul W, Crawford TO, Griffin JW, et al: Treatment of chronic inflammatory demyelinating polyneuropathy with cyclosporin-A, *J Neurol Neurosurg Psychiatry* 60:185–187, 1996.

180. Waterston JA, Brown MM, Ingram DA, et al: Cyclosporine A therapy in paraprotein-associated neuropathy, *Muscle Nerve* 15:445–448, 1992.

181. Barnett MH, Pollard JD, Davies L, et al: Cyclosporin A in resistant chronic inflammatory demyelinating polyradiculoneuropathy, *Muscle Nerve* 21:454–460, 1998.

182. Oksenhendler E, Chevret S, Leger JM, et al: PE and chlorambucil in polyneuropathy associated with monoclonal IgM gammopathy, *J Neurol Neurosurg Psychiatry* 59:243–247, 1995.

183. Wilson H, Lunn MPT, Schey S, et al: Successful treatment of IgM paraproteinaemic neuropathy with fludarabine, *J Neurol Neurosurg Psychiatry* 66:575–580, 1999.

184. Briani C, Zara G, Zambello R, et al: Rituximab-responsive CIDP, *Eur J Neurol* 11:788–791, 2004.

185. Renaud S, Gregor M, Fuhr P, et al: Rituximab in the treatment of polyneuropathy associated with anti-MAG antibodies, *Muscle Nerve* 27:611–615, 2003.

186. Renaud S, Fuhr P, Gregor M, et al: High-dose rituximab and anti-MAG associated polyneuropathy, *Neurology* 66:742–744, 2006.

187. Rudnicki SA, Harik SI, Dhodapkar M, et al: Nervous system dysfunction in Waldenström's macroglobulinemia: response to treatment, *Neurology* 51:1210–1213, 1998.

188. Kyle RA, Gertz MA: Systemic amyloidosis, *Crit Rev Oncol Hematol* 10:49–87, 1990.

189. Kyle RA, Greipp PR: Amyloidosis (AL): clinical and laboratory features in 229 cases, *Mayo Clin Proc* 58:665–683, 1983.

190. Simmons Z, Blaivas M, Aguilera AJ, et al: Low diagnostic yield of sural nerve biopsy in patients with peripheral neuropathy and primary amyloidosis, *J Neurol Sci* 120:60–63, 1993.

191. Kyle RA, Greipp PR: Primary systemic amyloidosis: comparison of melphalan and prednisone versus placebo, *Blood* 52:818–827, 1978.

192. Palladini G, Perfetti V, Obici L, et al: Association of melphalan and high-dose dexamethasone is effective and well tolerated in patients with ALS (primary) amyloidosis who are ineligible for stem cell transplantation, *Blood* 103:2936–2938, 2004.

193. Jaccard A, Moreau P, Leblond V, et al: High-dose melphalan versus melphalan plus dexamethasone for AL amyloidosis, *N Engl J Med* 357:1083–1093, 2007.

194. Wechalekar AD, Hawkins PN, Gillmore JD: Perspectives in treatment of AL amyloidosis, *Br J Haematol* 140:365–377, 2007.

195. Kyle RA, Kelly JJ, Dyck PJ: Amyloidosis and neuropathy. In Dyck PJ, Thomas PK, editors: *Peripheral Neuropathy*, 4th ed, Philadelphia, 2005, Saunders, pp 2427–2451.

196. Dispenzieri A, Suarez GA, Kyle RA: POEMS syndrome (osteosclerotic myeloma). In Dyck PJ, Thomas PK, editors: *Peripheral Neuropathy*, 4th ed, Philadelphia, 2005, Saunders, pp 2453–2469.

197. Kelly JJ, Kyle RA, Miles JM, et al: Osteosclerotic myeloma and peripheral neuropathy, *Neurology* 33:202–210, 1983.

198. Sung JY, Kuwabara S, Ogawara K, et al: Patterns of nerve conduction abnormalities in POEMS syndrome, *Muscle Nerve* 26:189–193, 2002.

199. Dispenzieri A, Kyle RA, Lacy MQ, et al: POEMS syndrome: definitions and long-term outcome, *Blood* 101:2496–2506, 2003.

200. Kuwabara S, Misawa S, Kanai K, et al: Neurologic improvement after peripheral blood stem cell transplantation in POEMS syndrome, *Neurology* 71:1691–1695, 2008.

201. Dispenzieri A, Moreno-Aspitia A, Suarez GA, et al: Peripheral blood stem cell transplantation in 16 patients with POEMS syndrome, and a review of the literature, *Blood* 104:3400–3407, 2004.

202. Mathew L, Talbot K, Love S, et al: Treatment of vasculitic peripheral neuropathy: a retrospective analysis of outcome, *Q J Med* 100:41–51, 2007.

203. Collins MP, Kissel JT: Neuropathies with systemic vasculitis. In Dyck PJ, Thomas PK, editors: *Peripheral Neuropathy*, 4th ed, Philadelphia, 2005, Saunders, pp 2335–2404.

204. Dyck PJ, Benstead TJ, Conn DL, et al: Nonsystemic vasculitic neuropathy, *Brain* 110:843–854, 1987.

205. Hawke SHB, Davies L, Pamphlett R, et al: Vasculitic neuropathy, *Brain* 114:2175–2190, 1991.

206. McCluskey L, Feinberg D, Cantor C, et al: "Pseudo-conduction block" in vasculitic neuropathy, *Muscle Nerve* 22:1361–1366, 1999.

207. Briemberg HR, Levin K, Amato AA: Multifocal conduction block in peripheral nerve vasculitis, *J Clin Neuromuscul Dis* 3:153–158, 2002.

208. Amato AA, Dumitru D: Acquired neuropathies. In Dumitru D, Amato AA, Zwarts MJ, editors: *Electrodiagnostic Medicine*, 2nd ed, Philadelphia, 2002, Hanley & Belfus, pp 937–1041.

209. Collins MP, Mendell JR, Periquet MI, et al: Superficial peroneal nerve/peroneus brevis muscle biopsy in vasculitic neuropathy, *Neurology* 55:636–643, 2000.

210. Collins MP, Periquet MI, Mendell JR, et al: Nonsystemic vasculitic neuropathy: insights from a clinical cohort, *Neurology* 61:623–630, 2003.

211. Vital C, Vital A, Canron M-H, et al: Combined nerve and muscle biopsy in the diagnosis of vasculitic neuropathy. A 16-year retrospective study of 202 cases, *J Peripher Nerve Syst* 11:20–29, 2006.

212. Burns TM, Schaublin GA, Dyck PJB: Vasculitic neuropathies, *Neurol Clin* 25:89–113, 2007.

213. Pagnoux C, Mahr A, Hamidou MA, et al: Azathioprine or methotrexate maintenance for ANCA-associated vasculitis, *N Engl J Med* 359:2790–2803, 2008.

214. Vrancken AFJE, Hughes RAC, Said G, et al: Immunosuppressive treatment for nonsystemic vasculitic neuropathy, *Cochrane Database Syst Rev* CD006050, 2007.

215. Kissel JT, Collins MP, Mendell JR: Vasculitic neuropathy. In Mendell JR, Kissel JT, Cornblath DR, editors: *Diagnosis and Management of Peripheral Nerve Disorders*, New York, 2001, Oxford University Press, pp 202–232.

216. Davies L, Spies JM, Pollard JD, et al: Vasculitis confined to peripheral nerves, *Brain* 119:1441–1448, 1996.

217. Griffin JW: Vasculitic neuropathies, *Rheum Dis Clin North Am* 27:751–760, 2001.

218. Apartis E, Leger JM, Musset L, et al: Peripheral neuropathy associated with essential mixed cryoglobulinemia: a role for hepatitis C virus infection? *J Neurol Neurosurg Psychiatry* 60:661–666, 1996.

219. Ciompi ML, Marini D, Siciliano G, et al: Cryoglobulinemic peripheral neuropathy: neurophysiologic evaluation in 22 patients, *Biomed Pharmacother* 50:329–336, 1996.

220. David WS, Peine C, Schlesinger P, et al: Nonsystemic vasculitic mononeuropathy multiplex, cryoglobulinemia, and hepatitis C, *Muscle Nerve* 19:1596–1602, 1996.

221. Steck AJ: Neurological manifestations of malignant and non-malignant dysglobulinaemias, *J Neurol* 245:634–639, 1998.

222. Gemignani F, Pevesi G, Fiocchi A, et al: Peripheral neuropathy in essential mixed cryoglobulinemia, *J Neurol Neurosurg Psychiatry* 55:116–120, 1992.

223. Vermeersch P, Gijbels K, Marien G, et al: A critical appraisal of current practice in the detection, analysis, and reporting of cryoglobulins, *Clin Chem* 54:39–43, 2008.

224. Khella SL, Frost S, Hermann GA, et al: Hepatitis C infection, cryoglobulinemia, and vasculitic neuropathy. Treatment with interferon alfa: case report and literature review, *Neurology* 45:407–411, 1995.

225. Lamprecht P, Gause A, Gross WL: Cryoglobulinaemic vasculitis, *Arthritis Rheum* 42:2507–2516, 1999.

226. Strunk J, Taborski U, Neeck G: Essential cryoglobulinaemic vasculitis with severe peripheral neuropathy and neurogenic muscular atrophy—including remission by cascade filtration, *Z Rheumatol* 61:733–739, 2002.

227. Lamprecht P, Lerin-Lozano C, Merz H, et al: Rituximab induces remission in refractory HCV associated cryoglobulinaemic vasculitis, *Ann Rheum Dis* 62:1230–1233, 2003.

228. Basse G, Ribes D, Kamar N, et al: Rituximab therapy for mixed cryoglobulinemia in seven renal transplant patients, *Transplant Proc* 38:2308–2310, 2006.

229. Braun A, Neumann T, Oelzner P, et al: Cryoglobulinaemia type III with severe neuropathy and immune complex glomerulonephritis: remission after plasmapheresis and rituximab, *Rheumatol Int* 28:503–506, 2008.

230. Harle JR, Disdier P, Pelletier J, et al: Dramatic worsening of hepatitis C virus-related cryoglobulinemia subsequent to treatment with interferon alpha, *JAMA* 274:126, 1995.

231. La Civita L, Zignego AL, Lombardini F, et al: Exacerbation of peripheral neuropathy during alpha-interferon therapy in a patient with mixed cryoglobulinemia and hepatitis B virus infection, *J Rheumatol* 23:1641–1643, 1996.

232. Scelsa SN, Herskovitz S, Reichler B: Treatment of mononeuropathy multiplex in hepatitis C virus and cryoglobulinemia, *Muscle Nerve* 21:1526–1529, 1998.

233. Cacoub P, Saadoum D: Hepatitis C virus infection induced vasculitis, *Clin Rev Allergy Immunol* 35:30–39, 2008.

234. Bennett RM, Bong DM, Spargo BH: Neuropsychiatric problems in mixed connective tissue disease, *Am J Med* 65:955–962, 1978.

235. Mellgren SI, Conn DL, Stevens JC, et al: Peripheral neuropathy in primary Sjögren's syndrome, *Neurology* 39:390–394, 1989.

236. Averbuch-Heller L, Steiner I, Abramsky O: Neurologic manifestations of progressive systemic sclerosis, *Arch Neurol* 49:1292–1295, 1992.

237. Hietaharju A, Jaaskelainen S, Kalimo H, et al: Peripheral neuromuscular manifestations in systemic sclerosis (scleroderma), *Muscle Nerve* 16: 1204–1212, 1993.

238. Brey RL, Holliday SL, Saklad AR, et al: Neuropsychiatric syndromes in lupus, *Neurology* 58:1214–1220, 2002.

239. Kissel JT, Collins MP: Vasculitic neuropathies and neuropathies of connective tissue disorders. In Katirji B, Kaminski HJ, Preston DC, editors: *Neuromuscular Disorders in Clinical Practice*, Boston, 2002, Butterworth-Heinemann, pp 669–702.

240. Griffin JW, Cornblath DR, Alexander E, et al: Ataxic sensory neuropathy and dorsal root ganglionitis associated with Sjögren's syndrome, *Neurology* 27:304–315, 1990.

241. Souayah N, Chong PS, Cros D: Acute sensory neuronopathy as the presenting symptom of Sjögren's syndrome, *J Clin Neurosci* 13:862–865, 2006.

242. Daniels TE, Whitcher JP: Association of patterns of labial salivary gland inflammation with keratoconjunctivitis sicca. Analysis of 618 patients with suspected Sjögren's syndrome, *Arthritis Rheum* 37:869–877, 1994.

243. Lee M, Rutka JA, Slomovic AR, et al: Establishing guidelines for the role of minor salivary gland biopsy in clinical practice for Sjögren's syndrome, *J Rheumatol* 25:247–253, 1998.

244. Malinow K, Yannakakis GD, Glusman SM, et al: Subacute sensory neuronopathy secondary to dorsal root ganglionitis in primary Sjögren's syndrome, *Ann Neurol* 20:535–537, 1986.

245. Chai J, Herrmann DN, Stanton M, et al: Painful small-fiber neuropathy in Sjögren's syndrome, *Neurology* 65:925–927, 2005.

246. Scheinberg L: Polyneuritis in systemic lupus erythematosus: review of the literature and report of a case, *N Engl J Med* 255:416–421, 1956.

247. Goldberg M, Chitanoundh H: Polyneuritis with albuminocytologic dissociation in the spinal fluid in systemic lupus erythematosus: report of a case with review of pertinent literature, *Am J Med* 27:342–350, 1959.

248. Molina JA, Benito-Leon J, Bermejo F, et al: Intravenous immunoglobulin therapy in sensory neuropathy associated with Sjögren's syndrome, *J Neurol Neurosurg Psychiatry* 60:699, 1996.

249. Asahina M, Kuwabara S, Asahina M, et al: D-Penicillamine treatment for chronic sensory ataxic neuropathy associated with Sjögren's syndrome, *Neurology* 51:1451–1453, 1998.

250. Chen WH, Yeh JH, Chiu HC: Plasmapheresis in the treatment of ataxic sensory neuropathy assciated with Sjögren's syndrome, *Eur Neurol* 45:270–274, 2001.

251. Caroyer JM, Manto MU, Steinfeld SD: Severe sensory neuronopathy responsive to infliximab in primary Sjögren's syndrome, *Neurology* 59:1113–1114, 2002.

252. Takahashi Y, Takata T, Hoshino M, et al: Benefit of IVIg for long-standing ataxic sensory neuronopathy with Sjögren's syndrome, *Neurology* 60:503–505, 2003.

253. Bastron J, Thomas J: Diabetic polyradiculopathy: clinical and electromyographic findings in 105 patients, *Mayo Clin Proc* 56:725–732, 1981.

254. Dyck PJB, Norell JE, Dyck PJ: Microvasculitis and ischemia in diabetic lumbosacral radiculoplexus neuropathy, *Neurology* 53:2113–2121, 1999.

255. Dyck PJB, Engelstand J, Norell J, et al: Microvasculitis in non-diabetic lumbosacral radiculoplexus neuropathy (LSRPN): similarity to the diabetic variety (DLSRPN), *J Neuropathol Exp Neurol* 59:525–538, 2000.

256. Dyck PJB, Norell JE, Dyck PJ: Non-diabetic lumbosacral radiculoplexus neuropathy: natural history, outcome and comparison with the diabetic variety, *Brain* 124:1197–1207, 2001.

257. Katz JS, Saperstein DS, Wolfe G, et al: Cervicobrachial involvement in diabetic radiculoplexopathy, *Muscle Nerve* 24:794–798, 2001.

258. Bradley WG, Chad D, Verghese JP: Painful lumbosacral plexopathy with elevated erythrocyte sedimentation rate: a treatable inflammatory syndrome, *Ann Neurol* 15:457–464, 1984.

259. Said G, Goulen-Goeau C, Lacroix C, et al: Nerve biopsy findings in different patterns of proximal diabetic neuropathy, *Ann Neurol* 35:559–569, 1994.

260. Verma A, Bradley WG: High-dose intravenous immunoglobulin therapy in chronic progressive lumbosacral plexopathy, *Neurology* 44:248–250, 1994.

261. Triggs WJ, Young MS, Eskin T, et al: Treatment of idiopathic lumbosacral plexopathy with intravenous immunoglobulin, *Muscle Nerve* 20:244–246, 1997.

262. Ogawa T, Taguchi T, Tanaka Y, et al: Intravenous immunoglobulin therapy for diabetic amyotrophy, *Intern Med* 40:349–352, 2001.

263. Filho JAF, Nathan BM, Palmert MR, et al: Diabetic amyotrophy in an adolescent responsive to intravenous immunoglobulin, *Muscle Nerve* 32:818–820, 2005.

264. Dyck PJB, Norell JE, Dyck PJ: Methylprednisolone may improve lumbosacral radiculoplexus neuropathy, *Can J Neurol Sci* 28:224–227, 2001.

265. Pascoe MK, Low PA, Windebank AJ, et al: Subacute diabetic proximal neuropathy, *Mayo Clin Proc* 72:1123–1132, 1997.

266. Parsonage M, Turner J: Neuralgic amyotrophy: the shoulder-girdle syndrome, *Lancet* 1:973–978, 1948.

267. Suarez GA, Giannini C, Bosch EP, et al: Immune brachial plexus neuropathy: suggestive evidence for an inflammatory-immune pathogenesis, *Neurology* 46:559–561, 1996.

268. Suarez GA: Immune brachial plexus neuropathy. In Dyck PJ, Thomas PK, editors: *Peripheral Neuropathy*, 4th ed, Philadelphia, 2005, Saunders, pp 2299–2307.

269. Tsairis P, Dyck PJ, Mulder D: Natural history of brachial plexus neuropathy, *Arch Neurol* 27:109–117, 1972.

270. Cruz-Martinez A, Barrio M, Arpa J: Neuralgic amyotrophy: variable expression in 40 patients, *J Peripher Nerv Syst* 7:198–204, 2002.

271. Van Alfen N, Van Engelen BGM: The clinical spectrum of neuralgic amyotrophy, *Brain* 129:438–450, 2006.

272. Malamut RI, Marques W, England JD, et al: Postsurgical idiopathic brachial neuritis, *Muscle Nerve* 17:320–324, 1994.

273. Haubenberger D, Rinner W, Auff E, et al: Global respiratory insufficiency due to proximal diabetic neuropathy, *J Neurol* 251:1536–1537, 2004.

274. Nakajima M, Fujioka S, Ohno H, et al: Partial but rapid recovery from paralysis after immunomodulation during early stage of neuralgic amyotrophy, *Eur Neurol* 55:227–229, 2006.

275. Wada Y, Yanagihara C, Nishimura Y, et al: A case of diabetic amyotrophy with severe atrophy and weakness of shoulder girdle muscles showing good response to intravenous immunoglobulin, *Diabetes Res Clin Pract* 75:107–110, 2007.

276. Hadjivassiliou M, Grunewald RA, Kandler RH, et al: Neuropathy associated with gluten sensitivity, *J Neurol Neurosurg Psychiatry* 77: 1262–1266, 2006.

277. Souayah N, Chin RL, Brannagan TH, et al: Effect of intravenous immunoglobulin on cerebellar ataxia and neuropathic pain associated with celiac disease, *Eur J Neurol* 15:1300–1303, 2008.

278. Hadjivassiliou M, Grunewald RA, Davies-Jones GAB: Gluten sensitivity as a neurological illness, *J Neurol Neurosurg Psychiatry* 72:560–563, 2002.

279. Luostarinen L, Himanen SL, Luostarinen M, et al: Neuromuscular and sensory disturbances in patients with well treated coeliac disease, *J Neurol Neurosurg Psychiatry* 74:490–494, 2003.

280. Brannagan TH, Hays AP, Chin SS, et al: Small-fiber neuropathy/neuronopathy associated with celiac disease: skin biopsy findings, *Arch Neurol* 62:1574–1578, 2005.

281. Chin RL, Tseng VG, Green PH, et al: Multifocal axonal polyneuropathy in celiac disease, *Neurology* 66:1923–1925, 2006.

282. Hadjivassiliou M, Kandler RH, Chattopadhyay AK, et al: Dietary treatment of gluten neuropathy, *Muscle Nerve* 34:762–766, 2006.

283. Kaplan JG, Pack D, Horoupian D, et al: Distal axonopathy associated with chronic gluten enteropathy: a treatable disorder, *Neurology* 38:642–645, 1988.

284. Pellecchia MT, Scala R, Perretti A, et al: Cerebellar ataxia associated with subclinical celiac disease responding to gluten-free diet, *Neurology* 53:1606–1608, 1999.

285. Cicarelli G, Della Rocca G, Amboni M, et al: Clinical and neurological abnormalities in adult celiac disease, *Neurol Sci* 24:311–317, 2003.

286. Burk K, Melms A, Schulz JB, et al: Effectiveness of intravenous immunoglobin therapy in cerebellar ataxia associated with gluten sensitivity, *Ann Neurol* 50:827–828, 2001.

287. Sander HW, Magda P, Chin RL, et al: Cerebellar ataxia and coeliac disease, *Lancet* 362:1548, 2003.

288. Dalmau J, Graus F, Rosenblum MK, et al: Anti-Hu associated paraneoplastic encephalomyelitis/sensory neuronopathy: a clinical study of 71 patients, *Medicine* 71:59–72, 1992.

289. Graus F, Keime-Guibert F, Rene R, et al: Anti-Hu associated paraneoplastic encephalomyelitis: analysis of 200 patients, *Brain* 124:1138–1148, 2001.

290. Voltz R, Dalmau J, Posner JB, et al: T-cell receptor analysis in anti-Hu associated paraneoplastic encephalomyelitis, *Neurology* 51:1146–1150, 1998.

291. Pellkofer H, Schubart AS, Hoftberger R, et al: Modelling paraneoplastic CNS disease: T-cells specific for the onconeuronal antigen PNMA1 mediate autoimmune encephalomyelitis in the rat, *Brain* 127:1822–1830, 2004.

292. Molinuevo JL, Graus F, Serrano C, et al: Utility of anti-Hu antibodies in diagnosis of paraneoplastic sensory neuropathy, *Ann Neurol* 44:976–980, 1998.

293. Oh S, Gurtekin Y, Dropcho EJ, et al: Anti-Hu antibody neuropathy: a clinical, electrophysiological, and pathological study, *Clin Neurophysiol* 116:28–34, 2005.

294. Camdessanche JP, Antoine JC, Honnorat J, et al: Paraneoplastic peripheral neuropathy associated with anti-Hu antibodies: a clinical and electrophysiological study of 20 patients, *Brain* 125:166–175, 2002.

295. Kuntzer T, Antoine JC, Steck AJ: Clinical features and pathophysiological basis of sensory neuronopathies (ganglionopathies), *Muscle Nerve* 30:255–268, 2004.

296. Llado A, Carpentier AF, Honnorat J, et al: Hu-antibody-positive patients with or without cancer have similar clinical profiles, *J Neurol Neurosurg Psychiatry* 77:996–997, 2006.

297. Keime-Guibert F, Graus F, Fleury A, et al: Treatment of paraneoplastic neurological syndromes with antineuronal antibodies (anti-Hu, anti-Yo) with a combination of immunoglobulins, cyclophosphamide, and methylprednisolone, *J Neurol Neurosurg Psychiatry* 68:479–482, 2000.

298. Uchuya M, Graus F, Vega F, et al: Intravenous immunoglobulin treatment in paraneoplastic neurological syndromes with antineuronal autoantibodies, *J Neurol Neurosurg Psychiatry* 60:388–392, 1996.

299. Darnell RB, DeAngelis LM: Regression of small-cell lung carcinoma in patients with paraneoplastic neuronal antibodies, *Lancet* 341:21–22, 1993.

300. Smitt PS, Grefkens J, de Leeuw B, et al: Survival and outcome in 73 anti-Hu positive patients with paraneoplastic encephalomyelitis/sensory neuronopathy, *J Neurol* 249:745–753, 2002.

Carlos A. Luciano, MD
Nivia Hernandez-Ramos, MD

15

Treatment and Management of Infectious, Granulomatous, and Toxic Neuromuscular Disorders

The disorders that fall under infectious, granulomatous, and toxic neuromuscular disorders are too numerous and broad to be covered comprehensively in a single chapter. To achieve the objectives of this book we focus on conditions that are seen more frequently and concentrate on the most important and relevant aspects of their management and treatment.

Infections of Nerve and Muscle

HIV Neuropathies and Myopathies

The advancements made in the treatment of human immunodeficiency virus (HIV) infection have resulted in marked changes in the neurologic complications associated with the disease (Boxes 15-1 and 15-2). HIV infection has turned into a chronic illness, with less immunosuppression, resulting in patients living longer but with prolonged exposure to multiple medications. The confluence of these factors has changed the incidence and prevalence of the known HIV-associated neurologic complications.[1-3] Peripheral neuropathies are the most common neurologic complications of HIV infection. The most common pattern of neuropathy is a distal symmetrical sensory neuropathy that can be associated with viral or immune mechanisms (HIV distal sensory polyneuropathy, or HIV-DSP) or with toxicity from antiretroviral agents (antiretroviral toxic neuropathy, or ATN), which can coexist. Other types of neuropathies that can be observed are acute and chronic forms of inflammatory demyelinating polyneuropathies (Guillain-Barré syndrome and chronic inflammatory demyelinating polyneuropathy [CIDP]), multiple mononeuropathies (mononeuritis multiplex), diffuse infiltrative lymphocytosis syndrome (DILS) neuropathy, and progressive polyradiculopathy.[4] The precise underlying mechanisms for these neuropathies are not well understood but include immune dysregulation from infection of macrophages and T cells with abnormal production of inflammatory cytokines and chemokines, neurotoxicity from viral proteins or antiretroviral medications, and, in some cases, infectious opportunistic agents.[5]

Involvement of skeletal muscle can also be observed in HIV-seropositive patients at the onset or more advanced stages of infection and at different stages of immunosuppression, and it can vary in its clinical and pathologic features. Similar to the HIV neuropathies, the HIV-associated myopathies can be associated with toxicity from antiretroviral medications, as is the case with zidovudine (AZT), or from alterations induced by the HIV infection per se. The principal types of nontoxic myopathies have been grouped as variants of HIV-associated myopathy or myositis: HIV polymyositis, which can be associated with the immune reconstitution inflammatory syndrome (IRIS); diffuse infiltrative inflammatory syndrome (DILS)-associated myositis; HIV-associated inclusion body myositis; and HIV-associated nemaline myopathy.[6] They are primarily distinguished by their pathologic features, and it is not clear if they represent a spectrum of the same complication or have different pathophysiologic mechanisms.[7] Other forms of myopathy are the toxic myopathies (AZT myopathy) and HIV-associated rhabdomyolysis. With the advent of highly active antiretroviral therapy (HAART) and better immunocompetence, some of these forms are now seen less frequently.

Diagnosis and Evaluation

As is the case in most neuromuscular diseases, the diagnosis of the various types of neuropathy and myopathies in HIV infection relies on a careful history and physical examination. It is important to have a basic understanding of some pertinent historical aspects of the various types of HIV-associated neuropathies. First, although this may be changing with the use of HAART, different types of neuropathies associated with HIV infection tend to be more prevalent in different stages of the disease.[8] The dysimmune types, demyelinating polyneuropathies and mononeuritis or mononeuritis multiplex, tend to be more prevalent in the early stages of the disease, while the immune system is still robust, and others such as HIV-DSP become more prevalent in the advanced stages of the disease. This implies that it is critical to determine the stage of HIV infection and degree of immunosuppression by measuring and recording the number of CD4+ T cells and the viral load (abundance of viral RNA). A careful assessment of medication exposure is equally important. The HIV myopathies are less common than the neuropathies and the typical HIV myositis can occur at any stage of infection. The demyelinating polyneuropathies, and in particular Guillain-Barré syndrome (GBS), tend to occur at the time of seroconversion or during the early stages of the HIV infection. More recently, since

---

Box 15-1 Classification of Peripheral Nerve Complications in HIV Disease

Early HIV Disease

Seroconversion-related neuropathies
Guillain-Barré syndrome
Mononeuropathies

Moderately Advanced HIV Disease

Chronic inflammatory demyelinating polyneuropathy
Mononeuritis multiplex
Diffuse infiltrative lymphocytosis syndrome
Syphilitic polyradiculopathy
Hepatitis C infection–related neuropathy
Human T-lymphotrophic virus infection type I–related neuropathy
Motor neuron disease syndrome

Advanced HIV Disease

Distal symmetrical sensory polyneuropathy
Autonomic neuropathy
HIV-related lumbosacral polyradiculopathy
Cytomegalovirus infection–related polyradiculopathy
Cytomegalovirus infection mononeuritis multiplex

Medication-Related Neuropathy

Antiretroviral drugs: didanosine, stavudine, and zalcitabine
Other drugs: ethambutol, HMG-CoA reductase inhibitors, isoniazid, paclitaxel (Taxol), thalidomide, vinblastine, and vincristine

HIV, human immunodeficiency virus; HMG-CoA, 3-hydroxy-3-methylglutaryl coenzyme A.
Reprinted with permission from Brew BJ: The peripheral nerve complications of human immunodeficiency virus (HIV) infection, *Muscle Nerve* 28:542–552, 2003.

Box 15-2 HIV-Associated Myopathies

HIV polymyositis
HIV-associated inclusion body myositis
HIV-associated nemaline myopathy
Myopathy and HIV-associated rhabdomyolysis
HIV cachexia

HIV, human immunodeficiency virus.

---

the introduction of HAART, GBS has been seen in association with IRIS.[9,10] The mononeuropathies and mononeuritis multiplex are less common and present more frequently as lesions of the facial nerve, lateral femoral cutaneous nerve of the thigh, median nerve at the wrist, or peroneal nerves. Facial neuropathies, unilateral or bilateral, are probably one of the more common presentations, again sometimes occurring during seroconversion. If the mononeuritis multiplex is present during the early stages of HIV infection, with less immunosuppression, it is associated with dysimmune processes or vasculitis, but if present with advanced immunosuppression it can be associated with cytomegalovirus (CMV).[11]

The most common symptoms with predominantly sensory neuropathies (HIV-DSP/ATN) are symmetrical distal painful dysesthesias, paresthesias, and numbness in the feet and toes that extend proximally as the neuropathy advances. Patients complain of tingling, burning, and aching pain in the toes and soles but any nonspecific discomfort in the feet and toes should trigger the suspicion in the clinician. The distinction between viral-associated and antiretroviral toxic neuropathy is difficult because clinically they are indistinguishable and they may often coexist. Suspicion for ATN should arise if the symptoms start shortly (within weeks) after

starting or increasing the dose of one of the suspect medications and if the symptoms improve or disappear after reducing the dose or discontinuing the suspect medication.[1] On the clinical examination, the most common findings are impaired distal sensation and reduced deep tendon reflexes, more prominently the Achilles tendon reflex. The latter reflex may appear normal but be relatively reduced when compared with the patellar reflex. Although patients may exhibit reduced pinprick sensation, in our experience and that of others,[2] decreased vibratory sensation at the toes is a more sensitive sign. Joint position sense is usually normal and weakness, if present, is limited to the distal foot muscles and is mild. In addition, patients may exhibit allodynia or hyperalgesia in the distal feet.

The clinical presentation of the acute and chronic demyelinating polyneuropathies is not different from the presentations seen in HIV seronegative patients. They are characterized by acute or progressive weakness, with or without prominent sensory symptoms, and reduced or absent reflexes. The mononeuropathies or mononeuritis multiplex cases usually present with a stepwise progression with multiple, often painful, mononeuropathies. The lumbosacral polyradiculopathy, which is usually seen in advanced immunosuppression with low CD4+ T-cell count, presents with lower back and radiating radicular pain, saddle anesthesia, and rapidly progressive weakness in the lower limbs with bladder dysfunction.

Muscle involvement in HIV infection is usually associated with subacute and symmetrical proximal muscle weakness, with involvement of the legs and, less often, the arms. Patients may complain of difficulty rising from a chair or climbing stairs and may indicate myalgias and decreased stamina. Two of the variants have some distinctive clinical features: myositis associated with diffuse infiltrative lymphocytosis syndrome (DILS myositis), which is associated with enlargement of the salivary glands and increased peripheral CD8+ lymphocytes, and HIV-associated inclusion body myositis (HIV-IBM), which may be clinically indistinguishable from sporadic IBM, with involvement of quadriceps and forearm muscles, except sometimes it is seen in younger patients.[12]

An important part of establishing the diagnosis of HIV-DSP/ATN relies on the exclusion of other causes or modifying factors for neuropathy. We usually order a comprehensive metabolic panel with fasting blood sugar to check for diabetes and liver or renal impairment. We also check vitamin B_{12} levels, perform thyroid function tests, and look for hepatitis C co-infection. Nerve conduction studies are helpful in establishing the diagnosis of HIV-DSP/ATN and in detecting neuropathy in patients with nonspecific symptoms in the feet. The typical pattern shows a predominantly sensory axonal polyneuropathy, although the study may be normal even in the presence of pain, given the possibility of predominant involvement of small sensory fibers. An inflammatory demyelinating polyneuropathy (AIDP or CIDP) will be suspected if motor weakness is a prominent feature. Nerve conduction studies (NCS) and needle electromyography (EMG) are an important part in the evaluation of these patients, because they provide objective information about sensory axonal loss and demyelination. In HIV-DSP, the typical features would be those of a length-dependent predominantly sensory polyneuropathy with loss of sensory axons in the distal lower extremities, resulting in reduced-amplitude sensory responses. Up to 25% of patients may have abnormal electrophysiologic findings without symptoms, and approximately 20% of patients with HIV-DSP have normal nerve conduction studies due to preferential involvement of small fibers.[13] We have also examined the value of the ratio of the superficial radial sensory amplitude to the sural sensory amplitude but have not found that this increases the detection of neuropathy.[14]

In addition to the clinical features, the serum creatine kinase (CK), the EMG examination, and the muscle biopsy are important tools in the evaluation of a patients suspected of having HIV-associated muscle involvement. In HIV myositis, the serum CK level can be markedly increased, up to 10 times the upper limit of normal, although it can also be elevated in AZT myopathy. The needle EMG typically shows increased spontaneous activity with fibrillation potentials and positive waves, as well as increased numbers of small-amplitude, short-duration polyphasic motor unit potentials, and this can be observed in the toxic and HIV-associated types. Not uncommonly the myositis and the distal sensory neuropathy coexist, as both are more common in the advanced stages. A muscle biopsy can be important in differentiating the toxic myopathy from the nontoxic subtypes. In zidovudine-associated myopathy, features of mitochondrial dysfunction are prominent, with numerous "ragged red" fibers, subsarcolemmal accumulation of red granular material, sparse, if any, endomysial inflammation, lipid accumulation, and paracrystalline mitochondrial inclusions on electron microscopy.[15] The typical biopsy in the patient with HIV myositis will show more prominent perimysial, endomysial, and perivascular inflammation, with varying degrees of necrosis, phagocytosis, and degeneration of muscle fibers.[7] In some patients abundant nemaline (rod) bodies can be observed and may be a predominant feature without inflammation, a finding used to define the nemaline subtype of HIV-associated myopathy. This observation has led to the suggestion that adult patients with nemaline myopathy on muscle biopsy should be tested for HIV infection. In DILS-associated myositis, typically there is a prominent CD8+ inflammatory infiltrate.

Because of the predominant involvement of small unmyelinated and myelinated fibers, the use of skin biopsies to study epidermal nerve fibers has been shown to be an important tool in the study of neuropathy in these patients. Skin biopsies are usually obtained in the lateral aspect of the distal leg and thigh. Studies examining epidermal innervation in adult HIV patients have shown that the density in epidermal nerve fibers is reduced in HIV patients compared to control subjects regardless of neuropathy status and is more reduced in patients with HIV-DSP.[16] However, in children and adolescent patients the epidermal nerve fiber density may be paradoxically increased.[17] Additional studies have shown that reduced epidermal nerve fiber densities in asymptomatic HIV patients may be a predictive factor for the development of neuropathy within 1 year.[18] Nerve biopsies are usually not necessary for the diagnosis of neuropathy in these patients, unless the patient has an asymmetrical or multifocal pattern that may suggest a vasculitic component.

Lumbar puncture with cerebrospinal fluid examination would be necessary in the context of a demyelinating polyneuropathy or a polyradiculopathy. Both acute and chronic demyelinating polyneuropathies show increased protein levels in the cerebrospinal fluid (CSF) but unlike the non-HIV demyelinating neuropathies, this is often, but not always, associated with a mild pleocytosis.[19] The progressive polyradiculopathy may show a polymorphonuclear pleocytosis, with increased protein and reduced CSF glucose.[4] In these cases, polymerase chain reaction (PCR) testing of the CSF for cytomegalovirus is necessary.

Treatment and Management
The basic principles for treatment of HIV neuropathies are mainly based on preventive strategies and symptomatic treatment. As with other toxic neuropathies and myopathies removal of the offending agent is a critical and important step for improvement or reversal of symptoms. In the case of ATN, however, in a phenomenon called *coasting*, symptoms may increase temporarily for 6 to 8 weeks after stopping the offending medication. This should not be confused with progression of the neuropathy. Also, because ATN often coexists with HIV-DSP, the symptoms may improve but may not disappear completely. The reduced incidence of HIV-DSP since the introduction of HAART supports the notion that proper treatment of the HIV infection, with reduction in viral loads and increased CD4 counts and avoiding neurotoxic antiretrovirals, can also result in improvement of the neuropathy, as some investigators suggested in the past.[19a] Careful follow-up by an HIV specialist is an integral part of the management of these patients.

Although there are no FDA-approved drugs for the treatment of HIV-DSP, some of the medications used in the management of painful dysesthesias and paresthesias in other neuropathies such as diabetic neuropathy have been used effectively. The clinician must be aware of the potential interactions with the antiretroviral medications and the multitude of other medications that HIV patients must take. Symptomatic treatment comprises mainly antidepressants and anticonvulsant medications. Among the various treatments for neuropathic pain that have proved effective, pregabalin and gabapentin are often preferred for their lack of interaction with the antiretroviral medications. Gabapentin has been shown to be effective in a few anecdotal reports and in one small placebo-controlled study at doses of 1200 mg, 2400 mg, and 3600 mg, depending on response.[20,21] A controlled study of pregabalin in painful HIV-DSP was recently completed but was inconclusive due to a high placebo response.[22] Lamotrigine has been used, but published reports have only shown efficacy in ATN and not in HIV-associated neuropathy as a separate entity. Memantine, an NMDA (N-methyl-D-aspartate) antagonist, was not effective in treating painful neuropathic symptoms in HIV-DSP.[23] Among the antidepressants that have been used in HIV-DSP, low-dose amitriptyline or nortriptyline continue to be used by neuro-AIDS specialists in spite of not being effective in a controlled study,[24] but the study may have been stopped prematurely.[25] Patients are usually started at a low dose (25 mg) in the evening and the dose is slowly titrated, to deal more effectively with sedation and anticholinergic side effects. Duloxetine is currently approved for the treatment of diabetic painful polyneuropathy, but its effectiveness and safety have not been reported in HIV-DSP. The recommended dose is 60 mg once a day, but to avoid nausea, the most common side effect, it is usually started at a low dose of 20 or 30 mg and slowly increased over a period of 2 weeks.

Topical capsaicin has been used in the past for painful neuropathic symptoms of HIV-DSP, but the need for frequent applications and initial exacerbation of pain limited its use. A new preparation of a high-concentration capsaicin dermal patch that provides at least 12 hours of relief after a single application shows promise as an additional treatment.[26] Smoked cannabis was also recently shown to be effective in relieving chronic neuropathic pain associated with HIV-DSP, although this is limited to states or countries where this therapy is legal.[27]

Although controlled studies specific for HIV-associated acute or chronic demyelinating polyneuropathies have not been performed, it is generally accepted that response to treatment is similar to non-HIV AIDP and CIDP.

Preferred treatment options for HIV-AIDP include intravenous gamma globulin at a dose of 0.4 g/kg/day for 5 days. Plasmapheresis is an alternative, but intravenous immunoglobulin (IVIg) is generally more accessible and does not require special expertise. For HIV-CIDP, oral prednisone will prevent relapses and improve strength, although caution must be taken in patients that have low CD4 counts to avoid further immunosuppression and interactions with protease inhibitors that will result in fluctuating prednisolone levels. Alternatives would also be regular courses of IVIg or plasmapheresis. The outcome of HIV-associated GBS is similar to HIV-seronegative GBS.[28]

Progressive polyradiculopathy is now rarely encountered since the introduction of HAART. Treatment is based on anti-CMV therapy and the initiation or optimization of HAART. The current therapies available are ganciclovir, valganciclovir, foscarnet, cidofovir, and fomivirsen. If CMV infection is suspected, the initial recommendations are for IV infusions of ganciclovir or foscarnet, twice daily as induction therapy, followed by IV maintenance therapy. In patients with severe disease, the use of two medications concomitantly is indicated. Patients may worsen during the first 2 weeks of therapy, but this does not indicate treatment failure.[25] Monitoring of CSF pleocytosis may be used as a marker of response to therapy. Maintenance therapy may be stopped once the CD4 counts have remained above 200 cells/μL and the viral loads have been reasonably suppressed for several months.[25]

Because of their relative rarity, there are no controlled studies of treatment for the HIV-associated myopathies. Treatment recommendations are based on anecdotal experience and from small case series and isolated case reports. The basic assumption for the nontoxic myopathies is that the manifestations are related to immune-mediated mechanisms associated with immune dysregulation in HIV infection. Based on this, investigators have used standard immunosuppressants with overall positive results.[7,29] HIV myositis can be treated with a short course of prednisone at a dose anywhere from 40 to 60 mg/day, as well as IVIg at dose of 2 g/kg given over 5 days. This should be given in conjunction with antiretroviral therapy to ensure adequate viral suppression. In HIV-associated nemaline myopathy, steroids, IVIg, and plasmapheresis have also being used with some success in a few cases.[30,31]

In the case of AZT-myopathy, discontinuing or reducing the dose of zidovudine and substituting with a nonmyotoxic antiretroviral agent usually results in improvement. The rapidity and degree of improvement depend on the severity of the myopathy at the time of discontinuation, but strength is usually improved within 4 to 6 weeks.[7] If strength does not improve, the possibility of a coexisting inflammatory component should be considered and a trial of steroids or IVIg may be of benefit.

West Nile Virus Neuroinvasive Disease

Over the past decade, West Nile virus (WNV), a mosquito-borne flavivirus, has been identified as an important infectious agent associated with epidemics of encephalitis and with involvement of the neuromuscular apparatus. Since it was first identified in the West Nile region of Uganda in 1937, this entity has spread to the Middle East and Eastern Europe and more recently to the United States, with the first cases identified in New York City in 1999.[32] The virus has continued to spread throughout the United States and has extended to Latin America and the Caribbean.[33]

The majority of cases of human infection are subclinical or, when symptomatic, can present as a febrile illness with malaise, myalgias, headaches, lymphadenopathy, gastrointestinal symptoms, and sometimes an associated maculopapular rash.[34] The incubation period after inoculation in most cases is 2 to 14 days, and older adults and immunosuppressed patients are at higher risk of having a more severe and complicated illness. Contrary to West Nile's clinical manifestations in the areas where it was originally described, where it usually results in a mild uncomplicated febrile illness (West Nile fever [WNF]), the more recent epidemics in the United States, Israel, and Eastern Europe have been associated with more prominent involvement of the nervous system. Only a minority of patients (<1%) develop neuroinvasive disease, although this disease can have a major impact on morbidity and mortality rates.[35–37] Clinically apparent WNV neuroinvasive disease can be categorized in three distinctive groups: WNV meningitis, WNV encephalitis, and WNV acute flaccid paralysis.[38,39] There can be substantial overlap between these presentations so that they can coexist. Patients with WNV meningitis will present with fever, stiff neck, and photophobia, classic signs of meningeal irritation. In addition, cranial nerve abnormalities, in particular unilateral or bilateral facial neuropathies, can be a frequent accompanying abnormality. Those with WNV encephalitis, in addition to signs of meningeal irritation, will present with altered level of consciousness, disorientation and confusion, and more focal signs of central nervous system (CNS) involvement such as seizures, ataxia, myoclonus, postural or kinetic tremors, and parkinsonism. These are less common features of other viral encephalitides and are seen more often in older (>50 years) patients.[38]

Patients with WNV acute flaccid paralysis (WNV-AFP) develop a rapid (24 to 48 hours) and progressive, usually asymmetrical paralysis caused by destruction of motor neurons in the anterior horn of the spinal cord. Although it is more commonly seen in patients in the context of WNV-meningoencephalitis, it may also present in the absence of fever or viral symptoms as an isolated clinical presentation.[40,41] The deep tendon reflexes are usually reduced or absent in the affected limb; a normal sensory examination points to an abnormality in the anterior horn cells. Although the pattern of weakness is usually asymmetrical, it can range from subjective weakness and disabling fatigue without objective weakness on examination to a monoparesis or a rapidly ascending flaccid quadriparesis with respiratory failure, clinically very similar to GBS.[36,40,42,43] Indeed, some cases of WNV infection have been associated with GBS, although this is a less common complication.[36] Dysarthria and dysphagia could be predictive of progression to respiratory failure. Loss of bladder function can be observed. On a long-term basis, the weakness usually persists, although the degree of improvement may vary depending on the severity of loss of motor neurons. Greater degrees of strength improvement are usually seen within the first 4 months after the infection.[36] Motor unit estimation (MUNE) may be useful in determining prognosis for recovery of strength in AFP.[44] In some instances, muscle weakness is rapidly reversible, implying that damage to the motor neurons may not necessarily be irreversible and that damage may occur in other segments of the motor unit such as the distal motor axons.[44]

WNV-AFP can usually be distinguished from typical GBS by the development of flaccid weakness during the symptomatic stage of viral infection, in contrast to GBS, in which symptoms typically develop 2 to 8 weeks after the viral infection. In addition, the presence of CSF pleocytosis, the meningoencephalitic symptoms, and the absence of sensory symptoms can be helpful distinguishing clinical features. The EMG-NCS can provide further evidence with the absence of demyelinating features.

Diagnosis and Evaluation

In suspected WNV infection, the diagnosis can be made by the detection of WNV-specific IgM from serum or CSF 8 to 21 days after onset. Before or after this time, titers may be undetectable or could have declined. To establish the diagnosis, it is usually required that a fourfold or higher increase in acute and convalescent antibody titers is documented. Because there can be cross-reaction with antibodies against other flaviviruses, determination of neutralizing antibody titers is usually required when only serum specimens are available.[34,45] Alternatively, PCR of CSF for viral RNA can be performed, although the sensitivity is lower. Other ancillary studies include CSF analysis, magnetic resonance imaging (MRI), and EMG/NCS. CSF analysis in WNV is notable for a pleocytosis with initial and often prolonged (>48 hours) predominance of polymorphonuclear neutrophils, changing later to a lymphocytic predominance, which is unusual for viral meningoencephalitides. The CSF protein is increased but the CSF glucose remains normal.[46] This pleocytosis differentiates WNV acute flaccid paralysis from GBS. The MRI is most often unremarkable, although in patients with WNV encephalitis, abnormally increased signal can be observed on T2-weighted, diffusion-weighted (DW), and fluid-attenuated inversion recovery (FLAIR) images in cerebral white matter, in the deep gray matter nuclei such as thalamus and basal ganglia, and in the brain stem.[47,48] In patients with AFP, there can also be increased signal in the anterior horns of the spinal cord in the T2-weighted images, an important finding indicating focal involvement of the motor neurons.[39,41,49] The EMG/NCS are an important component in the assessment of suspected WNV-AFP. These most often show decreased compound muscle action potential (CMAP) amplitudes with preserved motor conduction velocities and normal sensory nerve conduction studies. This picture is in the context of widespread denervation in weak limbs and paraspinal muscles, consistent with an anterior horn cell disorder.[40,42,50]

Treatment and Management

There is no specific antiviral treatment for infection with WNV at the present time, so a lot of the efforts have focused on prevention; information campaigns educating the public about protection measures during outdoor activities in the high-risk season, and the development of potential vaccines, have led these efforts. With respect to specific therapies most reports at present are anecdotal, although several controlled trials exploring these potential therapies are underway. Animal studies and some anecdotal reports in humans have shown benefit in patients with WNV-encephalitis, with passive transfer of anti-WNV antibodies using an IVIg preparation made with pooled blood from donors with high titers of anti-WNV antibodies (Omr-IgG-am, Omrix Biopharmaceuticals).[51,52] A randomized double-blind, placebo-controlled trial comparing Omr-IgG-am with U.S.-produced IVIg, has been completed and the results are pending. One of the critical issues is the timing of administration. Additional anecdotal reports have shown potential effectiveness with the use of interferon alfa-2b in patients with neuroinvasive WNV infection, including WNV-AFP.[53,54] The dose used in these reports was 3 million units, with an initial IV dose or only by subcutaneous injection, once per day for 14 days. High-dose steroids have been used successfully in one patient with WNV-AFP, although the role of steroids in the treatment of this complication remains to be proved.[55] In patients with WNV-AFP, physical and occupational therapy are probably important in preventing long-term complications in weak and immobilized limbs, although studies to this date have been limited to a few patients.[56,57]

The information available about the long-term outcome of infection with WNV suggests that there is a wide range of residual symptoms and deficits and that these, in general, are related to the severity of the initial infection, the age of the individual, and the presence of co-morbid conditions.[36,58–60] Studies among elderly patients have shown higher mortality rate in older individuals.[61] Patients with WNF and WNV meningitis have a more favorable outcome than those with encephalitis or AFP, although there is a high prevalence of subjective symptoms such as fatigue, weakness, and difficulty with concentration and memory.[58] In patients with WNV encephalitis, persistent and more prominent neurologic

sequelae can be observed; residual tremor parkinsonism and ataxia have been observed for months or more than 1 year after the original infection.[59] However, some patients, particularly if in good health prior to the illness, still recover to their premorbid level of functioning.[37] Patients with WNV-AFP appear to have the worse long-term outcome, with more prominent morbidity and mortality rates. As a group, worse outcome and increased mortality rates are seen in patients who develop respiratory failure, have more extensive weakness due to loss of motor neurons, and are older.[36,43] Mortality rates in patients with more severe involvement and in particular those with respiratory failure can range from 22% to 50%.[36,43] Less severe and more restricted weakness is associated with better recovery,[59] although some patients with severe weakness, including quadriplegia and respiratory failure, can recover to baseline strength.[36,44] Some studies have shown limited or absent recovery in very weak limbs, as one would expect with severe loss of motor neurons. In general, the outcome data to this date have shown that there is a spectrum of functional outcomes and that recovery is highly variable and difficult to predict on an individual basis.

Nervous System Lyme Disease (Lyme Neuroborreliosis)

Lyme disease is the most commonly reported vector-borne disease in the United States.[62] It is a multisystemic disease caused by infection with the spirochete Borrelia burgdorferi and acquired through the bite of ticks of the Ixodes complex (I. scapularis in the northeastern United States). The clinical condition was described originally in Europe and more recently was identified in the United States, where the spirochete causing the symptoms was first identified. The more common clinical presentations are different in Europe and the United States, and this has been associated with differences in the strains of Borrelia that predominate in each region.[63,64] In the United States, borreliosis is caused by B. sensu stricto and in Europe most cases are associated with B. garinni and B. afzelii, although B. sensu stricto is also found there. The infection has preferential involvement of the skin, heart, joints, and nervous system; hence, its common symptomatic manifestations of skin rash, carditis and cardiac conduction defects, arthralgias or frank arthritis, and meningoradiculoneuritis. When it involves the nervous system (Lyme neuroborreliosis), it primarily causes meningeal inflammation with a wide variety of manifestations affecting both the central nervous system and the peripheral nervous system. The characteristic triad of neuroborreliosis consists of meningitis, cranial neuropathies, and radiculitis,[65] although peripheral neuropathy (mononeuritis multiplex) and, more rarely, myositis can also be observed. We will focus our discussion around the more common manifestations.

Diagnosis and Evaluation

The diagnosis of Lyme neuroborreliosis is initially and foremost a clinical diagnosis, based on a precise history, a careful physical examination, and supportive laboratory tests. The history will be important to establish the appropriate geographic location, the seasonal preference, and the typical systemic and neurologic manifestations. In North America, about 95% of all infections occur in the northeastern states and north central states, from New Hampshire to Maryland, and in Minnesota and Wisconsin.[62] The infection is also prevalent in middle Europe and Scandinavia, and it occurs in Russia, China, and Japan.[66] Thus, it will be critical to determine if the patient resides or has traveled to an area where the disease is endemic. The seasonal aspect should be explored: Most infections occur from spring to autumn and are unlikely to happen during the winter months, when the tick is not active. Although most patients will not recall a tick bite, in a large proportion of patients it will be possible to establish the recent occurrence of a skin rash. This rash, the hallmark of Lyme disease in the United States, is a slowly expanding erythematous annular lesion, resembling a bull's-eye or a target, known as *erythema migrans*, occurring the first few weeks after infection. It is observed in 80% to 90% of patients in North America but in 50% or less of European patients.[63,64,66,67] The lesion is described as being at least 5 cm in diameter and could be multifocal. It is an early manifestation of the infection and in the context of systemic symptoms, such as fever, arthralgias, headache, chills, and malaise, would be strongly indicative of recent infection with *Borrelia* (stage 2). In Europe, erythema migrans is less common and more indolent, with milder systemic manifestations. European patients may present later in the course of the disease with another dermatologic manifestation, *acrodermatitis chronica atrophica*.[68] After the development of the erythema migrans, between 3% and 15% of patients with untreated Lyme borreliosis will develop neurologic symptoms, and these can result from central or peripheral nervous system involvement. Some investigators have divided the clinical manifestations into early and late stages.[69] There are two principal presentations of *Borrelia* infection of the nervous system (neuroborreliosis).[64,65] The most common presentation in the United States is subacute meningitis, with headache and meningismus, often with involvement of one or more of the cranial nerves, following within a few weeks to a few months the initial infection or the erythema migrans. The other major presentation, which is more common in Europe, is a painful radiculitis (Garin-Bujadoux-Bannwath syndrome) with a lymphocytic pleocytosis on CSF analysis. Cranial neuropathies are the most common focal neuropathies and can be observed in 40% to 70% of patients with early neuroborreliosis.[70,71] The most common cranial neuropathy is a facial (seventh cranial nerve) neuropathy, which accounts for about 70% to 80% of all cases.[70,72] The facial neuropathy is most commonly unilateral but can be bilateral in one third of the cases, as in sarcoidoisis and GBS. Although it is usually accompanied by meningeal inflammation, half of the patients with facial neuropathy may not have a lymphocytic pleocytosis, indicating that the nerve can be involved distal to the subarachnoid space. Other cranial neuropathies that have been described are neuropathies of the third (oculomotor), sixth (abducens), and eighth (vestibuloauditory) cranial nerves.[70]

The earliest neurologic manifestations typically occur within a few weeks of erythema migrans, which is a skin manifestation more commonly recognized in North America than in Europe. The painful radiculitis is most commonly seen in Europe and can present in up to 80% of patients with European neuroborreliosis. This is an acute painful radiculitis, worse at night, with painful dysesthesias, often described as lancinating in a dermatomal distribution.[64,65,71] The radiculitis can be in the cervical, thoracic, or lumbosacral distribution, may or not be associated with meningeal inflammation, and can be focal or multifocal and asymmetrical. Within days or weeks after the onset of the painful dysesthesias, patients may develop motor weakness in the affected root distribution, which if thoracoabdominal may be associated with abdominal protrusion.[73] Rarely, the radiculitis has been associated with spinal cord inflammation around the same segment, resulting in long tract signs, a sensory level, and sphincter abnormalities below the level of the involved segment. Brachial and lumbosacral plexopathies, mononeuritis multiplex, and a confluent mild distal axonal polyneuropathy have also been described, although they are less common.[65] Patients with untreated Lyme disease may present with a mild indolent chronic distal axonal polyneuropathy or polyradiculoneuropathy months to years after onset of disease.[69,74] This is characterized primarily by

symmetrical nonpainful paresthesias in a distal lower limb distribution or asymmetrical radicular pain. The most common finding is multimodal sensory loss, but only 60% of the patients will have objective abnormalities in the neurologic examination. Contrary to acute radiculoneuritis, this finding is not associated with cranial neuropathy, and a lymphocytic pleocytosis on CSF is usually absent. This neuropathy is usually mild and often requires electrophysiologic studies for detection. In European patients, chronic Lyme polyneuropathy is usually associated with acrodermatitis chronica atrophica.[75] The neuropathy preferentially affects the limb with the chronic skin changes and appears to be more painful and to affect motor fibers more commonly than the North American variety.

Laboratory diagnosis for neuroborreliosis relies on the detection of anti-*Borrelia* antibodies because the spirochete, if present in blood or CSF, is only present in low numbers and for a short time, it is difficult to isolate and culture, and the yield of PCR in CSF is low.[76] Current recommendations are for the use of a two-tier (two-step) approach, checking for *Borrelia*-specific antibodies using sonicate IgM and IgG enzyme-linked immunosorbent assay (ELISA) followed by Western blotting.[77] Serologic tests can be negative in the early stages of the infection, and thus if the patient has the characteristic clinical presentations (facial nerve palsy or radiculitis) with active or recent erythema migrans, treatment should be instituted in spite of the negative serologic test. Convalescent serum samples 2 weeks after the onset of symptoms should confirm the diagnosis. Additionally, positive antibody responses may last for extended periods, implying that a single positive test will not differentiate between an acute recent infection and a previous infection.

The demonstration of anti-*Borrelia* antibodies in serum or CSF does not constitute evidence of neuroborreliosis, because they may originate by passive transfer from blood, and many individuals from endemic areas have positive IgG and IgM antibodies in the absence of borreliosis or neuroborreliosis. To establish the presence of intrathecal synthesis of anti-*Borrelia* antibodies, and the diagnosis of neuroborreliosis, the use of an antibody index comparing proportions of CSF to serum antibodies has been recommended.[78–81] The index is defined as the ratio of IgG in the CSF to the IgG in serum, in relation to the total IgG in CSF and total IgG in serum. In a group of established cases of neuroborreliosis the index had a diagnostic sensitivity of 75% with a specificity of 97%.[78] A limitation of this assessment is the fact that an elevated CSF-to-serum ratio can persist for years after treatment.[82] In addition, patients with pure peripheral nerve syndromes may not have an increased intrathecal production of antibody.

Lumbar puncture for CSF analysis provides additional evidence of CNS involvement with meningeal inflammation. This typically shows a mild or moderate lymphocytic pleocytosis with a mildly increased protein concentration and normal glucose levels.[65,83] An increased IgG index and oligoclonal bands can also be observed. These findings could help differentiate other conditions with similar symptoms but without meningeal inflammation and may suggest the diagnosis of neuroborreliosis in patients with facial nerve palsies or painful radiculitis. As previously mentioned, some patients with strictly peripheral nervous system involvement may not have an associated pleocytosis or meningeal inflammation.[70,74]

EMG and NCS will help establish a radicular pattern of involvement and the presence of a mononeuritis multiplex or axonal polyneuropathy. Among the findings described in studies, there can be reduced-amplitude motor and sensory responses with preserved conduction velocities, consistent with an axonal polyneuropathy, and denervation in limb muscles extending to the paraspinal muscles consistent with a radicular lesion.[71,73,74,84] These findings may coexist.[84]

MRI findings are not specific for neuroborreliosis, and its role may be more to exclude alternative diagnoses or to establish parenchymal CNS involvement. MRI of peripheral neuroborreliosis may provide indirect confirmatory evidence of inflammation by showing enhancement of cranial nerves in patients with cranial neuropathies or enhancement of lumbosacral roots in patients with lumbosacral radiculitis (Bannwarth syndrome).[63]

Treatment and Management

The optimal approach and treatment for neuroborreliosis have been surrounded with some controversy, although current recommended regimens appear to be highly effective. An evidence-based review published by the American Academy of Neurology has shown that parenteral regimens with ceftriaxone and oral regimens with doxycycline are highly effective in both adult and pediatric neuroborreliosis.[85] Alternative parenteral choices can be cefotaxime or penicillin. Oral doxycycline has been shown to be as effective as parenteral ceftriaxone and has been used in Europe with success.[86] In the United States, doxycycline is considered an alternative choice for uncomplicated cases with facial neuropathies or radiculitis. Published studies have used treatment courses of 10 to 28 days, although the current recommendations are for a 14-day course; there appears to be no significant difference in the outcome. In Europe, parenteral regimens are favored in cases of parenchymal brain or spinal cord disease or cases that have failed oral treatment with doxycycline. Doxycycline is contraindicated in children younger than 8 years and in pregnant women. In these cases, amoxicillin or cefuroxime axetil are considered alternate choices. No benefit has been shown for prolonged treatment with antibiotics beyond 4 weeks or for the treatment of "post-Lyme" syndrome and so it is not recommended.[85,87] Clinicians should be aware that improvement after antibiotic therapy is slow and continues after completion of therapy. This pattern should not be confused with failure of treatment, which would be suspected only if new deficits or symptoms arise. Treatment failures with ceftriaxone and doxycycline may be seen, and alternative antibiotics may be considered in those instances. Nonsteroidal anti-inflammatory agents may be helpful for treating the myalgias, arthralgias, and headache associated with the systemic disease.[64] The use of steroids as part of the treatment, in particular for facial neuropathy, has not been shown to be either beneficial or detrimental and at the present time is not recommended.

The long-term outcome of neuroborreliosis largely depends on the pattern and severity of nervous system involvement, and effective treatment with antibiotics. In Europe, follow-up of patients without antibiotic therapy has shown no significant differences from those treated with antibiotics, suggesting that the host response appears to be effective and in the majority of cases the disease is self-limited even without antibiotic therapy.[88] In the United States, follow-up of patients not treated with antibiotics has shown that those with facial nerve paralysis, and possibly more widespread nervous system involvement, had more residual symptoms.[89] In patients with definite neuroborreliosis treated with antibiotics, a 5-year follow-up study showed that 75% had recovered completely and only 25% had some residual deficits.[90] Uncomplicated facial nerve paralysis has an excellent prognosis; close to 90% recover to normal or almost normal.[72,83] Some controversy exists about the presence of what has been called "chronic Lyme disease" or "post-treatment Lyme disease" with persistent nonspecific symptoms, including long-term fatigue and difficulty with concentration. Up to this date no convincing evidence of long-term infection or immune-mediated mechanisms has been found.[91–106]

Leprous Neuropathy

Leprosy continues to be one of the leading causes of peripheral neuropathy in the world, in spite of continuing decline in the number of cases of leprosy globally in recent years. Peripheral nerve damage can result from invasion of the infectious agent, *Mycobacterium leprae*, or from immunologically mediated reactions in the peripheral nerves.

The principal goal in the management of leprosy neuropathy is to prevent disability by early detection and treatment of peripheral nerve involvement. Detection of leprosy in the early stages is critical to prevent irreversible damage and long-standing disability. The onset of the disease is insidious, with an incubation period of 7 years on average, although it can range from 3 months to 40 years. The disease is classified based on the aggressiveness of the infection, which is a function of the host's cell-mediated immunity. The more restricted presentation is classified as tuberculoid leprosy and the more widespread and systemic form is classified as lepromatous leprosy; borderline leprosy manifests between tuberculoid and lepromatous. It is also classified according to the extent of skin involvement as multibacillary or paucibacillary leprosy.

The large majority of patients will exhibit both skin and peripheral nervous system abnormalities, although, less commonly, patients may present with a pure neural form that will require a high degree of suspicion and confirmatory tests for diagnosis. The three cardinal signs in leprosy neuropathy are (1) an anesthetic skin lesion, (2) enlarged nerves, and (3) evidence of acid-fast bacilli on skin biopsy.

The skin lesions are described as macules or plaques, with a raised border and hypopigmentation and with decreased sensation or anesthesia in the central portion. These lesions tend to be found more frequently on the trunk or abdomen but may occur in other locations. One must be aware, however, that up to 30% of skin lesions in leprosy do not exhibit sensory abnormalities.[107] The presence of enlarged nerves must be explored.

Involvement of peripheral nerves is different among the various forms of leprosy. In tuberculoid and borderline leprosy, the most common pattern of neuropathy is a mononeuritis multiplex. In lepromatous leprosy, nerve involvement is more widespread; a distal, symmetrical polyneuropathy pattern is more common. Because the bacterium favors cooler areas of the body, sensory loss may be observed in the chin, malar areas of the face, earlobes, buttocks, knees, and distal extremities. Negative sensory symptoms (numbness, anesthesia) are more common than positive sensory symptoms (paresthesias, pain).

Diagnosis and Evaluation

NCS are more sensitive at detecting peripheral nerve involvement than clinical examination. Among the electrodiagnostic tests, sensory nerve conduction studies, and in particular sensory amplitudes, as well as warm perception thresholds, are among the earliest abnormalities observed and are the most sensitive measures, even in the subclinical stages.[108] Motor nerve conductions can also be abnormal, even before clinical signs are apparent. Based on the frequency of involvement, nerve conduction studies should be performed in the ulnar, median, and superficial radial nerve in the upper limbs, and the peroneal, posterior tibial, and sural nerves in the lower limbs. The trigeminal and facial nerves should also be tested. The diagnosis can be made by demonstrating organisms in skin or nerve biopsy (Fig. 15-1) and the presence of serologic markers such as PGL-1 and PCR.

Treatment and Management

Treatment of leprosy and leprosy neuropathy involves both antibacterial therapy and strategies to limit inflammatory reactions. Current antibacterial treatment involves multidrug therapy (MDT)

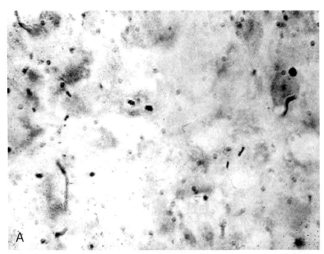

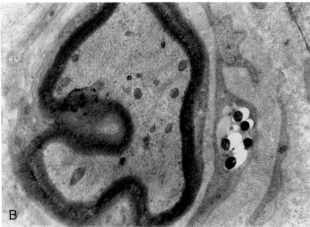

Figure 15-1 A, Leprosy in nerve. Acid-fast bacilli of leprosy (Ziehl-Neelsen stain, ×400). **B,** Leprosy in nerve. Lepra bacilli in Schwann cell cytoplasm on electron microscopy (×9,000). (**A,** Courtesy of Dr. A. Ciudad, Lima, Peru. **B,** Courtesy of Dr. S. Shankar, National Institute of Mental Health and Neurosciences, Bangalore, India.)

to prevent resistance, and varies between patients with paucibacillary or multibacillary disease. A current treatment recommendation for paucibacillary disease consists of 6 months of rifampicin (600 mg/day) and daily dapsone (100 mg). For multibacillary leprosy clofazimine (50 mg/day) is added and given for 12 months. Some clinicians may extend the treatment for 24 months if the medication is readily available and the patient has high bacterial loads. Patients are rendered noninfectious within 72 hours of treatment.

Treatment of leprosy may result in inflammatory reactions termed *type 1* and *type 2 reactions*. These immunologically mediated reactions may result in increased nerve damage and increased disability. With type 1 reactions, patients may observe enlargement of a preexisting skin lesion or the development of acute, painful nerve palsies. This reaction requires immediate treatment with prednisone at initial doses of 40 to 60 mg (1 mg/kg) lasting for 4 to 6 months and a higher dose if there is no improvement within 48 hours. Patients that have not responded to steroids after 6 weeks may be referred for surgical decompression (neurolysis). Patients with multiple or large lesions on the face may benefit from prophylactic steroids for 4 months at the start of MDT. Type 3 reactions (erythema nodosum leprosum) are mostly seen in lepromatous leprosy and will present with painful erythematous papules and systemic symptoms such as fever, uveitis, fatigue, and lymphadenopathy. It will also require prompt intervention with steroids at high

doses and often with repeated treatments. Thalidomide has also been recommended for the management of type 2 reactions, although this therapy may be complicated by the development of drug-induced neuropathy and must be used with caution.

Other Infectious Neuropathies and Myopathies

Human T-Lymphotrophic Virus

The human T-lymphotrophic virus type I (HTLV-I), and less commonly HTLV-II, are most commonly associated with a progressive spinal cord disorder and as the causative agents of HTLV-associated myelopathy/tropical spastic paraparesis (HAM/TSP), as well as adult T-cell leukemia. Although the most common neurologic presentation is the chronic progressive myelitis, it is known that patients may exhibit coexistent peripheral neuropathy and a myositis.[109] The neuropathy may be present in up to a third of patients with HAM/TSP but can be detected in about 6% of asymptomatic, HTLV-I–seropositive individuals. Clinically, patients with neuropathy present primarily with paresthesias or dysesthesias in the distal lower extremities, impaired vibration in the toes, and reduced (relative in the presence of hyperreflexia) or absent ankle reflexes, consistent with a distal sensory polyneuropathy. Patients with coexistent myositis will show prominent proximal muscle weakness and elevated serum CK levels. The diagnosis of HTLV-I/HTLV-II is made through ELISA-based antibody detection in serum and confirmed with Western blot or PCR for proviral DNA in peripheral blood mononuclear cells. There are no studies addressing treatment for the peripheral neuropathy in HTLV-I infection, although an inflammatory component, as is the case for HAM/TSP, is suspected. There is no established therapy for HAM/TSP, although a variety of treatments have been used. The only controlled studies have shown a benefit with interferon alfa, primarily in Japanese patients. Corticosteroids are probably the most commonly used, both by oral or intravenous route. Pulsed methylprednisolone (1 g/day for 3 days) has shown some benefit, although the benefit is probably greater in the early stages of the disease.[110] More recently, the possible benefit of valproic acid, as a histone deacetylase inhibitor, has been proposed as a novel method of treatment in HAM/TSP. HTLV-I–associated myositis has been treated with prednisone at 1 mg/kg/day and oral immunosuppressants such as azathioprine, although compared to seronegative polymyositis, patients appear to have a less optimal response.[111]

Other Viral Myopathies

Muscle involvement in the form of myalgias, myositis, or, in more severe cases, rhabdomyolysis, can be seen in a variety of other viral infections, in addition to HIV and HTLV-I viral infections. The most common causes of viral myositis in the United States are the influenza A and B viruses; myositis is more common with type B than with A.[112] Influenza infections are a seasonal problem most commonly presenting with signs and symptoms of an upper respiratory tract infection with systemic symptoms such as fever, headaches, and myalgias of varying severity that may appear before or at the same time as the systemic symptoms. In contrast to the typical myalgias, the myositis appears after the onset of fever and systemic symptoms (within a few days), is more restricted in distribution, and results in more severe pain. Clinically, it affects the calf muscles more frequently and prominently, causing pain, tenderness, and difficulty with ambulation. Myositis is more commonly seen in children than in adults and it tends to affect boys more often than girls.[113]

When present in adults, it is more severe. The diagnosis is based on the identification of influenza A or B infection and the suggestive clinical picture. CK levels are usually elevated, more in adults than in children. Muscle biopsy, although not usually performed, may reveal features of an acute necrotizing myositis. Treatment is mainly symptomatic, for the myositis usually appears after the infection is established and there is no evidence that antiviral agents or immunotherapy are beneficial for the myositis.[7,112] For the treatment of the underlying influenza, it is important to distinguish between A and B types and H3N2 or H1N1 subtypes for proper selection of antiviral agents. Rhabdomyolysis can also be seen with influenza infection and is more common with influenza A than B. Because of the danger of renal damage, rhabdomyolysis must be aggressively treated.

Parasitic Myositis

The most common parasitic infections of muscles include trichinosis, cysticercosis, and toxoplasmosis.

Trichinosis occurs from ingestion of improperly cooked meat contaminated with the nematode *Trichinella spiralis*. Although it is most commonly associated with ingestion of pork meat, more recently it has been associated with the ingestion of meat from wild animals, including bear, walrus, seal, cougar, and wild boar.[112] The clinical presentation includes a prodrome with gastrointestinal symptoms such as abdominal cramps, diarrhea, and vomiting, followed by fever, muscle soreness and tenderness, edema of the eyelids, subconjunctival hemorrhages, and eye pain. Examination can reveal muscle weakness that may include the intercostal muscles and diaphragm. Myocarditis may accompany the clinical picture, with persistent tachycardia, cardiac failure, and striking electrocardiographic changes. CNS manifestations can also occur. Laboratory testing shows eosinophilia, which may be as high as 50%, and elevation of serum CK, particularly in the acute stages of the disease. The EMG shows features of an inflammatory myopathy with fibrillations and myopathic changes. A muscle biopsy in affected muscles may help establish the diagnosis in the early clinical stages, when the serologic test is still negative. Findings in the muscle biopsy vary depending on the stage of infection and may show motile larvae, encapsulated calcified cysts, and inflammatory infiltrates with muscle fiber necrosis (Fig. 15-2).[114] The diagnosis may be confirmed,

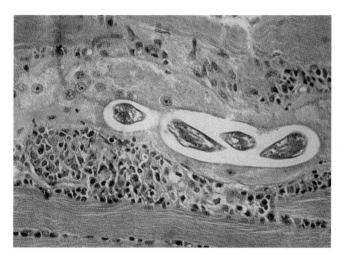

Figure 15-2 Trichinosis in muscle. Muscle fiber showing a parasite cyst in a case of trichinosis (hematoxylin and eosin, ×200). (Reprinted with permission from Bertorini TE: *Clinical Evaluation and Diagnostic Tests for Neuromuscular Disorders*. Woburn, MA: Butterworth-Heinemann, 2002.)

establishing the presence of antibodies in serum, with ELISA, fluorescent antibody test, or the bentonite flocculation assay.[112] In patients with mild infection, the recommended treatment is usually a combination of bed rest, analgesics, and antipyretics. Albendazole (400 mg twice a day for 8 days) or, alternatively, mebendazole may be used in the acute enteric stages of the disease to prevent further larval migration to the muscles. The drugs, however, are ineffective in treating the muscle infection. With more severe infections or myocarditis, corticosteroids (prednisone) are given in combination with the anthelmintic medications. Prevention by cooking meat properly and realizing that freezing does not kill all the trichina species are important parts in the management of this infection.

Cysticercosis is the systemic infection that results from the ingestion of undercooked pork meat contaminated with eggs from *Taenia solium*, the pork tapeworm. This is an important health problem in the developing world and is also seen in developed countries, particularly in immigrants from areas in which it is endemic. The larvae infect the CNS, muscle, eye, and subcutaneous tissue. The disease is often asymptomatic and is detected when cysticerci degenerate and cause inflammation in the CNS, resulting in seizures, or when it is detected incidentally on radiographs showing calcified cysts in muscle or CNS. There is a rare form of muscle involvement termed *pseudohypertrophic myopathy* that shows symmetrical enlargement and weakness of involved muscles that especially affects the calves.[112]

In addition to detecting the appropriate clinical picture and risk factors, the diagnosis is made on the basis of detection of the calcified cysts, for which computed tomography (CT), MRI, and ultrasound are often used. Biopsy of subcutaneous nodules can also be helpful in establishing the diagnosis. Confirmation of the diagnosis can be made using serologic tests, of which the ELISA is most helpful with CSF samples. The newer enzyme-linked immunoelectrotransfer blot (EITB) is preferred to ELISA because of its higher sensitivity and specificity, although it may be negative in patients with inactive lesions.[114] Stool sampling for ova and parasites is not very sensitive. The current preferred treatment is albendazole, at 15 mg/kg/day in two or three divided doses for 2 weeks, or praziquantel or niclosamide. Corticosteroids are commonly given concomitantly to control inflammatory responses produced by the dying cysts.

Toxoplasmosis is the infection caused by the ingestion of cysts of *Toxoplasma gondii*, in undercooked infected meat (most often pork or lamb), by consuming food items contaminated with sporocysts derived from cat feces, and transplacentally. In immunocompetent persons, the disease is usually asymptomatic or may present with a "mononucleosis-like" illness with fever, cervical adenopathy, myalgias, and malaise.[112] A polymyositis-like picture and myocarditis can develop in immunocompetent patients, although most symptomatic infections appear in individuals who are immunosuppressed, such as those with HIV infection or idiopathic CD4 lymphocytopenia. The disease may develop from primary infection or reactivation. Additional features that are sometimes seen are lymphadenopathy, hepatosplenomegaly, pneumonia, uveitis, chorioretinitis, and meningoencephalitis.

When there is muscle involvement, laboratory testing shows increased serum CK and EMG changes consistent with an inflammatory myopathy.

The diagnosis of toxoplasmosis can be made by serologic tests, by PCR, by demonstration of the organism histologically, or by isolation of the organism. The main challenge in the diagnosis is to determine if the infection has occurred recently or in the past. To differentiate between the two possibilities, patients undergo several serologic tests: the Sabin-Feldman dye test, which tests for IgG antibodies; ELISAs targeted at IgM, IgA, and IgE; and differential agglutination tests.[114]

In mild cases, treatment is not indicated because the disease is self-limited. In more severe cases, including those with myositis or that are immunosuppressed, treatment is indicated with a combination of pyrimethamine and sulfadiazine, or trisulfapyrimidines.[114] Since pyrimethamine is an antagonist of folic acid, folic acid supplementation should be given during treatment.

Granulomatous Diseases of Nerve and Muscle

Sarcoid Neuropathy and Myopathy

Sarcoidosis is a systemic disease of unknown etiology that is characterized by granulomatous involvement of many organs, including the central and peripheral nervous system. It is slightly more common in women and is more prevalent in North Americans of African ancestry and northern Europeans than in other groups.[97] Neurologic complications are infrequent; prevalence is between 5% and 10% of symptomatic neurologic involvement in patients with known sarcoidosis.[91,92,94,97,100] The most common neurologic manifestations of sarcoidosis are cranial neuropathies, leptomeningitis, granulomatous lesions in the brain or spinal cord with hypothalamic and pituitary dysfunction, and less commonly myopathy and radiculoneuropathies. Cranial neuropathies are seen in 50% to 80% of patients with neurosarcoidosis; facial nerve palsy is the most common and is present in 23% to 50% of patients.[97–99,105] Other cranial nerves, such as the optic nerve or the vestibuloauditory nerve, can also be affected.

Neuromuscular manifestations, besides facial neuropathies, are less common. Peripheral nerve involvement, including radiculopathies and radiculoneuropathies, occurs in approximately only 1% of patients with sarcoidosis.[92,94,97,100] There is a wide spectrum of presentations of peripheral nerve disease; polyradiculoneuropathies and axonal sensorimotor polyneuropathies are the most common.[93] Other presentations include a vasculitic mononeuritis multiplex, small fiber neuropathy, and a host of demyelinating neuropathies such as multifocal motor neuropathy and Guillain-Barré syndrome.

Muscle manifestations, including asymptomatic involvement, are more common than peripheral nerve or radicular symptoms. Asymptomatic muscle sarcoidosis can be seen in up to 50% of patients with sarcoidosis, although symptomatic muscle involvement is much rarer and usually seen in 1% to 2% of patients with sarcoidosis.[95,104,115]

Diagnosis and Evaluation
The diagnosis of neuromuscular sarcoidosis can be a dilemma due to the multitude of manifestations and the fact that they can occur in the absence of systemic sarcoidosis.

When neurologic symptoms appear in a patient with biopsy-proven sarcoidosis, the diagnosis can be made with more certainty, but symptoms that are initial manifestations or that develop in patients with inactive sarcoidosis represent a bigger challenge. It is important to be familiar with the potential presentations of neuromuscular sarcoidosis and to consider the possibility when other systemic symptoms and signs are present. The diagnosis is based on the detection of systemic manifestations, the suspicion from known patterns of involvement of the peripheral and central nervous system, and the detection of involvement in other tissues, preferably with tissue diagnosis.

Sarcoid myopathy usually presents in advanced stages of the disease and can manifest in three different forms: (1) acute myositis, (2) chronic myositis, and (3) nodular myositis. The most common

form is chronic myositis; acute and nodular myositis are less common and limited to isolated case reports in the literature. The chronic form usually presents in female patients older than 50 years with slowly progressive proximal weakness progressing over months to years.[94,102,103] Myalgias appear to be frequent, and the serum CK is usually normal or only mildly increased.

The diagnosis of sarcoid neuropathy or myopathy relies on the accurate detection of systemic involvement and pathologic confirmation in affected organs. Up to 50% of patients that present initially with neurosarcoid have systemic involvement. Evidence of systemic involvement should be sought by performing analysis to detect hypercalcemia, hypercalciuria, elevated immunoglobulins, or elevated serum or CSF levels of angiotensin-converting enzyme, although these tests are not confirmatory. Thoracic (lung, mediastinum) abnormalities are detected in 80% to 90% of patients with neurosarcoidosis, so imaging of the thorax should be performed in all patients. Radiologic tests should include a CT scan or MRI of the thorax. Alternative strategies include a gallium scan or, more recently, positron emission tomography (PET) scan has been used to identify areas of high yield for tissue diagnosis, including muscle. An evaluation for involvement of the eye, lung, skin, or other organs potentially involved should be performed.[99]

Pathologic evidence of sarcoidosis is usually required for diagnosis. In systemic sarcoidosis, lymph nodes and skin nodules are usually targeted for biopsy. Sarcoid muscle involvement may be established with a blind or directed muscle biopsy, and this may be abnormal, even in the absence of symptoms. The biopsy reveals noncaseating granulomas predominantly in connective tissue and perivascular distribution.[104] These are composed of epithelioid cells, lymphocytes, and multinucleated giant cells (Fig. 15-3). Fiber necrosis is unusual or not seen. Because these are focal lesions, serial sections of the muscle biopsy are recommended. Similarly, nerve biopsy can demonstrate noncaseating granulomas in the endoneurium, perineurium, or epineurium and may also show concurrent necrotizing vasculitis.[93,101] Skin biopsy has also provided evidence of small fiber involvement in some cases.

There are no specific findings in NCS and EMG for neuromuscular sarcoidosis, although this is still helpful in documenting peripheral nervous system involvement. In at least one study, NCS have shown

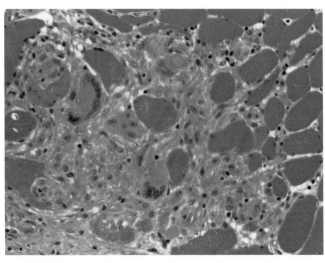

Figure 15-3 Sarcoidosis in muscle. Granuloma in muscle with lymphocytes, epithelioid cells, and giant cells (hematoxylin and eosin, ×200). (Reprinted with permission from Bertorini TE: *Neuromuscular Case Studies*. Woburn, MA: Butterworth-Heinemann, 2008.)

findings consistent with a predominant proximal, multifocal process; axonal changes are more common than demyelinating changes.[93] Needle EMG examination may be normal because the abnormalities are predominantly in the intervening connective tissue, or they may show myopathic changes in clinically symptomatic myopathy.

Treatment and Management

Because neuromuscular disease in sarcoidosis is rare, there are no randomized controlled clinical trials for the treatment of these complications and management is based on anecdotal reports or small series of cases. The goals of treatment are to prevent the fibrosis that may follow the chronic inflammation or the extension and progression of vascular damage when vasculitis is present. Steroids are the mainstay of treatment. Prednisone in doses of 0.5 to 1.0 mg/kg (40–60 mg/day) is usually used and has proved effective. The length of treatment varies with the severity of manifestations; a 2-week course followed by a tapering dose schedule is sufficient for a facial neuropathy, but longer courses are required for more extensive neuropathy or myopathy. As is the case in any patient being treated with steroids, evaluation for subclinical tuberculosis with purified protein derivative (PPD), or more importantly a chest radiograph, is mandatory prior to initiating therapy, as PPD could be negative even in infected cases. Prevention of osteoporosis with the use of calcium and vitamin D supplementation, or bisphosphonates in high-risk patients, should be instituted. Routine evaluations for hypertension, hyperglycemia, and cataract formation are an important part in the detection and management of side effects. In patients with refractory or relapsing disease, other immunosuppressive agents such as azathioprine, methotrexate, cyclosporine, mycophenolate mofetil, and cyclophosphamide have been used. Hydroxychloroquine has been used for long-term immunomodulation in neurosarcoidosis but is not a good choice in neuromuscular sarcoidosis because it may be associated with myopathy and neuropathy. A new and alternative approach for patients that are steroid intolerant or unresponsive has been the use of anti–tumor necrosis factor (TNF)-α therapy. Among the various alternatives, infliximab, a chimeric monoclonal antibody against TNF-α, has been used successfully in several patients with sarcoid myopathy. It is typically given as an intravenous bolus at a dose of 5 mg/kg initially every 2 weeks and then monthly for a target duration of 6 months. It can be associated with leukopenia and peripheral neuropathy, so caution and close monitoring should be performed in all patients. Because up to two thirds of patients with sarcoidosis go into spontaneous remission, it is sometimes arguable that all patients should be treated. Steroids have shown to be effective in peripheral neuropathy cases, but improvement is usually delayed and neuropathic symptoms may linger for a long time after treatment. For vasculitic neuropathy, corticosteroids and cytotoxic drugs have been the principal approaches for treatment.

Toxic Neuropathies and Myopathies

The expanded availability and use of medications, often in combination, has resulted in the detection of neuromuscular toxicities that were not seen during the initial trials in a small selected population, usually without coexistent diseases. Muscle and nerve toxicity are among the more prevalent toxicities seen with many of the commonly used medications, in part because the symptoms and signs are readily recognizable. Toxicity from industrial agents has declined in some countries due to the implementation of more effective surveillance and security programs; however, this is still an important source of neurotoxicity in developing countries. What follows is a discussion of the main issues associated with muscle and nerve toxicity from some industrial toxins and medications.

Toxic Neuropathies

Although medication-induced and other toxic neuropathies represent only a minority (about 4%) of all cases of neuropathy, it is critical to identify them because they are potentially reversible and may be the only sign of a previously unidentified toxic exposure that can be eliminated. Reports of possible associations between medications or toxins and the development of neuropathy are abundant, but objective evidence to establish causation is lacking in many of these reports. It is important to understand that exposure does not equal causation. Establishing the link between exposure and the presence of a polyneuropathy is a difficult task that requires the clinician to be familiar with medications with potential for neurotoxicity and with the systemic manifestations of industrial agents or other toxins that are known to cause neuromuscular toxicity. Clinicians should also be aware that patients with coexistent peripheral neuropathies, such as diabetic, alcoholic, or inherited neuropathies, are more susceptible to toxic insults and may develop earlier and more severe neuropathy.

The following discussion concentrates on the diagnosis and management of the most important of these agents where the evidence is clear and in a few newer agents that are highly suspect based on published reports.

Arsenic

Arsenic is a ubiquitous metal that occurs naturally, with unintentional chronic exposure resulting from the ingestion of contaminated ground water, from exposure in the metal smelting industry, pesticide manufacturing, burning of treated wood, and in non-Western traditional remedies, among others. It has also been used as a poison in suicide or homicide cases.[116]

The clinical presentation can vary depending on whether there is acute exposure of large amounts of arsenic or chronic low-grade exposure. In acute arsenic poisoning, patients often present initially with gastrointestinal symptoms, followed by an encephalopathy, renal failure, and later by ascending paralysis, with a picture similar to that for GBS. This later complication may develop days to weeks after acute exposure and is often associated with a protracted and incomplete recovery. The electrodiagnostic examination initially may show features consistent with segmental demyelination later followed by a distal, dying back, predominantly axonal polyneuropathy. In chronic arsenic poisoning, the systemic manifestations are more prominent. Patients present with a gradually progressive sensorimotor polyneuropathy, skin changes (palmar and plantar hyperpigmentation and hyperkeratosis), alopecia, and Mees lines. *Mees lines* are transverse lines that appear in the fingernails and toenails, although they are not specific for arsenic poisoning. Other clinical features are anorexia, weight loss, bone marrow suppression, hepatomegaly, and encephalopathy.[117,118]

Diagnosis and Evaluation

The diagnosis of arsenic poisoning is made from the combinations of clinical features and the determination of potential risk factors for exposure from a thorough history and investigation. In patients in whom arsenic poisoning is suspected, urinary arsenic excretion from a 24-hour urine collection is the most specific test. Blood arsenic levels are not used because levels can drop within 2 to 4 hours after ingestion. Care must be taken to differentiate inorganic arsenic, which is the neurotoxic form, from organic arsenic, which is present in seafood and is not toxic. Patients should avoid eating seafood for at least 4 days prior to the test. Fractionation is always important to determine if elevated arsenic is organic or inorganic. Evidence of multiorgan toxicity is assessed by performing a complete blood count with smear and a comprehensive metabolic panel. Abnormalities observed include pancytopenia, basophilic stippling, elevated hepatic enzymes, and renal insufficiency.[116,117,119] NCS can be helpful in establishing the pattern of neuropathy. In the acute form with massive exposure, as previously mentioned, there could be a demyelinating polyneuropathy. In the chronic form, the NCS show evidence of a distal axonal sensorimotor polyneuropathy. Chronic exposure can also be diagnosed from hair, nail, and skin samples.

Treatment and Management

Treatment of arsenic toxicity starts with the elimination of the exposure and incorporates chelation and supportive measures for acute exposure. In the patient at high risk for chronic exposure, periodic urinary arsenic levels are performed to monitor for toxicity. Normal urine arsenic levels (inorganic) for a 24-hour urine are less than 50 μg/L. Chelation is indicated in patients with severe symptoms after acute ingestion and elevated in inorganic urinary arsenic levels.[119] Chelation does not improve the recovery or progression of neuropathy unless given within hours of exposure. In the presence of acute neuropathy, the agents commonly used are dimercaprol (dimercaptopropanesulfonic acid, DMPS), penicillamine,[116,117,119] and succimer (dimercaptosuccinic acid, DMSA), which, although not approved for use in arsenic poisoning, appears less toxic than the others when used for lead poisoning.

Thallium

Thallium is another heavy metal used in the manufacture of lenses, semiconductors, insecticides, and rodenticides. The salts are tasteless, odorless, water soluble, and completely absorbed from the gastrointestinal tract, explaining their use as rodenticides and in intentional poisoning.

Diagnosis and Evaluation

Clinical manifestations depend on the dose, the age of the person exposed, and whether exposure is acute or chronic. The distinctive features are a rapidly developing polyneuropathy in the context of alopecia. The neuropathy is dominated by sensory symptoms with painful dysesthesias and paresthesias that occur within a week of exposure. Alopecia and Mees lines can also be observed and are features that occur later in the course. However, they are not helpful in the diagnosis of acute poisoning. It is important to know that not all patients with thallium poisoning develop alopecia and neuropathy. Early in the course, and with mild intoxication, small fiber involvement predominates, with both painful dysesthesias and dysautonomic features. Although sensory symptoms predominate in most cases, motor manifestations can also occur.

The diagnosis of thallium poisoning can be difficult given the rarity of the exposure and the nonspecific symptoms in the early stages. Hair analysis may provide early evidence of exposure. Darkening of the hair roots when examined under a microscope has been described as an early diagnostic feature.[117] NCS might show evidence of a sensory axonal polyneuropathy, although if small fiber involvement predominates, the studies early in the disease may be normal in spite of symptoms. The gold standard for diagnosis is the 24-hour urine collection.

Treatment and Management

The goal of treatment and management is to stop exposure and to increase elimination. Prussian blue (potassium hexacyanoferrate) is the most effective treatment at present, forming a complex with thallium and increasing its fecal excretion. The recommended dose is 3 g orally three times per day, although others advocate 250 mg/kg two times per day.[117] If Prussian blue is not available, activated charcoal has been recommended until Prussian blue does become available.

Lead

The other prototype for heavy-metal–induced neuromuscular toxicity can be absorbed through the gastrointestinal tract or inhaled and absorbed through the lungs. It is toxic in both its organic and inorganic forms. In children, it is more commonly associated with an encephalopathy, but in adults toxic exposure is more commonly associated with a peripheral neuropathy and less commonly with features of an encephalopathy. In adults, toxic exposure has been most commonly described through occupational exposure. Among those at risk for exposure are workers in lead acid battery manufacturing plants, metal ore smelters, individuals who work in the manufacture of glazed pottery and ceramics, those working with solders, and through consumption of bootleg liquor and some folk remedies.

Diagnosis and Evaluation

The clinical presentation of lead neuropathy in adults depends on whether there is acute exposure at high levels or chronic low-level exposure. With acute or subacute high-level exposure, patients present with an asymmetrical, predominantly motor neuropathy affecting the upper limbs more than the lower limbs and bilateral wrist drop as a typical feature. Sensory abnormalities in this presentation are usually not present. The neuropathy is often accompanied by systemic symptoms and signs such as abdominal pain, constipation, and anemia. Nephropathy and gout can also be observed. With chronic low-level exposure, it is more common to observe a distal sensorimotor polyneuropathy.[120] Hypertension is a common clinical sign observed in workers with chronic low-level exposure. Although in animal models the neuropathy is demyelinating, in humans the peripheral neuropathy is more of the axonal type.

For the diagnosis of lead-associated neuropathy, it is necessary to establish exposure corresponding to the development and progression of neuropathy and to document an abnormal content of lead in fluid or tissues. The best current screening test is venous blood lead levels. Recommendations for periodic testing in workers at risk for chronic lead exposure have been published.[121] Minor abnormalities in NCS have been seen with lead levels of 50 μg/dL or above, but clinically apparent neuropathy is usually not seen in individuals with levels below 80 μg/dL.[122] The electrodiagnostic findings are still debated; most studies show mild slowing of motor conduction velocities on a group basis (exposed vs. nonexposed) but many individual values fall within the range of normal.

Treatment and Management

Chelation therapy is usually given to adult patients who are symptomatic or have blood levels above 70 μg/dL. There is still some controversy about the optimal treatment for lead intoxication. One recommendation is to use oral succimer (DMSO) for patients with blood lead levels between 70 and 100 μg/dL. Patients with encephalopathy or levels greater than 100 μg/dL can be treated with intramuscular dimercaprol or oral succimer, followed by intravenous calcium disodium ethylenediaminetetraacetic acid (CaNa$_2$

EDTA).[117] Typically, after chelation therapy, a period of re-equilibration of 10 to 14 days is allowed and blood lead concentrations are then remeasured, to account for remobilization from bone stores.

Hexacarbon Neuropathy

Peripheral neuropathy has been associated with exposure to *n*-hexane and methyl-*n*-butyl ketone. These are hexacarbons present in industrial solvents, glues, spray paints, coatings, and silicones and associated with neurotoxicity in workers in printing plants, shoe factories, and furniture factories in the United States, Europe, and Asia. Both *n*-hexane and methyl-*n*-butyl ketone are metabolized in the liver to 2,5-hexanedione, which is the neurotoxic metabolite.[118] In more recent times, exposure and neurotoxicity has been associated with intentional inhalation of glue by "glue sniffers."[123]

n-Hexane exposure results in a peripheral neuropathy with distal sensory loss, atrophy, diminished or absent deep tendon reflexes, and autonomic dysfunction. With massive acute exposure, patients can present with a clinical picture mimicking GBS, similar to acute arsenic intoxication.[123] In these instances, motor nerve conduction studies can show conduction velocities in the demyelinating range. With chronic exposure, the more typical dying-back distal axonal sensorimotor neuropathy is usually observed. Concomitant degeneration of the distal corticospinal tracts and dorsal column can occur with chronic exposure and result in the presence of spasticity or signs of CNS involvement (central-peripheral-distal axonopathy). Impairment of color vision can also be observed with chronic exposure. The histopathologic hallmark is the presence of multifocal, giant axonal swellings in distal axons, secondary to abnormalities in axonal transport. Diagnosis is made based on the presence of exposure and evidence of neuropathy, with clinical findings of neuropathy and findings in NCS. Electrodiagnostic studies can show evidence of peripheral demyelination with motor conduction slowing and occasionally partial conduction block with coexistent axonal degeneration. Blood and urinary levels of 2,5-hexanedione (the common neurotoxic metabolite) can confirm current exposure.[119]

Treatment consists mainly of cessation of exposure. As in other toxic neuropathies, there can be transient worsening and progression weeks after exposure is stopped (coasting). The prognosis for recovery after cessation of exposure in chronic industrial exposure is usually favorable, but patients with massive exposure, such as glue sniffers, may have residual spasticity and weakness.

Alcoholic Neuropathy

Chronic alcoholism has been associated to both peripheral neuropathy and myopathy. The neuropathy is often asymptomatic, with a prevalence that has ranged from 12.5% to 48.6% of alcoholics, depending on the detection methods and criteria for neuropathy.[124] The etiology of neuropathy in alcoholics is most likely multifactorial, combining both toxic effects from alcohol and nutritional deficiencies. Although in the past there has been debate as to whether alcohol or thiamine deficiency is the cause of the observed neuropathy, recent data have shown that alcohol itself, in the absence of thiamine deficiency, can result in a painful small-fiber distal polyneuropathy.[125]

Diagnosis and Evaluation

The diagnosis is based on establishing the presence of neuropathy and chronic alcohol abuse. Unhealthy drinking is defined as more than three or four drinks per day or more than 10 g of alcohol per day. The clinical features of alcohol-associated polyneuropathy are variable and many patients are asymptomatic, so a careful assessment is of utmost importance. Symptoms are primarily sensory, and clinical presentations can range from a slowly progressive, predominantly sensory small-fiber distal polyneuropathy with painful dysesthesias to, most commonly, a mixed pattern with involvement of both large and small fibers.[126,127] Autonomic neuropathy may also be present and may be related to increased mortality rate. NCS may be normal if only small fibers are involved, although more typically they show a pattern of loss of sensory axons with abnormal sural sensory action potentials and conduction velocity as the most sensitive markers.[127]

Treatment and Management

Stopping alcohol consumption is the primary treatment for alcoholic polyneuropathy; some studies demonstrate recovery for mild to moderate alcoholic neuropathy after 4 to 5 years of abstinence. Based on the possibility of a nutritional component, a few studies have investigated the effect of vitamin supplementation for the treatment of alcoholic polyneuropathy. Short-term controlled studies have shown a beneficial effect from benfotiamine, a thiamine derivative with high bioavailability, with improvement in symptoms and sensory and motor measures.[128] In addition, some formulations with multiple B vitamins have also shown some efficacy in controlled studies.[129]

Medication-Induced Neuropathies

Numerous medications have been associated with the development of neuropathy, although in many, definite proof is lacking and there is still controversy about causation or simple association (Table 15-1). Because sensory neurons and axons are more sensitive to the toxic effects, the most common pattern of medication-induced neuropathy is a distal, symmetrical, length-dependent sensory polyneuropathy. Although less common, some drugs can preferentially affect dorsal root ganglion neurons or Schwann cells, resulting in sensory neuronopathies or demyelinating neuropathies. More recently, vasculitic neuropathies have also been reported with some immunomodulating agents, enlarging the spectrum of possible toxic mechanisms and clinical presentations of medication-induced neuropathy.

What follows is a brief discussion of some of the more commonly used drugs and relevant drug-induced neuropathies that may be encountered by a neurologist or neuromuscular specialist.

Chemotherapy-Associated Neuropathy

Since the basic principle of chemotherapy implies a process of controlled cytotoxicity, it is common for other nonmalignant cells, such as central or peripheral neurons, to be affected as innocent bystanders. Clinicians should be aware that susceptibility to the various agents can vary considerably, resulting in different temporal patterns and severity of toxicity in different patients. Chemotherapeutic agents that result in neuropathy typically interfere with DNA replication or with microtubule function or assembly. Similar to other toxic neuropathies, many patients exhibit the "coasting" phenomenon, with worsening of symptoms and signs even after completion of the chemotherapy course. Although a mild neuropathy may be the price to pay for effective cure of a malignancy, the impact in the quality of life should not be underestimated and prompt attention and intervention, if necessary, are warranted. Preexisting neuropathy such as diabetic or inherited neuropathy can increase the risk and result in a more severe grade of chemotherapy-induced neuropathy. Additionally, the possibility of a paraneoplastic neuropathy independent of the chemotherapy neurotoxicity should be an important consideration in patients undergoing treatment.

Table 15-1 Pharmacologic Toxins

Drug	Indication	Clinical Manifestation	Mechanism	Diagnostic Tests	Treatment
Antineoplastic Drugs					
Paclitaxel	Solid tumors of lung, breast, head and neck	Dose-dependent sensory > motor neuropathy; significant motor manifestations in severe cases	Polymerization of microtubules may interfere with axonal transport; also direct toxic effects on the axon	Sensory/motor axonal neuropathy on EMG; wallerian-like degeneration on nerve biopsy	Reduction of dose
Vincristine/ vinblastine	Lymphoma/ leukemia, some solid tumors	Dose-dependent sensory and automatic neuropathy; painful paresthesias in hands and feet	Interference with microtubule assembly presumably disrupts axonal transport	Sensory/motor axonal neuropathy on EMG; wallerian-like degeneration on nerve biopsy	Reduction of dose
Cisplatin	Small cell lung cancer, urogenital cancers	Sensory neuropathy/neuronopathy (sensory ataxia, areflexia, pain); may not show typical length dependence	Direct toxicity to DRG neurons	Loss of sensory potentials on NCV studies; loss of large myelinated fibers on sural nerve biopsy	Reduction of dose
Oxaliplatin	Colorectal cancer	Acute paresthesias and cold-induced cramping within hours of dose; chronic length-dependent polyneuropathy	Unknown; suspected acute symptoms are due to peripheral nerve hyperexcitability resulting from sodium channel opening	Electrodiagnostic studies show peripheral nerve afterdischarges and neuromyotonia	Reduction of dose; membrane-stabilizing drugs (anticonvulsants)
Amphiphilic Cationic Drugs					
Amiodarone	Ventricular arrhythmias	Sensory/motor neuropathy with areflexia and ataxia; not necessarily dose-related	Formation of drug-lipid complexes that are lysosome resistant and toxic	Demyelinating changes on NCV; nerve biopsy shows osmophilic granules in Schwann, endothelial, and perineurial cells	Cessation of drug
Chloroquine	Malaria (prophylaxis and treatment, connective tissue diseases	Neuromyopathy; may be motor predominant with significant weakness before sensory manifestations	Formation of drug-lipid complexes that are lysosome resistant and toxic	Vacuolar myopathy; osmophilic inclusions in Schwann, endothelial, and perineurial cells	Cessation of drug
Perhexiline	Angina pectoris (not used in United States)	Sensory/motor polyneuropathy with areflexia and autonomic features	Formation of drug-lipid complexes that are lysosome resistant and toxic	Osmophilic inclusions in Schwann, endothelial, and perineurial cells	Cessation of drug

Antiretrovirals				
Zalcitabine (ddC) Stavudine (d4T) Didanosine (ddI)	HIV infection	Painful, distal sensory polyneuropathy; sensory ataxia; more frequently seen in patients with AIDS; may complicate or uncover underlying HIV-associated neuropathy	Unknown; may interfere with mitochondrial function	NCV/EMG shows distal axonal polyneuropathy; nerve biopsy shows nonspecific axonal degeneration	Reduction in dose or cessation of drug
Miscellaneous				
Colchicine	Gout and other rheumatologic disorders	Neuromyopathy; paresthesias in hands and feet	Interferes with microtubule assembly, possibly affecting axonal transport	NCV/EMG shows mild length-dependent axonal neuropathy $\pm$ irritable myopathy; vacuolar myopathy in patients with renal failure	Cessation of drug
Thalidomide	Suppression of immune-mediated disorders	Distally predominant sensory/motor polyneuropathy	Unknown	NCV/EMG shows length-dependent sensory/motor axonal polyneuropathy	Cessation of drug
Dapsone	Antibiotic for leprosy and Pneumocystis pneumonia	Motor > sensory neuropathy; may affect hands disproportionately	Unknown	Motor axonal neuropathy	Cessation of drug
Pyridoxine (vitamin B_6)	Megavitamin therapy for various disorders	Sensory neuropathy/neuronopathy	Direct toxicity to DRG neurons	Pure sensory neuropathy	Cessation of exposure; late neuropathy may not be reversible

AIDS, acquired immunodeficiency syndrome; DRG, dorsal root ganglion; EMG, electromyography; HIV, human immunodeficiency virus; NCV, nerve conduction velocity.
With permission from Glass, J: Toxic neuropathy, from Johnson R, Griffin J, McArthur J (eds.): *Current Therapy in Neurologic Disease*, 7th ed. Philadelphia, 2006, Mosby.

Plant alkaloids such as taxanes, vinca alkaloids, and podo-phyllotoxins inhibit mitosis by interfering with microtubule synthesis and function, resulting in disruption of axonal transport. Vincristine is the vinca alkaloid most commonly associated with neuropathy. In the early stages, small-fiber sensory impairment and dysfunction predominate with distal painful dysesthesias and sensory loss. Autonomic dysfunction also can occur early with constipation, orthostatic hypotension, and impotence. With more severe neuropathy, patients can develop motor weakness, preferentially affecting extensor muscles in the upper and lower extremities. Although the neuropathy usually improves after exposure stops, recovery may be slow and residual symptoms may last indefinitely. One important aspect of the use of vincristine is increased susceptibility and more severe neurotoxicity in patients with an inherited neuropathy of the Charcot-Marie-Tooth type, or hereditary susceptibility to pressure palsies. Most reported cases, undiagnosed at the time of treatment, developed a severe neuropathy after only one or two doses of vincristine.[130]

The platinum-based agents such as cisplatinum, carboplatinum, and oxaliplatinum interfere with DNA replication and exert their neurotoxic effect in the dorsal root ganglion neurons. These agents may result in distal axonal dysfunction in the early stages or with lesser degrees of toxicity, and progression to a neuronopathy with continued exposure and more severe toxicity. Unfortunately, the severity of the neurotoxicity may not be apparent until late in the course of treatment or after it is finished, precluding more effective interventions. Cisplatinum exhibits more neurotoxicity than carboplatinum, although the clinical picture is similar. Patients complain of paresthesias and dysesthesias in the toes and feet, with proximal spread on accumulating exposure. Loss of dorsal root ganglion (DRG) neurons can result in a clinical picture of sensory neuronopathy with severely impaired proprioception and sensory ataxia. Oxaliplatinum results in unusual cold-induced paresthesias or dysesthesias and evidence of hyperexcitability with muscle contractions resembling neuromyotonia. This may be the result of a voltage-gated channelopathy provoked by the drug. The platinum-based compounds are the ones most commonly associated with worsening after discontinuation of therapy or "coasting" phenomenon.

The other group of antineoplastic agents that are commonly associated with peripheral neuropathy are the taxanes paclitaxel and docetaxel. These are used in the treatment of solid tumors and target the microtubullar system but, unlike the vinca alkaloids, not by inhibiting formation but by inhibiting disassembly and promoting polymerization. The neuropathy is dose-dependent (cumulative and individual cycle) and usually begins soon after treatment is initiated. Clinical symptoms are paresthesias and dysesthesias, most often with onset in the feet but possibly in hands and accompanied by perioral and tongue numbness. Toxicity is cumulative, and weakness will develop with continued exposure. Again, with more severe toxicity, symptoms and signs may persist after discontinuing exposure and may worsen after discontinuing therapy (coasting). Electrophysiologic studies usually show findings consistent with a symmetrical, length-dependent, axonal sensorimotor polyneuropathy. Among the newer antineoplastic agents, bortezomib, a proteasome inhibitor approved for the treatment of multiple myeloma, has shown preferential toxicity of small fibers, producing a painful, axonal small-fiber distal polyneuropathy in up to 30% of patients treated. Hypotensive episodes and paralytic ileus have also been reported. In patients with more severe toxicity, a demyelinating neuropathy has also been observed. In the majority of patients, symptoms resolve after stopping the medication. Laboratory assessment is aimed at excluding alternative or coexistent conditions associated with neuropathy and establishing the severity of the neuropathy. It usually includes standard laboratory tests for acquired neuropathies and EMG/NCS.

Treatment and Management

The approaches commonly used in the treatment and management of chemotherapy-induced neuropathy can be summarized as (1) prevention and neuroprotection, (2) reduction or elimination of exposure if possible, (3) pain management, and (4) supportive treatment with physical and occupational therapy.

In the absence of proven or established preventive or restorative therapies, supportive and symptomatic treatments are the mainstays of management at the present time. Several neuroprotective agents have been investigated in an effort to prevent or minimize neurotoxicity without affecting the antineoplastic effect. An excellent review of neuroprotection therapies during chemotherapy was published recently.[131] Although preliminary results for some of these neuroprotective agents have been promising, none are recommended until more rigorous controlled studies are performed. Among the various agents, glutathione, vitamin E, and glutamine have all been explored, with mixed results. Acetyl-L-carnitine has been used in doses of 1 g three times per day in patients with paclitaxel or platinum-associated neuropathy with positive results.[132] With oxaliplatin, investigators have successfully used calcium and magnesium infusions to prevent the cold-induced dysesthesias and muscle contractions.[133] Once symptoms are present and because neurotoxicity occurs in a dose-dependent manner and is cumulative, one of the most challenging issues is to decide whether to discontinue or reduce the dose of treatment at the expense of impaired efficacy or unsuccessful cure. Some investigators have suggested that at the moment a fixed deficit is detected, exposure should be stopped.[134] This should be carefully assessed in discussion with the oncologist and determined on an individual basis.

Pain management in chemotherapy-induced neuropathy has proved more challenging than in other painful neuropathies. Several anticonvulsants and antidepressants used in painful neuropathies, including amitriptyline, have not shown to be effective. Some investigators have reported successful management of oxaliplatin-induced neuropathic pain with low-dose venlafaxine or topiramate, although additional studies are needed.[132] Others have suggested the initial use of nonsteroidal anti-inflammatory agents and opioids as second-line agents.[135]

Tumor Necrosis Factor-α Antagonists

Some of the immunotherapies that have been recently developed and are currently in use for the treatment of autoimmune diseases have been associated with conflicting reports of improvement or development of peripheral neuropathy. Tumor necrosis factor-α (TNF-α) antagonists are increasingly in use for the treatment of rheumatoid arthritis, ankylosing spondylitis, and inflammatory bowel disease but have also been associated with development or worsening of other autoimmune diseases. There are reports of a wide variety of peripheral neuropathies associated with the use of TNF-α antagonists (infliximab, etanercept, adalimumab) including GBS, Miller-Fisher syndrome, chronic inflammatory demyelinating polyneuropathy, multifocal motor neuropathy with conduction block, vasculitic neuropathy, sensorimotor axonal polyneuropathy, and pure sensory neuropathy, during or after finishing treatment.[136] The proposed mechanisms are through both T-cell–mediated or antibody-mediated mechanisms or inhibition of axonal functions. Proper management of the neuropathy is not clear. Most patients have responded to standard immunotherapies or only by withdrawal of the medication, although this may take months. A long-term follow-up study has shown that some patients have remained stable with dose reduction only, implying that stopping the medication may not always be necessary for neuropathy control.[137]

Antiretroviral Agents

Among the antiretroviral agents used in the treatment of HIV infection, the ones most commonly associated with neuropathy during the pre-HAART era were the nucleoside analogs zalcitabine (ddC), didanosine (ddI), and stavudine (d4T).[138] More recently, some studies have suggested that the use of protease inhibitors, such as indinavir, saquinavir, and ritonavir, may be risk factors potentially associated with the development of neuropathy,[139–141] although this is still controversial.[142] Neurotoxicity is thought to be mainly through mitochondrial toxicity, given the antiretroviral agents' ability to inhibit mitochondrial polymerase gamma among other mitochondrial disruptive effects. As previously mentioned, it is not possible to distinguish antiretroviral toxic neuropathy (ATN) from HIV-associated neuropathy on clinical grounds only. The most important clue is the development of neuropathy within a short time, usually weeks to 6 months after the start of medication or an increase in dose. Some investigators have suggested that lactic acid levels may serve as a differentiating marker but this has not been validated. As with other toxic neuropathies, treatment of ATN is based on discontinuation of the offending agent, which has become more feasible given the expanded options for treatment. Several groups have studied the use of acetyl-L-carnitine (ALC) in doses that have ranged from 500 mg to 3 g/day, based on the hypothesis of mitochondrial toxicity. From the published results, it is appears that ALC may improve the painful neuropathic symptoms, although it is not clear that in the time frame studied, it resulted in regeneration or prevention of axonal loss.[143,144]

Lamotrigine was shown in one controlled study to be effective for ATN at target doses of 200 mg twice a day (400 mg/day) to 600 mg/day in those receiving enzyme-inducing drugs.[145] Lamotrigine was not effective as an adjunct treatment in patients who did not respond to gabapentin, tricyclics, or opioids.[146] The principal limitation is that it has to be started at a low dose (25 mg) and increased slowly over a period of 4 weeks to reduce the risk of skin rash.

Toxic and Medication-Induced Myopathies

Statin-Associated Myopathy

Statins or 3-hydroxy-3-methylglutaryl coenzyme A (HMG-CoA) reductase inhibitors have become the standard of care in treating hypercholesterolemia and are one of the most widely prescribed medications. Because hypercholesterolemia is a chronic condition, long-term use of these medications is often required. Myalgias and myotoxicity are among the most important treatment-limiting adverse effects, although other side effects such as constipation, flatulence, dyspepsia, and generalized gastrointestinal discomfort as well as elevated transaminase levels are also observed.[147]

There is considerable debate about the classification of the various degrees of myotoxicity associated with statin use. The American College of Cardiology/American Heart Association/National Heart, Lung, and Blood Institute have defined four myopathic syndromes related to the statins: statin myopathy, myalgia, myositis, and rhabdomyolysis.[148] Statin myopathy is characterized by diffuse muscle pain, tenderness, and weakness and occurs in approximately 1% to 5% of patients using statins. Myalgias are defined as muscle aches

or "weakness" without elevation of CK levels. Myalgias most often involve proximal muscles but they could also be generalized or focal. Myositis is defined as muscle symptoms with elevation of CK levels. Only 0.1% to 0.3% of those who receive monotherapy actually develop myositis. Rhabdomyolysis is muscle symptoms with substantial CK elevation (defined as CK elevation > ten times the upper limit of normal) and associated with creatinine elevation. Neuromuscular specialists and the subscribing authors find these definitions somewhat inaccurate because myalgia is strictly defined as muscle aches but not weakness, and myositis should imply that there is evidence of inflammation in the muscle biopsy, which is not part of the definition. As recently suggested by one neuromuscular specialist, it is possible to define statin myotoxicity into four main groups: (1) asymptomatic hyperCKemia, (2) myalgia with or without hyperCKemia, (3) muscle weakness with CK elevation, and (4) rhabdomyolysis.[149]

Although not clearly established, it is estimated that about 5% of all treated patients may exhibit asymptomatic elevations in CK levels.[149] In this group of patients, CK levels usually do not exceed 10 times the upper limit of normal and patients do not complain of myalgias or exhibit weakness. These patients are usually followed up clinically and with periodic laboratory evaluations. Patients with myalgias with or without CK elevation and without weakness can be changed to a statin with a lower potential for myotoxicity and followed clinically. Patients with CK elevations and weakness have become less common with increased awareness of the myotoxicity potential and the removal of cerivastatin (Baycol) from the market. In some patients, the onset of weakness sometimes cannot be temporally related to the exposure to statins, raising the question of a preexisting muscle disease being unmasked by the statin. Rhabdomyolysis is a more rare complication, with markedly increased CKs, myalgias, weakness, and myoglobinuria. This is a medical emergency and requires in-hospital management to prevent renal damage. This is most likely related to drug-drug interactions and is seen most often when combined with other medications such as amiodarone, gemfibrozil, and cyclosporine or colchicine. Co-administration of nicotinic acid, azole fungals, and macrolide antibiotics also increases the risk for developing myotoxicity. Clinicians should be thoroughly aware of drug interactions that increase the risk of myopathy and these should be recognized before starting patients on statins. This is most likely mediated through interactions with cytochrome P450 3A4 with resultant elevated levels of the statins, and most commonly associated with the lipid-soluble statins, atorvastin, lovastatin, and simvastatin.[150]

Clinicians should be aware that the myopathy can develop several weeks to years after starting treatment. One important possibility in patients with statin-myotoxicity is that of a preexisting elevation of the CK or undiagnosed muscle disease that has been unmasked by statin exposure. Baseline CK determinations prior to initiation of therapy may be helpful in identifying these patients, and clinicians should be aware of a possible heightened risk. Statins should be used cautiously and CK carefully monitored in patients with a history of myopathy and rhabdomyolysis.

In the evaluation of statin-associated myotoxicity, conditions that may mimic myopathy, such as claudication, peripheral neuropathy, amyotrophy, and lumbosacral radiculopathy, should be carefully excluded. There are several known risk factors associated with the development of statin-associated myopathy such as older age, higher doses, recent trauma, and coexisting diseases associated with myopathy (diabetes mellitus, hypothyroidism, hepatic dysfunction, and renal insufficiency).[151] Therefore, baseline liver, renal, and thyroid function tests should be done before starting patients on statins.

EMG performed in asymptomatic patients with elevated CK is usually normal. However, in patients with significant weakness, EMG may show spontaneous activity such as fibrillations, positive waves, and myotonic discharges and early recruitment.[152] The muscle biopsy, although rarely performed, usually shows nonspecific changes or, if severely affected, may show muscle fiber necrosis with phagocytosis and small regenerating fibers and an occasional "ragged red" fiber.[149,152] Currently there is no proven therapy to prevent or treat statin-induced myopathy. Based on the observation that coenzyme Q_{10} levels may be low, CoQ_{10} supplementation has been investigated with conflicting results. Concerns about the dose and power of the studies indicate that additional larger and more powered studies must be undertaken for a final result. In the interim, given CoQ_{10}'s relative safety, some investigators advocate its use at high doses, up to 800 mg/day.[149] In addition, muscle biopsies sometimes reveal inflammatory infiltrates, suggesting the possibility of an immune-mediated process and some investigators have advocated the use of immunotherapies such as IVIg in these patients, although this is not established practice.[149] Discontinuation of the statin or switching to a less myotoxic statin continues to be the mainstay of treatment. In patients with multiple medications, lowering the dose or switching to pravastatin, fluvastatin, or atorvastatin, which are not significantly metabolized by cytochrome P450 3A4 can be an option.[153] Physicians should not ignore patients' complaints. Patients should be examined and CK levels assessed if there is a suspicion. Patients can continue with the medication under close observation if symptoms are mild and tolerable, but the decision to continue with therapy should be in agreement with the patient after discussion of the potential risks and benefits. Statins should be discontinued if symptoms are moderate or severe or if CK levels increase to levels greater than 5 to 10 times the upper limit of normal. Patients should also be advised about the potential for heightened muscle disruption with vigorous exercise or prolonged dehydration.[150]

Steroid Myopathy

Steroid myopathy can result from both endogenous and exogenous corticosteroids and results in proximal muscle weakness and atrophy. Fluorinated glucocorticoids (triamcinolone > betamethasone > dexamethasone) have a greater propensity for producing weakness than the nonfluorinated ones.[152,154] There is a wide variability in dose and duration of glucocorticoid treatment among patients who develop weakness, although it is usually not seen at relatively low doses (i.e., 20 mg or less of prednisone daily).[149]

Clinically, weakness is usually more severe in the legs than the arms, and cranial-innervated muscles are spared. Patients usually exhibit other features of corticosteroid use such as cushingoid facies, fragile skin, or osteoporosis. The muscle weakness usually begins insidiously after chronic use of high-dose steroids, although some patients may develop an acute onset of severe generalized weakness, especially after receiving high doses of intravenous fluorinated steroids.[149] Serum CK and aldolase levels are usually normal. Muscle biopsy shows preferential atrophy of type 2 muscle fibers. Necrosis or inflammation is not observed. The mechanism for corticosteroid myopathy is not known.

The recommended treatment is to reduce the steroid dose to the lowest effective level and change to an alternate-day regimen. An additional strategy is to change to a nonfluorinated steroid.[154] Recovery is usually slow, and it may take months for full recovery to be observed. Ensuring adequate nutrition is important because

protein deprivation may accelerate the steroid-induced myopathic process. One common dilemma encountered by clinicians is to distinguish whether patients have become weaker due to exacerbation of their condition or due to the steroids. Sparing of neck flexors would suggest steroid myopathy, because these muscles are usually weak in the inflammatory myopathies. If the patient becomes weak when steroids are being tapered, the weakness is most likely due to relapse, but if the patient becomes weak while on high-dose steroids, then the cause is most likely steroid-induced myopathy. Serum CK levels, if elevated, would point toward an exacerbation, although the opposite (normal levels) may not be true. The needle EMG may also be helpful in distinguishing between exacerbation and steroid-induced weakness by documenting increased spontaneous activity (fibrillation and positive waves), which is a feature of inflammatory myopathy but not steroid myopathy.[152]

Alcoholic Myopathy

Although chronic alcohol consumption is mostly associated with neuropathy, it can cause many other significant problems such as liver cirrhosis, cardiomyopathy, and myopathy. Alcohol-induced muscle disease can result from either acute or chronic consumption, but it is mostly seen in patients with a long history of alcohol abuse. The severity of the muscle symptoms has been found to be proportional to the quantity of alcohol that is consumed. Several types of muscle disease are associated with alcohol consumption: (1) acute alcoholic myopathy, (2) acute hypokalemic myopathy, (3) chronic alcoholic myopathy, (4) asymptomatic alcoholic myopathy, and (5) alcoholic cardiomyopathy. Acute alcoholic myopathy, also known as acute necrotizing myopathy, occurs in approximately 1% of chronic alcoholics, usually associated with an episode of binge drinking. These patients develop weakness, myalgias, cramps, and edema. Their CK levels can increase considerably and they can develop myoglobinuria and rhabdomyolysis, which predisposes them to acute renal failure. Their muscle biopsies show necrosis of individual muscle fibers, all in the same stage of degeneration, and inflammatory infiltrates. However, the symptoms last only several weeks and are reversible after withdrawal. Alcohol can also induce hypokalemia, causing acute generalized weakness associated with low levels of potassium and elevated CK. Unlike acute alcoholic myopathy, patients do not present with myalgias, cramps, or edema. If a muscle biopsy is done during the acute presentation, vacuolar changes can be seen. Signs and symptoms are reversed with potassium correction. On electrophysiologic evaluation, both patients with acute alcoholic myopathy and those with acute hypokalemic myopathy can present with a primary myopathic process having normal or mildly abnormal NCS and increased insertional activity, with short-duration, low-amplitude motor unit action potentials on EMG.[152]

One third to two thirds of chronic alcoholics have chronic alcoholic myopathy,[155] making this the most frequent muscle abnormality in alcoholics of the various types discussed. Patients present with progressive proximal weakness and muscle atrophy that develops over the course of weeks to months. These patients have a normal or slightly elevated CK, and their muscle biopsies show predominant atrophy of type 2b fibers but no fiber necrosis.[156] Muscle strength improves on alcohol withdrawal, but complete recovery is usually not achieved. Asymptomatic alcoholic myopathy refers to the finding of elevated CK levels in alcoholic patients who do not complain of weakness and have no abnormalities on the neurologic examination. Lastly, alcoholic cardiomyopathy refers to the development of dilated cardiomyopathy due to chronic alcohol consumption. Alcohol cardiomyopathy resembles idiopathic dilated cardiomyopathy and is considered when other causes of idiopathic dilated cardiomyopathy have been ruled out.

Treatment of the various forms of alcohol-induced myopathy is primarily supportive, with hydration and correction of electrolyte abnormalities in the acute forms and efforts directed toward helping with the alcohol dependence to eliminate the toxic exposure.

Nucleoside Analog–Induced Myopathy

Among the various nucleoside analogs that have been developed as treatment for viral and retroviral infections, muscle toxicity has been most commonly observed with zidovudine (AZT, 3-azido-3′-deoxythymidine), stavudine (d4T), and fialuridine (FIAU).[149] Those myopathies associated with antiretroviral therapy are of particular importance due to their reversible nature if identified early and their importance as signs of mitochondrial toxicity. Zidovudine-associated myopathy is characterized by proximal muscle weakness 6 to 12 months after initiating treatment, myalgias in thighs and calves, fatigue, and variably increased serum CK.[149] The muscle biopsy reveals that features of mitochondrial dysfunction are prominent, with numerous "ragged red" fibers, subsarcolemmal accumulation of red granular material, sparse, if any, endomysial inflammation, lipid accumulation, many cytochrome-c oxidase (COX) negative fibers, and paracrystalline mitochondrial inclusions on electron microscopy. The precise mechanism of zidovudine myotoxicity is still debated but there is evidence for mitochondrial DNA depletion through inhibition of polymerase gamma; additionally, zidovudine-induced oxidative stress, direct inhibition of the mitochondrial bioenergetic machinery, mitochondrial L-carnitine deficiency, and impaired mitochondrial protein synthesis have also been proposed.[157] Zidovudine myopathy likely depends on cumulative drug dose and is therefore more common after high-dose, long-duration treatment. The frequency of zidovudine myopathy has decreased since lower doses have become the standard of therapy. Nowadays patients complain more frequently of fatigue and myalgia without clear weakness and atrophy. Blood measurements of CK and lactic acid may be helpful in symptomatic patients to differentiate from the immune-mediated HIV myositis. Treatment is based on removal of the offending agent, so switching to another nucleoside analog or antiretroviral agent, in the presence of symptoms and signs, is usually recommended. More recently and based on animal studies, uridine supplementation has been proposed as an alternative to be studied.[158]

Antimicrotubular Myopathy (Colchicine Myopathy)

Myopathies due to disruption of microtubule formation have been described with both colchicine and vincristine, although they are more common with the former agent. Both are also associated with a coexistent peripheral neuropathy in most cases. Colchicine is usually used for the treatment of gouty arthritis, although more recently it has also been used in the treatment of familial Mediterranean fever, Behçet's disease, and primary biliary cirrhosis. Its mechanism of action is through the interaction with tubulin and inhibition of polymerization of microtubules affecting mitosis and other microtubule-dependent functions in the cell. Disruption of this microtubular-dependent cytoskeletal network by colchicine is believed to result in the defective movement of lysosomes and the intracellular accumulation of autophagic vacuoles.[156] Myotoxicity is more commonly seen in older patients, ages 50 to 70 years, with mild renal insufficiency. Concomitant use of cyclosporine increases the risk of colchicine myotoxicity, and more recently, cases of rhabdomyolysis have been described with the concomitant use of statins.[159] Rarely, colchicine alone has been associated with rhabdomyolysis.[151] Patients most commonly present with proximal weakness of subacute onset associated with distal areflexia, myalgias, and elevated serum CK levels. There can also be mild elevation of serum CK in asymptomatic patients and more marked elevations in symptomatic patients. Patients commonly show signs and symptoms of a coexistent mild peripheral neuropathy. The nerve conduction studies typically show findings of a mild sensorimotor axonal polyneuropathy and prominent spontaneous activity (fibrillation and positive waves) with "myopathic" motor unit potentials in proximal muscles. Myotonic discharges may be prominent and may help to differentiate from other possibilities. The EMG changes are rapidly reversible upon discontinuation of the colchicine.[160] The muscle biopsy shows a vacuolar myopathy with accumulation of lysosomes and autophagic vacuoles without necrosis.

The mainstay of treatment is stopping colchicine at the first sign of myotoxicity. Weakness and EMG changes typically resolve promptly after it is discontinued. In order to prevent colchicine myopathy in patients with reduced creatinine clearances of 50 mL/min or less, it is recommended that the dose be no greater than 0.6 mg twice a day.[161] Colchicine should not be administered to patients with creatinine clearances below 10 mL/min or who require dialysis, because it is not removed by dialysis. A reduced dose of the medication is also recommended for patients with reduced muscle mass.

Chloroquine Neuromyopathy

Chloroquine is an antimalarial medication that at higher doses has been widely used for inflammatory conditions such as sarcoidosis, systemic lupus erythematosus, scleroderma, and rheumatoid arthritis. Its most notable side effect is retinal toxicity, but skin problems, anorexia, nausea, vomiting, diarrhea, dizziness, tinnitus, and headache are also seen. Less-common side effects include myasthenia-like syndrome, cardiomyopathy, and neuromyotoxicity.

The myopathy and neuropathy usually occur after long-term use (months or years) and at high doses above the daily 500 mg range. Clinically, patients present with slowly progressive, painless proximal weakness and atrophy, mostly notably in the lower extremities. The weakness may involve the trunk and the facial muscles if the medication is not discontinued.[156] Patients can also exhibit depressed deep tendon reflexes and distal sensory loss on examination. Serum CK is usually normal or only mildly elevated. In some instances, it may resemble acid maltase deficiency with respiratory failure and cardiomyopathy. Factors that may predispose patients to develop chloroquine myopathy include renal dysfunction and concomitant use of ciprofloxacin and nonsteroidal anti-inflammatory drugs. Nerve conduction studies may be normal or show findings consistent with a mild sensorimotor axonal polyneuropathy. The needle EMG shows increased insertional as well as spontaneous activity (fibrillations and positive waves), mostly in proximal limb muscles. Motor unit action potentials are mostly polyphasic with decreased amplitude and duration. Muscle biopsy shows involvement of type 1 fibers primarily with acid-phosphatase positive vacuoles in as many as 50% of the skeletal and cardiac muscle fibers.[152] With electron microscopy, these vacuoles are seen to contain myeloid debris and curvilinear structures identical to those seen in patients with neuronal ceroid lipofuscinosis. Hydroxychloroquine also produces a neuromyopathy, but toxicity is less severe. In case of both medications, the symptoms are relieved after discontinuation, although recovery may not be complete.

In addition to myopathy and neuropathy, some patients exposed to chloroquine have developed a myasthenia-like syndrome (as discussed above), with ptosis, extraocular muscle weakness, fatigue, and response to edrophonium.[162] This may present shortly after starting therapy or after weeks or months of treatment. It usually resolves promptly after discontinuation of the medication, although symptoms may recur if the medication is reintroduced.

Other Medications

Many other medications have been reported to cause neuropathy (see Box 15-1) and myopathy. Of these, amiodarone, a commonly used antiarrhythmic agent has been associated with CNS disorders characterized by tremors, ataxia, and optic neuropathy and with a peripheral neuropathy and a myopathy.[163,164] Amiodarone neuropathy could be predominantly demyelinating, axonal, or both. Clinical and biopsy findings in myopathy are nonspecific. Rare cases might develop rhabdomyolysis.[165]

Nerve biopsy on amiodarone neuropathy demonstrates loss of myelinated axons with regeneration and osmiophilic inclusions (Fig. 15-4).

The treatment is usually conservative and consists primarily of withdrawal of the medication.

Biologic Toxins

Many biologic toxins are the cause of central or peripheral nervous system complications. Some are discussed in previous chapters: tetanus (see Chapter 17), botulism, snake bites, and tick paralysis (see Chapter 18).

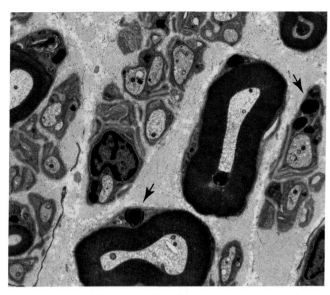

Figure 15-4 Amiodarone neuropathy. Electron microscopy on sural nerve biopsy showing osmiophilic inclusions in cytoplasm of Schwann cells (*arrows*) (×10,000). (Reprinted with permission from Bertorini TE: *Neuromuscular Case Studies*. Woburn, MA: Butterworth-Heinemann, 2008.)

Marine toxins can affect the central and peripheral nervous systems (Table 15-2).[166] Of these, ciguatera is the most common fish poisoning.[167] It results from the ingestion of a toxin in contaminated fish infected with the dinoflagellate *Gambierdiscus toxicus*, and the symptoms are caused by the activation of sodium channels.[168]

Table 15-2 Standard Treatments for Marine and Biologic Toxins

Indication	Drug/Treatment	Dose	Route	Serious Drug Side Effects
Ciguatera	Mannitol*	1 g/kg of a 20% solution	IV	Dehydration, hypotension, electrolyte imbalance
Tetrodotoxin ingestion	Pulmonary resuscitation	—	—	—
Scombroid poisoning	Cimetidine	300 mg	IV	Agitation, confusion, hallucinations, Steven-Johnson syndrome
	Diphenhydramine	10–50 mg	PO/IV/IM	Confusion, agitation, seizures
Pfiesteria	Cholestyramine	9 g qid for 2 weeks	PO	Constipation, pancreatitis
Jellyfish sting	Topical vinegar/hot water immersion 45–50° C, 113–120° F	—	—	—
	Antivenin (Chironex)	See package insert	IV/IM	Serum sickness, anaphylaxis
Venomous fish	Antivenin where available	See package insert	IV/IM	Serum sickness, anaphylaxis
	Heat therapy	—	—	—
Cone snail bite	Pulmonary resuscitation	—	—	—
Snake bites	Pulmonary resuscitation, hemodialysis with myotoxicity	—	—	—
Eastern coral snake bite	Coral snake antivenin	See package insert	IV/IM	Serum sickness, anaphylaxis
Viper bite	Crotalidae antivenin	See package insert	IV/IM	Serum sickness, anaphylaxis
Sea snake bite	Sea snake antivenin	See package insert	IV/IM	Serum sickness, anaphylaxis
Datura species poisoning	Physostigmine	0.5–2 mg; may repeat q 10–30 min prn	IM or slow IV (not > 1 mg/min IV)	Hypersalivation, dyspnea, seizures
Amanita phalloides mushroom poisoning	Liver transplant	—	—	—

Continued

Table 15-2 Standard Treatments for Marine and Biologic Toxins—Cont'd

Indication	Drug/Treatment	Dose	Route	Serious Drug Side Effects
Gyromitra mushroom poisoning	Pyridoxine	25 mg/kg over 15–30 min; may be repeated prn to a total dose of 15–20 g/day	IV	Peripheral neuropathy, neuronopathy, seizures, headache
Muscarine poisoning	Atropine	1–2 mg initially; repeat prn q 20–30 min	IV/IM	Cardiac arrhythmias, respiratory depression
Psilocybin poisoning	Haloperidol (Haldol)	2–10 mg	IM/IV	Neuroleptic malignant syndrome, cardiac arrhythmias
	Diazepam	2–5 mg	IV/PO	Sedation
Black widow spider bite	Latrotoxin antivenin; Calcium gluconate	See package insert Adults: 500–800 mg IV of 10% solution (5–8 mL) Infants and children: 60–100 mg/kg (0.6–2 mL/kg)	IV	Hypotension, cardiac arrest, confusion, cardiac arrhythmias, atrioventricular block
Tick paralysis	Remove tick			

*Normal saline solution is also useful.
From Stommel E, Watters M: Marine toxins and assorted biological toxins. In Johnson R, Griffin J, McArthur J, eds. *Current Therapy in Neurologic Disease*, 7th ed. Philadelphia, 2006, Mosby.

Poisoned patients develop pain, diarrhea, vomiting, myalgia, paradoxical reversal temperature sensation,[169] paresthesias, and mood disorders. These start 20 minutes to 24 hours after exposure. Common cardiac symptoms include bradycardia, tachycardia, and orthostatic hypotension, and some patients develop a polyneuropathy or a myopathy.

Electrophysiologic testing could be normal or could show slowing of sensory conduction velocity,[170] but the diagnosis is based mainly on the clinical history.

The treatment has been intravenous 25% mannitol 1 g/kg,[171] although a recent study showed that mannitol is not superior to normal saline infusions.[172] Gabapentin improves the paresthesias.[173]

References

1. Arenas-Pinto A, Bhaskaran K, Dunn D, Weller IV: The risk of developing peripheral neuropathy induced by nucleoside reverse transcriptase inhibitors decreases over time: evidence from the Delta trial, *Antivir Ther* 13:289–295, 2008.
2. Cherry CL, Skolasky RL, Lal L, et al: Antiretroviral use and other risks for HIV-associated neuropathies in an international cohort, *Neurology* 66:867–873, 2006.
3. Schifitto G, McDermott MP, McArthur JC, et al: Markers of immune activation and viral load in HIV-associated sensory neuropathy, *Neurology* 64:842–848, 2005.
4. Keswani SC, Luciano CA, Pardo CA, et al: The spectrum of peripheral neuropathies in AIDS. In Gendelman HE, Grant I, Everall IP, et al, editors: *Neurology of AIDS*, New York, 2005, Oxford University Press, pp 423–443.
5. McArthur JC, Brew BJ, Nath A: Neurological complications of HIV infection, *Lancet Neurol* 4:543–555, 2005.
6. Authier FJ, Chariot P, Gherardi RK: Skeletal muscle involvement in human immunodeficiency virus (HIV)-infected patients in the era of highly active antiretroviral therapy (HAART), *Muscle Nerve* 32:247–260, 2005.
7. Dalakas MC: Virus-related muscle diseases. In Engel AG, Francini-Armstrong C, editors: *Myology*, 3rd ed, vol 2, New York, 2004, McGraw-Hill, pp 1396–1404.
8. Luciano CA, Pardo CA, McArthur JC: Recent developments in the HIV neuropathies, *Curr Opin Neurol* 16:403–409, 2003.
9. Piliero PJ, Fish DG, Preston S, et al: Guillain-Barré syndrome associated with immune reconstitution, *Clin Infect Dis* 36:111–114, 2003.
10. Teo EC, Azwra A, Jones RL, et al: Guillain-Barré syndrome following immune reconstitution after antiretroviral therapy for primary HIV infection, *J HIV Ther* 12:62–63, 2007.
11. Ferrari S, Vento S, Monaco S, et al: Human immunodeficiency virus-associated peripheral neuropathies, *Mayo Clin Proc* 81:213–219, 2006.
12. Cupler EJ, Leon-Monzon M, Miller J, et al: Inclusion body myositis in HIV-1 and HTLV-1 infected patients, *Brain* 119(Pt 6):1887–1893, 1996.
13. Tagliati M, Grinnell J, Godbold J, Simpson DM: Peripheral nerve function in HIV infection: clinical, electrophysiologic, and laboratory findings, *Arch Neurol* 56:84–89, 1999.
14. Hernandez-Ramos N, Luciano CA, Jordan-Gonzalez M, et al: Electrophysiologic Markers of HIV Sensory Neuropathy: Sensitivity and Specificity, 7th Conference of the Specialized Neuroscience Research Programs, New York, NY, August 2008.
15. Dalakas MC, Illa I, Pezeshkpour GH, et al: Mitochondrial myopathy caused by long-term zidovudine therapy, *N Engl J Med* 322:1098–1105, 1990.
16. Polydefkis M, Yiannoutsos CT, Cohen BA, et al: Reduced intraepidermal nerve fiber density in HIV-associated sensory neuropathy, *Neurology* 58:115–119, 2002.
17. Luciano CA, Ebenezer G, Skolasky R, et al: Correlates of cutaneous hyper-innervation in pediatric/adolescent HIV sensory neuropathy, *Neurology* 66:A191, 2006.
18. Herrmann DN, McDermott MP, Sowden JE, et al: Is skin biopsy a predictor of transition to symptomatic HIV neuropathy? A longitudinal study, *Neurology* 66:857–861, 2006.
19. Brannagan TH 3rd, Zhou Y: HIV-associated Guillain-Barré syndrome, *J Neurol Sci* 208:39–42, 2003.
19a. Martin C, Solders G, Sönnerborg A, Hansson P: Antiretroviral therapy may improve sensory function in HIV-infected patients: a pilot study, *Neurology* 54:2120–2127, 2000.
20. Hahn K, Arendt G, Braun JS, et al: A placebo-controlled trial of gabapentin for painful HIV-associated sensory neuropathies, *J Neurol* 251:1260–1266, 2004.
21. La Spina I, Porazzi D, Maggiolo F, et al: Gabapentin in painful HIV-related neuropathy: a report of 19 patients, preliminary observations, *Eur J Neurol* 8:71–75, 2001.
22. Simpson DM, Schifitto G, Clifford DB, et al: Pregabalin for painful HIV neuropathy: a randomized, double-blind, placebo-controlled trial, *Neurology* 74:413–420, 2010.

23. Schifitto G, Yiannoutsos CT, Simpson DM, et al: A placebo-controlled study of memantine for the treatment of human immunodeficiency virus-associated sensory neuropathy, *J Neurovirol* 12:328–331, 2006.

24. Kieburtz K, Simpson D, Yiannoutsos C, et al: A randomized trial of amitriptyline and mexiletine for painful neuropathy in HIV infection. AIDS Clinical Trial Group 242 Protocol Team, *Neurology* 51:1682–1688, 1998.

25. Brew BJ: The peripheral nerve complications of human immunodeficiency virus (HIV) infection, *Muscle Nerve* 28:542–552, 2003.

26. Simpson DM, Brown S, Tobias J: Controlled trial of high-concentration capsaicin patch for treatment of painful HIV neuropathy, *Neurology* 70:2305–2313, 2008.

27. Abrams DI, Jay CA, Shade SB, et al: Cannabis in painful HIV-associated sensory neuropathy: a randomized placebo-controlled trial, *Neurology* 68:515–521, 2007.

28. Schleicher GK, Black A, Mochan A, Richards GA: Effect of human immunodeficiency virus on intensive care unit outcome of patients with Guillain-Barré syndrome, *Crit Care Med* 31:1848–1850, 2003.

29. Johnson RW, Williams FM, Kazi S, et al: Human immunodeficiency virus-associated polymyositis: a longitudinal study of outcome, *Arthritis Rheum* 49:172–178, 2003.

30. de Sanctis JT, Cumbo-Nacheli G, Dobbie D, Baumgartner D: HIV-associated nemaline rod myopathy: role of intravenous immunoglobulin therapy in two persons with HIV/AIDS, *AIDS Read* 18:90–94, 2008.

31. Dwyer BA, Mayer RF, Lee SC: Progressive nemaline (rod) myopathy as a presentation of human immunodeficiency virus infection, *Arch Neurol* 49:440, 1992.

32. Nash D, Mostashari F, Fine A, et al: The outbreak of West Nile virus infection in the New York City area in 1999, *N Engl J Med* 344:1807–1814, 2001.

33. Hayes EB, Komar N, Nasci RS, Montgomery SP, O'Leary DR, Campbell GL: Epidemiology and transmission dynamics of West Nile virus disease, *Emerg Infect Dis* 11:1167–1173, 2005.

34. Hayes EB, Sejvar JJ, Zaki SR, et al: Virology, pathology, and clinical manifestations of West Nile virus disease, *Emerg Infect Dis* 11:1174–1179, 2005.

35. Davis LE, DeBiasi R, Goade DE, et al: West Nile virus neuroinvasive disease, *Ann Neurol* 60:286–300, 2006.

36. Sejvar JJ, Bode AV, Marfin AA, et al: West Nile virus–associated flaccid paralysis outcome, *Emerg Infect Dis* 12:514–516, 2006.

37. Sejvar JJ, Haddad MB, Tierney BC, et al: Neurologic manifestations and outcome of West Nile virus infection, *JAMA* 290:511–515, 2003.

38. Debiasi RL, Tyler KL: West Nile virus meningoencephalitis, *Nat Clin Pract Neurol* 2:264–275, 2006.

39. Kramer LD, Li J, Shi PY: West Nile virus, *Lancet Neurol* 6:171–181, 2007.

40. Leis AA, Stokic DS, Webb RM, et al: Clinical spectrum of muscle weakness in human West Nile virus infection, *Muscle Nerve* 28:302–308, 2003.

41. Li J, Loeb JA, Shy ME, et al: Asymmetric flaccid paralysis: a neuromuscular presentation of West Nile virus infection, *Ann Neurol* 53:703–710, 2003.

42. Al-Shekhlee A, Katirji B: Electrodiagnostic features of acute paralytic poliomyelitis associated with West Nile virus infection, *Muscle Nerve* 29:376–380, 2004.

43. Saad M, Youssef S, Kirschke D, et al: Acute flaccid paralysis: the spectrum of a newly recognized complication of West Nile virus infection, *J Infect* 51:120–127, 2005.

44. Cao NJ, Ranganathan C, Kupsky WJ, Li J: Recovery and prognosticators of paralysis in West Nile virus infection, *J Neurol Sci* 236:73–80, 2005.

45. Petersen LR, Roehrig JT, Hughes JM: West Nile virus encephalitis, *N Engl J Med* 347:1225–1226, 2002.

46. Tyler KL, Pape J, Goody RJ, et al: CSF findings in 250 patients with serologically confirmed West Nile virus meningitis and encephalitis, *Neurology* 66:361–365, 2006.

47. Ali M, Safriel Y, Sohi J, et al: West Nile virus infection: MR imaging findings in the nervous system, *AJNR Am J Neuroradiol* 26:289–297, 2005.

48. Petropoulou KA, Gordon SM, Prayson RA, Ruggierri PM: West Nile virus meningoencephalitis: MR imaging findings, *AJNR Am J Neuroradiol* 26:1986–1995, 2005.

49. Jeha LE, Sila CA, Lederman RJ, et al: West Nile virus infection: a new acute paralytic illness, *Neurology* 61:55–59, 2003.

50. Marciniak C, Rosenfeld EL: Serial electrodiagnostic studies in West Nile virus-associated acute flaccid paralysis, *Am J Phys Med Rehabil* 84:904–910, 2005.

51. Haley M, Retter AS, Fowler D, et al: The role for intravenous immunoglobulin in the treatment of West Nile virus encephalitis, *Clin Infect Dis* 37:88–90, 2003.

52. Shimoni Z, Niven MJ, Pitlick S, Bulvik S: Treatment of West Nile virus encephalitis with intravenous immunoglobulin, *Emerg Infect Dis* 7:759, 2001.

53. Kalil AC, Devetten MP, Singh S, et al: Use of interferon-alpha in patients with West Nile encephalitis: report of 2 cases, *Clin Infect Dis* 40:764–766, 2005.

54. Sayao AL, Suchowersky O, Al-Khathaami A, et al: Calgary experience with West Nile virus neurological syndrome during the late summer of 2003, *Can J Neurol Sci* 31:194–203, 2004.

55. Pyrgos V, Younus F: High-dose steroids in the management of acute flaccid paralysis due to West Nile virus infection, *Scand J Infect Dis* 36:509–512, 2004.

56. Berner Y, Feldman J, Spigel D, et al: Rehabilitation of West Nile fever (WNF) encephalitis in elderly, *Arch Gerontol Geriatr* 41:15–21, 2005.

57. Marciniak C, Sorosky S, Hynes C: Acute flaccid paralysis associated with West Nile virus: motor and functional improvement in 4 patients, *Arch Phys Med Rehabil* 85:1933–1938, 2004.

58. Klee AL, Maidin B, Edwin B, et al: Long-term prognosis for clinical West Nile virus infection, *Emerg Infect Dis* 10:1405–1411, 2004.

59. Sejvar JJ: The long-term outcomes of human West Nile virus infection, *Clin Infect Dis* 44:1617–1624, 2007.

60. Watson JT, Pertel PE, Jones RC, et al: Clinical characteristics and functional outcomes of West Nile fever, *Ann Intern Med* 141:360–365, 2004.

61. Berner YN, Lang R, Chowers MY: Outcome of West Nile fever in older adults, *J Am Geriatr Soc* 50:1844–1846, 2002.

62. Bacon RM, Kugeler KJ, Mead PS: Surveillance for Lyme disease—United States, 1992–2006, *MMWR Surveill Summ* 57:1–9, 2008.

63. Hildenbrand P, Craven DE, Jones R, Nemeskal P: Lyme neuroborreliosis: manifestations of a rapidly emerging zoonosis, *AJNR Am J Neuroradiol* 30:1079–1087, 2009.

64. Pachner AR, Steiner I: Lyme neuroborreliosis: infection, immunity, and inflammation, *Lancet Neurol* 6:544–552, 2007.

65. Pachner AR, Steere AC: The triad of neurologic manifestations of Lyme disease: meningitis, cranial neuritis, and radiculoneuritis, *Neurology* 35:47–53, 1985.

66. Steere AC: Lyme disease, *N Engl J Med* 345:115–125, 2001.

67. Dandache P, Nadelman RB: Erythema migrans, *Infect Dis Clin North Am* 22:235–260, vi, 2008.

68. Mullegger RR, Glatz M: Skin manifestations of Lyme borreliosis: diagnosis and management, *Am J Clin Dermatol* 9:355–368, 2008.

69. Logigian EL, Kaplan RF, Steere AC: Chronic neurologic manifestations of Lyme disease, *N Engl J Med* 323:1438–1444, 1990.

70. Halperin JJ: Lyme disease and the peripheral nervous system, *Muscle Nerve* 28:133–143, 2003.

71. Thaisetthawatkul P, Logigian EL: Peripheral nervous system manifestations of Lyme borreliosis, *J Clin Neuromusc Dis* 3:165–171, 2002.

72. Halperin JJ: Facial nerve palsy associated with Lyme disease, *Muscle Nerve* 28:516–517, 2003.

73. Krishnamurthy KB, Liu GT, Logigian EL: Acute Lyme neuropathy presenting with polyradicular pain, abdominal protrusion, and cranial neuropathy, *Muscle Nerve* 16:1261–1264, 1993.

74. Logigian EL, Steere AC: Clinical and electrophysiologic findings in chronic neuropathy of Lyme disease, *Neurology* 42:303–311, 1992.

75. Kindstrand E, Nilsson BY, Hovmark A, et al: Peripheral neuropathy in acrodermatitis chronica atrophicans—a late *Borrelia* manifestation, *Acta Neurol Scand* 95:338–345, 1997.

76. Aguero-Rosenfeld ME, Wang G, Schwartz I, Wormser GP: Diagnosis of Lyme borreliosis, *Clin Microbiol Rev* 18:484–509, 2005.

77. Recommendations for test performance and interpretation from the Second National Conference on Serologic Diagnosis of Lyme Disease, *MMWR Morb Mortal Wkly Rep* 44:590–591, 1995.

78. Blanc F, Jaulhac B, Fleury M, et al: Relevance of the antibody index to diagnose Lyme neuroborreliosis among seropositive patients, *Neurology* 69:953–958, 2007.

79. Ljostad U, Skarpaas T, Mygland A: Clinical usefulness of intrathecal antibody testing in acute Lyme neuroborreliosis, *Eur J Neurol* 14:873–876, 2007.

80. Roos KL, Berger JR: Is the presence of antibodies in CSF sufficient to make a definitive diagnosis of Lyme disease? *Neurology* 69:949–950, 2007.

81. Stanek G, O'Connell S, Cimmino M, et al: European Union concerted action on risk assessment in Lyme borreliosis: clinical case definitions for Lyme borreliosis, *Wien Klin Wochenschr* 108:741–747, 1996.

82. Hammers-Berggren S, Hansen K, Lebech AM, Karlsson M: *Borrelia burgdorferi*–specific intrathecal antibody production in neuroborreliosis: a follow-up study, *Neurology* 43:169–175, 1993.

83. Halperin JJ: Nervous system Lyme disease, *Infect Dis Clin North Am* 22:261–274, vi, 2008.

84. Vallat JM, Hugon J, Lubeau M, et al: Tick-bite meningoradiculoneuritis: clinical, electrophysiologic, and histologic findings in 10 cases, *Neurology* 37:749–753, 1987.

85. Halperin JJ, Shapiro ED, Logigian E, et al: Practice parameter: treatment of nervous system Lyme disease (an evidence-based review): report of the Quality Standards Subcommittee of the American Academy of Neurology, *Neurology* 69:91–102, 2007.

86. Ljostad U, Skogvoll E, Eikeland R, et al: Oral doxycycline versus intravenous ceftriaxone for European Lyme neuroborreliosis: a multicentre, non-inferiority, double-blind, randomised trial, *Lancet Neurol* 7:690–695, 2008.

87. Halperin JJ: Prolonged Lyme disease treatment: enough is enough, *Neurology* 70:986–987, 2008.

88. Kruger H, Kohlhepp W, Konig S: Follow-up of antibiotically treated and untreated neuroborreliosis, *Acta Neurol Scand* 82:59–67, 1990.

89. Kalish RA, Kaplan RF, Taylor E, et al: Evaluation of study patients with Lyme disease, 10-20-year follow-up, *J Infect Dis* 183:453–460, 2001.

90. Berglund J, Stjernberg L, Ornstein K, et al: Five-year follow-up study of patients with neuroborreliosis, *Scand J Infect Dis* 34:421–425, 2002.

91. Baughman RP, Teirstein AS, Judson MA, et al: Clinical characteristics of patients in a case control study of sarcoidosis, *Am J Respir Crit Care Med* 164:1885–1889, 2001.

92. Burns TM: Neurosarcoidosis, *Arch Neurol* 60:1166–1168, 2003.

93. Burns TM, Dyck PJ, Aksamit AJ: The natural history and long-term outcome of 57 limb sarcoidosis neuropathy cases, *J Neurol Sci* 244:77–87, 2006.

94. Delaney P: Neurologic manifestations in sarcoidosis: review of the literature, with a report of 23 cases, *Ann Intern Med* 87:336–345, 1977.

95. Fayad F, Liote F, Berenbaum F, et al: Muscle involvement in sarcoidosis: a retrospective and followup studies, *J Rheumatol* 33:98–103, 2006.

96. Feder HM Jr, Johnson BJ, O'Connell S, et al: A critical appraisal of "chronic Lyme disease," *N Engl J Med* 357:1422–1430, 2007.

97. Hoitsma E, Faber CG, Drent M, Sharma OP: Neurosarcoidosis: a clinical dilemma, *Lancet Neurol* 3:397–407, 2004.

98. Joseph FG, Scolding NJ: Neurosarcoidosis: a study of 30 new cases, *J Neurol Neurosurg Psychiatry* 80:297–304, 2009.

99. Lower EE, Weiss KL: Neurosarcoidosis, *Clin Chest Med* 29:475–492, ix, 2008.

100. Oksanen V: Neurosarcoidosis: clinical presentations and course in 50 patients, *Acta Neurol Scand* 73:283–290, 1986.

101. Said G, Lacroix C, Plante-Bordeneuve V, et al: Nerve granulomas and vasculitis in sarcoid peripheral neuropathy: a clinicopathological study of 11 patients, *Brain* 125:264–275, 2002.

102. Scola RH, Werneck LC, Prevedello DM, et al: Symptomatic muscle involvement in neurosarcoidosis: a clinicopathological study of 5 cases, *Arq Neuropsiquiatr* 59:347–352, 2001.

103. Sepulveda-Sanchez JM, Villarejo-Galende A, Cabello A, et al: [Sarcoid myopathy. Report of two cases and review of the bibliography], *Rev Neurol* 41:159–162, 2005.

104. Silverstein A, Siltzbach LE: Muscle involvement in sarcoidosis. Asymptomatic, myositis, and myopathy, *Arch Neurol* 21:235–241, 1969.

105. Stern BJ, Krumholz A, Johns C, et al: Sarcoidosis and its neurological manifestations, *Arch Neurol* 42:909–917, 1985.

106. Stjernberg N, Cajander S, Truedsson H, Uddenfeldt P: Muscle involvement in sarcoidosis, *Acta Med Scand* 209:213–216, 1981.

107. Wilder-Smith EP, Van Brakel WH: Nerve damage in leprosy and its management, *Nat Clin Pract Neurol* 4:656–663, 2008.

108. van Brakel WH, Nicholls PG, Wilder-Smith EP, et al: Early diagnosis of neuropathy in leprosy-comparing diagnostic tests in a large prospective study (the INFIR Cohort Study), *PLoS Negl Trop Dis* 2:e212, 2008.

109. Araujo AQ, Silva MT: The HTLV-1 neurological complex, *Lancet Neurol* 5:1068–1076, 2006.

110. Croda MG, de Oliveira AC, Vergara MP, et al: Corticosteroid therapy in TSP/HAM patients: the results from a 10 years open cohort, *J Neurol Sci* 269:133–137, 2008.

111. Gilbert DT, Morgan O, Smikle MF, et al: HTLV-1 associated polymyositis in Jamaica, *Acta Neurol Scand* 104:101–104, 2001.

112. Crum-Cianflone NF: Bacterial, fungal, parasitic, and viral myositis, *Clin Microbiol Rev* 21:473–494, 2008.

113. Agyeman P, Duppenthaler A, Heininger U, Aebi C: Influenza-associated myositis in children, *Infection* 32:199–203, 2004.

114. Banker B: Parasitic myositis. In Engel A, Franzini-Armstrong C, editors: *Myology*, vol 2, New York, 2004, McGraw-Hill, pp 1419–1443.

115. Steininger C: Clinical relevance of cytomegalovirus infection in patients with disorders of the immune system, *Clin Microbiol Infect* 13:953–963, 2007.

116. Vahidnia A, van der Voet GB, de Wolff FA: Arsenic neurotoxicity—a review, *Hum Exp Toxicol* 26:823–832, 2007.

117. Ibrahim D, Froberg B, Wolf A, Rusyniak DE: Heavy metal poisoning: clinical presentations and pathophysiology, *Clin Lab Med* 26:67–97, viii, 2006.

118. London Z, Albers JW: Toxic neuropathies associated with pharmaceutic and industrial agents, *Neurol Clin* 25:257–276, 2007.

119. Kumar N: Industrial and environmental toxins. In Miller A, editor: *Continuum*, vol 14, Philadelphia, 2008, Lippincott Williams & Wilkins, pp 102–137.

120. Rubens O, Logina I, Kravale I, et al: Peripheral neuropathy in chronic occupational inorganic lead exposure: a clinical and electrophysiological study, *J Neurol Neurosurg Psychiatry* 71:200–204, 2001.

121. Kosnett MJ, Wedeen RP, Rothenberg SJ, et al: Recommendations for medical management of adult lead exposure, *Environ Health Perspect* 115:463–471, 2007.

122. Windebank A: Metal neuropathy. In Dyck P, Thomas P, editors: *Peripheral Neuropathy*, vol 2, Philadelphia, 2005, Saunders, pp 2527–2551.

123. Smith AG, Albers JW: *n*-Hexane neuropathy due to rubber cement sniffing, *Muscle Nerve* 20:1445–1450, 1997.

124. Vittadini G, Buonocore M, Colli G, et al: Alcoholic polyneuropathy: a clinical and epidemiological study, *Alcohol Alcohol* 36:393–400, 2001.

125. Koike H, Iijima M, Sugiura M, et al: Alcoholic neuropathy is clinicopathologically distinct from thiamine-deficiency neuropathy, *Ann Neurol* 54:19–29, 2003.

126. Koike H, Sobue G: Alcoholic neuropathy, *Curr Opin Neurol* 19:481–486, 2006.

127. Zambelis T, Karandreas N, Tzavellas E, et al: Large and small fiber neuropathy in chronic alcohol-dependent subjects, *J Peripher Nerv Syst* 10:375–381, 2005.

128. Woelk H, Lehrl S, Bitsch R, Kopcke W: Benfotiamine in treatment of alcoholic polyneuropathy: an 8-week randomized controlled study (BAP I Study), *Alcohol Alcohol* 33:631–638, 1998.

129. Peters TJ, Kotowicz J, Nyka W, et al: Treatment of alcoholic polyneuropathy with vitamin B complex: a randomised controlled trial, *Alcohol Alcohol* 41:636–642, 2006.

130. Weimer LH, Podwall D: Medication-induced exacerbation of neuropathy in Charcot Marie Tooth disease, *J Neurol Sci* 242:47–54, 2006.

131. Walker M, Ni O: Neuroprotection during chemotherapy: a systematic review, *Am J Clin Oncol* 30:82–92, 2007.

132. Malik B, Stillman M: Chemotherapy-induced peripheral neuropathy, *Curr Pain Headache Rep* 12:165–174, 2008.

133. Gamelin L, Boisdron-Celle M, Delva R, et al: Prevention of oxaliplatin-related neurotoxicity by calcium and magnesium infusions: a retrospective study of 161 patients receiving oxaliplatin combined with 5-fluorouracil and leucovorin for advanced colorectal cancer, *Clin Cancer Res* 10:4055–4061, 2004.

134. Windebank AJ, Grisold W: Chemotherapy-induced neuropathy, *J Peripher Nerv Syst* 13:27–46, 2008.

135. Kaley TJ, Deangelis LM: Therapy of chemotherapy-induced peripheral neuropathy, *Br J Haematol* 145:3–14, 2009.

136. Stubgen JP: Tumor necrosis factor-alpha antagonists and neuropathy, *Muscle Nerve* 37:281–292, 2008.

137. Lozeron P, Denier C, Lacroix C, Adams D: Long-term course of demyelinating neuropathies occurring during tumor necrosis factor-alpha–blocker therapy, *Arch Neurol* 66:490–497, 2009.

138. Youle M: HIV-associated antiretroviral toxic neuropathy (ATN): a review of recent advances in pathophysiology and treatment, *Antivir Ther* 10 (Suppl 2):M125–M129, 2005.

139. Lichtenstein KA, Armon C, Baron A, et al: Modification of the incidence of drug-associated symmetrical peripheral neuropathy by host and disease factors in the HIV outpatient study cohort, *Clin Infect Dis* 40:148–157, 2005.

140. Pettersen JA, Jones G, Worthington C, et al: Sensory neuropathy in human immunodeficiency virus/acquired immunodeficiency syndrome patients: protease inhibitor-mediated neurotoxicity, *Ann Neurol* 59:816–824, 2006.

141. Smyth K, Affandi JS, McArthur JC, et al: Prevalence of and risk factors for HIV-associated neuropathy in Melbourne, Australia 1993–2006, *HIV Med* 8:367–373, 2007.

142. Ellis RJ, Marquie-Beck J, Delaney P, et al: Human immunodeficiency virus protease inhibitors and risk for peripheral neuropathy, *Ann Neurol* 64:566–572, 2008.

143. Hart AM, Wilson AD, Montovani C, et al: Acetyl-L-carnitine: a pathogenesis based treatment for HIV-associated antiretroviral toxic neuropathy, *AIDS* 18:1549–1560, 2004.

144. Valcour V, Yeh TM, Bartt R, et al: Acetyl-L-carnitine and nucleoside reverse transcriptase inhibitor-associated neuropathy in HIV infection, *HIV Med* 10:103–110, 2009.

145. Simpson DM, McArthur JC, Olney R, et al: Lamotrigine for HIV-associated painful sensory neuropathies: a placebo-controlled trial, *Neurology* 60:1508–1514, 2003.

146. Silver M, Blum D, Grainger J, et al: Double-blind, placebo-controlled trial of lamotrigine in combination with other medications for neuropathic pain, *J Pain Symptom Manage* 34:446–454, 2007.

147. Evans M, Rees A: Effects of HMG-CoA reductase inhibitors on skeletal muscle: are all statins the same? *Drug Saf* 25:649–663, 2002.

148. Pasternak RC, Smith SC Jr, Bairey-Merz CN, et al: ACC/AHA/NHLBI Clinical Advisory on the Use and Safety of Statins, *Stroke* 33:2337–2341, 2002.

149. Dalakas MC: Toxic and drug-induced myopathies, *J Neurol Neurosurg Psychiatry* 80:832–838, 2009.

150. Baker SK, Samjoo IA: A neuromuscular approach to statin-related myotoxicity, *Can J Neurol Sci* 35:8–21, 2008.

151. Bannwarth B: Drug-induced musculoskeletal disorders, *Drug Saf* 30:27–46, 2007.

152. Walsh RJ, Amato AA: Toxic myopathies, *Neurol Clin* 23:397–428, 2005.

153. Klopstock T: Drug-induced myopathies, *Curr Opin Neurol* 21:590–595, 2008.

154. Ubogu E, Ruff R, Kaminski H: Endocrine myopathies. In Engel A, Franzini-Armstrong C, editors: *Myology*, 3rd ed, vol 2, New York, 2004, McGraw-Hill, pp 1713–1738.

155. Owczarek J, Jasinska M, Orszulak-Michalak D: Drug-induced myopathies. An overview of the possible mechanisms, *Pharmacol Rep* 57:23–34, 2005.

156. Sieb JP, Gillessen T: Iatrogenic and toxic myopathies, *Muscle Nerve* 27:142–156, 2003.

157. Scruggs ER, Dirks Naylor AJ: Mechanisms of zidovudine-induced mitochondrial toxicity and myopathy, *Pharmacology* 82:83–88, 2008.

158. Lebrecht D, Deveaud C, Beauvoit B, et al: Uridine supplementation antagonizes zidovudine-induced mitochondrial myopathy and hyperlactatemia in mice, *Arthritis Rheum* 58:318–326, 2008.

159. Baker SK, Goodwin S, Sur M, Tarnopolsky MA: Cytoskeletal myotoxicity from simvastatin and colchicine, *Muscle Nerve* 30:799–802, 2004.

160. Kuncl RW, Cornblath DR, Avila O, Duncan G: Electrodiagnosis of human colchicine myoneuropathy, *Muscle Nerve* 12:360–364, 1989.

161. Wilbur K, Makowsky M: Colchicine myotoxicity: case reports and literature review, *Pharmacotherapy* 24:1784–1792, 2004.

162. Robberecht W, Bednarik J, Bourgeois P, et al: Myasthenic syndrome caused by direct effect of chloroquine on neuromuscular junction, *Arch Neurol* 46:464–468, 1989.

163. Meier C, Kauer B, Müller U, Ludin HP: Neuromyopathy during chronic amiodarone treatment, A case report, *J Neurol* 220:231–239, 1979.

164. Fernando Roth R, Itabashi H, Louie J, et al: Amiodarone toxicity: Myopathy and neuropathy, *Am Heart J* 199:1223–1225, 1990.

165. Clouston PD, Donnelly PE: Acute necrotising myopathy associated with amiodarone treatment, *Aust N Z J Med* 19:483–485, 1989.

166. Lewis R: Ciguatera (fish poisoning). In Williamson J, Fenner P, Burnett J, Rifkin J, editors: *Venomous and Poisonous Marine Animals: A Medical and Biological Handbook*, Sidney, 1996, New South Wales University Press, pp 347–353.

167. Levine DZ: Ciguatera: current concepts, *J Am Osteopath Assoc* 95:193–198, 1995.

168. Bidard JN, Vijverberg HP, Frelin C, et al: Ciguatoxin is a novel type of Na^+ channel toxin, *J Biol Chem* 259:8353–8357, 1984.

169. Cameron J, Capra MF: The basis of the paradoxical disturbance of temperature perception in ciguatera poisoning, *J Toxicol Clin Toxicol* 31:571–579, 1993.

170. Cameron J, Flowers AE, Capra MF: Electrophysiological studies on ciguatera poisoning in man (Part II), *J Neurol Sci* 101:93–97, 1991.

171. Palafox NA, Jain LG, Pinano AZ, et al: Successful treatment of ciguatera fish poisoning with intravenous mannitol, *JAMA* 259:2740–2742, 1988.

172. Schnorf H, Taurarii M, Cundy T: Ciguatera fish poisoning: a double-blind randomized trial of mannitol therapy, *Neurology* 58:873–880, 2002.

173. Perez CM, Vasquez PA, Perret CF: Treatment of ciguatera poisoning with gabapentin, *N Engl J Med* 344:692–693, 2001.

William W. Campbell, Jr., MD

Treatment and Management of Segmental Neuromuscular Disorders

This chapter is devoted to focal disorders of the peripheral nervous system, including radiculopathies, plexopathies, and mononeuropathies. These conditions span a broad range of disorders, from radiculopathy due to Lyme disease and obturator neuropathy at the extremes of rarity to very common disorders such as cervical radiculopathy and carpal tunnel syndrome. This group of disorders makes up a large portion of neuromuscular medicine practice and only on a rare day will the neuromuscular clinician fail to see a patient with one of these conditions; on most days, this specialist is likely to see several. Intimate familiarity with the pathoanatomy, pathophysiology, clinical features, diagnosis, evaluation, and treatment of these conditions is necessary. This chapter is intended to provide a solid basis for acquiring the required expertise.

Radiculopathy

The intervertebral disk is the largest avascular structure in the body, depending for sustenance on the diffusion of nutrients across the endplate. The disks begin to desiccate and lose elasticity in the fifth and sixth decades; individuals in this age group are prone to intervertebral disk rupture. In the seventh to ninth decades, the tendency is to hardening and calcification, resulting in cervical spondylosis and spinal stenosis.

Clinical Pathoanatomy

Knowledge of the anatomic details of the spine and the spinal nerves is integral to managing patients with suspected radiculopathy. The vertebrae are separated by intervertebral disks, which are composed of an outer fibrous ring, the annulus fibrosus, and an inner gelatinous core, the nucleus pulposus (NP). The lateral recess is the corner formed by the pedicle, vertebral body, and superior articular facet. Hypertrophy of the facet can cause lateral recess stenosis.

The spinal nerve passes outward from the spinal canal through the intervertebral foramen, a passageway formed by the vertebral body anteriorly, pedicles above and below, and the facet mass and its articulation, the zygapophyseal joint, posteriorly. The uncovertebral joints (of Luschka), which are not true joints, are the points where the posterolateral surface of a cervical vertebra comes into apposition with a neighboring vertebra. Degenerative osteophytes projecting into the intervertebral foramen from the uncovertebral "joints" may narrow it and cause radiculopathy (Fig. 16-1).

The posterior longitudinal ligament (PLL) extends along the posterior aspect of the vertebral bodies and reinforces the disks posteriorly. The PLL is weak and flimsy and narrows as it descends. Disk herniations tend to occur posterolaterally, especially in the lumbosacral region, in part because of the lateral incompleteness of the PLL (Fig. 16-2). In the cervical region, the PLL may ossify and contribute to spondylotic narrowing. The ligamentum flavum extends along the posterior aspect of the spinal canal. It buckles and folds during neck extension and may also contribute to canal narrowing.

The static anatomy of the spine provides only a partial understanding of the changes that occur on motion. Direct measurements have shown that the pressure within the lumbar disk varies markedly with different postures and activities. It is lowest when lying supine, increases 400% on standing, and increases a further 50% when leaning forward. The pressure is 40% higher when sitting than standing. The higher pressure when sitting is clinically relevant, as patients with lumbosacral disk ruptures characteristically have more pain sitting than standing. Eating meals from the mantelpiece is virtually pathognomonic. The intradiscal pressure during a sit-up is astronomical.

The size of the intervertebral foramina decreases with extension and with ipsilateral bending. In extension, the facet joints draw closer together and the posterior quadrants of the spinal canal narrow. The longitudinal and flavum ligaments alternately stretch and buckle during flexion and extension. Tethering by the dentate ligaments accentuates the mechanical stresses laterally. Cervical roots stretch with flexion and may angulate at the entrance to the foramen. The intraspinal subarachnoid pressure varies with respiration and increases markedly with Valsalva or restriction of venous outflow. Like veins everywhere, the epidural and radicular veins change in size with posture and respiration. All these dynamic changes, which are especially relevant in the presence of disease, form the basis for clinical tests and historical questions useful for distinguishing the various causes for neck pain.

The annulus provides circumferential reinforcement for the disk; the spherical NP allows the vertebral bodies above and below to glide and slip across it, like a ball bearing. The NP is eccentrically

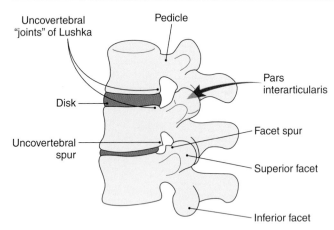

Figure 16-1 Lateral view of the cervical spine, showing the vertebral bodies separated by intervertebral disks, the pedicles merging into the facet joint with its superior and inferior facets, and intervening pars interarticularis. The facets are oblique in the cervical region, more vertical in the lumbosacral spine. The uncovertebral joints are not true joints, but just the opposing surfaces of the vertebral bodies. The uncovertebral processes may form osteophytes, or "spurs," which then project into the foramen.

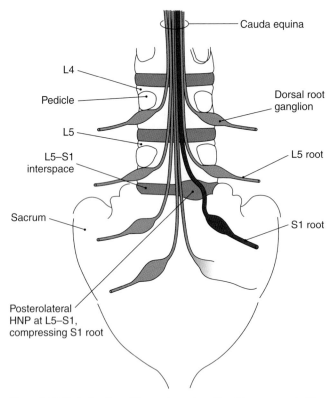

Figure 16-2 Posterior view of the cauda equina with exiting nerve roots. The nerve roots move laterally en route to their exit foramina. A posterolateral herniated nucleus pulposis (HNP) has compressed the S1 root as it passes by the L5–S1 interspace. The dorsal root ganglion lies well lateral and below, out of harm's way, so that the peripherally recorded sensory nerve action potential would not be affected. A central HNP at any interspace could affect multiple roots.

placed, closer to the posterior aspect of the disk. The relative thinness of the annulus posteriorly is another factor contributing to the tendency of disk herniations to occur in that direction.

The great majority of the weight-bearing function of a normal disk is borne by the NP, which contains proteoglycans,

macromolecules that heartily imbibe fluid. Early in life, the NP is 90% water, but it undergoes progressive desiccation over time. With desiccation of the NP and loss of compressibility, the annulus must assume more of the weight burden. This increased load, in the face of its own degenerative weakening, then makes the annulus prone to tears. Intradiscal proteoglycans are innocuous, but spilled into the epidural space in the course of disk rupture they can incite an inflammatory response. Other inflammatory mediators may be released by disk rupture, including the nitric oxide, prostaglandin E_2, and interleukin 6.

Spinal Roots

The spinal roots exit more or less horizontally in the cervical spine, although there is a slight downward slant. The downward slant increases through the thoracic region. When the cord terminates at the level of L1–2, the remaining roots drop vertically downward in the cauda equina to their exit foramina (see Fig. 16-2). In the cervical region, there is about a one segment discrepancy between the cord level and the spinous process, in the thoracic region about two segments, and in the lumbosacral region three to four segments. Therefore, the L5 nerve root exiting at the L5–S1 interspace has arisen as a discrete structure at L1–2 and had to traverse the interspaces at L2–3, L3–4, and L4–5 before exiting at L5–S1, sliding laterally all the while. So, the L5 root could be injured by a central disk at L2–3 or L3–4, a posterolateral disk at L4–5, or a far lateral disk or lateral recess stenosis at L5–S1. A posterolateral disk at L4–5 is the most likely culprit, but not the sole suspect. The clinician must correlate the clinical or electromyographic localization of a given root with the radiographic information to deduce the vertebral level involved and the proper course of action.

Pathology of Degenerative Spine Disease

With aging and recurrent micro- and macrotrauma, degenerative spine disease develops. This involves both the disk (degenerative disk disease, or DDD) and the bony structures and joints (degenerative joint disease, or DJD). These processes are separate but related. Together DDD and DJD are referred to as *spondylosis*.

Small tears in the annulus may cause nonspecific, nonradiating low back pain (LBP). More extensive tears lead to disk bulging or protrusion, in which the disk herniates but remains beneath the PLL. Frank ruptures breach the PLL and allow a full-blown herniation of the nucleus pulposus (HNP) into the epidural space. Most HNPs in the lumbosacral spine occur in a posterolateral direction; occasionally they are directly lateral or central (see Fig. 16-2). Which nerve roots are damaged depends largely on the direction of the herniation. In the face of disk herniation, the root may be damaged not only by direct compression but also by an inflammatory process induced by discal proteoglycans, ischemia due to pressure, and adhesions and fibrosis.

The anterior elements, vertebral body and pedicles, normally bear 80% to 90% of the weight. As degenerative changes advance with desiccation and loss of disk height, the posterior elements (facets, pars, and laminae) may come to carry up to 50% of the weight-bearing function. This increases the work of the posterior elements and accelerates their degenerative changes. They react to the increased weight-bearing role by becoming hypertrophic and elaborating osteophytes.

Osteoarthritis and synovitis of the facet joints is another source of problems. In response to the increased loading attendant on loss of disk height and shift of weight bearing posteriorly, the facet joints develop degenerative changes: laxity of the capsule, instability, subluxation, and bony hypertrophy with osteophyte formation. The friction induced by minor instability and microtrauma leads to the formation of osteophytes. In the cervical spine, there is the added element of hypertrophy of the uncinate processes and the development of uncovertebral spurs. Degenerative osteophytes arising simultaneously from the uncus and from the vertebral body end plate region may become confluent and create a spondylotic bar or ridge which stretches across the entire extent of the spinal canal. Like any arthritic joint, the facet may enlarge, impinging on the intervertebral foramen or the spinal canal, especially in the lateral recess. Loss of disk height causes the PLL and the ligamentum flavum to buckle and bulge into the canal. The degenerative changes in the disks and bony elements eventually may culminate in the syndrome of cervical spondylosis, with radiculopathy, myelopathy, or a combination of the two.

All these degenerative changes leave less room for the neural elements. In the sagittal plane, the average cervical spinal cord is about 8 mm and the average cervical spinal canal about 14 mm. A sagittal canal diameter less than 10 mm may put the spinal cord at risk. The epidural space is normally occupied primarily by epidural fat and veins. When disk herniations and osteophytes intrude into the space, the resultant clinical manifestations depend in large part on how much room there is to accommodate them. Patients with congenitally narrow canals and those who have undergone past spinal fusion procedures are at increased risk for developing spinal stenosis (Figs. 16-3 and 16-4). Compression of vascular structures may introduce an additional complication of cord or root ischemia.

Because of the varied pathologic processes involved, different types of radiculopathy occur in disk disease and spondylosis. The process is frequently multifactorial, involving some combination of disk herniation and spondylosis. The most straightforward clinical syndrome is unilateral "soft disk" rupture. A similar clinical picture can result from a foraminal osteophyte, a "hard disk" problem. Some patients have soft disk superimposed on hard disk involvement. It is clinically, radiologically, and sometimes surgically difficult to distinguish between soft disk and hard disk involvement. Osteophytes, spurs, and foraminal stenosis are more common than simple soft disk disease in the etiology of cervical radiculopathy (CR). In Radhakrishnan et al's series, soft disk disease (i.e., not present in

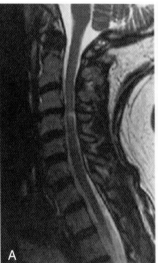
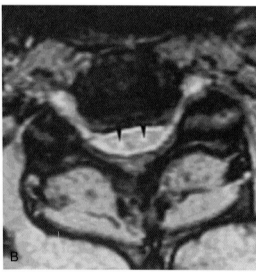

Figure 16-3 Cervical spondylotic myelopathy with myelomalacia. Sagittal (**A**) and axial (**B**), T2-weighted magnetic resonance images showing only moderate compression of the spinal cord at C3–4 level, and focal increased signal in the cord substance indicating that damage has occurred. On axial images this often has the appearance of "snake eyes" (*black arrowheads*) within the spinal cord. (From Adam A, Dixon AK, editors: *Grainger & Allison's Diagnostic Radiology*, 5th ed. London, 2008, Churchill Livingstone.)

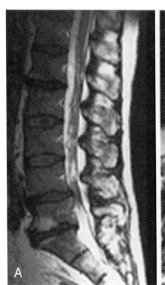
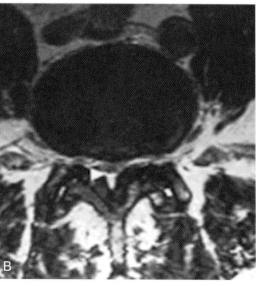

Figure 16-4 Degenerative spinal canal stenosis. Sagittal (**A**) and axial (**B**) T2-weighted magnetic resonance images of the lumbar spine showing a severe spinal canal stenosis at L4–5 with evidence of compression of the cauda equina, namely, obliteration of cerebrospinal fluid signal from the thecal sac at the site of compression (*white arrowhead*) and some redundant coiling of intrathecal spinal roots above. (From Adam A, Dixon AK, editors: *Grainger & Allison's Diagnostic Radiology*, 5th ed. London, 2008, Churchill Livingstone.)

association with significant spondylosis) was responsible in only 22%; the remainder had hard disk involvement or a combination.[1] A central HNP may compress the spinal cord.

Pathophysiology

The pathophysiology of radiculopathy is essentially the same regardless of etiology. Root compression due to HNP or spur tends to be concentrated on the distal portion of the root, proximal to the dorsal root ganglion (DRG). As with any nerve compression syndrome, the large myelinated fibers bear the brunt of the damage, and the degree of injury depends on the intensity and duration of the compressive force. Demyelination is the primary change with mild compression; more severe insults produce axon loss. Even with large lesions the damage is usually only partial. With recovery, remyelination and axon regrowth occur.

Electrodiagnosis

Electrodiagnosis will remain a mainstay in the evaluation of suspected radiculopathy for the foreseeable future. The general electrodiagnostic picture in radiculopathy includes normal motor and sensory conduction studies, with the needle electrode examination (NEE) disclosing abnormalities in a myotomal distribution, including the paraspinal muscles. Motor conduction abnormalities should reflect only axon loss, and even this is usually minimal. Sensory studies should be normal except for the very rare instance of an ectopic intraspinal dorsal root ganglion in the lumbosacral region.

The diagnosis of radiculopathy is based primarily on the NEE and primarily on the presence of fibrillation potentials. Normal muscles may contain complex or polyphasic potentials, and it is hazardous to diagnose radiculopathy on motor unit action potential (MUAP) changes in isolation unless there are flagrant abnormalities in a myotomal distribution, in which case fibrillation potentials will usually be present as well. For confident diagnosis, the abnormalities should involve at least two muscles sharing the same myotomal but different peripheral nerve innervations. The examination must be extensive enough to exclude a diffuse process.[2]

The timing of the study in relation to the onset of symptoms is pivotal. It generally requires 7 to 10 days for fibrillation potentials to appear in the paraspinal muscles, and 2 to 3 weeks in limb muscles. Reinnervation with disappearance of fibrillation potentials occurs in the same sequence after a variable delay. Thus, depending on the duration of the process, fibrillations could be found in any combination of limb and paraspinal muscles. The paraspinal findings are critical in the evaluation of radiculopathy patients, and it is important to specifically examine the muscles of the multifidus compartment.[3]

There are clear limitations of electromyography (EMG) in the diagnosis of radiculopathy, related to the multiple root innervation of most muscles, the variable relationship between the root level and the vertebral level of injury, the potential for reinnervation by collateral sprouts, the severity of the radicular lesion, and whether it involves axon loss or only demyelination. A normal study does not exclude radiculopathy.

Cervical Radiculopathy

A population-based study of CR provided a wealth of interesting information.[1] The incidence is highest at ages 50 to 54, with a mean age of 47 and a male predominance. Other series have also found a similar mean age and male predominance.[4] In the population-based study, there was a decline in incidence after age 60 (the patients are developing spondylosis and spinal stenosis). There was a history of physical injury or exertion in only 15%; the most common

precipitants were shoveling snow or playing golf. The onset was acute in half, subacute in a quarter, and insidious in a quarter, with the majority of patients symptomatic for about 2 weeks prior to diagnosis. Surgery was done in 26%. The disease tends to recur: 31% of patients had a previous history of CR and 32% had a recurrence during follow-up. At last follow-up, 90% of the patients had minimal to no symptoms. Others have noted this favorable long-term prognosis.

Clinical Signs and Symptoms

Two classic articles detail the history and examination findings in CR.[5,6] Yoss et al evaluated 100 patients with surgically confirmed single-level cervical radiculopathies (Table 16-1).[5] Murphey et al reviewed 648 cases of surgically treated single-level cervical radiculopathies.[6] Findings in terms of pain radiation and neurologic deficits were similar to those of Yoss et al. The Murphey series did emphasize the occurrence of pain in the pectoral region in 20% of their cases; they opined that neck, periscapular, and pectoral region pain was referred from the disk itself, and that arm pain was the result of nerve root compression.

In the Radhakrishnan series, cervicobrachial pain was present at the onset in 98% and was radicular in 65%.[1] Paresthesias were reported by 90%, almost identical to the Yoss series. Pain on neck movement was present in 98%, paraspinal muscle spasm in 88%, decreased reflexes in 84% (triceps 50%, biceps or brachioradialis 34%), weakness in 65%, and sensory loss in 33%. Employing their

Table 16-1 Clinical Findings in 100 Cervical Radiculopathy Patients

Clinical Finding	Highly Localizing to	Suggestively Localizing to
Pain only in neck and shoulder		C5
Presence of scapular/interscapular pain		C7 or C8
No pain below elbow		C5
Pain involving the posterior upper arm		C7
Pain involving the medial upper arm		C7 or C8
Paresthesias limited to the thumb	C6	
Paresthesias limited to index and middle	C7	
Paresthesias limited to ring and small	C8	
Whole hand paresthesias		C7
Depressed triceps reflex	C7 or C8	
Depressed biceps and brachioradialis reflexes	C5 or C6	
Weakness of spinatus	C5	
Weakness of deltoid	C5 or C6	
Weakness of triceps	C7	
Weakness of hand intrinsics	C8	
Sensory loss over thumb only		C6 or C7
Sensory loss involving middle finger	C7	
Sensory loss involving small finger	C8	

Modified from Yoss RE, Corbin KB, MacCarty CS, Love JG: Significance of symptoms and signs in localization of involved root in cervical disc protrusion, *Neurology* 7:673-683, 1957.

criteria, 45% of the patients were judged to have definite CR, 30% probable, and 25% possible. In a Cleveland Clinic series, 70% had motor and sensory symptoms, 12% had motor symptoms only, and 18% had sensory symptoms only.[7]

Localizing information in suspected CR is obtainable from the history, especially from patterns of pain radiation and paresthesias. Radiating pain on coughing, sneezing, or straining during a bowel movement is significant but seldom elicited. Increased pain on shoulder motion suggests nonradicular disease. Relief of pain by resting the hand atop the head is reportedly characteristic of CR (hand on head or shoulder abduction sign), but this phenomenon can occur with a Pancoast tumor.

Physical examination in patients with suspected CR should include an assessment of the range of motion of the neck and arm, a search for root compression signs, detailed examination of strength and reflexes, a screening sensory examination, and probing for areas of muscle spasm or trigger points.[8] The cervical spine range of motion is highly informative. Patients should be asked to put chin to chest and to either shoulder, each ear to shoulder, and to hold the head in full extension; these maneuvers all affect the size of the intervertebral foramen. Pain produced by movements that close the foramen suggest CR. Pain on the symptomatic side on putting the ipsilateral ear to the shoulder suggests radiculopathy, but increased pain on leaning or turning away from the symptomatic side suggests a myofascial origin. Radiating pain with the head in extension and tilted slightly to the symptomatic side is highly suggestive of CR; brief breath holding in this position will sometimes elicit the pain. The addition of axial compression (Spurling maneuver) does not seem to add much. Light digital compression of the jugular veins until the face is flushed and the patient is uncomfortable will sometimes elicit radicular symptoms: unilateral shoulder, arm, pectoral, or scapular pain or radiating paresthesias into the arm or hand (Viets or Naffziger sign). This is a highly specific but insensitive finding. An occasional patient has relief of pain with manual upward neck traction. Patients with a globally restricted cervical spine range of motion often have extensive degenerative disease. Patients with large disk ruptures or cervical spinal stenosis may have a positive Lhermitte sign on neck flexion.

Pain or limitation of motion of any upper extremity joint should signal the possibility of nonradicular disease. The patient should be asked to put the shoulder through a full active range of motion, touching the hand to the opposite shoulder and the opposite ear, then reaching behind as high between the scapulae as possible. Any pain or limitation of motion on the symptomatic side suggests bursitis, capsulitis, tendonitis, or impingement syndrome rather than CR as the cause of the patient's pain.

A focused but detailed strength examination should at least assess the power in the deltoids, spinatus, biceps, triceps, pronators, wrist extensors, abductor pollicis brevis, and interossei. The sensory examination should concentrate on the hand, and particularly assess touch, since the large, myelinated fibers conveying light touch are more vulnerable to pressure injury than the smaller fibers carrying pain and temperature. The reflex examination should include not only the standard upper extremity reflexes, but the knee and ankle jerks and plantar reflexes as well. Increased lower extremity reflexes and extensor plantar responses suggest myelopathy complicating the radiculopathy.

Based on the foregoing, Box 16-1 outlines the clinical data that favor the diagnosis of CR.

Evaluation and Diagnosis

Several different clinical syndromes may ensue from degenerative spine disease, including: simple, single-level radiculopathy; multilevel radiculopathy; cervical myelopathy; cervical radiculomyelopathy; and

Box 16-1 Features Favoring Cervical Radiculopathy as Opposed to Other Causes of Neck and Arm Pain

Age 35–60 years
Acute/subacute onset
Past history of cervical or lumbosacral radiculopathy
Cervicobrachial pain radiating to shoulder, periscapular region, pectoral region, or arm
Paresthesias in arm or hand
Pain on neck movement—especially extension or ipsilateral bending
Positive root compression signs
Radiating pain with cough, sneeze, or bowel movement
Myotomal weakness
Decreased reflex(es)
Dermatomal sensory loss
Pain relief with hand on top of head
Pain relief with manual upward traction

occasionally a central cord or Brown-Séquard syndrome. Rarely, radiculopathy results from other processes, such as tumor (e.g., neurofibroma, meningioma, metastasis), infection (e.g., Lyme disease, zoster, cytomegalovirus, syphilis), infiltration (e.g., meningeal neoplasia, sarcoidosis), or ischemia.[9] Diabetes commonly causes a lumbosacral radiculoplexopathy syndrome but can also frequently produce a painful thoracic radiculopathy often confused with herpes zoster and rarely a cervicobrachial radiculopathy.[10] With acute trauma, roots are sometimes injured along with the cervical spine or the brachial plexus, and in fact may be completely avulsed from the spinal cord in a severe brachial plexus injury. Acute and chronic inflammatory radiculoneuropathies commonly involve the roots.

A number of clinical conditions may be confused with CR, primarily brachial plexopathies, entrapment neuropathies, and non-neuropathic mimickers. The more common musculoskeletal conditions causing confusion include shoulder pathology (bursitis, tendinitis, impingement syndrome), lateral epicondylitis, and DeQuervain tenosynovitis. Cervical myofascial pain, facet joint disease, and cervical vertebral body disease can cause neck pain with referred pain to the arm. Patients with cervical strain due to whiplash rarely have radiculopathy. Lyme disease can cause meningitis and radiculitis, producing neck and arm pain. A rare patient with subarachnoid hemorrhage may present with neck pain without headache. Cervical epidural abscess or hematoma may present with neck pain and various neurologic signs. Pain can be referred to the neck, arm, or shoulder from the heart, lungs, esophagus, or upper abdomen.

A practice parameter was written by the AAEM Quality Assurance Committee lead authored by So, regarding EMG in CR. Because of indexing difficulty with PubMed the article is not retrievable but can be found at the American Association of Neuromuscular and Electrodiagnostic Medicine Web site: www.aanem.org (by members only) and in the 1999 *Muscle and Nerve* supplement issue.[11] The sensitivity of EMG for detecting abnormalities was in the range of 60% to 70%. The sensitivity is significantly higher in patients with motor involvement than in those with only pain or sensory abnormalities, and the yield increases with increasing severity of disease. Because EMG findings are rarely abnormal in normal subjects, the test is highly specific. There is generally a 65% to 85% correlation of EMG abnormalities with imaging and surgical findings. There is unanimity that C7 root lesions are the most common (±60%), C6 next most common (±20%), with C5 and C8 lesions making up about equal proportions of the remainder.[1,2,5–7]

The examiner should tailor EMG to probe the muscles most likely to be involved. In the absence of clear clinical direction, one must resort to a generic root screen. Choosing which muscles to study, and how many, has heretofore been a matter of personal opinion and preference. Recent investigations have provided some guidance. Lauder and Dillingham concluded that a screen of six limb muscles plus the paraspinals had a yield of 93% to 98%, and that examining more muscles made no significant additional contribution.[12] Levin et al studied 50 patients with surgically proven single-level cervical radiculopathies.[7] They found stereotyped patterns with C5, C7, and C8 lesions, but a variable pattern with C6 lesions which could resemble C5 or C7.

Plain cervical spine radiographs may show degenerative changes but are of little use in the diagnosis of a specific radiculopathy. Many asymptomatic patients have degenerative changes. Plain films, especially with flexion and extension views, may be useful in patients with more advanced disease to rule out any instability. Computed tomography (CT) is much more useful for visualizing bony detail but does not visualize neural structures unless contrast agent has been instilled (CT myelography). Plain myelography is rarely used. Magnetic resonance imaging (MRI) is the mainstay of diagnosis, although disk herniations are commonly observed on MRI in patients who have no symptoms, particularly in older patients. Careful clinical and electrodiagnostic correlation therefore remains essential.[8]

Treatment and Management

Treatment relies on three approaches: mechanical, medicinal, and surgical (Box 16-2). Nerve roots lying in the foramen normally enjoy freedom of movement through a small range. The size of the intervertebral foramen and the lateral recess changes dynamically with neck movement. The mainstay of conservative treatment is to reduce neck movement and increase the size of the foramen.

A soft cervical collar is usually helpful. For compressive CR, the collar should be worn "backward," with high side posterior to maintain neck in slight flexion and open the foramina. Hard collars cannot be turned around in this fashion and are not as useful for a radiculopathy syndrome as for myelopathy. The soft collar should be worn at night if tolerated; otherwise, the patient should use a cervical pillow. Prolonged use of a cervical collar may weaken neck muscles, so this method of treatment should be limited to a few weeks at most.

Cervical traction for 15 to 30 minutes three times a day is often very helpful; it distracts the spine, opens the foramina, and gives the involved root respite. An over-the-door home traction unit is adequate; referral to a physical therapist is unnecessary. The patient should start with a low weight (5–8 lb) and advance as tolerated

---

Box 16-2 Treatment of Cervical Radiculopathy

Soft cervical collar (backward)
Hard cervical collar in some situations
Cervical pillow for nighttime use
Cervical traction
Modality physical therapy (heat, ice, ultrasound)
Cervical epidural steroids
Selective foraminal steroid injection
Nonsteroidal anti-inflammatory drugs (NSAIDs)
Other analgesics for pain control as necessary
Surgical referral for
    Severe, unrelenting pain despite conservative therapy
    Strength Medical Research Council grade 4/5 or worse in any
      muscle
    Worsening motor deficit
    Evidence of myelopathy

---

to 12 to 15 lb. Too rapid a weight increase may cause neck or jaw soreness and limit compliance. It is theoretically best for the patient to face the door with the neck slightly flexed; the combination of flexion and distraction is more effective in opening the foramen. However, it is difficult to do anything but stare at the door during such treatment, and if facing away from the door appears equally efficacious for the individual patient, it is permissible and may improve compliance.

Modality physical therapy, or local heat or ice, may provide some relief of the axial pain component, but the effects seldom persist much beyond the individual treatment session. Cervical range-of-motion (ROM) exercises are of no benefit and may be harmful. Cervical epidural steroids or selective root injection with anesthetics or steroids may be useful; spinal manipulation is imprudent. Nonsteroidal anti-inflammatory drugs (NSAIDs) may decrease the radicular inflammatory component and relieve pain. Other analgesics are often necessary in addition, including occasional narcotics. When the neurologic deficit is moderate (Medical Research Council [MRC] grade 4+/5 in the most involved muscles), a course of oral steroids is reasonable (e.g., prednisone 60–100 mg/day for 7–10 days, tapering over next 7–10 days). Intensive conservative therapy is usually continued for 3 to 6 weeks, and if the patient is no better after that interval, surgical referral should be considered. Muscle relaxants add little and cause side effects of sedation and depression.

Consider surgical referral in patients with MRC strength of grade 4/5 or worse in any muscle or evidence of myelopathy or excruciating pain unresponsive to conservative treatment. In a population-based study, 26% required surgery. Newer microsurgical techniques are much less invasive than those used in the past.

The typical CR patient is significantly improved by 2 to 3 months; there is a generally favorable long-term prognosis; 90% have minimal to no symptoms on prolonged follow-up. When due to HNP, CR has a tendency to recur: 31% have a previous history of CR, and 32% have recurrence during follow-up.

Lumbosacral Radiculopathy

Although many patients suffer with sciatica at some time, clinically significant lumbosacral radiculopathy (LSR) occurs in only 4% to 6% of the population. Abnormalities on imaging studies are common in asymptomatic subjects and only loosely associated with symptoms and neurologic examination.[13–15] Recent studies using standing MRI may shed light on the matter.[16] There are numerous potential origins for low back pain (LBP). Most benign self-limited episodes of LBP arise from musculoligamentous structures, and discomfort is localized to the low back region. However, numerous pain-sensitive structures can underlie a clinical episode of LBP: the intervertebral disk, especially the outer fibers of the annulus; the facet joints; other bony structures; and spinal nerve roots. In addition, pain can be referred to the lower back from visceral structures in the abdomen and pelvis. The back may also be involved in systemic diseases, such as spondyloarthropathies.

Clinical Signs and Symptoms

Involvement of some of these pain-sensitive structures can produce referred pain that radiates to the extremity (buttock, hip, thigh) and can simulate the radiating pain of nerve root origin (Table 16-2). A study of 1,293 cases of LBP concluded that referred pain to the lower limb most often originated from sacroiliac and facet joints. Referred pain to the extremity occurred nearly twice as often as true radicular pain, and frequently mimicked the clinical presentation of radiculopathies.[17] Investigations have demonstrated that considerable

Table 16-2 Clinical Signs and Symptoms in Low Back Pain and Lumbosacral Radiculopathy

Disorder	Site of Involvement	Local Pain	Referred Radiating Pain	Radicular Radiating Pain	Pain Increased by	Pain Decreased by	+ Straight Leg Raising	Weakest Muscles	Decreased Reflex
L5 radiculopathy; HNP	L5 root-posterolateral HNP at L4–5	Back	Buttock, posterior thigh	Buttock, posterior thigh, lower leg, dorsum of foot, big toe	Sitting > standing, cough, sneeze, spinal flexion	Standing, lying	Yes	TA EHL, TP, EDL/EDB, PL, TFL, GMD	MHS
L5 radiculopathy; lateral recess syndrome	L5 root-lateral recess stenosis	Back	Buttock, posterior thigh	Buttock, posterior thigh, lower leg, dorsum of foot, big toe	Standing, extension	Spinal flexion	No		
S1 radiculopathy; HNP	S1 root-posterolateral HNP at L5–S1	Back	Buttock, posterior thigh	Buttock, posterior thigh, lower leg, heel, lateral foot/toes	Sitting > standing, cough, sneeze, spinal flexion	Standing, lying	Yes	Gastrocnemius, FDL, short toe flexors, decreased toe raises	Ankle, LHS
S1 radiculopathy; lateral recess syndrome	S1 root-lateral recess stenosis	Back	Buttock, posterior thigh	Buttock, posterior thigh, lower leg, heel, lateral foot/toes	Standing, extension	Spinal flexion	No		
Diskogenic pain	Intervertebral disk–torn annulus; internal disruption	Back	Buttock, posterior thigh	None	Sitting, spinal flexion	Lying	No	No weak muscles, possible splinting due to pain	None
Musculoligamentous pain	Muscular-ligamentous structures of low back	Back	Buttock, posterior thigh	None	Walking, bending, stooping, minor movements	Sitting or lying	Negative or equivocal, not radiating	No weak muscles	None
Nonorganic		Back + any other; often back + neck	None	None	No consistent pattern	No consistent pattern	Variable and nonorganic	None	None

EDB, extensor digitorum brevis; EDL, extensor digitorum longus; EHL, extensor hallucis longus; FDL, flexor digitorum longus; GMD, gluteus medius; HNP, herniated nucleus pulposus; LHS, lateral hamstrings; MHS, medial hamstrings; PL, peroneus longus; TA, tibialis anterior; TFL, tensor faciae latae; TP, tibialis posterior.

pain can be referred to the buttock and thigh with disease limited to the disk, the facet joint, or the sacroiliac joint.[18–20] A study of 92 patients with chronic LBP concluded that 39% had annular tears or other forms of internal disk disruption as the cause of their pain. No available clinical test differentiated between patients with internal disk disruptions and those with compressive radiculopathy.[21] A similar situation seems to exist with facet joint pain.[22,23] The first suggestion that a patient may have nerve root compression usually comes because of radiating pain into one or both lower extremities. Conservative therapy still usually suffices, even in patients with HNPs, and only 5% to 10% of patients ultimately need surgery.[24] Operative intervention is generally appropriate only when there is a combination of definite disk herniation shown by imaging studies, a corresponding syndrome of radicular pain, a corresponding neurologic deficit, and a failure to respond to conservative therapy.

Deyo et al reviewed the information that could be obtained from the history and physical examination in patients with LBP.[25] They suggest trying to answer three basic questions: Is there a serious, underlying systemic disease present? Is there neurologic compromise that might require further evaluation? Are there psychological factors leading to pain amplification? Factors that suggest the possibility of underlying systemic disease include a history of cancer, unexplained weight loss, pain lasting longer than 1 month, pain unrelieved by bed rest, fever, focal spine tenderness, morning stiffness, improvement in pain with exercise, and failure of conservative treatment.

The utility, or lack thereof, of various physical examination findings has been studied. The straight leg raising (SLR) test remains the mainstay in detecting radicular compression. The test is performed by slowly raising the symptomatic leg with the knee extended. Tension is transmitted to the nerve roots between about 30 and 70 degrees and pain increases. Pain at less than 30 degrees raises the question of nonorganicity, and some discomfort and tightness beyond 70 degrees is routine and insignificant. There are various degrees or levels of positivity. Ipsilateral leg tightness is the lowest level, pain in the back is more significant, and radiating pain in the leg is highly significant. When raising the good leg produces pain in the symptomatic leg (crossed straight leg raising sign), the likelihood of a root lesion is very high.

The positivity of the SLR should be the same with the patient supine or seated. If a patient with a positive supine SLR does not complain or lean backward when the extended leg is brought up while in the seated position (e.g., under the guise of doing the plantar response), it is suggestive of nonorganicity. The SLR can be enhanced by passively dorsiflexing the patient's foot just at the elevation angle at which the increased root tension begins to produce pain. A quick snap to the sciatic nerve in the popliteal fossa just as stretch begins to cause pain (bowstring sign, or popliteal compression test) accomplishes the same end. Patients with hip disease have pain on raising the leg whether the knee is bent or straight; those with root stretch signs only have pain when the knee is extended. Pain from hip disease is maximal when the hip is flexed, abducted, and externally rotated by putting the patient's foot on the contralateral knee and pressing down slightly on the symptomatic knee (Fabere test). There are other procedures for checking the sacroiliac joints.

The neurologic examination should include assessment of power in the major lower extremity muscle groups, but especially the dorsiflexors of the foot and toes, and the evertors and invertors of the foot. Plantar flexion of the foot is so powerful that manual testing rarely suffices. Having the patient do 10 toe raises with either foot is a better test. Sensation should be tested in the signature zones of the major roots. The status of knee and ankle reflexes is informative about the integrity of the L3–4 and S1 roots. There is no good reflex for the L5 root, but the hamstring reflexes are occasionally useful. The medial and lateral hamstrings are both innervated by both L5 and S1, but the medial hamstring tends to be more L5 and the lateral more S1. An occasional L5 radiculopathy produces a clear selective diminution of the medial hamstring reflex. In a patient with absent ankle jerks and a question of neuropathy, loss of the lateral hamstring with preservation of the medial helps confirm radicular disease. Preservation of the lateral hamstring jerk with an absent ankle jerk suggests a length dependent process (i.e., peripheral neuropathy).

Studies have found that only 8 of 27 physical tests investigated successfully discriminated between patients with chronic LBP and normal control subjects. The eight useful tests were pelvic flexion, total spinal flexion, total extension, lateral flexion, straight leg raising, spinal tenderness, bilateral active straight leg raising, and sit-up.[25] Tests for nonorganicity are very useful. Pain during simulated spinal rotation, pinning the patient's hands to the sides while passively rotating the hips back and forth (no spine rotation occurs as shoulders and hips remain in a constant relationship) suggests nonorganicity. Likewise, a discrepancy between the positivity of the SLR between the supine and seated position, pain in the back on pressing down on top of the head, widespread and excessive "tenderness," general overreaction during testing, and nondermatomal/nonmyotomal neurologic signs. The presence of three of these signs suggests, if not nonorganicity, at least embellishment.[25]

The major radicular syndromes include HNP, lateral recess stenosis, and spinal stenosis with cauda equina compression. Virtually all patients with radiculopathy have sciatica. The odds of a patient without sciatica having radiculopathy have been estimated at 1:1000.[25] The details of the sciatica are noteworthy, including the exact pattern of radiation, influence of body position and movement, and presence or absence of neurologic symptoms.

With HNP or lateral recess stenosis, leg pain usually predominates over back pain. With HNP the pain is typically worse when sitting, better when standing, better still when lying down, and generally worse in flexed than extended postures—all reflecting the known changes in intradiscal pressure that occur in these positions. With lateral recess stenosis, the pain is worse with standing or walking and relieved by sitting with the torso flexed or by lying down. Patients with HNP tend to have a positive SLR, but those with recess stenosis do not. The essence of the recess stenosis picture then is pain on standing, lack of pain on sitting, and a negative SLR. The essence of the HNP picture is pain worse on sitting, lessened with standing, and a positive SLR. Patients with HNP are usually in the 30 to 55 years age range; those with lateral recess stenosis a bit older. As with CR, pain may exacerbate with cough, sneeze, or Valsalva maneuver.

Evaluation and Diagnosis

As patients mature into the seventh decade and beyond, the liability to disk rupture decreases, but degenerative spine disease attacks in a different form. Osteophytic spurs and bars; bulging disks; thickened laminae and pedicles; arthritic, hypertrophied facets; and thickened spinal ligaments all combine to narrow the spinal canal and produce the syndrome of spinal stenosis. An extension posture contributes to spinal stenosis by causing narrowing of the foramina and dorsal quadrants, and buckling of the ligamentum flavum. Narrowing of the canal compresses neural and possibly vascular structures. Flexing the spine, as by leaning forward, stooping over, or sitting down opens the canal and decreases the symptoms.

Patients with spinal stenosis and neurogenic claudication experience pain, weakness, numbness, and paresthesias/dysesthesias when standing or walking. Symptoms decrease with sitting or bending forward. An occasional patient will have a bizarre symptom, such as spontaneous erections or fecal incontinence brought on by walking. Differentiation from vascular claudication is made by the wide distribution of symptoms, the neurologic accompaniments, and the necessity to sit down for relief. Vascular claudication tends to produce focal, intense, crampy pain in one or both calves and the pain subsides if the patient just stops and stands. Patients with vascular claudication have even more symptoms walking uphill, because of the increased leg work. Neurogenic claudication may decrease when walking uphill because of the increased spinal flexion in forward leaning. Patients with vascular claudication have as much trouble riding a bicycle as walking because of the leg work involved, whereas forward flexion on the bicycle opens up the spinal canal, allowing patients with neurogenic claudication to ride a bike with greater ease than they can walk.

An investigation of 68 patients with lumbar spinal stenosis found that pseudoclaudication, or neurogenic claudication, was the most common symptom, producing pain, numbness, or weakness on walking, frequently bilaterally and usually relieved by flexing the spine. Mild neurologic abnormalities occurred in a minority of patients. EMG showed one or more involved roots in 90% of patients.[26]

The vast majority of LSRs are due to degenerative spine disease. Other disease processes can occur and may require exclusion. Patients with acquired immunodeficiency syndrome (AIDS) may develop an acute lumbosacral (LS) polyradiculopathy with a rapidly progressive flaccid paraparesis and areflexia, frequently associated with sphincter disturbances, which is due to cytomegalovirus infection and responds to gancyclovir. Patients may develop back pain and radiculopathy with epidural abscess or hematoma, diffuse meningeal neoplasia, diabetes, and other conditions.[9]

Plain LS spine films are rarely helpful except in the setting of acute trauma or suspected infection or malignancy. Plain CT may be useful in patients who are unable to undergo MRI; when combined with intrathecal contrast, CT is highly accurate for detecting nerve root compression. Plain myelography is sometimes useful, particularly in patients unable to undergo MRI because of metallic fixation, and in those too obese to fit in an MRI scanner. MRI is the imaging procedure of choice in LSR, again with the caveat that many asymptomatic patients have this disease on MRI that is not clinically relevant.

Treatment and Management

Studies have clearly shown that bed rest is not efficacious in patients with nonspecific or mechanical low back pain.[27] There is less information about the role of bed rest in acute LSR, and brief, judicious bed rest may still be useful for short-term symptom control in patients who are in acute, severe pain. At the very least, if the patient remains up and active, he or she should avoid activities such as bending or lifting, which are known to increase intradiscal pressure. NSAIDs may be useful both for pain control and to help reduce acute radicular inflammation, although trials have not substantiated their usefulness compared to placebo. Opioids may be needed for pain relief in the acute situation. A short course of oral steroids is sometimes useful, although again this has not been studied definitively. Drugs used to treat neuropathic pain, such as tricyclic antidepressants, gabapentin, and similar agents, may be useful for the management of chronic radiculopathy, but there is little evidence that they are helpful in the acute situation.

Physical therapy such as back exercises should probably be avoided with an acute painful radiculopathy. After the acute stage has subsided, physical therapy may certainly be useful. However, if back exercises reproduce radicular pain, they should be stopped immediately. Numerous other nonoperative treatments are occasionally used, although demonstration of effectiveness in randomized trials is generally lacking. These treatments include transcutaneous electrical nerve stimulation, acupuncture, massage, spinal manipulation, epidural steroid injection, and selective transforaminal nerve root injection.

The vast majority of patients with acute LSR improve with time and conservative management, even when the disk herniation remains visible on MRI. Surgical referral should be prompt if the patient develops any evidence of cauda equina syndrome. Whether patients with more routine LSR benefit from surgery remains controversial, particularly with some of the aggressive and extensive procedures now commonly done. After 6 months, operated and nonoperated patients with simple LSR are doing about the same.[26]

Plexopathies

Numerous pathologic processes may affect either the brachial plexus (BP) or the lumbosacral plexus (LSP) (Box 16-3). Whereas the vast majority of radiculopathies are due to compression, the plexopathies may be caused by a number of different pathologic processes. The complex anatomy makes evaluation challenging (Fig. 16-5). The most common and clinically important of the brachial plexus disorders include neuralgic amyotrophy (acute brachial plexopathy or brachial plexitis); trauma, such as with missile and stab wounds or motor vehicle (especially motorcycle) accidents; neoplasms; postradiation plexopathy; obstetric palsies; postsurgical plexopathy; the "stinger" or "burner" phenomenon that frequently affects football players, which is likely a mild form of plexus injury; and thoracic outlet syndrome. Other causes include external compression (e.g., backpack or rucksack palsy), compression from an internal process (e.g., encroachment on the lower brachial plexus from a Pancoast tumor), or involvement in systemic processes such as systemic lupus erythematosus (SLE) or sarcoid, or iatrogenic plexopathy during cardiac surgery. The brachial plexus may rarely be involved in a number of other conditions, including lupus, lymphoma, Ehlers-Danlos syndrome, and infectious or parainfectious disorders. Some of these processes are by nature progressive.

With pressure injuries the same general rules apply as for other nerves. Mild lesions produce primarily demyelination and can cause severe clinical deficits but have an excellent prognosis. With plexopathies there may be the additional complication of disease progression. Many of the conditions which affect the plexuses are not static. Pancoast tumors continue to grow, radiation damage tends to progress, and systemic diseases such as SLE continue their activity. All these mechanisms of injury make the pathophysiology of plexopathies complex and the clinical evaluation challenging.

Evaluation and Diagnosis

The electrodiagnostic principles for both BP and LSP conditions are similar. From a clinical and electrodiagnostic standpoint the most common exercise is distinguishing plexopathy from radiculopathy. The NEE is the mainstay of diagnosis and localization, although sensory (more so than motor) conduction studies, late responses, and somatosensory evoked potentials (SEPs) can sometimes provide helpful information. The key feature is abnormalities in the distribution of some plexus component, a trunk or a cord, sparing the

Box 16-3 Causes of Brachial Plexopathy

Infectious/Parainfectious/Injections

Immunizations
Serum sickness
Botulinum toxin
Interleukin 2
Interferon
Heroin
Lyme disease
Erlichiosis
Herpes zoster
HIV infection
Epstein-Barr virus infection
Cytomegalovirus infection
Parvovirus infection
Yersiniosis

Hereditary

Hereditary neuralgic amyotrophy
Hereditary neuropathy with liability to pressure palsies (HNPP)
Ehlers-Danlos syndrome

Physical Injury

Radiation therapy
Cardiac surgery
Birth injury
Other postoperative plexopathies
Shoulder dislocation
Penetrating wounds
Axillary angiography
Clavicular nonunion
Prolonged burner

Other Causative Disorders/Conditions

Neuralgic amyotrophy
Thoracic outlet syndrome
Systemic lupus erythematosus
Pregnancy
Systemic vasculitis
Stretch
External pressure (e.g., backpack palsy, seat belts, Posey palsy)
Post–liver transplantation
Lymphoma
Metastatic disease
Pancoast tumor
Primary nerve tumors
Tattoos
Interscalene block
Myositis ossificans
Heparin therapy
Nodular fasciitis

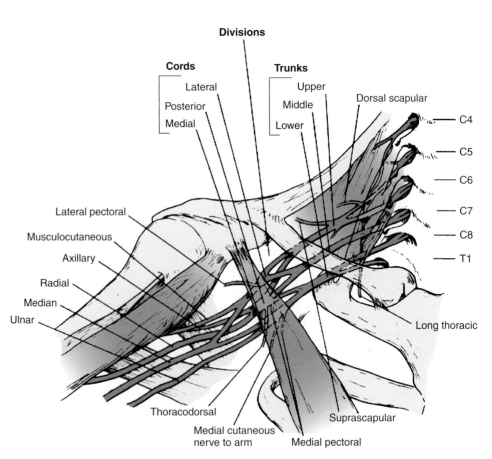

Figure 16-5 The brachial plexus. (From Canale ST, Beaty JH, editors: *Campbell's Operative Orthopaedics*, 11th ed. St. Louis, 2007, Mosby.)

paraspinals. The status of the sensory potentials is critical for distinguishing plexopathy from radiculopathy. In radiculopathy, the sensory potentials are normal; in plexopathy they are frequently absent or low in amplitude in the distribution of the affected plexus component (e.g., abnormal lateral antebrachial cutaneous in upper trunk or lateral cord plexopathies and abnormal medial antebrachial cutaneous in lower trunk or medial cord).

Imaging of the Plexus and Peripheral Nerves

MRI shows increasing promise as an imaging method for peripheral nerves and the plexuses. Although it is still not widely available, the growing body of literature documenting its utility suggests that in the future MRI will be widely used.[28,29] There is even the possibility of developing new contrast agents, such as gadofluorine M or gadofosveset trisodium, members of a new class of MRI contrast agents, that will cause nerves to enhance under some circumstances.[8,29] Imaging peripheral nerves currently requires the most advanced available technology, including high field strength MRI and dedicated radiofrequency coils (MHR neurography).[28]

MRI accomplishes two things in peripheral nerve and plexus lesions. It may show denervation changes in muscle that help define the distribution of the abnormality and localize the lesion to a particular nerve or branch. It can image muscles difficult or impossible to access by needle electromyography, such as the subscapularis. Alternatively, it may demonstrate a nerve lesion directly.

Recent technological advances now permit the ultrasonographic imaging of peripheral nerves using high-frequency "small-parts" transducers. Such high-resolution sonography (HRS) is being used increasingly in the evaluation of a variety of peripheral nerve abnormalities, including entrapment neuropathies and peripheral nerve trauma.[30,31]

Peripheral nerves have a characteristic ultrasonographic echotexture and other characteristics that allows differentiation between nerves, tendons, and blood vessels. By HRS, peripheral nerves typically show hypoechoic areas separated by hyperechoic foci. The hypoechoic areas are the nerve fascicles and the hyperechoic areas are epineurium. On longitudinal views, peripheral nerve shows a characteristic "tram-track" pattern due to reflection of the sound waves off the layers of epineurium that encase the nerve. This fascicular pattern is particularly clear in the median nerve, whereas the ulnar nerve tends to be more hypoechoic. HRS is particularly useful in the evaluation of peripheral nerve tumors.[32]

Although electrophysiology will remain the primary tool for aiding in the clinical evaluation of patients with focal neuropathies for the foreseeable future, it appears that HRS may be able to supplement or complement electrophysiologic testing for detection of focal peripheral nerve abnormalities.[32] In peripheral nerve trauma, because of the limitations of electrodiagnosis and the vagaries of anatomy, determination of the precise site of injury may remain uncertain. Critical information, such as whether or not a traumatized nerve is in continuity, the position of the proximal and distal stumps, and the presence or absence of a neuroma in continuity, until recently could be determined only by direct surgical inspection. Now both MRI and ultrasound may aid in clinical decision making. In a blinded proof-of-concept study, HRS was able to identify transected nerves in the upper extremity with 89% sensitivity and 95% specificity in fresh cadavers.[33] In patients with traumatic peripheral nerve injuries, HRS may be a useful tool in determining the precise localization of the injury site, the type of injury, the position of the stumps, and the presence of a neuroma.[33]

Disorders of the Brachial Plexus

Processes that affect the brachial plexus primarily include neuralgic amyotrophy (brachial plexitis, Parsonage-Turner syndrome), trauma, cancer, radiation, postoperative plexopathy, and true neurogenic thoracic outlet syndrome.

Neuralgic Amyotrophy

This condition has gone by a number of names, most frequently *brachial plexitis, Parsonage-Turner syndrome*, and *acute brachial plexus neuropathy. Neuralgic amyotrophy* (NA) is the currently preferred nosologic term.[4] Immune-mediated brachial plexus neuropathy (IBPN) was recently suggested as a better term.[34] Neuralgic amyotrophy is a fairly stereotyped clinical syndrome characterized by the acute onset of pain in the shoulder and upper arm, followed by weakness of variable severity, primarily affecting upper arm and shoulder muscles.[35] It runs a protracted course of slow, sometimes incomplete recovery, and sometimes as one arm is recovering the other is stricken. Recurrence is not rare. As in Guillain-Barré syndrome, many patients have some antecedent event, such as viral infection, immunizations, childbirth, or surgery, and the disease is thought to be immunologically mediated, although the precise mechanism remains uncertain. It has a predilection to affect young and middle-aged adults.

The pain in NA is a defining feature. It tends to begin abruptly and is very intense, often more severe at night, often over the lateral deltoid. After a variable interval, usually 3 to 10 days, weakness, often patchy, begins in the shoulder and upper arm, frequently as the pain is subsiding. The weakness is then followed by atrophy, often very severe. Occasionally, the weakness begins in, is limited to, or is maximal in a specific peripheral nerve distribution, classically the anterior interosseous or long thoracic nerve. Sensory loss is minimal or absent. The disease is frequently bilateral, and in approximately 20% of patients as the affected extremity is beginning to improve the other arm begins to develop the condition.[36]

Some cases of NA are familial. Patients with hereditary neuropathy with liability to pressure palsies (HNPP), which is a dominant condition due to mutation or deletion in the *PMP22* gene on chromosome 17, may develop recurrent brachial plexopathy, sometimes following minor trauma, which lacks the pain of NA and has a much better prognosis for recovery, with electrodiagnostic studies showing a picture more in keeping with demyelination and less in the way of axon loss. There are three other forms of familial NA unrelated to HNPP: HNA1, HNA2, and HNA3. All are dominant, only HNA1 is on chromosome 17. In a study of 246 NA patients, the 47 HNA patients had an earlier onset (28.4 versus 41.3 years), more attacks (mean 3.5 versus 1.5) and more frequent involvement of nerves outside the brachial plexus (55.8% versus 17.3%), a more severe maximum paresis, and a poorer eventual outcome.[37] Some HNA patients have unusual dysmorphic features. In one series, cleft palate was present in four individuals, hypotelorism was common, and there were unusual skinfolds and creases were observed on the necks of several individuals and on the scalp of one man (cutis verticis gyrata, a striking appearance). In three families, deep skin creases were present on the limbs of infants and toddlers who were subsequently affected with HNA.[38]

There appear to be other immunologically mediated brachial plexopathies. A painless form of brachial plexopathy has been reported as the only manifestation of chronic inflammatory demyelinating polyneuropathy (CIDP).[39] When brachial plexopathy is not accompanied by severe pain or followed by atrophy, the possibility of a primarily demyelinating and potentially treatable condition such as a restricted form of CIDP, multifocal motor neuropathy, or a similar condition should be considered in the differential diagnosis.[40,41]

Radiation and Neoplastic Plexopathies

Like radiation damage to other parts of the neuraxis, radiation plexopathy appears after a delay of months to years. This is also the time frame in which the radiation therapy (RT) may have kept a tumor at bay, either a primary nerve tumor such as a malignant neurofibrosarcoma or a local infiltrating neoplasm such as lymphoma or carcinoma of the breast or lung. The problem is to distinguish recurrent tumor from radiation plexopathy (RP), a difficult and important differential (Table 16-3). Pain can occur with either condition but is more likely to be an early and dominant symptom in neoplastic plexopathy (NP). Sensory dysfunction with numbness and paresthesias is more likely to be the predominant symptom with RP, but some patients have significant pain. Weakness and reflex changes occur in either condition. One study suggested that painless upper trunk lesions with lymphedema suggested radiation injury, and painful lower trunk lesions with Horner syndrome implied tumor infiltration.[42] Other studies also suggested that RP had an upper plexus and NP a lower plexus distribution, but this was not substantiated in subsequent investigations as a reliable differentiator because of the amount of overlap between the two groups.[4] Most patients in both groups have involvement of the lower trunk or the entire plexus.[43] Patients with RP are much more likely to have prominent fasciculations. The presence of myokymia on EMG is highly suggestive of RP, and is clearly the most useful electrodiagnostic discriminating feature.

Harper et al found that the presence or absence of pain as the presenting symptom, the temporal profile of the illness, a discrete mass on imaging studies, and myokymic discharges on EMG most reliably predicted the underlying cause of the plexopathy. Distribution of weakness was not useful in discriminating between the two groups.[43] A study of RP in 79 breast cancer patients from an oncologic rather than a neurologic viewpoint revealed that 35% developed RP. In 50% the process was panplexus, but of those with more focality, 18% had involvement of the upper trunk only, and only 4% the lower trunk. RP was more common after RT plus cytotoxic therapy than after RT alone. Most patients had no significant latency between RT and the onset of symptoms, raising the possibility of chemotherapy enhancement of radiation effects.[44] A painful, short latency

Table 16-3 Differential Diagnostic Points in Neoplastic versus Radiation-Induced Brachial Plexopathy

Neoplastic Plexopathy	Radiation Plexopathy
Horner's syndrome common	Horner's syndrome rare
Presents with pain	Presents with paresthesias
Pain is predominant symptom	Paresthesias and sensory loss are the predominant symptoms
More lower plexus (equivocal)	More upper plexus (equivocal)
Imaging study shows discrete mass	Imaging study is normal or shows only loss of tissue planes
Diffuse motor and sensory conduction abnormalities	Abnormal sensory nerve action potentials /normal motor neuron conduction velocities Conduction block across plexus Myokymia Fasciculation potentials Paraspinal fibrillations

brachial plexopathy may also occur during or after RT for Hodgkin disease.

Postoperative Brachial Plexopathy

Postoperative brachial plexopathies were noted to increase dramatically following the advent of modern open heart and coronary bypass surgical procedures. Postoperative plexopathies can occur as a presumably immunologically mediated event after procedures on parts of the body remote from the plexus. The most common situation by far is for plexopathy to follow coronary artery bypass graft (CABG) procedures. A number of injury mechanisms have been postulated, including hyperabduction of the arm, displacement of the clavicle, first rib fracture with plexus laceration, overzealous sternal spreading causing plexus stretch or compression of the plexus between the clavicle and first rib, and laceration of the plexus during attempted internal jugular (IJ) vein cannulation. Injuries continued to occur when the arms were routinely adducted at the patient's sides.

In a series of 421 CABG patients studied at the Cleveland Clinic, there was a 13% incidence of peripheral nervous system complications, and the majority (5%) were plexopathies.[45] The study analyzed 451 different variables. In 74% of the plexopathy patients, there was a correlation between the site of jugular cannulation and the side of the injury, suggesting inadvertent laceration or compression by hematoma. In four of the remaining six patients, an internal mammary graft was used. These grafts require greater sternal retraction, and seem more likely to stretch the plexus. So, either jugular cannulation or internal mammary grafting seemed to explain 21 of the 23 cases in this series. Blaming jugular cannulation has not gone unchallenged in the surgical literature.

In a large prospective study, 27 of 1000 patients developed postoperative brachial plexus injuries. Patients who underwent grafting of the internal mammary artery had a 10-fold increased incidence of plexus injury (10.6%) as compared with those who did not (<1%).[46] It appears that optimal positioning and the use of minimal retraction will lessen but not eliminate these injuries.

Most cases of post-CABG plexopathy appear to be traction injuries to the C8 anterior primary ramus rather that to the lower trunk or medial cord.[47] Horner syndrome may accompany the variable pain, numbness, and weakness. Induced hypothermia may play a role by increasing the susceptibility to nerve injury. The majority of deficits resolve within several weeks, suggesting that the predominant pathophysiology is demyelination.

Nerve compression injuries may also occur in this setting. In a Cleveland Clinic series, there were 5 ulnar neuropathies in the 421 patients.[45] In a prospective study of 20 patients undergoing CABG, conduction slowing of the ulnar nerve across the elbow was present in one third of the patients *preoperatively*, and conduction abnormalities developed in an additional 27% of the ulnar nerves postoperatively, all of which were *asymptomatic* and most of which resolved electrically on follow-up.[48] So, in addition to plexopathies, there appears to be a high incidence of mild, asymptomatic, and undetected ulnar neuropathies following CABG.

Traumatic Plexopathies

Traumatic plexopathies are primarily due to blunt or penetrating trauma or to stretch. Motorcyclists are particularly prone to upper plexus stretch when falling so that the shoulder and head are forced in opposite directions. Most traumatic plexopathies affect the supraclavicular portion or are diffuse. A frequent confounding injury is root avulsion, it which the stretch is severe enough to wrench one or more spinal roots from the cord. The plexus may also suffer external compression, as in backpack palsy or seat belt trauma, or be damaged in the course of shoulder dislocation or fracture of the clavicle. External compression palsies can be severe in susceptible individuals. The author once saw a young paratrooper in whom the initial manifestation of HNPP was an acute, severe backpack palsy. He stood, wearing an 80-lb rucksack, in preparation to jump, but the jump was delayed for 30 to 45 minutes because of wind conditions in the drop zone. In that span of time, he developed an acute, panplexus deficit and the left arm became flail. He jumped anyway! Recovery was prolonged and incomplete. Acute brachial plexus compression injury after drinking, akin to Saturday night radial nerve palsy, has been reported.[49]

Stretch injuries of the plexus occur during childbirth. These most often involve the upper plexus (Erb palsy) or the entire plexus, rarely the lower plexus alone (Klumpke palsy). High birth weight and complicated deliveries are predisposing factors. Some neonates have had fibrillation potentials detected in the first few days of life, suggesting an intrauterine mechanism of injury, such as compression by an amniotic band. Prognosis is generally good and the majority of patients make quick recoveries without specific treatment, suggesting the pathophysiology is often primarily demyelination. However, any kind of injury can occur, including severe axon loss and even root avulsion, and the injury often results in a devastating disability. For many years the injury was considered untreatable if it did not resolve on its own. In the 1970s and 1980s, J. Mallet in France revolutionized the management of these patients, showing that neonatal plexus injuries could be successfully repaired surgically, and separating patients who should have surgery from those who should be managed conservatively by their ability to perform certain motor functions at certain ages.[50] For example, the ability to get the hand to the mouth by 3 months generally indicated the patient would recover adequately without surgery.[51] Managing these children in the post-Mallet era with the availability of microneurosurgery, intraoperative nerve action potentials, nerve conduits, nerve grafts, and all the tools available in the twenty-first century is a very different proposition than in the past.[52,53]

The "stinger" or "burner" phenomenon is common in American football. Following a block or tackle, a player may develop sudden, intense, dysesthetic pain in the shoulder and arm. The injury is now thought to more likely involve the upper trunk of the plexus rather than the cervical roots. Traction when the head and neck are forcibly separated is one possibility, as in a mild form of the often devastating upper plexus injury that occurs in motorcyclists. A study at West Point showed that it is more likely that the symptoms result from the shoulder pad being forcefully pushed into Erb's point.[54] Some players have persistent symptoms, the "prolonged burner" syndrome.[55]

Thoracic Outlet Syndrome

Thoracic outlet syndrome (TOS) has a long and controversial history. First described by Kennier Wilson near the turn of the century, it was firmly established in the minds of physicians as a cause of acroparesthesias for more than 40 years before the medical community discovered the far more common entities of carpal tunnel syndrome (CTS) and CR. First rib resections for TOS are commonly performed in the United States, occasionally with disastrous results.[56,57] The likelihood of undergoing surgery may be related to the potential for reimbursement; first rib resections are very rare among Colorado Medicaid patients.[58]

Surgeons are still struggling to clearly define TOS as a clinical entity nearly 100 years after its original description.[59] The surgical

literature is inconsistent and often contradictory. In one center where TOS is felt to be common, 409 patients underwent TOS surgery in a 19-year span.[60] In contrast, one peripheral nerve surgeon believes surgery for TOS should be a rare event.[61] Jamieson et al find a TOS patient to operate on about every 2 weeks, but most electromyographers, who see patients with acroparesthesias and arm pain with high frequency, encounter one convincing case of TOS every 1 to 2 years.[60] Perceptions about the prevalence of TOS between surgeons and neurologists are at variance on the order of 100:1.[59,62]

There is substantial agreement about the entity of true neurogenic TOS (TNTOS): it is rare, most often due to compression of the lower trunk of the plexus by a cervical rib or band, and typically presents with medial arm pain, ulnar/C8 distribution sensory dysfunction, and thenar muscle wasting in a young woman.

The major problem arises with the entity now generally called *disputed neurogenic TOS* (DNTOS). Surgeons contend that 97% of the cases of TOS are of the neurologic type. Since there is agreement that TNTOS is rare, DNTOS accounts for the vast majority of cases.[63] The profusion of symptoms attributed to DNTOS—not only arm pain and numbness but also migraine headaches and a host of other complaints—challenges credulity.

One of the main criteria for the diagnosis, a positive Adson maneuver, was shown 50 years ago to be positive in 80% of normal asymptomatic individuals. The elevated arm stress test (EAST maneuver), touted for TOS, is frequently positive in patients with CTS and in normal control subjects. No confirmatory tests can reliably substantiate the diagnosis of DNTOS, which eludes all but clinical surgical evaluation, and can only be proved by surgical exploration, a self-fulfilling prophecy.

The droopy shoulder syndrome shares many similarities with DNTOS.[64] Some believe it accounts for most cases of TOS. Almost all droopy shoulder syndrome patients are slender young women with long graceful necks with horizontal or downsloping, rather than the normal slightly upsloping, clavicles. The T2 or lower vertebrae may be visible on lateral cervical spine films because of the low-lying shoulders. Electrodiagnostic studies are typically normal. Symptoms have been attributed to chronic brachial plexus stretch due to the low-hanging shoulders. Pain in the shoulder, arm, hand, and sometimes neck and head accompanied by paresthesias are the usual symptoms. Supraclavicular percussion and downward traction on the arms exacerbates, and passive elevation decreases, the symptoms. Treatment is with shoulder strengthening exercises. The prudence of separating droopy shoulder syndrome from other instances of DNTOS is debatable.

Evaluation and Diagnosis of Brachial Plexopathy

Electrodiagnostic assessment in plexopathies seeks to ascertain the distribution of the damage, the completeness of the lesion, the predominant pathophysiology, and whether or not there is an associated root avulsion. The findings vary with the severity and location of the lesion. Mild to moderate lesions would likely show normal motor conductions, low amplitude sensory nerve action potentials (SNAPs), delayed or absent late responses, and recruitment abnormalities on NEE in a distribution of a trunk or cord of the plexus, sparing the paraspinals. More severe lesions would typically show absent SNAPs and late responses, low compound muscle action potential (CMAP) amplitude in affected muscles, possibly with motor nerve conduction velocity (NCV) slowing in proportion to axon loss, with more severe MUAP abnormalities and fibrillations on NEE.

If there is root avulsion, the dorsal root ganglion and the peripheral processes remain intact and the peripherally recorded sensory potentials remain normal in the face of clinical anesthesia in the same distribution and marked motor abnormalities. However, it is difficult to avulse a root without some associated plexus stretch. Myelography may show a traumatic meningocele in root avulsion, but both false positive and false negative studies occur. The correlation between the myelographic and the neurophysiologic data was only 50% in one study.[65]

The electrodiagnostic picture in TNTOS is characteristic. Patients have a low-amplitude or absent ulnar SNAP, a low-amplitude median CMAP recorded from the thenar muscles, generally normal conduction velocities except for slowing in proportion to axon loss, delayed or absent median and ulnar F wave responses, and chronic neurogenic MUP changes in the distribution of the lower trunk, sparing the paraspinals. The medial antebrachial cutaneous SNAP is abnormal more frequently than the ulnar SNAP.[4] The reason for the paradoxical involvement of ulnar sensory and median motor fibers is unclear but may be related to the internal fascicular anatomy and selective fascicular vulnerability of the lower trunk.

Conduction slowing across the plexus with stimulation at Erb's point was touted for many years, after the publication of Urschel and Razzuk, as the best method of electrically demonstrating the pathology in TOS.[66] The technique failed utterly in the hands of most EMG operators. Wilbourn and Lederman later exposed this research as fraudulent, and the Urschel paper was retracted, accompanied by editorial comment regarding ethics in research and followed by a flurry of correspondence. To this day, there is still no convincing evidence that such across-plexus conduction studies have any value. Other techniques, especially SEPs, have been advocated but also proved disappointing, likely due largely to the rarity of compression of neural structures in suspected TOS.

Neuralgic amyotrophy produces a stereotyped clinical syndrome, a spotty axon loss pattern on NEE and abnormal SNAPs.[35] Myokymia and the absence of pain suggest radiation plexopathy in the patient with a history of cancer and radiotherapy. Traumatic plexopathies can follow stretch, external pressure, and penetrating wounds; lower trunk lesions occur in 5% to 10% of patients undergoing coronary artery bypass grafts. Electrodiagnosis can help in determining the pathophysiology, distribution, and completeness of the lesion, and in ruling out root avulsion. True neurogenic thoracic outlet syndrome has a characteristic clinical and electrodiagnostic picture. The disputed neurogenic form of TOS is muddy clinically and electrodiagnostically.

In NA, MRI may show muscle denervation changes and exclude other pathology, such as rotator cuff disease, that may mimic NA clinically.[29] Denervation in the distribution of the suprascapular nerve, particularly with concomitant changes in the axillary nerve distribution, are particularly characteristic. No abnormality of the brachial plexus itself has so far been reported. In other lesions of the brachial plexus, such as neoplasms, the MRI of course demonstrates the pathology directly. The brachial plexus is too deep and complex for ultrasound to play much of a role in diagnosis at the present time. It is commonly used to aid in the placement of blocks and catheters for regional anesthesia.

Treatment and Management of Brachial Plexopathy

There is no specific treatment for most nontraumatic brachial plexopathies. In neuralgic amyotrophy, steroids may help alleviate the severe pain but do not improve the weakness or change the eventual outcome. Physical and occupational therapy are useful to maintain joint mobility, maintain strength in uninvolved muscles, and improve function. Surgical exploration is sometimes done when the distinction between neoplastic and radiation-induced plexopathy

cannot be made noninvasively. Radiotherapy is usually given when tumor has invaded the plexus.

Treatment for traumatic brachial plexopathy is primarily surgical. See earlier discussion of traumatic plexopathy due to birth injury. In adults, exploration is usually carried out at about 3 months if there have been no signs of recovery. Careful preoperative evaluation to exclude root avulsion is mandatory before exploration. Intraoperative nerve action potentials are often used to help distinguish reparable from irreparable damage. Repair usually involves end-to-end neurorrhaphy or grafting. Even under the best of circumstances the outcome is often poor. There is movement gaining momentum to forgo direct repair of the plexus in favor of nerve transfers.[67] Nerve transfers employ other intact motor nerves that have a minor function to reinnervate critical muscles. The distal end of a freshly cut normal nerve is joined to the distal stump of an injured nerve. A variation is to join selected fascicles from a normal nerve to an injured nerve. For instance, fascicles of the ulnar nerve may be implanted into the musculocutaneous nerve or biceps muscle in order to gain elbow flexion (Oberlin procedure).

Disorders of the Lumbosacral Plexus

Processes that affect the lumbosacral plexus primarily include diabetes, cancer, and radiation. There is a syndrome of idiopathic lumbosacral plexopathy (LSP) which may be analogous to neuralgic amyotrophy involving the brachial plexus, but with some important differences. A simplified version of the relevant anatomy is shown in Figure 16-6.

Diabetic Amyotrophy

In diabetic amyotrophy (DA), diabetes involves the lumbosacral plexus and roots. Like neuralgic amyotrophy, diabetic amyotrophy has a stereotyped clinical presentation. The typical patient is older, with type

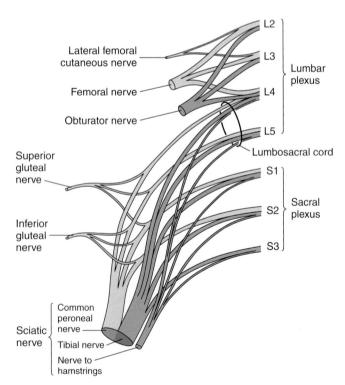

Figure 16-6 The lumbosacral plexus. (From Canale ST, Beaty JH, editors: *Campbell's Operative Orthopaedics*, 11th ed. St. Louis, 2007, Mosby.)

2 diabetes, usually mild, and occasionally not previously diagnosed. Symptoms begin subacutely with pain in one hip or thigh that becomes severe. Weakness of the hip flexors, gluteal muscles, and quadriceps ensues, and the patient begins to lose weight, often 20 lb or more. Pain continues, the quadriceps atrophies, and the knee jerk disappears. Similar but milder pain, weakness, and atrophy occur on the opposite side. At its zenith, the patient has painful, bilateral but asymmetrical, weakness and wasting of the thighs along with substantial weight loss. The process eventually stabilizes and a slow and occasionally incomplete recovery follows over months to a couple of years.[68]

The clinical deficit most often involves the lumbar plexus diffusely. The sacral plexus is minimally involved or spared, though patients sometimes develop a mild foot drop. Examination shows bilateral but asymmetrical weakness and wasting of the hip flexors, adductors, gluteal muscles, hamstrings, and quadriceps. The knee jerk is usually absent, often with preservation of the ankle reflexes. Sensory loss is minimal or absent. The differential diagnosis primarily includes high lumbar HNP, involving L2, L3, or L4. Diabetic amyotrophy is sometimes referred to as *proximal diabetic neuropathy*; there is evidence that it may be due to an underlying vasculitic or immune process and may respond to immunoglobulin therapy.[69,70] This is also discussed in Chapter 20.

Radiation and Neoplastic Plexopathies

Neoplasms may metastasize to the LSP or directly invade it. The most common tumors are colorectal, breast, and cervical carcinomas, sarcomas, and lymphomas. As with the brachial plexus, RT given as treatment for the tumor may itself damage the plexus and it is common to be faced with distinguishing neoplastic lumbosacral plexopathy (NLSP) from radiation lumbosacral plexopathy (RLSP).

Patients with NLSP typically present with insidious pelvic or lumbosacral pain with variable radiation into the leg, followed by paresthesias, sensory loss, and weakness, with weakness in a unilateral, multiroot distribution, sensory loss, and reflex asymmetry. Leg edema and a palpable mass are occasionally present. The process may affect the upper, lower, or entire plexus.[71] Radiation plexopathy usually presents after a long latency period, mean 6.5 years, with progressive asymmetrical leg weakness.[68] Pain is present at onset in only 10% of these patients and occurs at some time in the course in only 50%. Weakness is bilateral in most. Prognosis is poor in either condition.

Lumbosacral Plexopathy

Whether there is a primary, spontaneous "plexitis" affecting the LSP analogous to the entity of neuralgic amyotrophy of the brachial plexus has been a matter of conjecture. If so, it occurs at only a fraction of the incidence of the upper extremity condition. Bradley et al described six patients with a painful lumbosacral plexopathy associated with a high sedimentation rate and which responded to immunosuppression. An immunologically mediated process with an ischemic mechanism was suspected.[72] Chronic inflammatory demyelinating polyneuropathy involving the LSP has been reported, responsive to immunoglobulin therapy.[73] In a patient with a presumed diagnosis of atypical multifocal motor neuropathy, a condition that characteristically affects the upper extremities, causing severe proximal leg weakness responsive to immunoglobulin therapy, the diagnosis was suggested by conduction block of the unaffected tibial nerve.[74] A syndrome identical to DA in nondiabetics can occur rarely and is probably immunologically mediated.[47] Retroperitoneal hematomas, either due to a condition such as hemophilia or

disseminated intravascular coagulation, or, most commonly, to the use of anticoagulants are a common cause of lumbosacral plexus injury. Other causes of LSP include aortic aneurysm, amyloidosis, sarcoidosis, trauma, and obstetric injury.[75–78]

Evaluation and Diagnosis

The electrodiagnostic picture in DA is one of axon loss in a lumbar plexus distribution.[4] Paraspinal fibrillations are frequently present and do not necessarily indicate structural radiculopathy because the condition is by its nature a radiculoplexopathy. Helpful EMG findings in RLSP include paraspinal fibrillations (50%), fasciculations (35%), and myokymia. In a study of 20 patients with RLSP, myokymia was present in 60% compared to none of 21 patients with NLSP. Paraspinal fibrillations probably result from RT damage to roots, and this condition has also been called a radiculoplexopathy.

Imaging studies, especially CT and MRI, are helpful in the diagnosis of structural plexopathies, such as retroperitoneal hematoma or neoplasm. At other times imaging can be outright misleading, as in showing evidence of lumbosacral spine disease, common even in asymptomatic older patients, in a patient who clinically has DA and whose subsequent course of slow, spontaneous resolution or response to immunoglobulins, clearly demonstrates that the acute condition was not due to a structural radiculopathy.

Treatment and Management

Discrete hematomas should be evacuated and invasive tumors should be irradiated. Except for these two instances there is no specific treatment for lumbosacral plexopathy; intravenous immunoglobulin (IVIg) is often given empirically when lumbosacral plexopathy occurs for no apparent reason.

Focal Neuropathies

Focal neuropathies may result from compression, entrapment, ischemia, stretch, direct trauma such as lacerations and missile wounds, involvement in fractures or dislocations, and other processes. The terms *compression* and *entrapment* are often used more or less interchangeably, sacrificing some accuracy. *Compression neuropathy* refers to nerve damage due to pressure applied to a nerve, whatever the source. The term *entrapment neuropathy* is appropriate when the pressure is exerted by some anatomic or pathoanatomic structure, such as the transverse carpal ligament in carpal tunnel syndrome (CTS). All entrapment neuropathies are compression neuropathies, but not all compression neuropathies are due to entrapment. Entrapment neuropathies are all chronic conditions; compression neuropathies due to externally applied pressure can develop acutely over several hours (postoperative ulnar neuropathy, tourniquet paralysis, Saturday night radial nerve palsy), subacutely over days to weeks (peroneal neuropathy at the fibular head due to prolonged bed rest or a short leg cast), or chronically over months to years (ulnar neuropathy in the retroepicondylar groove). In some instances, a nerve is injured by relatively low force applied repetitively over a long period of time (retroepicondylar ulnar neuropathy, ulnar neuropathy at the wrist due to bicycling, peroneal neuropathy at the fibular head due to habitual leg crossing). Almost any nerve in the body can be compressed or entrapped, and by definition involvement is limited to the distribution of a single peripheral nerve.

Pathology and Pathophysiology of Compression/Entrapment Neuropathies

At the most minimal levels of nerve compression, reversible symptoms without accompanying structural changes, the familiar "falling asleep" sensation, is the primary manifestation. Referred to as *acute*, or *rapidly reversible*, *physiologic block*, these symptoms are due to nerve ischemia. Transient symptoms in some entrapment syndromes, such as the nocturnal paresthesias in CTS, may have an ischemic component. Although ischemic infarction of nerve clearly occurs, as in vasculitis, in most instances of compression or entrapment the predominant clinical manifestations are primarily related to pathologic changes in the myelin sheath or axon directly due to pressure; ischemia seems to play a relatively minor role in most instances. In certain acute and chronic compression syndromes in which axon loss is disproportionate to the apparent level of applied pressure or to the accompanying demyelination, ischemia may be a significant factor.[6]

Pathologic changes involving the myelin sheath are the earliest indication of pressure applied to a nerve. Low levels of force produce selective paranodal demyelination, greater levels of force cause myelin loss along a longer section of the nerve, involving both paranodal and internodal sections, referred to as segmental demyelination. Depending on the length of the segment involved, conduction velocity may simply slow or conduction may fail entirely, producing conduction block. Not all nerve fibers are equally susceptible to pressure injury. In experimental compression, large fibers are more susceptible than small, and peripheral fibers more vulnerable than central ones. In addition, different fascicles within a nerve at a given point exhibit different susceptibility to pressure injury, mostly reflecting the relationship between the fascicle's position within the nerve and the force vectors being applied. Several problematic phenomena are probably explicable on this basis of selective fascicular vulnerability, including sparing of the forearm flexors with ulnar lesions at the elbow, different degrees of involvement of different hand muscles in ulnar neuropathy, and lumbrical sparing in CTS. Selective fascicular vulnerability creates another level of difficulty in the evaluation of focal neuropathies, and the traditional concept of focal neuropathies as transverse lesions with equal involvement of all fibers below the level of the lesion needs revision.

Peripheral nerves have significant potential for repair and recovery.[79] After nerve compression is relieved, or proceeding pari passu with chronic repetitive trauma, nerve repair occurs. Axolemmal and partially digested myelin proteins are mitogenic for Schwann cells and induce proliferation and elaboration of myelin. Remyelination after purely demyelinating processes occurs over a period of several weeks to several months. Generally, myelin repair is complete within 12 weeks. With axonal damage recovery is much more protracted. Reinnervation after axon loss occurs by sprouting, which has two patterns. In the periphery, intact axons adjacent to injured ones rapidly send collateral sprouts to denervated muscle fibers. At the site of injury, the intact stump of the injured axon forms growth cones which attempt to span any gap present and regenerate the axon. If the growth cones can span the gap and regenerating axons can find their way into a Schwann cell tube, reinnervation is enhanced. Axons then grow at a rate of about 1 to 3 mm/day from the injury site to the target. When intraneural fibrosis prevents axons from spanning the gap, the proliferating fibers form a chaotic mass of disorganized, contorted axons known as a traumatic neuroma. A neuroma in continuity is one formed on a nerve which remains grossly intact but is severely disrupted internally.

As attempts at repair and regeneration occur at the injury site, important changes are occurring in the target organs. Muscle fibers deprived of innervation and not promptly rescued by collateral sprouts undergo neurogenic atrophy. After some period of time, atrophic fibers are replaced by fat and fibrosis. As a general rule, muscle fibers which have not been reinnervated within 12 to 18 months begin to undergo irreversible changes.

Traumatic nerve injuries can be classified by several systems. Seddon's system, the most commonly used classification scheme, divides nerve injuries into three types: neurapraxia, axonotmesis, and neurotmesis. In neurapraxia, the injury involves only the myelin. Although the initial deficit may be severe, recovery is rapid and generally complete within 12 weeks. In axonotmesis there is discontinuity of axons. The nerve trunk remains intact and in continuity, and regenerating axons can find their way into surviving endoneurial tubes. Axonotmesis is almost invariably associated with at least some degree of neurapraxia. In neurotmesis, the nerve is discontinuous. Supporting elements as well as axons are disrupted, and the nerve is separated into a proximal and distal stump with an intervening gap of variable width. Regenerating axons must first span any gap present and find the distal stump before reinnervation can proceed. Sunderland added two useful subclasses of axonotmesis. In a third-degree injury, there is endoneurial fibrosis which inhibits regeneration and results in variably incomplete recovery. In a fourth-degree injury, nerve continuity is maintained only by scar formation and there is no effective reinnervation. The Sunderland first-, second-, and fifth-degree lesions correspond to Seddon's neurapraxia, axonotmesis, and neurotmesis.

In neurapraxia there is no axonal loss. Recovery occurs over days to weeks and there is no Tinel sign at the site of the lesion. With a second-degree injury, axonal regeneration produces a Tinel sign at the injury site which then advances distally at the average rate of 1 inch per month. With a third-degree injury, the Tinel also advances, but ultimate recovery is incomplete and aberrant reinnervation may occur. Unfortunately, an advancing Tinel sign is associated with significant functional recovery in only 50% of cases. With a fourth-degree injury, the Tinel sign never advances beyond the injury site and no recovery occurs. Fifth-degree (neurotmetic) injuries are associated with lacerating or rupture injuries and the proximal and distal stumps are not in continuity. Neither fourth- nor fifth-degree lesions improve without surgery.

Focal Neuropathy Syndromes

CTS, ulnar neuropathy at the elbow, peroneal neuropathy at the knee, and retrohumeral radial neuropathy make up the majority of focal neuropathies, but virtually any nerve in the body can be compressed or entrapped (Table 16-4). Many other interesting and important focal neuropathies occur, some of which are summarized in Table 16-5. Several excellent monographs and other publications discuss these less common syndromes.[4,80]

Carpal Tunnel Syndrome

Clinical Pathoanatomy

The median nerve crosses from the distal forearm to the hand through the carpal tunnel. The walls and floor of the tunnel are formed by the carpal bones and the roof by the transverse carpal ligament (TCL). The TCL evolves from the antebrachial fascia at about the level of the wrist crease and extends 4 to 6 cm into the palm. The passageway is narrowest 2.0 to 2.5 cm distal to its origin, which corresponds to the

Table 16-4 Common Compression or Entrapment Neuropathies

Condition	Clinical Features	Treatment
Carpal tunnel syndrome	Pain in hand/wrist/forearm; numbness in hand especially at night or provoked by certain activities, weakness, occasional atrophy of thenar muscles, clumsiness	Wrist splints, nonsteroidal anti-inflammatory drugs, low-dose oral prednisone, steroid injection into carpal tunnel, avoid inciting activities, surgery (open or endoscopic) with failure to respond to conservative therapy or for significant or progressing motor deficit
Ulnar neuropathy at the elbow	Typically presents with numbness and tingling of ring and small fingers dependent on elbow position, pain not a prominent feature, with progression weakness of ulnar hand intrinsic muscles develops, often with atrophy of interossei and evolution of a claw deformity; some cases follow clear elbow trauma, most are idiopathic	Elbow pads (wrestler's or hockey player's) to avoid pressure on ulnar groove and to avoid prolonged elbow flexion; soft, cloth pads (e.g., Heelbo) not usually sufficient; avoid activities that produce pressure on the ulnar groove or require prolonged or repetitive elbow flexion; high incidence of spontaneous resolution; consider surgery for significant or progressive motor deficit
Retrohumeral radial neuropathy	Typically due to prolonged pressure on radial nerve in or near spiral groove presenting with wrist and finger drop; eventual complete recovery is typical	No specific treatment; need splints to maintain finger extension and physical therapy to maintain joint motion
Common peroneal neuropathy at the fibular head	Compression of the nerve where it lies superficially as it crosses the fibular head; prolonged squatting or focal pressure are usual precipitants; foot drop is the usual presentation, primary differential diagnosis consideration is L5 radiculopathy	No specific treatment; physical therapy to maintain joint mobility, ankle-foot orthosis for ambulation safety; knee pads rarely useful; failure of deficit to improve, or worsening of deficit, raises possibility of mass lesion in the region of the fibular tunnel and may require surgical exploration
Meralgia paresthetica (compression or entrapment of the lateral femoral cutaneous nerve)	Pain, numbness, and tingling of the lateral thigh, usually brought on my weight gain or wearing tight garments, belts, or other paraphernalia that compress the nerve in the region of the anterior superior iliac spine and lateralmost aspect of the inguinal ligament	Weight loss, avoidance of constricting garments and other things that cause pressure near the anterior superior iliac spine

Table 16-5 Clinical Features of Some Uncommon Focal Neuropathies

Syndrome	Clinical Features
Posterior interosseous neuropathy	Finger drop without wrist drop; pure motor; entrapment in the region of the supinator muscle
Median neuropathy due to supracondylar spur	Median entrapment by the ligament of Struthers running from distal humeral spur to medial epicondyle
Pronator teres syndrome	Main trunk median entrapment at the level of the pronator teres; motor and sensory dysfunction
Anterior interosseous neuropathy	Entrapment just distal to the pronator teres after anterior interosseous nerve leaves the main trunk; motor dysfunction only
Ulnar neuropathy at the wrist	Various combinations of motor and sensory dysfunction depending on precise location of lesion, external pressure frequently a factor (e.g., bicyclist's palsy)
Tarsal tunnel syndrome	Entrapment behind medial malleolus; pain and sensory dysfunction in sole of foot
Meralgia paresthetica	Lateral femoral cutaneous nerve entrapment near anterior superior iliac spine; pain/numbness in lateral thigh; obesity and tight garments predispose
Femoral neuropathy	May be injured at the inguinal ligament, in the pelvis or within the psoas muscle; hip/thigh weakness with decreased knee jerk and sensory loss in saphenous distribution (medial lower leg)
Suprascapular neuropathy	May be injured or entrapped at suprascapular or spinoglenoid notch, often associated with vigorous exercise, may be involved in neuralgic amyotrophy
Obturator neuropathy	May be injured in pelvic fracture or mass or compressed by obturator hernia or injured during hip replacement; difficulty stabilizing the hip joint
Sciatic neuropathy	May be injured in the hip/gluteal region by trauma, pelvic mass, or hip surgery; may be injured in the thigh by blunt or penetrating trauma; involvement of the short head of the biceps femoris by electromyography is the diagnostic clue to most sciatic neuropathies

usual site of median nerve compression.[81,82] Lying with the median nerve in the canal are the eight tendons of the flexor digitorum profundus and superficialis and the tendon of the flexor pollicis longus, surrounded by a complex synovial sheath.

The palmar cutaneous branch of the median nerve leaves the main trunk 5 to 8 cm proximal to the wrist crease. It travels through its own separate passageway in the TCL and provides sensation to the thenar eminence; it does not traverse the carpal tunnel. Loss of sensation over the thenar eminence is not part of CTS and suggests a lesion proximal to the wrist. After exiting the tunnel, the median nerve gives off its recurrent thenar motor branch, which curves backward and radially to innervate the thenar muscles.

Entrapment of the median nerve beneath the TCL is often brought on or exacerbated by excessive hand/wrist/finger movements; the combination of repetitive finger flexion with wrist motion seems to be the most hazardous ergonomic stress. Both vocational and recreational activities (e.g., gardening, metal scavenging, fly fishing, refinishing furniture, knitting/needlepoint, karate) can incite or aggravate the condition. CTS can rarely result from mass lesions narrowing the passageway (e.g., ganglion, osteophyte, lipoma, aneurysm, anomalous muscle). Numerous systemic conditions predispose to CTS, including rheumatoid arthritis, diabetes mellitus, chronic renal insufficiency, hypothyroidism, amyloidosis, myeloma, and pregnancy.

Clinical Signs and Symptoms

CTS produces a characteristic clinical picture of hand pain, numbness, and paresthesias (all usually more severe at night), along with varying degrees of weakness.[83] Proximal upper extremity pain, usually in the forearm but sometimes as far as the shoulder, is less typical but not uncommon. Many patients initially complain of "whole hand" symptoms. The reason for the nocturnal exacerbation of symptoms remains obscure, but the diagnosis should remain suspect in the absence of this feature.

Findings on examination vary with the severity of the condition. Patients with mild CTS may have normal findings on physical examination, or trivial sensory loss over the fingertips. The earliest sensory loss seems to occur over the volar tip of the middle finger. Patients with more advanced disease have more easily demonstrable sensory loss and frequently have weakness of the thenar muscles. Patients with severe involvement demonstrate thenar atrophy and dense sensory loss. Such patients with longstanding, untreated end-stage CTS often have surprisingly few symptoms. Provocative tests, such as the Tinel sign, Phalen's sign, carpal compression maneuver, and the flick sign have proved disappointing, with high proportions of false positive and false negative results.[84,85]

Evaluation and Diagnosis

The most common differential diagnostic exercise is between CTS and CR, most often at C6. Neck and shoulder pain, weakness in C6 innervated muscles, reflex changes, sensory loss restricted to the thumb, the absence of nocturnal paresthesias, and reproduction of the paresthesias with root compression maneuvers all favor CR. Other conditions occasionally meriting consideration include proximal median neuropathy, neurogenic thoracic outlet syndrome, and upper brachial plexopathy. Various musculoskeletal conditions, especially de Quervain tendonitis, can cause hand and wrist pain suggestive of CTS.

The electrodiagnosis of CTS has been recently reviewed.[86] The earliest electrodiagnostic change is prolongation of the median SNAP latency. The 8 cm palm to wrist technique is more sensitive than wrist/finger studies because of the shorter segment of unaffected nerve included.[87] Abnormal NAP amplitude or latency, while

the earliest detectable abnormality, is not localizing. With more severe involvement there is loss of NAP amplitude, prolongation of the motor distal latency, and the development of denervation in thenar muscles.

A minority of patients with a clinical diagnosis of CTS have normal electrodiagnostic evaluations, from 10% to 40% depending on the technique. Numerous special techniques have been proposed to detect the cases missed by the usual methods. But since each procedure carries its own incidence of false positive results, performing multiple tests in an attempt to diagnose CTS may do more to increase the false positive rate than make any real contribution to the diagnosis in problem cases.[88] The most significant recent advance in the electrodiagnosis of CTS has been the development of the combined sensory index, or "Robinson index."[89] This is a summary index of the differences in latency between the median and ulnar palmar latencies, the median and ulnar latencies to the ring finger, and the median and radial latencies to the thumb. It is highly sensitive and specific for CTS.

Because CTS is common and the median nerve at the wrist is easy to image by MRI, the literature on MRI findings in CTS is more extensive than for any other nerve. Various findings have been reported, including abnormal T2 signal in the nerve, proximal nerve enlargement, flattening distally and anterior bowing of the TCL. Nevertheless, at the current time, the accuracy of nerve conduction studies remains superior to that of MRI.[29] This conclusion was reached based on routine conduction studies, excluding advanced and superior techniques such as the combined sensory index.

There is a growing body of literature regarding ultrasound in the evaluation of CTS. The typical finding is enlargement of the median nerve at the wrist crease, documented via a number of parameters. Sonography is simple to perform, but its place in the diagnostic armamentarium is yet to be determined. In a prospective study of 207 patients with a clinical diagnosis of CTS, Visser and colleagues found the accuracy of sonography to be similar to that for electrodiagnostic studies.[90] In one study designed to determine whether HRS can be an alternative method to NCS in the diagnosis of CTS, it was found that sensitivity was similar between HRS and NCS, but specificity was significantly lower for HRS; the investigators concluded that sonography is not accurate enough to replace NCS for the diagnosis of CTS.[91]

Treatment and Management

Initial attempts at treatment should involve trying to identify predisposing vocational or avocational activities that may be inducing or aggravating the symptoms (Box 16-4). The ergonomonics of CTS have been studied extensively. The greatest ergonomonic stress is activities that involve repetitive flexion and extension of the wrist accompanied by flexion and extension of the fingers. This activity is prone to induce flexor tendon tenosynovitis, which is well recognized to be associated with CTS. Occupational activities likely

---

Box 16-4 Treatment of Carpal Tunnel Syndrome

Avoidance of aggravating/inciting activities
Wrist splints (worn constantly until better, then at night only)
Nonsteroidal anti-inflammatory drugs (NSAIDs)
Low-dose oral steroids
Steroid injection
Carpal tunnel release
  Open
  Endoscopic
No evidence to support use of pyridoxine

to induce CTS include those requiring heavy use of the hands, such as carpentry, bricklaying, and other manual labor. The most frequently blamed activity is use of a computer, however, almost everyone in the modern world uses a computer and patients developed CTS regularly when the PC was the dream of a handful of zealots. The patient should stop suspicious activities for a trial period consistent with the limits of their employment. Avocational activities that may cause CTS include such things as heavy gardening, woodworking, metal scavenging, knitting and crocheting, and many others.

Splints are clearly helpful. The splint should be lightweight and neutral or slightly dorsiflexion in position. If the patient is only having occasional nocturnal symptoms, then wearing the splint only at night is acceptable. If the patient is having symptoms more than three or four nights per week, multiple times per night, or having symptoms during the day, then an effective strategy is to have the patient wear the splint day and night for the first few weeks, and to drop back to nighttime use only when the symptoms have improved.

Several types of medications are used in CTS; none are especially useful. NSAIDs are used to combat the tenosynovitis but have not been shown to be very helpful. Some physicians use pyridoxine despite the fact there is not one scintilla of evidence to support its use and it can cause neuropathy if used chronically at a dose as low as 200 mg/day (and is sold over the counter in capsules with doses as high as 500 mg). Any physician foolish enough to use this homeopathic remedy is duty bound not to cause harm with it! Low-dose prednisone at a dose of 20 mg for 1 week and 10 mg for 1 week has been shown to be of benefit.[92]

If immobilization, NSAIDs, and low-dose prednisone are not useful, many physicians proceed to a steroid injection, using 20 mg or equivalent or methylprednisolone and 1 mL of 1% lidocaine. In a prospective study, local steroid injection resulted in long-term improvement in nerve conduction parameters, symptom severity, and functional scores in patients with mild CTS.[93] Details on how to perform an injection are given elsewhere. Anyone administering an injection should be very familiar with the technique. Rarely, an injection is given when CTS is considered likely but the clinical picture is ambiguous and the electrodiagnostic picture is not definitive.

Conservative therapy is most likely to be effective when the CTS is relatively acute, developing over days or weeks due to tenosynovitis developing in response to an identifiable activity, such as putting in the spring garden, knitting a large afghan, or heavy work on the weight bench. More long-standing CTS is much less likely to respond to conservative therapy and more likely to need surgical decompression.

There are two surgical approaches: open and endoscopic. There are advantages and disadvantages to each. Conventional wisdom has been that complications are higher with the endoscopic procedure, but there is less postoperative pain and an earlier return to work. A recent review left much of this conventional wisdom in doubt and seriously questioned the wisdom of the endoscopic approach.[94]

Proximal Median Neuropathies

The median nerve may be compressed just proximal to the elbow by an anomalous structure, the ligament of Struthers, which runs from a congenital supracondylar spur down to the medial epicondyle; decompression involves the main trunk of the median nerve. The median nerve may be involved in the region of the pronator teres muscles, typically as it passes between the superficial and deep heads of the muscle (pronator teres syndrome). The deficit may involve the main trunk of the median or only the anterior interosseous nerve (AIN), depending upon the exact anatomy. Whether the pronator

teres is involved again depends upon the exact anatomy; most often it is spared. The AIN may be compressed by fibrous bands or other anomalous structures in the region of the pronator muscle (see Table 16-5). The AIN is commonly involved in neuralgic amyotrophy, and in fact neuralgic amyotrophy may present as an AIN mononeuropathy.

Ulnar Neuropathy at the Elbow

Ulnar neuropathy at the elbow (UNE) is the second most common compression neuropathy after CTS.

Clinical Pathoanatomy

After descending without branches through the upper arm, the nerve traverses the retroepicondylar groove between the medial epicondyle (ME) and olecranon process (OP). The nerve then passes beneath the humeroulnar aponeurotic arcade (HUA), a dense aponeurosis joining the humeral and ulnar heads of origin of the flexor carpi ulnaris (FCU), which typically lies 1.0 to 2.5 cm distal to a line connecting the ME and the OP.[95] After passing under the HUA, the nerve runs through the belly of the FCU, then exits through the deep flexor pronator aponeurosis lining the deep surface of the muscle 4.0 to 6.0 cm beyond the ME.

Anatomic factors account for much of the susceptibility of the ulnar nerve to injury at the elbow. The lack of protective covering over the nerve in its course through the ulnar groove accounts for its susceptibility to external pressure. This is particularly pronounced in patients with a low body mass index (BMI), who have an increased risk of developing UNE.[96] Repetitive flexion and extension may predispose to UNE because of the dynamic changes in the nerve's passageway with motion. With elbow joint derangement due to trauma or arthritic changes, the nerve's vulnerability increases even further. Valgus deformities increase the stretch on the nerve with elbow flexion, and osteophytic overgrowth further narrows an often already narrow passageway. The nerve may be entrapped at the HUA or at the point of exit from the FCU.[4]

A number of problems arise in the differential diagnosis of suspected UNE. There are at least three potential sites of ulnar compression in the region of the elbow: the ulnar groove, the HUA, and the exit site from the FCU. The clinical manifestations of disease at the wrist, elbow, and more proximal sites can be similar. The nerve's branching pattern limits both clinical and electrodiagnostic localization. Selective vulnerability may produce varying degrees of involvement of different fascicles.[97] Forearm muscles are often spared in lesions at the elbow.

A terminology morass has grown out of imprecision in the use of terms such as *tardy ulnar palsy* and *cubital tunnel syndrome*. *Tardy ulnar palsy* was first used to describe UNE developing after remote elbow trauma, generally after an old fracture or dislocation. It soon degenerated into a nonspecific, generic term for any ulnar neuropathy at the elbow, on the weak presumption that remote trauma must have occurred but the patient simply couldn't recall it. Feindel and Stratford coined the term *cubital tunnel syndrome* (*cubit* is Latin for elbow or forearm) to refer to patients with compression of the nerve by the HUA.[98] They were attempting to define a subgroup of "tardy ulnar palsy" patients who suffered from a focal entrapment by the FCU aponeurosis, and who could be spared a transposition procedure and managed with simple release of the aponeurotic arcade. As with tardy ulnar palsy, the term *cubital tunnel syndrome* soon degenerated into a useless, nonspecific, generic label for any UNE as the term increasingly grew in popularity with few bothering to read the original paper. Many clinicians, even neurologists, neurosurgeons, and orthopedists, now use *cubital tunnel syndrome* the way their predecessors not many years ago used *tardy ulnar palsy*: to refer to any UNE. All these terms except *UNE* now invite confusion and miscommunication and should be stricken from the lexicon. Curiously, some physicians who insist on using the term *median neuropathy at the wrist* instead of *carpal tunnel syndrome* are comfortable referring to cubital tunnel syndrome, a situation that would undoubtedly cause Mr. Spock to arch an eyebrow.

Clinical Signs and Symptoms

The physical examination of a patient with suspected UNE should include detailed assessment of strength, sensation, and reflexes, and examination of the elbow for range of motion and deformity. Weakness of nonulnar C8 muscles is the usual clue to disease involving the lower brachial plexus or C8 root. This finding should in turn prompt further examination of the cervical spine and a check for Horner syndrome. Weakness in the ulnar innervated long finger flexors and FCU may help separate UNE from a more distal lesion, though normal strength in these muscles is still entirely consistent with an elbow level lesion. Ulnar neuropathy is not the only condition that can cause hand clawing.

A careful sensory examination can be rewarding. The cutaneous field of the ulnar nerve does not extend more than a few centimeters proximal to the wrist crease. Involvement of the distribution of the medial antebrachial cutaneous nerve over the medial forearm excludes UNE, because this nerve runs anterior to the ME and not through the ulnar groove. Impaired sensation over the dorsum of the hand establishes the location of the lesion as proximal to the takeoff of the dorsal cutaneous branch, but sparing of the dorsal cutaneous territory does not exclude UNE because of possible selective sparing of its fascicles. Involvement of the palmar cutaneous branch distribution likewise suggests a proximal lesion. Splitting of the ring finger fairly reliably excludes plexopathy and radiculopathy.

Impaired elbow range of motion or a valgus deformity strongly suggests UNE. Reproduction of symptoms with elbow flexion and ulnar groove pressure can be informative. Examining for subluxation is seldom helpful, as this is a common phenomenon in normal individuals. Eliciting a Tinel sign can be useful, but many normal patients exhibit Tinel signs over all their nerves; only the presence of a disproportionately active Tinel sign over the clinically suspect ulnar nerve has any localizing value.

Evaluation and Diagnosis

Lesions of the brachial plexus and lower cervical roots cause signs and symptoms occasionally difficult to distinguish from UNE. Patients with anterior horn cell disease and other myelopathies may develop small hand muscle wasting resembling that seen in UNE. The sensory symptoms of UNE can mimic those of CR, plexopathy, and ulnar lesions at the wrist or upper arm.

The mainstay of the evaluation of suspected UNE is electrodiagnosis. However, the ulnar is a difficult nerve to study and there are persistent problems with sensitivity and specificity, especially in inexperienced hands. The Practice Parameter of the American Association of Neuromuscular and Electrodiagnostic Medicine is an exhaustive discussion of the matter of ulnar electrodiagnosis.[99] The summary recommendations are listed in Box 16-5. A 2003 review article provides a nice summary.[100]

Subsequent studies have shown that the optimal distance for screening for UNE, considering both sensitivity and specificity, is significantly less than the standard 10 cm, perhaps as low as 4 to 6 cm; considering in addition the likely locations of focal lesions, the best distance is 6 to 8 cm.[101] For precise diagnosis and localization, the

---

Box 16-5 Evaluation of Ulnar Neuropathy at the Elbow*

1. When using moderate elbow flexion (70–90 degrees from horizontal), a 10-cm across-elbow (AE) distance, and surface stimulation and recording, the following abnormalities suggest a focal lesion involving the ulnar nerve at the elbow. The most important criterion is the presence of multiple internally consistent abnormalities. Multiple abnormalities are more convincing than isolated abnormalities, which raise the possibility of artifact or technical mishap.
   a. Absolute motor nerve conduction velocity (NCV) from AE to below-elbow (BE) of less than 50 m/sec.
   b. An AE to BE segment greater than 10 m/sec slower than the BE to wrist (W) segment.
   c. A decrease in compound muscle action potential (M wave) negative peak amplitude from BE to AE greater than 20%.
   d. A significant change in M wave configuration at the AE site compared to the BE site.
2. If routine motor studies are inconclusive, the following procedures may be of benefit:
   a. Nerve conduction studies (NCS) recorded from the first dorsal interosseous (FDI) muscle.
   b. An inching or short segment study.
3. Needle examination should include the FDI, the most frequently abnormal muscle, and ulnar innervated forearm flexors. Neither changes limited to the FDI, nor sparing of the forearm muscles, exclude an elbow lesion. If ulnar innervated muscles are abnormal, the examination should be extended to include nonulnar C8/medial cord/lower trunk muscles to exclude brachial plexopathy and the cervical paraspinals to exclude radiculopathy.

*Synopsis of the recommendations of the Practice Parameter of the American Association of Neuromuscular and Electrodiagnostic Medicine.

---

utility of short segment incremental studies at 1 or 2 cm has been demonstrated repeatedly since the original descriptions.[102–104] Keeping the elbow warm during ulnar conduction studies is vital and will markedly decrease the incidence of false positive studies.[105]

MRI of the ulnar nerve at the elbow has proved more useful than in CTS. In UNE, the sensitivity is said to be as high as 95%, compared to 60% to 75% for routine NCS. Studies reaching this conclusion did not rely on advanced conduction techniques such as short segment incremental studies.[29] There are potential problems with the claim of 95% sensitivity, beginning with the long ago established entity of asymptomatic enlargement of the ulnar nerve in the groove and the concept of subclinical ulnar neuropathy.[106,107]

Ultrasound of the ulnar nerve is growing in popularity, but it remains to be determined whether it adds a significant element to the diagnosis. Beekman et al prospectively examined the correlations between the clinical characteristics, electrophysiologic features, and sonographic ulnar-nerve diameter in 102 patients with UNE and concluded that routine NCS had a sensitivity of 78%, and the addition of sonography increased this to 98%. There has been a recent flurry of publications on this topic, including the establishment of reliable reference values for ulnar nerve measurements.[30,108,109] In one personal case, MRI and ultrasound showed marked enlargement of the ulnar nerve in the groove in a patient who clinically had medial epicondylitis from bowling (daily, for money, a hustler) but not one scintilla of clinical or electrodiagnostic evidence of ulnar neuropathy.[106,107] Caution is required before relying too heavily on either MRI or ultrasound abnormalities as the sole findings in the diagnosis of UNE.

Treatment

Patients with UNE may improve with conservative treatment (Box 16-6). De Jesus and Steiner followed a group of patients managed nonsurgically for periods up to 4 years.[110] At follow-up, 46% were normal after nonoperative management and 15% were significantly improved. The likelihood of spontaneous recovery was greatest in those patients with the mildest electrophysiologic abnormalities. Dellon et al prospectively evaluated 128 patients with UNE managed nonoperatively.[111] Just 11% of those with symptoms only eventually had surgery as compared with 33% of those with mild to moderate abnormalities on examination and 62% of those with more severe abnormalities. The presence of persistent paresthesias, abnormal two-point discrimination, and any degree of muscle wasting moved patients into the category of likely eventual surgery. Electrodiagnostic abnormalities were not found to have predictive value. A history of elbow injury significantly worsened the outcome.

Patients who require ulnar nerve surgery may undergo any of several procedures, depending largely on the preference and habits of the surgeon. Complications are unlikely with simple decompression of the HUA. Anterior transposition is usually safe, but can go terribly awry. Most ulnar nerve disasters occur in patients who have undergone transposition. Although debate continues, evidence increasingly seems to favor in situ decompression as just as efficacious and with a lower incidence of complications compared to transposition.[94] An endoscopic method for in situ decompression has been developed.

Ulnar Neuropathy Not at the Elbow

The ulnar nerve may be entrapped by the medial intramuscular septum, the so-called arcade of Struthers, most typically in a patient who has had ulnar transposition with an inadequate proximal release. The nerve may be entrapped at its point of exit from the flexor carpi ulnaris muscle in the upper forearm, more rarely in the distal forearm.[112,113] Ulnar neuropathy at the wrist occurs in Guyon's canal. There are several subtypes, and the deficit depends upon the exact site of compression, varying from involvement of the entire nerve in proximal Guyon's canal compression to involvement of only the deep ulnar branch producing a pure motor deficit with more distal compression.

Radial Neuropathy

Acute compression of the radial nerve in the retrohumeral spiral groove, frequently referred to as *Saturday night* or *bridegroom's palsy*, results from sustained compression over a period of several hours during sleep or a drug- or alcohol-induced stupor. Weakness involves all muscles distal to the triceps, which receives its innervation from a branch arising proximal to the spiral groove. The most prominent complaint and finding is wrist drop. Sensory loss is usually present in the superficial radial nerve distribution. Confusion commonly arises on two points: (1) because of mechanical factors, the interossei cannot exert normal power in the face of finger drop and may seem weak and (2) weakness of thumb abduction occurs

due to dysfunction of the radial innervated abductor pollicis longus. The apparent weakness of the interossei and of thumb abduction may befuddle the unwary and cause mislocalization. The primary differential diagnostic considerations include C7 radiculopathy, posterior interosseous nerve palsy, and lesions involving the middle trunk or posterior cord of the brachial plexus. The radial nerve seems particularly prone to involvement in systemic vasculitis.

Common Peroneal Neuropathy at the Fibular Head

In its arc across the fibular head, the peroneal nerve is superficial and vulnerable to external compression, and peroneal neuropathy at the knee most often develops in the setting of external pressure. The nerve may also be susceptible to stretch injury or entrapment at its point of passage through the fibrous arch at the origin of the peroneus longus muscle (the "fibular tunnel").

Habitual leg crossing is the classic cause of peroneal neuropathy at the knee, but external pressure damage may come from a variety of potential sources. Other causes include prolonged squatting, and sudden, forceful plantar flexion or inversion of the ankle. Rarely, a mass lesion, such as a ganglion or peripheral nerve tumor may compress the nerve, or it may suffer entrapment at the fibular tunnel.

The most important element in the workup is the medical detective work necessary to detect the mechanism of compression or stretch. In most patients, a meticulous history will uncover a likely explanation. Searching for a dimple, discoloration, or callus over the fibular head may help confirm an external pressure mechanism. Failure to find a satisfactory explanatory mechanism of injury, failure of the neuropathy to resolve, or progression of the deficit under observation raises the possibility of mass lesion or fibular tunnel entrapment.

The most common differential diagnostic exercise is between common peroneal neuropathy at the fibular head (CPNFH) and L5 radiculopathy in the patient with foot drop. The presence of back and leg pain, weakness of foot inversion, positive root stretch signs, and depression of the medial hamstring reflex favor radiculopathy. The absence of pain, weakness limited to ankle eversion and foot/toe dorsiflexion, and preservation of the medial hamstring reflex favor CPNFH.

In rare patients, sciatic neuropathy, deep peroneal neuropathy, or lumbosacral plexopathy may simulate CPNFH. Patients with sciatic neuropathy have involvement of the short head of the biceps femoris on EMG; otherwise, it is clinically difficult to distinguish proximal sciatic neuropathy from peroneal neuropathy. Patients with superficial peroneal neuropathy, a rarity, only have involvement of the foot evertors. In deep peroneal neuropathy, the peroneus longus and brevis are spared, foot eversion is clinically intact, and the deficit depends on the exact level of the lesion. In deep peroneal neuropathy due to anterior tarsal syndrome, there is no foot drop and involvement is limited to deep peroneal innervated intrinsic foot muscles. A number of generalized conditions may require consideration, especially if foot drop is bilateral, including generalized neuropathies, motor neuron disease, and several types of primary muscle disease (e.g., distal myopathy, inclusion body myositis, myotonic dystrophy, and scapuloperoneal syndromes).

The standard electrodiagnostic technique is to record from the extensor digitalis brevis or tibialis anterior muscle while stimulating the peroneal nerve above and below the fibular head (FH) searching for focal slowing, temporal dispersion, or conduction block. When stimulating in the popliteal fossa, there is a significant chance of inadvertent spread of the stimulus current to the tibial nerve, which produces spurious and confusing M-wave amplitude variations. Because of the dictates of the "10 cm rule" (see earlier discussion under ulnar neuropathy), many EMG operators stimulate below the FH and then measure at least 10 cm into the popliteal fossa. Again, there is a tradeoff of experimental error against lesion detection, and the proximal stimulation in this instance can become frankly problematic because of stimulus spread. To detect spread, in addition to noting changes in M-wave amplitude and waveform, it is useful to observe the motion of the foot. Peroneal stimulation will produce an extension/eversion movement. Tibial stimulation will produce plantar flexion. If both nerves are being stimulated, the foot will simply "quiver" and move neither up nor down.

CPNFH can produce almost any combination of demyelination and axon loss, which may involve any of the target muscles to different degrees. The M-wave amplitude with stimulation below the FH, compared with laboratory reference values or the contralateral leg, provides an index of the degree of axon loss. The difference in M-wave amplitude with below FH versus above FH stimulation reflects the degree of demyelinating neurapraxia. Slowing across the FH indicates the CV in demyelinated but not blocked fibers. Which of these features is paramount is a matter of debate.

The superficial peroneal (SP) SNAP is very useful in evaluating CPNFH. Although some mild, demyelinating lesions may spare the SP SNAP, with lesions causing any significant axon loss this potential will be reduced in amplitude or absent. In contrast, the most common process mimicking CPNFH, L5 radiculopathy, should leave a robustly normal SP SNAP.

Needle electromyography should focus not only on peroneal innervated muscles but also on nonperoneal L5 muscles, such as the tibialis posterior and flexor digitorum longus, and should always include the short head of the biceps femoris. Because the short head of the biceps is the only peroneal innervated muscle lying proximal to the FH, any abnormality there suggests a lesion above the midthigh. Because a lesion severe enough to cause neurapraxia or significant conduction slowing is usually severe enough to damage at least a few axons, some, occasionally many, fibrillation potentials can be seen in peroneal innervated muscles even with a primarily demyelinating CPNFH. The M-wave amplitude and SP SNAP amplitude are better indicators of the extent of axon loss.

MRI may be useful in defining the distribution of muscle denervation and distinguishing peroneal neuropathy from radiculopathy, but it has not been reported to show abnormalities of the peroneal nerve itself.[29] There is only limited information regarding the utility of sonography.[114]

There is no specific treatment for CPNFH except to remove any persistent or recurrent compression, avoid prolonged squatting, and eliminate other such etiologic factors. If there has been no substantial axon loss, the nerve should remyelinate with good recovery. If there has been axon loss, recovery is likely to be incomplete and sometimes the patient is left with a foot drop. If the neuropathy progresses under observation after predisposing factors have been eliminated, consideration should be given to surgical exploration to exclude nerve sheath tumor and to decompress the fibular tunnel.

References

1. Radhakrishnan K, Litchy WJ, O'Fallon WM, Kurland LT: Epidemiology of cervical radiculopathy. A population-based study from Rochester, Minnesota, 1976 through 1990, *Brain* 117:325–335, 1994.
2. Wilbourn AJ, Aminoff MJ: AAEE minimonograph #32: the electrophysiologic examination in patients with radiculopathies, *Muscle Nerve* 11:1099–1114, 1988.
3. Haig AJ, Moffroid M, Henry S, et al: A technique for needle localization in paraspinal muscles with cadaveric confirmation, *Muscle Nerve* 14:521–526, 1991.
4. Campbell WW: *Essentials of Electrodiagnostic Medicine*, Baltimore, 1998, Williams & Wilkins.
5. Yoss RE, Corbin KB, MacCarty CS, et al: Significance of symptoms and signs in localization of involved root in cervical disc protrusion, *Neurology* 7:673–683, 1957.
6. Murphey F, Simmons JCH, Brunson B: Surgical treatment of laterally ruptured cervical disc: review of 648 cases, 1939–1972, *J Neurosurg* 38:679–683, 1996.
7. Levin KH, Maggiano HJ, Wilbourn AJ: Cervical radiculopathies: comparison of surgical and EMG localization of single root lesions, *Neurology* 46:1022–1025, 1996.
8. Abbed KM, Coumans JV: Cervical radiculopathy: pathophysiology, presentation, and clinical evaluation, *Neurosurgery* 60(1 Suppl 1):S28–S34, 2007.
9. Naftulin S, Fast A, Thomas M: Diabetic lumbar radiculopathy: sciatica without disc herniation, *Spine* 18:2419–2422, 1993.
10. Katz JS, Saperstein DS, Wolfe G, et al: Cervicobrachial involvement in diabetic radiculoplexopathy, *Muscle Nerve* 24(6):794–798, 2001.
11. So YT, Weber CF, Ball RD, et al: The electrodiagnostic evaluation of patients with suspected cervical radiculopathy: literature review on the usefulness of needle electromyography, *Muscle Nerve* 22(Suppl 8):S213–S221, 1999.
12. Lauder TD, Dillingham TR: The cervical radiculopathy screen: optimizing the number of muscles studied, *Muscle Nerve* 19:662–665, 1996.
13. Jensen MC, Brant-Zawadzki MN, Obuchowski N, et al: Magnetic resonance imaging of the lumbar spine in people without back pain, *N Engl J Med* 331:69–73, 1994.
14. Wipf JE, Deyo RA: Low back pain, *Med Clin North Am* 79:231–246, 1995.
15. Carrino JA, Lurie JD, Tosteson AN, et al: Lumbar spine: reliability of MR imaging findings, *Radiology* 250(1):161–170, 2009.
16. Alyas F, Connell D, Saifuddin A: Upright positional MRI of the lumbar spine, *Clin Radiol* 63(9):1035–1048, 2008.
17. Bernard TN Jr, Kirkaldy-Willis WH: Recognizing specific characteristics of nonspecific low back pain, *Clin Orthop* (217):266–280, 1987.
18. Milette PC, Fontaine S, Lepanto L, Breton G: Radiating pain to the lower extremities caused by lumbar disk rupture without spinal nerve root involvement, *AJNR Am J Neuroradiol* 16:1605–1613, 1995; discussion, 1614–1615.
19. Schwarzer AC, Aprill CN, Bogduk N: The sacroiliac joint in chronic low back pain, *Spine* 20:31–37, 1995.
20. Schwarzer AC, Aprill CN, Derby R, et al: The relative contributions of the disc and zygapophyseal joint in chronic low back pain, *Spine* 19:801–806, 1994.
21. Schwarzer AC, Aprill CN, Derby R, et al: The prevalence and clinical features of internal disc disruption in patients with chronic low back pain, *Spine* 20:1878–1883, 1995.
22. Schwarzer AC, Aprill CN, Derby R, et al: Clinical features of patients with pain stemming from the lumbar zygapophysial joints. Is the lumbar facet syndrome a clinical entity? *Spine* 19:1132–1137, 1994.
23. Nath S, Nath CA, Pettersson K: Percutaneous lumbar zygapophysial (facet) joint neurotomy using radiofrequency current, in the management of chronic low back pain: a randomized double-blind trial, *Spine* 33(12):1291–1297, 2008.
24. Deyo RA, Loeser JD, Bigos SJ: Herniated lumbar intervertebral disk, *Ann Intern Med* 112:598–603, 1990.
25. Deyo RA, Rainville J, Kent DL: What can the history and physical examination tell us about low back pain? *JAMA* 268:760–765, 1992.
26. Hall S, Bartleson JD, Onofrio BM, et al: Lumbar spinal stenosis. Clinical features, diagnostic procedures, and results of surgical treatment in 68 patients, *Ann Intern Med* 103:271–275, 1985.
27. Kinkade S: Evaluation and treatment of acute low back pain, *Am Fam Physician* 75(8):1181–1188, 2007.
28. Amrami KK, Felmlee JP, Spinner RJ: MRI of peripheral nerves, *Neurosurg Clin North Am* 19(4):559–572, 2008.
29. Hof JJ, Kliot M, Slimp J, Haynor DR: What's new in MRI of peripheral nerve entrapment? *Neurosurg Clin North Am* 19(4):583–595, vi, 2008.
30. Cartwright MS, Shin HW, Passmore LV, et al: Ultrasonographic findings of the normal ulnar nerve in adults, *Arch Phys Med Rehabil* 88(3):394–396, 2007.

31. Chloros GD, Cartwright MS, Walker FO, et al: Sonography and electrodiagnosis in carpal tunnel syndrome diagnosis, an analysis of the literature, *Eur J Radiol* 71(1):141–143, 2009.

32. Martinoli C, Bianchi S, Gandolfo N, et al: US of nerve entrapments in osteofibrous tunnels of the upper and lower limbs, *Radiographics* 20(Spec No):S199–S213, 2001; discussion, S213.

33. Cartwright MS, Chloros GD, Walker FO, et al: Diagnostic ultrasound for nerve transection, *Muscle Nerve* 35(6):796–799, 2007.

34. Amato AA, Russell JA: *Neuromuscular Disorders*, New York, 2008, McGraw-Hill.

35. Subramony SH: AAEE case report #14: neuralgic amyotrophy (acute brachial neuropathy), *Muscle Nerve* 11:39–44, 1988.

36. van Alfen N: The neuralgic amyotrophy consultation, *J Neurol* 254(6): 695–704, 2007.

37. van Alfen N, van Engelen BG: The clinical spectrum of neuralgic amyotrophy in 246 cases, *Brain* 129(Pt 2):438–450, 2006.

38. Jeannet PY, Watts GD, Bird TD, et al: Craniofacial and cutaneous findings expand the phenotype of hereditary neuralgic amyotrophy, *Neurology* 57 (11):1963–1968, 2001.

39. Amato AA, Jackson CE, Kim JY, et al: Chronic relapsing brachial plexus neuropathy with persistent conduction block, *Muscle Nerve* 20(10): 1303–1307, 1997.

40. Dionne A, Brunet D: A case of Lewis-Sumner syndrome with conduction abnormalities only in the brachial plexus and roots, *Muscle Nerve* 34(4): 489–493, 2006.

41. Veltkamp R, Krause M, Schranz C, et al: Progressive arm weakness and tonic hand spasm from multifocal motor neuropathy in the brachial plexus, *Muscle Nerve* 28(2):242–245, 2003.

42. Kori SH, Foley KM, Posner JB: Brachial plexus lesions in patients with cancer: 100 cases, *Neurology* 31(1):45–50, 1981.

43. Harper CM Jr, Thomas JE, Cascino TL, et al: Distinction between neoplastic and radiation-induced brachial plexopathy, with emphasis on the role of EMG, *Neurology* 39:502–506, 1989.

44. Olsen NK, Pfeiffer P, Mondrup K, et al: Radiation-induced brachial plexus neuropathy in breast cancer patients, *Acta Oncol* 29:885–890, 1990.

45. Lederman RJ, Breuer AC, Hanson MR, et al: Peripheral nervous system complications of coronary artery bypass graft surgery, *Ann Neurol* 12:297–301, 1982.

46. Vahl CF, Carl I, Muller-Vahl H, Struck E: Brachial plexus injury after cardiac surgery. The role of internal mammary artery preparation: a prospective study on 1000 consecutive patients, *J Thorac Cardiovasc Surg* 102: 724–729, 1991.

47. Wilbourn AJ: Plexopathies, *Neurol Clin* 25(1):139–171, 2007.

48. Watson BV, Merchant RN, Brown WF: Early postoperative ulnar neuropathies following coronary artery bypass surgery, *Muscle Nerve* 15:701–705, 1992.

49. Marchini C, Zambito MS, Cavagna E, et al: Saturday night brachial plexus palsy, *Neurol Sci* 28(5):279–281, 2007.

50. Mallet J: [Obstetrical paralysis of the brachial plexus. 3. Conclusions], *Rev Chir Orthop Reparatrice Appar Mot* 58(Suppl 1):201–204, 1972.

51. van der Sluijs JA, van Doorn-Loogman MH, Ritt MJ, et al: Interobserver reliability of the Mallet score, *J Pediatr Orthop B* 15(5):324–327, 2006.

52. Piatt JH Jr: Birth injuries of the brachial plexus, *Clin Perinatol* 32(1):39–vi, 2005.

53. Piatt JH Jr: Birth injuries of the brachial plexus, *Pediatr Clin North Am* 51(2):421–440, 2004.

54. Markey KL, Di Benedetto M, Curl WW: Upper trunk brachial plexopathy. The stinger syndrome, *Am J Sports Med* 21:650–655, 1993.

55. Speer KP, Bassett FH III, : The prolonged burner syndrome, *Am J Sports Med* 18(6):591–594, 1990.

56. Wilbourn AJ: Thoracic outlet syndrome surgery causing severe brachial plexopathy, *Muscle Nerve* 11:66–74, 1988.

57. Cherington M, Happer I, Machanic B, et al: Surgery for thoracic outlet syndrome may be hazardous to your health, *Muscle Nerve* 9:632–634, 1986.

58. Rosomoff HL, Fishbain D, Rosomoff RS: Chronic cervical pain: radiculopathy or brachialgia. Noninterventional treatment, *Spine* 17:S362–S366, 1992.

59. Wilbourn AJ: Thoracic outlet syndromes: a plea for conservatism, *Neurosurg Clin North Am* 2:235–245, 1991.

60. Jamieson WG, Chinnick B: Thoracic outlet syndrome: fact or fancy? A review of 409 consecutive patients who underwent operation, *Can J Surg* 39:321–326, 1996.

61. Mackinnon SE, Patterson GA, Novak CB: Thoracic outlet syndrome: a current overview, *Semin Thorac Cardiovasc Surg* 8:176–182, 1996.

62. Katirji B, Hardy RW Jr, : Classic neurogenic thoracic outlet syndrome in a competitive swimmer: a true scalenus anticus syndrome, *Muscle Nerve* 18:229–233, 1995.

63. Roos DB, Wilbourn AJ, Hachinski V: The thoracic outlet syndrome is underrated/overdiagnosed, *Arch Neurol* 47:327–330, 1990.

64. Swift TR, Nichols FT: The droopy shoulder syndrome, *Neurology* 34:212–215, 1984.

65. Trojaborg W: Clinical, electrophysiological, and myelographic studies of 9 patients with cervical spinal root avulsions: discrepancies between EMG and x-ray findings, *Muscle Nerve* 17:913–922, 1994.

66. Urschel HCJ, Razzuk MA: Management of the thoracic-outlet syndrome, *N Engl J Med* 286:1140–1143, 1972.

67. Slutsky DJ, Hentz VR: *Peripheral Nerve Surgery*, Philadelphia, 2006, Churchill Livingstone.

68. Chokroverty S, Sander HW: AAEM case report #13: diabetic amyotrophy, *Muscle Nerve* 19:939–945, 1996.

69. Ogawa T, Taguchi T, Tanaka Y, et al: Intravenous immunoglobulin therapy for diabetic amyotrophy, *Intern Med* 40(4):349–352, 2001.

70. Baba M: Diabetic amyotrophy or proximal diabetic neuropathy an immune-mediated condition? *Intern Med* 40(4):273–274, 2001.

71. Jaeckle KA, Young DF, Foley KM: The natural history of lumbosacral plexopathy in cancer, *Neurology* 35:8–15, 1985.

72. Bradley WG, Chad D, Verghese JP, et al: Painful lumbosacral plexopathy with elevated erythrocyte sedimentation rate: a treatable inflammatory syndrome, *Ann Neurol* 15:457–464, 1984.

73. Hernalsteen D, Cosnard G, Peeters A, Duprez T: Lumbar plexus involvement with chronic inflammatory demyelinating polyneuropathy (CIDP): a variant case of the generic disorder, *JBR-BTR* 88(6):322–324, 2005.

74. Maurer M, Stoll G, Toyka KV: Multifocal motor neuropathy presenting as chronic progressive proximal leg weakness, *Neuromuscul Disord* 14(6): 380–382, 2004.

75. Plecha EJ, Seabrook GR, Freischlag JA, et al: Neurologic complications of reoperative and emergent abdominal aortic reconstruction, *Ann Vasc Surg* 9:95–101, 1995.

76. Antoine JC, Baril A, Guettier C, et al: Unusual amyloid polyneuropathy with predominant lumbosacral nerve roots and plexus involvement, *Neurology* 41:206–208, 1991.

77. Zuniga G, Ropper AH, Frank J: Sarcoid peripheral neuropathy, *Neurology* 41:1558–1561, 1991.

78. Feasby TE, Burton SR, Hahn AF: Obstetrical lumbosacral plexus injury, *Muscle Nerve* 15:937–940, 1992.

79. Campbell WW: Evaluation and management of peripheral nerve injury, *Clin Neurophysiol* 119(9):1951–1965, 2008.

80. Campbell WW: Diagnosis and management of common compression and entrapment neuropathies, *Neurol Clin North Am* 15:549–567, 1997.

81. Kimura J: The carpal tunnel syndrome: localization of conduction abnormalities within the distal segment of the median nerve, *Brain* 102:619–635, 1979.

82. Rosenbaum RB, Ochoa JL: *Carpal Tunnel Syndrome and Other Disorders of the Median Nerve*, 2nd ed, Boston, 2002, Butterworth-Heinemann.

83. Ross MA, Kimura J: AAEM case report #2: the carpal tunnel syndrome, *Muscle Nerve* 18:567–573, 1995.

84. Stewart JD: *Focal Peripheral Neuropathies*, 2nd ed, New York, 1993, Raven Press.

85. Hansen PA, Micklesen P, Robinson LR: Clinical utility of the flick maneuver in diagnosing carpal tunnel syndrome, *Am J Phys Med Rehabil* 83 (5):363–367, 2004.

86. Robinson LR: Electrodiagnosis of carpal tunnel syndrome, *Phys Med Rehabil Clin North Am* 18(4):733–746, vi, 2007.

87. Jablecki CK, Andary MT, Floeter MK, et al: Practice parameter: electrodiagnostic studies in carpal tunnel syndrome. Report of the American Association of Electrodiagnostic Medicine, American Academy of Neurology, and the American Academy of Physical Medicine and Rehabilitation, *Neurology* 58(11):1589–1592, 2002.

88. Rivner MH: Statistical errors and their effect on electrodiagnostic medicine, *Muscle Nerve* 17:811–814, 1994.

89. Robinson LR, Micklesen PJ, Wang L: Strategies for analyzing nerve conduction data: superiority of a summary index over single tests, *Muscle Nerve* 21(9):1166–1171, 1998.

90. Visser LH, Smidt MH, Lee ML: High-resolution sonography versus EMG in the diagnosis of carpal tunnel syndrome, *J Neurol Neurosurg Psychiatry* 79(1):63–67, 2008.

91. Kwon BC, Jung KI, Baek GH: Comparison of sonography and electrodiagnostic testing in the diagnosis of carpal tunnel syndrome, *J Hand Surg [Am]* 33(1):65–71, 2008.

92. Herskovitz S, Berger AR, Lipton RB: Low-dose, short-term oral prednisone in the treatment of carpal tunnel syndrome, *Neurology* 45:1923–1925, 1995.

93. Agarwal V, Singh R, Sachdev A, et al: A prospective study of the long-term efficacy of local methyl prednisolone acetate injection in the management of mild carpal tunnel syndrome, *Rheumatology (Oxford)* 44(5):647–650, 2005.

94. Toussaint CP, Zager EL: What's new in common upper extremity entrapment neuropathies, *Neurosurg Clin North Am* 19(4):573–581, vi, 2008.

95. Campbell WW, Pridgeon RM, Riaz G, et al: Variations in anatomy of the ulnar nerve at the cubital tunnel: pitfalls in the diagnosis of ulnar neuropathy at the elbow, *Muscle Nerve* 14:733–738, 1991.

96. Landau ME, Barner KC, Campbell WW: Effect of body mass index on ulnar nerve conduction velocity, ulnar neuropathy at the elbow, and carpal tunnel syndrome, *Muscle Nerve* 32(3):360–363, 2005.

97. Campbell WW, Pridgeon RM, Riaz G, et al: Sparing of the flexor carpi ulnaris in ulnar neuropathy at the elbow [see comments], *Muscle Nerve* 12:965–967, 1989.

98. Feindel W, Stratford J: The role of the cubital tunnel in tardy ulnar palsy, *Can J Surg* 1:287–300, 1958.

99. Campbell WW: Guidelines in electrodiagnostic medicine. Practice parameter for electrodiagnostic studies in ulnar neuropathy at the elbow, *Muscle Nerve Suppl* 8:S171–S205, 1999.

100. Kern RZ: The electrodiagnosis of ulnar nerve entrapment at the elbow, *Can J Neurol Sci* 30(4):314–319, 2003.

101. Landau ME, Barner KC, Campbell WW: Optimal screening distance for ulnar neuropathy at the elbow, *Muscle Nerve* 27(5):570–574, 2003.

102. Campbell WW, Pridgeon RM, Sahni KS: Short segment incremental studies in the evaluation of ulnar neuropathy at the elbow, *Muscle Nerve* 15:1050–1054, 1992.

103. Kanakamedala RV, Simons DG, Porter RW, et al: Ulnar nerve entrapment at the elbow localized by short segment stimulation, *Arch Phys Med Rehabil* 69:959–963, 1988.

104. Visser LH, Beekman R, Franssen H: Short-segment nerve conduction studies in ulnar neuropathy at the elbow, *Muscle Nerve* 31(3):331–338, 2005.

105. Landau ME, Barner KC, Murray ED, et al: Cold elbow syndrome: spurious slowing of ulnar nerve conduction velocity, *Muscle Nerve* 32(6):815–817, 2005.

106. Neary D, Ochoa J, Gilliatt RW: Sub-clinical entrapment neuropathy in man, *J Neurol Sci* 24:283–298, 1975.

107. Neary D, Eames RA: The pathology of ulnar nerve compression in man, *Neuropath Appl Neurobiol* 1:69–88, 1975.

108. Yoon JS, Walker FO, Cartwright MS: Ultrasonographic swelling ratio in the diagnosis of ulnar neuropathy at the elbow, *Muscle Nerve* 38(4):1231–1235, 2008.

109. Yoon JS, Hong SJ, Kim BJ, et al: Ulnar nerve and cubital tunnel ultrasound in ulnar neuropathy at the elbow, *Arch Phys Med Rehabil* 89(5):887–889, 2008.

110. De JP Jr, Steiner JC: Spontaneous recovery of ulnar neuropathy at the elbow, *Electromyogr Clin Neurophysiol* 16(2–3):239–248, 1976.

111. Dellon AL, Hament W, Gittelshon A: Nonoperative management of cubital tunnel syndrome: an 8-year prospective study, *Neurology* 43:1673–1677, 1993.

112. Campbell WW, Pridgeon RM, Sahni SK: Entrapment neuropathy of the ulnar nerve at its point of exit from the flexor carpi ulnaris muscle, *Muscle Nerve* 11:467–470, 1988.

113. Campbell WW: AAEE case report #18: ulnar neuropathy in the distal forearm, *Muscle Nerve* 12:347–352, 1989.

114. Lo YL, Fook-Chong S, Leoh TH, et al: High-resolution ultrasound as a diagnostic adjunct in common peroneal neuropathy, *Arch Neurol* 64(12):1798–1800, 2007.

*Pushpa Narayanaswami, MD**

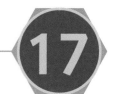

Treatment and Management of Disorders of Neuromuscular Hyperexcitability

Muscle pain, stiffness, and cramps are symptoms frequently seen in neuromuscular practice. The differential diagnosis of these symptoms is wide and includes systemic disorders, neurologic disorders involving the pyramidal or extrapyramidal systems, and neuromuscular disorders (Box 17-1). The neuromuscular disorders that manifest with muscle stiffness, cramps, and muscle pain as the predominant symptoms are referred to as the "syndromes of neuromuscular hyperexcitability." They include central disorders such as stiff-person syndrome, syndromes of peripheral nerve hyperexcitability such as neuromyotonia (including Isaacs syndrome and its variant, Morvan syndrome) and cramp fasciculation syndrome, skeletal muscle channelopathies that manifest clinically as the nondystrophic myotonias and the periodic paralyses, and other disorders affecting the muscle such as rippling muscle disease. The metabolic myopathies and Brody disease are disorders of muscle that are associated with exercise-induced muscle stiffness and cramps (see Box 17-1).[1] As a group, these disorders are rare. However, a working knowledge of these diseases is important for several reasons: genetic implications in some, autoimmune and potentially paraneoplastic causes in others, and the need for monitoring for potentially fatal cardiac arrhythmias or other systemic complications in yet others. This review discusses the clinical features, diagnosis, and treatment of the syndromes of neuromuscular hyperexcitability (Fig. 17-1).

Central Disorders

Stiff-Person Syndrome

In 1956, Moersch and Woltman described a syndrome characterized by "progressive fluctuating muscular rigidity and muscle spasms" without other neurologic signs.[2] Since this initial description, atypical forms of the disorder have been reported, including the stiff-leg syndrome (SLS) and progressive encephalomyelitis with rigidity (PER).[3] The discovery of autoantibodies to glutamic acid decarboxylase (GAD) by Solimena et al in 1988 confirmed the autoimmune nature of the disorder, and forms the basis for immunotherapy in stiff-person syndrome (SPS).[4]

---

*Dedicated to my children, Shruti and Varun, who put up with my long hours and erratic schedule patiently.

Diagnosis and Evaluation

Classical SPS presents with the insidious onset of muscle rigidity, usually beginning symmetrically in the lumbar and thoracic paraspinal muscles and the proximal lower extremity muscles. The disorder affects both sexes equally, typically with onset between 30 and 50 years of age. Episodic muscle spasms are superimposed on the rigidity. These spasms, along with difficulty in bending the trunk because of the rigidity, may cause unexplained falls. The gait becomes slow, stiff, and careful, partly to avoid falling. Breathing difficulty may occur due to stiffness in the thoracic muscles and resultant restriction of chest movements. The spasms may be precipitated by movement, auditory or tactile stimuli, or by emotion. They are often painful, and typically begin with an abrupt jerk followed by a more sustained, tonic contraction that slowly subsides over seconds to minutes. "Status spasticus" or sustained generalized spasms that may last as long as 2 weeks has been described.[5] Stiffness and spasms fluctuate during the day and improve or disappear in sleep. Spasms may be severe enough to cause femoral fractures, joint subluxation or ankylosis, and herniation of abdominal contents.[6–10] Although most descriptions of SPS report sparing of the facial muscles, others make note of facial muscle involvement with a "tight-faced" or "pursed-lipped" expression that may limit speech, mask-like facies, risus sardonicus, and dysphagia.[9,11] Reflex painful spasms initiated by swallowing, resulting in weight loss, have been reported.[12] Autonomic dysfunction, with hyperthermia, diaphoresis, pupillary dilation, tachycardia, tachypnea, and hypertension may be seen. Repeated muscle spasms accompanied by autonomic dysfunction necessitating intensive care management have been reported.[13] Rhabdomyolysis may result as a complication of the muscle spasms and rigidity.[14] Sudden death has been reported in about 10% of patients.[15,16]

About 10% to 25% of patients with SPS have coexisting epilepsy.[5,17] Other conditions that are associated with SPS include insulin-dependant diabetes mellitus, autoimmune thyroiditis, pernicious anemia, celiac disease, and, rarely, systemic lupus erythematosus.[5,13,18–21] SPS may be a paraneoplastic phenomenon in about 5% of patients.[22–24] Malignancies associated with paraneoplastic SPS include breast cancer, small cell lung cancer, thymoma, adenocarcinoma of the celon, and Hodgkin's disease.[22,25–28,29,30] SPS has been described following autologous bone marrow transplant and interferon treatment for multiple myeloma.[31]

Box 17-1 Disorders Associated with Muscle Pain, Stiffness, and Cramps

1. Corticospinal tract dysfunction
2. Extrapyramidal disorders: akinetic–rigid syndromes (Parkinson's disease and parkinsonian syndromes, progressive supranuclear palsy) other degenerative disorders, dystonia
3. Anterior horn cell disorders
   a. Stiff-person syndrome and variants
   b. Myelopathies: traumatic, ischemic, spinal arteriovenous malformation, spondylotic, neoplastic
   c. Toxins: tetanus, black widow spider venom, strychnine
4. Peripheral nerve disorders
   a. Tetany: hypocalcemia, hypomagnesemia, alkalosis
   b. Neuromyotonia
   c. Cramps: postexertion, dehydration/salt depletion, pregnancy, denervation (motor neuron disease, neuropathies), idiopathic
5. Disorders of muscle
   a. Myotonic disorders: myotonia congenita, paramyotonia congenita, myotonic dystrophy (DM1), proximal myotonic myopathy (DM2), Schwartz-Jampel syndrome

b. Metabolic myopathies: deficiencies of myophosphorylase (McArdle's disease), phosphofructokinase (Tarui's disease), phosphorylase b kinase, phosphoglycerate mutase, phosphoglycerate kinase, lactate dehydrogenase
c. Rippling muscle disease
d. Brody's disease
e. Inherited disorders causing weakness and muscle contractures: rigid spine syndrome, Emery-Dreifuss muscular dystrophy, Bethlem myopathy
f. Acquired diseases of muscle: inflammatory myopathies, endocrine myopathies (hypothyroidism, Addison's disease)
6. Contractures
   a. Bony (ankylosis)
   b. Soft tissue (Volkmann's ischemic contracture)

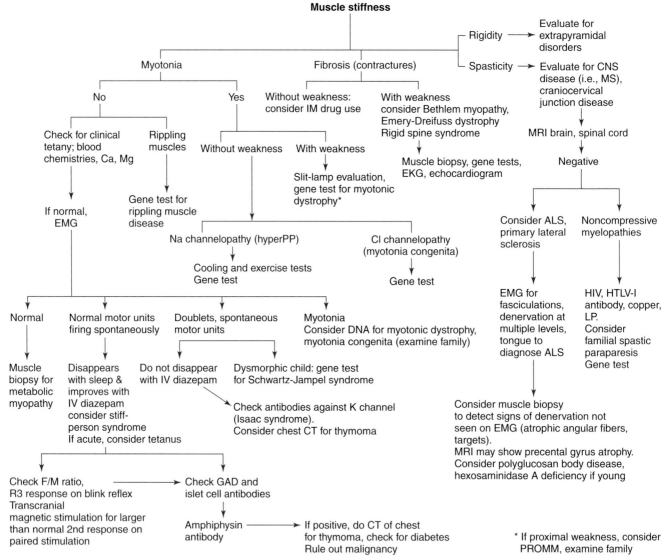

Figure 17-1 Evaluation of a patient presenting with muscle stiffness. ALS, amyotrophic lateral sclerosis; Ca, calcium; Cl, chloride; CNS, central nervous system; CT, computed tomography; EKG, electrocardiogram; EMG, electromyogram; F/M ratio, F-response to M-response amplitude ratio; GAD, glutamic acid decarboxylase; HIV, human immunodeficiency virus; HTLV-1, human T-lymphotrophic virus-1; IM, intramuscular; IV, intravenous; K; potassium; LP, lumbar puncture; Mg, magnesium; MRI, magnetic resonance imaging; MS, multiple sclerosis; PP, periodic paralysis; PROMM, myotonic dystrophy type 2 (DM2). (Edited and reproduced with permission from Bertorini TE: *Clinical Evaluation and Diagnostic Tests for Neuromuscular Disorders*, Philadelphia, 2002, Butterworth-Heinemann, Fig. A1.7.)

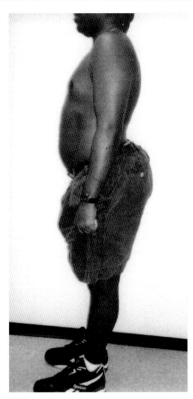

Figure 17-2 Prominent lumbar lordosis in a patient with stiff-person syndrome. (From Bertorini TE: *Clinical Evaluation and Diagnostic Tests for Neuromuscular Disorders*, Philadelphia, 2002, Butterworth-Heinemann, Fig. 2.3B.)

On examination, there is increased tone in the paraspinal muscles. The continuous muscle contractions give rise to a board-like, rigid appearance of the abdomen while co-contraction of the abdominal and paraspinal muscles gives rise to the typical exaggerated lumbar lordosis that is an almost universal finding in individuals with SPS (Fig. 17-2). Exaggerated tendon reflexes and loss of abdominal cutaneous reflexes may be seen.[9,13] Although tone may be increased in a diffuse fashion in the extremities, cog-wheel rigidity and spasticity are absent. The Babinski sign has been described in a few patients.[5] Extrapyramidal, lower motor neuron, sensory, and sphincter abnormalities are absent.[24]

Brown and Marsden[32] classify patients with rigidity and spasms of central origin into classical "stiff man" syndrome and the "stiff man plus" syndromes. They suggest that the "stiff man plus" syndromes have a poorer response to treatment and worse prognosis as compared to classical SPS. The "stiff man plus" syndromes include *progressive encephalomyelitis with rigidity (PER)*, *jerking stiff-man syndrome*, and *stiff-leg syndrome*. PER is characterized by a subacute course, rigidity, myoclonus, brain stem involvement, pyramidal signs, and a poor prognosis with survival less than 3 years. The other two syndromes, jerking stiff-man syndrome and stiff-leg syndrome, are chronic and, unlike PER, do not manifest long tract signs. In jerking stiff-man syndrome, the picture is dominated by brain stem myoclonus involving the extremities. The jerks may be severe enough to compromise respiration.[33] Brown and Marsden differentiated jerking stiff-man syndrome from PER by the time course of the disorder, but it is uncertain if they actually represent different entities. In stiff-leg syndrome, the clinical picture is dominated by spasms and rigidity of the limbs, most frequently the lower limbs. This condition has also been termed the *stiff-limb syndrome* (SLS).[34-36]

Focal rigidity of a lower extremity associated with quadriceps myoclonus has been reported as a paraneoplastic syndrome associated with small cell lung cancer.[37] It has been suggested that SLS predominantly involving the upper extremity should raise suspicion for paraneoplastic SPS.[10,38]

Although this classification into SPS and "stiff man plus" syndromes is based on differences in clinical presentation, there appears to be considerable overlap between these syndromes. SPS evolving into a clinical picture resembling PER has been described.[39] In their series, Dalakas et al found that patients who presented initially with stiffness in a limb progressed to develop generalized symptoms.[5] PER associated with anti-GAD antibodies has been reported.[40,41] Thus, it seems plausible that these clinically discrete disorders may simply reflect a spectrum of autoimmune disorders associated with anti-GAD antibodies.

SPS is a clinical diagnosis supported by autoantibody testing and the electrodiagnostic features described next. The neurologic examination can distinguish between SPS and other disorders causing muscle stiffness and spasms. Diagnostic criteria for SPS proposed by Lorish et al are summarized in Box 17-2.[18] Electrodiagnostic testing is useful in establishing a diagnosis of SPS and differentiating it from other disorders that present with muscle stiffness. Routine motor and sensory nerve conduction studies (NCS) are normal. On needle electromyography (EMG) of involved muscles, continuous activation of motor unit action potentials (MUAPs) that persists despite attempts at relaxation is observed. The MUAPs appear normal with a normal firing pattern. The continuous motor activity is abolished by sleep, general anesthesia, peripheral nerve block, and benzodiazepines.[42] There is co-contraction of agonist and antagonist muscles during voluntary movement, instead of the normal pattern of agonist activation and antagonist relaxation.[24] The silent period is normal, in contrast to chronic tetanus, in which the silent period

---

Box 17-2 Diagnosis of Stiff-Person Syndrome

Clinical Features[17]

Progressive stiffness and rigidity of the axial muscles with slow progression to involve proximal limb muscles
Hyperlordosis or other abnormal axial postures
Superimposed episodic spasms precipitated by tactile stimuli, voluntary movement, noise or emotional stress
Normal intellect, absent brain stem; pyramidal, extrapyramidal, lower motor neuron, and sensory signs or sphincter disturbances
Clinical response to benzodiazepines

Electrodiagnostic Features

Electromyography (EMG): continuous motor unit activity in at least one axial muscle; abolished by sleep, general anesthesia, peripheral nerve block, and benzodiazepines; co-contraction of agonist and antagonist muscles during voluntary movement
Normal silent period
Blink reflex: R1 response occurs both ipsilaterally and contralaterally, and a third response, R3, occurs bilaterally with stimulus intensity above the detection threshold

Laboratory Features

Antibodies to glutamic acid decarboxylase (GAD)
Anti-amphiphysin antibodies
Antibodies to the α_1-subunit of the glycine receptor

Additional Diagnostic Workup

Screen for diabetes, thyroid disease, malignancy

Adapted from Espay AJ, Chen R: Rigidity and spasms from autoimmune encephalomyelopathies: stiff-person syndrome, *Muscle Nerve* 34:677–690, 2006.

in involved muscles is absent.[43,44] The R1 response of the blink reflex occurs both ipsilaterally and contralaterally, and a third response, R3, occurs bilaterally with stimulus intensity above the detection threshold.[45]

Antibodies to GAD are detected in the serum as well as cerebrospinal fluid (CSF) of 65% to 85% of patients with SPS. The antibodies detected in CSF represent intrathecal synthesis. These antibodies are directed against two isoforms of GAD, 65 kDa and 67 kDa.[4,46,47] Most patients have antibodies to the 65 kDa isoform. In a study by Dalakas and colleagues, very high titers of antibody were present in the serum of patients with SPS (7.5–215 μg/mL) as compared to control patients with other autoimmune neuromuscular disorders or type 1 diabetes mellitus. The antibody titers were 50-fold lower in patients with diabetes mellitus (0–1,760 ng/mL). Two patients, each with myasthenia gravis and dermatomyositis, had detectable GAD antibodies in the serum, albeit at much lower titers than the SPS patients (100–265 ng/mL). GAD antibodies were absent in the CSF of eight disease control subjects in this study, suggesting that CSF antibodies to GAD are specific for SPS.[48] Although it has been suggested that CSF testing for GAD antibodies may be important to confirm the diagnosis of SPS, the clinical criteria and high titers of serum GAD antibodies are probably sufficient in the vast majority of cases. These antibodies have also been described in PER and SLS, suggesting that these disorders may be related pathogenetically to SPS.[40,49,50] The antibodies are not useful in predicting disease severity, and antibody titers do not correlate with disease duration.[51]

Antibodies to the synaptic membrane protein amphiphysin have been described in patients with paraneoplastic SPS.[23] Murinson and Guarnaccia recently reviewed 11 cases of SPS associated with antibodies to amphiphysin, and compared them with 116 anti-GAD–positive SPS patients. Patients with amphiphysin antibodies were older and female and the majority had breast cancer. The pattern of stiffness was different in these patients with prominent involvement of the arms and neck. Diabetes was infrequent in these patients.[52] This pattern is in keeping with prior observations that a paraneoplastic cause should be suspected in SPS involving the upper extremities. Other antibody associations include a case of paraneoplastic PER associated with anti-Ri antibodies.[53] There is one report of PER associated with antibodies to gephyrin, a cytosolic protein that is concentrated at the postsynaptic membranes of inhibitory synapses in association with γ-aminobutyric acid (GABA) receptors. This patient had an undifferentiated mediastinal tumor.[54] Very recently, Hutchinson et al reported a patient with PER associated with antibodies to the α_1-subunit of the glycine receptor. In this patient, the antibodies were present at the onset of the illness, higher during clinical relapse, and absent after immunosuppressive treatment.[55]

The diagnostic evaluation of SPS is incomplete without screening for underlying malignancy with appropriate imaging and other tests for cancer screening. Malignancy is only infrequently associated with anti-GAD antibody positive SPS; the cancer associations include thymoma, myeloma, Hodgkin's disease, breast cancer, and renal cell cancer.[27,36,56,57] However, in women with SPS predominantly involving the upper extremities and neck or in the presence of amphiphysin antibodies, a comprehensive search for breast cancer and, if negative, lung cancer is appropriate.[52] Finally, magnetic resonance imaging of the spine is indicated in patients with SLS, since focal lesions of the spinal cord including intrinsic cord tumors, syringomyelia, spinal cord ischemia, and trauma have been reported to cause an SPS-like picture.[58–62]

Treatment and Management

There are two approaches to the treatment of SPS: (1) symptomatic treatment of the rigidity and muscle spasms with medications that potentiate GABA-ergic inhibitory neurotransmission, and (2) immunomodulation (Table 17-1). Agents that have been used for symptomatic therapy include diazepam and other benzodiazepines, baclofen, sodium valproate, levetiracetam, vigabatrin, tiagabine, gabapentin, clonidine, and tizanidine.[7,45,63–70] However, there are few controlled trials of these medications. Vigabatrin is available in the United States only through a special restricted distribution program for approved indications because of the risk of permanent visual loss. High doses of diazepam, up to 100 mg/day, may be required. Intrathecal baclofen may be more effective than oral baclofen.[71,72] However, a small double-blind, placebo-controlled trial of intrathecal baclofen in three patients revealed clinical improvement in only one patient, although all patients showed improvement in electrophysiologic parameters.[73] Low doses of continuous intravenous propofol (10 μg/kg/min) were used successfully to control severe spasms as a bridge to intrathecal baclofen in one patient.[74] Botulinum toxin A injections into the paraspinal and limb muscles have improved spasms and rigidity in two small studies.[75,76] Tricyclic antidepressants and levodopa may worsen stiffness.[77] Rapid withdrawal of therapy can cause life-threatening worsening of symptoms.[78]

Several immunomodulating agents have been utilized in the treatment of SPS. Prednisone has been reported to improve symptoms in some cases, but not others.[41,79–82] Plasmapheresis has both ameliorated clinical symptoms and reduced antibody titers in several case reports of SPS and in isolated case reports of PER.[83–87] Shariatmadar and Noto suggested that antibody-negative patients may not respond as well to plasma exchange. However, this was a study of only two antibody-negative patients, and Nakamagoe et al reported a good response to plasma exchange in an antibody-negative patient.[88,89] A randomized, placebo-controlled, cross-over trial in 16 GAD antibody–positive SPS patients demonstrated significant improvement in stiffness scores in patients who received intravenous immunoglobulin (IVIg) compared with placebo. Duration of benefit ranged from 6 weeks to 1 year.[90] Baker et al reported a good response and lasting remission with rituximab in one patient with GAD antibody–positive SPS.[91] Treatment of an underlying malignancy followed by immunotherapy results in significant improvement in paraneoplastic SPS.[22,94] A recent study of SPS associated with amphiphysin antibodies suggests that this syndrome may respond better to corticosteroids and treatment of an underlying malignancy.[52]

Tetanus

Tetanus is an infectious disease characterized by central nervous system hyperexcitability, resulting in muscle rigidity and spasms. The causative organism, *Clostridium tetani* is a gram-positive anaerobic bacterium normally present in spore form in the gastrointestinal tract of mammals and in soil. When these spores gain access to damaged human tissue, they transform into the vegetative form and produce the toxins tetanospasmin and tetanolysin. The primary toxin is tetanospasmin, a neurotoxin that is transported to the spinal cord and brain stem by retrograde axonal transport, where it irreversibly inhibits the release of glycine and GABA at inhibitory synapses.[95] This results in disinhibition, initially affecting the alpha motor neurons and subsequently the preganglionic autonomic neurons and causing the clinical signs of the disease. The role of the second toxin, tetanolysin, in the pathogenesis of the disease is not

Table 17-1 Treatment of Stiff-Person Syndrome

Medication	Daily Dose	Comments
Symptomatic Treatment		
Diazepam	Up to 100 mg in three doses	Avoid abrupt withdrawal; pregnancy category C
Clonazepam	2.5–18 mg in three doses	Pregnancy category D
Sodium valproate	600 mg–2 g in three doses	Fatal hepatoxicity, pancreatitis, teratogenesis, low platelet counts, tremor Monitor liver function tests, platelet count and amylase at baseline and frequently at least during the first 6 months
Levetiracetam	2000 mg in two doses	Risk of suicidality, hepatotoxicity, pancytopenia; pregnancy category C
Tiagabine	6 mg in two to four doses	Sedation, dizziness, gastrointestinal side effects; pregnancy category C
Gabapentin	300–3600 mg in three doses	Risk of suicidality, Stevens-Johnson syndrome, sedation, ataxia; pregnancy category C
Vigabatrin*	2–3 g	Diplopia, abnormal color perception, visual field defects, optic atrophy, and changes in retinal pigmentation
Baclofen	10–100 mg in two or three doses orally	Weakness, somnolence; pregnancy category C
Clonidine	0.0025 mg/kg in two doses	Sedation; pregnancy category C
Immunotherapy		
Prednisone	25–80 mg	Monitor blood pressure, blood glucose, electrolytes, cataracts, glaucoma, osteoporosis, reactivation of pulmonary tuberculosis
Intravenous immunoglobulin	1 g/kg/day for 2 days	Aseptic meningitis, renal failure Monitor blood pressure, creatinine during infusions; pregnancy category C
Plasmapheresis	Four exchanges of 3 L over 8 days	
Rituximab	375 mg/m^2	Fatal infusion reactions, progressive multifocal leukoencephalopathy, hematologic toxicity; pregnancy category C

*Available only through a special restricted distribution program because of the risk of permanent visual loss.
Adapted from Espay AJ, Chen R: Rigidity and spasms from autoimmune encephalomyelopathies: stiff-person syndrome, *Muscle Nerve* 34:686, 2006. Copyright © 2006 Muscle and Nerve; with permission of John Wiley & Sons, Inc.

completely understood, but it is thought to cause local tissue damage and make conditions for bacterial multiplication favorable.[96,97]

Diagnosis and Evaluation

Tetanus is preceded by an obvious antecedent injury in most patients. These injuries include penetrating injuries, burns, gangrene, ulcers, unsterile intramuscular or subcutaneous injections, neonatal tetanus due to umbilical stump infections, septic abortions, and surgical procedures especially with necrotic infections involving bowel flora. However, injuries may be trivial and not serious enough to seek medical attention in up to 50% of patients. In a small percentage of patients there is no antecedent injury.[98,99] The average incubation period is about 3 to 21 days, but varies from 1 day to several months depending on the site of the wound, reflecting the distance that the toxin must travel to the nervous system.[100–102] The onset time, from the first symptom to the first spasm is about 1 to 7 days. Shorter incubation periods and onset times are associated with more severe disease.[98,102]

The disease is characterized by tonic muscle rigidity, intermittent muscle spasms, and dysautonomia. In most patients, the disease is *generalized*. Early symptoms include irritability, restlessness, tachycardia, and diaphoresis. Trismus or "lockjaw" due to rigidity of the masseters is often the presenting symptom. Spasm of the facial muscles gives rise to the characteristic facies, "risus sardonicus" or sardonic smile. The rigidity and spasms spread caudally to involve all muscles. Retraction of the head and opisthotonus result from rigidity of the neck and truncal muscles. Superimposed on the rigidity are intermittent spasms, either spontaneous or triggered by external stimuli such as noise, light, or touch. Spasms may be strong enough to cause fractures. Sudden generalized spasms result in opisthotonus, adduction at the shoulders, flexion at the elbows and wrists, and extension of the lower extremities, associated with a rise in body temperature. Consciousness is preserved throughout the illness, and the rigidity and spasms are intensely painful.[100] Respiratory failure may occur due to several factors: chest wall rigidity and spasm, airway obstruction due to pharyngeal and laryngeal spasms, and aspiration pneumonia. The most important direct cause of death is respiratory failure.[102] Autonomic dysfunction may manifest as diaphoresis and cardiovascular instability.[98,103,104] After the first 2 weeks of the illness, once the spasms and respiratory function stabilize, dysautonomia becomes a major cause of mortality.[105]

Local tetanus is the term used to describe a more limited form of the disease characterized by rigidity and spasms restricted to one limb or body region. Local tetanus has a milder course but often progresses to become generalized.[106] Localized tetanus resulting from head injuries and involving the cranial nerves is referred to as *cephalic tetanus*. It is defined as trismus associated with paralysis of one or more cranial nerves. Cephalic tetanus tends to progress to generalized tetanus in about two thirds of the cases.[107] *Tetanus neonatorum*, or neonatal tetanus, presents in the first 2 weeks of birth with feeding difficulty and convulsions and is due to poor umbilical stump care in the newborns of unimmunized mothers.[108] Last, rare cases of "chronic tetanus" that have a prolonged nonfulminant course over months have been reported.[109,110]

Tetanus is a clinical diagnosis. Other disorders that may present with muscle rigidity and spasms include tetany, SPS, dystonic reactions, strychnine poisoning, and rabies. Wound cultures often do not detect *C. tetani*. The absence of serum antibodies to tetanus supports the diagnosis but does not exclude it. Tetanus has been reported in individuals with antibody titers in the protective range.[111] Electrophysiologic studies in patients with chronic tetanus reveal an increase in the F-response amplitude to M-response amplitude ratio (F/M ratio). The silent period is usually absent but may be normal.[44,109,112,113] Motor units are usually normal; the spasms are characterized by involuntary bursts of motor unit activity.[42]

Treatment and Management

Three principles guide the management of tetanus: (1) control of active *C. tetani* infection to stop further production of toxin, (2) neutralization of circulating toxin, (3) supportive care. Penicillin G is the traditional antibiotic of choice, in a dose of 100,000 to 200,000 IU/kg/day in 4 to 6 divided doses intravenously for 7 to 10 days. However, the GABA-antagonistic properties and epileptogenic effects of intravenous penicillin have raised concerns about the use of penicillin in tetanus.[114] More recently, metronidazole has been considered the antibiotic of choice at a dose of 400 mg rectally or 500 mg intravenously every 6 hours for 7 to 10 days. Ahmadsyah and Salim reported a lower mortality rate in patients treated with metronidazole as compared to penicillin. In a large study by Yen and colleagues, although mortality rate was no different in patients treated with metronidazole or penicillin, patients treated with metronidazole required fewer muscle relaxants and sedatives.[115,116] Alternative antibiotics include erythromycin, tetracycline, chloramphenicol, and clindamycin.[96,117] Wound débridement is essential to eliminate the anaerobic environment that encourages the growth of *C. tetani*.

Tetanus toxin that is bound to the central nervous system cannot be neutralized. However, human tetanus immune globulin is routinely used in a dose of 3000 to 6000 units intramuscularly to neutralize circulating toxin.[118] A Brazilian randomized controlled study compared intrathecal tetanus immunoglobulin to the intramuscular route in 128 patients with tetanus. In this study, patients treated with intrathecal immunoglobulin had a shorter duration of spasms and hospitalization as well as a reduced need for assisted respiration as compared to those who received intramuscular immunoglobulin. It is not clear, however, whether tetanus immune globulin or human lyophilized immunoglobulin was used.[119]

Supportive care includes the treatment of muscle rigidity and spasms and treatment of dysautonomia. Several agents have been used in the supportive care of tetanus, but controlled trials are few. Benzodiazepines serve the dual purpose of controlling spasms and rigidity and reducing autonomic instability. Diazepam is most commonly utilized, and large doses may be required, up to 3 to 8 mg/kg/day. The large doses, combined with the long half-life (72 hours) and the presence of active metabolites commonly results in respiratory depression.[102] Midazolam, 5 to 15 mg/hour, and propofol 20 to 80 mg/hour intravenously have also been used with success in several reports.[120–122] Other agents used for sedation include phenobarbital, morphine, and chlorpromazine.[123–125] Intravenous ketamine (2 mg/kg) alternating with diazepam has been used in one case report of cephalic tetanus with severe laryngospasm.[126]

Neuromuscular blockade is used when sedation is inadequate to control the spasms. Pancuronium has been used to induce neuromuscular blockade, but has the disadvantage of potentially worsening autonomic dysfunction due to catecholamine reuptake inhibition.[127] Vecuronium has the advantage of minimal cardiovascular side effects, but is short acting and requires continuous infusion.[128]

Dantrolene has been reported to be useful in controlling spasms without need for neuromuscular blockade in one case.[129] Intrathecal baclofen, 500 to 2000 µg/day has also been found to be useful in controlling muscle spasms. Coma and respiratory depression were the most frequent adverse events. Meningitis occurred in 3 of 14 patients in one study.[130–132]

Although sedation is the first line in the management of dysautonomia, several other specific agents have been used to control hypertension and tachycardia. It has been suggested that morphine is useful in the management of dysautonomia because it does not worsen cardiovascular instability.[125,133] Beta blockade with propranolol does not appear to be beneficial; on the contrary, it may cause hypotension, pulmonary edema, and even sudden death.[99,134] Labetalol is also not recommended for similar reasons.[135] Esmolol infusion was used with success in a single case report.[136] Small series and case reports of the use of clonidine, atropine, and epidural or spinal bupivacaine are available.[137–140] Magnesium sulfate has had utility in the control of spasms and management of dysautonomia.[141,142] In a randomized double-blind controlled trial of magnesium sulfate (40 mg/kg over 30 minutes followed by an infusion at 1.5–2 g/hour) compared to placebo in 256 patients, magnesium sulfate reduced the requirement for other drugs to treat spasms as well as the need for verapamil to treat cardiovascular instability.[143] In a recent prospective study, intravenous magnesium sulfate alone was effective in only milder cases of tetanus; more severe cases required additional sedatives.[144]

Ancillary care includes early tracheostomy and ventilatory support, management of tracheal secretions, nutritional support, often necessitating gastrostomy tube placement, prophylaxis of deep venous thrombosis, management of nosocomial infections, and prevention of decubiti and gastrointestinal stress ulcerations. Corticosteroids were found to reduce mortality in an open labeled study of 63 patients with severe tetanus.[145] Administration of tetanus toxoid in three doses at least 2 weeks apart is recommended because the disease does not confer immunity.

Disorders of Peripheral Nerve Hyperexcitability

Neuromyotonia

Neuromyotonia is a disorder of generalized peripheral nerve hyperexcitability (PNH) characterized by sustained motor unit activity. The terminology used in the literature for clinical syndromes that are associated with neuromyotonia is quite varied and includes *continuous muscle fiber activity* and *Isaacs syndrome*, among others.[146] To add to the confusion, the term *neuromyotonia* is also used for the EMG finding of continuous irregular bursts of single motor units firing as doublets, triplets, or multiplets firing at very high intraburst frequencies of up to 150 to 300 Hz. The clinical syndrome of neuromyotonia may be associated with the EMG finding of neuromyotonia or myokymia, as described later, and should be distinguished from the EMG finding of neuromyotonia.

Neuromyotonia may be hereditary or acquired. Box 17-3 details a clinical classification of neuromyotonia. In the following review, the term *Isaacs syndrome* is used synonymously with *autoimmune acquired neuromyotonia*. Hereditary syndromes of PNH due to mutations in the *voltage-gated potassium channel (VGKC)* gene have been described. The PNH in these cases is usually associated with episodic ataxia with myokymia (EA-1) or neonatal epilepsy. In EA-1, mutations in the *KCNA1* gene have been identified. Mutations in the *KCNQ2* gene have been reported in patients with

Box 17-3 Clinical Classification of Neuromyotonia

1. Autoimmune
   a. Associated with VGKC antibodies: Isaacs syndrome and Morvan's syndrome
   b. Paraneoplastic: thymoma, small cell lung cancer, lymphoma, plasmacytoma with IgM paraproteinemia
   c. Associated with peripheral neuropathy: idiopathic, CIDP, Guillain-Barré syndrome
   d. Associated with other autoimmune disorders: myasthenia gravis, diabetes mellitus, hypo/hyperthyroidism, Addison's disease, SLE, systemic sclerosis, rheumatoid arthritis, celiac disease, pernicious anemia, amyloidosis
2. Non–immune-mediated
   a. Drugs and toxins: gold, d-penicillamine, oxaliplatin, mercury, timber rattlesnake venom
   b. Associated with motor neuron disease
3. Hereditary
   a. Associated with episodic ataxia with myokymia (EA-1)
   b. Associated with neonatal epilepsy
   c. Associated with hereditary neuropathy (HMSN 1a, HNPP)
   d. Schwartz-Jampel syndrome

CIDP, chronic inflammatory demyelinating polyneuropathy; HMSN, hereditary motor sensory neuropathy; HNPP, hereditary neuropathy with predisposition to pressure palsies; SLE, systemic lupus erythematosus; VGKC, voltage-gated potassium channel.
Adapted from Maddison P: Neuromyotonia, *Clin Neurophysiol* 117:2118–2127, 2006, with permission from Dr. Maddison and the Editor, *Clinical Neurophysiology.*

neonatal epilepsy and PNH.[147,148] A family with a mutation in the *KCNA1* gene with varying clinical phenotypes including PNH without episodic ataxia has been described.[149] Similarly, one patient with PNH without neonatal epilepsy and a mutation in the *KCNQ2* gene has been reported.[150] An Italian family with neuromyotonia without mutations in the *KCNA1, KCNA6,* or *KCNQ2* genes suggests that other hitherto unrecognized mutations may exist.[151]

Neuromyotonia may occur in isolation or develop in association with peripheral neuropathies, both hereditary and acquired. It may also appear as a paraneoplastic disorder in association with small cell carcinoma of the lung, thymoma, and rarely, thyroid carcinoma and lymphoma.[152–158] Nine percent of patients with acquired neuromyotonia had autoimmune myasthenia gravis (MG) in one study.[158] Drugs such as gold, penicillamine, and oxaliplatin, and toxins such as mercury have also been causally associated with neuromyotonia.[155,159–162] One patient with human immunodeficiency virus infection and neuromyotonia and one with idiopathic hypoparathyroidism and neuromyotonia have been reported.[163,164] There are isolated reports of neuromyotonia associated with systemic sclerosis and following bone marrow transplantation.[165,166] A recent report of a patient who developed neuromyotonia following recovery from VGKC-antibody associated limbic encephalitis emphasizes the expanding spectrum and clinical overlap in the autoimmune channelopathies.[167]

Vernino et al suggest that acquired neuromyotonia (Isaacs syndrome and its variant, Morvan syndrome), cramp fasciculation syndrome, and acquired rippling muscle disease are a "continuum of autoimmune neuromuscular hyperexcitability."[158] Rippling muscle disease, a myopathy with muscle hyperexcitability, is described in the following section. The acquired forms of PNH (acquired neuromyotonia [Isaacs syndrome and Morvan syndrome] and cramp fasciculation syndrome) are characterized by an autoimmune etiology and are associated with antibodies to the VGKC.[168,169]

Diagnosis and Evaluation
Isaacs Syndrome

Isaacs syndrome (acquired autoimmune neuromyotonia) is defined by the presence of continuous muscle fiber hyperactivity that manifests with muscle stiffness, fasciculations, and continuous vermiform movements across muscles (myokymia) that have been likened to a bag of worms under the skin (Table 17-2). The disorder may present in children or adults and develops insidiously. Infantile onset has

Table 17-2 Clinical Features of Isaacs Syndrome and Cramp Fasciculation Syndrome

Disorder	Symptoms and Signs	Electromyography/Nerve Conduction Studies	Autoantibodies	Treatment
Isaacs syndrome	Muscle stiffness, fasciculations Continuous vermiform movements that disappear with neuromuscular blockade, persist in sleep and after general anesthesia, and have a variable response to peripheral nerve block Hyperhidrosis, muscle hypertrophy. Abnormal postures of hands and feet Hallucinations/insomnia (Morvan syndrome)	*Routine NCS:* After-discharges following CMAP or F/H waves *EMG:* Myokymia or neuromyotonia; may be accentuated by hyperventilation or ischemia; fibrillations and fasciculations may be seen	VGKC antibodies in 40%–60% Ganglionic AChR antibodies (14%), striational antibodies	*Symptomatic:* Phenytoin, carbamazepine, sodium valproate, baclofen, gabapentin, diazepam, acetazolamide, mexiletene. *Immunosuppressive:* Prednisone, azathioprine, plasma exchange, intravenous immunoglobulin
Cramp fasciculation syndrome	Muscle aching, stiffness, cramps (painful muscle contractions precipitated by movement, relieved by stretching) Fasciculations on examination	*NCS:* Afterdischarges seen only with repetitive nerve stimulation *EMG:* Cramp discharges and fasciculations; neuromyotonia, myokymia, fibrillations absent	VGKC antibodies in 20%–30% Ganglionic AChR antibodies (6%), striational antibodies	Carbamazepine, prednisone

AChR, acetylcholine receptor; CMAP, compound muscle action potential; VGKC, voltage-gated potassium channel.

been reported.[170,171] The movements are usually seen in distal and proximal limb muscles, but may also involve the axial muscles, face, and tongue.[155,172] Rare involvement of laryngeal muscles resulting in dysphonia and dyspnea has been reported.[173] Persistent contraction of muscles results in abnormal postures with flexion or extension of the hands and feet, resembling carpopedal spasm. Other features include muscle cramps that may worsen following voluntary muscle contraction. Hyperhidrosis and muscle hypertrophy are frequently present and are attributed to the continuous muscle fiber activity. Treatment with phenytoin sodium resulted in reduction in muscle fiber activity as well as muscle hypertrophy in one patient.[174] "Pseudomyotonia" is a clinical diagnostic feature of neuromyotonia but is seen only in about a third of the patients. It refers to delayed muscle relaxation after voluntary contraction without percussion myotonia and is so termed to differentiate it from myotonia that originates in the muscle membrane. It commonly affects hand grip. Hart et al reported weakness in approximately 30% of their patients. The weakness usually involved the most overactive muscles. Tendon reflexes may be normal or absent.[169,172,175] The continuous muscle activity persists during sleep and general anesthesia and has a variable response to peripheral nerve block but is abolished by neuromuscular blockade with curare, establishing the peripheral nerve origin of the disorder.[175] Prolonged post-operative paralysis due to hypersensitivity to a nondepolarizing muscle relaxant, rocuronium, has been reported, with attendant implications regarding safety of anesthesia.[176] The association of neuromyotonia and encephalopathy in the form of hallucinations and insomnia is referred to as Morvan's syndrome or Morvan's fibrillary chorea. VGKC antibodies have been reported in Morvan's syndrome.[177–179] Neuromyotonia has also been described after recovery from VGKC antibody associated limbic encephalitis.[167] Focal myokymia involving the face has been reported as an autoimmune syndrome associated with VGKC antibodies, expanding the clinical spectrum of VGKC-antibody-mediated syndromes.[180]

Cramp-Fasciculation Syndrome

Tahmoush et al reported nine patients with a syndrome of PNH characterized by muscle aching and cramps—termed cramp-fasciculation syndrome (see Table 17-2). They defined cramps as painful muscle contractions precipitated by movement and relieved by stretching.[181] Although cramp-fasciculation syndrome (CFS) is usually benign, rare instances of CFS progressing to amyotrophic lateral sclerosis have been reported.[182] Hart et al, in an excellent study, emphasize the fact that neuromyotonia or Isaacs syndrome and CFS appear to be different only quantitatively; that is, the symptoms appear to be more severe and more widespread in patients with Isaacs syndrome as compared to those with CFS. In their study, the EMG was used to differentiate between these two syndromes, as discussed in the following paragraphs.[169]

Laboratory evaluation of patients with PNH should include tests for other autoimmune disorders such as diabetes mellitus and thyroid dysfunction. Serum creatine kinase (CK) may be elevated. Oligoclonal bands may be detected in spinal fluid.[155] Imaging of the chest for thymoma and lung cancer is important. The tumors may precede or follow the diagnosis of peripheral nerve hyperexcitability and in the study by Hart et al, lung tumors were detected as long as 4 years after the diagnosis of PNH. Hence, serial computed tomography of the chest may be indicated.[169]

Hart et al reported the presence of anti-VGKC antibodies in approximately 40% of patients with acquired neuromyotonia and 28% of patients with CFS. In their study, the majority of patients with VGKC antibody had an underlying thymoma. There was no correlation between the antibody titer and symptom severity or

EMG features.[169] Vernino et al reported a patient with CFS and MG associated with thymoma. This patient had ganglionic and muscle acetylcholine receptor (AChR) antibodies, but VGKC antibodies were not detected.[183] In a subsequent study by Vernino and Lennon, VGKC antibodies were more frequently detected in Isaacs syndrome than in CFS (54% vs. 16%). In addition, 14% of patients with neuromyotonia and 6% with CFS had antibodies to the ganglionic AChR. Either VGKC or ganglionic AChR antibodies were present in 63% of patients with neuromyotonia and in 22% with CFS. Other autoantibodies detected in these conditions included striational antibodies and muscle AChR antibodies. The authors suggest that Isaacs syndrome and CFS are part of a spectrum of channelopathies with a common autoimmune pathogenesis. They recommend that patients with PNH should have assays for VGKC, muscle AChR, ganglionic AChR, and striational antibodies, and perhaps other neuronal nuclear and cytoplasmic antibody markers of thymoma and small cell lung cancer.[158]

The diagnosis of Isaacs syndrome and CFS is based on the clinical features in combination with the EMG findings described here. The electrophysiologic terms that have been used to describe the spontaneous activity seen in Isaacs syndrome include *neuromyotonic discharges* and *myokymic* discharges. Electromyographically, neuromyotonia refers to continuous irregular bursts of single motor units firing as doublets, triplets, or multiplets. The intraburst frequency is 150 to 300 Hz. Bursts may be short or last a few seconds, with abrupt onset and termination. The amplitude often wanes. The bursts may be spontaneous, precipitated by needle movement, or nerve percussion. Myokymic discharges seen on EMG are similar except that the intraburst frequency of the discharges is lower at 5 to 150 Hz. These bursts repeat at regular or irregular intervals, semirhythmically, followed by a few seconds of silence. The interval between bursts depends on the length of the bursts, longer bursts firing less frequently. Electrophysiologically, both neuromyotonia and myokymia are felt to represent a continuum of the same abnormality, as are the clinical syndromes of neuromyotonia and myokymia.[158,184] Fibrillations and fasciculations may also be noted. The spontaneous activity persists in sleep, is unchanged or diminished by peripheral nerve block, and disappears after neuromuscular blockade with curare. The discharges may be accentuated by hyperventilation or ischemia. NCS may reveal an underlying peripheral neuropathy. In addition, afterdischarges are often seen following the compound motor action potential or after the F or H wave on routine NCS.[42,170,184]

In CFS, unlike in Isaacs syndrome, afterdischarges occur only after repetitive nerve stimulation and not after a single stimulus. The EMG findings are less prominent, and patients usually have fasciculations and cramp discharges. Myokymia, neuromyotonia, and fibrillations are usually absent.[170] Benatar et al studied repetitive nerve stimulation of motor nerves with supramaximal stimuli at 1, 5, 10, and 30 Hz in patients with CFS. Afterdischarges consisting of individual potentials following the train of stimuli were seen in patients with the clinical phenotype of CFS. At 10 Hz stimulation, the test had a sensitivity of 79% and a specificity of 88%.[185] In a subsequent study, Harrison et al found that tibial nerve repetitive stimulation correctly classified the presence or absence of CFS in 75% of patients.[186]

Treatment and Management
Isaacs Syndrome

Systematic studies of symptomatic therapy in Isaacs syndrome and CFS are lacking. However, the effect of several drugs has been described in case reports or small series (see Table 17-2). Agents evaluated include phenytoin, carbamazepine, sodium valproate, baclofen, gabapentin, diazepam, acetazolamide, and mexiletene.[155,156,181,187–191] Although symptomatic relief may be achieved to varying degrees with these medications, immunosuppressive therapy has been found useful in achieving long-term remission. Newsom-Davis and Mills used plasma exchange or a combination of prednisone (60–80 mg on alternate days) and azathioprine (1.5–2.5 mg/kg daily) in three of their five patients, with improvement in two. Plasma exchange has been noted to be successful in other case reports as well, either alone or in combination with oral immunosuppressants.[155,187,192]

Ho and Wilson reported successful treatment of one patient with acquired neuromyotonia and thymoma with IVIg.[193] Another patient failed to respond after six plasma exchanges and could not tolerate steroids and azathioprine, but had good benefit from IVIg.[194] Ishii et al treated one patient with Isaacs syndrome with plasma exchange, which achieved remission of symptoms for about 5 months. With subsequent IVIg treatment, dysphagia worsened and dyspnea appeared. EMG revealed an increase in continuous muscle fiber activity. The symptoms improved after another plasma exchange.[195] Van den Berg et al made a similar observation in one patient with neuromyotonia associated with thymoma, in whom IVIg at 0.4 g/kg for 5 days was ineffective. A subsequent course of plasma exchange five times a week for 2 weeks resulted in a dramatic improvement in symptoms within 2 days.[196] It has been suggested that the worsening of symptoms following IVIg administration in Isaacs syndrome may be due to an IVIg-mediated increase in intracellular calcium and subsequent muscle cramps. Additionally, plasma exchange may be more effective than IVIg in reducing autoantibody titers.[196,197] Although sparse, the data seem to suggest that plasma exchange may be more effective than IVIg in the treatment of Isaacs syndrome.

Cramp-Fasciculation Syndrome

The optimal treatment of CFS is not known. In their initial report, Tahmoush et al noted a "fair to good" response to carbamazepine titrated up to effect, with a maximum dose of 1600 mg/day. Treatment with prednisone 25 to 30 mg/day improved cramps in one patient with MG, CFS, and thymoma (see Table 17-2).[181,183]

Primary Disorders of Muscle

Rippling Muscle Disease

Rippling muscle disease (RMD) is a myopathy with hyperexcitability of the muscle. Torbergsen is credited with the initial description of this disorder in five affected members in a family over three generations.[198] Subsequently, Ricker et al described two German families with the disorder and introduced the term *rippling muscle disease*.[199] Further work has established that most cases of the disorder are autosomal dominant, although autosomal recessive and sporadic cases have been reported.[200–203]

The phenotype of RMD has recently expanded to include acquired forms of the disorder with an autoimmune etiopathogenesis, most often associated with MG (Box 17-4). Interestingly, in one patient, the rippling muscle phenomenon seemed to improve with worsening of MG.[158,183,204–206] Rare cases of acquired RMD without MG have been reported; one patient developed autoimmune hemolytic anemia a year after the onset of RMD, and another developed malignant lymphoma 3 years after the onset of RMD.[207,208] Schulte-Mattler et al have reported a patient with RMD with

Box 17-4 Classification of Rippling Muscle Disease

Hereditary

Autosomal dominant, chromosomal locus 1q41–42 (gene defect unknown)
Autosomal dominant, chromosomal locus 3p25 (caveolin-3 gene)
Autosomal recessive, chromosomal locus 3p25 (caveolin-3 gene)

Acquired

Sporadic, due to de novo mutations in the caveolin-3 gene
Autoimmune: associated with myasthenia gravis, thymoma, lymphoma, and other autoimmune disorders

inflammatory changes and IgG deposits on the sarcolemma on muscle biopsy, and serum antibodies to striated muscle and titin. In this patient, as well as in some of the other reported patients with MG and RMD, thymoma was present.[183,204,206,209] One patient with sporadic RMD unmasked by simvastatin therapy has been reported. This patient developed MG about a year after the onset of RMD.[210]

Diagnosis and Evaluation

The disease usually presents in the first two decades. In an excellent review of 46 individuals from two families, Vorgerd et al found that the age of onset ranged from 5 to 54 years (mean 22 years). In this series, patients presented with muscle stiffness that was most pronounced in the proximal lower extremities and sometimes mildly painful. Slowness of movements after a period of rest and muscle cramping were other features. Muscle pain, cramps, or stiffness were induced by exercise in some patients, while in others muscle cramps occurred when standing and walking after a period of rest and disappeared with continuing exertion.[211,212]

On examination, there are three main signs: the rippling phenomenon, muscle mounding, and percussion-induced rapid muscle contractions. The rippling phenomenon is elicited by forceful muscle contraction followed by abrupt relaxation, such as forceful extension of the knee followed by abrupt flexion, or forceful flexion of the elbow followed by abrupt extension. This induces slow rolling movements across the muscle. The mechanical stretch appears to be a stimulus to muscle rippling. The speed of muscle rippling has been shown to be 0.6 m/sec, about 10 times slower than muscle fiber conduction velocity.[199,211] Muscle mounding is characterized by a visible localized swelling of muscles that is elicited by tapping the muscle at various intensities and may be painful. It may be generalized or confined to a few muscles. When generalized, it seems to be most prominent in the deltoid, biceps brachii, brachioradialis, extensor digitorum, thenar muscles, and quadriceps. Slight muscle percussion may result in instant, pronounced contraction that may be sustained for several seconds, termed percussion-induced rapid muscle contractions (PIRC). PIRC may be elicited in all extremity muscles and the sternomastoid. They are usually painless and do not habituate. Other features of RMD include muscle hypertrophy that may be focal, typically involving the calf, or generalized. Mild proximal muscle weakness may be seen.[199,211] There is a peculiar tendency to toe-walk, especially on awakening in the morning or after a prolonged period of rest. The toe-walking improves after several minutes of walking and has been attributed to disproportionate stiffness of the calf muscles.[199,211,213] Recurrent myoglobinuria has been reported.[211,214]

Vorgerd et al used the following diagnostic criteria for RMD in their study: (1) PIRC in at least two muscles of the upper and two muscles of the lower extremity in the presence of normal tendon reflexes; (2) at least one of the following: muscle mounding, muscle rippling, or elevated serum CK. In their series, PIRC was the most reliable clinical sign of RMD. PIRC and muscle mounding are uniformly present in RMD, whereas muscle rippling is seen in only about two thirds of patients, despite the fact that the disease bears the name of the phenomenon.[211] Greenberg suggests that the absence of PIRC may distinguish acquired RMD associated with MG from genetic RMD.[206] The clinical course is relatively mild and either nonprogressive or slowly progressive.[200,211]

The first RMD genetic locus identified was 1q41 by Stephan and colleagues in 1994 in a large Oregon family. However, the same genetic defect was not detected in the two German families previously reported by Ricker, indicating genetic heterogeneity.[199,215] Betz et al identified mutations in the caveolin-3 gene on chromosome 3p25 in patients with autosomal dominant RMD.[216] A caveolin-3 mutation has also been reported in a sporadic case of RMD.[203] Finally, homozygous mutations of the caveolin-3 gene have been reported in autosomal recessive RMD.[217,218] The spectrum of "caveolinopathy" thus includes four distinct but sometimes overlapping autosomal dominant diseases: limb girdle muscular dystrophy (LGMD type 1c), hyperCKemia, RMD, and distal myopathy. Most often, a mutation within a family seems to cause a similar phenotype, although a few reports suggest that there may be overlapping phenotypes within a family.[219–221] The same caveolin-3 mutation may also cause different phenotypes in different families.[222] All the mutations reduce the expression of caveolin-3 on the muscle membrane.

The diagnostic evaluation of patients with suspected RMD includes estimation of serum CK levels, which are often significantly elevated (3–30 fold).[214] Routine laboratory tests are otherwise usually normal. Thyroid function testing is indicated, because the muscle mounding seen in RMD is reminiscent of the "myoedema" described in hypothyroidism. Muscle and ganglionic AChR antibodies, VGKC antibodies and striated muscle antibodies may be detected in patients with the autoimmune form of RMD.[158,183] Radiologic evaluation for thymoma is appropriate, especially in non-familial cases.

In RMD, needle EMG is usually completely normal; however, increased insertional activity has been reported. The muscle rippling, mounding, and PIRC, which are the diagnostic clinical signs, are electrically silent.[211] Increased insertional activity and spontaneous high-frequency motor unit discharges during the muscle rippling have been reported in patients with the autoimmune form of RMD.[158,183] So et al suggest that the familial form of RMD can be differentiated from acquired or autoimmune RMD by the electrical silence of rippling muscle seen in the former.[213] This does not appear to be a consistent observation. Greenberg, in a review of acquired RMD, noted that in five of eight patients with acquired RMD and MG, the muscle ripple was electrically silent. He also noted that most of the patients with electrically silent muscle rippling had high titers of muscle AChR antibodies, although the significance of this finding is unclear.[206] Muscle biopsy has been reported to be normal on routine stains, although nonspecific features such as fiber size variation have been described. A vacuolar myopathy has been reported.[223] Inflammatory changes have been reported in acquired RMD.[183,205,206,209] On immunostaining, there is reduction or absence of sarcolemmal caveolin-3. Additionally, a secondary reduction in dysferlin may be seen in both genetic and acquired forms of the disease. It has been suggested that a mosaic pattern of immunostaining for caveolin-3, with some fibers revealing reduced staining and others demonstrating normal staining, is suggestive of immune-mediated rather than hereditary RMD.[209,214] Electron microscopy revealed T-tubular dilatation and loss of "caveolae," the

invaginations of the sarcolemmal membrane, in one patient.[209] Caveolin-3 DNA sequencing is commercially available and may be used in place of muscle biopsy in patients with suspected genetic RMD.

Treatment and Management

Literature on the treatment of RMD is sparse, given the rarity and the benign nature of the disorder. The rippling phenomenon and PIRC do not seem to affect quality of life.[214] Medications that have been reported to be useful include dantrolene and nifedipine. Phenytoin and tocainide have been ineffective.[199,224] Isolated case reports ascribe no response to carbamazepine, tizanidine, and mexiletene.[203,206] Immune-mediated RMD may respond to immunosuppressive therapy with azathioprine or prednisone, or to treatment of an underlying thymoma.[183,204–206,208] In an interesting report of a family with autosomal dominant RMD, Madrid et al noted that early-onset toe-walking was a prominent feature. In their study, two patients underwent surgical Achilles tendon lengthening, resulting in prolonged resolution of toe-walking. However, the role of this procedure in routine management of patients with RMD is uncertain.[225] Pyridostigmine may worsen muscle rippling.[205] This may be important in the management of patients with RMD coexisting with MG. It may be prudent to discuss the risk for exertional myoglobinuria with patients. Although the halothane contracture test has been reported to be positive in one patient with RMD, the risk of malignant hyperthermia is unknown.[200]

Muscle Channelopathies

Ion channels subserve several essential functions including excitability of nerve/muscle membranes. The channelopathies are disorders that result from abnormal ion channel function. The channelopathies that result in skeletal muscle hyperexcitability and weakness include two related groups of disorders: the nondystrophic myotonias and the periodic paralyses. These disorders were the first conditions wherein a genetic defect in voltage-gated ion channel function was identified. Other skeletal muscle channelopathies such as malignant hyperthermia, central core disease, and congenital myasthenic syndromes[226] present with weakness or fatal anesthetic complications, and are not discussed in this review. Malignant hyperthermia is discussed in Chapter 10. The molecular genetics of the nondystrophic myotonias and periodic paralyses are summarized in Table 17-3.[227] A detailed discussion of the genetics and mechanisms of channel dysfunction is beyond the scope of this review.

Nondystrophic Myotonias

Myotonia refers to the impaired relaxation of muscle following voluntary contraction. Although myotonic dystrophy is the most common myotonic syndrome (see Chapter 19), the prominent symptom in patients with myotonic dystrophy is weakness rather than myotonia. In contrast, the primary clinical manifestation of the nondystrophic myotonias is myotonia. Two major disorders compose the family of the nondystrophic myotonias: myotonia congenita (MC) and paramyotonia congenita (PMC).

Diagnosis and Evaluation
Myotonia Congenita

Patients with myotonia congenita present with muscle tightness, cramps, or pain. They may also notice difficulty in relaxing muscles after contraction, such as difficulty in releasing handgrip after a handshake. Muscles may "lock up" when sudden activity is attempted, resulting in falls. The stiffness improves with repeated

Table 17-3 The Skeletal Muscle Channelopathies

Disorder	Inheritance	Affected Channel	Chromosomal Locus	Gene
Myotonia congenita (Thomsen disease)	Autosomal dominant	Chloride	7q35	CLCN1
Myotonia congenita (Becker disease)	Autosomal recessive	Chloride	7q35	CLCN1
Hyperkalemic periodic paralysis	Autosomal dominant	Sodium	17q23	SCN4A
Paramyotonia congenita	Autosomal dominant	Sodium	17q23	SCN4A
Potassium aggravated myotonias*	Autosomal dominant	Sodium	17q23	SCN4A
Hypokalemic periodic paralysis 1	Autosomal dominant	L-type calcium	1q32	CACNA1S
Hypokalemic periodic paralysis 2	Autosomal dominant	Sodium	17q23	SCN4A
Hypo/hyperkalemic periodic paralysis	Autosomal dominant	Auxiliary potassium channel subunit (MiRP2)	11q13–14	KCNE3
Anderson-Tawil syndrome	Autosomal dominant	Potassium	17q	KCNJ2

*The potassium-aggravated myotonias include myotonia fluctuans, myotonia permanens, and acetazolamide responsive myotonia.

contractions of the muscle group involved (the "warm-up" phenomenon). The disorder may be autosomal dominant (Thomsen disease) or recessive (Becker disease). It may be useful to note here that the eponym Becker disease used for autosomal recessive MC is distinct from late-onset dystrophinopathy or Becker muscular dystrophy.

Thomsen disease presents in infancy or early childhood, usually in the first 2 years of life, but tends to be milder than the recessive form (Becker disease). Infants may be noted to have difficulty in eye opening after a crying spell. Falls may occur due to leg stiffness. Facial myotonia may cause chewing and swallowing difficulty. Muscle hypertrophy may be noted, but muscle weakness is usually not a feature. The face and arms tend to be more involved than the legs.

Becker disease is the only autosomal recessive skeletal muscle channelopathy. It usually presents later than Thomsen disease, in the first or even the second decade, but the myotonia tends to be more severe. The disease progresses slowly until 30 to 40 years of age and then appears to stabilize. The legs are more severely involved than the face or arms, and severe myotonia of the lower extremities may result in disability. Severe myotonic episodes may be associated with transient muscle weakness, especially in the hands. There may also be episodes of transient generalized muscle weakness, often occurring on attempts to get up from a recumbent position after rest. Mild, fixed distal weakness may develop.[228–230]

On examination, myotonia can be elicited by voluntary contraction of a muscle followed by attempts at relaxation, as after making and releasing a fist ("grip myotonia"). Tightly closing the eyes for a few seconds results in difficulty opening them, eyelid myotonia. Myotonia can also be elicited on percussion of muscles, such as the thenar eminence, with a percussion hammer, causing a muscle contraction that persists for several seconds. With the forearm extended and the wrist flexed, striking the extensor muscles of the forearm with a percussion hammer elicits sustained extensor posturing of the wrist similar to PIRC in RMD. Myotonia displays the "warm-up phenomenon" in that it improves with repeated voluntary contraction. There is often muscle hypertrophy, usually more prominently in the lower limbs.

Paramyotonia Congenita

In contrast to MC, paramyotonia congenita (PMC) is characterized by myotonia that worsens with exercise. The "warm-up" phenomenon does not occur; in contrast, myotonia worsens with repeated voluntary contraction. Another characteristic feature of PMC is worsening of myotonia with cold exposure. The disorder manifests

at birth or in early infancy and tends to predominantly affect the face, tongue, and arms. Cold exposure may not only aggravate myotonia, but also cause focal or generalized weakness that may persist for several hours even after warming. Some patients may also have episodic weakness, an overlap syndrome with hyperkalemic periodic paralysis. Symptoms tend to be nonprogressive.[228–230]

The differential diagnosis of MC and PMC includes myotonic dystrophy, because mild phenotypes of myotonic dystrophy may not have prominent dystrophic features early in the illness. Careful examination for the typical facies of myotonic dystrophy, premature cataracts, diabetes, and cardiac conduction defects should be performed.

Potassium-Aggravated Myotonias

The potassium-aggravated myotonias (PAM) comprise a group of potassium-sensitive disorders that manifest with myotonia similar to MC without episodic weakness, in contrast to the periodic paralyses. Unlike MC, these disorders are caused by SCNA4 sodium channel mutations similar to PMC. PAM may be distinguished from autosomal dominant MC, which it closely resembles, by a worsening of the myotonia with potassium ingestion.[231] The PAMs include *myotonia fluctuans*, *myotonia permanens*, and *acetazolamide responsive myotonia*.

In *myotonia fluctuans*, patients have myotonia that fluctuates and varies in severity. Additional features include increased myotonia induced by exercise occurring after a delay of several minutes, presence of the "warm-up phenomenon," and eyelid paramyotonia. Episodes of weakness following cold exposure, hyperkalemia, or exercise do not occur. Patients may be asymptomatic for days and then spontaneously experience marked stiffness of facial and limb muscles.[228,232] Patients with *myotonia permanens* have almost constant, severe myotonia without weakness. The myotonia is aggravated by potassium but not by cold. Myotonia of the respiratory muscles may occur, resulting in hypoxia.[228,233] *Acetazolamide responsive myotonia* presents in childhood with painful muscle stiffness involving predominantly the face and hands. Myotonia is provoked by fasting, potassium, and exercise and is alleviated by a high carbohydrate meal. Episodic weakness does not occur.[228,234]

Schwartz-Jampel Syndrome

Although Schwartz-Jampel syndrome (SJS) is not a channelopathy, it bears brief mention in the differential diagnosis of the non-dystrophic myotonias. This is a rare disorder characterized by short stature, skeletal deformities, a characteristic facies, muscle stiffness, and myotonia. The disease manifests in the first year of life, and motor development may be delayed. Patients have congenital blepharophimosis, masklike or "stiff" face, micrognathia, low-set ears, low hairline, high arched palate, short neck, pigeon chest, contractures, spinal deformities, hip dysplasias, and osteochondroplasia on radiographs. Muscle hypertrophy, particularly involving proximal muscles, is common; the distal muscles may become progressively atrophic. Action and percussion myotonia are present, and continuous muscle activity in the form of rippling movements may be seen in limb muscles. Tendon reflexes may be diminished. Cataract formation, laryngeal stridor, and high-pitched voice have been reported. The disease is slowly progressive to adulthood and then stabilizes. A rare neonatal form has been termed *SJS2*. SJS2 presents at birth with feeding and respiratory difficulty, stiffness, and myotonia. Episodes of malignant hyperthermia may be seen, resulting in early death. Skeletal deformities may be detected even prenatally.[235–237] SJS is usually inherited as an autosomal recessive trait, but rare autosomal dominant inheritance has been reported.[238] The genetic locus is on chromosome 1p35–36, on the gene *HSPG2* encoding perlecan, a heparan sulfate proteoglycan found in basement membranes.[239,240]

Laboratory evaluation in the nondystrophic myotonias and SJS may reveal mild elevation of serum CK. In patients with paramyotonia congenita or hyperkalemic periodic paralysis overlap, serum potassium may be elevated during attacks. Other routine laboratory tests are usually normal. Electrodiagnostic testing is the mainstay of diagnosis. Routine motor and sensory NCS are normal. The most prominent abnormality is the presence of myotonic discharges on needle EMG. These discharges comprise spontaneous painless bursts of repetitively firing potentials that wax and wane both in amplitude and frequency (the "dive bomber" discharges). The potentials fire at a rate of 20 to 80 Hz and are of two types: brief (less than 5 msec) biphasic spike potentials that resemble fibrillation potentials, or positive waves 5 to 20 msec in duration that resemble positive sharp waves.[241] The discharges may be evoked by needle movement and percussion. They may also occur as afterdischarges following voluntary activity. Repeated contractions decrease the discharges in MC, the electrophysiologic equivalent of the warm-up phenomenon, whereas the discharges become more prominent after repeated contractions in PMC.[242] These discharges are present in most limb muscles. Continuous myotonia may obscure examination of volitional motor units. Motor unit morphology and recruitment are usually normal, although myopathic features

with early recruitment of brief small amplitude motor units may be seen in recessive MC. In PMC, cooling the limb can evoke fibrillation potentials, worsen myotonia and eventually cause electrical inexcitability. In SJS, EMG reveals continuous high-frequency discharges at rest that increase with needle movement, percussion, or voluntary activation. The discharges resemble neuromyotonia rather than myotonia, and are abolished by neuromuscular blockade with curare or succinylcholine in some, but not all, cases.[236,243] Myotonic discharges are reported in some cases.[244,245] It has been suggested that abnormal muscle membrane excitability as well as peripheral nerve excitability may be present in SJS.[238]

Other tests that may be useful in the diagnosis of nondystrophic myotonias include repetitive nerve stimulation and the exercise tests. Repetitive nerve stimulation at 5 to 10 Hz results in a decremental response, but this is not specific for a myotonic disorder. The decremental response in myotonia has been attributed to transient inexcitability of the muscle membrane, rather than a disorder of neuromuscular transmission.[246,247] Exercise testing is useful in confirming the diagnosis as well as differentiating the various skeletal muscle channelopathies. (See Appendix 17-1 at the end of the chapter for exercise test protocols.) The short exercise test (SET) results in a transient decrease in the amplitude of the compound motor action potential (CMAP) in MC. In PMC, CMAP amplitude may either increase or decrease during the SET. However, on repeated trials of the SET, the CMAP amplitude decreases in PMC, but does not change in MC. Thus, an increase in CMAP amplitude during the SET or a progressive decrease in CMAP amplitude when the SET is repeated suggests PMC rather than MC. The long exercise test (LET) may result in decreased CMAP amplitude in PMC but seems to be less useful in MC (Table 17-4). The effect of cold on PMC has been used during electrodiagnostic evaluation by recording the CMAP before and after cooling the limb to 20° C for 15 to 30 minutes. In PMC, a CMAP decrement greater than 50% is typically observed. Postexercise fibrillations and myotonia are abolished, and voluntary recruitment of MUAPs is decreased. These features are not seen in MC.[248–250] In an elegant study, Fournier et al identified five EMG patterns that correlate with subgroups of mutations in the skeletal muscle channelopathies. They suggest that these patterns may be used as guides for molecular diagnosis. They also describe postexercise myotonic potentials (PEMP), defined as several potentials of decreasing amplitude that follow the CMAP evoked by a single supramaximal stimulus after short duration exercise.

Table 17-4 Electrodiagnostic Features of the Nondystrophic Myotonias and the Periodic Paralyses

Diagnostic Feature	Disorder-Specific Finding			
	MC	**PMC**	**HyperPP**	**HypoPP**
CMAP after SET				
First trial	Transient decrease	Increase/decrease	Increase	No change
Repeat trials	No change	Gradual decrease	Gradual increase	No change
CMAP after LET				
Immediate amplitude change	No change/slight decrease	Decrease	Increase	No change
Late amplitude change	None	Decrease	Decrease	Decrease
Needle EMG: myotonic discharges	+++	+++	+ or −	−
SET sensitivity (%) (95% CI)	83 (53–100)	100 (81–100)	83 (53–100)	0 (0–23)
LET sensitivity (%) (95% CI)	25 (1–50)	89 (76–100)	93 (81–100)	84 (72–97)

CI, confidence interval; CMAP, compound motor action potential; EMG, electromyography; HyperPP, hyperkalemic periodic paralysis; HypoPP, hypokalemic periodic paralysis; LET, long exercise test; MC, myotonia congenita; PMC, paramyotonia congenita; SET, short exercise test.

Adapted from Fournier E, Arzel M, Sternberg D, et al: Electromyography guides toward subgroups of mutations in muscle channelopathies, *Ann Neurol* 56: 650–661, 2004. Copyright © 2004 *Annals of Neurology*; with permission from John Wiley and Sons, Inc.

They disappear 10 to 30 msec after completion of exercise. These potentials are seen in MC, PMC, and PAM, but not in the periodic paralyses.[251] Table 17-4 summarizes the electrodiagnostic features of the nondystrophic myotonias and the periodic paralyses.

Muscle biopsy is usually not necessary for the diagnosis of the nondystrophic myotonias. If biopsy is performed, the muscle may be normal or may demonstrate mild myopathic features. Absence of type 2b muscle fibers is a characteristic of MC. A vacuolar myopathy may be seen in PMC patients who have hyperkalemic periodic paralysis.[228] In SJS, muscle biopsy may be normal, may demonstrate mild nonspecific features, or may show mild to moderate dystrophic changes.[243–245] Genetic testing is available commercially for MC but not for PMC. Genetic testing for myotonic dystrophy may be necessary in patients where the diagnosis is uncertain and the gene test for the *CLCN1* mutation is negative. Genetic testing for SJS is available in specialized centers. Recently, the ability of muscle magnetic resonance imaging to measure ion fluxes in vivo has been applied to muscle channelopathies. An increase in Na^{23} signal intensity and edema-like changes on T2-weighted images have been described in PMC.[252]

Treatment of Nondystrophic Myotonias

Many patients with nondystrophic myotonia have mild symptoms that do not require treatment except avoiding precipitating factors such as cold exposure. If the myotonia is severe enough to necessitate treatment, antiepileptic medications and antiarrhythmic agents that block muscle sodium channels may be useful. In an early randomized double blind study comparing procainamide, quinine, and prednisone, where patients received all three medications, 15 of 20 patients who received procainamide and 15 of 19 patients taking prednisone improved. Only 6 of 20 patients improved with quinine.[253] Phenytoin, tocainide, procainamide, flecainide, propafenone, and mexiletene have been used in the symptomatic treatment of myotonia.[254–257] A single-blind study of antiarrhythmic drugs suggested that mexiletene and tocainide were the most potent antimyotonic agents, but the use of tocainide was limited by hematologic side effects.[258] Tocainide is no longer available owing to risks of bone marrow toxicity and interstitial lung disease. Propafenone was effective in a single case of PMC.[257] Dantrolene may also be useful. Mexiletene is probably used most frequently. It can sometimes be useful in preventing the transient weakness that may accompany severe myotonia in recessive MC. It is usually started at doses of 150 mg daily and increased to efficacy, with a maximum dose of 300 mg three times daily. Lightheadedness, diarrhea, and dyspepsia are the major adverse effects. An electrocardiogram (ECG) should be performed prior to initiation of mexiletene to evaluate conduction abnormalities and the QT interval.[228] Mexiletene is proarrhythmic and is contraindicated in the presence of second- or third-degree atrioventricular block. It should be used with caution in patients with first-degree atrioventricular block, sinus node dysfunction, or intraventricular conduction defects. Blood counts, liver function tests, and ECG should be monitored during treatment. Acetazolamide may be useful in some cases of PMC. In a study of seven patients with MC and two with PMC, all patients improved with acetazolamide. One patient with PMC developed quadriparesis 12 hours after acetazolamide.[230,259] The nondystrophic myotonias may be associated with prolonged recovery times after general anesthesia, and propofol and depolarizing neuromuscular blockade may worsen myotonia.[260] Patients should be advised of this risk.

Mexiletene may be useful for the symptomatic treatment of myotonia in patients with myotonia fluctuans.[228,232] The myotonia and pain of acetazolamide responsive myotonia respond to acetazolamide, as the name implies. Acetazolamide is started at 125 mg/day and increased, if necessary, to 250 mg three times a day. Mexiletene may also be helpful. It has been suggested that a therapeutic trial of acetazolamide is appropriate in patients with a clinical syndrome resembling MC who complain of pain.[228,234]

Treatment of SJS is directed at the symptom of stiffness. Isolated reports of improvement with phenytoin, carbamazepine, procainamide, and diazepam have been published.[237,238,244] Botulinum toxin has been used for blepharophimosis.[261]

Periodic Paralysis

The primary periodic paralyses (PP) are disorders of skeletal muscle excitability due to inherited ion channel dysfunction. They present with episodic weakness and disturbances in serum potassium concentration. They are classified as hypokalemic or hyperkalemic based on the serum potassium level during attacks or response to potassium. Anderson-Tawil syndrome is a rare autosomal dominant disorder characterized by the triad of periodic paralysis, cardiac arrhythmias, and skeletal malformations.[262]

Diagnosis and Evaluation
Hyperkalemic Periodic Paralysis

Hyperkalemic periodic paralysis (HyperPP) is characterized by recurrent episodes of generalized or focal muscle weakness, which occur in association with elevated serum potassium levels. The disease is inherited as an autosomal dominant trait with a high degree of penetrance and is due to mutations in the sodium channel gene *SCN4A* on chromosome 17q23. It usually manifests in the first decade in infancy or childhood. Episodes are triggered by high potassium foods and may occur when the patient is resting about 20 to 30 minutes after exercise. Cold, emotional stress, fasting, and pregnancy may also trigger attacks. Attacks usually occur in the morning but may occur at any time of the day. The muscle weakness may vary in severity. Weakness usually starts in the lower extremities and spreads to the trunk and upper extremities. Respiratory and bulbar muscles are usually spared, although there are rare reports of involvement of these muscles during a severe attack. Attacks last from less than an hour up to 2 hours and may be shortened by mild exercise. On rare occasions, the weakness may persist for days. Reflexes are diminished or absent during attacks and are normal in between attacks. The frequency of the episodes is variable; some patients have daily attacks, but the frequency tends to diminish with age. In between attacks, electromyographic myotonia is described in 50% to 75% of patients, but clinical myotonia is seen in less than 20%. Lid lag and eyelid myotonia may be evident on examination. Some patients develop a fixed proximal muscle weakness that does not appear to be related to the frequency of episodes.[228–230,263–265] One family with HyperPP and malignant hyperthermia linked to the *SCN4A* locus has been reported.[266] Diagnostic criteria for HyperPP are summarized in Box 17-5.

Hypokalemic Periodic Paralysis

Hypokalemic periodic paralysis (HypoPP) is the most frequent form of PP. Although it is inherited as an autosomal dominant trait, one third of cases are sporadic and the penetrance in women is only 50%, so a family history may not be present. About 70% of patients with HypoPP have mutations in the gene encoding the calcium channel CACNA1S on chromosome 1q32, *HypoPP-1*. In 10% of patients, the disorder is due to mutations in the gene encoding the sodium channel SCN4A on chromosome 17q23, *HypoPP-2*. In a recent study, Matthews et al found that mutations in any one of

Box 17-5 Diagnostic Criteria for Primary Hyperkalemic Periodic Paralysis

1. Two or more attacks of muscle weakness with documented serum potassium >4.5 mEq/L
2. One attack of muscle weakness in the proband and one attack of weakness in one relative with documented serum potassium >4.5 mEq/L in at least one attack
3. Three of six clinical or laboratory features as outlined below:
   a. Onset before third decade of life
   b. Duration of attack (muscle weakness involving one or more limbs) <2 hours
   c. Positive triggers (exercise, stress)
   d. Myotonia
   e. Positive family history or genetically confirmed skeletal sodium channel mutation
   f. Positive McManis short exercise test
4. Exclusion of other causes of hyperkalemia (renal, adrenal, thyroid dysfunction; potassium-sparing diuretic use)

From Sansone V, Meola G, Links T, et al: Treatment for periodic paralysis, *Cochrane Database Syst Rev* 1, 2008. With permission from Dr. Sansone; Copyright Cochrane Collaboration, reproduced with permission.

several arginine residues in the voltage sensing segments of the α-subunits of either *CACNA1S* or *SCN4A* with resultant charge loss of the voltage sensors underlies the clinical phenotype of HypoPP, the "gating pore cation leak hypothesis."[266a] The disorder typically presents in late childhood or adolescence, slightly later than HyperPP, although it may rarely present as late as the second decade. Often, the patient awakens in the morning with weakness. These attacks are often triggered by strenuous physical activity or a carbohydrate-rich meal the previous day. Attacks may also be precipitated by sodium-rich foods, alcohol ingestion, cold, intercurrent viral infections, lack of sleep, menstruation, and certain medications (beta agonists, corticosteroids, and insulin). Some patients report a prodrome of paresthesias, fatigue, and behavioral and cognitive changes the day before an attack. Attacks of flaccid paralysis are longer than those in HyperPP, lasting hours to days, and tend to be more severe but are less frequent than those of HyperPP. Weakness may be generalized or focal; when generalized, the lower limbs are affected before the upper extremities. Bulbar, extraocular, respiratory, and sphincter muscles are usually spared. Similar to HyperPP, reflexes are diminished or absent during the attack. Sensation is normal. As with HyperPP, attack frequency varies but tends to diminish with age. In between attacks, patients are normal and do not usually have myotonia. A fixed weakness may develop after repeated attacks.[228,229,264,265] Box 17-6 lists the diagnostic criteria for HypoPP.

Andersen-Tawil Syndrome

The triad of periodic paralysis, ventricular arrhythmias, and skeletal dysmorphisms defines Andersen-Tawil syndrome (ATS), a rare autosomal dominant disorder caused by mutations in the gene for the inward rectifying potassium channel *KCNJ2* on chromosome 17q23.[267] The dysmorphisms seen in ATS include clinodactyly or syndactyly, low-set ears, mandibular hypoplasia, and hypertelorism. Short stature may be associated. Scoliosis, high-arched palate, brachydactyly, ptosis, single palmar crease, vaginal atresia, and unilateral dysplastic kidney have all been reported in ATS. The facial dysmorphisms that are a clue to the diagnosis of ATS may be mild and easily overlooked. Episodes of paralysis and cardiac arrhythmia begin

in early childhood. Although patients may have either hypokalemic or hyperkalemic paralysis, potassium loading typically will provoke attacks. A proximal myopathy is often associated. The initial presentation may be due to ventricular arrhythmias, especially bidirectional ventricular tachycardia. The expression of the disorder varies widely within families, with some family members having only asymptomatic QT interval prolongation on ECG or minimal dysmorphisms.[229,230,262,268,269] A distinct pattern of neurocognitive impairment characterized by deficits in executive functioning and abstract reasoning has been described in patients with ATS.[270]

Secondary Periodic Paralysis

Secondary forms of PP and thyrotoxic PP (discussed later) should be considered in the differential diagnosis of HyperPP and HypoPP, especially when there is no family history, or if the first attack of weakness occurs in adulthood. Secondary hyperkalemia as a result of an underlying endocrinopathy such as Addison disease, hyporeninemic hypoaldosteronism, treatment with potassium supplements or potassium-sparing diuretics, and chronic renal failure may cause generalized weakness. In these instances, serum potassium levels typically are greater than 7 mEq/L. Clinical or electrical myotonia is not seen in these patients.[228,271] Secondary causes of hypokalemia include thyrotoxicosis, renal tubular acidosis, Bartter syndrome, hyperaldosteronism, chronic diuretic use, licorice ingestion, corticosteroid use, amphotericin B toxicity, and laxative abuse.

In this context, *thyrotoxic PP* deserves brief mention. The paralysis develops in the setting of hyperthyroidism in genetically predisposed individuals, especially of Asian or Hispanic heritage, although it is increasingly reported in patients from varied racial and ethnic backgrounds. The clinical features of thyrotoxic PP are otherwise similar to those for HypoPP.[228]

Laboratory testing between attacks of PP is typically normal. During an attack, serum potassium is elevated in *HyperPP*. However, the potassium level may be within the normal range or may correct early in the attack, and it is only when the potassium level is rechecked after the weakness improves that a relative increase in potassium during attacks becomes apparent. The name *potassium sensitive periodic paralysis* has been suggested for HyperPP to reflect

Box 17-6 Diagnostic Criteria for Primary Hypokalemic Periodic Paralysis

1. Two or more attacks of muscle weakness with documented serum potassium <3.5 mEq/L
2. One attack of muscle weakness in the proband and one attack of weakness in one relative with documented serum potassium <3.5 mEq/L in at least one attack
3. Three of six clinical or laboratory features as outlined below:
   a. Onset in the first or second decade of life
   b. Duration of attack (muscle weakness involving one or more limbs) >2 hours
   c. Positive triggers (carbohydrate-rich meal, rest after exercise, stress)
   d. Improvement with potassium intake
   e. Positive family history or genetically confirmed skeletal calcium or sodium channel mutation
   f. Positive McManis short exercise test
4. Exclusion of other causes of hypokalemia (renal, adrenal, thyroid dysfunction; renal tubular acidosis; diuretic and laxative abuse)

From Sansone V, Meola G, Links T, et al: Treatment for periodic paralysis, *Cochrane Database Syst Rev* 1, 2008. With permission from Dr. Sansone; Copyright Cochrane Collaboration, reproduced with permission.

the relative, rather than absolute, increase in potassium levels that trigger attacks.[228] ECG is an important ancillary investigation in patients with a suspected episode of PP. Tall T waves are seen in HyperPP.

In *HypoPP*, serum potassium levels are usually low (less than 3 mEq/L) during attacks. During episodes of HypoPP, ECG reveals flattening of T waves, which precedes their disappearance, followed by the appearance of U waves and prolonged PR and QT intervals.

Electrophysiologic testing is not always possible during the acute attacks, but if performed, motor NCS reveal reduced CMAP amplitudes. Needle EMG may reveal spontaneous activity with fibrillations and positive sharp waves during the attack, but when the weakness is complete, the muscle is electrically silent. In between attacks, EMG may reveal myotonia in HyperPP. Some patients with HypoPP may have myopathic features on EMG. Both the short (SET) and long (LET) exercise tests may be abnormal in PP (see Appendix 17-1 for test protocols). In *HyperPP*, the SET reveals an increment in CMAP amplitude. Repeated SET demonstrates a gradual increase in CMAP amplitude. The LET results in an increment in the CMAP amplitude. In *HypoPP*, the SET does not seem to be as useful, whereas the CMAP amplitude decreases during the LET. Table 17-4 summarizes the electrodiagnostic features of the nondystrophic myotonias and PP.

Serum CK is usually elevated in all forms of PP during the episodes of weakness and returns to normal with resolution of weakness. Thyroid function studies and other workup for secondary causes should be performed, especially in cases without family history or with onset of symptoms in adulthood. In ATS, a prolonged QT interval is seen on ECG in about 80% of patients.[228] Muscle biopsy is usually not necessary for diagnosis. If performed, the presence of a vacuolar myopathy or tubular aggregates supports a diagnosis of PP. Genetic testing is commercially available for both HypoPP and HyperPP but may not detect a mutation in all patients.

Provocative Tests

Oral potassium loading may precipitate an attack of weakness in *HyperPP*. After an overnight fast, potassium chloride 0.05 g/kg in a sugar-free solution is given orally over 3 minutes. Muscle strength and serum potassium are monitored every 15 minutes for 2 hours and then every 30 minutes for the next 2 hours. If hyperkalemia (>6.5 mEq/L) is persistently noted for more than 1 hour, intravenous glucose or insulin and glucose may be used to lower potassium.

If weakness develops, it usually resolves over several hours. If the test does not induce weakness, it can be repeated at another sitting with a higher dose of potassium chloride, 0.1 to 0.15 g/kg.[272] Exercise and a high carbohydrate meal the day before the provocative test may be useful in provoking an attack.

In *HypoPP*, episodes of weakness can be precipitated by glucose/insulin loading. After an overnight fast, an oral glucose load of 1.5 g/kg is given over 3 minutes. Muscle strength, serum potassium, and glucose levels are monitored every 30 minutes for 3 hours, then every hour for 2 hours. If weakness develops, 30 to 60 mEq of potassium chloride is given orally every 15 to 30 minutes until the serum potassium level reaches baseline level. If oral potassium is not tolerated because of vomiting, potassium chloride, 35 mEq/L in 5% mannitol, may be used intravenously to reverse the hypokalemia. ECG monitoring and close medical supervision are necessary during the tests, and they should not be performed in patients with cardiac or renal dysfunction. These provocative tests are infrequently performed now because of the potential risks of cardiac arrhythmias and the time-consuming nature of the tests.[272]

Treatment and Management of Periodic Paralysis

The management of PP is three-pronged and consists of avoidance of triggers, use of pharmacologic agents for preventing attacks, and treatment of acute attacks. Dietary measures include avoidance of potassium-rich foods in HyperPP and high carbohydrate meals in HypoPP. Lifestyle modifications include avoidance of triggers such as fasting or strenuous exercise (Table 17-5).

In *HyperPP*, thiazide diuretics (hydrochlorothiazide 25–50 mg daily) are useful in *preventing attacks* and are often chosen as the first line of therapy. The carbonic anhydrase inhibitors are probably the preferred first choice of prophylactic therapy in *HypoPP*. Patients who do not tolerate or respond to them may benefit from potassium-sparing diuretics such as triamterene 25 to 100 mg/day or spironolactone 25 to 100 mg/day.[228] The efficacy of oral potassium supplementation, which is often intuitively used in HypoPP, remains unproved.

The carbonic anhydrase inhibitors acetazolamide and dichlorphenamide are frequently used *prophylactically* for both HyperPP and HypoPP.[272-275] A randomized, double-blind, placebo-controlled cross-over trial of dichlorphenamide found that it was effective in preventing episodes of weakness in both HyperPP and HypoPP.[273] A trial comparing dichlorphenamide with

Table 17-5 Treatment of Periodic Paralysis

Disorder	Prophylactic Therapy	Treatment of Acute Attacks*	Diet and Lifestyle
Hyperkalemic periodic paralysis	Hydrochlorothiazide 25–50 mg/day Acetazolamide up to 1500 mg/day in two or three doses Dichlorphenamide 50–100 mg twice daily	*Early in the attack*: Acetazolamide or hydrochlorothiazide orally or inhaled β-agonist, e.g., albuterol *Mild hyperkalemia*: Oral or intravenous glucose *Severe hyperkalemia*: Intravenous insulin and glucose	Avoid potassium-rich foods Avoid triggers such as fasting or strenuous exercise
Hypokalemic periodic paralysis	Acetazolamide up to 1500 mg/day in two or three doses Dichlorphenamide 50–100 mg twice daily Triamterene 25–100 mg/day Spironolactone 25–100 mg/day Oral potassium supplementation?	*Mild hypokalemia*: Oral potassium 0.25 mEq/kg repeated every 30 min *Severe hypokalemia*: Intravenous potassium chloride 0.05–0.1 mEq/kg or 20–40 mEq in 5% mannitol	Avoid high-carbohydrate meals Avoid triggers such as fasting or strenuous exercise

*Cardiac monitoring is recommended in both forms of periodic paralysis during acute attacks.

acetazolamide versus placebo is ongoing. Some patients with HypoPP may experience worsening of symptoms with acetazolamide.[276] Dalakas and colleagues reported improvement in interepisode muscle weakness after treatment with dichlorphenamide in three patients who were resistant to or worsened by acetazolamide, but the optimal treatment of myopathy associated with PP is unknown.[277] Acetazolamide is usually started at 125 mg daily and increased in 125-mg increments to a maximum dose of 1500 mg daily in two or three divided doses. The dose of dichlorphenamide is 50 to 100 mg twice daily. Adverse effects associated with carbonic anhydrase inhibitors include perverted taste, perioral and extremity paresthesias, nausea, anorexia, and kidney stones.

Treatment and Management of Acute Attacks

Acute attacks of HyperPP may be aborted by a single dose of acetazolamide, a thiazide diuretic, or an inhaled beta-adrenergic agonist such as albuterol if used early.[278,279] Mild hyperkalemia is managed with oral carbohydrates or intravenous glucose. In more severe hyperkalemia, intravenous insulin with glucose may be needed.[272] Acute attacks of HypoPP are managed with oral potassium supplementation (0.25 mEq/kg) repeated every 30 minutes until strength improves. In severe cases, intravenous potassium chloride (0.05–0.1 mEq/kg or 20–40 mEq in 5% mannitol) may be used. For both types of PP, cardiac monitoring is essential.[272]

Treatment and Management of Andersen-Tawil Syndrome

In ATS, carbonic anhydrase inhibitors may be useful in preventing acute episodes of weakness. Since attacks may be hypo- or hyperkalemic, it is useful to define the potassium level during the attack in individual patients to manage both the cardiac conduction abnormalites and weakness effectively. The recognition and management of ventricular arrhythmias are important. There are not many studies of optimal management of arrhythmias in ATS, but it has been suggested that conventional antiarrhythmics may not be effective. Amiodarone and imipramine have been noted to be useful in anecdotal reports. Recently, flecainide has been shown to be useful in the treatment of ventricular arrhythmias and tachycardia-induced cardiomyopathy. Cardioverter-defibrillator implantation may be necessary.[230,262,278,280–284]

Thyrotoxic PP, unlike familial PP, may not respond to carbonic anhydrase inhibitors. Beta blockers may be useful in reducing the frequency and severity of attacks. Treatment of thyrotoxicosis abolishes the attacks, which may recur if the hyperthyroid state recurs.[228]

Brody Disease

In 1969, Brody described a disorder characterized by increasing impairment of relaxation during exercise.[285] In 1986, Karpati et al characterized the disorder in four patients from two families. These patients experienced exercise-induced stiffness and cramping in the limbs, first appearing in childhood. Exercise such as deep knee bends or opening and closing the hand resulted in progressive stiffening of the exercised muscles with difficulty in relaxing them. Sarcoplasmic calcium adenosine triphosphatase (SR Ca^{2+} ATPase) was reduced in type 2 muscle fibers in these patients, thus impairing ATP-dependent calcium transport. Progressive impairment of muscle relaxation occurs during exercise, owing to accumulation of myofibrillar calcium. Since type 2 fast-twitch muscle fibers appear to be selectively involved in this disorder, symptoms occur during phasic exercise. During the delayed relaxation after exercise, the muscle is electrically silent, thus differentiating this condition from the

myotonic disorders. The differential diagnosis includes metabolic myopathies such as McArdle disease that are associated with exercise-induced contractures that are electrically silent. However, the delayed relaxation in Brody disease is much shorter in duration and painless.[286] A mutation in the *ATP2A1* gene on chromosome 16p that encodes the fast-twitch isoform of SR Ca^{2+} ATPase has been identified in this disorder.[287] Treatment is unknown. Dantrolene and nifedipine were not useful in one case.[286]

Metabolic Myopathies

Several metabolic myopathies present clinically with muscle cramps, exercise-induced muscle contractures and myoglobinuria (see Box 17-1). These disorders are discussed elsewhere.

References

1. Ahmed SN, Bertorini TE, Narayanaswami P, et al: Clinical approach to a patient presenting with muscle stiffness, *J Clin Neuromuscul Dis* 4:150–160, 2003.
2. Moersch FP, Woltman HW: Progressive fluctuating muscular rigidity and spasm ("stiff-man" syndrome); report of a case and some observations in 13 other cases, *Proc Staff Meet Mayo Clin* 31:421–427, 1956.
3. Barker RA, Revesz T, Thom M, et al: Review of 23 patients affected by the stiff man syndrome: clinical subdivision into stiff trunk (man) syndrome, stiff limb syndrome, and progressive encephalomyelitis with rigidity, *J Neurol Neurosurg Psychiatry* 65:633–640, 1998.
4. Solimena M, Folli F, Denis-Donini S, et al: Autoantibodies to glutamic acid decarboxylase in a patient with stiff-man syndrome, epilepsy, and type I diabetes mellitus, *N Engl J Med* 318:1012–1020, 1988.
5. Dalakas MC, Fujii M, Li M, et al: The clinical spectrum of anti-GAD antibody-positive patients with stiff-person syndrome, *Neurology* 55:1531–1535, 2000.
6. Asher R: A woman with the stiff-man syndrome, *Br Med J* 1:265–266, 1958.
7. Cohen L: Stiff-man syndrome. Two patients treated with diazepam, *JAMA* 195:222–224, 1966.
8. O'Connor DDJ: Stiff man syndrome, *Br Med J* 1:645, 1958.
9. Gordon EE, Januszko DM, Kaufman L: A critical survey of stiff-man syndrome, *Am J Med* 42:582–599, 1967.
10. Rosin L, DeCamilli P, Butler M, et al: Stiff-man syndrome in a woman with breast cancer: an uncommon central nervous system paraneoplastic syndrome, *Neurology* 50:94–98, 1998.
11. Levy LM, Dalakas MC, Floeter MK: The stiff-person syndrome: an autoimmune disorder affecting neurotransmission of gamma-aminobutyric acid, *Ann Intern Med* 131:522–530, 1999.
12. Cuturic M, Harden LM, Kannaday MH, et al: Stiff-person syndrome presenting as eating disorder: a case report, *Int J Eat Disord*, Feb 22, 2010 [Epub ahead of print].
13. Meinck HM, Thompson PD: Stiff man syndrome and related conditions, *Mov Disord* 17:853–866, 2002.
14. Petzold GC, Marcucci M, Butler MH, et al: Rhabdomyolysis and paraneoplastic stiff-man syndrome with amphiphysin autoimmunity, *Ann Neurol* 55:286–290, 2004.
15. Mitsumoto H, Schwartzman MJ, Estes ML, et al: Sudden death and paroxysmal autonomic dysfunction in stiff-man syndrome, *J Neurol* 238:91–96, 1991.
16. Goetz CG, Klawans HL: On the mechanism of sudden death in Moersch-Woltman syndrome, *Neurology* 33:930–932, 1983.
17. Martinelli P, Montagna P, Pazzaglia P, et al: Electrophysiological findings in a case of stiff man syndrome associated with epilepsy and nocturnal myoclonus, *Riv Neurol* 48:479–491, 1978.
18. Lorish TR, Thorsteinsson G, Howard FM Jr: Stiff-man syndrome updated, *Mayo Clin Proc* 64:629–636, 1989.
19. Raju R, Foote J, Banga JP, et al: Analysis of GAD65 autoantibodies in stiff-person syndrome patients, *J Immunol* 175:7755–7762, 2005.

20. Goeb V, Dubreuil F, Cabre P, et al: Lupus revealing itself after a stiff-person syndrome, *Lupus* 13:215, 2004.
21. Munhoz RP, Fameli H, Teive HA, et al: Stiff person syndrome as the initial manifestation of systemic lupus erythematosus, *Mov Disord* 25: 516–517, 2010.
22. Folli F, Solimena M, Cofiell R, et al: Autoantibodies to a 128-kd synaptic protein in three women with the stiff-man syndrome and breast cancer, *N Engl J Med* 328:546–551, 1993.
23. De Camilli P, Thomas A, Cofiell R, et al: The synaptic vesicle-associated protein amphiphysin is the 128-kD autoantigen of stiff-man syndrome with breast cancer, *J Exp Med* 178:2219–2223, 1993.
24. Espay AJ, Chen R: Rigidity and spasms from autoimmune encephalomyelopathies: stiff-person syndrome, *Muscle Nerve* 34:677–690, 2006.
25. Werbrouck B, Meire V, De Bleecker JL: Multiple neurological syndromes during Hodgkin lymphoma remission, *Acta Neurol Belg* 105: 48–50, 2005.
26. Tanaka H, Matsumura A, Okumura M, et al: Stiff man syndrome with thymoma, *Ann Thorac Surg* 80:739–741, 2005.
27. Ferrari P, Federico M, Grimaldi LM, Silingardi V: Stiff-man syndrome in a patient with Hodgkin's disease. An unusual paraneoplastic syndrome, *Haematologica* 75:570–572, 1990.
28. Dropcho EJ: Antiamphiphysin antibodies with small-cell lung carcinoma and paraneoplastic encephalomyelitis, *Ann Neurol* 39:659–667, 1996.
29. Schmidt C, Freilinger T, Lieb M, et al: Progressive encephalomyelitis with rigidity and myoclonus preceding otherwise asymptomatic Hodgkin's lymphoma, *J Neurol Sci* 291:118–120, 2010.
30. Liu YL, Lo WC, Tseng CH, et al: Reversible stiff person syndrome presenting as an initial symptom in a patient with colon adenocarcinoma, *Acta Oncol* 49:271–272, 2010.
31. Clow EC, Couban S, Grant IA: Stiff-person syndrome associated with multiple myeloma following autologous bone marrow transplantation, *Muscle Nerve* 38:1649–1652, 2008.
32. Brown P, Marsden CD: The stiff man and stiff man plus syndromes, *J Neurol* 246:648–652, 1999.
33. Leigh PN, Rothwell JC, Traub M, et al: A patient with reflex myoclonus and muscle rigidity: "jerking stiff-man syndrome," *J Neurol Neurosurg Psychiatry* 43:1125–1131, 1980.
34. Brown P, Rothwell JC, Marsden CD: The stiff leg syndrome, *J Neurol Neurosurg Psychiatry* 62:31–37, 1997.
35. Gurol ME, Ertas M, Hanagasi HA, et al: Stiff leg syndrome: case report, *Mov Disord* 16:1189–1193, 2001.
36. Silverman IE: Paraneoplastic stiff limb syndrome, *J Neurol Neurosurg Psychiatry* 67:126–127, 1999.
37. Roobol TH, Kazzaz BA, Vecht CJ: Segmental rigidity and spinal myoclonus as a paraneoplastic syndrome, *J Neurol Neurosurg Psychiatry* 50:628–631, 1987.
38. Schmierer K, Valdueza JM, Bender A, et al: Atypical stiff-person syndrome with spinal MRI findings, amphiphysin autoantibodies, and immunosuppression, *Neurology* 51:250–252, 1998.
39. Gouider-Khouja N, Mekaouar A, Larnaout A, et al: Progressive encephalomyelitis with rigidity presenting as a stiff-person syndrome, *Parkinsonism Relat Disord* 8:285–288, 2002.
40. Burn DJ, Ball J, Lees AJ, et al: A case of progressive encephalomyelitis with rigidity and positive antiglutamic acid decarboxylase antibodies [corrected], *J Neurol Neurosurg Psychiatry* 54:449–451, 1991.
41. Meinck HM, Ricker K, Hulser PJ, et al: Stiff man syndrome: clinical and laboratory findings in eight patients, *J Neurol* 241:157–166, 1994.
42. Auger RG: AAEM minimonograph #44: diseases associated with excess motor unit activity, *Muscle Nerve* 17:1250–1263, 1994.
43. Mamoli B, Heiss WD, Maida E, et al: Electrophysiological studies on the "stiff-man" syndrome, *J Neurol* 217:111–121, 1977.
44. Struppler A, Struppler E, Adams RD: Local tetanus in man. Its clinical and neurophysiological characteristics, *Arch Neurol* 8:162–178, 1963.
45. Meinck HM, Ricker K, Conrad B: The stiff-man syndrome: new pathophysiological aspects from abnormal exteroceptive reflexes and the response to clomipramine, clonidine, and tizanidine, *J Neurol Neurosurg Psychiatry* 47:280–287, 1984.

46. Solimena M, De Camilli P: Autoimmunity to glutamic acid decarboxylase (GAD) in stiff-man syndrome and insulin-dependent diabetes mellitus, *Trends Neurosci* 14:452–457, 1991.
47. Solimena M, Folli F, Aparisi R, et al: Autoantibodies to GABA-ergic neurons and pancreatic beta cells in stiff-man syndrome, *N Engl J Med* 322:1555–1560, 1990.
48. Dalakas MC, Li M, Fujii M, et al: Stiff person syndrome: quantification, specificity, and intrathecal synthesis of GAD65 antibodies, *Neurology* 57:780–784, 2001.
49. Warren JD, Scott G, Blumbergs PC, et al: Pathological evidence of encephalomyelitis in the stiff man syndrome with anti-GAD antibodies, *J Clin Neurosci* 9:328–329, 2002.
50. Saiz A, Graus F, Valldeoriola F, et al: Stiff-leg syndrome: a focal form of stiff-man syndrome, *Ann Neurol* 43:400–403, 1998.
51. Rakocevic G, Raju R, Dalakas MC: Anti-glutamic acid decarboxylase antibodies in the serum and cerebrospinal fluid of patients with stiff-person syndrome: correlation with clinical severity, *Arch Neurol* 61: 902–904, 2004.
52. Murinson BB, Guarnaccia JB: Stiff-person syndrome with amphiphysin antibodies: distinctive features of a rare disease, *Neurology* 71:1955–1958, 2008.
53. McCabe DJ, Turner NC, Chao D, et al: Paraneoplastic "stiff person syndrome" with metastatic adenocarcinoma and anti-Ri antibodies, *Neurology* 62:1402–1404, 2004.
54. Butler MH, Hayashi A, Ohkoshi N, et al: Autoimmunity to gephyrin in stiff-man syndrome, *Neuron* 26:307–312, 2000.
55. Hutchinson M, Waters P, McHugh J, et al: Progressive encephalomyelitis, rigidity, and myoclonus: a novel glycine receptor antibody, *Neurology* 71:1291–1292, 2008.
56. Hagiwara H, Enomoto-Nakatani S, Sakai K, et al: Stiff-person syndrome associated with invasive thymoma: a case report, *J Neurol Sci* 193:59–62, 2001.
57. Schiff D, Dalmau J, Myers DJ: Anti-GAD antibody positive stiff-limb syndrome in multiple myeloma, *J Neurol Oncol* 65:173–175, 2003.
58. Lourie H: Spontaneous activity of alpha motor neurons in intramedullary spinal cord tumor, *J Neurosurg* 29:573–580, 1968.
59. Rushworth G, Lishman WA, Hughes JT, et al: Intense rigidity of the arms due to isolation of motoneurones by a spinal tumour, *J Neurol Neurosurg Psychiatry* 24:132–142, 1961.
60. Tarlov IM: Rigidity in man due to spinal interneuron loss, *Arch Neurol* 16:536–543, 1967.
61. Penry JK, Hoefnagel D, Van den Noort S, et al: Muscle spasm and abnormal postures resulting from damage to interneurones in spinal cord, *Arch Neurol* 3:500–512, 1960.
62. Davis SM, Murray NM, Diengdoh JV, et al: Stimulus-sensitive spinal myoclonus, *J Neurol Neurosurg Psychiatry* 44:884–888, 1981.
63. Kuhn WF, Light PJ, Kuhn SC: Stiff-man syndrome: case report, *Acad Emerg Med* 2:735–738, 1995.
64. Spehlmann R, Norcross K, Rasmus SC, et al: Improvement of stiff-man syndrome with sodium valproate, *Neurology* 31:1162–1163, 1981.
65. Ruegg SJ, Steck AJ, Fuhr P: Levetiracetam improves paroxysmal symptoms in a patient with stiff-person syndrome, *Neurology* 62:338, 2004.
66. Vermeij FH, van Doorn PA, Busch HF: Improvement of stiff-man syndrome with vigabatrin, *Lancet* 348:612, 1996.
67. Murinson BB, Rizzo M: Improvement of stiff-person syndrome with tiagabine, *Neurology* 57:366, 2001.
68. Vasconcelos OM, Dalakas MC: Stiff-person syndrome, *Curr Treat Options Neurol* 5:79–90, 2003.
69. Miller F, Korsvik H: Baclofen in the treatment of stiff-man syndrome, *Ann Neurol* 9:511–512, 1981.
70. Sechi G, Barrocu M, Piluzza MG, et al: Levetiracetam in stiff-person syndrome, *J Neurol* 255:1721–1725, 2008.
71. Penn RD, Mangieri EA: Stiff-man syndrome treated with intrathecal baclofen, *Neurology* 43:2412, 1993.
72. Piovano C, Piattelli M, Spina T, et al: The stiff-person syndrome. Case report, *Minerva Anestesiol* 68:861–865, 2002.
73. Silbert PL, Matsumoto JY, McManis PG, et al: Intrathecal baclofen therapy in stiff-man syndrome: a double-blind, placebo-controlled trial, *Neurology* 45:1893–1897, 1995.

74. Hattan E, Angle MR, Chalk C: Unexpected benefit of propofol in stiff-person syndrome, *Neurology* 70:1641–1642, 2008.

75. Davis D, Jabbari B: Significant improvement of stiff-person syndrome after paraspinal injection of botulinum toxin A, *Mov Disord* 8:371–373, 1993.

76. Liguori R, Cordivari C, Lugaresi E, et al: Botulinum toxin A improves muscle spasms and rigidity in stiff-person syndrome, *Mov Disord* 12:1060–1063, 1997.

77. Meinck HM, Conrad B: Neuropharmacological investigations in the stiff-man syndrome, *J Neurol* 233:340–347, 1986.

78. Murinson BB, Vincent A: Stiff-person syndrome: autoimmunity and the central nervous system, *CNS Spectr* 6:427–433, 2001.

79. Harding AE, Thompson PD, Kocen RS, et al: Plasma exchange and immunosuppression in the stiff man syndrome, *Lancet* 2:915, 1989.

80. Piccolo G, Cosi V, Zandrini C, et al: Steroid-responsive and dependent stiff-man syndrome: a clinical and electrophysiological study of two cases, *Ital J Neurol Sci* 9:559–566, 1988.

81. McEvoy KM: Stiff-man syndrome, *Mayo Clin Proc* 66:300–304, 1991.

82. Blum P, Jankovic J: Stiff-person syndrome: an autoimmune disease, *Mov Disord* 6:12–20, 1991.

83. Hayashi A, Nakamagoe K, Ohkoshi N, et al: Double filtration plasma exchange and immunoadsorption therapy in a case of stiff-man syndrome with negative anti-GAD antibody, *J Med* 30:321–327, 1999.

84. Hao W, Davis C, Hirsch IB, et al: Plasmapheresis and immunosuppression in stiff-man syndrome with type 1 diabetes: a 2-year study, *J Neurol* 246:731–735, 1999.

85. Fogan L: Progressive encephalomyelitis with rigidity responsive to plasmapheresis and immunosuppression, *Ann Neurol* 40:451–453, 1996.

86. Brashear HR, Phillips LH 2nd: Autoantibodies to GABAergic neurons and response to plasmapheresis in stiff-man syndrome, *Neurology* 41:1588–1592, 1991.

87. Vicari AM, Folli F, Pozza G, et al: Plasmapheresis in the treatment of stiff-man syndrome, *N Engl J Med* 320:1499, 1989.

88. Shariatmadar S, Noto TA: Plasma exchange in stiff-man syndrome, *Ther Apher* 5:64–67, 2001.

89. Nakamagoe K, Ohkoshi N, Hayashi A, et al: Marked clinical improvement by plasmapheresis in a patient with stiff-man syndrome: a case with a negative anti-GAD antibody, *Rinsho Shinkeigaku* 35:897–900, 1995.

90. Dalakas MC, Fujii M, Li M, et al: High-dose intravenous immune globulin for stiff-person syndrome, *N Engl J Med* 345:1870–1876, 2001.

91. Baker MR, Das M, Isaacs J, et al: Treatment of stiff person syndrome with rituximab, *J Neurol Neurosurg Psychiatry* 76:999–1001, 2005.

92. Katoh N, Matsuda M, Ishii W, et al: Successful treatment with rituximab in a patient with stiff-person syndrome complicated by dysthyroid ophthalmopathy, *Intern Med* 49:237–241, 2010.

93. Dupond JL, Essalmi L, Gil H, et al: Rituximab treatment of stiff-person syndrome in a patient with thymoma, diabetes mellitus and autoimmune thyroiditis, *J Clin Neurosci* 17:389–391, 2010.

94. David C, Solimena M, De Camilli P: Autoimmunity in stiff-man syndrome with breast cancer is targeted to the C-terminal region of human amphiphysin, a protein similar to the yeast proteins, Rvs167 and Rvs161, *FEBS Lett* 351:73–79, 1994.

95. Curtis DR, De Groat WC: Tetanus toxin and spinal inhibition, *Brain Res* 10:208–212, 1968.

96. Bleck TP: Pharmacology of tetanus, *Clin Neuropharmacol* 9:103–120, 1986.

97. Bleck TP: Tetanus: pathophysiology, management, and prophylaxis, *Dis Mon* 37:545–603, 1991.

98. Cook TM, Protheroe RT, Handel JM: Tetanus: a review of the literature, *Br J Anaesth* 87:477–487, 2001.

99. Edmondson RS, Flowers MW: Intensive care in tetanus: management, complications, and mortality in 100 cases, *Br Med J* 1:1401–1404, 1979.

100. Weinstein L: Tetanus, *N Engl J Med* 289:1293–1296, 1973.

101. Patel JC, Mehta BC: Tetanus: study of 8,697 cases, *Indian J Med Sci* 53:393–401, 1999.

102. Farrar JJ, Yen LM, Cook T, et al: Tetanus, *J Neurol Neurosurg Psychiatry* 69:292–301, 2000.

103. Rhee P, Nunley MK, Demetriades D, et al: Tetanus and trauma: a review and recommendations, *J Trauma* 58:1082–1088, 2005.

104. Kokal KC, Dastur FD, Mahashur AA, et al: Disordered pulmonary function in tetanus, *J Assoc Physicians India* 32:691–695, 1984.

105. Trujillo MH, Castillo A, Espana J, Manzo A, Zerpa R: Impact of intensive care management on the prognosis of tetanus. Analysis of 641 cases, *Chest* 92:63–65, 1987.

106. Dutta TK, Padmanabhan S, Hamide A, et al: Localised tetanus mimicking incomplete transverse myelitis, *Lancet* 343:983–984, 1994.

107. Jagoda A, Riggio S, Burguieres T: Cephalic tetanus: a case report and review of the literature, *Am J Emerg Med* 6:128–130, 1988.

108. Roper MH, Vandelaer JH, Gasse FL: Maternal and neonatal tetanus, *Lancet* 370:1947–1959, 2007.

109. Risk WS, Bosch EP, Kimura J, et al: Chronic tetanus: clinical report and histochemistry of muscle, *Muscle Nerve* 4:363–366, 1981.

110. Wakasaya Y, Watanabe M, Tomiyama M, et al: An unusual case of chronic relapsing tetanus associated with mandibular osteomyelitis, *Intern Med* 48:1311–1313, 2009.

111. Crone NE, Reder AT: Severe tetanus in immunized patients with high anti-tetanus titers, *Neurology* 42:761–764, 1992.

112. Rich J, Sabin T, Cros D: Focal tetanus, *Muscle Nerve* 1177, 1992.

113. Garcia-Mullin R, Daroff RB: Electrophysiological investigations of cephalic tetanus, *J Neurol Neurosurg Psychiatry* 36:296–301, 1973.

114. Walker AE, Johnson HC: Principles and practice of penicillin therapy in diseases of the nervous system, *Ann Surg* 122:1125–1135, 1945.

115. Ahmadsyah I, Salim A: Treatment of tetanus: an open study to compare the efficacy of procaine penicillin and metronidazole, *Br Med J (Clin Res Ed)* 291:648–650, 1985.

116. Yen LM, Dao LM, Day NPJ: Management of tetanus: a comparison of penicillin and metronidazole. In *Symposium of Antimicrobial Resistance in Southern Vietnam*, 1997.

117. Chambers HF, Sande MA: Antimicrobial agents. In Hardman JG, Limbird LE, editors: *The Pharmacological Basis of Therapeutics*, New York, 1996, McGraw-Hill Health Professions, pp 1029–1225.

118. Alfery DD, Rauscher LA: Tetanus: a review, *Crit Care Med* 7:176–181, 1979.

119. Miranda-Filho D de B, Ximenes RA, Barone AA, et al: Randomised controlled trial of tetanus treatment with antitetanus immunoglobulin by the intrathecal or intramuscular route, *BMJ* 328:615, 2004.

120. Orko R, Rosenberg PH, Himberg JJ: Intravenous infusion of midazolam, propofol and vecuronium in a patient with severe tetanus, *Acta Anaesthesiol Scand* 32:590–592, 1988.

121. Gyasi HK, Fahr J, Kurian E, et al: Midazolam for prolonged intravenous sedation in patients with tetanus, *Middle East J Anesthesiol* 12:135–141, 1993.

122. Borgeat A, Popovic V, Schwander D: Efficiency of a continuous infusion of propofol in a patient with tetanus, *Crit Care Med* 19:295–297, 1991.

123. Jenkins MT, Luhn NR: Active management of tetanus based on experiences of an anesthesiology department, *Anesthesiology* 23:690–709, 1962.

124. Prys-Roberts C, Corbett JL, Kerr JH, et al: Treatment of sympathetic over-activity in tetanus, *Lancet* 1:542–545, 1969.

125. Rie MA, Wilson RS: Morphine therapy controls autonomic hyperactivity in tetanus, *Ann Intern Med* 88:653–654, 1978.

126. Obanor O, Osazuwa HO, Amadasun JE: Ketamine in the management of generalised cephalic tetanus, *J Laryngol Otol* 122:1389–1391, 2008.

127. Buchanan N, Cane RD, Wolfson G, et al: Autonomic dysfunction in tetanus: the effects of a variety of therapeutic agents, with special refernce to morphine, *Intensive Care Med* 5:65–68, 1979.

128. Fassoulaki A, Eforakopoulou M: Vecuronium in the management of tetanus. Is it the muscle relaxant of choice? *Acta Anaesthesiol Belg* 39:75–78, 1988.

129. Tidyman M, Prichard JG, Deamer RL, et al: Adjunctive use of dantrolene in severe tetanus, *Anesth Analg* 64:538–540, 1985.

130. Saissy JM, Demaziere J, Vitris M, et al: Treatment of severe tetanus by intrathecal injections of baclofen without artificial ventilation, *Intensive Care Med* 18:241–244, 1992.

131. Engrand N, Guerot E, Rouamba A, et al: The efficacy of intrathecal baclofen in severe tetanus, *Anesthesiology* 90:1773–1776, 1999.

132. Santos ML, Mota-Miranda A, Alves-Pereira A, et al: Intrathecal baclofen for the treatment of tetanus, *Clin Infect Dis* 38:321–328, 2004.

133. Rocke DA, Wesley AG, Pather M, et al: Morphine in tetanus—the management of sympathetic nervous system overactivity, *S Afr Med J* 70:666–668, 1986.

134. Buchanan N, Smit L, Cane RD, et al: Sympathetic overactivity in tetanus: fatality associated with propranolol, *Br Med J* 2:254–255, 1978.

135. Wesley AG, Hariparsad D, Pather M, Rocke DA: Labetalol in tetanus. The treatment of sympathetic nervous system overactivity, *Anaesthesia* 38:243–249, 1983.

136. King WW, Cave DR: Use of esmolol to control autonomic instability of tetanus, *Am J Med* 91:425–428, 1991.

137. Dolar D: The use of continuous atropine infusion in the management of severe tetanus, *Intensive Care Med* 18:26–31, 1992.

138. Gregorakos L, Kerezoudi E, Dimopoulos G, et al: Management of blood pressure instability in severe tetanus: the use of clonidine, *Intensive Care Med* 23:893–895, 1997.

139. Southorn PA, Blaise GA: Treatment of tetanus-induced autonomic nervous system dysfunction with continuous epidural blockade, *Crit Care Med* 14:251–252, 1986.

140. Shibuya M, Sugimoto H, Sugimoto T, et al: The use of continuous spinal anesthesia in severe tetanus with autonomic disturbance, *J Trauma* 29:1423–1429, 1989.

141. James MF, Manson ED: The use of magnesium sulphate infusions in the management of very severe tetanus, *Intensive Care Med* 11:5–12, 1985.

142. Attygalle D, Rodrigo N: Magnesium as first line therapy in the management of tetanus: a prospective study of 40 patients, *Anaesthesia* 57:811–817, 2002.

143. Thwaites CL, Yen LM, Loan HT, et al: Magnesium sulphate for treatment of severe tetanus: a randomised controlled trial, *Lancet* 368:1436–1443, 2006.

144. Mathew PJ, Samra T, Wig J, et al: Magnesium sulphate for treatment of tetanus in adults, *Anaesth Intensive Care* 38:185–189, 2010.

145. Paydas S, Akoglu TF, Akkiz H, et al: Mortality-lowering effect of systemic corticosteroid therapy in severe tetanus, *Clin Ther* 10:276–280, 1988.

146. Isaacs H: A syndrome of continuous muscle-fiber activity, *J Neurol Neurosurg Psychiatry* 24:319–325, 1961.

147. Eunson LH, Rea R, Zuberi SM, et al: Clinical, genetic, and expression studies of mutations in the potassium channel gene *KCNA1* reveal new phenotypic variability, *Ann Neurol* 48:647–656, 2000.

148. Dedek K, Kunath B, Kananura C, et al: Myokymia and neonatal epilepsy caused by a mutation in the voltage sensor of the *KCNQ2* K+ channel, *Proc Natl Acad Sci U S A* 98:12272–12277, 2001.

149. Kinali M, Jungbluth H, Eunson LH, et al: Expanding the phenotype of potassium channelopathy: severe neuromyotonia and skeletal deformities without prominent episodic ataxia, *Neuromusc Disord* 14:689–693, 2004.

150. Wuttke TV, Jurkat-Rott K, Paulus W, et al: Peripheral nerve hyperexcitability due to dominant-negative *KCNQ2* mutations, *Neurology* 69:2045–2053, 2007.

151. Falace A, Striano P, Manganelli F, et al: Inherited neuromyotonia: a clinical and genetic study of a family, *Neuromusc Disord* 17:23–27, 2007.

152. Caress JB, Abend WK, Preston DC, et al: A case of Hodgkin's lymphoma producing neuromyotonia, *Neurology* 49:258–259, 1997.

153. Vasilescu C, Alexianu M, Dan A: Neuronal type of Charcot-Marie-Tooth disease with a syndrome of continuous motor unit activity, *J Neurol Sci* 63:11–25, 1984.

154. Partanen VS, Soininen H, Saksa M, et al: Electromyographic and nerve conduction findings in a patient with neuromyotonia, normocalcemic tetany and small-cell lung cancer, *Acta Neurol Scand* 61:216–226, 1980.

155. Newsom-Davis J, Mills KR: Immunological associations of acquired neuromyotonia (Isaacs' syndrome). Report of five cases and literature review, *Brain* 116(Pt 2):453–469, 1993.

156. Odabasi Z, Joy JL, Claussen GC, et al: Isaacs' syndrome associated with chronic inflammatory demyelinating polyneuropathy, *Muscle Nerve* 19:210–215, 1996.

157. Hahn AF, Parkes AW, Bolton CF, et al: Neuromyotonia in hereditary motor neuropathy, *J Neurol Neurosurg Psychiatry* 54:230–235, 1991.

158. Vernino S, Lennon VA: Ion channel and striational antibodies define a continuum of autoimmune neuromuscular hyperexcitability, *Muscle Nerve* 26:702–707, 2002.

159. Reeback J, Benton S, Swash M, et al: Penicillamine-induced neuromyotonia, *Br Med J* 1:1464–1465, 1979.

160. Gil R, Lefevre JP, Neau JP, et al: Morvan's fibrillary chorea and acrodynic syndrome following mercury treatment, *Rev Neurol (Paris)* 140:728–733, 1984.

161. Mitsumoto H, Wilbourn AJ, Subramony SH: Generalized myokymia and gold therapy, *Arch Neurol* 39:449–450, 1982.

162. Saadati H, Saif MW: Oxaliplatin-induced hyperexcitability syndrome in a patient with pancreatic cancer, *JOP* 10:459–461, 2009.

163. Garea MJ, Aparicio-Blanco M, Espino P, et al: Syndrome of continuous muscle fiber activity in a human immunodeficiency virus-infected patient, *Neurology* 50:1506–1507, 1998.

164. Zambelis T, Licomanos D, Leonardos A, Potagas C: Neuromyotonia in idiopathic hypoparathyroidism, *Neurol Sci* 30:495–497, 2009.

165. Liguori R, Vincent A, Avoni P, et al: Acquired neuromyotonia after bone marrow transplantation, *Neurology* 54:1390–1391, 2000.

166. Benito-Leon J, Miguelez R, Vincent A, et al: Neuromyotonia in association with systemic sclerosis, *J Neurol* 246:976–977, 1999.

167. Takahashi H, Mori M, Sekiguchi Y, et al: Development of Isaacs' syndrome following complete recovery of voltage-gated potassium channel antibody-associated limbic encephalitis, *J Neurol Sci* 275:185–187, 2008.

168. Shillito P, Molenaar PC, Vincent A, et al: Acquired neuromyotonia: evidence for autoantibodies directed against K+ channels of peripheral nerves, *Ann Neurol* 38:714–722, 1995.

169. Hart IK, Maddison P, Newsom-Davis J, et al: Phenotypic variants of autoimmune peripheral nerve hyperexcitability, *Brain* 125:1887–1895, 2002.

170. Auger RG, Daube JR, Gomez MR, et al: Hereditary form of sustained muscle activity of peripheral nerve origin causing generalized myokymia and muscle stiffness, *Ann Neurol* 15:13–21, 1984.

171. Thomas NH, Heckmatt JZ, Rodillo E, et al: Continuous muscle fibre activity (Isaacs' syndrome) in infancy: a report of two cases, *Neuromusc Disord* 4:147–151, 1994.

172. Maddison P: Neuromyotonia, *Clin Neurophysiol* 117:2118–2127, 2006.

173. Jackson DL, Satya-Murti S, Davis L, et al: Isaacs' syndrome with laryngeal involvement: an unusual presentation of myokymia, *Neurology* 29:1612–1615, 1979.

174. Zisfein J, Sivak M, Aron AM, et al: Isaacs' syndrome with muscle hypertrophy reversed by phenytoin therapy, *Arch Neurol* 40:241–242, 1983.

175. Thompson PD: Stiff people. In Marsden CD, Fahn S, editors: *Movement Disorders*, Oxford, 1994, Butterworth-Heinemann, pp 373–405.

176. Ginsburg G, Forde R, Martyn JA, Eikermann M: Increased sensitivity to a nondepolarizing muscle relaxant in a patient with acquired neuromyotonia, *Muscle Nerve* 40:139–142, 2009.

177. Lee EK, Maselli RA, Ellis WG, et al: Morvan's fibrillary chorea: a paraneoplastic manifestation of thymoma, *J Neurol Neurosurg Psychiatry* 65:857–862, 1998.

178. Liguori R, Vincent A, Clover L, et al: Morvan's syndrome: peripheral and central nervous system and cardiac involvement with antibodies to voltage-gated potassium channels, *Brain* 124:2417–2426, 2001.

179. Barber PA, Anderson NE, Vincent A: Morvan's syndrome associated with voltage-gated K+ channel antibodies, *Neurology* 54:771–772, 2000.

180. Gutmann L, Tellers JG, Vernino S: Persistent facial myokymia associated with K+ channel antibodies, *Neurology* 57:1707–1708, 2001.

181. Tahmoush AJ, Alonso RJ, Tahmoush GP, et al: Cramp-fasciculation syndrome: a treatable hyperexcitable peripheral nerve disorder, *Neurology* 41:1021–1024, 1991.

182. de Carvalho M, Swash M: Cramps, muscle pain, and fasciculations: not always benign? *Neurology* 63:721–723, 2004.

183. Vernino S, Auger RG, Emslie-Smith AM, et al: Myasthenia, thymoma, presynaptic antibodies, and a continuum of neuromuscular hyperexcitability, *Neurology* 53:1233–1239, 1999.

184. Gutmann L: Myokymia and neuromyotonia 2004, *J Neurol* 251:138–142, 2004.

185. Benatar M, Chapman KM, Rutkove SB: Repetitive nerve stimulation for the evaluation of peripheral nerve hyperexcitability, *J Neurol Sci* 221: 47–52, 2004.

186. Harrison TB, Benatar M: Accuracy of repetitive nerve stimulation for diagnosis of the cramp-fasciculation syndrome, *Muscle Nerve* 35:776–780, 2007.

187. Ansell J, Kirby S, Benstead T: A case of Isaacs' syndrome with associated central nervous system findings, *Muscle Nerve* 20:1324–1327, 1997.

188. Vasilescu C, Alexianu M, Dan A: Valproic acid in Isaacs-Mertens syndrome, *Clin Neuropharmacol* 10:215–224, 1987.

189. Wasserstein PH, Shadlen MN, Dorfman LJ: Successful treatment of neuromyotonia with mexiletene, *Neurology* 42:270, 1992.

190. Celebisoy N, Colakoglu Z, Akbaba Y, et al: Continuous muscle fibre activity: a case treated with acetazolamide, *J Neurol Neurosurg Psychiatry* 64:256–258, 1998.

191. Dhand UK: Isaacs' syndrome: clinical and electrophysiological response to gabapentin, *Muscle Nerve* 34:646–650, 2006.

192. Martinelli P, Patuelli A, Minardi C, et al: Neuromyotonia, peripheral neuropathy and myasthenia gravis, *Muscle Nerve* 19:505–510, 1996.

193. Ho WK, Wilson JD: Hypothermia, hyperhidrosis, myokymia and increased urinary excretion of catecholamines associated with a thymoma, *Med J Aust* 158:787–788, 1993.

194. Alessi G, De Reuck J, De Bleecker J, et al: Successful immunoglobulin treatment in a patient with neuromyotonia, *Clin Neurol Neurosurg* 102:173–175, 2000.

195. Ishii A, Hayashi A, Ohkoshi N, et al: Clinical evaluation of plasma exchange and high dose intravenous immunoglobulin in a patient with Isaacs' syndrome, *J Neurol Neurosurg Psychiatry* 57:840–842, 1994.

196. van den Berg JS, van Engelen BG, Boerman RH, et al: Acquired neuromyotonia: superiority of plasma exchange over high-dose intravenous human immunoglobulin, *J Neurol* 246:623–625, 1999.

197. Van Engelen BG, Benders AA, Gabreels FJ, et al: Are muscle cramps in Isaacs' syndrome triggered by human immunoglobulin? *J Neurol Neurosurg Psychiatry* 58:393, 1995.

198. Torbergsen T: A family with dominant hereditary myotonia, muscular hypertrophy, and increased muscular irritability, distinct from myotonia congenita Thomsen, *Acta Neurol Scand* 51:225–232, 1975.

199. Ricker K, Moxley RT, Rohkamm R: Rippling muscle disease, *Arch Neurol* 46:405–408, 1989.

200. Torbergsen T: Rippling muscle disease: a review, *Muscle Nerve* (Suppl 11): S103–S107, 2002.

201. Van den Bergh PY, Gerard JM, Elosegi JA, et al: Novel missense mutation in the caveolin-3 gene in a Belgian family with rippling muscle disease, *J Neurol Neurosurg Psychiatry* 75:1349–1351, 2004.

202. Koul RL, Chand RP, Chacko A, et al: Severe autosomal recessive rippling muscle disease, *Muscle Nerve* 24:1542–1547, 2001.

203. Vorgerd M, Ricker K, Ziemssen F, et al: A sporadic case of rippling muscle disease caused by a de novo caveolin-3 mutation, *Neurology* 57:2273–2277, 2001.

204. Ansevin CF, Agamanolis DP: Rippling muscles and myasthenia gravis with rippling muscles, *Arch Neurol* 53:197–199, 1996.

205. Muller-Felber W, Ansevin CF, Ricker K, et al: Immunosuppressive treatment of rippling muscles in patients with myasthenia gravis, *Neuromusc Disord* 9:604–607, 1999.

206. Greenberg SA: Acquired rippling muscle disease with myasthenia gravis, *Muscle Nerve* 29:143–146, 2004.

207. Takagi A, Kojima S, Watanabe T, et al: Rippling muscle syndrome preceding malignant lymphoma, *Intern Med* 41:147–150, 2002.

208. Ashok Muley S, Day JW: Autoimmune rippling muscle, *Neurology* 61:869–870, 2003.

209. Schulte-Mattler WJ, Kley RA, Rothenfusser-Korber E, et al: Immune-mediated rippling muscle disease, *Neurology* 64:364–367, 2005.

210. Baker SK, Tarnopolsky MA: Sporadic rippling muscle disease unmasked by simvastatin, *Muscle Nerve* 34:478–481, 2006.

211. Vorgerd M, Bolz H, Patzold T, et al: Phenotypic variability in rippling muscle disease, *Neurology* 52:1453–1459, 1999.

212. Perez AS, Bertorini TE, Narayanaswami P: A woman with spontaneous focal muscle movements, *J Clin Neuromusc Dis* 8:35–44, 2006.

213. So YT, Zu L, Barraza C, et al: Rippling muscle disease: evidence for phenotypic and genetic heterogeneity, *Muscle Nerve* 24:340–344, 2001.

214. Aboumousa A, Hoogendijk J, Charlton R, et al: Caveolinopathy—new mutations and additional symptoms, *Neuromusc Disord* 18:572–578, 2008.

215. Stephan DA, Buist NR, Chittenden AB, et al: A rippling muscle disease gene is localized to 1q41: evidence for multiple genes, *Neurology* 44: 1915–1920, 1994.

216. Betz RC, Schoser BG, Kasper D, et al: Mutations in *CAV3* cause mechanical hyperirritability of skeletal muscle in rippling muscle disease, *Nat Genet* 28:218–219, 2001.

217. Traverso M, Bruno C, Broccolini A, et al: Truncation of caveolin-3 causes autosomal-recessive rippling muscle disease, *J Neurol Neurosurg Psychiatry* 79:735–737, 2008.

218. Kubisch C, Ketelsen UP, Goebel I, et al: Autosomal recessive rippling muscle disease with homozygous *CAV3* mutations, *Ann Neurol* 57:303–304, 2005.

219. Fischer D, Schroers A, Blumcke I, et al: Consequences of a novel caveolin-3 mutation in a large German family, *Ann Neurol* 53:233–241, 2003.

220. Woodman SE, Sotgia F, Galbiati F, et al: Caveolinopathies: mutations in caveolin-3 cause four distinct autosomal dominant muscle diseases, *Neurology* 62:538–543, 2004.

221. Yabe I, Kawashima A, Kikuchi S, et al: Caveolin-3 gene mutation in Japanese with rippling muscle disease, *Acta Neurol Scand* 108:47–51, 2003.

222. Cagliani R, Bresolin N, Prelle A, et al: A *CAV3* microdeletion differentially affects skeletal muscle and myocardium, *Neurology* 61:1513–1519, 2003.

223. Sadeh M, Berg M, Sandbank U: Familial myoedema, muscular hypertrophy and stiffness, *Acta Neurol Scand* 81:201–204, 1990.

224. Mion CC, Tsanaclis AM, Lusvarghi E, et al: [Increased muscular irritability syndrome: treatment with nifedipine. Report of a case], *Arq Neuropsiquiatr* 42:72–76, 1984.

225. Madrid RE, Kubisch C, Hays AP: Early-onset toe walking in rippling muscle disease due to a new caveolin-3 gene mutation, *Neurology* 65: 1301–1303, 2005.

226. Kullmann DM, Hanna MG: Neurological disorders caused by inherited ion-channel mutations, *Lancet Neurol* 1:157–166, 2002.

227. Jurkat-Rott K, Lehmann-Horn F: Human muscle voltage-gated ion channels and hereditary disease, *Curr Opin Pharmacol* 1:280–287, 2001.

228. Saperstein DS: Muscle channelopathies, *Semin Neurol* 28:260–269, 2008.

229. Ryan AM, Matthews E, Hanna MG: Skeletal-muscle channelopathies: periodic paralysis and nondystrophic myotonias, *Curr Opin Neurol* 20:558–563, 2007.

230. Davies NP, Hanna MG: The skeletal muscle channelopathies: basic science, clinical genetics and treatment, *Curr Opin Neurol* 14:539–551, 2001.

231. Heine R, Pika U, Lehmann-Horn F: A novel *SCN4A* mutation causing myotonia aggravated by cold and potassium, *Hum Mol Genet* 2: 1349–1353, 1993.

232. Lennox G, Purves A, Marsden D: Myotonia fluctuans, *Arch Neurol* 49:1010–1011, 1992.

233. Rudel R, Lehmann-Horn F: Paramyotonia, potassium-aggravated myotonias and periodic paralyses. 37th ENMC International Workshop, Naarden, The Netherlands, 8–10, Dec. 1995, *Neuromusc Disord* 7: 127–132, 1997.

234. Trudell RG, Kaiser KK, Griggs RC: Acetazolamide-responsive myotonia congenita, *Neurology* 37:488–491, 1987.

235. Al-Gazali LI, Varghese M, Varady E, et al: Neonatal Schwartz-Jampel syndrome: a common autosomal recessive syndrome in the United Arab Emirates, *J Med Genet* 33:203–211, 1996.

236. Cao A, Cianchetti C, Calisti L, de Virgiliis S, Ferreli A, Tangheroni W: Schwartz-Jampel syndrome. Clinical, electrophysiological and histopathological study of a severe variant, *J Neurol Sci* 35:175–187, 1978.

237. Nicole S, Topaloglu H, Fontaine B: 102nd ENMC International Workshop on Schwartz-Jampel syndrome, 14–16, December 2001, Naarden, The Netherlands, *Neuromusc Disord* 13:347–351, 2003.

238. Pascuzzi RM, Gratianne R, Azzarelli B, et al: Schwartz-Jampel syndrome with dominant inheritance, *Muscle Nerve* 13:1152–1163, 1990.

239. Nicole S, Ben Hamida C, Beighton P, et al: Localization of the Schwartz-Jampel syndrome (SJS) locus to chromosome 1p34–p36.1 by homozygosity mapping, *Hum Mol Genet* 4:1633–1636, 1995.

240. Nicole S, Davoine CS, Topaloglu H, et al: Perlecan, the major proteoglycan of basement membranes, is altered in patients with Schwartz-Jampel syndrome (chondrodystrophic myotonia), *Nat Genet* 26:480–483, 2000.

241. AAEE glossary of terms in clinical electromyography, *Muscle Nerve* 10:G1–G60, 1987.

242. Fuglsang-Frederiksen A: The role of different EMG methods in evaluating myopathy, *Clin Neurophysiol* 117:1173–1189, 2006.

243. Taylor RG, Layzer RB, Davis HS, et al: Continuous muscle fiber activity in the Schwartz-Jampel syndrome, *Electroencephalogr Clin Neurophysiol* 33:497–509, 1972.

244. Huttenlocher PR, Landwirth J, Hanson V, et al: Osteo-chondro-muscular dystrophy. A disorder manifested by multiple skeletal deformities, myotonia, and dystrophic changes in muscle, *Pediatrics* 44:945–958, 1969.

245. Aberfeld DC, Hinterbuchner LP, Schneider M: Myotonia, dwarfism, diffuse bone disease and unusual ocular and facial abnormalities (a new syndrome), *Brain* 88:313–322, 1965.

246. Aminoff MJ, Layzer RB, Satya-Murti S, et al: The declining electrical response of muscle to repetitive nerve stimulation in myotonia, *Neurology* 27:812–816, 1977.

247. Brown JC: Muscle weakness after rest in myotonic disorders; an electrophysiological study, *J Neurol Neurosurg Psychiatry* 37:1336–1342, 1974.

248. Miller TM: Differential diagnosis of myotonic disorders, *Muscle Nerve* 37:293–299, 2008.

249. Nielsen VK, Friis ML, Johnsen T: Electromyographic distinction between paramyotonia congenita and myotonia congenita: effect of cold, *Neurology* 32:827–832, 1982.

250. Subramony SH, Malhotra CP, Mishra SK: Distinguishing paramyotonia congenita and myotonia congenita by electromyography, *Muscle Nerve* 6:374–379, 1983.

251. Fournier E, Arzel M, Sternberg D, et al: Electromyography guides toward subgroups of mutations in muscle channelopathies, *Ann Neurol* 56:650–661, 2004.

252. Koltzenburg M, Yousry T: Magnetic resonance imaging of skeletal muscle, *Curr Opin Neurol* 20:595–599, 2007.

253. Leyburn P, Walton JN: The treatment of myotonia: a controlled clinical trial, *Brain* 82:81–91, 1959.

254. Ricker K, Haass A, Hertel G, Mertens HG: Transient muscular weakness in severe recessive myotonia congenita. Improvement of isometric muscle force by drugs relieving myotomic stiffness, *J Neurol* 218:253–262, 1978.

255. Rudel R, Dengler R, Ricker K, et al: Improved therapy of myotonia with the lidocaine derivative tocainide, *J Neurol* 222:275–278, 1980.

256. Rosenfeld J, Sloan-Brown K, George AL Jr: A novel muscle sodium channel mutation causes painful congenital myotonia, *Ann Neurol* 42:811–814, 1997.

257. Alfonsi E, Merlo IM, Tonini M, et al: Efficacy of propafenone in paramyotonia congenita, *Neurology* 68:1080–1081, 2007.

258. Kwiecinski H, Ryniewicz B, Ostrzycki A: Treatment of myotonia with antiarrhythmic drugs, *Acta Neurol Scand* 86:371–375, 1992.

259. Griggs RC, Moxley RT 3rd, Riggs JE, Engel WK: Effects of acetazolamide on myotonia, *Ann Neurol* 3:531–537, 1978.

260. Russell SH, Hirsch NP: Anaesthesia and myotonia, *Br J Anaesth* 72:210–216, 1994.

261. Vargel I, Canter HI, Topaloglu H, et al: Results of botulinum toxin: an application to blepharospasm Schwartz-Jampel syndrome, *J Craniofac Surg* 17:656–660, 2006.

262. Tawil R, Ptacek LJ, Pavlakis SG, et al: Andersen's syndrome: potassium-sensitive periodic paralysis, ventricular ectopy, and dysmorphic features, *Ann Neurol* 35:326–330, 1994.

263. Plassart E, Reboul J, Rime CS, et al: Mutations in the muscle sodium channel gene (*SCN4A*) in 13 French families with hyperkalemic periodic paralysis and paramyotonia congenita: phenotype to genotype correlations and demonstration of the predominance of two mutations, *Eur J Hum Genet* 2:110–124, 1994.

264. Jurkat-Rott K, Lehmann-Horn F: Paroxysmal muscle weakness: the familial periodic paralyses, *J Neurol* 253:1391–1398, 2006.

265. Venance SL, Cannon SC, Fialho D, et al: The primary periodic paralyses: diagnosis, pathogenesis and treatment, *Brain* 129:8–17, 2006.

266. Moslehi R, Langlois S, Yam I, et al: Linkage of malignant hyperthermia and hyperkalemic periodic paralysis to the adult skeletal muscle sodium channel (*SCN4A*) gene in a large pedigree, *Am J Med Genet* 76:21–27, 1998.

266a. Matthews E, Labrum R, Sweeney MG, et al: Voltage sensor charge loss accounts for most cases of hypokalemic periodic paralysis, *Neurology* 72:1544–1547, 2009.

267. Plaster NM, Tawil R, Tristani-Firouzi M, et al: Mutations in Kir2.1 cause the developmental and episodic electrical phenotypes of Andersen's syndrome, *Cell* 105:511–519, 2001.

268. Sansone V, Griggs RC, Meola G, et al: Andersen's syndrome: a distinct periodic paralysis, *Ann Neurol* 42:305–312, 1997.

269. Andersen ED, Krasilnikoff PA, Overvad H: Intermittent muscular weakness, extrasystoles, and multiple developmental anomalies. A new syndrome? *Acta Paediatr Scand* 60:559–564, 1971.

270. Yoon G, Quitania L, Kramer JH, et al: Andersen-Tawil syndrome: definition of a neurocognitive phenotype, *Neurology* 66:1703–1710, 2006.

271. Evers S, Engelien A, Karsch V, et al: Secondary hyperkalaemic paralysis, *J Neurol Neurosurg Psychiatry* 64:249–252, 1998.

272. Griggs RC: Periodic paralysis and myotonia. In Griggs RC, Mendell JR, Miller RG, editors: *Evaluation and Treatment of Myopathies*, Philadelphia, 1995, FA Davis, pp 318–354.

273. Tawil R, McDermott MP, Brown R Jr, et al: Working Group on Periodic Paralysis: Randomized trials of dichlorphenamide in the periodic paralyses, *Ann Neurol* 47:46–53, 2000.

274. Resnick JS, Engel WK, Griggs RC, et al: Acetazolamide prophylaxis in hypokalemic periodic paralysis, *N Engl J Med* 278:582–586, 1968.

275. Griggs RC, Engel WK, Resnick JS: Acetazolamide treatment of hypokalemic periodic paralysis. Prevention of attacks and improvement of persistent weakness, *Ann Intern Med* 73:39–48, 1970.

276. Sternberg D, Maisonobe T, Jurkat-Rott K, et al: Hypokalaemic periodic paralysis type 2 caused by mutations at codon 672 in the muscle sodium channel gene *SCN4A*, *Brain* 124:1091–1099, 2001.

277. Dalakas MC, Engel WK: Treatment of "permanent" muscle weakness in familial hypokalemic periodic paralysis, *Muscle Nerve* 6:182–186, 1983.

278. Davies NP, Hanna MG: The skeletal muscle channelopathies: distinct entities and overlapping syndromes, *Curr Opin Neurol* 16:559–568, 2003.

279. Hanna MG, Stewart J, Schapira AH, et al: Salbutamol treatment in a patient with hyperkalaemic periodic paralysis due to a mutation in the skeletal muscle sodium channel gene (*SCN4A*), *J Neurol Neurosurg Psychiatry* 65:248–250, 1998.

280. Chun TU, Epstein MR, Dick M 2nd, et al: Polymorphic ventricular tachycardia and KCNJ2 mutations, *Heart Rhythm* 1:235–241, 2004.

281. Gould RJ, Steeg CN, Eastwood AB, et al: Potentially fatal cardiac dysrhythmia and hyperkalemic periodic paralysis, *Neurology* 35:1208–1212, 1985.

282. Fox DJ, Klein GJ, Hahn A, et al: Reduction of complex ventricular ectopy and improvement in exercise capacity with flecainide therapy in Andersen-Tawil syndrome, *Europace* 10:1006–1008, 2008.

283. Pellizzon OA, Kalaizich L, Ptacek LJ, et al: Flecainide suppresses bidirectional ventricular tachycardia and reverses tachycardia-induced cardiomyopathy in Andersen-Tawil syndrome, *J Cardiovasc Electrophysiol* 19:95–97, 2008.

284. Bokenkamp R, Wilde AA, Schalij MJ, Blom NA: Flecainide for recurrent malignant ventricular arrhythmias in two siblings with Andersen-Tawil syndrome, *Heart Rhythm* 4:508–511, 2007.

285. Brody IA: Muscle contracture induced by exercise. A syndrome attributable to decreased relaxing factor, *N Engl J Med* 281:187–192, 1969.

286. Karpati G, Charuk J, Carpenter S, et al: Myopathy caused by a deficiency of Ca^{2+}-adenosine triphosphatase in sarcoplasmic reticulum (Brody's disease), *Ann Neurol* 20:38–49, 1986.

287. Odermatt A, Taschner PE, Khanna VK, et al: Mutations in the gene-encoding SERCA1, the fast-twitch skeletal muscle sarcoplasmic reticulum Ca^{2+} ATPase, are associated with Brody disease, *Nat Genet* 14:191–194, 1996.

Appendix 17-1. Exercise Tests for Periodic Paralysis

Short Exercise Test (Streib, 1987; Fournier et al, 2004)

1. The hand to be tested is rested for 10 minutes before testing.

2. The hand is immobilized, and CMAPs are recorded over the ADM with surface electrodes and supramaximal stimulation of the ulnar nerve at the wrist.

3. Baseline CMAP is recorded every 60 seconds for 2 minutes.

4. The ADM is maximally contracted by forceful abduction of the fifth digit against resistance for 10 seconds.

5. The CMAP is recorded again immediately after exercise and every 10 seconds until no change in amplitude is observed.

6. The test may be repeated three times with 60 seconds of rest between trials.

7. The percentage change in amplitude is calculated as follows:

Increase = 100 × (greatest amplitude after exercise − amplitude before exercise)/amplitude before exercise

Decrease = 100 × (greatest amplitude after exercise − smallest amplitude after exercise)/greatest amplitude after exercise

The normal limit for amplitude increase is less than 20% and for amplitude decrease is less than 10%.

Long Exercise Test (McManis et al, 1986; Kuntzer et al, 2000)

1. The hand to be tested is rested for 10 minutes before testing.

2. The hand is immobilized, and CMAPs are recorded over the ADM with surface electrodes and supramaximal stimulation of the ulnar nerve at the wrist.

3. Baseline CMAP is recorded every 60 seconds for 2 minutes.

4. The ADM is maximally contracted by forceful abduction of the fifth digit against resistance for 5 minutes with 3- to 5-second rest periods every 30 seconds.

5. The CMAP is recorded every minute post-exercise for 50 minutes or until no change in amplitude is noted for 5 minutes.

6. The percentage change in CMAP amplitude is calculated as for the short exercise test.

Normal limit for amplitude increase is less than 30% and for amplitude decrease is less than 41%.

References

Fournier E, Arzel M, Sternberg D, et al: Electromyography guides toward subgroups of mutations in muscle channelopathies, *Ann Neurol* 56:650–661, 2004.

Kuntzer T, Flocard F, Vial C, Kohler A, et al: Exercise test in muscle channelopathies and other muscle disorders, *Muscle Nerve* 23:1089–1094, 2000.

McManis PG, Lambert EH, Daube JR: The exercise test in periodic paralysis, *Muscle Nerve* 9:704–710, 1986.

Streib EW: AAEE minimonograph #27: Differential diagnosis of myotonic syndromes, *Muscle Nerve* 10:603–605, 1998.

ADM, abductor digiti minimi; CMAP, compound motor action potential.

Shin J. Oh, MD

18

Treatment and Management of Disorders of the Neuromuscular Junction

Disorders of the neuromuscular junction include myasthenia gravis (MG), Lambert-Eaton myasthenic syndrome (LEMS), botulism, congenital myasthenic syndrome (CMG), tick-paralysis, snakebite myasthenia, organophosphate poisoning (OPP), and hypermagnesemia-induced paralysis.

In preparing this chapter, I reviewed all the major existing literature on the management and treatment of these diseases and analyzed critically the data for evidence-based information. The literature includes review articles and large case series from Medline and Cochrane reviews. In accord with the evidence-based data, the studies are categorized into four classes: class I, randomized controlled trials available; class II, controlled trials without randomization, or randomized trials with small patient numbers; class III, uncontrolled trials; and class IV, case series. This classification and the recommendations are based on guidance provided by the European Federation of Neurological Societies (EFNS) scientific task force,[1] which have been modified slightly from the 2002 American Academy of Neurology guidelines.[2]

Principles of the therapeutic guidelines are formulated largely on the best available evidence-based data, and the rating of recommendations is derived from the evidence-based classification: level A (established as effective, ineffective, or harmful) requires at least one convincing class I study or at least two consistent, convincing class II studies; level B (probably effective, ineffective, or harmful) requires at least one convincing class II study or overwhelming class III evidence; and level C (possibly effective, ineffective, or harmful) requires at least two convincing class III studies. The European Task Force adopted a "good practice point" recommendation when there was a uniform consensus among the experts, although there was inadequate evidence for a formal recommendation.[3] Usually this recommendation was based on class IV data. When there was no consensus among the experts, therapeutic guidelines and recommendations were made on the basis of my personal experience or my personal choice for the best possible regimen.

Myasthenia Gravis

Myasthenia gravis (MG) is due to an antibody-induced postsynaptic defect in the neuromuscular junction, producing exertion-induced weakness or easy fatigability and, commonly, oculobulbar palsy. Electron microscopic studies show simplification of the postsynaptic folds at the neuromuscular junction, which is induced by the acetylcholine receptor (AChR) antibody.

MG is the most common disorder of the neuromuscular junction. The prevalence of MG is approximately 5 to 10 per 100,000 population. The disease affects all ages. In the 1970s and 1980s, two peaks were identified in MG: young women and older men. In more recent studies, an upsurge of MG has been noted in older patients, especially men, whereas female predominance was maintained in younger patients.[4]

With the advent and widespread use of immunotherapy, and improvement in respiratory care and intensive care unit (ICU) management during MG crisis over the past 30 years, the prognosis of MG patients has improved vastly. In a Danish population-based study, the overall 3-, 5-, 10-, and 20-year survival rates were 85%, 81%, 69%, and 63%, respectively.[5] Most MG patients can be returned to a full, productive life with adequate therapy.

There is considerable evidence indicating an autoimmune mechanism in the pathogenesis of MG. The strongest evidence is seen in experimental autoimmune myasthenia gravis (EAMG). Within 2 weeks of injection of AChR antigen purified from electric eels, animals develop weakness which is reversed by edrophonium. Their electrophysiologic and pharmacologic responses are identical to those in human MG. The thymus seems to be the major organ initiating AChR antibody formation in MG, which eventually damages the postsynaptic fold.

MG is characterized by a fluctuating weakness of skeletal muscles with remissions and exacerbations. Classically, weakness becomes worse with exertion or exercise, and oculobulbar symptoms are common, being seen in 90% of MG patients. Frequently, such patients complain of droopy eyelids, diplopia, swallowing or speech difficulty, and proximal muscle weakness. In 85% of patients, MG becomes generalized, usually within 3 years. Rarely, respiratory difficulty is the initial symptom. Exertion-induced weakness (myasthenic or fatigable weakness) can be documented on examination by repetitive exercise.

The diagnosis of MG is based on history and clinical findings. It is confirmed by the edrophonium test, the AChR antibody (AChR-Ab) test, the muscle-specific kinase antibody (MuSK-Ab) test, repetitive nerve stimulation (RNS) test, and single-fiber electromyography (SFEMG).

Diagnosis and Evaluation

The diagnosis of MG is easily confirmed by the intravenous edrophonium test, a short-acting acetylcholinesterase inhibitor (AChEI).[6] Dramatic improvement is noted within 1 minute after injection. This test is positive in 95% of MG patients. The edrophonium test is still the most helpful, simple, and rapid test for diagnosis of MG. To perform an adequate edrophonium test, placebo injection and objective measurement of two or three clinical parameters are crucial. Placebo injection has been helpful in sorting out many pseudo-MG patients in whom both the edrophonium test and placebo test were positive. A positive edrophonium test has also been reported in other diseases. Understandably, it is positive in penicillamine-induced MG and in MG unmasked or precipitated by drugs. The edrophonium test was positive in 89% of overlap MG/LEMS patients, in 37% of patients with LEMS, and in 27% of those with botulism. Among the congenital myasthenic syndromes, patients with endplate acetylcholine receptor deficiency and choline acetyltransferase deficiency (familial infantile myasthenia) showed positive results. A false negative edrophonium test may be seen in ocular MG, especially when ophthalmoplegia is severe or when it is too minimal for objective measurement. In such cases, the prostigmine test is often positive. A positive edrophonium test is less common in MuSK-Ab-positive MG than in other forms of MG, being positive in one half of cases. Since 1979, a simple and inexpensive "ice-pack test" (application of ice over one eye for 5 minutes) was found to be positive for ocular MG.[7] This test was evaluated in patients with MG, normal individuals, and a few patients of third nerve palsy, and was positive only for MG in 90% of cases.

The serum AChR antibody has become a more specific test for MG, though it is positive in 70% to 95% (averaging 85%) of cases.[8] False positive responses have rarely been reported in disease. However, the titer is not correlated with disease severity. MuSK-Ab was positive in 20% to 49% of the cases of seronegative generalized MG, with an average rate of 36%.[9] MuSK-Ab is negative in ocular MG. MuSK-Ab should be tested in all AChR-Ab-negative cases.

Other objective diagnostic tests include the RNS test and the SFEMG.[10]

The RNS test is the time-honored test for the neuromuscular transmission (NMT) disorders and offers the advantages of relative simplicity and rapid results. Though certain patterns on the RNS test are indicative of MG, it is less specific than the AChR-Ab assay. The distinct advantages of the RNS test over the AChR-Ab assay are that this test can provide a rapid and objective diagnosis of MG and can be used serially for evaluation of severity of disease. The RNS test is positive in 75% of cases when the distal muscles (usually hand muscles) and proximal muscles (usually facial and trapezius muscles) are tested together. The most common types of RNS abnormalities are those typical of postsynaptic NMT blocks: (1) normal compound muscle action potential (CMAP) amplitude, (2) normal or minimal postexercise fatigue (PEF), (3) decremental response at low-rate stimulation (LRS), (4) normal or decremental response at high-rate stimulation (HRS), and (5) post-tetanic facilitation (PTF) followed by post-tetanic exhaustion (PTE) (Figs. 18-1 and 18-2). Among these, the decremental response at LRS is the most common and characteristic RNS finding in MG. In MuSK-Ab-positive MG (MuSK-MG), RNS test of limb muscle had a relatively low yield (25%–57%), but RNS test of facial muscles showed a decrement in 85% of cases. This is because of the predominant involvement of faciobulbar muscles in MuSK-MG.

SFEMG is the single most sensitive diagnostic test for MG, being positive in 77% to 100% of cases with an average rate of 95%. The test is so sensitive that Stalberg and Trontelj concluded that the diagnosis of MG can be abandoned if abnormal jitter is not present in a weak muscle.[11] The classic SFEMG pattern in MG is characterized by a definite increase in jitter with or without neuromuscular blocking. For obvious reasons, the SFEMG is most useful in "double" seronegative MG cases in which the RNS test was negative. In mild generalized and ocular MG, in which the

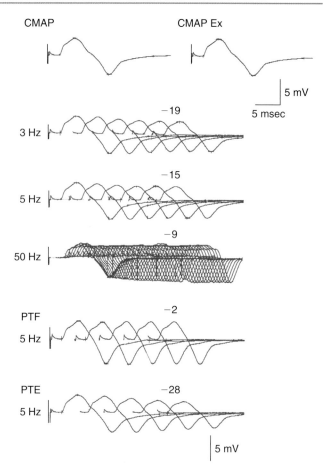

Figure 18-1 Typical repetitive nerve stimulation pattern in the abductor digiti quinti muscle in mild myasthenia gravis. Normal compound muscle action potential (CMAP) amplitude at rest and after exercise (CMAP Ex). Decremental response (−19% at 3 Hz and −15% at 5 Hz) at low-rate stimulation. Normal response at high-rate stimulation (50 Hz). Post-tetanic facilitation (PTF, 5 Hz stimulation immediately after 50 Hz stimulation) and post-tetanic exhaustion (PTE, 5 Hz stimulation 4 minutes after 50 Hz stimulation) are present.

RNS test and AChR-Ab are often normal, this test can be the crucial means of confirming the diagnosis of MG. In none of our MG patients were all three tests found to be negative. Thus, MG can be confidently ruled out if all three tests are negative.

Treatment and Management

In 2006, the EFNS Task Force published consensus guidelines for the treatment of autoimmune neuromuscular transmission disorders.[3] In general, we will follow these consensus guidelines with some modification. There are two main modes of treatment in MG: (1) symptomatic treatment and (2) immunotherapy.

Symptomatic Treatment
Acetylcholinesterase Inhibitors (AChEIs)
The mainstay of symptomatic treatment is AChEIs, which are effective in almost all cases. A poorer response was reported in MuSK-MG: one series showed nonresponsiveness in 71% of 14 patients.[12]

AChEIs inhibit the breakdown of ACh at the neuromuscular junction, increase the availability of ACh to stimulate AChR, and facilitate muscle activation and contraction. AChEIs used in MG bind reversibly to AChE as opposed to organophosphate AChEIs, which bind irreversibly (Table 18-1). These drugs cross the blood-brain barrier poorly and generally remain in the extracellular space.

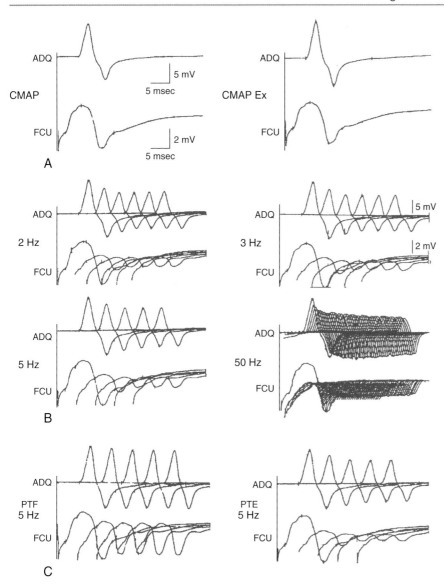

Figure 18-2 Typical repetitive nerve stimulation (RNS) pattern in the abductor digiti quinti (ADQ) and flexor carpi ulnaris (FCU) muscles in severe myasthenia gravis (MG). **A,** Normal compound muscle action potential (CMAP) at rest and after exercise (CMAP Ex). **B,** Decremental response at low-rate stimulation (2, 3, 5 Hz) and at high-rate stimulation (50 Hz). **C,** Post-tetanic facilitation (PTF) and post-tetanic exhaustion (PTE) are also present.

Adverse effects of AChEIs are caused by the increased concentration of ACh at both nicotinic and muscarinic synapses. The common muscarinic effects are gut hypermotility (diarrhea and stomach cramps), increased sweating, salivation, and, when severe, bradycardia. The main nicotinic adverse effects are fasciculation and sometimes muscle cramps. Muscarinic effects are relieved by oral atropine (the usual dose is 0.4 mg two or three times a day), glycopyrrolate (Robinul, usual dose 1 mg or 2 mg two or three times a day), or 5 mg diphenoxylate with atropine (Lomotil), which has no effect on the neuromuscular junction. Glycopyrrolate is better for this purpose because it does not enter the brain and so will not cause blurring of vision or toxic delirium expected with a high dose of atropine. However, it does not dry up secretions as well as atropine. Lomotil can be obtained without a prescription. It is important to tell patients in advance about the possible side effects of AChEIs and to provide relief with glycopyrrolate or atropine so that they will not be alarmed about them. These side effects are the most common reason MG patients provide for not taking AChEIs.

The most serious side effect of AChEIs is cholinergic weakness and crisis, which are due to too much AChEI medication. This can lead to overaccumulation of ACh at the neuromuscular junction, producing sustained endplate depolarization without any time for repolarization (depolarization block). This was a common phenomenon before immunotherapy in MG and was one of the well-known causes of MG crisis. Cholinergic crisis is extremely rare these days because higher doses of AChEIs are no longer used, but it has been observed in MuSK-MG patients at the usual dose of AChEIs for MG.[12]

Although these drugs have been used extensively since 1935, when Walker used prostigmine as the first miracle drug for MG,[13,14] there have been no placebo-controlled randomized studies for these drugs. However, case series demonstrate an objective and marked clinical effect (class IV evidence). Among the various AChEIs, Mestinon (pyridostigmine) is the most commonly used drug because of the 6-hour duration of the drug effect. The starting dose is 60 mg three to four times a day, depending on symptoms, usually given in the daytime. At night pyridostigmine TS is the preferred agent because of its slow-release benefit. Pyridostigmine syrup is used for children or for patients with difficulty swallowing pills. Parenteral use of AChEIs is necessary on rare occasions such as during a postoperative period or during MG crisis. Intravenous pyridostigmine should be given at about one thirtieth of the oral dose. In my practice, I have not used the intramuscular or

Table 18-1 Pharmacologic Properties of Acetylcholinesterase Inhibitors (AChEIs)

Drug	Dosage/Form	Equivalent Doses	Time to Onset, Peak, and Duration of Effect	Initial Dose (adults)	Side Effects	Other Comments
Pyridostigmine bromide (Mestinon tablet)	60 mg/tablet	60 mg	*Onset:* 30 min *Peak:* 1–2 hr *Duration:* 3–5 hr	60 mg tid in daytime, up to 1 g/day	Most common side effect: GI symptoms	
Pyridostigmine bromide TS (extended-release tablet; Mestinon TS)	180 mg/tablet	180 mg	*Onset:* 30–60 min *Duration:* 6–10 hr	180 mg at night up to 360 mg/day	Less than pyridostigmine tablet	Absorption is erratic
Pyridostigmine bromide syrup (liquid; Mestinon syrup)	60 mg/5 mL	5 mL	*Onset:* 30 min *Peak:* 1–2 hr *Duration:* 3–5 hr	60 mg tid in daytime, up to 1 g/day	Same as pyridostigmine tablet	Patient who has swallowing difficulty
Pyridostigmine bromide (Regonol) IV	5 mg/mL (2 mL or 5 mL ampule)	2 mg	*Onset:* 2–5 min *Duration:* 3–5 hr	1–2 mg q2–3 h, administer slowly	Cardiac dysrhythmia	During MG crisis
Neostigmine bromide (Prostigmine tablet)	15 mg/tablet	15 mg	*Onset:* 30 min *Duration:* 2–3 hr	15 mg qid in daytime, up to 150 mg/day	More GI side effects than pyridostigmine	Patients allergic to pyridostigmine
Neostigmine methylsulfate (Prostigmine solution) SC, IM	0.5 mg/mL 1 mg/mL 2.5 mg/mL	1 mg	*Onset:* 20–30 min *Duration:* 2–3 hr	0.5–1 mg q3h up to 10 mg/day		
Neostigmine methylsulfate (Prostigmine solution) IV	0.5 mg/mL 1 mg/mL 2.5 mg/mL	0.5 mg	*Onset:* 4–8 min *Duration:* 2–3 hr	0.5 mg administered slowly every hour up to 10 mg/day		
Ambenonium chloride (Myetelase)	10 mg/tablet 25 mg/tablet	10 mg	*Duration:* 6–8 hour	10 mg bid up to 100 mg/day	Fewer GI side effects than pyridostigmine, headache	Patients allergic to pyridostigmine
Edrophonium chloride (Tensilon)	10 mg/mL		*Onset:* immediate *Duration:* 2–5 min	2–10 mg IV/IM		Used for diagnostic test

GI, gastrointestinal; IM, intramuscular; IV, intravenous; SC, subcutaneous.

intravenous forms of AChEIs in recent years. Neostigmine (prostigmine) is an alternative choice of AChEIs in patients who are allergic to pyridostigmine. It has a slightly shorter duration of action and slightly greater muscarinic effects. Ambenonium (Mytelase) has been suggested as the last resort for patients who cannot take pyridostigmine or prostigmine for whatever reason.

The optimal dose is determined by the balance between clinical improvement and adverse effects and can vary over time with concomitant treatment. Dose adjustment should be gradual and achieved usually with the help of the patient. The patient's report of definite improvement following AChEI intake or the physician's assessment of the patient's condition at its peak of effectiveness is a reliable index of appropriate dose and effectiveness. The latter is almost impossible for nonhospitalized patients. Thus, the patient should be taught to adjust the dose. The maximal daily dose of pyridostigmine is 1 g. If a patient needs more than 720 mg (12 tablets) of pyridostigmine for control of MG symptoms, we recommend immunotherapy. Patients with mild disease can often be managed adequately with AChEIs alone. In patients receiving immunotherapy, symptoms can be controlled with AChEIs.

Another symptomatic agent, ephedrine, increases ACh release. This can be used for relief of fatigue as an adjunctive symptomatic treatment at a dose of 25 mg of ephedrine sulfate two to three times a day. This drug has been banned by the Food and Drug

Administration (FDA) in the United States for safety reasons. Ephedrine also has been found useful in some congenital myasthenic syndromes. Ephedrine is one of the medicines used to treat asthma. Interestingly, other asthma medications have a mild positive effect on MG, such as theophylline and terbutaline.

Immunotherapy
Because MG is an autoimmune disease, it is natural to treat this disorder with various immunotherapies, including immunosuppressive therapy, immunomodulating therapy, and thymectomy.

Immunosuppressive Therapy
Steroids
In a large nonrandomized study, remission or marked improvement was reported in 63% to 82% of patients with generalized MG and in 66% to 86% of those with ocular MG who were treated with oral corticosteroids, usually prednisone (class IV evidence) (Table 18-2).[15] The efficacy has been established in double-blind, placebo-controlled trials with methylprednisolone, but not with prednisone. In a randomized, double-blind trial of IV methylprednisolone (10 patients) versus placebo (9 patients) for generalized MG (Table 18-3), the second group showed a 7.2 times greater improvement in muscle strength than the placebo group after 2 weeks of treatment, indicating

Table 18-2 Literature Review of Nonrandomized Studies of Various Immunosuppressants Used in the Treatment of Myasthenia Gravis (MG)

Study	Total No. of Patients	No. (%) of Patients with Good Overall Improvement		Other Information
		Improvement	Remission	
Steroids				
Brunner (1972)[16]	9	9		Multiple short course of methylprednisone Severe MG
Arsura (1985)[17]	15	12		IV MP followed by oral prednisone
Pascuzzi (1984)[18]	116	61 (52.6%) marked	32 (27.6%)	
Sghirlanzoni (1984)[19]	60	18 (30.0%) marked	25 (41.7%)	
Cosi (1991)[20]	142	42 (29.6%) marked	48 (33.8%)	
Evoli (1992)[21]	104	44 (42.3%) marked	41 (39.4%)	
Bu (2000)[22]	600	95%		151 generalized; 449 pure ocular
Kupersmith (1996)[23]	32	21 (66%)		Ocular MG
Sommer (1997)[24]	45	19 (86%)		Ocular MG
Azathioprine (AZA)				
Matell (1976)[25]	26	78%		Unresponsive to steroid or ACTH
Mertens (1981)[26]	78	91%		Alone, in combination with steroid, thymectomy, or both
Matell (1987)[27]	99	72% (38% marked)		Alone, in combination with steroid, thymectomy or both
Witte (1984)[28]	18	15 (83%)		Alone for >6 months
Kuks (1991)[29]	41	41 (100%)		Alone or with prednisone for >3 yr
Mantegazza (1988)[30]	32	75%		Alone
	57	70%		With prednisone
Heckmann (2001)[31]			50%	2-yr class 2 study Early high-dose prednisone vs. 16% in low-dose control
Cyclophosphamide (CPP)				
Perez (1981)[32]	47		47 (100%)	With steroid in 33; thymectomy in 5; at 3 yr
Cyclosporine A (CsA)				
Goulon (1998)[33]	10	8 (80%) marked		12-mo open-label trial Severe MG, unresponsive to AChEI or thymectomy plus steroid or AZA
Bonifati (1997)[34]	9	7 (78%) marked		2-yr open-label trial Unresponsive to thymectomy, AZA, and steroid
Lavrnic (2005)[35]	52	44 (85%) marked		30-mo open label trial Severe MG unresponsive to thymectomy, steroid, and AZA
Mycophenolate mofetil				
Cos (2000)[36]	22	15 (68%)		2- to 18-mo open-label trial 3/5 alone; 4/7 unresponsive to AZA; 7/10 with steroid
Ciafaloni (2001)[37]	12	8 (67%) marked		6-mo open-label trial Unresponsive to AZA, steroids, CsA for <6 mo
Chaudhry (2001)[38]	32	19 (59%)		Alone in 4; 28 on other immunosuppresants
Meriggiori (2003)[39]	85	73%		48 thymectomy; 66 with CsA, steroid, AZA, MTX
Tacrolimus				
Konishi (2003)[40]	19	7 (37%)		16-wk open-label study: thymectomy and steroid
	12	8 (67%)		2-yr treatment

Continued

Table 18-2 Literature Review of Nonrandomized Studies of Various Immunosuppressants Used in the Treatment of Myasthenia Gravis (MG)—Cont'd

Study	Total No. of Patients	No. (%) of Patients with Good Overall Improvement		Other Information
		Improvement	Remission	
Kawaguchi (2004)[41]	17	12 (71%)		Open-label trial Mean follow-up 19.2 mo
Ponseti (2005)[42]	79		69 (87%) Pharmacologic	Open-label trial Severe MG Thymectomy, steroid, and CsA Mean follow-up 2.5 yr
Etanercept				
Rowin (2004)[43]	11	6 (55%)		Open-label trial

AChEI, acetylcholinesterase inhibitor; ACTH, adrenocorticotropic hormone; IV, intravenous.

Table 18-3 Literature Review of Randomized Studies of Various Immunotherapies for Myasthenia Gravis (MG)

Study	Agent	Method(s)	Intervention(s)	Outcome	Notes
Steroids					
Mount (1964)[44]	ACTH (n = 43)	RCT, PC	ACTH (580 units) 8 days vs. placebo	No evidence of efficacy of ACTH	Ocular MG
Howard (1976)[45]	Prednisone (n = 13)	RCT, DB, PC	Prednisone 100 mg (n = 6) on alternate day vs. placebo (n = 7)	No significant difference In 6 months 3 improved on placebo and 3 on prednisone	Small number for statistical analysis
Lindberg (1998)[46]	Methylprednisone (MP)	RCT, DB, PC	2 g MP IV for 2 days (n = 10) vs. placebo (n = 10)	Significant improvement in IV MP at 2 weeks Improved in 8 of 10 in MP and in 1 of 9 in placebo	Mean duration of improvement 8 weeks
Bromberg (1997)[47]	Prednisone (n = 10)	RCT	Prednisone 60 mg daily (n = 5) vs. AZA 2.5 mg/kg daily (n = 5)	No difference in improvement Improvement in 4 of 7 in prednisone and in 1 of 3 in AZA	Small number for statistical analysis
Schuchardt (2004)[48]	MP (n = 33)	RCT	MP 1–1.5 mg/kg for 14 days vs. 3 g IVIg daily for 5 days	No difference between 2 groups at day 14	MG with exacerbation
Immunosuppressants					
Gajdos (1993)[49]	Azathioprine (AZA) (n = 41)	RCT, unblind	AZA 3 mg/kg daily plus initial prednisone (n = 21) vs prednisone (n = 20) 1 mg/kg daily	No difference in remission or marked improvement between 2 groups at 1, 2, and 3 years	Prednisone treatment for months in AZA group
Palace (1998)[50]	AZA (n = 34)	RCT, blind	AZA 2.5 mg daily (n = 15) vs. placebo (n = 19) All patients on prednisone 1.5 mg/kg or 100 mg on alternate days	No difference between 2 groups at 12 months Significant reduction of prednisone dose in AZA at 36 months (0 in AZA vs. 40 mg in placebo)	Prednisone-sparing effect
De Feo (2002)[51]	Cyclophosphamide (CPP) (n = 23)	RCT, DB	CPP 0.5 g/m² of body surface IV monthly (n = 12) vs. placebo (n = 11) All patients on prednisone more than 50 mg initially	No significant difference between 2 groups in 12 months	IV every other month after the first 6 months
Tindall (1987)[52]	Cyclosporine A (CsA) (n = 20)	RCT, DB, PC	Cyclosporine (6 mg/kg daily) (n = 10) vs. placebo (n = 10)	Significant greater increase in QMG score in CsA at 6 and 12 months	
Tindall (1993)[53]	Cyclosporine (n = 39)	RCT, DB	Cyclosporine (5 mg/kg daily) plus prednisone 60–100 mg on alternate day (n = 20) vs. prednisone plus placebo (n = 19)	Significant greater increase in QMG score in CsA plus prednisone at 6 months	No steroid-sparing effect

Table 18-3 Literature Review of Randomized Studies of Various Immunotherapies for Myasthenia Gravis (MG)—Cont'd

Study	Agent	Method(s)	Intervention(s)	Outcome	Notes
Nagane (2005)[54]	Tacrolimus (n = 34)	RCT, unblind	Tacolimus 3 mg/day plus steroids (n = 18) vs. no tacrolimus plus steroid (n = 16) Plasmapheresis is given if necessary to either group	Significantly less number of treatment with plasmapheresis plus high-dose IV MP in tacrolimus during early- and follow-up phase treatment at 1 year The period of early-phase treatment is significantly shorter in tacrolimus The oral prednisone dose is significantly lower in tacrolimus	Reduction in need for other immunotherapy, to include steroid-sparing effect
Meriggiolo (2003)[55]	Mycophonolate mofetil (MM) (n = 14)	RCT, DB	MM (n = 7) vs. placebo (n = 7). Cyclosporine, prednisone, or no immunosuppresants in either group	No difference between two groups Improvement in 1 in each group	
Sanders (2008)[56]	MM (n = 80)	RCT, DB	MM (2.5 g daily) (n = 41) vs. placebo (n = 39) All on prednisone 20 mg/day	No difference in QMG score change at 3 months	
Sanders (2008)[56]	MM (n = 176)	RCT, DB	MM (2 g/day) (n = 88) vs. placebo (n = 88) All on prednisone 20 mg/day for 1 mo	No difference in QMG score change at 9 months	
Immunomodulating Therapies					
Gajdos (1983)[57]	Plasma exchange (PE) (n = 14)	RCT	Prednisone (n = 7) vs. prednisone plus PE (n = 7) PE: 3 PE over a 10-day period with PE once a week if necessary All on prednisone 1 mg/kg/day for 1 month	No difference in muscle strength score change at 1 month or 1 year Significantly less relapse in prednisone: 1 in prednisone vs. 8 in PE in 1 year	4 in each group in MG crisis
Gajdos (1997)[58]	Intravenous immunoglobulin (IVIg) (n = 87)	RCT	3 PEs vs. IVIg 2 g/kg or IVIg 1.2 g/kg	No difference in MM score change at day 15.	MG exacerbation
Gajdos (2005)[59]	IVIg (n = 173)	RCT	IVIg 1 g/kg vs. IVIg 2 g/kg	No difference in MM score change at day 15	MG exacerbation
Ronager (2001)[60]	IVIg (n = 12)	RCT, crossover	IVIg 0.4 g/kg for 3 days plus 5 PE vs. opposite schedule	No difference in QMG change 7 days after treatment	
Wolfe (2002)[61]	IVIg (n = 12)	RCT	IVIg 1 g/kg for 2 days vs. 5% albumin for 3 days	No difference in QMG change day 42	
Zinman (2007)[62]	IVIg (n = 51)	RCT, DB, PC	IVIg 1 g/kg for 2 days vs. 5% dextrose for 2 days	Significance in QMG change and postintervention status in IVIg at day 14	Treatment effect maintained for 28 days after infusion

ACTH, adrenocorticotropic hormone; DB, double blind; IV, intravenous; PC, placebo-controlled; RCT, randomized controlled trial.

significant short-term benefit from steroids. A randomized, double-blind trial of prednisone (six patients) versus placebo (seven patients) in generalized MG showed no significant difference in improvement at 6 months. This study lacks credence because of the small number of patients in each group. In a randomized controlled trial of methylprednisolone versus intravenous immunoglobulin (IVIg), no significant difference was noted at day 14, indicating that methylprednisolone is as effective as IVIg. Thus, steroids are useful as short-term immunosuppressants (class II). Long-term use of steroids is associated with many adverse effects, including weight gain, fluid retention, diabetes, psychosis, glaucoma, cataract, gastrointestinal bleeding, and osteoporosis. Steroids should be used ideally as short-term (60 mg/day for 3–4 months) immunosuppressants, though the long-term usage of steroids is not unusual. The risk of osteoporosis is reduced by giving bisphosphonate (class IV).

Oral prednisone is recommended as the first drug of choice when immunosuppressive drugs are necessary in MG (class IV) because steroids are known to induce the earliest onset of improvement among

Table 18-4 Pharmacologic Properties of Various Immunotherapies

Drug/Therapy	Mechanism of Action	Time to Onset, Peak Effect	Contraindication(s)
Steroids	Inhibit activation and antigen processing of T cells Decrease number of circulating T cells Increase muscle AChR synthesis	*Onset*: 2–3 days *Peak*: 3–6 mo	Severe diabetes
Azathioprine (AZA)	Purine antagonist Inhibit T cell and B cell proliferation	*Onset*: 4–10 mo *Peak*: 1–2 yr	Pregnancy, TPMT deficiency, liver failure, cancer
Mycophenolate mofetil (MM)	Purine antagonist Inhibit T cell and B cell proliferation	*Onset*: 4 wk–10 mo (mean, 11 wk) *Peak*: 8–26 mo (mean, 7 mo)	Pregnancy
Cyclosporine	Calcineurin inhibitor Decrease IL-2 production in T cells	*Onset*: 1 wk–8 mo	Severe hypertension, renal failure
Tacrolimus	Calcineurin inhibitor Prevents IL-2 transcription in T cells	*Onset*: 2 wk–4 mo *Peak*: 4 mo–2 yr	Pregnancy, renal failure, severe diabetes
Cyclophosphamide (CPP)	Alkylating agent Nonspecific cell cycle inhibitor, more effect on B cells	*Onset*: 2 mo *Peak*: 3–12 mo	Pregnancy, cancer, impaired bone marrow function
Rituximab	Chimeric human-murine monoclonal CD20 antibody Reduce B cell activation and proliferation	*Onset*: 1–2 mo *Peak*: 7 mo	Cardiac disease
Plasma exchange	Removal of AChR antibody	*Onset*: 1 day *Peak*: 2 wk *Duration*: 1–3 mo	Coronary artery disease, coagulopathy
Intravenous immunoglobulin (IVIg)	Neutralize the blocking effects of MG IgG antibodies to AChR	*Onset*: 5 days	Renal failure

AChR, acetylcholine receptor; MG, myasthenia gravis; TPMT, thiopurine methyltransferase.

the various immunosuppressants. Controversy exists regarding the most prudent method of initiating therapy (high-dose daily, high-dose on alternate day (AD), or low-dose AD, with a gradually increasing regimen). A low dose (20–30 mg) is recommended by those who believe that some patients develop steroid worsening, including MG crisis, in 4 to 10 days on higher doses (class IV) (Table 18-4). The low dose is gradually increased to a high dose over a few weeks' time. An initial high dose (>60 mg/day) is recommended by those, including this author, who believe that improvement is more rapid with a high-dose daily regimen, and that steroid worsening represents the natural worsening of MG in a patient whose disease is unstable. I personally believe that steroid worsening is exaggerated and extremely rare these days now that we use a smaller daily dose of AChEIs. Thus, I recommend an initial high-dose regimen unless there is a compelling reason not to do so. Once the maximal benefit or pharmacologic remission is achieved, owing to the potential adverse effects with prolonged use of steroids, the dose should be slowly reduced to the minimum effective dose or withdrawn and the simultaneous use of a long-term immunosuppressant be initiated.

Azathioprine

Azathioprine (AZA) is extensively used as an immunosuppressant. The onset of therapeutic response may be delayed for 4 to 10 months, and maximal effect is obtained in 1 to 2 years. AZA is usually well tolerated but idiosyncratic flu-like symptoms or gastrointestinal disturbances including pancreatitis occur in 10% of patients, usually within the first few days of treatment. Side effects may include bone marrow suppression and hepatotoxicity, which usually responds to drug reduction or withdrawal. When the white blood

cell count falls below 4000 mm³, the dose should be reduced; if it is below 3000 mm³, AZA should be discontinued. Matell's study showed that the incidence of malignancy was not increased over 22 years of AZA treatment.[63]

There are several observational series of AZA treatment which showed 70% to 100% improvement with AZA alone, or in combination with other treatment, mostly steroids (class IV).[15] One study comparing early "high-dose" immunosuppression with AZA and prednisone resulted in 50% of patients achieving remission after 2 years, compared with a remission rate of only 16% in those on a "low-dose" regimen.

One large double-blind, randomized study[50] has demonstrated the efficacy of AZA as a steroid-sparing agent with a better outcome in patients on a combination of AZA and steroids than in patients treated with steroids alone (class I). In a randomized, unblinded trial of AZA plus initial prednisone versus prednisone alone, no difference was found in remission or marked improvement between two groups after 1 to 3 years of long-term treatment.

Because AZA has been associated with relatively few treatment failures and a steroid-sparing effect in two randomized controlled trials (class I), we do recommend AZA as the first choice long-term immunosuppressant drug. Some prefer to start AZA together with steroids to allow tapering of steroids to the lowest dose possible. The usual recommended daily dose is 150 mg. (Please see Chapter 7 for further details of this and other immunosuppressant drugs.)

Cyclophosphamide

In one observational study in 42 patients who were given cyclophosphamide (CPP) with duration of treatment from 2 to

37 months, remission was achieved in 58% of patients within 1 year, in 85% of patients within 2 years of treatment, and in 100% of patients within 32 months of treatment.[15] In a randomized, double-blind trial of CPP plus prednisone versus prednisone plus placebo in generalized MG,[51] CPP significantly improved muscle strength at 12 months, but not at 6 months. The CPP-treated patients were on significantly lower doses of prednisone at 6 months and 12 months. Thus, this study showed that CPP is clinically effective in generalized MG, and that it has a steroid-sparing effect (class II). The usual oral dose of CPP was 5 mg/kg/day (usual initial dose, 150 mg/day). CPP can be given via monthly pulse therapy at an IV dose of 1 g/m^2/month. High-dose CPP (50 mg/kg/day for 4 days) followed by granulocyte colony-stimulating factor was also used to "reboot" the immune system in refractory MG.[64] In three MG patients who were unresponsive to plasma exchange, thymectomy, and conventional immunosuppressants, remission was achieved. In view of the relatively high risk of toxicity, including bone marrow suppression, opportunistic infections, bladder toxicity, sterility, and neoplasm, this drug is recommended as the last choice of immunosuppressants for patients who are intolerant of, or unresponsive to, other immunosuppressants. The usual recommended oral daily dose is 150 mg.

Cyclosporine A

Cyclosporine A (CsA) is the first agent used in treating MG that showed a definite benefit in a randomized, controlled trial. Three observational studies in severe MG unresponsive to thymectomy, AZA, or steroid showed marked improvement in 75% to 80% of patients within 1 to 3 years of treatment. One placebo-controlled, double-blind, randomized study in 20 patients for 6 months with an open extension (class I) showed significantly improved strength and reduction in AChR antibody titer compared with the placebo group at 6 and 12 months. Another controlled, double-blind, randomized, study with 39 patients showed significantly improved muscle strength at 6 months in the CsA-plus-prednisone group compared with the placebo-plus-prednisone group, but a steroid-sparing effect was not observed. Thus, two randomized, controlled trials have shown that CsA is clinically effective in generalized MG. The initial daily dose is 4 to 6 mg/kg/day with monitoring of drug levels. Because of significant side effects of nephrotoxicity, hypertension, and malignancy, it should be considered only in patients intolerant of or unresponsive to AZA (level B recommendation). The usual recommended dose is 200 mg/day. Other common side effects include hypertrichosis, gingival hyperplasia, myalgia, and "flu-like" symptoms. Nonsteroidal anti-inflammatory drugs should be avoided together with CsA because they increase nephrotoxicity.

Mycophenolate Mofetil

Two open-label trials and two observational studies in MG patients unresponsive to steroid, AZA, or CsA showed a 59% to 73% improvement in 2 to 18 months of treatment. Improvement occurred in monotherapy as well as in combination with other immunosuppressants. Two randomized, double-blind trials of mycophenolate mofetil (MM) plus steroids versus steroid plus placebo for generalized MG failed to demonstrate any efficacy of MM at 3 months or 9 months. Another small randomized, double-blind trial of MM plus either CsA, prednisone, or no immunosuppressants versus placebo plus either CCA, prednisone, or no immunosuppressants also did not show any benefit of MM. Though MM has been reported not to be efficacious in randomized, controlled trials in generalized MG, this drug is well tolerated with a relatively good adverse-effect profile.[56]

The adverse effects of MM were usually mild: nausea, headache, or diarrhea. Serious adverse effects such as infections and hematopoietic suppression were rare. One advantage of MM compared with other immunosuppressants is a lower carcinogenic tendency: the kidney transplant patients on mycophenolate mofetil had a smaller incidence of cancer in the long-term follow-up. Lymphoma was reported as a rare complication. The European Task Force recommends MM as the second-line long-term therapy in MG patients intolerant of or unresponsive to AZA (level B recommendation). This view might have to be modified in view of negative results in two randomized controlled studies. The usual recommended daily dose is 1.5 g.

Tacrolimus

Although tacrolimus and CsA act in a similar fashion, the potency of tacrolimus appears to be 10 to 100 times greater than that of CsA. Tacrolimus at 3 mg/day for MG is 20% of the dose given to organ transplant patients. One 4-month open-label study showed an improvement in 37% of cases. Three observational studies of longer than 19 months' duration showed improvement in 67% to 71% of patients and pharmacologic remission in 87% of patients. A randomized, unblinded, non-placebo-controlled trial of tacrolimus plus steroids with or without plasma exchange (PE) versus no tacrolimus plus steroids with or without PE showed a significantly fewer number of treatments with PE plus high-dose intravenous methylprednisolone (IVMP), a significantly shorter period of early-phase treatment, and significantly lower prednisone doses in the tacrolimus-treated groups.[54] Thus, this study showed that tacrolimus reduces the need for other immunotherapy, indicating that this drug is effective in generalized MG. Tacrolimus seems to be relatively safe at the doses used in MG, so it should be recommended as a third-line treatment for patients who are intolerant of or unresponsive to AZA. Common side effects of the drug include hypertension, renal insufficiency, hyperkalemia, headache, and hyperglycemia. It may have carcinogenic properties. The usual recommended daily dose is 3 mg.

Methotrexate

The European Task Force recommends methotrexate as a second-line drug because it has been well studied in other autoimmune disorders.[3] However, there is no good randomized or nonrandomized study in MG to support this recommendation. We recommend this drug as the last choice if all other immunosuppressants fail or cannot be taken. One advantage of this medication is its one-time weekly administration. The initial starting dose is 7.5 mg weekly, with a maximum weekly dose of 30 mg. The usual recommended weekly dose is 7.5 mg.

Rituximab

There are several promising case reports of improvement of refractory MG with rituximab. Aside from the success of rituximab as a steroid-sparing agent in refractory MG patients, several case reports have also demonstrated clinical improvement and a reduction in AChR antibodies or MuSK antibodies.[15] However, this drug needs to be evaluated more extensively against current immunosuppressants before it can be recommended. In addition, the current prohibitive cost of this drug is a major drawback. Common infusion-related side effects of rituximab are fever, chills, nausea, vomiting, flushing, and bronchospasm. Other more serious side effects include neutropenia and increased risk of infection.

Immunomodulating Therapies
Plasma Exchange

Plasma exchange (PE), or plasmapheresis, removes antibodies from patient serum by membrane filtration or centrifugation. Patients typically undergo five sessions of PE at 20 to 50 mL/kg body weight per session over a span of 2 weeks. The plasma is separated from blood cells using membrane filtration or centrifugation, and then the blood cells are reinfused into another vein with diluted albumin, colloids, or crystalloids while plasma is removed. The onset of improvement is within the first week and the effect lasts 1 to 3 months. Side effects are associated with the insertion of the intravenous catheter and hypotension. Although PE has been extensively used as the treatment of choice in acute MG exacerbation, there is no randomized, double-blind control study for the short-term or long-term benefit.[20] There are two nonrandomized, controlled studies. One study in 1979 compared six patients who received PE over 2 to 2.5 weeks and six patients who were assigned to a control group. None of the control group improved, whereas all treated patients improved strikingly. Another study in 1979 compared the long-term effect in severe MG patients treated with PE plus immunosuppressive drugs and seven patients treated with immunosuppressants alone. PE was associated with short-term improvement in all seven patients. At 6 to 12 months clinical outcome, as well as AChR antibody titer decline, were similar in both groups. Many observational studies showed short-term clinical improvement in 65% to 100% of cases. Cochrane research revealed only one eligible controlled trial.[65] The aim of this trial was to compare the long-term effect of prednisone (seven patients) versus prednisone plus PE (seven patients). No difference was observed in the muscle strength score change at 1 month or 1 year between the two groups, but there was significantly less relapse in the prednisone group. Thus, this trial failed to demonstrate any long-term benefit of prednisone and PE versus prednisone alone. On the basis of these findings, the National Institutes of Health (NIH) consensus of 1986 states the following: "PE can be useful in strengthening patients with MG before thymectomy and during the postoperative period. It can also be valuable in lessening symptoms during initiation of immunosuppressants and during an acute crisis" (class IV). Therefore, sham controlled trials would be unethical. Cochrane review (2008)[65] concluded that there are no adequate randomized controlled trials to establish whether PE improves the long- or short-term outcome from MG, but many case series report short-term benefit from PE in MG, especially in myasthenic crisis.[49] Repeated PE is thus not recommended as a treatment to obtain a continuous and lasting immunosuppression in MG.

Intravenous Immunoglobulin

IVIg is a fractionated blood product consisting primarily of IgG, derived from 3000 to 10,000 human plasma donors. The mechanism of action of IVIg is complex, including almost all aspects of the immune system. The most relevant mechanisms for MG are the neutralizing effect of commercial polyclonal IgG on the blocking of myasthenic IgG antibodies to nicotinic AChR and the inhibiting effect on the production of autoantibodies by inhibiting the body's ability to produce globulin. IVIg is relatively easier to administer than PE. The usual IVIg dose is 0.4 to 1 g/kg body weight given over 2 to 5 days. After infusion, serum IVIg levels increase fivefold, then decline by 50% in 72 hours and return to pretreatment levels after 21 to 28 days. Severe reactions from IVIg are rare. The most serious reactions so far reported include anaphylactic reaction, hepatitis C outbreak, aseptic meningitis, acute renal failure, hemolysis, and cerebral infarction.[66] Anaphylactic reaction following IVIg has been reported in patients with selective IgA deficiency due to IgG or IgE antibodies to IgA; IgA deficiency occurs in about 1 of every 200 to 800 persons. Thus, IgA deficiency is the only contraindication for the use of IVIg, and the IgA level should be checked when IVIg therapy is

considered. If IVIg has to be given in IgA-deficient patients, a product with anti-IgA should be infused (e.g., Gamimmune and Gammagard). An outbreak of hepatitis C was last reported with IVIg in early 1994. Death from acute renal failure in diabetic patients has been reported. Aseptic meningitis has become the most common troublesome side effect for clinicians, seen in about 11% of patients.

Most other reactions are mild and self-limiting and are associated with too-rapid infusion of IVIg. In a review of seven nonrandomized observational studies with 10 participants or more, Jongen and associates reported an overall rate of improvement of 76% (90/119) with a median of 87% (range 48% to 92%).[67] In the only randomized, controlled trial comparing IVIg (1 g/kg for 2 days) with placebo (5% dextrose for 2 days), there was a significant improvement in quantitative MG score (QMG) in favor of the IVIg group on day 14. Importantly, this effect was not observed in mild MG but was significant in moderate to severe MG. Other randomized, controlled trials showed no difference in improvement between PE and IVIg, or between IVIg 1 g/kg and 2 g/kg regimens. A further, yet underpowered, trial showed no significant difference between IVIg and oral methylprednisolone. Recently, IVIg was proposed as a maintenance therapy for MG. IVIg 2 g/kg over 5 days was followed by 0.4 g/kg once monthly or once every 6 weeks in one trial in 10 patients with severe generalized MG and another in 11 patients with severe MG with bulbar palsy. All patients were unresponsive to steroid and immunosuppressants. All patients improved after 1 year in one study and after a mean period of 20 months in another study. Cochrane review concluded that IVIg is effective in severe MG exacerbation in one randomized, controlled trial, but that there is insufficient evidence from randomized trials to determine whether IVIg is efficacious in chronic MG.[68]

On the basis of these findings, we recommend the use of IVIg in preference to PE for acutely worsening MG (class I), for the preparation of weak patients for surgery including thymectomy (class IV), and as an adjuvant to immunosuppressive therapy to minimize the long-term side effects of oral immunosuppressants and maintain improved status. In MuSK-MG, a retrospective multicenter study in 52 patients showed a poorer outcome with IVIg than for PE (class IV).[69]

Thymectomy

In 1939, Blalock et al reported the remission of generalized MG in a 21-year-old woman after removal of a cystic thymic tumor and subsequently performed thymectomy on MG patients without thymoma.[70] They found hyperplasia in the thymus gland and reported improvement in at least half their patients. Since these reports, thymectomy has been accepted widely as a form of treatment for MG. So far, there have been no randomized, controlled studies for thymectomy in MG. At this writing, a multicenter randomized, controlled study is under way to answer this question.

The Quality Standard Subcommittee of the American Academy of Neurology reviewed 28 articles from 1953 to 1998 describing outcomes in 21 MG cohorts with or without thymectomy.[71] Most series used the trans-sternal approach, and a few series used the transcervical approach. The follow-up ranged from 3 to 28 years. All studies compared the outcome between thymectomized and nonthymectomized MG patients (class II). Most studies are retrospective analyses of cases. There were a number of methodologic problems in the studies, including definition of remission, the selection criteria, matched design, medical therapy, and data on AChR-Ab. They calculated the median relative rate of outcome by dividing the thymectomy group's crude rate of achieving the outcome by the nonthymectomy group's crude rate and compared these rates between the two groups. Eighteen of 21 cohorts showed improvement in thymectomized patients compared with nonthymectomized patients. Those undergoing thymectomy were twice as likely to achieve medication-free remission, 1.6 times as likely to become asymptomatic, and 1.7 times as likely to improve. A subgroup analysis using a single confounding variable yielded additional results: severe cases were 3.7 times more likely to achieve remission after thymectomy than those without surgery (0.007); in the male subgroup the relative outcome decreased by a median of 25% ($P < 0.043$); and in a generalized subgroup, there was a tendency of improvement ($P = 0.06$). Controlled trials did not provide convincing evidence that one thymectomy technique was superior to another. Gronseth and Barohn[71] concluded that the benefit of thymectomy in nonthymomatous autoimmune MG has not been established conclusively and made a statement as practice recommendation that, for patients with nonthymomatous autoimmune MG, thymectomy is recommended as an option to increase the probability of remission or improvement (class II). Their recommendation is supported by the European Task Force with the specification that patients with generalized MG and AChR antibodies are the group most likely to benefit (level B recommendation).

At this time, the indication for thymectomy in AChR-Ab-negative patients is controversial. Two retrospective cohort studies showed a comparable response among AChR-Ab-positive and AChR-Ab-negative groups.[72,73] In MuSK-MG, several small retrospective studies showed no benefit with thymectomy.[9]

Age is another controversial subject in the debate over thymectomy. Thymectomy is often avoided in children because of the theoretical possibility of impairing the developing immune system. However, reports of thymectomy in children as young as 2 to 3 years of age have shown favorable results without adverse effects on the immune system. Thymectomy has been largely discouraged in late-onset MG (>55 years of age), mainly because of frequent observation of an atrophic, involuted thymus. One series showed a less favorable outcome of thymectomy in late-onset MG: post-thymectomy improvement was transitory and no longer detectable at 2 years after thymectomy (class IV). The patient's age at MG onset was a more important factor than the age at thymectomy.[74] They also concluded that outcome comparison between uncontrolled studies does not provide conclusive evidence of the superiority of one technique over another.

In comparing the various surgical approaches, Sonett and Jaretzki[75] employed the Kaplan-Meier life table analysis at 5 years and concluded that the combined transcervical-trans-sternal, extended trans-sternal, extended cervical, and video-assisted thoracoscopic extended thymectomy (VATET) procedures appear to produce, more or less, the same percentage (40%–55%) of remission at 5 years. It appears that the more thorough the removal of all tissue that may contain thymus, the better the longer-term results. Therefore, conceptually, the combined transcervical-trans-sternal thymectomy best fulfills these criteria.

Alternatively, we support an aggressive extended trans-sternal thymectomy in the hands of experienced surgeons. It predictably removes all but a possible small amount of the thymic variations in the neck, has less risk of injury to recurrent laryngeal nerves, has produced good results, and at this time is probably the most commonly performed procedure. Accordingly, in the hands of surgeons experienced with these techniques, the extended transcervical thymectomy and the VATET thymectomy (bilateral thoracoscopic thymectomy combined with a formal neck exploration) appear to be acceptable alternatives.

Sonett and Jaretzki stated that it is far preferable to leave behind small amounts of suspected thymus, or even likely thymus, tissue than to injure the recurrent laryngeal, the left vagus, or the phrenic nerve.[75] Injuries to these nerves can be devastating to a patient with MG.

Perioperative mortality rates were higher in patients undergoing thymectomy before 1970, with commonly reported rates being between 5% and 15%. After 1970, reported mortality rates in studies reviewed here were consistently less than 1%.

On the basis of this information, we believe that thymectomy is indicated in any early-onset (<60 years of age) generalized MG patients whose symptoms are not satisfactorily controlled with AChEIs alone (level B recommendation). Thymectomy induces long-term improvement and remission. About 33% of patients will achieve remission in the first 3 years after thymectomy and 50% within 5 years. Thymectomy produces a stable remission by eliminating thymic centers. The effects are delayed because of the long life-span of the existing pool of small immunocompetent lymphocytes.

Treatment of the Specific Subtypes of Myasthenia Gravis

Myasthenic Crisis
Myasthenic crisis (MC) is a life-threatening complication of MG. Traditionally, it is defined as respiratory failure due to worsening MG, requiring intubation and mechanical ventilation (MGFA class V). Here we define MC as a respiratory failure due to worsening MG requiring mechanical ventilation, to accommodate noninvasive mechanical ventilation which was introduced as a treatment mode for serious respiratory failure in MG.[76] About 15% to 20% of patients with MG experience an MC at some point in the course of their disease, but often in the first year of illness. Patients with MuSK-MG have a higher risk of MC because of predominant bulbar weakness.[9]

MC is caused by severe weakness of respiratory muscles, upper airway muscles (bulbar myasthenia), or both. It occurs in AChR-Ab-positive, MuSK-positive, and DSN (double seronegative) MG. Infections are known to be the most common precipitating factor for MC, accounting for 38% of cases in one series. Thymoma was observed in 32% of cases of MC and may be a risk factor in one series.[76] Other rare recognized precipitating factors for crisis are surgery, pregnancy, and medications (Box 18-1). Excessive dosing with AChEIs can potentially increase weakness due to depolarization blockade at the neuromuscular junction. Previously it was customary to differentiate between cholinergic crisis and MC by edrophonium test in MC patients with a known diagnosis of MG who were taking high doses of AChEIs. Cholinergic crisis is rare in today's practice because high doses of AChEI are not used anymore.

Diagnosis of MC in patients with an established diagnosis of MG is relatively easy. Respiratory failure was reported to be the first manifestation of MG in 14% to 18% of MG patients. In these cases, the diagnosis of MG is based on the clinical findings and should be confirmed by edrophonium test, RNS test, or, rarely, SFEMG. The diagnostic sensitivity of the RNS test in MC is about 94%.

Clinical Signs of Myasthenic Crisis
Prompt recognition of impending respiratory paralysis is the key to successful management of MC. Features of impending MC include severe bulbar weakness, marginal vital capacity (20 to 25 mL/kg), weak cough with difficulty clearing secretions from the airway, or paradoxical breathing while supine. These patients should be admitted to the Intensive Care Unit (ICU) and monitored closely. They should receive no food or liquid by mouth to prevent aspiration. Careful observation and bedside measurements (pulse rate, blood pressure, oximetry, vital capacity, tidal volume, peak inspiratory and expiratory pressure) are more important than repeated monitoring of blood gases. The 20/30/40 rule (vital capacity < 20 mL/kg, or 1 L; peak inspiratory pressure > −30 cm H_2O; and peak

Box 18-1 Drugs/Factors Associated with Unmasking or Aggravating Myasthenia Gravis (MG)*

Definite Association

Drugs/factors that are known to induce autoimmune MG and thus are contraindicated in patients with MG
  Alpha interferon
  Bone marrow transplantation
  D-Penicillamine
Drugs/factors that are known *definitely* to unmask or aggravate MG and thus should be avoided in patients with MG
  Botulinum toxin, type A (Botox)
  Antibiotics—ketolide (telithromycin [Ketek])
  Depolarizing and nondepolarizing neuromuscular blocking agents
  Iatrogenic hypermagnesemia including that due to magnesium sulfate

Probable Association

Drugs/factors that are known to unmask or aggravate MG in more than two cases and thus are not recommended for use in patients with MG; if used, then close monitoring is required
  Antibiotics
    Aminoglycosides: gentamicin, kanamycin, netilmycin, neomycin, streptomycin
    Fluoroquinolones: ciprofloxacin, ofloxacin
    Other antibiotics: bacitracin, colistin, polymyxin
  Cardiovascular drugs
    Beta blockers: propranolol
    Verapamil
    Procainamide
    Statins
  Quinolones: chloroquine, fluoroquinolone antibiotics, quinidine, quinine
  Iodinated contrast media
  Ophthalmologic medication: timolol maleate eyedrops
  Anticonvulsants: phenytoin
  Psychotrophic medication: lithium carbonate

Possible Association

Drugs/factors that are known to unmask or exacerbate MG in one or two cases and thus can be used safely in most patients with MG, with close monitoring recommended
  Antibiotics: amino acid antibiotics, ampicillin, azithromycin, clarithromycin, clindamycin, erythromycin, imipenem and cilastatin sodium, macrolides, nitrofurantoin, pyrantel pamoate, ritonavir, sulfonamides, tetracyclines, vancomycin
  Beta blockers: accubutol, oxprenolol, practolol
  Other cardiac drugs: bretylium, propafenone HCl, trimethaphan
  Anticonvulsant medications: carbamazepine, ethosuximide, gabapentin, trimethadione
  Ophthalmologic medications: betaxolol hydrochloride, echothiophate, proparacaine, tropicamide
  Psychotropic medication: phenothiazide
  Other medicines neurologists often prescribe: riluzole, glatiramer acetate, methocarbamol, trihexyphenidyl (Artane)
  Miscellaneous drugs/agents: fludarabine, cisplatin, interleukin, carnitine, nitcotine patch, diatrizoate meglumine, chlorine gas

*For further information, consult www.myasthenia.org/docs/MGFA_Medicationsand.

Box 18-2 Principles of Management of Myasthenic Crisis

1. Provide airway assistance and ventilation: This step is most critical; *always* intubate when in doubt
2. Discontinue AChEIs initially
3. Remove and treat precipitating factors
4. Routine monitoring
   Cardiac monitoring
   Oximetry
   Pulmonary function monitoring: forced vital capacity, peak inspiratory pressure and expiratory pressure, every 2–4 hours
4. General medical care
   Institute prophylaxis for deep vein thrombosis with low-molecular-weight heparin
   Identify and treat infection
   Identify and treat cardiac arrhythmia and congestive heart failure
5. Initiate specific treatment for MG
   Plasma exchange (removal of 2 to 3 L of plasma volume on each session × 5)
   Alternatively, IVIg (0.4 mg/kg/day × 5)
   High-dose steroid (prednisone 1 mg/kg/day)
   Start a low-dose AChEI when the patient gets stronger and benefit is found with trial

AChEI, acetylcholinesterase inhibitor; IVIg, intravenous immunoglobulin; MG, myasthenia gravis.

intubation and mechanical ventilation in MG, but the experience is still relatively limited. One retrospective study[77] showed that, in 14 (58%) of 24 patients initially treated with BiPAP, endotracheal intubation was avoided, and patients treated with BiPAP had shorter stays in the ICU and in the hospital than those treated initially with intubation. The only predictor of BiPAP failure was a PCO_2 level exceeding 45 mm Hg on BiPAP initiation. This study suggests the possibility that some patients with MC or impending crisis might be managed with BiPAP ventilation.[77]

Treatment of Myasthenia Gravis

To date, the treatment of MG during MC is based on clinical consensus, not on evidence-based data (Box 18-2). There is a general agreement among the experts that high-dose steroids in combination with plasma exchange or immunoglobulin are the cornerstone of MG treatment during MC.

There have been a few treatment trials in MC, and both plasma exchange and IVIg are comparable in terms of efficacy on the basis of clinical evidence. Because response to PE is more predictable and a good clinical response to PE in some myasthenic patients refractory to IVIg was reported,[78] many experts take the view that PE is probably more effective than IVIg in MC.[79–81] Thus, PE has become the most commonly used immunotherapy for MC. In one retrospective multicenter review of 54 episodes of MC, PE had a superior outcome for ventilatory status at 2 weeks and functional outcome at 1 month, despite a higher complication rate with PE.

IVIg represents an alternative short-term immunomodulating therapy for myasthenic crisis in patients who are poor candidates for PE owing to various medical reasons, including vascular access problems, septicemia, and cardiac failure. The wider availability and ease of administration of IVIg makes it an automatic choice as the first-line therapy for MC in patients who have difficult access to medical centers which can perform PE.

Steroids are the drug of choice as the immunotherapeutic agent for maintaining an improved status by PE or IVIg because an initial stable improvement is achieved within weeks (average 13–39 days) of beginning steroid treatment in contrast to months with other

expiratory pressure < 40 cm H_2O) is probably the most helpful guide to decide when intubation is necessary. In MC, the clinician should anticipate the need for respiratory assistance rather than deal with emergency intubation ("when in doubt, intubate").

Noninvasive mechanical ventilation with bilevel positive airway pressure (BiPAP) ventilation has been used as an alternative to immunosuppressants.[82] Most experts recommend high-dose (1 mg/kg) prednisone daily as the initial regimen.

Intravenous pyridostigmine infusion at 1 to 2 mg/hour has been advocated in patients during crisis by Berroushot et al.[83] In 63 episodes of MC treatment in an acute care setting with pyridostigmine ($n = 24$), pyridostigmine and prednisolone ($n = 18$), and PE alone ($n = 23$), they did not find any significant differences in short-term efficacy, comparable long-term outcome, and side effect profile between the different regimens. Based on these results, they advocated an approach tailored to the individual patient, considering the precrisis condition of the patient and the precipitating factors of MC. However, because of possible cardiac complications, sometimes fatal cholinergic crisis, and excessive secretions,[84] most experts recommend discontinuing pyridostigmine during crisis (drug holiday) and reinstituting it orally when patients are getting stronger and the benefit is found after trial. This is usually around the extubation time. Some believe that a drug holiday heightens the patients' sensitivity to AChEIs.[82] The usual recommendation is to start at a low dose (60 mg every 8 hours enterally), gradually increasing to a dose that produces a clear benefit.

Immunosuppressants are usually not recommended because the improvement with these agents is generally not seen for several months. They may be used in place of prednisone, however, when steroid therapy is contraindicated, but not for myasthenic crisis. There is no indication for thymectomy during MC.

Respiratory Management and Treatment

This management is also discussed in Chapter 2. When intubation is performed, nasotracheal intubation is preferred, as nasotracheal tubes are more comfortable than orotracheal tubes. A tracheostomy should be considered for patients requiring more than 2 weeks of mechanical ventilation.

Weaning trials should begin after patients demonstrate a clear trend of improved respiratory muscle strength. The general guideline is the 10/20/40 rule: vital capacity above 10 mL/kg, maximum negative inspiratory force below -20 cm H_2O, and peak positive expiratory force greater than 40 cm H_2O.

The three most common complications are fever, pneumonia, and atelectasis. Aggressive treatment for pneumonia and atelectasis is mandatory.

Mortality rates in MC had declined from over 40% in the early 1960s to approximately 5% in the 1970s, due in large part to improvement in respiratory care and ICU management. Current statistics still report a 4% mortality rate despite newer treatments and better intensive medical care, indicating no documented improvement in fatality rates over the last several decades. All deaths were ascribed to severe medical co-morbidity. The two most common causes of death in MC were cardiac arrhythmia and infections.

Ocular Myasthenia Gravis

Pyridostigmine was usually effective for ptosis, but not for double vision, a more troublesome symptom. Steroid was effective in ocular MG (OMG) as well as in generalized MG. AZA was also used as the second-line immunosuppressive medication. Oral steroid produced improvement in 66% to 85% of OMG patients.[85] However, a permanent remission was associated with steroid in only 10% of patients.

A major question in the treatment of OMG is whether steroid or immunosuppressant drugs may prevent the development of generalized MG. In 49% to 69% of patients, OMG worsened into generalized MG (GMG). This occurred within 2 years in 50% to 88% of cases; in AChR-Ab-positive OMG, this conversion occurred in 45% to 71% of cases.

Retrospective analyses suggested reduced rates of generalization with steroid in four studies and azathioprine in one study. Only 7% to 17% of OMG patients treated with prednisone developed GMG compared with 36% to 83% in patients not treated with immunosuppressants. In OMG patients treated with azathioprine, GMG developed in 16% within 2 years and in 23% within 4 years. There is no randomized, controlled trial to support this finding.[85]

Thymectomy is not generally indicated in OMG because of its benign course. Two case series claimed its benefits (class IV): no generalization in 18 patients in 26 months and "cure" in 51% of 61 patients, with a 9-year mean follow-up.[86]

MuSK-Ab-Positive Myasthenia Gravis

MuSK is a surface receptor that plays an essential role in the clustering of AChR during development. MuSK-Ab-positive MG (MuSK-MG) was first reported in 2001. MuSK-Ab is negative in ocular MG. MuSK-Ab has been reported to be positive in 0% in Norway to 49% in Turkey, with a mean frequency of approximately 36% of generalized AChR-Ab-negative MG.[9] MuSK-MG is predominantly observed in females.[87] Age at onset is usually younger. Patients tend to have more severe forms of MG and crisis is commoner in MuSK-MG. Prominent cranial and bulbar weakness is the most consistent pattern. Profound facial and tongue atrophy has been observed in some of these cases. Predominant neck, shoulder, and respiratory involvement but without ocular weakness was another rare manifestation.

A positive edrophonium test is less common in MuSK-MG than in other forms of MG, being positive in half the cases. RNS test of limb muscles had a relatively low yield (25%–57%) in MuSK-MG, but RNS test of facial muscles showed a decrement in 85% of cases. This percentage of decrement is of greater magnitude than in the other two forms. Thus, including facial muscles in the RNS protocol is important when evaluating patients suspected of having MuSK-MG. Many series reported a relatively low yield of abnormality with the SFEMG in the limb muscles, but when the proximal and cranial muscles were added for the study, this test was abnormal in the majority of MuSK-MG patients.

The clinical response to anticholinesterase agents in MuSK-MG has generally been disappointing. With a standard pyridostigmine dose, unresponsiveness, actual worsening, or intolerance manifested by severe muscarinic and nicotinic side effects is common. Most patients need one or a combination of immunotherapeutic agents. Among the various immunotherapies, steroid and plasma exchange seem to evoke the best responses.[69] However, the general impression is that MuSK-MG is relatively refractory to standard treatment because finding the right combination of immunotherapy is time-consuming and difficult.

Pregnancy

The course of MG during pregnancy is unpredictable: approximately one third of patients remain the same, one third improves, and the remaining one third worsens.[88] Worsening of MG symptoms is more likely in the first trimester and the puerperal periods and is possibly related with an increased level of α-fetoprotein (α-FP), which is known to block the binding of AChR-Ab to AChR. The clinical state of MG at the beginning of pregnancy or in a previous pregnancy does not predict the concurrence of exacerbation or remission during gestation. MG does not cause any adverse effect on the course of pregnancy. The coexistence of MG and preeclampsia, though rare, may produce high morbidity and mortality rates for these mothers and fetuses. Magnesium sulfate, the drug of choice in the treatment of preeclampsia, is contraindicated in MG because hypermagnesemia inhibits the release of ACh at the neuromuscular junction and worsens MG muscle weakness, causing a severe myasthenic crisis.

Management of Myasthenia Gravis

Patients have to be more frequently evaluated for possible worsening of MG throughout pregnancy. Screening for asymptomatic bacteriuria should be regularly performed and appropriate treatment of urinary tract infections is required, because infection is a known cause for MG worsening and crisis. Pregnant women with MG should carefully monitor fetal movement and seek medical advice as soon as they find it reduced. If indicated, fetal ultrasound evaluations should be done to detect any sign of the fetal akinesia sequence.

Oral AChEIs are the drugs of choice for symptomatic treatment of MG and can be used alone in mild cases of MG. Pyridostigmine is considered to be safe during pregnancy when used at the recommended dosage of less than 1000 mg (14 tablets) a day.

Steroids are the drugs of choice for immunotherapy because they present little if any teratogenic risk to the fetus; only a slight increase in the incidence of cleft palate has been reported. Another advantage of steroid is that it works much faster than many immunosuppressants in achieving a stable course of MG. All other immunosuppressants should be avoided before and during pregnancy whenever possible because of potential teratogenic effects.

PE or IVIg can be and has been used as an effective treatment for severe worsening of MG or crisis during pregnancy without any major complication. Thymectomy during pregnancy has no role because of its delayed effect and possible surgical risk.

Management of Myasthenia Gravis during Labor and Delivery

Most deliveries can safely be completed vaginally.[88] Epidural anesthesia is preferred for vaginal and surgical delivery because many myasthenic patients are sensitive to many anesthetic agents.[89] Local anesthetics can be used, but high doses should be avoided because they may interfere with neuromuscular transmission. Lidocaine is the recommended local anesthetic because it is an aminoacylamide and is not affected by AChEIs. Women taking steroids during pregnancy should continue the treatment during labor, and a stress dose should be given (an extra intramuscular [IM] dose of 50–100 mg of prednisone at the first stage of labor, or Solu-Medrol 200 mg IV drip during labor).

During the second stage of labor, which involves the voluntary expulsive effort, the patient may become exhausted and require immediate AChEIs. Neostigmine (1.5–2.0 mg IM or 0.5 mg IV every 3–4 hours) is preferred to pyridostigmine. Contrary to expert recommendation, many MG women prefer cesarean section for delivery of the baby because of an overall increased rate of delivery complications and a higher rate of intervention during delivery.[90]

Neonatal Myasthenia Gravis

Neonatal MG (NMG) is a syndrome that occurs in 10% to 20% of newborns of a myasthenic mother shortly after birth. NMG is reported in all types of MG. Symptoms develop most commonly 12 to 48 hours after birth and include generalized weakness, hypotonia, difficulty feeding, feeble cry, ptosis, facial paresis, and respiratory distress. NMG usually resolves within 3 weeks but occasionally persists for as long as 4 months. This spontaneous improvement is most likely due to gradual degradation of the maternally derived IgG in a newborn baby. NMG symptoms usually respond to

AChEIs, and ventilatory support should be used as necessary until the weakness resolves.

Arthrogryposis Multiplex Congenita

Maternal MG is a rare cause of arthrogryposis multiplex congenita (AMC), which consists of nonprogressive multiple congenital joint contracture developing in utero from lack of fetal movements caused by maternal AChR antibodies to fetal AChR.

Breastfeeding

The American Academy of Pediatrics classifies pyridostigmine and steroids as compatible with breastfeeding and methotrexate as contraindicated during breastfeeding.[91] Though there is no firm data for the safety of other immunosuppressants, generally breastfeeding is not recommended.

Thymoma

Thymoma is an epithelial neoplasm of the thymus and represents the most common primary neoplasm of the anterior superior mediastinum. The majority of thymomas are completely encapsulated, but in one third of cases there may be invasion of the tumor capsule or the surrounding structure (invasive thymoma or malignant thymoma).

MG is common in thymoma (T-MG), occurring in approximately 44% of patients. Conversely, 10% to 15% of MG patients have thymoma. Thymoma occurs in MG at any age. However, it is much more common among middle-aged and older patients. MG tends to be more severe in patients with thymoma than early-onset MG subgroup and has a poorer prognosis than MG without thymoma, requiring long-term immunotherapy with prednisone, AZA, or other immunosuppressive drugs.

When the diagnosis of T-MG is established, thymoma should be removed surgically ensuring radical excision. The removal of the thymoma does cure the thymic neoplasia in most cases, but MG symptoms usually continue after thymectomy.

The pharmacologic treatment of T-MG is not different from nonparaneoplastic MG, except for administration of tacrolimus, which should be considered in difficult cases. Tacrolimus, an immunosuppressant and enhancer of ryanodine receptor (RyR)-related sarcoplasmic calcium release, is beneficial in MG patients with RyR antibodies that in theory might block the RyR. It seems to have a purely symptomatic effect in addition to its immunosuppressive effects. Because most patients with T-MG have RyR antibodies, tacrolimus may act specifically in T-MG patients.

The first antibodies described in MG in 1960 were the striational muscle (SM) antibodies and the main antigens were later identified as titin and RyR. In patients with thymoma alone, 24% had antibodies. When MG and thymoma were present, 80% to 90% had antibodies; in MG without tumor, 38% had antibodies.[92] There is a correlation between the titer of SM antibody and the likelihood of a thymoma. The appearance of thymic enlargement on the computed tomography (CT) scan and a high titer of AS antibody make the diagnosis of thymoma virtually certain. More specific striational muscle antibody tests against titin and RyR have become available in recent years. Approximately 95% and 70% of thymoma MG patients have titin and RyR antibodies, respectively,[93] and 58% and 6% of late-onset MG patients have titin and RyR antibodies, respectively. Titin- and RyR-antibody tests and CT scan of the mediastinum share similar sensitivity for thymoma in MG. Skeie and Romi claimed that the presence of titin and RyR antibodies in an MG patient younger than 60 years strongly suggests a thymoma, and the absence of such antibodies at any age strongly excludes thymoma.[93]

Treatment of thymoma is determined after the lesion has been staged (class III). In general, complete surgical resection of the tumor is the preferred treatment. This is the treatment of choice in stage I tumor (noninvasive thymoma), given the very low recurrence rate. In invasive thymoma (stages II, III, and IV), adjuvant radiation therapy is recommended to inhibit recurrence of tumor.

Radiation Therapy

Mediastinal irradiation at a dose ranging from 45 to 55 Gy was performed postoperatively in patients with invasive thymoma. This therapy has been used for a long period of time and most experts agree that adjuvant radiotherapy (presurgical, postsurgical, or both) may improve the prognosis of these patients.

Chemotherapy was carried out according to standard cisplatin-based protocols consisting of doxorubicin (50 mg/m^2 IV day 1)/cyclophosphamide (500 mg/m^2 IV day 1)/cisplatin (50 mg/m^2 IV day 1) or etoposide (100 mg/m^2 IV days 1–3)/cisplatin (80 mg/m^2 IV day 1); cycles were repeated every 3 weeks. At this time, this treatment is controversial as to whether the chemotherapy regimen is superior alone or in combination with radiation therapy.

Tumor surveillance was performed by CT scan every 1 to 2 years along with periodic tests of the serologic marker for thymoma, striate muscle antibody.

Preoperative Therapy for Thymoma Surgery

Unless there is a compelling medical indication, there is no reason to rush to surgery. My recommendation is to stabilize these patients' MG status first with an aggressive therapy, including steroids, plasma exchange, and IVIg, before subjecting them to surgery.

Drugs and Agents Unmasking or Aggravating Myasthenia Gravis

Many drugs and agents are known to unmask MG or aggravate MG symptoms.[94,95] Except for penicillamine, no drugs are absolutely contraindicated in patients with MG or LEMS. Drugs and agents are listed in Box 18-1 as definite, probable, and possible in the order of probability of cause.

General Guidelines for Therapeutic Management of Myasthenia Gravis

There are many regimens for the therapeutic management of MG. Treatment regimens vary among physicians from different parts of the world and even among different centers from the same country. Steroids are popular in the United States, while AZA is preferred in Europe and tacrolimus in Japan (Table 18-5).

The guidelines presented here are the University of Alabama at Birmingham protocol based on the general consensus, best knowledge, and the UAB experience and should be used as general, rather than strict, guidelines (Fig. 18-3).

Once the diagnosis of MG is established, AChEIs are used for symptomatic treatment in all MG patients, and thymoma, when found, should be removed by thymectomy. CT scan of the mediastinum without contrast agent is the image of choice for thymoma. When MG symptoms are not well controlled with AChEIs alone at a maximal daily recommended dose (<1 g/day), steroids are chosen as the first-line immunosuppressive therapy, mainly for short-term immunotherapy. However, steroids may be used as long-term therapy if pharmacologic remission can be achieved with a minimal dose (less than 10 mg of prednisone a day) without undue side effects. If MG symptoms are not well controlled with AChEIs and steroids within a reasonable time (6 months), AZA is chosen as the second-line immunosuppressive therapy, mainly for long-term therapy or to reduce the dose of steroids. For the third-line immunosuppressive therapy, we prefer MM because of minimal side-effect profile, not based on the best evidence. CsA and tacrolimus are the fourth-line immunosuppressive therapy. The choice of CsA or tacrolimus depends on one's experience. CPP is the least preferred immunosuppressive therapy because of serious

Table 18-5 Evidence-Based Class and Recommendation of Various Immunotherapies

Drug/Therapy	Evidence Class*	Recommendation(s)
AChEIs	Class IV	Symptomatic treatment
Steroids	Class II	First-line immunotherapy agent. Mainly for short-term use. For long-term use if the dose can be reduced to a level at which side reactions are negligible.
Azathioprine (AZA)	Class I	Second-line immunotherapy. Mainly for long-term use. Can be used to reduce the steroid dose, or for patients unresponsive to or intolerant of steroids.
Cyclosporine	Class I	Fourth-line immunotherapy. Mainly for long-term use. For patients intolerant of or unresponsive to steroids or AZA.
Cyclophosphamide	Class II	Last-choice agent for long-term immunotherapy. For patients unresponsive to or intolerant of steroids, AZA, cyclosporine, or tacrolimus.
Myocophenolate mofetil	Class IV	Third-line immunotherapy. Mainly for long-term use. This can be used as an additional agent to any long-term immunosuppressant.
Tacrolimus	Class I	Fourth-line immunotherapy. For patients unresponsive to or intolerant of steroid, AZA, or cyclosporine.
Plasma exchange	Class III	Indicated for severe MG, acute exacerbation, and MG crisis. For patients unresponsive to or intolerant of IVIg.
IVIg	Class I	Indicated for severe MG and acute exacerbation and used as adjunctive immunotherapy agent to maintain an improved status. For patients unresponsive to or intolerant of plasma exchange.
Thymectomy	Class II	Any patient with early-onset generalized MG who needs immunotherapy is candidate.

*Evidence class I: randomized controlled trials available; class II: controlled trials without randomization or randomized trial with small patient number; class III: uncontrolled trials; class IV: case series.
AChEIs, acetylcholinesterase inhibitors; IVIg, intravenous immunoglobulin; MG, myasthenia gravis.

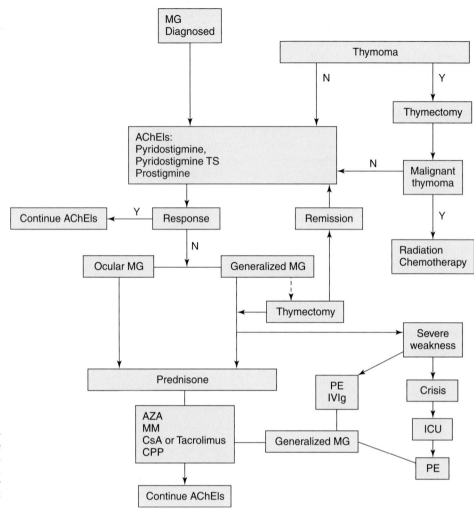

Figure 18-3 Treatment algorithm in myasthenia gravis (MG). AChEIs, acetylcholine esterase inhibitors; AZA, azathioprine; CPP, cyclophosphamide; CsA, cyclosporine A; ICU, intensive care unit; IVIg, intravenous immunoglobulin; MM, mycophenolate mofetil; N, no; PE, plasma exchange; TS, time span; Y, yes.

potential side effects, not based on the best evidence. We prefer MM as an adjunct agent to any long-term immunosuppressant because of minimal side-effect profile, not based on the best evidence, and thus is the last choice of immunosuppressive therapy.

We believe that thymectomy is indicated in any early-onset MG (<60 years of age) patients in whom generalized MG is not satisfactorily controlled with AChEIs alone (class IV). This is done with the understanding that thymectomy induces long-term improvement and remission. Thymectomy should be done when MG is stable.

Plasma exchange is the treatment of choice for MG crisis. PE and IVIg are recommended for rapidly worsening MG patients for short-term improvement (class III for PE and class I for IVIg). Intermittent IVIg can also be used as an adjuvant to long-term immunosuppressive therapy (class IV), a definite advantage of IVIg over PE.

Lambert-Eaton Myasthenic Syndrome

Lambert-Eaton myasthenic syndrome (LEMS) is an autoimmune disease clinically characterized by easy fatigability, proximal leg weakness, paucity of oculobulbar symptoms, and hyporeflexia. The main defect in this disorder is the insufficient release of ACh at the presynaptic membrane, possibly induced by the antibodies against voltage-gated calcium channels (VGCCs). A recent study showed that this antibody was found in 52% of LEMS patients for the N type and in 90% of LEMS patients for the P/Q type.[96]

The clinical, electrophysiologic, and pharmacologic differences between MG and LEMS are given in Table 18-6. The clinical diagnosis of LEMS is almost always elusive. According to our experience, it can mimic MG, myopathy, motor neuropathy, conversion reaction, or lumbar radiculopathy. Clinical suspicion is the key for the diagnosis of LEMS. The most common symptoms are easy fatigability and leg weakness. The classic clinical triad of LEMS includes proximal leg weakness, hyporeflexia or areflexia, and cholinergic dysautonomia (dry mouth, impotence, and orthostatic hypotension). A transient improvement in muscle strength and reflexes immediately after brief exercise is classically observed in these patients. These findings, if observed, are pathognomonic of LEMS. This facilitation is most easily detected in moderately affected muscles, often the deltoid or iliopsoas muscles. This is the clinical counterpart of postexercise facilitation (PEF) on the RNS test. Unfortunately, these are not common observations, being noted in one out of three cases, according to our experience.[97] Thus, when LEMS is suspected, these simple bedside tests are extremely helpful for confirmation of the disease. With brief exercise and tetanic nerve stimulation, more calcium is available at the presynaptic membrane, which increases ACh release, subsequently improving neuromuscular transmission. This is an explanation for postexercise improvement of muscle strength or reflexes.

LEMS is a pivotal example of a paraneoplastic neurologic syndrome. From the first description of LEMS, its association with

Table 18-6 Differences between Myasthenia Gravis and Lambert-Eaton Myasthenic Syndrome

	Myasthenia Gravis	Lambert-Eaton Myasthenic Syndrome
Sex	F:M = 2:1	F:M = 2:3
Presenting signs	Weakness of ocular, bulbar, and facial muscles	Weakness of proximal leg muscles
Exertion	Exertional weakness	Transient improvement after brief exercise followed by weakness
Reflexes	Normal	Reduced or absent
Tumor	Thymoma in 16% of cases	Small cell carcinoma of the lung in 50% of cases
Basic defect	Postsynaptic defect	Presynaptic defect
RNS test		
CMAP		
At rest	Normal	Low
After exercise	No change	Marked increase
Low-rate stimulation	Decremental response	Decremental response
High-rate stimulation	Normal or decrement	Incremental response
Antibodies	AChR-ab (+) in 85%	VGCC-ab (+) in 90%
Drugs	AChEls	Guanidine, aminopyridine
Immunotherapies	Steroids, immunosupressants, plasmapheresis, and IVIg	Steroids, immunosupressants, plasmapheresis, and IVIg
Thymectomy	Effective	Not indicated

CMAP, compound muscle action potentials; RNS, repetitive nerve stimulation.

small cell cancer of the lung (SCLC) has been well known. As noted previously, an earlier study showed that 73% of LEMS patients had SCLC, whereas a more recent study showed this association in only 50% of cases, suggesting a trend toward a lower tumor frequency in recent years. Certainly, a smoking history is a risk factor for LEMS because it is a risk factor for SCLC. It is estimated that LEMS occurs in about 3% of patients with SCLC. Though other tumors have been reported to be associated with the disease, most cancer associated with it is due to SCLC. A recent study suggested that lymphoproliferative disorders may constitute another risk group for LEMS.

LEMS is a disease of the elderly, with the most common age of onset of symptoms being about 60 years of age. Paraneoplastic LEMS typically develops in the middle-aged to elderly and was originally seen more commonly in men. More recent studies showed less male predominance. Our latest series showed a 1:1 ratio. Paraneoplastic LEMS was clearly more common in males, whereas autoimmune LEMS was more frequent in females. In subjects younger than 30 years of age, the chance of cancer association was small. Usually the discovery of LEMS preceded that of cancer by several months to years. In all cases, cancer developed within 4 years following diagnosis of LEMS. Thus, it is important to do a workup for occult cancer, especially SCLC, at the time of diagnosis of LEMS and serially thereafter, as noted. There are no clinical and electrophysiologic differences that distinguish paraneoplastic LEMS from autoimmune LEMS. According to our experience, cancer is less likely associated with LEMS if the patient is a young female and if cancer is not found within 4 years after the diagnosis of LEMS is made.

The diagnosis of LEMS can only be confirmed by the RNS test.

Diagnosis and Evaluation

The RNS test in LEMS is characterized by a presynaptic NMT block: (1) low CMAP, (2) dramatic PEF, (3) decremental response at LRS, (4) marked incremental response at high-rate stimulation (HRS), and (5) prominent PTF but less prominent PTE (Fig. 18-4).[10] Low CMAP has been noted in 95% of cases in this disorder. In many

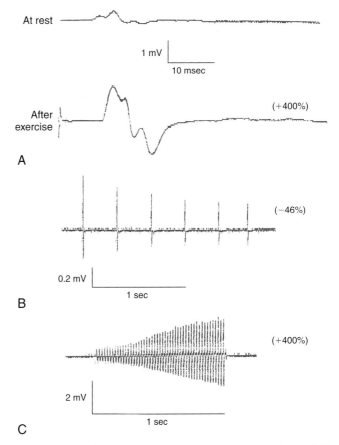

Figure 18-4 Typical repetitive nerve stimulation pattern in the abductor digiti quinti muscle in Lambert-Eaton myasthenic syndrome. **A,** Low compound muscle action potential amplitude at rest, marked incremental response (+400%) after 30 seconds of exercise. **B,** Decremental response (−46%) at low-rate stimulation (3 Hz). **C,** Marked incremental response (+400%) at high-rate stimulation (50 Hz).

patients, it is extremely low. The most dramatic increase in the CMAP amplitude after exercise (PEF) has been noted in this disease. Lambert et al (1961) observed a 120% to 1800% increase in the CMAP amplitude in LEMS patients.[98] This is in contrast to a 15% increase for normal individuals and a 94% increase for MG patients. Thus, a more than 100% increase in the CMAP amplitude after exercise is considered to be typical of LEMS. In our series, PEF was not observed in 27% of patients because of lack of cooperation or severe weakness of the hand muscles. Thus, although this test alone is not sufficient to rule out LEMS, it is a simple and relatively painless procedure that should be performed in all suspected cases because it is abnormal in a majority of LEMS patients. In almost all cases, a decremental response has been noted at LRS. In our series, a decremental response was present in 93% of cases.[10] The most dramatic facilitation at HRS was seen in this disease. In all cases, there was an incremental response at HRS, ranging from 100% to 4000%. A more than 100% incremental response at HRS is almost pathognomonic of LEMS. Our recent study showed that a more than 60% increment in PEF or at HRS is sufficient for the diagnosis of LEMS. This study also showed that the RNS test is more typical of LEMS and more abnormal in the seropositive LEMS group, and that the classic triad (low CMAP amplitude, decrement at LRS, and increment at PEF or HRS) is rare in the seronegative group.[100]

P/Q type VGCC antibody is positive in 90% of LEMS patients. Measurement of VGCC antibodies is helpful in the diagnosis. The workup should also include a CT scan of the chest for small cell carcinoma of the lung and, if negative, more extensive workup could be necessary particularly searching for breast and ovarian tumors in females. If cancer is not found, an autoimmune etiology should be considered and patients should be studied for other autoimmune disorders.

Treatment and Management

Symptomatic Treatment

In contrast to MG, in which symptomatic improvement is achieved by AChEIs, which increase the availability of ACh at the postsynaptic membrane, in LEMS symptomatic improvement is achieved by two agents that increase a release of ACh at the presynaptic membrane.

Guanidine

Guanidine acts on the presynaptic neuromuscular junction by increasing the number of ACh quanta released from the immediately available pool on nerve impulse by blocking potassium channels and thus prolonging the nerve terminal action potential or by a facilitating effect on the nerve terminal calcium channels.[101] Thus, this is an ideal for symptomatic treatment of LEMS and has been used since 1966. It was mostly studied in case reports and has not been studied in randomized trials. Guanidine was used in about 50 LEMS cases and clinical improvement was reported in most cases. Two papers describe a larger series, both of nine patients. Improvement ranged from "slight to dramatic." Electrophysiologic improvement was also reported in two studies. In the RNS test, all parameters improved in all tested cases. However, the most definite improvement was in the CMAP amplitude. SFEMG showed improvement in two of three tested cases.[102]

The most common side effects are gastrointestinal symptoms and distal paresthesia. Such reactions are known to occur even at very low doses and are usually mild and transient. Moreover, gastrointestinal troubles induced by guanidine are easily controlled by antacids or atropine. Thus, these problems alone are not an indication for discontinuation of treatment. In one series, gastrointestinal symptoms were the most common side effects, as observed in 50% of cases, and medication had to be discontinued in a few cases.

The most common serious side effects of guanidine are hematologic abnormalities and renal insufficiency. In most reported cases, hematologic abnormalities developed in the early course of the high-dose therapy and were reversible. Norris et al's study in motor neuron disease, which is probably the largest series of guanidine trials, reported five cases (2.5%) of bone marrow suppression among 200 patients.[103] This finding emphasizes the importance of routine monthly blood tests during the first few months in guanidine-treated patients until a safe dose level is established.

In contrast, less commonly reported guanidine-induced renal insufficiency tended to develop after longer use (mean duration: 26 months) and with a dose higher than 1000 mg/day in three cases. It is most likely to be irreversible. Up to this time, there has been no reported case of guanidine-induced renal insufficiency with a total daily dose of guanidine less than 1000 mg/day.

Low-dose guanidine (less than 1000 mg a day) was used together with pyridostigmine in nine LEMS patients who participated in an open trial.[102] Mean treatment duration was 3 years, during which time three participants stopped taking guanidine due to persistent gastrointestinal side effects. Combination treatment was beneficial in terms of muscle strength and electrophysiologic CMAP amplitude measurements in all nine participants. There were no reported serious side effects. Another study described the successful change of daily low-dose guanidine therapy (10 mg/kg) into an alternate-day regimen, after the patient had developed neutropenia on the daily dose. These observations suggest that the effect of guanidine is dose-dependent with minor side effects at 5 to 10 mg/kg/day and at a ceiling dose of 30 mg/kg/day.

Aminopyridine

Aminopyridine, a potassium channel blocker, increases ACh release at the presynaptic level by prolonging the duration of nerve action potential at central, autonomic, and neuromuscular synapses.

4-Aminopyridine (4-AP) was used for the symptomatic treatment of LEMS in open trials in nine patients, who experienced clinical and electrophysiologic improvement.[104] However, seizures occurred in two patients. The threat of serious central nervous system (CNS) side effects has thus limited the use of 4-AP, a drug known to cross the blood–brain barrier and result in epileptogenic effects in animals.

3,4-Diaminopyridine (3,4-DAP) has been shown in animals to be more potent in improving neuromuscular transmission and less convulsant than 4-AP. In addition, it has an advantage over 4-AP because it crosses the blood–brain barrier less readily, resulting in fewer CNS side effects. The first use of 3,4-DAP was in three patients with LEMS without lung cancer, and clinical and electrophysiologic improvement was noted in all three patients. Since then, the clinical effectiveness of 3,4-DAP in LEMS has been consistently well documented in repeated case reports and one open trial in more than 70 cases.[104]

So far there have been three randomized, placebo-controlled trials of 3,4-DAP in patients with LEMS. McEvoy et al found a significant dose-related improvement with 3,4-DAP in three independent measurements (neurologic disability score, isometric strength testing, and CMAP amplitude) in 12 patients in a randomized, double-blind cross-over study.[105] Sanders et al found a significantly greater improvement in two measurements (QMG score and the summated CMAP) in 12 3,4-DAP patients in comparison with 14 placebo patients in a prospective randomized study.[106] Oh et al reported a significant improvement in all listed primary endpoints (subjective symptoms, LEMS classification, muscle strength score, QMG score, and CMAP) in a double-blind, placebo-controlled, cross-over trial of 3,4-DAP compared with placebo in seven patients.[107]

The usual effective dose of 3,4-DAP in LEMS is 20 to 60 mg/day[101] and the ceiling dose is 60 mg/day. The drug is well tolerated with only mild side effects as long as the dose is kept below 60 mg/day. Patients notice the onset of effect less than 30 minutes after taking a dose, and benefit from a single dose, which lasts for 2.5 to 4 hours. Many patients notice a cumulative effect of fixed doses, with the maximum response occurring 3 to 4 days after a dose change. DAP effects begin to wear off after less than 8 hours following the last dose and have cleared entirely in less than 2 days. Mild side effects include perioral or acral parethesias, lightheadedness, epigastric distress, nausea, anxiety, and insomnia.[101] The only major side reactions reported so far have been seizures in three patients on a 100 mg daily dose,[108] chorea in one patient after 5 years of continuous use,[104] and cardiac arrest from iatrogenic overdose (360 mg/day) of the medication. Lundh et al reported drug tolerance to 3,4-DAP in three patients after several months of treatment.[104] The responsiveness to the drug was restored after a few weeks of "drug holiday," which was confirmed by repeated EMG testing. Because of the possible serious side effects of guanidine and 4-aminopyridine,[99] 3,4-DAP was preferred for treatment in LEMS. In Europe, 3,4-DAP has become the mainstay of symptomatic treatment of LEMS and was approved for LEMS in 2009.

AChE Inhibitors

Pyridostigmine has been used for symptomatic treatment in more than 80 cases since 1953, when the first case of LEMS was reported. The edrophonium test was reported to be positive in 37% of tested cases in LEMS, which is understandable in view of the clinical similarity between MG and LEMS. As in MG, repeated doses at 4-hour intervals are used. Several papers describe monotherapy with pyridostigmine as having no effect on clinical signs or symptoms. A double-blind, placebo-controlled, cross-over study found significant improvement of CMAP amplitude and muscle strength with IV administration of 3,4-DAP but not with pyridostigmine. A minimal to moderate response was reported in five patients among more than 80 treated cases in an extensive review.[101] Thus, there seems to be a consensus in available literature that AChE inhibitors alone are ineffective in LEMS. On the other hand, two studies from centers with extensive experience in LEMS treatment showed that pyridostigmine alone can be effective in mild LEMS cases. In our study of 14 patients who had symptomatic treatment longer than 3 months, pyridostigmine alone (180–1200 mg/day) was used to maximum benefit in six patients, including two who could not take guanidine because of adverse side effects.[102] We found that, in some mild LEMS cases, pyridostigmine alone is enough to induce a satisfactory symptomatic improvement when LEMS is stable with immunotherapy or anticancer therapy.[108] Lundh et al tested the oral administration of pyridostigmine, 3,4-DAP, and combinations of both drugs on consecutive days as the test protocol.[104] They found only slight improvement at 60 mg and a more clear-cut effect at 120 mg on the clinical tests as well as in the CMAP in the test protocol. They reported that a few of 19 LEMS patients did well on pyridostigmine alone.

A combined therapy of pyridostigmine and guanidine or 3,4-DAP seems to be a favored treatment at many centers. As discussed previously, we preferred a liberal use of pyridostigmine and low-dose guanidine (less than 1000 mg/day) for LEMS. Several reports suggest a potentiation of the therapeutic effect of 3,4-DAP with pyridostigmine. Lundh et al reported that addition of pyridostigmine to 3,4-DAP improved the step test performance, though it did not significantly improve the limb elevation tests or CMAP, and that many patients benefited from combined treatment with both

drugs.[104] In McEvoy et al's study, 4 of 12 patients had pyridostigmine added to DAP during the follow-up period.[105] In Sanders et al's series, 25 patients participated in an open-label DAP trial.[106] All but three improved by at least two QMG score points, usually with pyridostigmine. In Tim's study, 53 patients were treated with DAP and pyridostigmine, with 79% reporting functional improvement.[109] These findings indicate that, in practice, many patients on 3,4-DAP need additional pyridostigmine to maintain an improved status in LEMS.

Immunotherapy
Considering that LEMS is an autoimmune disorder, immunotherapy should be the mainstay of treatment. IVIg is the only therapy in which a rigorous controlled study showed effectiveness.[110]

Immunosuppressive Therapy
Clinical improvement with steroids was first reported in 1969 in one patient after 2 weeks of treatment with prednisone. Three other patients were reported to show clinical improvement with a high dose of prednisone: onset of improvement within 2 weeks and maximal improvement in 3 to 4 months. In Tim's series, nine (28%) of 32 patients showed moderate improvement with prednisone.[109] A combination of steroid therapy with AZA was reported to be more effective than prednisone monotherapy.[111] Three of six non-cancer LEMS patients achieved almost complete remission of symptoms within a year of beginning treatment with prednisone and AZA. The remaining three patients also improved but to a lesser degree (two patients were intolerant of AZA and received prednisone alone). Similar improvements were seen in resting CMAP amplitudes. Because of concern about its carcinogenic properties, AZA is not recommended for paraneoplastic LEMS. In this connection, MM may be an alternative: the kidney transplant patients on MM had a lower incidence of cancer in the long-term follow-up. So far there has not been any trial with other immunosuppressants in LEMS. Most experts recommend immunosuppressive treatment in patients who are unresponsive to symptomatic treatment and specific tumor therapy. Newsom-Davis prefers prednisone for paraneoplastic LEMS and prednisone combined with AZA for nonparaneoplastic LEMS.[112]

Immunomodulating Therapy
One randomized, double-blind, placebo-controlled study showed a significant improvement in myometric strength and a significant decline in serum VGCC antibody titers with IVIg compared with placebo in nine patients compared with placebo.[110] One gram of IVIg was given during 2 consecutive days. The beneficial effect on strength was maximal 2 to 4 weeks after treatment. VGCC titer decreased rapidly in the first week and became normal after 3 weeks.

Several studies reported a marked clinical improvement in LEMS patients after treatment with either PE or IVIg: four studies dealing with one to nine patients receiving PE and five studies dealing with three patients on IVIg.[108] In Tim's study, a marked improvement was reported in 2 (11%) of 19 patients with PE and in 7 (41%) of 17 patients with IVIg.[109] They stated that the benefit was transient with PE or IVIg.

In the best open trial study of PE, serial clinical and CMAP amplitude assessment was done in nine patients over 0.5 to 2.5 years.[111] Eight of nine patients showed a short-term clinical and EMG improvement with PE. The improvement in muscle strength developed after a longer time interval (about 10 days) than was the case with MG, where the response was typically evident within 2 days.[111] This suggests a slower turnover rate of VGCCs as compared with

AChR-Ab. Improvement peaked at 2 weeks and subsided by 6 weeks. PE and IVIg are indicated in severely weak patients.

Tumor Treatment in Lambert-Eaton Myasthenic Syndrome

Unlike other paraneoplastic neurologic syndromes, which are usually resistant to any therapy, LEMS is known to be consistently responsive to immunotherapy or anticancer therapy.[113] Thus, treatment of cancer is of paramount importance in paraneoplastic LEMS. Successful cancer treatment may result in remission or otherwise in improvement as noted in several case reports and two small series. Tumors are implicated as the initial site of VGCC antibody production in paraneoplastic LEMS.[101] Therefore, treatment of the tumor, especially its surgical removal, would presumably reduce or even eliminate the antigenic driving of the autoantibody response. Aggressive therapy for cancer is recommended. A small retrospective study showed that 7 of 11 paraneoplastic-LEMS patients surviving specific tumor therapy by more than 2 months subsequently showed progressive improvement in their neurologic symptoms, and 3 patients had improvement followed by a relapse. Specific tumor therapy in a small retrospective series resulted in recovery from LEMS within 6 to 12 months.[113] This was confirmed by a parallel recovery in the CMAP amplitudes, which in all patients studied had returned to the normal range within 6 to 12 months of starting therapy. The specific tumor therapy included chemotherapy, surgical resection, and local radiation therapy. Chemotherapy is the first choice in SCLC and this will have an additional immunosuppressive effect. The standard regimen for the treatment of SCLC is combination chemotherapy with cisplatin and etoposide (EP regimen). Anthracyclin-based regimens with CPP, doxorubicin, and vincristine (CAV regimen) have also been widely used. Thoracic radiation therapy and prophylactic cranial radiation therapy are also offered to patients with limited-stage disease who respond to chemotherapy. Despite a high chemosensitivity and trials with different combinations of therapy, SCLC remains associated with a poor long-term survival. Less than 10% of the patients survive longer than 2 years.[114] A recent study showed a significant prolonged survival in 15 SCLC LEMS patients compared to matched SCLC patients without LEMS. These findings suggest that the autoimmune response elicited by the tumor might help to slow down the growth of the SCLC.

Drugs Aggravating Lambert-Eaton Myasthenic Syndrome

Competitive neuromuscular blocking agents such as *d*-tubocurarine and pancuronium, magnesium agents, diltiazem, verapamil, ofloxacin, botulinum toxin, and muscle relaxants are reported as aggravating LEMS in isolated cases.[101] Varenicline (Chantix) and cephalexin unmasked LEMS in one case each. Many drugs which induce or aggravate MG may also aggravate LEMS.

General Guidelines for the Therapeutic Management of Lambert-Eaton Myasthenic Syndrome

The guidelines presented here are the UAB protocol based on the general consensus, the best knowledge, and UAB experience and should be used as general guidelines, rather than strict directives (Fig. 18-5).

Once the diagnosis of LEMS is established, 3,4-DAP is the drug of choice for symptomatic treatment (class I). This will virtually always produce symptomatic improvement. If 3,4-DAP is not available, certainly guanidine HCl is an alternative choice, usually along with a liberal dose of pyridostigmine (class VI; label B). Some LEMS patients find that the addition of pyridostigmine to 3,4-DAP treatment is beneficial.

The next important workup at the time of diagnosis of LEMS is to confirm the SCLC because it is found in half the LEMS patients at the time of or within 2 years of diagnosis. The best diagnostic test for SCLC is a high-resolution chest CT scan and possibly also a bronchoscopy and 18-fluorine fluro-2-deoxyglucose positron emission tomography (FDG-PET) scan if the CT scan is negative. This is especially important for patients with a high risk of SCLC (history of smoking and older patients). Follow-up should be continued with a CT scan every 6 months for at least 4 years.

Once the diagnosis of SCLC is established, treatment of cancer will be implemented in its own right, but an added benefit is that it induces an improvement of LEMS symptoms. Chemotherapy is the first choice in SCLC because it has an additional immunosuppressive effect. The presence of LEMS in a patient with SCLC is known to improve survival.

If symptomatic treatment is insufficient, the next step is immunosuppressive therapy, usually with high-dose steroid (class IV) regardless of whether the patient has SCLC. When remission has been obtained in LEMS, the prednisone dose should be tapered to the minimum required to maintain remission. As a long-term immunosuppressive medication, AZA is the first choice for autoimmune LEMS (class IV). However, for paraneoplastic LEMS, this agent is not recommended because of the concern about the carcinogenic property of AZA. In this connection, MM may be an alternative (level C).

For the second-line choice for long-term immunosuppressive medication, one can choose IVIg (intermittent use) (class I). CsA and MM are other alternatives.[115] However, this recommendation is based on MG, not on LEMS. Personally, none of our patients needed CsA or MM for long-term immunosuppression.

For patients with severe LEMS, IVIg is the treatment of choice because it is shown to be beneficial in short-term treatment (class I). PE may be an alternative treatment if IVIg is not effective (class IV).

Respiratory and bulbar muscle weakness, rare in LEMS, can occasionally be life-threatening. In patients with such severe weakness, PE can produce a short-term benefit when given as a 5-day course (class IV).

Botulism

Botulism is an uncommon, but a potentially life-threatening neuroparalytic syndrome caused by a potent neurotoxin produced by *Clostridium botulinum*. Botulism is both an old and an emerging disease. The classic foodborne botulism was first reported more than 100 years ago and new forms of botulism were added in the 20th century with the newest addition of Botox-induced botulism.

C. botulinum is a gram-positive spore-forming anaerobic bacterium found in soil throughout the world. Spores of *C. botulinum* are ubiquitous and not dangerous in themselves when ingested. When spores germinate in an anaerobic environment, they produce botulinum toxin, one of the most potent neurotoxins in human beings. It has been estimated that doses as small as 0.05 to 0.1 µg can cause death. Unlike the toxin, which is heat-labile, the spores are relatively heat-resistant. A temperature of 120° C may be required to kill the spores, although heating at 85° C inactivates the toxin.

Eight strains of *C. botulinum* are known to produce antigenically distinct toxins (A, B, C1, C2, D, E, F, and G). In human subjects, A, B, and E strains are almost always involved, and the F strain is

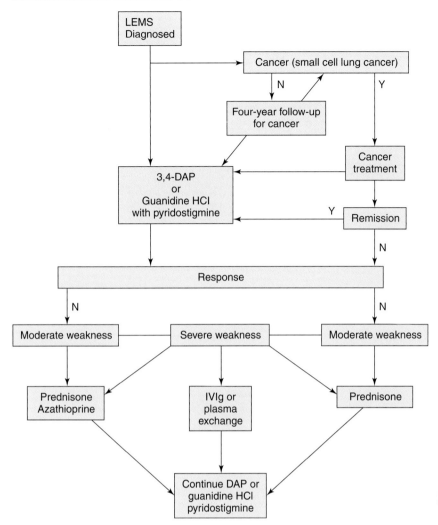

Figure 18-5 Treatment algorithm in Lambert-Eaton myasthenic syndrome (LEMS). 3,4-DAP, 3,4-diaminopyridine; IVIg, intravenous immunoglobulin; N, no; Y, yes.

extremely rare. Recent studies show that recovery time from paralysis in type A poisoning is longer than that from type E.[116]

Six distinct clinical syndromes have been described: (1) foodborne botulism, (2) infant botulism, (3) wound botulism, (4) adult variant of "infant botulism," (5) Botox-induced botulism, and (6) inhalational botulism.

Among these, the first three syndromes are clinically more important because the latter three syndromes are rare. (See Table 18-7 for botulism subtypes.)

Types of Botulism

Foodborne Botulism

Foodborne botulism is caused by ingestion of preformed toxins in foods that have not been canned or preserved properly. European cases most commonly are associated with type B contamination of home-processed meats, but Alaskan, Canadian, and Japanese outbreaks often involve type E toxin in preserved seafood.[117] By far, home-processed foods are responsible for most (94%) outbreaks of foodborne botulism in the United States. In the United States, vegetables are the most commonly implicated foods in types A and B outbreaks, and fish or fish products are responsible for type E outbreaks. The toxin type most often responsible for foodborne botulism corresponds well with the geographic distribution of the toxinogenic species. Most of the type A outbreaks have occurred

west of the Mississippi River, and most of the type B outbreaks occurred in the East. Most type E poisoning was distributed around the Great Lakes and in Alaska. Toxin A produces a more severe illness than type B, and type E is least severe.

Botulinum toxin is primarily absorbed by the upper gastrointestinal tract, but toxin reaching the lower small bowel and colon may be slowly absorbed, thus perhaps accounting for the delayed onset and prolonged duration of symptoms seen in many patients with clinical botulism. The mortality rate is around 3% to 5% at present.

Infant Botulism

Infant botulism was first described in 1976 and is the most common form of botulism in the United States at this time, exceeding the foodborne botulism. Infant botulism results from toxin produced in vivo from the intestinal colonization of C. botulinum in infants younger than 6 months. The infant intestinal tract often lacks both the protective bacterial flora and the Clostridium-inhibiting bile acids found in the normal adult intestinal tract. Type B is more common than type A in infant botulism. Clinical features in these infants included acute onset of constipation, poor sucking, weak cry, hypotonia, and muscle weakness. Loss of head control was particularly striking. Ophthalmoplegia, ptosis, flaccid facial expression, pooled oral secretions, dysphagia, and a weak gag reflex were frequent. With adequate supportive care, most infants recovered in weeks or months

Table 18-7 Clinical, Diagnostic, and Therapeutic Features of Subtypes of Botulism

Feature	Food Botulism	Wound Botulism	Infant Botulism
Prevalence	Rare	Mainly in injection drug users Most common in California	Most common form in the United States Infants <6 months of age
Source of infection	Ingestion of preformed toxin in the ingested food	Toxin from organisms in the wound	Toxin from organisms in the infant intestine
Fever	Absent	May be present if other infections are present	Absent
Incubation	6 hr–8 days	4–14 days	3–30 days
Gastrointestinal symptoms	May be present: nausea and vomiting	Absent	Almost always: constipation
Sensory deficit	Absent	Unilateral sensory deficits may be present	Absent
Botulinum toxin in serum	Present	Present	Rarely present
Diagnosis	Toxin in serum; toxin and *Clostridium botulinum* in food and its container, gastric contents, vomitus and feces	Toxin in serum Toxin and *C. botulinum* in wound	Toxin or *C. botulinum* in feces
Treatment	Trivalent antitoxin Laxative or enema	Wound débridement Antibiotics for other bacteria Trivalent antitoxin	Intravenous botulinum immunoglobulin (BIG-IV)

without sequelae. The mortality rate (1%) was low compared to foodborne botulism (5%). On rare occasions (5%), infants may show a recurrence of symptoms.

Wound Botulism

Wound botulism is caused by systemic spread of the toxin produced by *C. botulinum* in the anaerobic milieu of abscess and is associated with trauma, surgery, subcutaneous heroin injection (recently, black tar injection), and sinusitis from intranasal cocaine abuse. Through 1992, only one to three cases of wound botulism were reported in the United States each year. Since 1992, the number of cases of wound botulism has increased dramatically. Nearly all these new cases have occurred in heroin-injection drug users, mostly from California. Two thirds of these cases were type A and almost one third were type B. The mortality rate was about 10%.

Adult Variant of Infant Botulism

Similar in pathogenesis to infant botulism, this form occurs in older children and adults with an abnormal bowel condition such as colitis, following an intestinal bypass procedure, or in association with other conditions that may create local or widespread disruption in the normal intestinal flora. These cases were associated with a prolonged latent period of up to 47 days after ingestion before onset of symptoms. A diagnostic clue is abnormality in the gastrointestinal tract, as described earlier. The finding of *C. botulinum* in the feces of adult patients is almost always associated with clinical botulism.

Iatrogenic Botulism

Subclinical neuromuscular transmission abnormality was discovered by SFEMG in distant muscles in patients with cervical dystonia who had received Botox treatment. Dysphagia is the most common complication of Botox injection. A case of brachial plexus neuropathy was reported following Botox injection. A few cases of frank but mild botulism were reported following injection of botulinum toxin for cosmetic or therapeutic purposes. Mostly these were from Dysport (British) botulinum toxin.

Inhalation Botulism

To date, three human cases have been the result of inadvertent inhalation of toxin by laboratory workers.

Pathophysiology

Botulinum toxins interfere with the release of ACh at the cholinergic transmission sites of the peripheral nervous system. As a rule, neuromuscular block is most prominent at these sites, producing paralysis of extraocular, bulbar, and limb muscles. Because of the involvement of the parasympathetic nervous system, autonomic dysfunction is common but less prominent and includes pupillary abnormality, paralytic ileus, urinary retention, diminution of secretions, and orthostatic hypotension. Dysautonomia is more commonly observed in type B botulism and neuromuscular block in type A.

Diagnosis and Evaluation

Clinical Manifestations

The hallmark of botulism is an acute descending symmetrical motor paralysis first affecting muscles supplied by the cranial nerves. Presenting complaints generally consisted of oculobulbar symptoms: ptosis, blurred or double vision, dysphagia, or dysarthria. These symptoms were usually followed by descending weakness and dyspnea. Dyspnea should be regarded as a warning sign of impending respiratory failure, which may require ventilatory support. Dysautonomic symptoms including dryness of the mouth, pupillary abnormalities, and ileus were frequently seen. Dilatation of the pupils was found in fewer than 50% of patients. Deep tendon reflexes were frequently depressed symmetrically or absent. Conspicuously absent was any objective sensory disturbance despite profound motor abnormality. Thus, the clinical features mimicked those of myasthenia gravis and the descending form of Guillain-Barré syndrome (GBS). In myasthenia, dysautonomic findings are lacking and reflexes are preserved. In GBS, an ascending weakness is the classical presentation and the spinal fluid protein is invariably high. In botulism, the spinal fluid protein is normal. In Fisher syndrome, a variant of the descending form of GBS, 90% of patients have autoantibodies to the GQ1b antibody in acute-phase sera.

Electrodiagnostic Features

Electrophysiologic studies are extremely helpful in the diagnosis of botulism. Because the RNS test provides the only relatively specific responses in botulism, this test has been found to be the most convincing objective evidence of botulism until microbiologic confirmation is achieved. In all cases of botulism accompanied by muscle weakness, the RNS test showed some abnormalities. The most characteristic RNS abnormalities are those of presynaptic NMT blocks: low CMAP amplitude, decremental response at LRS, and incremental response at HRS (Fig. 18-6). The most consistent electrophysiologic abnormality is an incremental response at HRS, followed by a low CMAP amplitude to a single stimulation in a clinically affected muscle. Decremental response at LRS is infrequent. Small-amplitude short-duration (SASD) motor unit action potentials (MUAPs) typical of myopathy are characteristic findings in the needle EMG. Fibrillations are observed in about 50% of cases. SFEMG typically showed increased jitter and blocking, which became less marked at the higher rate of discharge.

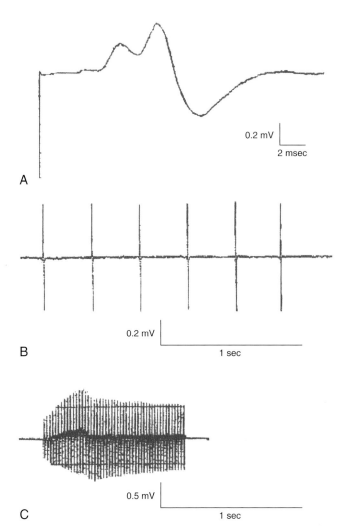

0.2 mV

2 msec

A

0.2 mV

1 sec

B

0.5 mV

1 sec

C

Figure 18-6 Typical repetitive nerve stimulation pattern in the abductor digiti quinti muscle in infant botulism. **A,** Low amplitude compound muscle action potential at rest. **B,** Normal response at low-rate stimulation (3 Hz). **C,** Incremental response (+114%) at high-rate stimulation (50 Hz).

Diagnosis

The most important clue in the diagnosis of botulism is a high index of suspicion on the basis of history and examination. A cluster of two or more patients with compatible symptoms of botulism are essentially pathognomonic of foodborne botulism, because the illnesses that resemble botulism do not produce outbreaks. Every case of botulism is a public health emergency, and the clinician should report the suspected case to the 24-hour emergency telephone number of the state health department or the Centers for Disease Control and Prevention (CDC) 24-hour botulism consultancy service (770-488-7100, the CDC Emergency Operations Center).

Diagnosis of botulism is confirmed either by detection of toxin in the serum or identification of C. botulinum organism or toxin in food or container (foodborne botulism), in tissue (wound botulism), and any gastrointestinal fluid or excretes (infant botulism or foodborne botulism). Confirmation of the diagnosis can be made in almost 75% of cases.[117] Early cases are more likely to be diagnosed by toxin assay, whereas late-onset cases are more likely to have a positive culture. If the delay in securing serum samples is more than 2 days after ingestion of the toxin, the chance of obtaining a positive test is less than 30%.[116] Only 36% of stool cultures are positive after 3 days. Laboratory confirmation of toxin presence is via a mouse bioassay, and identification of the toxin type is performed by mouse toxin neutralization test. From the time that mice are injected, final results may not be available for 24 hours or even 48 hours. In foodborne botulism, the toxin is found in serum in 39% of cases, in stool in 24% of cases, and organisms are found in cultures of stool in 55% of cases. In infant botulism, stools or enema fluid is the specimen of diagnostic choice, as serum was only rarely toxin-positive. In wound botulism, the diagnosis is confirmed by toxin in serum or by toxin or C. botulinum organisms in wound specimens. In the adult variant of infant botulism, organism may be detected in stool and toxin in serum for up to 119 days following the onset of symptoms.

Treatment and Management

Intensive Supportive Care

The most important treatment for severe botulism is an intensive supportive care with special attention to respiratory status (good practice) (see Fig. 18-3). During the first half of the 20th century in the United States, the mortality rate among patients with botulism was 60% to 70%, even when equine antitoxin was administered in heroic doses.[118] Since then, the mortality rate decreased precipitously, until it reached the current rate of 3% to 5%. This was largely due to modern intensive supportive care, principally mechanical ventilation. Thus, any patient with clinical findings or history suggestive of botulism should be hospitalized immediately and meticulously monitored for signs of respiratory failure. Mechanical ventilation should be instituted at the earliest sign of respiratory failure. Paralysis due to botulism can be protracted, lasting weeks to months, and intensive care is required during this period of recovery.

Trivalent Equine Botulism Antitoxin

Though trivalent equine botulism antitoxin has been available in the United States since 1940, its efficacy has never been evaluated in a controlled trial. The best data in this regard are from two retrospective case studies.[119,120]

Tacket and associates analyzed the clinical data on 132 cases of type A foodborne botulism reported to the CDC between 1973 and 1980.[119] The clinical data were collected from the patients' clinicians by completion of questionnaires. Eighty-seven percent received antitoxin sometime during their course. The mortality rate was 19%. Patients who had received trivalent equine antitoxin were found to have a lower mortality rate (10–15% vs. 46%) and a shorter course (10–41 days vs. 56 days in the hospital) than those who did not receive antitoxin; and patients who received antitoxin in the first 24 hours after onset had a shorter course (10 days vs. 41 days in hospital) but about the same fatality rate (10% vs. 15%) as those who received antitoxin later (class III).

In type A wound botulism, Sandrock and Murin analyzed the long-term outcome in 20 consecutive patients from 1991 to 1998 in one university hospital and showed that prompt (<12 hours after presentation) antitoxin administration was associated with a decreased likelihood of developing respiratory failure (57% vs. 85%), and neither antibiotic administration nor surgical débridement appeared to affect the course of the disease (class IV). Their data were not statistically significant.[120]

Thus, these studies suggest at best that early administration (<24 hours after onset) of equine trivalent antitoxin to adult patients with foodborne and wound botulism was associated with improved outcome. This is because antitoxin neutralizes only toxin molecules that are yet unbound to nerve endings. Approximately 6% of adults with foodborne botulism had anaphylaxis or serum sickness when treated with one or two vials of equine botulism antitoxin and, thus, such treatment is not suitable for infants.

Human Botulism Immune Globulin

Human botulism immune globulin (BIG) intravenous (BIG-IV) has been available in the United States since 2006 and its efficacy was proved by a randomized, double-blind, placebo-controlled trial and later open-label study in infant botulism.[121]

Arnon et al[121] performed a 5-year, randomized, double-blind, placebo-controlled trial in California, of BIG-IV in 122 infants with suspected (and subsequently laboratory-confirmed) infant botulism (74 caused by type A C. botulinum toxin, and 47 by type B toxin); a single intravenous infusion of BIG-IV (50 mg/kg of body weight [1 mL/kg]) was given within 3 days after hospital admission. This was tested against placebo immune globulin. Sixty-three patients received the placebo immune globulin, and 59 patients received BIG-IV. They found that, as compared with the control group in the randomized trial, infants treated with BIG-IV had a reduction in the mean length of the hospital stay, the primary efficacy outcome measure, by 3.1 weeks. BIG-IV treatment also reduced the mean duration of intensive care by 3.2 weeks, the mean duration of mechanical ventilation by 2.6 weeks, the mean duration of tube or intravenous feeding by 6.4 weeks, and the mean hospital charges per patient day by $88,600. The efficacy was statistically significant (class I).

In an open-label study on 382 patients with laboratory-confirmed infant botulism, infants treated with BIG-IV within 7 days of admission had a mean length of hospital stay of 2.2 weeks, and early treatment within 3 days of admission shortened the mean length of stay significantly more than did later (4–7 days) treatment (class I). The only adverse effect perhaps related with BIG-IV was a transient, blush-like erythematous rash. Another advantage of BIG-IV is a longer half-life (28 days in vivo compared with 6 days in trivalent botulinum toxin) and thus a larger capacity to neutralize botulinum toxin. A single infusion will neutralize for at least 6 months all botulinum toxin that may be absorbed from the colon of an infant.

BIG-IV is a safe and effective treatment for infant botulism type A and type B. Treatment should be given as soon as possible after hospital admission and should not be delayed for confirmatory testing of feces or enema. Baby BIG is available as public-service orphan drug in the United States. (Information on this drug may be obtained at www.infantbotulism.org and by telephone from the CDHS Infant Botulism Treatment and Prevention Program at 510-231-7600.)

Guanidine and 3,4-DAP

These drugs increase the release of ACh from the nerve terminal, which theoretically should improve the strength of muscles. More than 20 patients were treated with guanidine hydrochloride. Varying degrees of clinical improvement were reported. It has been most effective in overcoming paralysis of limb and extraocular muscles, less effective for respiratory paralysis and autonomic dysfunction. 3,4-DAP was tried in two cases, with improvement in one and none in the other. Thus, in view of the mixed results of improvement and less effectiveness for respiratory paralysis, they are not a substitute for medical management in an intensive care unit.

Antibiotics

The effectiveness of antibiotic therapy is unproved by clinical trial, but it is widely used and recommended for wound botulism, because of the risk of polymicrobial infection. In cases of leukocytosis when fever, an abscess, or cellulitis is present, it is a good practice to treat the patient with an antibiotic. One study showed that the final outcome is not affected by antibiotic treatment.[71] However, penicillin G (3 million units IV every 4 hours in adults) or metronidazole (500 mg IV every 8 hours) in penicillin-allergic patients is usually recommended. The use of aminoglyocides is contraindicated, because they have been reported to induce neuromuscular blockade, potentiating the effects of the toxin in these patients.

Toxin Removal Treatment

This treatment is aimed mainly at removing unabsorbed toxin from the gastrointestinal tract in foodborne botulism or from the wound in wound botulism (good practice point). In foodborne botulism, laxatives, enemas, or other cathartics may be given, provided no significant ileus is present. Magnesium salt-containing cathartics are not recommended because the slowly absorbed ion will potentially aggravate the neuromuscular block in botulism. Magnesium is known to reduce ACh from the presynaptic membrane. Patients presenting with wound botulism should undergo an extensive débridement, even if the wound appears unimpressive, to remove the source of toxin (good practice). In one study, surgical débridement did not affect the course of disease.[120]

General Guidelines for Therapeutic Management

Any patients with a history, symptoms, and clinical signs suspicious for botulism should be hospitalized immediately and closely monitored for signs of respiratory failure. If needed, ventilatory support should be provided (Fig. 18-7).

Once the diagnosis of botulism is clinically suspected, physicians should call their state health department's emergency 24-hour telephone or the CDC to report suspected botulism cases, arrange for a clinical consultation, and if indicated, request release of botulism antitoxin.

The only specific treatment for botulism is administration of botulinum antitoxin. Antitoxin injection following CDC guidelines should be given early in the course of illness, ideally sooner than 24 hours after onset of symptoms because the antitoxin neutralizes only toxin molecules that

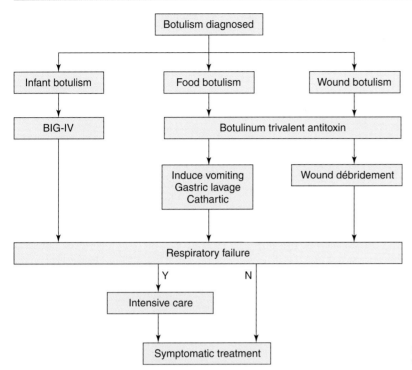

Figure 18-7 Treatment algorithm in botulism. BIG-IV, intravenous botulinum immunoglobulin; N, no; Y, yes.

are yet unbound to nerve endings. This is the best method to prevent respiratory failure and the need for mechanical ventilation.

Before treatment with antitoxin, one has to obtain 10 to 15 mL of serum, 25 to 50 g of feces, and possibly 25 to 50 mL of fluid from gastric aspiration. Also, one has to collect and refrigerate a similar quantity of suspected food samples for testing. In constipated patients, a gentle saline enema may be required to obtain fecal specimens. In wound botulism, wound tissue is obtained for culture and toxin.

Two botulism antitoxin therapies are available in the United States. Trivalent equine botulism antitoxin is used to treat children older than 1 year of age and adults; BIG-IV is used for infants younger than 1 year of age. In food and wound botulism, trivalent botulism antitoxin (one vial [10,000 IU of antibodies against toxin types A, B, and E]) diluted 1:10 with saline, administered IV over 30 to 60 minutes is recommended. Skin test for hypersensitivity should be done before the antitoxin injection following the CDC guideline. In infant botulism, BIG-IV should be given (50 mg/kg [1 mL/kg] IV infusion; 25 mg/kg/hour IV [0.5 mL/kg/hour]) at the initial infusion rate (0–15 minutes), not to exceed an infusion rate of 50 mg/kg/hour (1 mL/kg/hour).[117] This is obtained from the California Department of Health Services (24-hour telephone: 510-540-2646) (Box 18-3).

In foodborne botulism, laxatives, enemas, and other cathartics may be given to remove the toxin from the gut. In wound botulism, wound débridement is recommended and antibiotics are widely used (good practice).

Congenital Myasthenic Syndromes

Congenital myasthenic syndrome (CMS) refers to the heterogeneous groups of hereditary congenital disorders of the neuromuscular junctions. Various forms of CMS have been described in the past decade and new syndromes are added almost every year (Table 18-8; CMS subtypes). Recent studies showed that many cases of CMS are

Box 18-3 Protocols for Clinicians Evaluating Suspected Cases of Botulism

Clinicians evaluating a suspected case of botulism should immediately seek clinical consultation and should administer antitoxin as follows:

For suspected foodborne botulism or botulism of unknown source, the state health department should be contacted via its 24-hour emergency telephone number. If there is no response, then the Centers for Disease Control and Prevention Director's Emergency Operations Center should be contacted at 770-488-7100.

For suspected infant botulism occurring in any state, the California Department of Health Services Infant Botulism Treatment and Prevention Program should be contacted at 510-540-2646.

now known to be due to mutations in genes for presynaptic membrane, synaptic basal lamina, and postsynaptic proteins.[122]

Diagnosis and Evaluation

Clinical Manifestation
Most disorders manifest at birth by definition, but some patients are not evaluated until later in childhood or adult life because the symptoms are mild or not recognized. A positive family history is consistent with the diagnosis of CMS, but a negative family history does not exclude autosomal recessive or even dominant inheritance. Most cases of CMS are inherited by an autosomal recessive pattern except one: the classic slow-channel syndrome has an autosomal dominant inheritance. On examination, the most important clue to a NMT disorder is increasing weakness on sustained exertion (myasthenic weakness) involving ocular, bulbar, and limb muscles. There are some findings suggestive of specific forms of CMS: scoliosis and delayed pupillary light reflex in acetylcholinesterase (AChE) deficiency, selective severe weakness of cervical muscles and of wrist

Table 18-8 Congenital Myasthenic Syndromes

Type	Clinical Features	Electrophysiology	Genetics	Endplate Defects	Treatment
Presynaptic Defects	**The least common**				
ChAT deficiency CMS-EA Familial infantile myasthenia	Hypotonia, respiratory failure at birth, episodic apnea and crisis, improvement with age	Decrement at LRS after prolonged exercise or continous repetitive stimulation at moderate stimulation rate (10–15 Hz)	ChAT	Normal	AChEI: improvement
Paucity of ACh vesicles and decreased quantal release	Ptosis and bulbar weakness in childhood	Decreased quantal release Decrement at LRS		Marked reduction in synpatic vesicles	AChEI: improvement
Congenital LEMS	Hypotonia, areflexia Respiratory failure	Classic triad of LEMS		Normal	Guanidine, 3,4-DAP
Synaptic Defects	**The second most common**				
Endplate AChE deficiency	Early onset; variable severity; general muscle weakness/severe axial muscle involvement Absent pupillary response	Repetitive discharge in CMAP Deremental response at LRS and HRS	COLQ	Small nerve terminals; degenerated junctional fold	Worse with AChEI Ephedrine: improvement
Postsynaptic Defects	**The most common**				
AChR deficiency	Early onset, variable severity; fatigue; typical MG features	Decremental response to RNS; decreased MEPP amplitude	Autosomal recessive Epsilon subunit mutation is most common Many different mutations	Increased length of endplates; variable synaptic folds	AChEI: improvement
Slow channel syndrome (SCCMS)	Most common; forearm extensor weakness; onset 2nd to 3rd decade; variable severity	Repetitive discharge; decrement at LRS and HRS; prolonged channel opening and MEPP duration	Autosomal dominant Alpha, beta, epsilon AChR mutations	Excitotoxic endplate myopathy; decreased AChRs	Quinidine Fluoxetine Anti-AChE: worse
Fast channel syndrome	Early onset; moderately severe; typical MG feature	Decremental response in RNS Brief and infrequent channel opening; opposite of channel syndrome	Autosomal recessive	Normal endplate	AChEI/3,4-DAP: improvement
Rapsyn deficiency	Early onset: arthrogryposis, episodic apnea and crisis, hypotonia Late onset: typical MG features		RAPSN; N88K mutation is common		AChEI/3,4-DAP
MuSK deficiency	Ptosis, respiratory distress since birth		MuSK mutation		3,4-DAP: improved
Sodium channel	Ptosis and weakness with episodic respiratory and bulbar paralysis	Low CMAP amplitude and decrement at 2 Hz stimulation after 10–50 Hz repetitive stimulation for 1 or more min	SCN4A mutation		Pyridostigmine/ acetazolamide
Limb girdle CMS	Limb girdle weakness	Decremental response	Exon 7 of the Dok-7 in some cases	CK may be elevated Tubular aggregate in some	AChEI
Plectin deficiency	Progressive myopathy and fatigability in ocular, facial, and limb muscles	Decremental response at LRS		Fibronecrosis and regeneration in addition to other abnormality	3,4-DAP: improved

AChE, acetylcholinesterase; AChEI, acetylcholinesterase inhibitor; AChR, acetylcholine receptor; ChAT, choline acetyltransferase; CMAP, compound muscle action potential; CMS, congenital myasthenic syndrome; CMS-EA, CMS, congenital myasthenic syndrome with episodic apnea; 3,4-DAP, 3,4-diaminopyridine; HRS, high-rate stimulation; LEMS, Lambert-Eaton myasthenic syndrome; LRS, low-rate stimulation; MEPP, miniature endplate potential; MG, myasthenia gravis; MuSK, muscle-specific kinase; RNS, repetitive nerve stimulation.

and finger extensor muscles in endplate AChE deficiency and slow-channel syndrome, lack of ocular muscle involvement in AChE deficiency, slow-channel syndrome or familial limb girdle myasthenia, and hyporeflexia in congenital LEMS. A positive edrophonium test is consistent with the diagnosis of CMS, but a negative test does not rule out CMS, because this test is negative in patients with endplate AChE deficiency, and in familial infantile myasthenia between attacks of weakness. Responsiveness to AChE inhibitors is present in many patients with CMS, but not in endplate AChE deficiency and slow-channel syndrome.

RNS Test

The diagnosis must be supported by a decremental response at LRS in at least one muscle or by abnormal jitter and blocking on SFEMG, according to Engel (1994).[123] The decremental response may be absent in familial infantile myasthenia between attacks. In these cases a decremental response can be elicited by prolonged 10 Hz stimulation or by exercise for several minutes before 2 Hz stimulation. Repetitive discharges are typically observed in two forms: endplate AChE deficiency and slow-channel CMS (SCCMS). The LEMS pattern has been reported in congenital LEMS.

Diagnosis

Diagnosis of CMS can be made on the basis of the classic triad: myasthenic symptoms since birth, exertion-induced weakness on examination, negative AChR-Ab and MuSK-Ab, and decremental response at LRS. The clinical history and examination, edrophonium response, and RNS test findings can provide sufficient information for a specific diagnosis of CMS in some cases (see Table 18-8), but detailed microphysiologic, ultrastructural, and histochemical studies are required for accurate diagnosis and classification. These latter studies can be performed in only a few centers in the world. Conventional muscle biopsy and routine histochemical studies show no major abnormalities except for a type I fiber predominance and occasional minor nonspecific myopathic changes. Serum creatine kinase (CK) is normal or slightly elevated.[124]

Treatment and Management

AChE Inhibitors

An AChE inhibitor, mainly pyridostigmine, has been used as the first drug of choice in CMS historically because of the similarity between MG and CMS. It has been effective in most cases except two: SCCMS and endplate AChE deficiency. In fact, AChE inhibitor worsens symptoms in these types of CMS. There has not been any systemic study of the benefit of AChE inhibitors. Clinical improvement was documented in case studies. Examples of CMS responding to pyridostigmine are CMS due to ChAT deficiency, paucity of the synaptic vesicles and decreased quantal release, fast-channel syndrome, rapsyn mutation, AChR deficiency, and sodium-channel syndrome.

Ephedrine

Felice and Relva reported the effects of treatment with ephedrine 25 mg twice a day in three CMS patients.[125] All three patients had longstanding and variable weakness, substantial decremental responses to the RNS test, a positive family history, absent AChR antibody, clinical worsening on oral AChE inhibitors, and subjective improvement on ephedrine 25 mg/day. In an open study in three patients, all admitted to mild improvement in strength and stamina while on ephedrine but failed to show any significant improvement in forced vital capacity (FVC), muscle strength, hand dynamometer readings, or RNS test.[125] The subtype of CMS was not identified.

Considering their clinical worsening on oral AChE inhibitors, it is possible that these patients had slow-channel syndrome or AChE deficiency.

3,4-Diaminopyridine (DAP)

This drug acts by blocking K^+ conductance and increasing nerve terminal ACh release at the nerve terminal. There were two reports on 3,4-DAP in CMS:

Palace et al[126] studied 16 patients in open prospective trials, and four of them in a double-blind cross-over trial; current AChE inhibitors were continued. All patients had fatigable muscle weakness, EMG evidence of abnormal neuromuscular transmission (decrement > 10% at 3 Hz stimulation or jitter > 53 μsec on SFEMG), and absence of AChR-Ab. Most patients had onset of disease early in life and showed a relatively stable state. The subtype of CMS was not identified. Assessment was performed before entry into the study, and at the end of each month of treatment. Measurements included myometry, FVC, a timed walk of 30 m reversing direction at the half-way point, and a timed drink of 150 mL of water. Between 5 and 20 mg of 3,4-DAP was given orally three or four times daily. In an open prospective study for the group as a whole, there was a highly significant increase in muscle strength ($P < 0.001$, $n = 16$), and in individual paired comparisons, 13 out of 16 showed significant improvement. In a double-blind cross-over trial in four patients 3,4-DAP or placebo was given for 1 month. The patients could often guess from the perioral and distal limb paresthesia whether the preparation was 3,4-DAP or placebo. Each of the four patients improved significantly on the 3,4-DAP in mean muscle strength, with P-values ranging from 0.01 to 0.002. They concluded that 3,4-DAP, either alone or combined with AChE inhibitors, may be a useful additional treatment in congenital LEMS.

Anlar et al[127] studied the benefit of 3,4-DAP in 11 CMS patients in a double-blind, placebo-controlled, cross-over study. Diagnostic criteria for CMS were identical to Palace's criteria. 3,4-DAP or placebo was given for 7 to 10 days with a 1-week washout period between the two drugs. The daily dose varied between 10 and 80 mg according to the patient's age and response; it was adjusted by daily increments of 5 to 10 mg until optimal or maximal dose was achieved. Examination parameters included strength of limb muscles, eye movement, ptosis, a timed walk of a distance of 20 m, inspiratory capacity, and deep knee-bending. A change of at least 20% of the baseline value was considered significant. Significant clinical improvement was observed in 5 of 11 CMS patients, and with placebo, in 3 of 11. Thus, this study did not show any significant benefit of 3,4-DAP over placebo. Extraocular movements were more likely to improve. The patients who benefited from 3,4-DAP were at least partially responsive to AChE inhibitors. Considering that AChE inhibitors was allowed in Palace's study,[126] one cannot completely rule out the effect of AChE inhibitors in the 3,4-DAP study in CMS. Thus, my conclusion is that 3,4-DAP is not effective by itself, but may have an added benefit to AChE inhibitors in congenital MG.

Fluoxetine (Prozac)

Harper et al found that fluoxetine significantly shortened at 5 μM/L and nearly normalized at 10 μM/L the prolonged opening bursts of slow-channel CMS AChR expressed in fibroblasts.[128] They studied its effects in two patients who were allergic to quinidine with up to 80 to 120 mg of fluoxetine per day over 3 years (serum fluoxetine + norfluoxetine levels 8 to 11 μM/L). Both patients showed subjective and objective improvement by quantitative muscle strength testing using the neuropathy impairment score and EMG. The CMAP increased by 58% to 120% and the decrement improved dramatically at 50-Hz stimulation, decreasing from 72% to 4% in one case and from 67% to 28% in the other. In one patient, the repetitive CMAP was less prominent with treatment. They interpreted that the progressive improvement on fluoxetine is similar to that observed in SCCMS patients treated with quinidine and likely corresponds to gradual repair of the endplate myopathy.

Quinidine

Harper et al found that levels of quinidine sulfate attainable in clinical practice shortened the opening episodes of genetically engineered mutant SCCMS receptors in vitro and treated six SCCMS patients with quinidine sulfate (QS) in an open-label trial, using objective clinical measurement of muscle strength and RNS test as endpoints.[178] One patient became allergic to quinidine after 7 days. One patient with borderline baseline respiratory failure developed nocturnal hypoventilation after 3 months of QS therapy (900 mg/day; serum level 2.0– mg/mL), which was significantly improved on a combination of QS (800 mg/day) and nocturnal oxygen under positive pressure. The remaining patients tolerated the drug well and after 30 days of continuous therapy showed statistically significant improvement in muscle strength and in the decrement of the CMAP at HRS. Acutely, the peak effect was observed 60 to 90 minutes after a single 200 mg dose of QS. Quinidine sulfate was administered orally at a dose of 200 mg three times daily. After the first weeks, the dose was gradually increased to maintain a serum level of 1.0 to 2.5 μg/mL. The usual dose required for long-term therapy was QS 600 to 900 mg/day. They concluded that QS appeared to be a safe and effective treatment in most patients with SCCMS but that it should be used with caution because of potential adverse effects, such as drug allergy, exacerbation of weakness at concentrations higher than 5 μg/mL, and the possible development of respiratory failure in patients with borderline baseline respiratory function.

General Guidelines for Therapeutic Management

Since the Mayo group has the most experience in treatment of congenital MS, the treatment guidelines in CMSs are based on their latest recommendations.[129]

In principle, CMSs that decrease the synaptic response to ACh are best treated with drugs that augment cholinergic stimulation, namely AChE inhibitors (pyridostigmine) and, in some cases, 3,4-DAP. AChE inhibitors increase the number of AChRs activated by each quantum by inhibiting ACh breakdown. 3,4-DAP increased the number of quanta released by nerve impulses. By contrast, CMSs that increased the synaptic response, SCCMS, were treated with long-lived open-channel blockers of AChR, namely quinidine and fluoxetine. Thus, theoretically, pyridostigmine should be effective in most CMSs because most patients have CMSs that decrease the synaptic response to ACh.

According to Engel and Sine,[129] special consideration applies to the following CMS:

1. Choline acetyltransferase (ChAT) deficiency is treated prophylactically with an oral pyridostigmine to prevent respiratory crises, and with parenteral prostigmine methylsulfate during respiratory crises.

2. In endplate AChE deficiency, it is important to avoid cholinergic agonists, because they make symptoms worse. Anecdotal reports suggest that ephedrine mitigates the disease.

3. SCCMS is treated with quinidine sulfate or fluoxetine. Both medications act as long-lived open-channel blockers of AChR and gradually improve the disease.

4. Fast-channel syndrome patients, and especially those without AChR deficiency, respond well to combined therapy with pyridostigmine and 3,4-DAP.

5. Patients with rapsyn deficiency respond to pyridostigmine, and some derive striking further benefit from the use of 3,4-DAP.

6. A patient with sodium channel myasthenia showed improved endurance on treatment with pyridostigmine; additional therapy with acetazolamide, which is known to mitigate periodic paralysis attributed to $Na_v1.4$ mutations, prevented further attacks of respiratory and bulbar weakness.

Tick Paralysis

Tick paralysis, also known as tick toxicosis, is a rare human neuromuscular disorder. Tick paralysis is the only tick-borne disease that is not caused by an infectious organism but is due to a neurotoxin from the salivary glands of ticks. It can be fatal if the attached tick is not found and removed.[130,131] Thus, it is important to consider tick paralysis as a differential diagnostic possibility in any children presenting with acute generalized flaccid weakness.

Epidemiology

Tick bites are common but tick paralysis is extremely rare. Most tick bites do not result in disease. Though it has a world-wide distribution, most of the reported cases were from the entire eastern Australia or North American *Ixodes holocyclus*, especially in the Pacific Northwest, the Rocky Mountain states, and the Southeastern United States.[132] This geographic localization is largely because of the vectors.[133]

More than 60 different species of tick have been associated with tick paralysis. The most important species causing human disease are the Australian paralysis tick in Australia, and the *Dermacentor* species in North America: *Dermacentor andersoni* (Rocky mountain wood tick) in the Northeast and *Dermacentor variabilis* (American dog tick) in the Southeast.

Tick paralysis usually occurs in spring and summer when nymphs and adults are actively feeding. Children aged 10 years and younger are most commonly affected, especially girls.[134] Men are more commonly affected in the adult group. Long hair in young girls, which provides camouflage for feeding ticks and the greater exposure of adult men to tick-infested environments may explain this gender difference. The most frequent tick locations are the scalp, behind the ears, the neck, and the groin.[135] Only the adult female tick produces the toxin responsible for causing tick paralysis.

Pathophysiology

Tick paralysis is caused by a toxin, a paralytic agent, secreted into a host through saliva from the salivary glands of feeding female ticks.[136,137] A toxin from the *Ixodes* species is named "holocyclotoxin" because Stone found this toxin in the saliva of the *Ixodid holocyclus* female tick.[137] Kaire[136] isolated holocyclotoxin and induced tick paralysis in mice and dogs by injecting one of three principal extracts.[135] Animals treated with an antiserum did not develop clinical disease. Though the precise details of the cellular mechanism of a toxin in tick paralysis have not been delineated, there is consensus that a decrease of acetylcholine release at the presynaptic membrane is responsible for tick paralysis,[136] possibly secondary to the action of toxin at the terminal axons.

Diagnosis and Evaluation

Clinical Manifestations

The clinical presentation of tick paralysis is very similar to that of Guillain-Barré syndrome (GBS). In general, Australian tick paralysis

Table 18-9 Differences between North American and Australian Tick Paralysis

Feature	North American Cases	Australian Cases
Vectors	*Dermacentor andersoni* *Dermacentor variabilis*	*Ixodes holycyclus*
Nonresponsive pupils	Rare	More common
Cranial nerve involvement	Rare	More common
Progression of symptoms	Usually begin to remit as soon as tick is removed	Often progress for 24–48 hours after tick removal
Recovery after tick removal	Generally ≤24 hours	Can be prolonged for days to weeks
Antiserum therapy	Never used	Occasionally used
Duration of observation	Shorter	Longer

appears to be more severe than North American tick paralysis (Table 18-9).

The classic presentation is acute symmetrical ascending areflexic flaccid paralysis that evolves over hours to days, sometimes preceded by prodromal symptoms, including paresthesias, irritability, fatigue, and myalgias.[133,138] Symptoms usually begin 2 to 6 days after tick attachment. The initial neurologic symptoms are usually unsteadiness of gait followed by falling and then complete inability to walk. Then, paralysis quickly ascends to involve the arms, cranial and respiratory muscles, causing oculomotor paralysis, bulbar weakness, and respiratory failure.[131] Neurologic examination shows a varying degree of weakness in limb muscles, usually greater in the lower extremities than in the upper, and associated typically with absent or decreased reflexes. Sensorium remains clear in the absence of untreated respiratory failure. When cranial nerves are involved, facial diplegia, bulbar palsy, and ophthalmoplegia may be present. In some cases, respiratory failure may occur requiring ventilatory support. Pupillary involvement may be present, more commonly in Australia.[131] Sensory examination is usually normal despite the sensory complaints, but mild proprioception loss has been reported.[131]

Atypical cases have been reported. Acute cerebellar syndrome without any significant muscle weakness, facial palsy as the predominant symptom, and brachial plexus neuropathy were reported.

Electrophysiologic Findings
A low CMAP amplitude is the most striking abnormality and is seen in all tested nerves in upper and lower extremities, the most severe reduction being in the lower extremities. Motor NCVs are normal or mildly slow. Sensory nerve conduction is generally normal. RNS test in a few cases showed response at low and high rates of stimulation. Rapid improvement has been documented in the CMAP amplitude. This corresponds to the rapid clinical improvement seen within hours or days after removal of the tick.

Laboratory Findings
Routine blood tests were normal. CSF was consistently normal. This finding is in notable contrast to GBS, in which CSF protein was typically high. Mild transient elevation of CK was reported in one Australian patient.[131]

Diagnosis
There is no laboratory test to diagnose tick paralysis. The most important factor in the diagnosis of tick paralysis is a high index of suspicion. This disorder should be included in the differential diagnosis of GBS and Fisher syndrome. In every child with ascending paralysis developing in spring and summer, a tick should be searched for. Misdiagnosis of GBS can be costly in view of an expensive IVIg treatment as reported in a few patients.[131,134,138] High spinal fluid protein and slow nerve conduction velocity should help identify GBS. The edrophonium test was normal in one single case.[139]

Treatment and Management
Tick paralysis is cured by quickly finding and removing the engorged tick. The tick is best removed by grasping it as close to the skin as possible and applying firm steady pressure. The entire tick has to be removed. Once the tick is removed, the patient's rapid recovery is the rule in North American cases. In Australian patients, a continued progression of weakness for a few days is not unusual but eventual recovery is the rule. Antitoxin, a hyperimmune serum prepared from dogs, the usual treatment for paralyzed animals, has been used sparingly and only in severely ill Australian patients because of the risk of acute reactions and serum sickness.[131] Limited data (class IV) are available on its use in human patients. If the tick is not found and removed, respiratory failure ensues. If this occurs, standard ICU care with ventilatory support is critical. Mortality rate in the era predating modern ICU care was 10% to 12%. A 1999 review of a series of 33 patients from Washington State collected between 1946 and 1996 reported two deaths (6%) during the 1940s.[130]

Snakebite Myasthenic Syndrome

The victims of snakebites are mainly from the rural population who are bitten during field work and when sleeping outdoors. Most snakes are not venomous and are harmless. Some venomous snakes rarely bite and many venomous snakes make a dry bite. Neurotoxic envenomation by snakes is common in some parts of the world and may lead to fatal respiratory failure. Four families of poisonous snakes (Elapidae, Atractaspididae, Colubridae, Viperidae) are responsible for most envenomations. Cobras, vipers, and kraits are the principal cause of snakebite deaths in India, Sri Lanka, and Southeast Asia. Thus, most research on this subject is from these countries.

Snake venoms contain complex mixtures of enzymes, polypeptide toxins including neurotoxins, procoagulants, and hemorrhagins, producing failure of several organs.[140] The percentage of combined organ failures varies depending on the family of poisonous snakes. Among these, neurotoxicity, blood coagulability, and acute renal failure are three major problems in snake envenomation.

Envenomed patients usually have fang marks at the site of the bite, local pain, swelling, and discoloration of the bite site, local tender lymphadenopathy, and abdominal pain.[141] A systemic consumption coagulopathy may develop within 1 to 2 hours of the bite in many patients. Renal failure may ensue in some patients and requires peritoneal dialysis.

Snakebite myasthenic syndrome is a reversible syndrome characterized by descending paralysis, as noted in myasthenia gravis. Neuromuscular paralysis may set in within an hour after a bite. In one series, the onset of neuromuscular paralysis occurred within 30 minutes to 4 hours.[142] Neuromuscular paralysis lasted up to 10 days, with fatigability lasting for 12 days.[141] Fatigability, ptosis, double vision, and external ophthalmoplegia were common findings.

These were followed by facial and bulbar palsy producing dysphagia and dysphonia and by proximal muscle weakness. Respiratory failure was seen in severe cases, necessitating mechanical ventilation, and was reported in 2% to 18% of cases in two series.[141,142] The majority of these patients were bitten by the krait.[142,143] Assisted ventilation with intermittent positive pressure was required usually for 18 to 48 hours. The pupils were spared. Reflexes were normal and sensory function was preserved. Death from snakebite was extremely rare, usually due to consumption coagulopathy.

Pathophysiology

Historically, snake venom neurotoxins have been known to produce effects similar to those of curare and myasthenia gravis (MG). Snakebite myasthenic syndrome arises from the action of two major groups of toxins: presynaptic neurotoxins and postsynaptic neurotoxins (Box 18-4). The best known presynaptic toxins are beta-bungarotoxin, taipoxin, and crotoxin. Among postsynaptic toxins, the best known is alpha-bungarotoxin. Though there might be some difference in degree depending on the species of snake, snakebite myasthenic syndrome is due to combined presynaptic and postsynaptic neuromuscular blockade. This explains the conflicting observations on the edrophonium test results and anticholinesterase benefit in these disorders. The edrophonium test showed no positive response in one study,[142,143] a positive response in seven of eight other tested cases, and a positive response in a placebo-controlled study in eight patients with cobra bites.[144] Clinical trials testing anticholinesterase drugs have demonstrated both favorable and unfavorable results.[141] Considering all the data available, it appears that the presynaptic block is more influential in snakebite myasthenic syndrome.

As rare neurotoxin syndromes, myokymia caused by the bite of a timber rattlesnake (*Crotalus horridus*), rhabdomyolysis from a Russell's viper, and dysautonomia from a Malayan krait have been reported.

Diagnosis and Evaluation

Electrophysiologic Findings

Sensory nerve conduction was completely normal. In motor nerve conduction, terminal latency, NCV, and F-wave latencies were all normal. Low CMAP was observed in severe cases. There may have been a progressive decrease in the CMAP in the first 2 to 4 days after envenomation, paralleling the clinical deterioration. Needle EMG showed motor unit potentials (MUPs) were normal. Fibrillation was detected in all four severe cases but not in milder ones.[143] SFEMG during the recovery phase from illness revealed markedly increased jitter and blocking in all of three tested cases.[144] In the RNS test, the CMAP amplitude was normal and low in severe cases.[143] A decremental response at the low rate stimulation was rare and reported only in severe cases. In contrast, a decremental response at the high rate of stimulation (30–50 Hz) was common, most marked around 6 days after the bite, and more often seen in milder cases. Sanmuganathan claimed that this is the distinct pattern for SBMS.[141] Connolly observed that the decrement, which was never more than mild at rest, was enhanced dramatically 5 to 30 seconds following exercise or tetanic stimulation.[145] These effects lasted up to 30 minutes. This pattern is distinctive and probably reflects the severely depleted numbers of vesicles seen in the motor terminals on electron microscopy.

Diagnosis

Diagnosis of snakebite myasthenic syndrome is not very difficult in the endemic areas such as Southeastern Asia. An extensive diagnostic workup is generally unnecessary, since most patients are fully aware of prevalence of snakebites. Differentiation between nonvenomous and venomous snakebites is beyond the scope of this chapter. In general, the presence of local pain, swelling, and discoloration and regional lymphadenopathy permit early recognition of a venomous snakebite. Ptosis, double vision, difficulty opening the mouth, and protruding the tongue are usual early signs of snakebite myasthenic syndrome. Enzyme-linked immunosorbent assay (ELISA) for detection of snake venoms is generally available in Australia and other nations to aid in determining the specific snake species involved in a bite. These kits identify venom in the victim's blood, urine, and wound aspirate.[140]

Treatment and Management

Specific antivenin treatment is the mainstay of hospital treatment for venomous snakebites. There is no universal consensus in regard to AChEIs usage in SBMS. In cases of respiratory failure, supportive ventilatory care should be provided. In addition to SBMS, there are other life-threatening complications of snake envenomation: hypovolemic shock, coagulopathy, and acute renal failure. These have to be diagnosed and treated appropriately. Often these other complications are the cause of death in venomous snakebites.

Antivenins

Specific antivenins should be used in accordance with local guidelines as soon as systemic poisoning, including neurotoxicity, is apparent but should be administered in a medical facility (expert consensus). Some antivenins are specific for the venom of one species, whereas other are polyvalent against the venoms of all snakes of a particular geographic area (in the United States, antivenin Crotalidae polyvalent (ACP); in Australia, tiger snake antivenom). Antivenins used in the past 35 years have been equine-derived. Antivenin is administered intravenously but should be administered in a facility where acute anaphylaxis and serum sickness can be treated. Physicians should be present for antivenin administration, and epinephrine and antihistamine should be at the bedside. In a retrospective study, the rate of acute allergic reaction with ACP administration ranged from 23% to 56%, with even higher rates for delayed serum sickness. Ideally, antivenin should be administered within 4 hours after snakebite, but it is effective for at least the first

---

Box 18-4 Toxin in Snakebite Myasthenic Syndromes

Presynaptic Toxin*	Postsynaptic Toxin
Binds to motor nerve terminals causing an early depletion of synaptic vesicle and delayed degeneration of the motor nerve terminal	Irreversible binding to the alpha subunit of the acetylcholine receptor
Presynaptic block Beta-bungarotoxin (krait) Notexin (tiger snake) Taipoxin (Taipan) Crotoxin (Brazilian rattlesnake) Gamma-bungarotoxin (krait)	Postsynaptic block Alpha-bungarotoxin (Elapidae family): producing irreversible block Cobra toxin: producing reversible block
Tensilon test result: Negative	Tensilon test result: Positive
More lethal than postsynaptic toxins	Antivenin is effective AChEI: Effective if Tensilon test result is positive

*Usually contains phospholipase A2 activity responsible for myotoxicity.
AChEI, anticholinesterase inhibitor.

24 hours. Antivenin is known to be effective against postsynaptic neurotoxins.[146] It accelerates dissociation of the toxin from the postsynaptic receptor. Presynaptic toxins have no response to antivenin. In recent years, ovine (sheep-derived) antivenin has been approved. A prospective study showed that ovine antivenin had a significantly lower incidence of adverse reactions, with nearly all events being mild to moderate.[147,148] Its use is still limited because of availability and expense, but it is likely to soon replace equine antivenin.

AChE Inhibitors

Experimentally, the neuromuscular blocking activity of snake-venom fractions can sometimes be reversed by AChEIs,[149] but clinical trials have demonstrated conflicting results, both favorable and unfavorable. Unfortunately, these trials have been uncontrolled, and most have lacked objective data. Watts et al conducted a placebo-controlled, double-blind, cross-over trial of intravenous edrophonium in 10 SBMS patients with cobra bites and found significantly more improvement in ptosis and duration of upward gaze after edrophonium than after placebo (class II).[144] Further, they also found that this test accurately predicted the eventual response to neostigmine. They controlled neurologic signs and symptoms by careful titration of the amount of neostigmine for each patient, beginning with 25 µg/kg of body weight per hour delivered by continuous infusion. No additional antivenin was given to any patient. No severe reactions were observed. Abdominal pain was the most frequent effect and was easily controlled with atropine. Watts et al's dramatic experience with the edrophonium test and subsequent good response with neostigmine was most likely due to their selection of patients with cobra bites. Cobra toxin is known to be a postsynaptic blocker. The edrophonium test has been used by some to identify SBMS patients who are likely to respond to anticholinesterase medications (class IV).[142] Six out of seven patients with a positive response to the edrophonium test, who were treated with oral neostigmine, made a full recovery within 8 days. It is reasonable to offer anticholinesterase therapy to those who demonstrate a positive response to the edrophonium test.

Supportive Treatment

Artificial respiratory support is mandatory and lifesaving if respiratory failure occurs (good practice point). Respiratory failure caused by venom neurotoxins may be difficult to reverse with antivenin. This may be because antivenin is known to be more effective against postsynaptic neurotoxins.[146] It accelerates dissociation of the toxins from the postsynaptic receptor. Intermittent positive pressure ventilation with or without tracheostomy is often needed. It may be used alone or combined with antivenin and neostigmine-atropine. 3,4-Diaminopyridine was also reported to reverse respiratory paralysis.[149] Artificial respiratory support was often required for 14 to 48 hours in cases of krait and cobra bites and was required for more than 10 weeks in an Australian snakebite case.[140] That patient eventually recovered.

Organophosphate Intoxication

Organophosphate (OP) poisoning is a major global health problem with 1 million serious accidental and 2 million suicidal poisonings due to insecticides worldwide every year.[150] Of these, some 200,000 die, with most deaths occurring in developing countries including India and Sri Lanka. OP poisoning is the most common mode of suicidal poisoning in India. Thus, most studies are from these countries. Though the possibility is small, the potential use of organophosphates in "nerve gas" (e.g., tabun [GA], sarin [Gb], soman [GD]) in chemical warfare continues to be a serious concern.

Pathophysiology

Organophosphates are a class of compounds that inhibit cholinesterases, including acetylcholinesterase (AChE). Organophosphates cause toxicity from their absorption through the skin, mucous membranes, and respiratory tract following accidental exposure, or from the gastrointestinal tract following suicidal ingestion.[150]

Following the release of acetylcholine (ACh) in response to a nerve impulse and subsequent depolarization of ACh receptors at the postsynaptic membrane, ACh is quickly hydrolyzed by AChE, allowing for the repolarization of the postsynaptic membrane. OP, by inhibiting AChE, results in excessive accumulation of ACh at the various cholinergic receptors: the pre- and postganglionic parasympathetic and sympathetic nervous system, central nervous system, and neuromuscular junctions. ACh stimulates muscarinic and nicotinic receptors resulting in acute cholinergic syndrome, including excessive pulmonary secretions, muscle weakness, and CNS depression. Binding of OP with AChE is initially reversible, but after the passage of time this binding becomes irreversible due to aging of AChE. Following inhibition, recovery of this enzyme occurs slowly at a rate of about 1% per day.[151] Restoration of AChE occurs by spontaneous rephosphorylation of the enzyme and by new enzyme synthesis.

Clinical Manifestations

OP poisoning leads to three distinct main syndromes: acute cholinergic crisis, intermediate syndrome (IMS), and OP-induced delayed polyneuropathy (OPIDPN) (Table 18-10).

Acute Cholinergic Crisis

OPs being inhibitors of esterases, particularly AChE, lead to acute cholinergic syndrome. Clinical effects from acute poisoning can be separated into those affecting the autonomic nervous system (ANS), the neuromuscular junction, and CNS categories. Increased parasympathetic muscarinic activity results in the classic SLUDGE (salivation, lacrimation, urination, defecation, gastric secretions, and emesis) or DUMBBELS (defecation, urination, miosis, bronchorrhea, bradycardia, emesis, lacrimation, salivation) syndromes. Miosis is a commonly recognized feature of OP poisoning and is reportedly present in 65% to 95% of cases.[150] Excess nicotinic stimulation at the neuromuscular junction is responsible for rapid depolarization with muscle fasciculations, followed by receptor blockade manifesting as weakness or paralysis. Paralysis can occur during acute cholinergic syndrome or several days after acute cholinergic syndrome. Paralysis may lead to respiratory failure, requiring mechanical ventilation, and is thought to be the most common cause of death in acute OP poisoning. Paralysis usually resolves within 48 to 72 hours, but complete clinical recovery may take up to a week after exposure to OP. CNS effects are from excessive nicotinic and muscarinic stimulation in the brain. Commonly reported symptoms are agitation, depressed mental status, coma, and seizure. Seizures are more commonly associated with the chemical nerve agents.[150]

Intermediate Syndrome

After the resolution of cholinergic effects in acute cholinergic crisis, but before the onset of OPIDPN, a myasthenia-like syndrome can occur owing to prolonged action of ACh on the nicotinic receptors. This is termed intermediate myasthenic syndrome (IMS). The incidence of IMS was reported to be between 5% and 65% of patients with OP poisoning. Symptoms typically occurred 1 to 3 days after the acute cholinergic crisis and were characterized by weakness in the neck and proximal muscles, less often in the ocular, bulbar, and respiratory muscles. Reflexes were absent in 50% cases in one

Table 18-10 Pathophysiologic and Clinical Features of Various Syndromes in Organophosphate Poisoning

Feature	Acute Cholinergic Crisis	Intermediate Syndrome	OPIDPN
Frequency		11%–68%	1.5%
Pathophysiology	Excessive ACh at the CNS, ANS, and neuromuscular junction (muscarinic syndrome)	Excessive ACh at neuromuscular junction (nicotinic syndrome)	Phosphorylation and aging of neuropathy target esterase in nervous system
Time to onset		1–3 days after acute cholinergic crisis	1–4 weeks after exposure
Clinical features	SLUDGE Neuromuscular paralysis CNS symptoms: agitation decreased mental status, coma, and seizure	Myasthenic syndrome: weakness of the proximal and neck, followed by cranial nerve palsy and rarely respiratory failure	Predominantly motor polyneuropathy followed by spastic myelopathy
Electrophysiology	Repetitive discharge Decrement-increment at 30–50 Hz stimulation	Repetitive discharge Decrement or decrement-increment at 30–50 Hz stimulation Needle EMG: normal	Axonal motor neuropathy Needle EMG: fibrillation/positive sharp waves
Recovery	Typically in 2–3 days	Typically in 4–18 days	Slow recovery
Treatment	Atropine Diazepam for seizure Oximetherapy	Respiratory care	Physical therapy

ACh, acetylcholine; ANS, autonomic nervous system; CNS, central nervous system; EMG, electromyography; OPIDPN, organophosphate-induced delayed neuropathy; SLUDGE (salivation, lacrimation, urination, defecation, gastric distress, emesis).

series.[152] IMS is distinguished from acute cholinergic crisis by the absence of other muscarinic symptoms and lack of response to atropine. It is also distinguished from OPIDPN in that the latter affects distal muscles and spares the cranial nerves and respiratory muscles. Prolonged suppression of AChE is seen during this stage. Full recovery occurs eventually in 4 to 18 days. No specific therapy has been shown to be beneficial in the treatment or prevention of IMS. Recognition of IMS, however, is critically important, as respiratory failure can be fatal without adequate ventilatory care. The mainstay of treatment is respiratory support in the form of mechanical ventilation. Atropine is not effective in this syndrome.

Organophosphate-Induced Delayed Polyneuropathy
OPIDPN is common following exposure to OP compounds that have weak AChE activity (e.g., triorthocresylphosphate). However, exposure to commonly available OP compounds that have strong AChE activity is distinctly uncommon.[152] OPIDPN is the result of phosphorylation and aging of a protein found in nervous tissue known as neuropathy target esterase (NTE), which is present in the brain, spinal cord, and the peripheral nerves. Symptoms of OPIDPN begin 1 to 4 weeks after exposure, long after cholinergic signs have worn off. The earliest symptoms are paresthesia and calf pain, soon followed by weakness in the distal muscles of the legs over a 2-week period. Examination showed a predominantly motor length-dependent polyneuropathy with weakness of the distal limb muscles. Clinical involvement of the corticospinal tract and the dorsal columns becomes apparent when the peripheral neuropathy improves. No treatment is currently available for OPIDPN. Over time patients may regain some function. Other neurobehavioral changes and some extrapyramidal symptoms were also reported as some of the chronic neurologic sequelae persisting after cessation of exposure.

Diagnosis and Evaluation

Electrophysiologic Findings
Motor NCV and distal latencies are normal even in severely paralyzed patients.

Needle EMG was done in 18 cases of IMS. None showed fibrillation or PSW; MUPs were normal.[153] In OPIDPN, however, axonal motor neuropathy was found in NCS, and needle EMG showed fibrillations and positive sharp wave (PSW).[154]

The RNS test shows a rather distinct pattern indicative of an excessive cholinergic state: (1) repetitive discharges in the CMAP with a single stimulation, and (2) a decrement-increment phenomenon with a high rate of stimulation (10–50 Hz). These are due to depolarization block due to an excess ACh. The CMAP with repetitive discharges is the earliest and most frequent abnormality of excessive ACh regardless of the severity of poisoning. Therefore, this is the most sensitive indicator of the action of ACh at the endplate. Repetitive discharges are also seen in pyridostigmine intoxication, such as cholinergic crisis in MG and two congenital myasthenic syndromes: slow-channel myasthenic syndrome and AChE deficiency. With progression of weakness, the decrement-increment response, a unique abnormality seen only in the excessive cholinergic state, follows. Unlike MG, the decrement is maximal by the second stimulus and this is followed by a gradual increment.

These various RNS abnormalities are useful in staging the severity of OP poisoning and following its progress.[154,155] The CMAP with repetitive discharges is seen early and is virtually always present. The decrement-increment phenomenon occurs next in the course of intoxication and may be associated with minimal or no clinical weakness. The decrement response occurs with more severe intoxication. The degree of decrement in the decrement response may reflect the severity of weakness, and the subsequent improvement in the decrement heralds the onset of clinical recovery.[154]

Diagnosis
The diagnosis of OP poisoning is made on clinical grounds: a history of exposure to OP and clinical features of cholinergic excess. Confirmation of OP poisoning is based on the measurement of cholinesterase activity. Typically, the results are not readily available. Although erythrocyte and plasma (pseudo) cholinesterase levels can

both be used, the erythrocyte cholinesterase test is the more accurate of the two measurements because it reflects better the AChE found in neural synapses. On the other hand, plasma cholinesterase is easier to assay and is more readily available. The usefulness of these tests is further limited by the lack of good correlation with severity of clinical illness, considerable interindividual variation, and the effects of other disease states. Thus, it appears that, at best, the tests can be useful as a marker of OP exposure.[150] Field and fast methods using paper strips are also available in India.[151]

Treatment and Management

The World Health Organization (WHO) and Eddleston et al[156] urge restriction of the use of class I pesticides (extremely toxic). They urge a ban or major restriction on the use of class I pesticides and reduction of pesticide use to a minimal number of less hazardous compounds.[157] In 1981, Jordan banned Parathion use and the number of poisoning autopsies in Amman fell from 50 a year in 1981 to below 10 in 1983–1985.[157] In Samoa, the same results occurred after banning Paraquat. Wadia recommends banning of aluminum phosphide and high-concentration formulations as the first step in preventing the high mortality rate of OP poisoning in India.[157]

During acute cholinergic crisis, the mainstay of medical therapy includes atropine, pralidoxime (2-PAM), and benzodiazepines.

Acute Management

During acute cholinergic crisis, the initial therapy should be the immediate removal of patients from further OP exposure and aggressive use of atropine as an antidote to counter the muscarinic effects of ACh. All cases require aggressive decontamination with complete removal of the patient's clothes and vigorous irrigation of the affected area. In cases of OP ingestion, the position statement by the American Academy of Clinical Toxicology and European Association of Poison Centers and Clinical Toxicologists states that gastric lavage should be considered only if a poisoned patient presents within 1 hour of ingestion of a potentially toxic amount. However, gastric lavage is routinely used, particularly in developing countries.[158] Apparently this is due to a lack of any good studies to settle this issue. In warfare, potential use of OP requires the availability of gas masks.

Atropine

Atropine is primarily effective in treating the muscarinic effects of OP poisoning, especially in its effects on bronchial secretions, It has no effect on the neuromuscular junctions. Atropine crosses the blood-brain barrier and counters the effects of excess ACh on the extrapyramidal system. Thus, atropinization is the most important mode of treatment during acute cholinergic crisis and can be achieved with the judicious use of atropine. As many as 30 dose schedules of atropine have been cited by different authors. Atropinization, once achieved, should be maintained for 3 to 5 days, depending upon the compound involved. The endpoint of atropinization is pulmonary secretions. Tachycardia and mydriasis must not be used to limit or to stop subsequent doses of atropine. According to the most frequently cited schedule, the recommendation is to begin IV atropine at 2 to 5 mg in adults or 0.05 mg/kg in children. This should be given for 3 to 5 minutes until pulmonary secretions clear.[150] An alternative to repeated doses of atropine is a continuous infusion (0.02–0.08 mg/kg/hour) after the initial bolus has been given.[150] Glycopyrrolate (Robinul) may be considered as an alternative to atropine when the patient develops too much central anticholinergic delirium or agitation. Glycopyrrolate does not enter the brain and so will not cause toxic delirium, but it does not dry up secretions as effectively as atropine.

Oximes

Cholinesterase reactivators (oximes) should be theoretically effective as an antidote for OP poisoning. Oximes work by removal of the phosphoryl group from the inhibited AChE enzyme, resulting in enzyme reactivation. When given before aging (permanent inhibition of the cholinesterase enzyme), oximes are generally regarded as effective treatments in reversing nicotinic signs. Pralidoxime (PAM) is the most commonly used oxime worldwide. However, a meta-analysis of various trials did not conclusively prove the efficacy of PAM.[158,159] Unfortunately, in the trials that were analyzed, PAM was used in doses lower than that recommended by WHO.[160] A recent trial reported from India showed beneficial effects with high doses of PAM in patients with moderately severe OP poisoning, particularly when it was given within 2.5 hours of exposure.[161] The initial dose was 2 g of PAM (as the iodide salt) followed by 1 g every hour as an infusion for 48 hours, and then 1 g every 4 hours until recovery.

Diazepam

Seizures from OP poisoning are rare. Although seizures are more commonly associated with the chemical nerve agents, in one case series of pesticide poisoning seizures occurred in as many as 13% of patients.[162] Seizures from OP poisoning are thought to be initiated by increased ACh levels and are atropine-responsive. Ongoing seizure activity is due to subsequent glutamate release and is not responsive to atropine. Diazepam, which is known to potentiate effects of gamma-aminobutyrate (GABA) and facilitate inhibitory GABA neurotransmission, has been effectively used for control of OP poisoning. It now appears that diazepam may also be beneficial in patients without seizures, in whom it may protect the CNS and reduce mortality rate.[153] The usual dose is 5 to 15 mg IV every 5 to 10 minutes as needed.

Hypermagnesemia-Induced Paralysis

Hypermagnesemia is an uncommon clinical finding, and symptomatic hypermagnesemia is even less common. This disorder is rare because the normal kidney is able to eliminate excess magnesium by rapidly reducing its tubular reabsorption to almost negligible amounts.[163]

The most common cause of hypermagnesemia is renal failure. The ingestion of magnesium-containing medications (e.g., antacids, cathartics) can exacerbate the condition. In the treatment of eclampsia, hypermagnesemia is induced deliberately and sometimes can be symptomatic.

Normally, the serum magnesium level is 1.5 to 2.5 mEq/L. Above 5 mEq/L, deep-tendon reflexes are depressed. Reflexes are usually absent at levels of 9 to 10 mEq/L, and weakness is usually seen in that range. At levels greater than 14 mEq/L, there may be severe cardiac arrhythmias or respiratory failure.

Magnesium impairs neuromuscular transmission primarily by reducing ACh release. Calcium entry into the presynaptic terminal is necessary for ACh release, and magnesium competitively blocks calcium entry. Thus, hypermagnesemia produces a presynaptic block.

Diagnosis and Evaluation

Muscle weakness in hypermagnesemia resembles LEMS, with hyporeflexia and limb weakness usually sparing the extraocular muscles.

In two reported cases of weakness due to hypermagnesemia, electrophysiologic findings resembled those of LEMS: low CMAP amplitude, incremental response (186%–300%) after exercise, decremental response at LRS, and incremental response (254%) at HRS.

A diagnosis of hypermagnesemia is suspected in the right clinical set-up, confirmed by the serum level of magnesium.

Treatment and Management

Because magnesium-induced weakness is almost always iatrogenic, prevention is usually possible. Avoidance of magnesium-containing compounds in patients with renal failure is the most important preventive measure. Treatment of hypermagnesemia depends on the severity of the clinical manifestations. In mild cases, discontinuation of magnesium or furosemide 20 to 80 mg/daily orally may be all that is required. In serious weakness, IV calcium gluconate (100–300 mg calcium IV diluted in 150 mL of 5% dextrose in water [D_5W] over 10 minutes) will usually produce prompt improvement.

References

1. Bainin M, Barnes M, Baron JC, et al: Guidance for the preparation of neurological management guidelines by EFNS scientific task forces-revised recommendations, *Eur J Neurol* 11:577–581, 2004.
2. Franklin GM, Zahn CA: American Academy of Neurology. AAN clinical practice guidelines: above the fray, *Neurology* 59(7):975–976, 2002.
3. Skeie GO, Apostolski S, Evoli A, et al: Guidelines for the treatment of autoimmune neuromuscular transmission disorders, *Eur J Neurol* 2010 April 12, [Epub ahead of print].
4. Keesey JC: Clinical evaluation and management of myasthenia gravis, *Muscle Nerve* 29:484–505, 2004.
5. Christensen PB, Jensen TS, Tsiropoulos I, et al: Mortality and survival in myasthenia gravis, *J Neuro Neurosurg Psychiatry* 64:78–83, 1998.
6. Oh SJ, Cho HK: Endophonium responsiveness not necessarily diagnostic of myasthenia gravis, *Muscle Nerve* 13(3):187–191, 1990.
7. Ertaş M, Araç M, Kumral K, et al: Ice test as a simple diagnostic aid for myasthenia gravis, *Acta Neurol Scand* 89:227–229, 1994.
8. Vincent A, McConville J, Farrugia ME, et al: Antibodies in myasthenia gravis and related disorders, *Ann N Y Acad Sci* 998:324–335, 2003.
9. Wolfe GI, Trivedi JR, Oh SJ: Clinical review of muscle-specific tyrosine kinase-antibody positive myasthenia gravis, *J Clin Neuromuscul Dis* 8: 217–224, 2007.
10. Oh SJ: *Electromyography. Neuromuscular Transmission Studies*, Baltimore, 1988, Williams & Wilkins.
11. Stalberg E, Trontelj JV: The study of normal and abnormal neuromuscular transmission with single fibre electromyography, *J Neurosci Methods* 74 (2):145–154, 1997.
12. Hantanaka Y, Hemmi S, Morgan MB, et al: Nonresponsiveness to anticholinesterase agents in patients with MuSK-antibody-positive positive MG, *Neurology* 65:1508–1509, 2005.
13. Walker MB: Case showing the effect of prostigmine on myasthenia gravis, *Proc R Soc Med* 28:759–761, 1935.
14. Keesey JC: Contemporary opinions about Mary Walker, a shy pioneer of therapeutic neurology, *Neurology* 51:1433–1439, 1998.
15. Sthasivam S: Steroids and immunosuppressant drugs in myasthenia gravis, *Nat Clin Pract Neurol* 4:317–327, 2008.
16. Brunner NG, et al: Corticosteroids in the management of severe generalized myasthenia gravis. Effectiveness and comparison with corticotrophin therapy, *Neurology* 22:603–610, 1972.
17. Arsura EL, et al: High-dose intravenous methylprednisolone in myasthenia gravis, *Arch Neurol* 42:1149–1153, 1985.
18. Pascuzzi RM, et al: Long-term corticosteroid treatment of myasthenia gravis: report of 116 patients, *Ann Neurol* 15:291–298, 1984.
19. Sghirlanzoni A, et al: Myasthenia gravis: prolonged treatment with steroids, *Neurology* 34:170–174, 1984.
20. Cosi V, et al: Effectiveness of steroid treatment in myasthenia gravis: a retrospective study, *Acta Neurol Scand* 84:33–39, 1991.
21. Evoli A, et al: Long-term results of corticosteroid therapy in patients with myasthenia gravis, *Eur Neurol* 32:37–43, 1992.
22. Bu B, et al: A prospective study of effectiveness and safety of long-term prednisone therapy in patients with myasthenia gravis [Chinese], *Zhonghua Shen Jing Ge Za Zhi* 33:28–31, 2000.
23. Kufersmith MJ, Moster M, Bhuiyan S, et al: Beneficial effects of corticosteroids on ocular myasthenia gravis, *Arch Neurol* 53:802–804, 1996.
24. Sommer N, Sigg B, Melms A, et al: Ocular myasthenia gravis: response to long-term immunosuppressive treatment, *J Neurol Neurosurg Psychiatry* 62:156–162, 1997.
25. Matell G, et al: Effects of some immunosuppressive procedures in myasthenia gravis, *Ann N Y Acad Sci* 274:659–676, 1976.
26. Mertens HG, Hertel G, Reuther P, et al: Effect of immunosuppressive drugs (azathioprine), *Ann N Y Acad Sci* 377:691–699, 1981.
27. Matell G: Immunosuppressive drugs: azathioprine in the treatment of myasthenia gravis, *Ann N Y Acad Sci* 505:589–594, 1987.
28. Witte AS, et al: Azathioprine in the treatment of myasthenia gravis, *Ann Neurol* 15:602–605, 1984.
29. Kuks JBM, et al: Azathioprine in myasthenia gravis: observations in 41 patients and a review of literature, *Neuromuscul Disord* 1:423–431, 1991.
30. Mantegazza R, et al: Azathioprine as a single drug or in combination with steroids in the treatment of myasthenia gravis, *J Neurol* 235:449–453, 1988.
31. Heckmann JM, et al: High-dose immunosuppressive therapy in generalized myasthenia gravis—a 2-year follow-up study, *S Afr Med J* 91:765–770, 2001.
32. Perez MC, et al: Stable remissions in myasthenia gravis, *Neurology* 31:32–37, 1981.
33. Goulon M, et al: Results of a one-year open trial of cyclosporine in ten patients with severe myasthenia gravis, *Transplant Proc* 20(3 Suppl 4):211–217, 1988.
34. Bonifati DM, Angelini C: Long-term cyclosporine treatment in a group of severe myasthenia gravis patients, *J Neurol* 244:542–547, 1997.
35. Lavrnic D, et al: Cyclosporine in the treatment of myasthenia gravis, *Acta Neurol Scand* 111:247–252, 2005.
36. Cos L, et al: Mycophenolate mofetil (MyM) is safe and well tolerated in myasthenia gravis (MG), *Neurology* 54(Suppl 3):A137, 2000.
37. Ciafaloni E, et al: Mycophenolate mofetil for myasthenia gravis: an open-label pilot study, *Neurology* 56:97–99, 2001.
38. Chaudhry V, et al: Mycophenolate mofetil: a safe and promising immunosuppressant in neuromuscular diseases, *Neurology* 56:94–96, 2001.
39. Meriggioli MN, et al: Mycophenolate mofetil for myasthenia gravis: an analysis of efficacy, safety, and tolerability, *Neurology* 61:1438–1440, 2003.
40. Konishi T, et al: Clinical study of FK506 in patients with myasthenia gravis, *Muscle Nerve* 28:570–574, 2003.
41. Kawaguchi N, et al: Low-dose tacrolimus treatment in thymectomised and steroid-dependent myasthenia gravis, *Curr Med Res Opin* 20:1269–1273, 2004.
42. Ponseti JM, et al: Long-term results of tacrolimus in cyclosporine- and prednisolone-dependent myasthenia gravis, *Neurology* 64:1641–1643, 2005.
43. Rowin J, Meriggioli MN, Tuzun E, et al: Etanercept treatment in corticosteroid depdendent myasthenia gravis, *Neurology* 55:1062–1063, 2000.
44. Mount FW: Corticotropin in treatment of ocular myasthenia, *Arch Neurol* 11:114–124, 1964.
45. Howard FM Jr, et al: Alternate-day prednisone: preliminary report of a double-blind controlled study, *Ann N Y Acad Sci* 274:596–607, 1976.
46. Lindberg C, et al: Treatment of myasthenia gravis with methylprednisolone pulse: a double blind study, *Acta Neurol Scand* 97:370–373, 1998.
47. Bromberg MB, et al: Randomized trial of azathioprine or prednisolone for initial immunosuppressive treatment of myasthenia gravis, *J Neurol Sci* 150:59–62, 1997.
48. Schuchardt V, Kohler W, Hund E, et al: A randomized, controlled trial of high-dose intravenous immunoglobulin versus methylprednisolone in moderate exacerbations of myasthenia gravis: final analysis after early termination (unpublished data). Cited in Schneider-Gold C, Gajdos P, Toyka KV, et al: Corticosteroids for myasthenia gravis. *Cochrane Database Syst Rev*. 2: CD 002828, 2005.
49. Gajdos P, Simon N, De Rohan-Chabot P, et al: Long term effects of plasma exchange in myasthenia gravis. Results from a randomized study (Effet a long terme des echanges plasmatiques au cours de la myasthenia. Resultat d'une etude randomisee), *Presse Med* 12(15):939–942, 1983.
50. Palace J, Neusome-Davis J, Lecky B: A randomized double-blind trial of prednisolone alone or with azathioprine in myasthenia gravis. Myasthenia gravis study group, *Neurology* 50:1778–1783, 1998.
51. De Feo LG, et al: Use of intravenous pulsed cyclophosphamide in severe, generalized myasthenia gravis, *Muscle Nerve* 26:31–36, 2002.
52. Tindall RSA, et al: Preliminary results of a doubleblind, randomized, placebo-controlled trial of cyclosporine in myasthenia gravis, *N Engl J Med* 316:719–724, 1987.

53. Tindall RS, et al: A clinical therapeutic trial of cyclosporine in myasthenia gravis, *Ann N Y Acad Sci* 681:539–551, 1993.

54. Nagane Y, et al: Efficacy of low-dose FK506 in the treatment of myasthenia gravis—a randomized pilot study, *Eur Neurol* 53:146–150, 2005.

55. Meriggioli MN, et al: Mycophenolate mofetil for myasthenia gravis: a double-blind, placebo-controlled pilot study, *Ann N Y Acad Sci* 998:494–499, 2003.

56. Sanders DB, Hart IK, Mantegazza R, et al: An international, phase III, randomized trial of mycophenolate mofetil in myasthenia gravis, *Neurology* 71:400–406, 2008. Muscle study group: A trial of mycophenolate mofetil with prednisone as initial immunotherapy in myasthenia gravis, *Neurology* 71:394–399, 2008.

57. Gajdos P, Simon N, De Rohan-Chabot P, et al: Long term effects of plasma exchange in myasthenia gravis. Results from a randomized study [Effet à long terme des échanges plasmatiques au cours de la myasthénie. Résultat d'une étude randomisée], *Presse Méd* 12(15):939–942, 1983.

58. Gajdos P, Chevret S, Clair B: Clinical trial of plasma exchange and high dose immunoglobulin in myasthenia gravis, *Ann Neurol* 41(6):789–796, 1997.

59. Gajdos P, Tranchant C, Clair B, et al: Treatment of myasthenia gravis exacerbation with intravenous immunoglobulin 1g/kg versus 2g/kg: a randomized double blind clinical trial, *Arch Neurol* 62(11):1689–1693, 2005.

60. Ronager J, Ravnborg M, Hermansen I, Vorstrup S: Immunoglobulin treatment versus plasma exchange in patients with chronic moderate to severe myasthenia gravis, *Artif Organs* 25(12):967–973, 2001.

61. Wolfe GI, Barohn RJ, Foster BM, et al: Randomized, controlled trial of intravenous immunoglobulin in myasthenia gravis, *Muscle Nerve* 26 (4):549–552, 2002.

62. Zinman L, Ng E, Bril V: IV immunoglobulin in patients with myasthenia gravis, *Neurology* 68:837–841, 2007.

63. Matell G: Immunosuppressive drugs: azathioprine in the treatment of myasthenia gravis, *Ann N Y Acad Sci* 505:589–594, 1987.

64. Drachman DB, Jones RJ, Brodsky RA: Treatment of refractory myasthenia: "rebooting" with high-dose cyclosphosphamide (see comment), *Ann Neurol* 53(1):29–34, 2003.

65. Gajos P, Chevret S, Toyka K: Plasma exchange for myasthenia gravis, *Cochrane Database Syst Rev* (4):CD002275, 2008.

66. Oh SJ: Intravenous immunoglobulin therapy in neuromuscular disease: emerging therapy in the 1990's, *J KAMA* 2:47–55, 1996.

67. Jongen JL, van Doorn PA, van der Mech FG: High-dose intravenous immunoglobulin therpay for myasthenia gravis, *J Neurol* 245(1):26–31, 1998.

68. Gajdos P, Chevret S, Toyka K: Intravenous immunoglobulin for myasthenia gravis, *Cochrane Database Syst Rev* (1):CD002277, 2008.

69. Pasnoor M, Wolfe GI, Nations S, et al: Clinical findings in MuSK-antibody positive myasthenia gravis: a U.S. experience, *Muscle Nerve* 41:370–374, 2010.

70. Blalock A, Mason MF, Morgan HJ, et al: Myasthenia gravis and tumors of the thymic regions, report of a case in which tumor was removed, *Ann Surg* 110:554–561, 1939.

71. Gronseth GS, Barohn RJ: Practice parameter: thymectomy for autoimmune myasthenia gravis (an evidence based review): report of the Quality Standards Subcommittee of the American Academy of Neurology (see comments), *J Neurol* 55(1):7–15, 2000.

72. Yuan HK, Huan BS, Kung SY, et al: The effectiveness of thymectomy on seronegative generalized myasthenia gravis, *Acta Neurol Scand* 115: 181–184, 2007.

73. Guillermo GR, Tellez-Zenteno JF, Weder-Cisneros N, et al: Response of thymectomy: clinical and pathological characteristics among seronegative and seropositive myasthenia gravis patients, *Acta Neurol Scand* 109:217–221, 2004.

74. Romi F, Gilhus NE, Varhaug JE, et al: Thymectomy and antimuscle antibodies in non-thymomatous myasthenia gravis, *Ann N Y Acad Sci* 998:481–490, 2003.

75. Sonett JR, Jaretzki A III: Thymectomy for nonthymomatous myasthenia gravis. A critical analysis, *Ann N Y Acad Sci* 1132:325–328, 2008.

76. Thomas CE, Nayer SE, Gungor Y, et al: Myasthenic crisis: clinical features, mortality, complications and risk factors for prolonged intubation, *Neurology* 48:1253–1260, 1997.

77. Seneviratne J, Mandrekar J, Wijdicks EFM, et al: Noninvasive ventilation in myasthenic crisis, *Arch Neurol* 65:54–58, 2008.

78. Stricker RB, Kwiatkowska BJ, Habis JA, Kiprov DD: Myasthenic crisis. Response to plasmapheresis following failure of intravenous gamma-globulin, *Arch Neurol* 50(8):837–840, 1993.

79. Jani-Acsadi A, Lisak RP: Myasthenic crisis: guidelines for prevention and treatment, *J Neurol Sci* 161:127–133, 2007.

80. Chaudhuri A, Behan PO: Myasthenic crisis, *Q J Med* 102:97–107, 2009.

81. Qureshi AI, Choudhry MA, Akbar MS, et al: Plasma exchange versus intravenous immunoglobulin treatment in myasthenic crisis, *Neurology* 52:629–632, 1999.

82. Beinberg MB, Cater O: Corticosteroid use in the treatment of neuromuscular disorders: empirical and evidence-based data, *Muscle Nerve* 30:20–37, 2004.

83. Berroushot J, Barumann I, Kalishewski P, et al: Therapy of myasthenic crisis, *Crit Care Med* 25:1228–1235, 1997.

84. Bedlack RS, Sanders DB: How to handle myasthenic crisis. Essential steps in patient care (see comment), *Postgrad Med* 107(4):211–214, 2000.

85. Antonio-Santos AA, Eggenberger ER: Medical treatment options for ocular myasthenia gravis, *Curr Opin Ophthalmol* 19:468–478, 2008.

86. Luchanok U, Kaminski H: Ocular myasthenia: diagnosis and treatment recommendations and the evidence base, *Curr Opin Neurol* 21:8–15, 2008.

87. Oh SJ: Muscle-specific receptor tyrosine kinsase antibody positive myasthenia gravis: Current status, *J Clin Neurol* 5:53–64, 2009.

88. Ferrero S, Esposito F, Biamonti M, et al: Myasthenia gravis during pregnancy, *Expert Rev Neurother* 8:979–988, 2008.

89. Ciafaloni E, Massey JM: Myasthenia gravis and pregnancy, *Neurol Clin* 22:771–782, 2004.

90. Hoff JM, Daltveit AK, Gilhus N: Myasthenia gravis: consequences for pregnancy, delivery, and the new born, *Neurology* 61:458–460, 2003.

91. Committee on Drugs, American Academy of Pediatrics: The transfer of drugs and other chemicals into human breast milk, *Pediatrics* 93:137–150, 1994.

92. Rivner MH, Swift TR: Thymoma: diagnosis and management, *Semin Neurol* 10:83–88, 1990.

93. Skeie GO, Romi F: Paraneoplastic myasthenia gravis: immunological and clinical aspects, *Euro J Neurol* 15:1029–1033, 2008.

94. Wittbrodt ET: Drugs and myasthenia gravis. An update, *Arch Intern Med* 157(4):399–408, 1997.

95. Howard JF: Adverse drug effects on neuromuscular transmission, *Semin Neurol* 10:89–102, 1990.

96. Lennon VA, Lambert EH: Autoantibodies bind solubilized calcium channel-omega-conotoxin complexes from small cell lung carcinoma: a diagnostic aid for Lambert-Eaton myasthenic syndrome, *Mayo Clin Proc* 64(12):1498–1504, 1989.

97. Odabasi Z, Demirci M, Kim DS, et al: Postexercise facilitation of reflexes is not common in Lambert-Eaton myasthenic syndrome, *Neurology* 59(7): 1085–1087, 2002.

98. Lambert EH, Rooke ED, Eaton LM, Hodgson CH: Myasthenic syndrome occasionally associated with bronchial neoplasm: neurophysiological studies. In Viets HR, editor: *Myasthenia Gravis*, Springfield, IL, 1961, Charles C Thomas, pp 88–116.

99. Oh SJ: Diverse electrophysiological spectrum of the Lambert-Eaton myasthenic syndrome, *Muscle Nerve* 12:464–469, 1989.

100. Oh SJ, Hatanaka Y, Claussen GC, et al: Electrophysiological differences in seropositive and seronegative Lambert-Eaton myasthenic syndrome, *Muscle Nerve* 35:178–183, 2007.

101. Verschuuren II, Wirtz PW, Titulaer MJ, et al: Available treatment options for the management of Lambert-Eaton myasthenic syndrome, *Expert Opin Pharmacother* 7:1323–1336, 2006.

102. Oh SJ, Kim DS, Head TC, Claussen GC: Low-dose quinidine and pyridostigmine: relatively safe and effective long-term symptomatic therapy in Lambert-Eaton myasthenic syndrome, *Muscle Nerve* 1146–1152, 1997.

103. Norris FH, Calanchini PR, Fallat RJ, et al: The administration of guanidine in amyotrophic lateral sclerosis, *Neurology* 24:721–728, 1974.

104. Lundh H, Nilsson O, Rosen I, et al: Practical aspects of 3, 4-diaminopyridine treatment of the Lambert-Eaton myasthenic syndrome, *Acta Neurol Scand* 88 (2):136–140, 1993.

105. McEvoy KM, Windebank AJ, Daube JA, et al: 3, 4Diaminopyridine in the treatment of Lambert Eaton syndrome, *N Engl J Med* 321:1567–1571, 1989.

106. Sanders DB, Howard J Jr, Massey JM: 3, 4-Diaminopyridine in Lambert-Eaton myasthenic syndrome and myasthenia gravis, *Ann N Y Acad Sci* 681:588–590, 1993.

107. Oh SJ, Hatanaka Y, Claussen G, Morgan M: 3,4-Diaminopyridine is effective over placebo in a randomized double cross-over drug study, *Muscle Nerve* 48:795–808, 2009.

108. Oh SJ, Kim DS, Kwon KH, Tseng A, Mussell H, Claussen GC: Wide spectrum of symptomatic treatment in Lambert-Eaton myasthenic syndrome, *Ann N Y Acad Sci* 841:827–831, 1998.

109. Tim RW, Massey JM, Sanders DB: Lambert-Eaton myasthenic syndrome: electrodiagnostic findings and response to treatment, *Neurology* 54:2176–2178, 2000.

110. Bain PG, Motomura M, Newsom-Davis J, et al: Effects of intravenous immunoglobulin on muscle weakness and calcium-channel autoantibodies in the Lambert-Eaton myasthenic syndrome, *Neurology* 47(3):678–683, 1996.

111. Newsom-Davis J, Murray N: Plasma exchange and immunosuppressive drug treatment in the Lambert Eaton myasthenic syndrome, *Neurology* 34:480–485, 1984.

112. Newsom-Davis J: A treatment algorithm for Lambert-Eaton myasthenic syndrome, *Ann N Y Acad Sci* 841:817–822, 1998.

113. Chalk CH, Murray NM, Newsom-Davis J, et al: Response of the Lambert-Eaton myasthenic syndrome to treatment of associated small-cell lung carcinoma, *Neurology* 40(10):1552–1556, 1990.

114. Maddison P, Newsom-Davis J, Mills KR, et al: Favorable prognosis on Lambert-Eaton myasthenic syndrome and small-cell carcinoma, *Lancet* 353:117–118, 1999.

115. Maddison P, Newsom-Davis J: Treatment for Lambert-Eaton myasthenic syndrome, *Cochrane Database Syst Rev* (2):CDO03279, 2005.

116. Cherington M: Botulism: update and review, *Semin Neurol* 24:155–163, 2004.

117. Talliac PP, Kim J, Bessman E: CBRNE-Botulism, *E Med.* The last update April 10, 2008.

118. Sobel J: Botulism, *Clin Infect Dis* 41:1167–1173, 2005.

119. Tacket CO, Shandera WX, Mann JM, et al: Equine antitoxin use and other factors that predict outcome in type A foodborne botulism, *Am J Med* 76:794–798, 1984.

120. Sandrock CE, Murin S: Clinical predictors of respiratory failure and long-term outcome in black tar heroin-associated with botulism, *Chest* 120:562–566, 2001.

121. Arnon SS, Schechter R, Maslanka SE, et al: Human botulism immune globulin for the treatment of infant botulism, *N Engl J Med* 354:462–471, 2006.

122. Engel AG, Ohno K, Sine SM: Congenital myasthenic syndromes: progress over the past decade, *Muscle Nerve* 27(1):4–25, 2003.

123. Engel AG: Congenital myasthenic syndromes, *Neurol Clin* 12(2):401–437, 1994.

124. Abicht A, Lochmuller H: Congenital myasthenic syndromes, *Gene Rev.* Last revision: 9/16/2006.

125. Felice KJ, Relva GM: Ephedrine in the treatment of congenital myasthenic syndrome, *Muscle Nerve* 19:799–800, 1996.

126. Palace J, Wiles CM, Newsom-Davis J: 3, 4-Diamonopyridine in the treatment of congenital (hereditary) myasthenia, *J Neurol Neurosurg Psychiatry* 54:1069–1072, 1991.

127. Anlar B, Varli K, Ozdirim E, Mevlut E: 3,4-Diaminopyridine in childhood myasthenia: double-blind placebo-controlled trial, *J Child Neurol* 11:458–461, 1996.

128. Harper CM, Fukodome T, Engel AG: Treatment of slow channel congenital myasthenic syndrome with fluoxetine, *Neurology* 60:1710–1713, 2003.

129. Engel AG, Sine SM: Current understanding of congenital myasthenic syndrome, *Curr Opin Pharmacol* 5:308–321, 2005.

130. Dworkin MS, Shoemaker PC, Anderson DE: Tick paralysis: 33 human cases in Washington State, 1946–1996, *Clin Infect Dis* 29:1435–1439, 1999.

131. Grattan-Smith PJ, Morris JG, Johnston HM, et al: Clinical and neurophysiological features of tick paralysis, *Brain* (12):1975–1987, 1997.

132. Gentile DA, Lang JE: Tick-borne diseases. In Auerbach PS, editor: *Wilderness Medicine*, 4th ed, St. Louis, 2001, Mosby, pp 769–806.

133. Edlow JA, McGillicuddy DC: Tick paralysis, *Infect Dis Clin North Am* 22:397–413, 2008.

134. Schmitt NM, Bowmer EJ, Greson JD: Tick paralysis in British Columbia, *Can Med Assoc J* 100:417–421, 1969.

135. Mumhaghan MF: Site and mechanism of tick paralysis, *Science* 131:418–419, 1960.

136. Kaire GH: Isolation of tick paralysis toxin from *Ixodes holocyclus*, *Toxicon* 4:91–97, 1966.

137. Stone BF, Commins MA, Kemp DJ: Artificial feeding of the Australian paralysis tick, *Ixodes holocyclous* and collection of paralyzing toxin, *Int J Parasitol* 13:447–454, 1983.

138. Vedanarayanan V, Sorey WH, Subramony SH: Tick paralysis, *Semin Neurol* 24:2181–2184, 2004.

139. Swift TR, Igacio OJ: Tick paralysis: electrophysiological studies, *Neurology* 25:1130–1133, 1975.

140. Minton SA: Neurotix snake envenoming, *Semin Neurol* 10:52–61, 1990.

141. Sanmuganathan PS: Myasthenic syndrome of snake envenomation: a clinical and neurophysiological study, *Postgrad Med J* 74:596–599, 1998.

142. Seneviratne U, Dissanayake S: Neurological manifestations of snake bite in Sri Lanka, *J Postgrad Med* 48:275–278, 2002.

143. Singh G, Pannu HS, Chawla PS, et al: Neuromuscular transmission failure due to common Krait (*Bungarus caeruleus*) envenomation, *Muscle Nerve* 22:1637–1643, 1999.

144. Watt G, Theakston RDG, Hayes CG, et al: Positive response to edrophonium in patients with neurotoxic envenoming by cobras (*Naja naja philippinensis*), *N Engl J Med* 315:1444–1448, 1986.

145. Connolly S, Trevett AJ, Nwokolo NC, et al: Neuromuscular effects of Papuan Taipan snake venom, *Ann Neurol* 38:916–920, 1995.

146. Harris JB, Goonetilleke A: Animal poisons and the nervous system. What the neurologist needs to know, *J Neurol Neurosurg Psychiatry* 75:iii40–iii46, 2004.

147. Juckett G, Hancocx JG: Venomous snakebites in the United States. Management, review and update, *Am Fam Phys* 65:1367–1377, 2002.

148. Ariaratnam CA, Sjostrom L, Rzaierk Z, et al: An open, randomized comparative trial of two antivenoms for the treatment of envenoming by Sri Lankan Russel's viper (*Daboia russeili russelii*), *Trans R Soc Trop Med Hyg* 95:74–80, 2001.

149. Watt G, Smith CD, Kaewsupo A, et al: 3, 4-Diaminopyradine reverses respiratory paralysis induced by a presynaptically active snake venom and its major neurotoxin, *Trans R Soc Trop Med Hyg* 88:243–246, 1994.

150. Rusyniak DE, Nanagas KA: Organophosphate poisoning, *Semin Neurol* 24:197–204, 2004.

151. Singh S, Sharma N: Neurological syndromes following organophosphate poisoning, *Neurol India* 48:308–313, 2000.

152. Wadia RS, Sadagopan C, Amin RB, et al: Neurological manifestations of organophosphorous insecticide poisoning, *J Neurol Neurosurg Psychiatry* 37:841–847, 1974.

153. Wadi RS, Chitra S, Amin RB, et al: Electrophysiological studies in acute organophosphate poisoning, *J Neurol Neurosurg Psychiatry* 50:1442–1448, 1987.

154. Gutmann L, Besser R: Organophosphate intoxication: pharmacologic, neurophysiological, clinical, and therapeutic considerations, *Semin Neurol* 10:45–51, 1990.

155. Jayawardane P, Dawson AH, Weerasinghe V, et al: The spectrum of intermediate syndrome following acute organophosphate poisoning: a prospective cohort study from Sri Lanka, *PLoS Med* 5:e147, 2008.

156. Eddleston M, Szinicz L, Eyer P, et al: Oximes in acute organophosphorus pesticide poisoning: a systemic review of clinical trials, *Q J Med* 95(5):275–283, 2002.

157. Wadia RS: Treatment of organophosphate poisoning, *Indian J Crit Care Med* 7:85–87, 2003.

158. Peter JV, Moran JL, Graham P: Oxime therapy and outcomes in human organophosphate poisoning: an evaluation using meta-analytic techniques, *Crit Care Med* 34:502–510, 2006.

159. Buchley NA, Eddleston M, Szincz L: Oximes for acute organophosphate pesticide poisoning, *Cochrane Database Syst Rev* CDO05085, 2005.

160. Aggarwal P, Jamshed N: What's new in emergencies, trauma, and shock? Snake envenomation and organophophate poisoning in the emergency department, *J Emerg Trauma Shock* 1:59–62, 2008.

161. Pawar KS, Bhoite RR, Pillary CP, et al: Continous pralidoximine infusion versus repeated bolus injection to treat organophosphrus pesticide poisoning: a randomized controlled trail, *Lancet* 368:2136–2141, 2006.

162. Rusyniak DE, Nanagas KA: Organophosphate poisoning, *Semin Neurol* 24:197–204, 2004.

163. Krendal DA: Hypermagnesemia and neuromuscular transmission, *Semin Neurol* 10:42–45, 1990.

*Diana M. Escolar, MD, Peter O'Carroll, MD,
and Robert Leshner, MD*

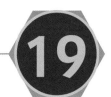

Treatment and Management of Muscular Dystrophies

Muscular dystrophies have long been recognized as inherited disorders, characterized by progressive skeletal muscle degeneration and weakness. These diseases are known to have autosomal dominant, recessive, or X-linked inheritance. Clinical observations initially led to classification into six groups: Duchenne-like, Emery-Dreifuss type, limb-girdle type, facioscapulohumeral peroneal type, distal myopathies, and oculopharyngeal type.[1] The expanding genetic and molecular understanding of the muscular dystrophies has further complicated their classification. An updated classification system for these disorders is shown in Table 19-1.

The underlying molecular defects responsible for these disorders are found throughout the cellular structure, including extracellular matrix structural proteins (laminin-2, collagen type VI) and glycosylation enzymes (fukutin-related protein [FKRP], protein-O-mannosyl transferases 1 and 2 [POMT1 and POMT2], protein-O mannose β1,2-N-acetylglucosaminyltransferase 1 [POMGNT1]), transmembrane- and sarcolemma-associated proteins (dystrophin, sarcoglycans, dystroglycan, caveolin-3, β1- and α7-integrins, dysferlin), cytoplasmatic proteases and ligases (calpain-3, tripartite motif-containing 32 [TRIM32]), cytoplasmic proteins associated with organelles and sarcomeres (titin, myotilin, fukutin, telethonin), and nuclear membrane proteins (lamin, emerin). These diseases have provided a window to better understanding of sarcolemmal organization and the underlying muscle biology responsible for the structure and maintenance of normal muscle cell function. The relationships between these proteins are complex; the function of each of the defective proteins, including the most investigated one, dystrophin, is not entirely known. Structural, enzymatic, and signaling dysfunctions provide the basis for the pathophysiology that has been associated with these disorders. Figure 19-1 shows a current depiction of the muscle membrane as well as other areas of the muscle fiber associated with muscular dystrophies.

Dystrophinopathies

Dystrophinopathies are a group of dystrophies resulting from mutations in the dystrophin (*DMD*) gene, located on the short arm of the X chromosome in the Xp21 region.[2] Duchenne muscular dystrophy (DMD) is the most common dystrophinopathy and represents a complete absence of the subsarcolemmal protein dystrophin. Becker muscular dystrophy (BMD), which is rarer, involves a decrease in the quantity or quality of the dystrophin protein. This gives rise to a milder disease with variable severity and time of clinical onset.

Duchenne and Becker Muscular Dystrophies

The clinical and pathologic features of DMD were first described in 1851 by Edward Meryon, an English physician, in a communication about eight boys in three British families who had the disease. Several years later, in 1868, the French neurologist Guillaume-Benjamin Duchenne described the same syndrome in detail, and it ultimately would bear his name. Several other meticulous descriptions of the disease can be found in the early literature.

Molecular Pathogenesis

The *DMD* gene consists of 86 exons (including seven promoters linked to unique first exons), which make up only 0.6% of the gene. The gene, which spans a genetic distance of more than 2.5 million base pairs,[3] is the largest isolated human gene.

More than 90% of boys with DMD have an absence of dystrophin corresponding to an "out-of-frame" mutation that disrupts normal dystrophin transcription.[4] These mutations cause a premature stop codon and early termination of mRNA transcription. As a result, an unstable RNA is produced that undergoes rapid decay, leading to the production of nearly undetectable concentrations of truncated protein. If the mutation is one that does not stop transcription, an "in-frame" deletion, the BMD phenotype occurs, with abnormal dystrophin protein.[5] This reading frame hypothesis holds for more than 90% of cases and is commonly used both to confirm diagnosis of dystrophinopathies and to differentiate between DMD and BMD.

Exceptions occur in approximately 10% of patients. Out-of frame deletions affecting exons 3-7, 5-7, 3-6, or downstream at exons 51, 49-50, 47-52, 44, or 45 can result in a milder BMD phenotype. The most common underlying explanation for the presence of at least some dystrophin in these patients is a process called *exon skipping*, which occurs via alternative splicing.[6,7] In these BMD patients the carboxy-terminus is always preserved.[8] The involved exons are generally thought to encode noncritical areas of the protein so that when they are skipped, a shortened but still functional dystrophin protein is produced. Exon skipping is also the underlying mechanism for the revertant fibers (a few scattered muscle fibers showing dystrophin staining in muscle biopsies) seen in approximately 50% of DMD boys.[9] The limited expression of dystrophin results in a

Table 19-1 Pathophysiological Classification of Muscular Dystrophies

Disease	Gene Locus	Gene Product	Mode of Inheritance
Limb-girdle Muscular Dystrophy (LGMD) Caused by Sarcolemma or Cytosolic Protein Defects			
Duchenne/Becker MD	Xp21	Dystrophin	XR
LGMD 1A	5q22	Myotilin	AD
LGMD 1B	1q21.2	Lamin A/C	AD
LGMD 1C	3p25	Caveolin 3	AD
LGMD 1D	7q	?	AD
LGMD 1E	6q23	?	AD
LGMD 1F	7q32	?	AD
LGMD 1G	4q21	?	AD
LGMD 1H	3p23	?	AD
LGMD 2A	15q15	Calpain 3	AR
LGMD 2B/Myoshi myopathy	2p13.1	Dysferlin	AR
LGMD 2C	13q12	Gamma-sarcoglycan	AR
LGMD 2D	17q21	Alpha-sarcoglycan	AR
LGMD 2E	4q12	Beta-sarcoglycan	AR
LGMD 2F	5q33	Delta-sarcoglycan	AR
LGMD 2G	17q11.2	Telethonin (TCAP)	AR
LGMD 2H	9q31-q33	Tripartite motif-containing 32 (TRIM32)	AR
LGMD 2I	13q13.3	Fukutin-related protein (FKRP)	AR
LGMD 2J/Tibial muscular dystrophy	2q31	Titin	AR/AD
LGMD 2K	9q34.1	Protein-O-mannosyltranseferase (POMT1)	AR
LGMD 2L	11p14.3	ANO5	AR
LGMD 2M	9q31	Fukutin	AR
LGMD 2N	14q24	POMT2	AR
Congenital Muscular Dystrophy (CMD) Secondary to Glycosylation Disorder			
Fukuyama MD (syndromic)	9q31	Fukutin	AR
Muscle-eye-brain disease (syndromic)	1p34.1	Protein O-linked mannose β1,2-N-acetylglucosaminyltransferase (POMGnT1)	AR
Walker-Warburg syndrome (syndromic)	9q34.1	Protein-O-mannosyltranseferase (POMT1)	AR
MDC 1A (merosin-negative CMD)	6q22-23	Laminin-α2 (merosin)	
MDC 1B (merosin-positive CMD)	1q42	?	AR
MDC 1C	19q13.3	Fukutin-related protein (FKRP)	AR
MDC 1D	22q12.3-q13.1	LARGE	AR
Other Congenital Muscular Dystrophies			
CMD with early rigid spine (RSS)	1p36	Selenoprotein N-1	AR
CMD with *ITGA7* mutations	12q	Integrin α7	AR
Ullrich syndrome/Bethlem myopathy	21q22.3 (A1, A2) 2q37 (A3)	Collagen VI α1, α2, and α3	AD
Muscular Dystrophies Secondary to Nuclear Envelope Defects			
Emery-Dreifuss MD X1	Xq28	Emerin	XR
Emery-Dreifuss MD X2	q21.2	Lamin A/C	AD
Emery-Dreifuss MD X3	1q21.2	Lamin A/C	R
Emery-Dreifuss MD X4	6q25	Synaptic nuclear envelope protein 1 (SYNE1; Nesprin-1)	AD
Emery-Dreifuss MD X5	14q23	SYNE2	AD
Emery-Dreifuss MD X6	Xq26	Four-and-a-half-LIM protein 1 (FHL1)	AR/AD
Muscular Dystrophies Secondary to RNA Metabolism Defects			
Myotonic dystrophy 1 (DM1)	19q13.3	Myotonic dystrophy-associated protein kinase (DMPK)	AD
Myotonic dystrophy 2 (DM2)	3q21	Zinc finger, nucleic acid binding protein (ZNF9)	AD

Table 19-1 Pathophysiological Classification of Muscular Dystrophies—Cont'd

Disease	Gene Locus	Gene Product	Mode of Inheritance
Other Muscular Dystrophies of Unknown Mechanism			
Facioscapulohumeral dystrophy (FSHD)	4q35	FRG-1 (FSH region gene 1)	AD
Oculopharyngeal MD	14q11.2-q13	PABPN1	AD

Also see Table 12-2.
AD, autosomal dominant; AR, autosomal recessive; X, X-linked recessive.

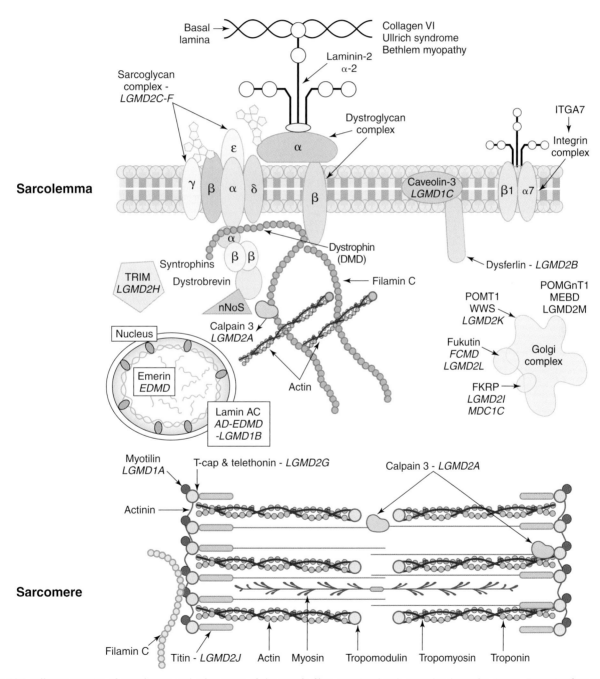

Figure 19-1 Different proteins of sarcolemma and other areas of the muscle fiber associated with muscular dystrophy. EDMD, Emery-Dreifuss muscular dystrophy; FCMD, fukuyama congenital muscular dystrophy; FKRP, fukutin-related protein; ITGA7, integrin, alpha7; LGMD, limb-girdle muscular dystrophy; LGMD2M, limb-girdle muscular dystrophy 2M; MEBD, muscle-eye-brain disease; nNOS, neuronal nitric oxide synthase; POMGnT1, protein O-linked mannose β1,2-N-acetylglucosaminyltransferase; POMT, protein O-mannosyltransferase; TRIM, tripartite motif; WWS, Walker-Warburg syndrome.

slower progression of muscle weakness compared with the usual Duchenne phenotype.[2,10–12] This process is therefore an appealing target for therapy in dystrophinopathies, because pharmacologic induction of exon skipping in DMD patients should produce some quantity of dystrophin and may alleviate the severity of the disease (see discussion of Treatment and Management in this chapter).

Approximately 60% of cases of Duchenne and Becker muscular dystrophy are the result of deletions.[13–17] Deletions can occur almost anywhere in the *DMD* gene, but two hotspots have been identified. The most commonly mutated region includes exons 45-55 with the genomic breakpoint (i.e., the endpoint of where the deletions actually occurs) lying within intron 44. The second region includes exons 2-19 with genomic breakpoints commonly found in introns 2 and 7.[18–21] The other 40% of cases result from small mutations (point mutations resulting in frame-shift or nonsense mutations) or duplications. There is a great deal of variability between the size and type of mutations, how they effect transcription, and the clinical phenotype of the disease. The Leiden database (http://www.dmd.nl/) is a useful resource for phenotype/genotype correlation in cases in which genetic testing and phenotype do not appear to be clearly correlated.

The incidence of DMD has been estimated at approximately in 3300 male births.[22,23] The most common mode of inheritance is X-linked recessive, but approximately 30% of cases are spontaneous mutations with no demonstrable family history.[23–26] Males are primarily affected, but females may manifest symptoms of DMD if they also exhibit skewed X-inactivation, wherein the abnormal X chromosome is expressed in an excessively abnormal proportion.[27–30]

Pathophysiology
Dystrophin Protein
The normal *DMD* gene creates a 14-kb dystrophin mRNA that encodes dystrophin, a 427-kDa protein. Dystrophin localizes to the subsarcolemmal region in skeletal and cardiac muscle and composes 0.002% of total muscle protein.[31–33] Dystrophin binds to the cytoskeletal actin and to the cytoplasmic tail of the transmembrane dystrophin-glycoprotein complex (DGC) protein β-dystroglycan, and through this to α-sarcoglycan, thus forming a link from the cytoskeleton to the extracellular matrix (see Fig. 19-1). The dystrophin protein is also found in brain, smooth muscle, and retina.

Primary and Secondary (Downstream) Events
Muscle cell death (by apoptosis and necrosis) in the muscular dystrophies is conditional on endogenous biochemical mechanisms and reflects a propensity that varies between muscles and changes with age (Fig. 19-2).[34] Although dystrophin deficiency is the primary cause

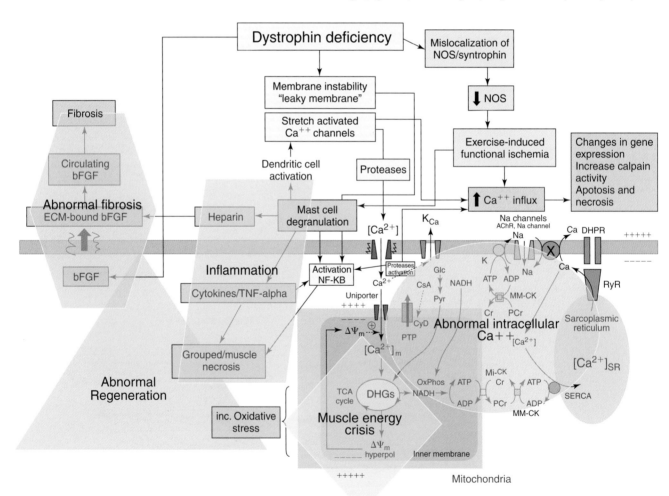

Figure 19-2 Events in the pathogenesis of muscle necrosis in Duchenne muscular dystrophy. ADP, adenosine diphosphate; ATP, adenosine triphosphate; bFGF, basic fibroblast growth factor; DHGs, dehydrogenases; DHPR, dihydropyridine receptor; ECM, extracellular matrix; MM-CK, MM fraction of creatine kinase; NADH, nicotinamide adenosine dinucelotide (reduced); NOS, nitric oxide synthase; SERCA, sarcoplasmic/endoplasmic Ca²⁺ ATPase; SR, sarcoplasmic reticulum; TCA, tricarboxylic acid cycle; TNF, tumor necrosis factor.

of DMD, multiple secondary pathways are responsible for the progression of muscle necrosis, the abnormal fibrosis, and the failure of regeneration that results in a progressively worsening clinical status. The literature is rich in evidence supporting oxidative radical damage to myofibers,[35–38] inflammation,[39–45] abnormal calcium homeostasis,[36,46–50] myonuclear apoptosis,[51–57] abnormal fibrosis, and failure of regeneration.[58–66] The following is a brief summary of the current understanding of how these processes occur.

Mechanical Membrane Fragility

Dystrophin is a link between the intracellular cytoskeleton and the extracellular matrix. The carboxy-terminal of dystrophin is attached to the sarcolemma, the surface membrane of striated muscle cells,[67–70] binding to β-dystroglycan[71] and through this to other dystrophin-associated glycoproteins, and to α-dystroglycan, which links the sarcolemma to the extracellular matrix.[72] When dystrophin is not present, the disconnection of contractile proteins from β-dystroglycan results in loss of β- and α-dystroglycan and the DGC from the sarcolemma. This disruption results in membrane fragility and abnormal permeability, particularly to calcium ions.

Abnormal Permeability to Calcium and Chronic Increase in Intracellular Calcium

In addition to the membrane disruption theory, there is accumulating evidence that abnormal Ca^{2+} handling may be related to direct dystrophin regulation of mechanosensitive transient receptor potential (TRP) channels[47,73] as well as abnormal intracellular Ca^{2+} cycling.[74–76]

The deregulation of Ca^{2+} channels is seen in abnormal function of voltage-insensitive or "stretch-activated" Ca^{2+} channels, a subfamily of the TRP channels.[77] These stretch-activated channels are abnormally active under mechanical stimulation in myotubes of *mdx* mice (murine model of DMD), resulting in an increase in intracellular calcium.[73,78,79]

The L-type, voltage-gated Ca^{2+} channels also appear to be abnormal in the absence of dystrophin; it has been shown that the Ca^{2+} currents in response to an action potential are much smaller in *mdx* mice than in normal controls. A disrupted direct or indirect linkage of dystrophin with these channels may be crucial for proper excitation-contraction coupling, initiating Ca^{2+} release from the sarcoplasmic reticulum.

The abnormal intracellular Ca^{2+} levels result in abnormal activation of Ca^{2+}-activated proteases (i.e., calpain) with subsequent abnormal degradation of intracellular proteins, which probably contributes to the abnormal functioning of the calcium leak channels.[80] Recent evidence shows that exercise worsens the abnormalities in calcium homeostasis in *mdx* mice.[81] This finding supports the clinical observation that eccentric exercises in DMD are deleterious and exacerbate muscle weakness.[82,83] Calcium also accumulates in mitochondria, contributing to cell dysfunction by affecting energy production.[46]

Abnormal Immunologic Response

A persistent inflammatory response is observed in dystrophic skeletal muscle. Mechanical stretch can abnormally activate nuclear factor kappa-beta (NF-κB), resulting in increased expression of the inflammatory cytokines interleukin-1β and tumor necrosis factor-alpha (TNF-α).[84] The extracellular environment is marked by an increased presence of inflammatory cells (i.e., macrophages) and elevated levels of various inflammatory cytokines (i.e., TNF-α, transforming growth factor-beta [TGF-β]). The presence of these substances, which lead to successful muscle repair in healthy muscle, may promote muscle wasting and fibrosis in dystrophic muscle.

Many of these immune response pathways are known to be blocked by prednisone, which is known to slow progression of the disease. These include induction of the transcription of NF-κB inhibitor, which keeps NF-κB in the inactive state; and decreased production of pro-inflammatory cytokines and induction of genes that inhibit cyclo-oxygenase-2, adhesion molecules, and other inflammatory mediators.

Abnormal Signaling Functions

Mounting evidence shows that the dystroglycan complex has important muscle cell signaling functions, and its integrity is essential for muscle cell viability.[85] These functions include transmembrane signaling (through β-dystroglycan), docking of signal transduction molecules (i.e., caveolin-3), and interaction with or regulation of other transmembrane complexes (i.e., integrins). When the dystroglycan complex is disassociated from the sarcolemma, there is a disruption of the cell signaling involved in regulating apoptosis[85] and in the metabolism of reactive oxygen species.[36,37,84,86–88]

Another abnormality of cell signaling is likely the underlying explanation for the "vascular" theory of DMD pathogenesis, supported in the past by morphologic evidence of muscle fiber group necrosis occurring very early in the disease, presumably secondary to ischemia. Recent findings show that the mislocalization and reduction of neuronal nitric oxide synthase (nNOS) in dystrophic muscle affects smooth vessel vasodilation in response to alpha-adrenergic stimuli in exercise,[89] resulting in muscle ischemia.[90] Dystrophin-associated α-syntrophin appears to be essential for the membrane localization of nNOS.[89]

Abnormal Fibrosis and Muscle Regeneration

Fibrosis (excessive deposition of endomysial and perimysial extracellular matrix) is a known secondary phenomenon to chronic muscle inflammation and fiber degeneration in DMD.[44] However, the amount of fibrosis in DMD seems disproportionate to the clinical severity in the earlier stages of the disease. Observation of this fact spurred the idea that fibrosis may also occur independent from muscle necrosis and degeneration. Evidence suggests that both enhanced fibrinogenesis and decreased fibrinolysis[91] are implicated in the development of muscle fibrosis in DMD. It has been established that expression of the fibrogenic cytokine TGF-β1 is increased in the muscle of DMD patients[59] and in serum samples of individuals with DMD.[92]

Diagnosis and Evaluation

Clinical Characteristics

Duchenne Muscular Dystrophy

Neuromuscular Involvement

Muscle fiber necrosis with elevated muscle calcium levels and a high serum creatine kinase (CK) enzyme level can be found in infancy in patients with DMD,[93] but the clinical manifestations are typically not recognized until at least age 3 years. This discrepancy represents a potential therapeutic window in which early interventions could theoretically prevent or delay the onset of symptoms. Walking often begins later than in normal children, and affected boys experience more falling than expected. Gait abnormality often becomes apparent by age 3 to 4 years, leading to clinical evaluation. Muscle weakness presents initially in neck flexor muscles, with power being less than antigravity. As a result, the child turns on his side when getting up from a supine position on the floor, which is the initial sign of the Gowers maneuver. Hypertrophy of calf muscles becomes prominent by age 3 or 4 years (Fig. 19-3). Hypertrophy of other muscles, including the vastus lateralis, infraspinatus, deltoid, and less frequently the gluteus maximus, triceps, and masseter muscles, may also

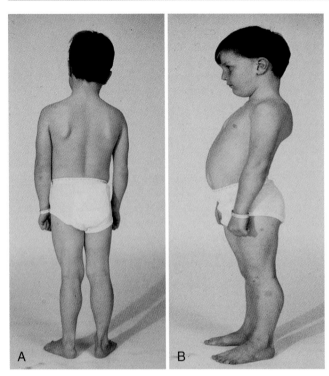

Figure 19-3 A child with Duchenne muscular dystrophy. Notice winging of the scapulae (**A**), hypertrophy of the calf muscles, and prominent lordosis (**B**).

develop. Muscle mass is usually decreased in later stages in the pectoral, peroneal, and anterior tibial muscles.

Because of hip girdle weakness, untreated patients exhibit the Gowers sign by age 5 or 6 years. The patient assumes a locked-leg, buttocks-first position followed by pushing off the floor with the hands, literally pushing the trunk erect by bracing the arms against the anterior thighs. Patients also tend to rock from side to side when walking, producing the waddling gait that is typical in older boys with the disease. Climbing stairs also becomes difficult with disease progression, and eventually distal muscles of the arms and legs become weak.

Accelerated deterioration in strength and balance often results from intercurrent disease or surgically induced immobilization. A wheelchair is required when ambulation is no longer possible, typically near the end of the first decade in untreated DMD and about 3 to 10 years later in steroid-treated DMD. After loss of ambulation, contractures become more pronounced in the lower extremities; they also soon involve the shoulders, and kyphoscoliosis may develop. Cardiac and respiratory involvement often occurs in this later disease stage as well.

Adolescent patients manifest increasing weakness and are unable to perform routine daily tasks with their arms, hands, and fingers. The head may progressively flex forward as extensor neck muscles lose strength. Lower facial muscles may be involved in the advanced phase.

Respiratory Involvement

Pulmonary function becomes compromised because of weakness of intercostal and diaphragmatic muscles and severe scoliosis. It occurs later in the disease in nonambulatory boys and is the primary cause of mortality in DMD. Muscle weakness affects all aspects of lung function, including mucociliary clearance, gas exchange at rest and during exercise, and respiratory control during wakefulness and sleep.[94] It is important to recognize that DMD is often associated with sleep disordered breathing, which could be asymptomatic or only mildly symptomatic. Respiratory complications and their treatment are discussed in greater detail in Chapter 2.

Cardiac Involvement

Boys with DMD are at risk for cardiomyopathy, especially if they have deletion of exons 48 to 53.[95] Mild degrees of cardiac compromise in DMD may occur in up to 95% of boys.[96] Chronic heart failure may affect up to 50%.[96,97] Sudden cardiac failure can occur, especially during adolescence. In one series of 19 patients, autopsies revealed that 84% had demonstrable cardiac involvement.[98] Cardiac complications and their management are discussed further in Chapter 3.

Neuropsychological Involvement

Overall, the IQ curve in boys with DMD is shifted to the left.[99] The mean IQ score in one study was 83 (range, 46 to 134). Other studies have not been able to prove a difference in overall IQ.[100–103] Recently, it has become evident that certain cognitive areas (i.e., verbal memory) are more affected than others in DMD.[102]

Other Organ Involvement

Rarely, gastrointestinal tract involvement associated with smooth muscle dysfunction causes megacolon, volvulus, abdominal cramping, and malabsorption.[104]

Clinical Characteristics of Becker Muscular Dystrophy

Becker muscular dystrophy is present in 3 to 6 per 100,000 male births.[105] The onset of weakness is later than in the Duchenne type, usually seen after age 7 years and often in the second decade; the disease is also marked by lordosis, calf hypertrophy, and other features of DMD of a milder phenotype (Fig. 19-4). The course is prolonged into adulthood, often with a normal life span. Ambulation is typically maintained beyond age 30 years. CK level is usually between 2000 and 20,000 U/L but may be in the normal range for mildly affected males. Because these patients can be asymptomatic for decades, they commonly are misdiagnosed as having liver disorder

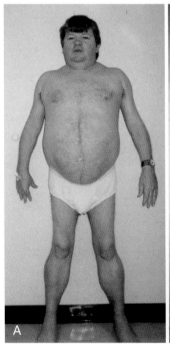
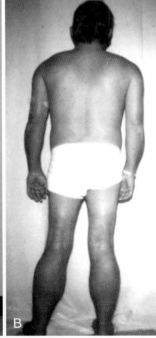

Figure 19-4 An adult patient with Becker muscular dystrophy. **A,** Patient's front; **B,** patient's back. Notice the prominent calf muscles.

when routine laboratory values show elevated transaminases (AST and ALT), which are elevated in parallel with serum CK levels. At times, the BMD diagnosis is made after many years of gastrointestinal follow-up for elevated transaminases, until someone thinks of measuring the CK, which comes back extremely elevated. The patient may have undergone liver biopsies to no avail. Pseudohypertrophy, proximal hip weakness resulting in the Gowers sign, and electrocardiogram (ECG) abnormalities associated with DMD are also common to BMD.

Chromosome Xp21 Microdeletion Syndromes

The Xp21 microdeletion syndromes are a series of syndromes that include DMD, Aland Island eye disease, adrenal hypoplasia, glycerol kinase deficiency, retinitis pigmentosa (*RP3*), mental retardation (*MRX1*), and ornithine transcarbamylase deficiency. The combination of these conditions led to the discovery of the *DMD* gene on Xp21.[106]

Female DMD Carriers and Manifesting Carriers

Carrier females are heterozygous with a normal *DMD* gene on one X chromosome and a mutant gene on the other. More than 90% of female carriers are asymptomatic. However, variable degrees of muscle weakness may be seen with skewed X-inactivation, in which more than half of the mutant X chromosomes are operant in muscle cells. Such cells are prone to degeneration. If a large number of abnormal muscle fibers are present in a given muscle, that muscle may display weakness. The degree of strength from one muscle to another may vary from normal strength to significant weakness.

Signs and symptoms of female dystrophinopathy include muscle weakness, myopathic findings on muscle biopsies, elevated CK levels, and partial absence of dystrophin in muscle.[107] Symptoms manifest in about one fifth of DMD carriers.[108] The diagnosis should be considered in women with elevated CK levels and muscle weakness, even in the absence of a positive family history for DMD.[109]

Duchenne muscular dystrophy carriers appear to have an increased incidence of cardiomyopathy. Studies have shown an incidence of asymptomatic cardiomyopathy ranging from 8% to 48% in adult DMD carriers[108,110,111] and from 0% to 15% in DMD carrier girls under age 16 years.[112]

Clinical Laboratory Tests

In DMD, serum CK is greatly elevated, typically from 10,000 to 30,000 U/L, early in the course of the disease. Gaps in the sarcolemma allow efflux of the enzyme into the circulation. Serum CK levels can vary greatly with activity and decrease as muscle mass is lost with disease progression. There is no correlation between the serum CK level and clinical severity in DMD, and use of CK levels as a surrogate marker of treatment response is not well supported. Because of the leakage of intracellular muscle proteins, other muscle isoenzymes also increase in the circulation. These include aldolase, lactate dehydrogenase, ALT, and, to a lesser degree, AST.

Genetic Testing

Genetic testing for DMD and BMD is widely available, especially for the deletions in the two "hot spots" of the gene. The screening of only 19 exons by multiplex polymerase chain reaction (PCR) identifies approximately 98% of all deletions.[19] Southern Blot analysis is utilized to predict if the deletion, when in the rod domain, will shift the reading frame, and thus is conclusive for DMD or BMD. However, when the deletions are in the first 25 exons, there are enough exemptions to the "reading frame" rule[112a] that muscle biopsy is necessary to determine with accuracy whether the patient has Duchenne or Becker muscular dystrophy. This technique is very

effective for the molecular diagnosis of common deletions (60% of patients); however, it cannot be used to identify duplications, other point mutations, intronic mutations, or to genotype female carriers. Other diagnostic approaches, such as quantitative PCR[113,114] or multiplex amplifiable probe hybridization,[115] might be used for accurate diagnosis and for carrier testing. With more recent technology, it is now possible to screen the entire *DMD* gene to search for the specific molecular defects responsible for the other 40% of DMD and BMD.

Muscle Biopsy

Histology of DMD muscle demonstrates fiber size variation, degenerating and regenerating fibers, clusters of smaller fibers, endomysial fibrosis, and a few scattered lymphocytes. Large, opaque fibers are prominent on modified Gomori-Wheatley trichrome staining (Fig. 19-5). As the disease progresses, muscle fibers are lost and replaced with fat and connective tissue. Fiber typing with adenosine triphosphatase histochemistry is less distinct than expected. Oxidative histochemistry is maintained. Absence of immunoreactivity for dystrophin with monoclonal antibodies against the C-terminal, rod domain, and N-terminal are necessary for accurate diagnosis of DMD (Fig. 19-6). Quantitative dystrophin analysis by immunoblot

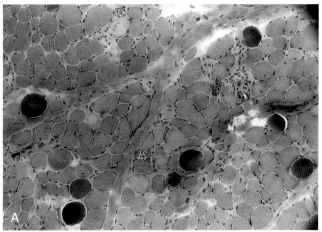

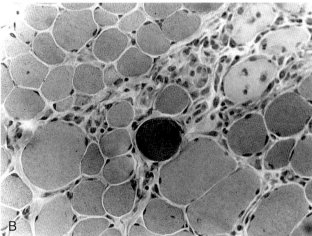

Figure 19-5 A, A trichrome-stained section of a muscle biopsy from a patient with Duchenne muscular dystrophy showing necrosis, opaque fibers, mildly increased endomysial connective tissue, and variation in muscle fiber size (×200). **B,** Higher magnification (×400) showing fiber atrophy, hypertrophy and necrosis, and interstitial infiltrates of mononuclear cells. (Reproduced with permission from Bertorini T: "Muscular Dystrophies" in Pourmond's *Neuromuscular Diseases, Expert Clinicians' Views,* Boston, 2001, Butterworth-Heinemann.)

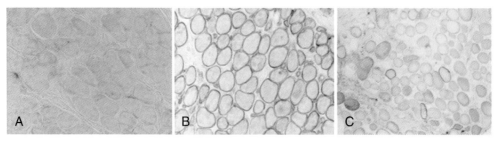

Figure 19-6 Muscle biopsy of Duchenne muscular dystrophy showing staining for dystrophin with absence of the protein (**A**) compared with control muscle (**B**) showing normal staining for dystrophin and muscle atrophy. (**C**) An area of the muscle biopsy showing scattered revertant fibers that stain positive for dystrophin (×200).

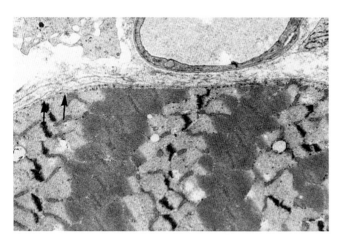

Figure 19-7 Electromicrograph of a specimen from a 6-year-old child with Duchenne muscular dystrophy revealing sarcolemma (cell wall) disruption (*arrows*) with redundant membranes (×10,800). (Reprinted with permission from Escolar D: "Muscular Dystrophies" in *Pediatric Neurology Principles & Practice*, Philadelphia, 2006, Mosby.)

is more accurate for diagnosis than immunostaining, with dystrophin value being less than 5% in DMD patients. On electron microscopy, gaps in the sarcolemma with preservation of the basement lamina are seen in nonnecrotic fibers (Fig. 19-7).

Histologic findings in BMD are similar to but less pronounced than those in DMD. The sarcolemmal gaps are not as readily seen. Using monoclonal antibodies directed to separate regions of dystrophin, immunoreactivity over the sarcolemma shows a variety of staining patterns, ranging from intact to absent, with one or more antibodies.[116]

Treatment and Management

In DMD and BMD, multidisciplinary care involving physicians (neurologists, physiatrists, orthopedic surgeons, cardiologists, and pulmonary medicine specialists), physical and occupational therapists, nutritionists, exercise physiologists, and social workers is important for the overall well-being of the child and the family.

Pharmacologic Treatment

Daily prednisone stabilizes or improves the strength of boys with DMD and is the only proven treatment for this disease. The benefits of this drug were first reported in an open trial of 2 mg/kg/day,[117] later reinforced by other open design trials[118,119] and subsequent double-blinded, placebo-controlled trials.[120–122] The most effective dose is 0.75 mg/kg/day. There is a dose-response effect, with the lowest effective dose being 0.3 mg/kg/day.[120] Effects on strength can be observed as soon as 10 days after treatment starts, with a peak at 3 months and then a stabilization period.[123] In a 3-year follow-up

study, improvement was maintained in those children who were kept on doses of at least 0.5 or 0.6 mg/kg/day.[121] DMD boys treated with prednisone from an earlier age usually remain ambulatory into their teens, have less incidence of scoliosis[124,125] and contractures,[126] and maintain normal or near-normal respiratory function.[125,127–129]

Despite the evidence in favor of daily prednisone, a source of major concern for patients and physicians are the numerous potential side effects caused by this treatment. Most commonly seen are increased appetite and weight gain, irritability, hirsutism, cushingoid features, and decreased linear growth.[130] In this young population, diabetes, hypertension, ulcers, and infections are rare. Steroid-induced osteoporosis is difficult to assess in DMD, because baseline osteoporosis might be present secondary to decreased activity.[131–133]

Deflazacort, a corticosteroid not available in the United States, has similar benefits to prednisone but causes less weight gain and cushingoid features, though it appears to have an increased predisposition to asymptomatic cataract formation.[127,128,130,134–136] Suggested dosage is 0.9 to 1.2 mg/kg/day. Because of its unavailability, some patients import the drug from other countries. This should only be recommended for those DMD patients who are already overweight before treatment and in a more advanced stage of the disease. Lower dose regimens, including alternate-day corticosteroids and treatment for the first 10 days of the month, have not demonstrated sustained efficacy.[121,137]

Accumulating evidence suggests that treatment of DMD should start as soon as the diagnosis is made,[129,138,139] but early corticosteroids are associated with significant decrease in linear growth. However, this might be a mechanical advantage for DMD boys. A pilot study of 10 mg/kg given over 2 consecutive days of the week (Friday and Saturday) showed that DMD boys improved muscle strength and function while maintaining linear growth, and they did not have increased body mass index compared with untreated DMD boys.[140] A larger study comparing both dosing regimens was completed by the Cooperative International Neuromuscular Research Group (CINRG) at the end of 2007. Preliminary results were presented at scientific meetings, but the results of this trial have not yet been published. This study will clarify many questions associated with both regimens concerning appropriate onset of treatment at different stages of the disease and the side effects of steroids in this specific population.

Obesity is often a major problem in DMD, even if no steroids are used. For uncertain reasons, patients gain excessive weight, which often becomes apparent before ambulation is lost. The obesity becomes more prominent after confinement to a wheelchair. Boredom, diminished physical activity, and depression may lead to inappropriate food intake,[141] and rigorous measures are required to forestall weight gain. Obesity reduces the period of walking capability, hastens scoliosis, and fosters respiratory and cardiac insufficiency. Therefore, if steroid treatment is offered, these patients need to follow a restricted caloric intake diet to prevent excessive weight gain. A diet high in proteins, fresh fruits, and vegetables and low in fat and carbohydrates is ideal. A nutritionist should be part of the medical team of a DMD boy receiving long-term steroid treatment.

Other immunosuppressive medications have mixed results in DMD. Azathioprine demonstrated no benefit,[122] but cyclosporin A showed evidence of efficacy in DMD in an uncontrolled trial.[142,143] At 5 mg/kg/day, it showed improvement in strength in a test on an isolated muscle.

A randomized, controlled, blinded trial of creatine monohydrate and glutamine supplementation in ambulatory DMD patients (ages 5 to 11 years) was also negative based on manual muscle testing (primary outcome). However, there were consistent and clear trends toward improvement in isometric muscle strength in older patients with creatine, and increased function in younger children with creatine and glutamine.[144] Other studies have shown increase in muscle strength and body mass index with creatine in DMD.[145,146] No significant side effects were seen with doses of 5 g/day for at least 6 months.[144]

Another open label pilot study conducted by CINRG demonstrated a possible beneficial effect of coenzyme Q10 as an add-on to traditional corticosteroid therapy. These results have not yet been published.

A regimen of prednisone 0.75 mg/kg/day for 10 days alternating with 10-day steroid-free periods is currently being utilized by some physicians in Europe. One retrospective study of this regimen was perfomed[147]; the benefit over daily or high-dose weekend schedules is unclear. A direct prospective comparison of all three regimens would be useful.

Current Research in Pharmacologic Approaches

Better understanding of the pathophysiology of dystrophinopathies has provided three main areas of interest for researchers: (1) manipulation of the *DMD* gene with either repair or replacement; (2) up-regulation of proteins that may compensate for a lack of dystrophin; and (3) pharmacologic manipulation of the downstream events that occur when dystrophin is absent or reduced (Fig. 19-8). Several approaches at these different levels have been investigated, and more are currently being evaluated. Most of the preclinical experiments have been performed in the mouse model of muscular dystrophy (*mdx*), but overall there have been mixed results in the transfer of results from mouse to human.

Gene Repair or Replacement

A small percentage of patients with DMD have nonsense mutations that promote premature translational termination of the dystrophin protein. The result is a small unstable protein that gets rapidly degraded. A new pharmacologic approach to treat DMD aims to "skip" these premature stop codons.

Gentamicin, an aminoglycoside antibiotic, has been investigated based on its binding of the ribosome causing "read-through" of premature stop codon (nonsense) mutations. It was tried first in the *mdx* model of DMD[148] and then in a clinical trial on four DMD/BMD patients.[149] Although the *mdx* experiments showed positive dystrophin in approximately 15% of previously negative muscle fibers,[148] the human trial was unable to duplicate this finding.

An unrelated drug with a similar mechanism of action (forced read-through of premature stop codon mutations), PTC124 (Ataluren) is currently under investigation in DMD boys. This oral medication can cause suppression of premature stop codons at much lower doses (from 10-fold to 100-fold lower) than gentamicin.[150] A randomized, placebo-controlled, dose-finding phase II study was recently stopped because the study failed to show statistically significant improvement in its primary outcome, the 6-minute walk test (6 MWT). Results of the study have not yet been published.

Another approach to gene repair includes the delivery to dystrophin-deficient cells of RNA-DNA oligonucleotides that target the specific mutation and revert it to the normal sequence (chimeroplasts),[151] or the delivery of antisense RNA molecules to dystrophin-deficient cells so that semi-functional dystrophin can be produced.[152–156] This method forces the splicing machinery of the cell to skip the *DMD* gene exon that contains the gene mutation, which results in the full translation of dystrophin mRNA (minus the mutant exon) into an "in-frame" semi-functional dystrophin protein. A recent trial of an antisense oligonucleotide (PRO051) injected into the tibialis anterior muscles of four DMD patients demonstrated evidence of some sarcolemmal dystrophin in 64% to 97% of muscle fibers. The quantitative ratio of dystrophin to laminin-α2 was 17% to 35% of that seen in controls.[157] A phase II/III systemic delivery of PRO051 by subcutaneous infection in DMD is ongoing. A recent study showed that long-term administration of antisense oligonucleotides into the paraspinal muscles of *mdx* mice reduced dystrophy-related kyphosis. Systemic delivery of another type of AON with a different chemistry

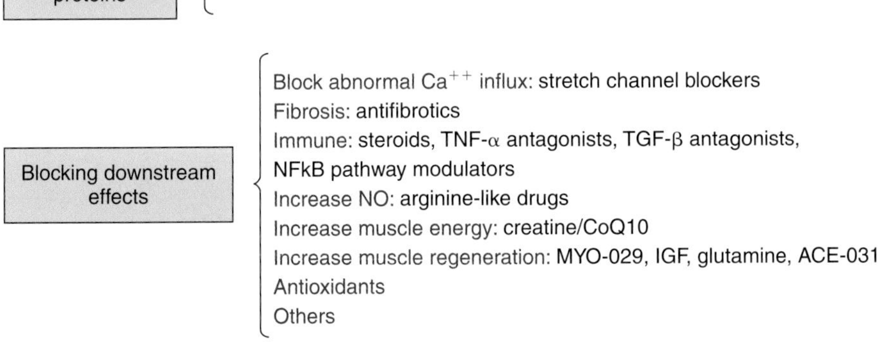

Gene repair or replacement	DNA (gene editing ex vivo with AON, then autologous cell transplantation)
	Gene replacement (AAV, myoblast transfer)
	RNA splicing (exon skipping with AON)
	Translation: stop codon read through (AON, AG, other antibiotics, PTC124 [Ataluren])

| Upregulation of compensatory proteins | Utrophin, α-dystrobrevin, α-7 integrin, GALNAc, NOS, etc. |

Blocking downstream effects	Block abnormal Ca^{++} influx: stretch channel blockers
	Fibrosis: antifibrotics
	Immune: steroids, TNF-α antagonists, TGF-β antagonists, NFkB pathway modulators
	Increase NO: arginine-like drugs
	Increase muscle energy: creatine/CoQ10
	Increase muscle regeneration: MYO-029, IGF, glutamine, ACE-031
	Antioxidants
	Others

Figure 19-8 Different treatment approaches in Duchenne muscular dystrophy, including gene repair, replacement, and upregulation of compensatory proteins and modification of downstream effects. AAV, adeno-associated virus; AG, aminoglycosides; AON, antisense oligonucleotides; PTC124, (Ataluren); ATb, antibiotic; CoQ10, coenzyme Q10; DNA, deoxyribonucleic acid; GALNAc, N-acetylgalactosamine; IGF, insulin-like growth factor; MYO-029, NFkB, nuclear factor κB; NO, nitric oxide; NOS, nitric oxide synthase; RNA, ribonucleic acid; TGF, transforming growth factor; TNF, tumor necrosis factor.

backbone (morpholino) in dystrophic dogs restored dystrophin and produced clinical improvement, opening the doors for trials in humans.[158,159] The first morpholino AON proof of concept trial, also targeting exon 51, has been completed in DMD boys. The local intramuscular injection of this AON showed significant increased dystrophin in muscle biopsies.[159a] A systemic intravenous administration phase II trial is ongoing.

Another area of interest is the delivery of functional mini-*DMD* genes to replace the missing dystrophin, using adeno-associated viral (AAV) vectors. Dystrophin can be produced, the immune response can be prevented, and improved function and pathology in young and older animals has been achieved.[160–163] An important hurdle was crossed when systemic delivery of an AAV6 vector with a mini-*DMD* gene was achieved in the older *mdx* mouse.[164] Recent attempts at vector-mediated mini-*DMD* gene expression in GRMD (Golden Retriever muscular dystrophy) dogs have caused a significant immune response; therefore, a canine mini-dystrophin gene was developed and was investigated in *mdx* mice before transfer into GRMD dogs was attempted. The canine mini-dystrophin gene caused expression of dystrophin, improved both fibrosis and central nucleation, and improved the plasma membrane integrity of myofibers in *mdx* mice.[165] The first U.S. clinical trial of mini-*DMD* gene transfer into humans began in 2006 and is currently underway.

Finally, the transfer of myoblasts and other stem cells have been studied as an attempt to introduce the normal *DMD* gene, but these approaches have not yet been very encouraging.[165] Myoblast transplants were tried in DMD boys with no success,[166–169] although they were effective in *mdx* mice.[170] New muscle cell precursor populations have since been identified, including the recently described "satellite side population (SP) cells,"[171] which may be the precursors of the muscle-repair "satellite cells." In *mdx* mice, these SP cells have been more efficient in engrafting into muscle fibers than the more mature cells used in previous trials, and the mice demonstrated extensive muscle regeneration and dystrophin production.

Up-regulation of Compensatory Proteins

Although the ultimate target for a cure in DMD is normalized expression of dystrophin, several other structural proteins have been proven to have at least a modifying effect on the disease. Utrophin is a sarcolemmal protein with a structure very similar to that of dystrophin. Transgenic overexpression of both truncated and full-length utrophin protein in *mdx* mice has demonstrated a significant improvement in phenotype.[172–174] Up-regulation of utrophin by pharmacologic means has been investigated. Prednisone is known to up-regulate utrophin; arginine also has been shown to do the same.[175] At least one drug is in development for future studies.

The α7β1-integrin protein is an alternative to the DAG, attaching the muscle fiber to laminin in the basal lamina. Transgenic expression of this protein in dystrophin- and utrophin-deficient mice has shown improvements in life expectancy and a reduction of muscle pathology.[176]

Poloxamer 188 (P188) is an amphiphilic polymer that acts as a synthetic sealant by localizing into damaged portions of membranes.[177] A recent study in *mdx* mice showed strong evidence of improvement in cardiomyopathy when P188 was administered.[178] However, similar results have not been reliably achieved in skeletal muscle.[179]

Several other types of proteins have shown the ability to compensate for the loss of dystrophin outside the arena of structural integrity. For instance, myostatin, the protein that negatively regulates muscle growth, has been targeted as a potential modulator of dystrophinopathies. Early studies on myostatin inhibition in mice were encouraging,[180] but an initial human trial using anti-myostatin antibodies did not demonstrate clinical effectiveness.[181] Efforts have also been focused on a related protein, follistatin, which is an endogenous inhibitor of myostatin. The transgenic expression of follistatin has demonstrated increased muscle mass and a decrease in signs of disease on histology in *mdx* mice.[182]

A correlation has been observed between calcium-dependent protease (calpain) activity in dystrophic muscle and muscle necrosis.[183] Calpastatin is a specific endogenous inhibitor of two types of calpain, and transgenic overexpression of calpastatin has demonstrated a reduction in muscle necrosis.[184]

As indicated above, the absence of dystrophin results in mislocalization of the nNOS protein and its absence from the membrane. Transgenic expression of nNOS in *mdx* mice has demonstrated reduced inflammation and necrosis in both skeletal and cardiac muscle.[185]

Modification of Downstream Events

After an almost 15-year gap in which all efforts were focused on a definite cure with gene therapy, there has been an explosion of clinical studies to evaluate new pharmacologic approaches to treat DMD. The CINRG has completed several clinical trials for DMD over the past 2 years, besides the creatine study mentioned above. A study comparing daily prednisone (0.75mg/kg/day) against a weekly pulse of 10 mg/kg divided over 2 days had the objective of determining if a different dose schedule could be as effective as daily prednisone but with lesser side effects. This study was also designed to evaluate the effect of steroids on bone density and behavior after 1 year of treatment. There was equal randomization to younger and older patient groups, so that the study could suggest if efficacy and side effect profile differs by age or stage of disease. The results of this study have not yet been published.

Novel pharmacologic approaches at modifying downstream events associated with dystrophinopathies are also under investigation and development.

Intracellular Calcium

L-type voltage-dependent calcium channel blockers such as diltiazem and verapamil have shown some benefit in *mdx* mice, including decreased CK levels and decreased permeability of the sarcolemma in the diaphragm.[186] However, to date no human trials have demonstrated significant benefit of this drug class in DMD.[187]

Blockage of stretch-activated channels has been achieved by the nonselective TRP blockers gadolinium and streptomycin, as well as by the selective cationic TRP blocker GsMTx4 (spider venom toxin), and has resulted in normalization of intracellular calcium and muscle force generation ex vivo in *mdx* mouse muscle.[188,189] Furthermore, treatment of *mdx* mice with oral streptomycin resulted in decreased muscle necrosis, which opens the door for clinical translation.[188]

Pentoxifylline, a phosphodiesterase inhibitor, has recently been demonstrated to counteract the voltage-independent calcium channel overactivity in *mdx* mice[190] and has shown increased resistance to exercise in *mdx* mice and increased tetanic tension of strips of diaphragm muscle taken from treated mice. Pentoxifylline also has antifibrotic, anti-inflammatory, and antioxidant actions. A pilot study looked at the effect of pentoxifylline in young (ages 4 to 7 years), steroid-naive DMD boys. A liquid, immediate-release formulation was used, with a dose of 20 mg/kg. The main purpose of the study was to evaluate safety of the drug in this young child population and to determine any effect on overall muscle strength. A larger, controlled study evaluated the effect of adding pentoxifylline (long-release, FDA-approved form) to steroid-treated DMD boys age 7 and older. Both studies have been presented in scientific meetings, but have not yet been published.

Dantrolene, which inhibits calcium release from the sarcoplasmic reticulum, has been shown to improve function in *mdx* mice and in a small clinical trial decreased muscle spasms and CK in patients with DMD.[191]

Abnormal Immune Response

The inflammation activated NF-κB pathway is a potentially favorable target for treatment. Genetic alteration of various members of this pathway in *mdx* mice have shown favorable results, as has the administration of a soluble inhibitor of the pathway.[192] Blockade of the related TNF-α pathways has also produced favorable results in mice.[193] The beneficial effects of prednisone in DMD are thought to be partly related to inhibition of this pathway.

Abnormal Signaling Functions

Efforts to ameliorate the effects of reactive oxygen species are currently under investigation. One promising compound along these lines is idebenone (SNT-MC17), which incorporates into the mitochondrial membrane, improving respiratory chain function and inhibiting lipid peroxidation and thus decreasing oxidative stress. When given presymptomatically and long term to *mdx* mice, it prevented cardiac diastolic dysfunction and the development of lethal acute heart failure.[194]

Another approach being studied is the activation of the nitric oxide (NO) pathway, which is impaired in DMD. A compound named HCT 1026 combines NO activation with nonsteroidal anti-inflammatory activity. The administration of this drug improved morphologic and functional features of *mdx* mice.[195] Similar NO donor compounds have been shown to cause a down-regulation of the histone deacetylase HDAC2 in dystrophic muscle.[196] This finding may represent a role for such proteins in the pathogenesis of Duchenne muscular dystrophy.

Abnormal Fibrosis and Muscle Regeneration

The abnormal fibrosis seen in DMD muscle is targeted by a novel drug called *halofuginone*. This compound inhibits TGF-β mediated collagen production. The *mdx* mice given halofuginone showed increased muscle cell proliferation; improved limb, cardiac, and respiratory function; and better recovery from exercise.[197]

A class of drugs called *deacetylase inhibitors* has demonstrated possible utility in DMD; in *mdx* mice, trichostatin A showed increased myofiber size and improved resistance to exercise-induced degeneration as well as decreased fibrosis and normalized muscle architecture.[198] The presumed mechanism of action is an up-regulation of the myostatin inhibitor, follistatin. This group of drugs is readily available in clinical practice and includes valproic acid and phenylbutyrate. Another approach to increase muscle size and decrease fibrosis has now reached the clinical arena. A soluble activin type II receptor attached to the Fc portion of the human gammaglobulin (ACE031) effectively binds circulating myostatin and other negative regulators of muscle growth and fibroblast growth and results in increased lean muscle mass, decreased fibrosis, and increased strength and function in the mdx mouse (Acceleron Pharma, unpublished data). A Phase II clinical trial in DMD boys has been initiated.

The angiotensin II type 1 receptor blocker, losartan, has also recently been shown to improve muscle regeneration and function in *mdx* mice via antagonism of TGF-β activity.[199]

Respiratory Care

Patients with DMD or BMD eventually progress to have ineffective cough and decreased ventilation, leading to pneumonia, atelectasis, and respiratory insufficiency in sleep and while awake.[94] These complications are generally preventable with careful follow-up and assessments of respiratory function. Patients with DMD should have routine immunizations by a primary care physician as recommended for well children by the American Academy of Pediatrics. In addition, these patients should receive the pneumococcal vaccine and annual influenza vaccine.

A polysomnographic study with continuous CO_2 monitoring is the best way to assess the need for ventilatory support. Pulse oximetry, especially during the awake state, is suboptimal. The decisions regarding long-term ventilation, be it invasive or noninvasive, should involve the patient, caregivers, and medical teams. Physicians have a legal and ethical responsibility to disclose treatment options and must avoid using their own perceptions of quality of life as the main factor in deciding whether to offer this type of information.[200] End of life decision-making should be discussed earlier based on all possible information available to the patient. Further details of respiratory management are provided in Chapter 2.

Cardiac Management

Although ECG abnormalities are common in DMD, the best correlation of cardiac involvement with prognosis is by measuring left ventricular dysfunction by echocardiography.[202] Recent guidelines for the study of cardiac involvement in DMD have been published.[203,204] These recommend that DMD patients have an ECG and echocardiography at the time of diagnosis, at every 2 years up to age 10 years, and subsequently every year. The early, preventive use of ACE inhibitors and later β-blockers is recommended.[203,204] Cardiac management is discussed in more detail in Chapter 3.

Drug Precautions

Use of anticholinergic drugs and ganglionic blocking agents should be avoided because of their tendency to decrease muscle tone. Patients with DMD may be susceptible to malignant hyperthermia, and proper evaluation and preparation before administration of general anesthesia are recommended.[213] Cardiotoxic drugs, such as halothane, should not be used, and caution is advised in undertaking general anesthesia.[214] Details are further discussed in Chapter 10.

Rehabilitation

No large prospective studies have been performed to evaluate the role of physical therapy, stretching exercises, use of braces, or type of physical activity in DMD. Thus, the evidence is lacking for solid recommendations. These approaches are described further in Chapter 8.

Contractures

Active range-of-motion exercises supplemented by passive stretching are important to prevent contractures. Nighttime stretching orthoses (similar to the static ankle-foot orthosis, but with a hinge at the ankle and adjustable straps) are useful and should be recommended at age 5 to 6 years. A standing board tilted up 20 degrees may be used for 20 minutes twice a day to provide constant stretching of the Achilles tendons. Keeping the heel cords stretched through vigorous passive stretching by parents and physical therapists helps maintain better gait mechanics. This program requires stretching of the tensor fascia lata, hamstrings, knee flexors, and ankle plantar flexors. If strenuous stretching is not effective, surgical release of tight heel cords may be beneficial,[201] even if the quadriceps and gastrocnemius muscle groups are both less than antigravity in strength. In the latter case, long leg bracing can be offered to keep some ambulation after contractures are corrected. Mobilization in a walking cast immediately after surgery is essential to prevent loss of strength. Temporary bracing after surgery is necessary for optimal results after tenotomy procedures. Hip flexion contractures may benefit from surgical release followed by application of long leg braces. Resection of the fascia lata (Rideau procedure) may be beneficial for some patients.[201]

Scoliosis

Nearly all patients with DMD develop scoliosis after losing independent ambulation. The use of solid seat and back inserts in properly fitted wheelchairs is helpful in preventing scoliosis by keeping truncal posture erect. For some boys, long leg braces can be fitted to allow braced upright daily standing to prevent curvature. Baseline back x-ray films to document the degree of curvature if scoliosis begins to develop should be obtained for comparison with future films. The use of steroids, perhaps because it prolongs ambulation beyond the growth spurt of the early teen years, delays or prevents scoliosis, even if the child is eventually wheelchair bound.[124,126] Surgical management of scoliosis and other orthopedic complications is discussed in Chapter 9.

Genetic Counseling

Duchenne and Becker muscular dystrophies are inherited in an X-linked recessive manner; the risk to the siblings of a proband depends on the carrier status of the mother. Carrier females have a 50% chance of transmitting the *DMD* mutation in each pregnancy. Sons who inherit the abnormal gene will be affected, whereas daughters will be carriers. Males with DMD do not reproduce. However, males with BMD and X-linked dilated cardiomyopathy may reproduce. All of their daughters will be carriers but none of the sons will inherit their father's *DMD* mutation. Prenatal testing for pregnancies at risk is possible. Until the molecular genetics of DMD and BMD were understood, the diagnosis of maternal and female sibling carriers was based on pedigree analysis and indirect assays. These included serum CK level determinations,[205,206] the occasional finding of histologic abnormalities in muscle obtained from carriers,[207] and in vitro muscle ribosomal protein synthesis.[208–210] Today, the specific molecular characterization of a proband makes genetic counseling much easier. If a specific mutation is found in a boy with DMD or BMD, genetic testing of the mother or sister looking for the exact mutation will determine if she is a carrier, and appropriate counseling can be done for further pregnancies. When DNA analysis in the proband is not informative, muscle biopsy of the fetus can be used to make the diagnosis.[211] Study of muscle from male fetuses with DMD show morphologic changes by the second trimester, especially greater muscle nuclear size when compared with fetuses of the same gestational age.[212] Immunoreaction for dystrophin is absent. When a deletion or specific mutation in the *DMD* gene has been demonstrated in another family member, the deletion may be looked for in fetal issue or earlier in chorionic villus. This means that intrauterine diagnosis is possible by 7 weeks' gestation in suspect male embryos.

Emotional and Behavioral Management

Dysthymic disorder and major depressive disorder can occur in DMD boys, especially in the adolescent.[215,216] An affected boy's preoccupation with self and subsequent withdrawal may lead many families to seek counseling. Depression may be seen in a boy who has lost an older brother or close friend to DMD. Depression is often associated with intellectual limitation, which may induce low tolerance for frustration and overstress other manifestations of emotional immaturity. Psychological evaluation and counseling may be necessary. Neuropsychological screening for intellectual deficits and behavioral problems is ideally done as the boy enters school and should be repeated in preadolescence.

Limb-Girdle Muscular Dystrophies

The limb-girdle muscular dystrophies (LGMD) are characterized by progressive muscle weakness of the large muscles around the shoulder and pelvic girdles (Fig. 19-9). The recent identification of individual causative mutations has led to a more thorough picture of the phenotype, but a confusing nomenclature has developed. The initial classification of these disorders was based on the mode of inheritance, dividing them into autosomal dominant (type 1: LGMD1), autosomal recessive (type 2: LGMD2), and X-linked forms. With the expanding list of identified genes, we now have a list of eight dominant forms (LGMD1A to LGMD1H), and fourteen recessive forms (LGMD2A to LGMD2N). An integrated classification taking into account the type and localization of the proteins was recently proposed.[1] The following is a summary of some of the better understood limb-girdle dystrophies.

Limb-Girdle Muscular Dystrophy 1C: Caveolinopathy

Caveolins are small transmembrane proteins with intracellular domains that undergo extensive oligomerization to form membrane complexes known as *caveolae*. Skeletal muscle disorders result from mutations in the gene that encodes caveolin 3 (*CAV3*), localized to chromosome 3p25. This protein interacts with nNOS and the dystrophin-associated protein complex via the intracellular portion of β-dystroglycan.[217,218] The disease can present in childhood with a range of symptoms from simple exertional myalgias to slowly progressive weakness, calf hypertrophy, and CK elevation. *CAV3* mutations are also associated with autosomal dominant rippling muscle disease.

Limb-Girdle Muscular Dystrophy 2A: Calpainopathy

This childhood-onset LGMD has been reported as the most frequent autosomal recessive LGMD in several series.[219–222] The abnormal protein, calpain 3, is a nonlysosomal intracellular, muscle-specific, Ca^{2+}-activated neutral protease.[223] LGMD 2A was the first form of limb-girdle dystrophy identified that is caused by deficiency of a nonstructural protein.

The calpain 3 gene (*CAPN3*) is located to chromosome 15q15.1–q21.1 and consists of 24 exons extending over a genomic region of

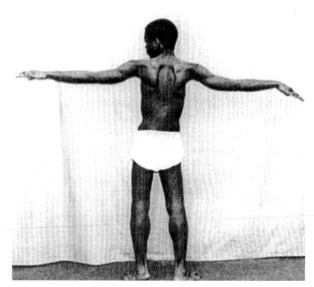

Figure 19-9 A patient with limb-girdle muscular dystrophy showing wasting of the thigh muscles and winging of the scapulae.

50 kb.[224,225] Homozygous null-null mutations appear to have the most severe phenotype, in terms of earlier wheelchair need, whereas a heterozygous missense mutation has the milder phenotype.[226]

CAPN3 appears to be a cytoskeleton modulator with an important role in muscle maturation.[227] One current hypothesis is that calpain could have a protective effect and be involved in muscle detoxification, preventing a degradation of the muscle fiber.[228] It may also play a role in intracellular signaling pathways, and its deficiency might be associated with myonuclear apoptosis by deregulation of the NF-κBα inhibitor/NF-κB pathway.[229]

Under normal circumstances, *CAPN3* undergoes rapid autocatalytic activity after translation.[230] During the short minutes (less than 5 minutes in muscle cultures) that the protein is present, it is in a resting state unless it becomes activated by signaling mechanisms.[231] The autocatalytic activity resides in a Ca^{2+}-sensitive region between domains II and III of the protein.

LGMD2A has a characteristic phenotype in approximately 64% of genetically confirmed patients. Interfamilial and intrafamilial variability, though, is not uncommon.[228] Age of symptom onset is between 2 and 49 years, with a mean age of presentation of about 14 years (±8).[226] The disease causes symmetric weakness of the pelvic and shoulder girdle muscles. Cardiac muscle is not affected. Scapular winging can be seen early.[232] Most patients, regardless the age of onset, become wheelchair bound about 25 years after symptom onset. The CK level is elevated by 5-fold to 20-fold. Cognition is not impaired.

The diagnosis of calpainopathy is based on a typical phenotype, a muscle biopsy showing Western blot abnormalities and a genetic test showing two mutations on two alleles. The combination of a typical phenotype with an abnormal Western blot in muscle biopsy (at least 2 abnormal bands) brings the probability of being calpainopathy to 90%.[226] However, if one of these tests is missing, the probability of accurate diagnosis is reduced to about 75%.[226] A 20% to 40% false-negative rate on Western blot in these patients indicates that genetic sequencing should be pursued when there is clinical suspicion.[226,233]

Muscle pathologic findings are positive for necrosis, regeneration, altered myofibrillar architecture, increased centrally placed nuclei, fibrosis, fiber type I predominance, and normal immunoreactivity for dystrophin and α-sarcoglycan. Mild inflammation can also be seen.

Limb-Girdle Muscular Dystrophy 2B: Dysferlinopathy

Mutations in the dysferlin gene (*DYSF*) on chromosome 2p13 cause distinct phenotypes of muscular dystrophy: limb-girdle muscular dystrophy type 2B (LGMD2B), Miyoshi myopathy (MM), or juvenile-onset distal posterior compartment myopathy, as well as distal anterior compartment myopathy, which are known collectively by the term *dysferlinopathy*. These conditions represent 1% of recessive LGMD and about 33% of distal LGMD.

The *DYSF* gene encodes a 230-kDa protein with widespread expression in tissues such as skeletal muscle, cardiac muscle, kidney, placenta, lung, and brain. Immunohistochemical studies show that, in skeletal muscle, dysferlin is located at the plasma membrane, as well as in cytoplasmic vesicles.[234]

This new class of muscular dystrophy is distinct in its pathogenesis in that the defect lies in the maintenance, not the structure, of the plasma membrane. Histopathologic and immunohistochemical studies in these patients show absence of dysferlin.[235] In addition, a very active inflammatory and degenerative process is characteristic in this disease and can lead to a misdiagnosis of polymyositis. The features of the immune response are different, though, with macrophages more common than T cells, perivascular and interstitial infiltrates consisting of CD8+ and CD4+ cells without B cells, and overexpression of major histocompatibility complex class I on muscle fibers.[236]

There are two common phenotypes, LGMD2B and the distal posterior compartment myopathy or MM, both presenting in the second decade of life.[237] Two other phenotypes, distal anterior compartment and scapuloperoneal types, can also be seen earlier.[238] The patients show normal early developmental milestones and no signs in childhood with a slowly progressive muscle weakness and wasting starting in the early to late teens.[239] The MM phenotype typically begins in the calves (Fig. 19-10) with later development of proximal weakness. LGMD 2B phenotype shows a predominantly proximal muscular dystrophy. Affected individuals have pelvic girdle muscle weakness, with lower limbs abducted and externally rotated and hyperlordosis as a result of hip muscle weakness.

Diagnosis of dysferlinopathy is based on the absence of dysferlin expression on immunoblots or cryostat sections as well as on exclusion of dystrophinopathy, sarcoglycanopathy, calpainopathy, and caveolinopathy. The diagnosis of dysferlinopathy can also be made by measuring dysferlin expression in peripheral blood mononuclear cells by immunoblot analysis, which shows excellent correlation with muscle biopsy findings.[240] This test is available commercially.

Limb-Girdle Muscular Dystrophies 2C, 2D, 2E, 2F: Sarcoglycanopathies

The sarcoglycanopathies are a family of autosomal recessive disorders often presenting with an early and severe phenotype. The four sarcoglycans comprise a tetrameric complex of membrane proteins that contributes to the stability of the plasma membrane cytoskeleton and facilitates the association of dystrophin with the dystroglycans. The four sarcoglycan genes (alpha, beta, gamma, and delta) are related to each other structurally and functionally, but each has a discrete chromosomal location. Mutations in each gene may produce partial or complete loss of the entire complex.[241] Patients with sarcoglycanopathies were initially delineated from children with a severe Duchenne-like presentation who proved dystrophin positive and in whom autosomal recessive inheritance was likely.[242] The term *severe childhood autosomal recessive*

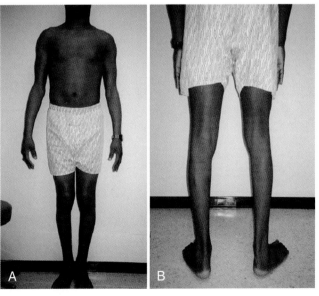

Figure 19-10 A patient with Miyoshi myopathy: front (**A**); back (**B**). Notice prominent atrophy of the posterior distal compartment muscles.

muscular dystrophy (SCARMD) was employed to describe these children, some of whom were later found to be deficient in a 50-kD dystrophin-associated protein, the gene for which was localized to chromosome 13q12, the locus for gamma-sarcoglycan.[243,244] Sister proteins were identified,[245] and the phenotypes associated with sarcoglycanopathies broadened to include less severely involved children.

Before investigating a child for sarcoglycanopathy, primary dystrophinopathy must be excluded. Less than 5% of boys with a Duchenne/Becker phenotype will prove to have a sarcoglycanopathy or other limb-girdle muscular dystrophy, and young girls with a "Duchenne/Becker" phenotype are nearly as likely to be manifesting carriers of a dystrophinopathy as to have an alternative diagnosis.[246]

Immunostaining of muscle with anti-sarcoglycan antibodies is the standard screening for new cases of sarcoglycanopathy. Muscle biopsies of patients with primary dystrophinopathy will show reduced sarcoglycan immunoreactivity. Therefore, both dystrophin and sarcoglycan immunostaining must be done on the same muscle tissue.

Limb-Girdle Muscular Dystrophy 2I: Fukutin-related Protein (FKRP) Deficiency

A recently characterized disorder, LGMD2I is one of the most common LGMDs, representing from 11% to 19% of all LGMDs in different series.[228,247,248]

The disease is caused by a mutation in the *FKRP* gene on chromosome 19q13.3.[249] The most common mutation is a single point (826C>A) missense mutation in one allele (>90%), causing a Leu276Ileu (C826A) change.[250] Disease severity correlated with a mutation on the second allele.

Age of onset ranges from 0.5 to 27 years, with 61% of patients presenting before age 5 years. These patients present with either a DMD phenotype, caused by heterozygous mutations, or with late-onset limb-girdle syndrome in those with homozygous mutations. The clinical course varies, usually involving weakness and wasting of the shoulder girdle muscles and proximal extremities, with significant calf hypertrophy and elevated serum CK, the increase ranging from 5-fold to 70-fold. Other clinical presentations have been described, including exercise-induced myalgias, isolated myalgias, cramps, and dilated cardiomyopathy with or without muscle weakness.[247] In some series, patients presented with muscle pain and myoglobinuria as the earliest presenting symptoms.[248] Cardiac and respiratory involvement are relatively common in the heterozygous, earlier presentation cases, occurring in approximately 30% of patients, at times while they are still ambulatory.[251,252]

Genetic sequencing of the *FKRP* gene from peripheral blood is commercially available, so diagnosis can be easily confirmed. Muscle biopsy shows characteristic dystrophic changes, with muscle fiber size variation, muscle fiber necrosis and regeneration, and mild increase in connective tissue. The most consistent abnormality is a secondary abnormal laminin-2 immunostaining. Most patients also have a marked decrease in immunostaining of muscle alpha-dystroglycan and a reduction in its molecular weight on Western blot analysis.[249,250]

Limb-Girdle Muscular Dystrophy 1A, 2G, and 2J: Sarcomeric Proteins Deficiency

Limb-Girdle Muscular Dystrophy 1A (Myotilinopathy)
LGMD1A was the first autosomal dominant limb-girdle dystrophy to be linked to a specific gene locus. Initial clinical observations of the co-segregating of two rare diseases in a family with muscular dystrophy and Pelger-Huet anomaly[253] and of a family in West

Virginia with proximal weakness and nasal dysarthria[254] were followed years later by linkage studies localizing the gene to chromosome 5q31–q33[255] and the discovery of the first of several missense mutations in the gene coding for the sarcomeric protein myotilin.[256]

Myotilin has been implicated in other diseases, including having a causal role in some cases of myofibrillar myopathy[257,258] and a secondary role in central core disease and nemaline myopathy.[259]

The diagnosis in new patients is challenging. Immunostaining of myotilin could be normal. A history of slowly progressive limb-girdle weakness with a family history consistent with autosomal dominant transmission may be obtained, but the incidence of spontaneous mutation is unknown. The findings of heel cord contracture, nasal dysarthria, mild to moderate elevation of CK, and muscle biopsy findings of Z-line streaming and autophagic vacuoles should increase clinical suspicion. Mutation analysis of the myotilin (*MYOT*) gene is needed for a definitive diagnosis.

Limb-Girdle Muscular Dystrophy 2G (Telethonin)
Telethonin is a small 19-kD sarcomeric protein expressed in skeletal and cardiac muscle.[260] Its gene maps to 17q11–12, and it is seen only in a small cohort of Brazilian families, presenting as a mainly proximal myopathy with onset from ages 9 to 15 years. Muscle biopsy revealed degenerating and regenerating muscle fibers and rimmed vacuoles.[261] Future patients can be screened with immunohistochemical techniques using anti-telethonin antibodies.

Limb-Girdle Muscular Dystrophy 2J (Titin)
Titin is a giant structural sarcomeric protein with a molecular weight of more than 3800 kD. The largest human protein, it forms the third filament system in striated muscle along with actin and myosin. Single titin molecules span half sarcomeres from Z disks to M lines in skeletal and cardiac muscle. Titin contributes to sarcomere assembly and passive tension of myofibrils as well as serving sensor and signaling functions.[262,263] Titin serine kinase phosphorylates telethonin, the protein implicated in LGMD2G.

Mutations in the titin (*TTN*) gene on chromosome 2q31 most often produce autosomal dominant tibial muscular dystrophy, a distal muscular dystrophy of mid-adult life with prominent involvement of the tibialis anterior and toe extensor muscles.[264] This disorder is most commonly seen in persons of Finnish descent.

Other Distal Muscular Dystrophies

A group of dystrophies with predominantly distal involvement that do not fall into the classification of limb-girdle muscular dystrophy are listed in Table 19-2 (pp 363–364) (Fig. 19-11).

Emery-Dreifuss Muscular Dystrophy

Both the X-linked and autosomal dominant forms of Emery-Dreifuss muscular dystrophy result from mutations in genes coding for nuclear envelope proteins. The X-linked form of Emery-Dreifuss (XL-EDMD or EMD1) is caused by mutations of the *EMD* gene located at Xq28, which encodes a 34-kD ubiquitously expressed nuclear envelope protein, emerin.[265] Approximately 95% of mutations producing XL-EDMD are null mutations associated with a complete absence of emerin in skeletal muscle, as well as smooth muscle, skin fibroblasts, leukocytes, and exfoliative buccal cells.

Autosomal dominant Emery-Dreifuss (AD-EDMD or EMD2) and autosomal recessive or sporadic Emery-Dreifuss muscular

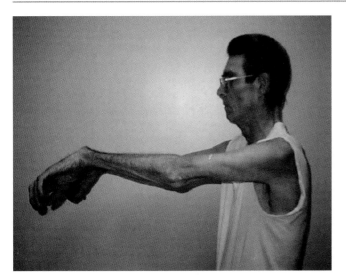

Figure 19-11 A patient with Welander distal myopathy. Notice the distal forearm wasting and wrist drop.

dystrophy (EMD3) result from mutations of the *LMNA* gene located on 1q21, which encodes two nuclear envelope proteins, lamins A and C.[266] Lamin A/C are alternatively spliced products of the same gene and comprise part of the nuclear lamina; they interact with chromatin and other proteins of the inner nuclear membrane, including emerin.[267] Mutations of the *LMNA* gene producing the AD-EDMD phenotype are missense mutations that allow translation of full-length lamin A/C. Immunostaining of lamin A/C is therefore not reliable for confirmation of the diagnosis of AD-EDMD.[268] The diagnosis of lamin A/C disorders requires DNA sequencing or mutation scanning.[269-271]

New mutations have been found to explain the 40% of EMD patients that did not present with the most common emerin or lamin AC mutations, expanding the genetic heterogeneity of the EMD phenotype. EMD4 and EMD5 decribed in few families are caused by mutations in the synaptic nuclear envelope protein 1 (SYNE1) and 2 (SYNE2).[271a] EMD6, caused by mutation in the X-linked four-and-a-half-LIM protein 1 (FHL1) gene, is inherited as an AR or sporadic form.[271b]

Although XL-EDMD and AD-EDMD usually share a similar phenotype, wide clinical variation, with poor genotype-phenotype correlation has been documented in both forms.[269,272,273] Interfamilial and intrafamilial phenotypic variability may exist in those sharing identical mutations.

The onset of contractures occurs early in the disease in the first or second decade and often precedes clinically significant weakness. Contractures are most prominent at the elbows, Achilles tendons, and posterior cervical muscles (Fig. 19-12A).[274] Upper extremity contractures often precede axial and lower extremity deformities. The arms are held in a semi-flexed position. The feet are set in equinus, often with associated toe walking. Posterior cervical contractures preclude full neck flexion (Fig. 19-12B). Contractures usually remain disproportionate to the degree of weakness[268] and may be the major factor in functional impairment. Muscle weakness is relatively mild and slowly progressive. The distribution of motor deficits is humeroperoneal with upper extremity (biceps, triceps, and spinal muscles) occurring earlier than leg weakness (tibialis anterior and peroneal muscles). Pseudohypertrophy is not seen and helps clinically differentiate XL-EDMD from dystrophinopathy (e.g., Becker muscular dystrophy).

Cardiac symptoms may include palpitations, syncope, and diminished exercise tolerance. Supraventricular arrhythmias, atrioventricular conduction block, ventricular arrhythmias, and restrictive or dilated cardiomyopathy may evolve. The risk of ventricular dysfunction and arrythmias is greater in the autosomal dominant than in the X-linked form,[275,276] but symptomatic cardiomyopathy may occur in women heterozygous for null emerin mutations. Cardiac symptoms usually evolve after the second decade.

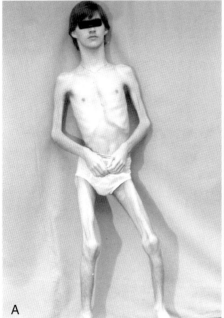

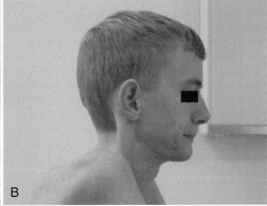

Figure 19-12 A, A patient with Emery-Dreifuss muscular dystrophy with diffuse muscle atrophy and prominent contractures. (Reprinted from T. Bertorini, "Muscular Dystrophies" in Pourmand's *Neuromuscular Diseases, Expert Clinicians' Views*, Boston, 2001, Butterworth-Heinemann.) **B,** A patient with Emery-Dreifuss muscular dystrophy, with significant neck extensor contractures limiting neck flexion. (Reprinted from Escolar D: Muscular Dystrophies, in *Pediatric Neurology Principles & Practice*, Philadelphia, 2006, Mosby.)

Treatment and Management

The management and treatment of LGMDs is in many ways similar to that for DMD, particularly when the disorders present in children. This includes the management of pulmonary complications, contractures, bracing, physical therapy and rehabilitation, and scoliosis surgery when indicated. Several LGMDs affect the heart as well, with management similar to that in DMD, sometimes requiring transplantation. Of particular importance is the management of Emery-Dreifuss muscular dystrophy, in which the severe cardiac complications and prominent contractures necessitate early, aggressive treatment.

Specific treatment is not currently available for any of these disorders. In some LGMDs, particularly sarcoglycanopathies, the use of gene therapy may be an option in the future. The small molecular weight of the coding sequences for sarcoglycans makes AAV transfer a feasible approach, and results have been favorable in the rodent model of the disease.[277] Actually, in LGMD2D, gene therapy by a local injection restores alpha sarcoglycan and increases muscle fiber size.[277a] Many of the treatments under investigation for the treatment of DMD may also be of benefit in some of these diseases. Of great interest are drugs or other approaches that might inhibit fibrosis, promote nerve regeneration, or inhibit muscle atrophy.

In some cases, the use of steroids has shown some benefit. These drugs have demonstrated a marked benefit in LGMD2L and LGMD2I (fukutin- and FKRP-associated), and some reported benefit in LGMD2D (alpha-sarcoglycan deficient).[278,279] In dysferlinopathies, despite the pronounced inflammatory response seen on muscle biopsy, steroids are not beneficial and might worsen the clinical course. Unfortunately, because of the limited number of patients with each particular disease, the performance of randomized, controlled clinical trials similar to those in DMD is difficult. Therefore, decisions regarding the use of steroids in LGMDs should be considered on a case-by-case basis.

Facioscapulohumeral Muscular Dystrophy

Facioscapulohumeral muscular dystrophy (FSHD) is inherited as an autosomal dominant disorder with high penetrance and variable expression. From 10% to 30% of cases represent new mutations.[280] Prevalence is estimated at 1 in 20,000. FSHD1A is associated with chromosome locus 4q35 and a sequence of repeats named D4Z4.[281] Healthy individuals have 11 to 100 repeats on both alleles, whereas patients with FSHD1A have 1 to 10 repeats on one allele.[282] An inverse correlation exists between the D4Z4 region size and disease severity,[280] with the largest deletions resulting in severe, congenital FSHD.[283,284]

Commercially available testing of the 4q35 region is the most specific and sensitive diagnostic test for FSHD1A. Subtelomeric translocations between chromosomes 4q35 and 10q26 occur relatively frequently in the general population and may complicate molecular diagnosis. In 5% of FSHD patients, a 4q35 deletion is not identified, suggesting that at least one additional genetic disorder, designated FSHD1B, produces the FSHD phenotype.[285]

Clinical Features

Clinical diagnostic criteria have been established by the FSHD Consortium.[286] This group specifies autosomal dominant inheritance, bifacial weakness, and weakness of either the scapular stabilizers or ankle dorsiflexor muscles. Supporting criteria include asymmetry of motor deficits (a finding far more common in FSHD than any other muscular dystrophy); sparing of deltoid, neck flexor, and calf muscles; and

involvement of wrist extensors and abdominal muscles. High-frequency hearing loss and retinal vasculopathy (Coats' disease) are additional supportive findings. Exclusion criteria include eyelid ptosis, extraocular muscle weakness, skin rash, elbow contractures, cardiomyopathy, sensory loss, neurogenic changes on muscle biopsy, and myotonia or neurogenic motor unit potentials on needle electromyography.

Weakness of the orbicularis oculi is usually asymptomatic but may be appreciated by observing incomplete burying of the eyelashes with forced eyelid closure and the ease with which the closed eyelids can be pried apart. A history of "sleeping with the eyes open" may be offered by a parent or spouse. Facial weakness may not be symmetric (Fig. 19-13).

Weakness of scapular fixation is evidenced by scapular winging accentuated by arm elevation in a forward plane (Fig. 19-14). The

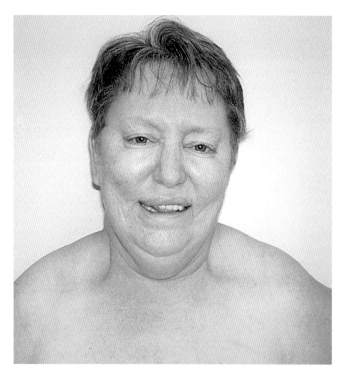

Figure 19-13 A patient with facioscapulohumeral muscular dystrophy with asymmetric facial weakness.

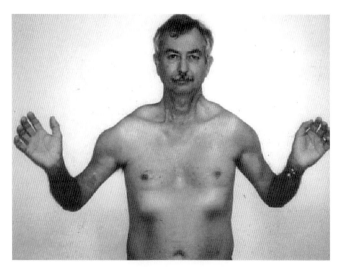

Figure 19-14 A patient with facioscapulohumeral muscular dystrophy, showing wasting of the biceps and the trapezius muscle with prominence of the scapulae protruding upward.

scapulae ride high on the back, producing the illusion of hypertrophied trapezius muscles. Arm abduction is impaired in the face of normal power and bulk of the deltoid muscles. Wasting of the biceps and triceps with preservation of deltoid and forearm muscles yields a "Popeye" configuration to the arms. Wasting of the clavicular head of the pectoral muscles produces a reversal of the axillary folds with a deep upward slope. Weakness of lower abdominal muscles may result in a pot belly when standing and a positive Beevor's sign (cephalad movement of the umbilicus with neck flexion) when the patient lies supine.

Lower extremity weakness is usually first noted in the ankle dorsiflexors with compromised heel walking or overt foot drop. Atrophy is most prominent in the tibialis anterior. Preservation or hypertrophy of the extensor digitorum brevis muscle clinically excludes a neurogenic etiology for the foot drop. Axial paraspinal muscle weakness may result in marked lumbar lordosis, especially in childhood-onset FSHD patients.

Congenital onset of FSHD has been associated with mental retardation and epilepsy in children with the largest D4Z4 deletions (EcoRI fragment size of 10kb; .i.e., less than 10 repeats). The congenital-onset, or infantile, phenotype is severe and rapidly progressive, accompanied by sensorineural hearing loss and Coats' disease.[287–289] Marked shoulder and pelvic girdle weakness is present before age 6 years with loss of ambulation by age 15 years. The condition may be mistaken for Möbius syndrome. Profound weakness of facial muscles, including extraocular muscles, is typical (Fig. 19-15).

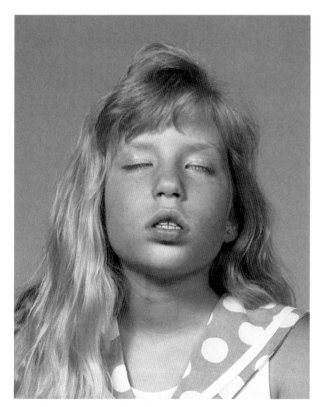

Figure 19-15 Early onset of infantile form of facioscapulohumeral muscular dystrophy manifests with incomplete eyelid closure and lack of facial expression. (Reprinted with permission from Escolar D: Muscular Dystrophies, in *Pediatric Neurology Principles & Practice*, Philadelphia, 2006, Mosby.)

Diagnosis and Evaluation

Results of CK determinations are either normal or slightly elevated; CK levels more than five times laboratory norms suggests an alternative diagnosis. Genetic testing has largely replaced electrodiagnostic and muscle biopsy evaluations in suspect FSHD patients. Electromyography (EMG) studies of moderately weak muscles reveal brief, low-amplitude motor unit action potentials consistent with myopathy; sparse fibrillations reflecting muscle fiber necrosis can also be noted. However, the needle EMG examination may be normal in clinically powerful muscles. Muscle biopsy findings are often nonspecific, with occasional small angular fibers, necrotic fibers, and regenerating "lobulated" fibers. A modest increase in the percent of hypertrophic type II muscle fibers may be seen. Foci of inflammatory cell in a perivascular or endomysial distribution are commonly encountered and on occasion may lead to a pathologic misdiagnosis of polymyositis, particularly in younger patients.[290]

Treatment and Management

Because no proven specific treatments are available for FSHD, the main therapeutic approaches are adaptive and protective. Ankle-foot orthoses for foot drop are commonly utilized. Orthopedic scapular fixation may improve upper extremity function,[291,292] but the gain may be short lived. Musculoskeletal and joint pain is common and may require nonsteroidal anti-inflammatory drugs (NSAIDs) or antidepressants if chronic. Routine auditory and ophthalmologic screening is recommended, especially in infantile-onset FSHD, in which Coats' disease is most often seen. Respiratory complications should be kept in mind, and routine measurement of forced vital capacity should be performed on those patients with severe weakness or kyphoscoliosis.

Unlike muscular dystrophies associated with sarcolemmal proteins, the muscle fibers in FSHD are not prone to damage as a result of exercise. Multiple studies, in fact, demonstrate beneficial effects of both strength training and aerobic exercise in FSHD.[293,294] Care should be taken, however, to avoid injury to weakened joints.

The beta-adrenergic agonist albuterol has been shown to improve muscle mass but has little effect on function,[295] a finding supported by a study examining the use of both albuterol and strength training.[296] Therapeutic trials of corticosteroids have been disappointing.[297] Data derived from a trial of creatine that included FSHD patients showed no benefit for this subgroup.[145] The clinical trial of the myostatin antibody (MYO-029) discussed in the DMD section of this chapter showed no benefits in function or strength in FSHD either.[181]

Several strategies are being considered as possible treatment approaches for FSHD in the future. Because patients with FSHD demonstrate hypomethylation in the D4Z4 region, folic acid and vitamin B_{12} have been evaluated as possible treatments since they contribute to DNA methylation. Initial studies have not shown clear benefit.[298] Alternative methods of myostatin inhibition are also being investigated, as is the case in other dystrophic diseases.[282] Finally, the autologous delivery of unaffected myoblasts or mesangioblasts is under consideration as a potential approach for therapy.[282]

Myotonic Dystrophy

Myotonic Dystrophy Type 1

Type 1 myotonic dystrophy (DM1) is an autosomal dominant disorder with multisystem involvement. DM1 is the second most common of the muscular dystrophies, affecting 1 in 8000 individuals.

It is the most prevalent of the dystrophies in adults. Skeletal, smooth, and cardiac muscles are affected, as well as the eye, endocrine, and central nervous systems. Clinical signs and symptoms are variable, including among affected family members, with a spectrum ranging from asymptomatic to severe.

Molecular Genetics

Type 1 myotonic dystrophy is caused by a mutation in the length of a CTG trinucleotide repeat in the 3' untranslated region of the myotonic dystrophy protein kinase (*DMPK*) gene on chromosome 19q. The normal gene has between 5 and 36 CTG trinucleotide repeats. Minimally affected individuals have as few as 50 copies; severely affected DM patients may have thousands of repeats.[299] The CTG repeat gene shows marked intergenerational and somatic instability in patients with DM1 when the repeat is expanded to more than approximately 55 repeats.[300] Virtually all children with the most severe congenital phenotype have inherited the *DMPK* allele from their mothers. In fact, the sex of the transmitting parent is an important factor that determines DM allele size in the offspring.

The pathophysiologic mechanism of disease in myotonic dystrophy has been recently described as one mediated by "toxic RNA."[301] The repeat expansion of *DMPK* is actually outside of any coding region, and the protein product is therefore normal. However, the RNA transcript itself (a CUG expanded repeat) is thought to form a hairpin structure that accumulates in the nucleus,[302] leading to dysfunction of the RNA binding proteins MBNL1 and CUGBP1.[303,304] These proteins normally regulate the alternative splicing of pre-RNA. When this process is misregulated, a "spliceopathy" of the muscle chloride channel and insulin receptor occurs, making abnormal versions of these gene products and leading to the myotonia and insulin resistance seen in DM1.[304–306] Cardiac conduction disturbances in DM1 appear to be mediated by mutant RNA increasing the expression of NKX2-5, a cardiac transcription factor.[307]

Clinical Features

The clinical presentation of DM1 is highly variable among patients and within families. Congenital DM1 is most commonly seen in infants born to mothers with *DMPK* expansion alleles of 600 or more CTG repeats. Symptoms are often noted before birth. Reduced fetal movement and polyhydramnios are warning signs. There is an increased incidence of breech presentation. At delivery, marked hypotonia, generalized weakness, and inefficient respiration are noted. Characteristic facies with a tented upper lip indicating facial diplegia is seen in nearly all infants. Arthrogryposis, most often producing talipes equinovarus deformity, is common. Life-threatening respiratory insufficiency requiring mechanical ventilator support may portend an ominous long-term prognosis.

Classic DM1 is most likely to develop in the second to fourth decade (Fig. 19-16) in patients with CTG repeat lengths of 100 or more. Teenagers and young adults may complain of "stiffness" as the first symptom of myotonia. Difficulty with fine motor skills such as handwriting and complaints referrable to distal upper extremity weakness and grip-induced myotonia follow. Evolution of lower limb distal weakness progresses to foot drop and inability to skip or vertically leap. Typical myopathic facies (also described as *hatchet facies*) with temporal muscle wasting and eyelid ptosis give a "dull" appearance (Fig. 19-17).

Nonskeletal muscle signs and symptoms require close clinical attention. Cardiac conduction defects tend to evolve after age 30 years, but early cardiac screening with ECG is needed to detect those patients with progressive atrioventricular conduction block, a significant cause of early death in patients with classic DM1.[308]

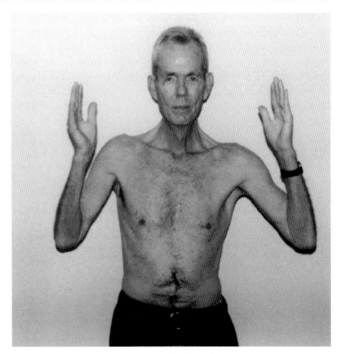

Figure 19-16 An adult patient with myotonic dystrophy. Note wasting of the temples, anterior neck, and forearm muscles.

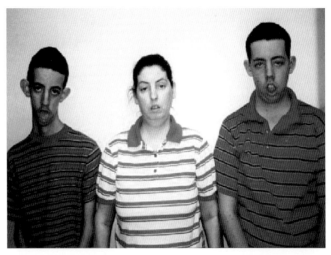

Figure 19-17 A family with myotonic dystrophy. A mildly affected mother and her two sons with markedly elongated face and temporal wasting.

Smooth muscle dysfunction may produce dysphagia, constipation, or diarrhea. Hypokinesis of the small and large bowel may produce pseudo-obstruction or megacolon. Impaired sphincter of Oddi function predisposes to cholelithiasis. Endocrinopathies, including hyperinsulinism with glucose intolerance and impaired growth hormone secretion, are usually asymptomatic.[309] Gonadal atrophy and reduced fertility are common but usually evolve after the prime reproductive years. An underappreciated complication of classic DM1 is hypersomnia, often found in association with both central and obstructive sleep apnea.[310] Men may exhibit frontal balding beginning in their late teens. Christmas tree cataracts can be detected with slit-lamp examination beginning in the teens. Women with classic DM1 are at risk for obstetric complications, including spontaneous miscarriage; failure of progression of labor, necessitating cesarean section; and postpartum hemorrhage.[311] Worsening of motor impairment rarely accompanies pregnancy. All patients with classic DM1 require added precautions when undergoing surgery. Sensitivity to sedatives and inhalation anesthesia mandates close observation in the recovery room. Blunted responses to hypercarbia and hypoxemia may be partially responsible for postanesthetic complications.

Diagnosis and Evaluation

The universal availability of DNA testing for patients suspected of having DM1 has made other diagnostic investigations obsolete. Lymphocyte DNA assay for the CTG expansion repeat in the *DMPK* gene is nearly 100% accurate. PCR analysis is performed to detect up to 100 repeats; Southern blot analysis is used to quantitate CTG expansions of greater length. "False negatives" have proven to represent other diseases, most commonly DM2.

Older diagnostic techniques for the identification of DM1 are of historical interest. They include needle EMG, which demonstrates waxing and waning high-frequency discharges typical of true myotonia. CK levels are normal or slightly elevated. Muscle biopsy in older children and adults reveals type I muscle fiber atrophy, increased numbers of internal nuclei, and ring fibers. The muscle biopsy in infants with congenital DM1 show poor fiber type differentiation, and peripheral halos of many fibers void of oxidative activity. None of these morphologic findings are pathognomonic for DM1.

Myotonic Dystrophy Type 2 (DM2)

Shortly after the discovery that myotonic dystrophy was caused by a CTG trinucleotide repeat expansion in the *DMPK* gene, reports appeared that some patients with typical clinical features of this disorder showed neither the CTG repeat expansion nor localization to 19q13.3.[312] Some of these patients manifest weakness in a proximal greater than distal distribution; the term *proximal myotonic myopathy* (PROMM) was coined to describe this newly appreciated disorder.[313,314] Further phenotype-genotype investigations localized the disease to 3q21[315] and shortly thereafter the gene was localized to the zinc finger protein 9 (*ZNF9*) gene and a CCTG repeat sequence expansion in intron 1 of this gene was discovered.[316] The toxic accumulation of RNA theory described above also applies to the CCTG transcript of this repeat.[316]

These manifest both proximal motor deficits as well as findings typical for classic myotonic dystrophy. The majority of patients with DM2 present in their adult years, but patients as young as age 8 years have demonstrated symptoms. Importantly, no congenital phenotype has yet been reported.[317,318] DM1 and DM2 share common findings of myotonia, early cataracts, frontal balding, and cardiac involvement. DNA studies provide the means for definitive classification of affected patients.

Treatment and Management

Patients diagnosed with myotonic dystrophy require education about their disease and an explanation of the phenomenon of anticipation (especially for young women of child-bearing age). Periodic pulmonary function studies and ECGs should begin in the second decade and cardiology consultation obtained liberally throughout the lives of these patients for symptoms suggestive of arrhythmias, syncope or presyncope, or progressive ECG changes. Routine ophthalmologic examination is recommended to screen for cataracts.

Myotonia is not the most serious complication of DM, although it can exacerbate disability. Trials of drugs such as phenytoin (100 mg two to three times per day), carbamazepine (600 to 800 mg/day), or mexiletine (150 to 200 mg three times per day) may be helpful for treatment of myotonia in selected patients, but their safety and efficacy have not been studied in long-term randomized, controlled trials.[319] These are all sodium channel blockers, and their use could exacerbate weakness in these patients. Furthermore, mexiletine should be avoided in patients with second- and third-degree heart block, which are not uncommon in these diseases. Muscle pain is a common complaint in patients with DM2 and may respond to NSAIDs, gabapentin, or tricyclic antidepressants.

Lethargy and fatigue may suggest central or obstructive sleep apnea. If sleep studies are negative, empiric trials of stimulant medications may be helpful for these symptoms. Patients undergoing surgery should make both surgeon and anesthesiologist aware of their neuromuscular disorder, limit the use of sedative agents, and anticipate a prolonged period of observation in the recovery room.

Ankle-foot orthoses help address distal lower limb weakness and foot drop. Lesser degrees of distal leg weakness can be helped by well-supported, high-topped athletic shoes. At later stages, the use of walkers or wheelchairs may become necessary.

The infant with congenital DM1 requires a multidisciplinary approach with occupational, physical, and speech therapy services. Nutritional consultation and trials of various food consistencies are often helpful. Parents and teachers should anticipate cognitive impairment and learning disabilities and monitor for symptoms of attention deficit disorder.

Future Targets for Specific Treatment in Myotonic Dystrophy

Because of the presumed causative nature of mutant RNA in myotonic dystrophy, this and the mechanisms affected by it are appealing targets for therapy. The most direct approach would be elimination of the mutant RNA itself. Approaches using either ribozyme or antisense RNAs designed to degrade mutant *DMPK* alleles have shown some promise in myoblasts.[320,321] A study on murine models demonstrated that exon skipping with antisense oligonucleotides could achieve normal chloride channels with improvement of myotonia.[322] Other approaches of interest are manipulation of the expression of the RNA binding proteins MBNL1 and CUGBP1, which are affected by the accumulation of the mutant RNA.[323]

The progressive muscle wasting in DM1 appears to be secondary to a defect in muscle anabolism.[324,325] This has led to the study of anabolic agents as possible treatments for the disease. Testosterone[326] and creatinine[327,328] have not shown any benefit. Dehydroepiandrosterone (DHEA) has been shown to improve strength in a small pilot study.[329] Studies of compounds including recombinant human insulin-like growth factor, a strong stimulator of anabolism, are currently underway.[323]

Oculopharyngeal Muscular Dystrophy

Oculopharyngeal muscular dystrophy (OPMD) is an autosomal dominant, adult-onset disease. The gene has been mapped to chromosome 14q11.2-q13, and the disease is caused by a trinucleotide repeat (GCG) expansion. This repeat occurs in the coding region of the polyalanine binding protein-nuclear 1 (*PABPN1*) gene. Histopathology demonstrates small angulated fibers, rimmed vacuoles in muscle fibers, and intranuclear inclusions consisting of mutated aggregates of PABPN1.[330]

OPMD typically presents after age 50 years.[331] Many affected individuals of French Canadian descent are traced to a single ancestor from France,[332] although it can also occur in other ethnic groups.

OPMD is recognized in the fourth to sixth decade by onset of ptosis, partial extraocular muscle paresis, dysphagia, and tongue weakness. Proximal upper and lower extremity muscle weakness (see Fig. 1-5D) slowly develops. Serum CK level may be normal or mildly elevated.

Progressive oculopharyngeal dysfunction was described in Greek siblings, ages 11 and 14 years, who both had rimmed vacuoles; one had cytoplasmic and intranuclear tubulofilamentous inclusions 25 nm in diameter on muscle biopsy.[333] Another childhood-onset oculopharyngeal syndrome presented with intestinal pseudo-obstruction.[334] These may be examples of recessively inherited conditions similar to dominantly inherited OPMD.

Treatment and Management

Several specific therapies are under investigation in OPMD cells and in animal models of OPMD. Trehalose is a disaccharide chemical chaperone that has been shown to decrease PABPN1 aggregates and improve muscle weakness.[335] Antibodies to different epitopes of *PABPN1* have been identified that, when expressed intracellularly, can prevent and reduce aggregations of PABPN1.[336] Doxycycline has been shown to delay and lessen the severity of symptoms in a murine model as well as reduce PABPN1 aggregates.[337] A human trial is underway that will examine the utility of autologous satellite cell therapy in *OPMD*.[338]

Due to the unavailability of specific therapies, adaptive measures are of most benefit currently for OPMD patients. These include the treatment of ptosis either surgically or with eyelid crutches. For diplopia, Fresnel prisms might be helpful in some patients. Speech therapy consultation and close monitoring of swallowing function are also important.

Congenital Muscular Dystrophy

The congenital muscular dystrophies (CMD) are a heterogeneous group of autosomal recessive disorders characterized by hypotonia, weakness, and variable degrees of muscle contractures. They are normally classified into syndromic (with brain and eye abnormalities) and nonsyndromic types. Within these broad classifications considerable phenotypic variation exists, and clinical differences may be more quantitative than qualitative. However, evidence supports genetically distinct bases for the different CMD subgroups. The summed incidence of all forms of CMD is approximately 1 in 21,500.[339] Signs and symptoms are evident in the newborn period or the first few months of life. Serum CK is usually elevated. Muscle biopsy abnormalities suggesting a myopathic or dystrophic process, including variation in muscle fiber size, necrotic and regenerating fibers, and an increase in endomysial connective tissue, establish a working diagnosis of CMD. Delineation of a precise diagnosis requires integration of muscle and systemic findings, immunostaining or Western blot of extracellular proteins, and DNA testing when available.

Nonsyndromic Congenital Muscular Dystrophies

The most common of the nonsyndromic types is merosin-negative congenital muscular dystrophy (MDC1A). Merosin is the heavy α2 chain of laminin-2 (LAMA2). The laminins are heterotrimeric proteins that influence cell adhesion, growth, and migration. LAMA2 is expressed in the basement membrane of muscle fibers, Schwann cells of intramuscular nerves, and at neuromuscular junctions. LAMA2 promotes myotube stability and inhibits apoptosis.[340] Patients with complete absence of merosin present as hypotonic infants with limb weakness, normally more prominent than bulbar or respiratory impairment, and multiple joint contractures (Fig. 19-18A). On magnetic resonance imaging, white matter abnormalities, seen as increased signal on T2-weighted images, involve the centrum semiovale.[341] Epilepsy occurs frequently, even in patients with normal intellect.[342] Absence of immunohistochemical staining for the laminin α2 chain on snap frozen muscle biopsy tissue provides confirmation of the diagnosis of merosin deficiency (Fig. 19-18B). Prenatal diagnosis of merosin-deficient CMD is possible by direct mutation analysis of chorionic villus biopsy material or linkage analysis. Direct immunostaining of trophoblasts from chorionic villus samples with laminin α2 chain antibodies provides an additional method for prenatal diagnosis.

Another nonsyndromic CMD is the merosin-positive group (MDC1B). The majority of patients with normal merosin expression or partial merosin deficiency presenting with a CMD phenotype have other genetic disorders that do not link to 6q. They share a similar, but usually milder clinical course than merosin-negative children.

CMD due to FKRP deficiency (MDC1C) usually presents at birth or in the first few weeks of life with hypotonia and leg muscle hypertrophy. CK values are greatly increased (1000 to 10,000 IU/L). Children follow a regressive course that may include cardiomyopathy. Immunohistochemical staining reveals partial merosin deficiency and severely reduced alpha-dystroglycan. The reduced molecular weight of alpha-dystroglycan on Western blot indicates that defective glycosylation is important in the pathophysiology of MDC1C. The genetic defect maps to 19q13.3, and DNA testing is commercially available.

CMD with integrin α-7 deficiency is a rare disorder that has been discovered in the analysis of large groups of patients with undefined congenital myopathies. The muscle biopsies of three patients showed deficiency of this protein with different mutations in the *ITGA7* gene on chromosome 12q13.[343]

CMD with early rigid spine syndrome is another rare form seen in consanguineous Moroccan, Turkish, and Iranian families that demonstrate mutations in the gene on chromosome 1p35–46 coding for selenoprotein.[344] An American family has also been described demonstrating a phenotype of infantile hypotonia, cervical muscle weakness, and early spinal rigidity with scoliosis that maps to the same locus on 1p.[345]

Ullrich CMD is caused by autosomal recessive mutations in any of three genes encoding collagen VI, an extracellular matrix protein.[346,347] The protein is composed of three alpha peptide chains, which are encoded by two genes on chromosome 21q22.3 and one gene on chromosome 2q37. The disease presents with infantile weakness, hypotonia, and early severe proximal joint contractures with hyperlaxity of distal joints.[348] The distal laxity may be replaced by progressive flexion contractures of the wrists, fingers, and ankle. Serum CK is usually normal or only slightly elevated. Muscle biopsy shows nonspecific myopathic or dystrophic changes with reduced or absent collagen VI immunostaining.[349]

Bethlem myopathy, also due to mutations in collagen VI genes, was first described as a benign myopathy with autosomal dominant inheritance.[350] Clinical features are much more variable than in Ullrich CMD. Patients usually have proximal weakness in early childhood and may demonstrate the Gowers sign. More severe cases may present in neonates with hypotonia, foot deformities, torticollis, and arthrogryposis. Unlike Ullrich CMD, weakness is usually nonprogressive, but contractures may develop late in the first decade in the ankles, elbow flexors, and finger flexors.

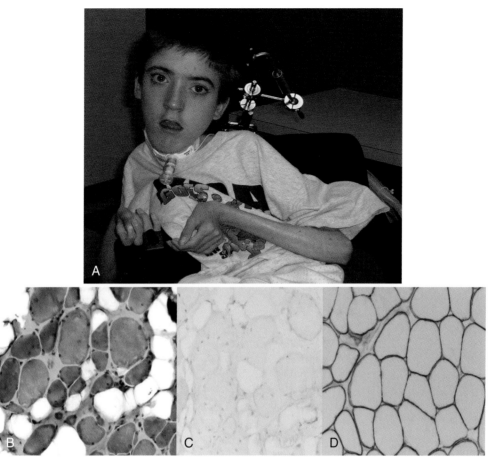

Figure 19-18 A, A patient with merosin-deficient congenital muscular dystrophy. The patient has a tracheotomy, prominent contractures, and scoliosis. **B,** Muscle biopsy from the same patient stained modified with trichrome. Note the fiber atrophy, increased endomysial connective tissue, and fat (×400). **C,** Note the lack of merosin compared with a normal control (**D**). (A, Reprinted with permission from Bertorini T: *Neuromuscular Case Studies*, Philadelphia, 2008, Butterworth-Heinemann.)

Table 19-2 Distal Muscular Dystrophies

Type and Eponym	Gene Localization	Gene Product	Initial Weakness	Serum CK Level	Biopsy
Late adult-onset, predominantly in hands (Welander) (AD)	2p13	Unknown	Hands: finger/wrist extensors	Normal or slightly elevated	Myopathic: vacuoles in most cases
Late adult-onset, predominantly in legs					
IIa. Finnish (Tibial, Udd) (AD)	2q31	Titin	Legs; anterior compartment	Normal or slightly elevated	Vacuolar myopathy, sarcolemmal disruption, accumulation of myofibrillar proteins
IIb. Markesbery-Griggs* (AD)	10q22.3-23.2	ZASP	Legs: anterior compartment	Normal or slightly elevated	As above but fewer vacuoles
Early adult-onset, anterior compartment in legs (Nonaka type, quadriceps-sparing, HIBM2) (AR; some sporadic)	9p1q1	GNE: glucosamine (UDP-N-acetyl)-2-epimerase/N-acetylman-nosamine kinase	Legs: anterior compartment	Increased, usually <5× normal	Vacuolar myopathy
HIBM with Paget disease and frontotemporal dementia (AD)	9p13-p12	Valosin-containing protein (VC)	Legs: mainly anterior compartment	Normal or slightly elevated	Vacuolar myopathy
HIBM-3 (AD)	17p13-1	MyHC-IIa: type IIa myosin heavy chain	Variable presentation	Normal in children, elevated in adults	Vacuolar myopathy

Continued

Table 19-2 Distal Muscular Dystrophies—Cont'd

Type and Eponym	Gene Localization	Gene Product	Initial Weakness	Serum CK Level	Biopsy
Early adult-onset posterior compartment in legs (Miyoshi) (AR)	2p13	Dysferlin (allelic to LGMD 2B)	Legs: posterior compartment	Increased, 10–150× normal	Myopathic, necrosis, no vacuoles; dysferlin deficiency
Early adult-onset (Laing) (AR)	14q11	Myosin heavy chain 7	Legs: anterior compartment; neck flexors	Slightly increased, <3× normal	Moderate myopathic changes; no vacuoles
Distal myopathy with vocal cord and pharyngeal weakness (onset in fourth to sixth decades) (AR)	5q31	Matrin 3	Legs: anterior compartment; finger extensors may first be involved	Normal to moderately increased	Vacuolar myopathy
Myofibrillar myopathy (AD, sporadic) (onset in childhood to fifth decade)	2q35 (AP.AR) 11q21-23 (AD) 5q22.3-3.13(AR) 10q22.3-23.2(AD) 7q32.1(AD) 1p36 (AR)	Desmin Crystallin αB CAP myotilin ZASP Filamin C Selenoprotein N1	Hands or legs, some with scapuloperoneal	Moderately increased, <5× normal	Myopathic, usually with vacuoles; subsarcolemmal granules or cytoplasmic bodies; accumulation of desmin and other myofibrillar proteins
Others					
Some caveolinopathies	3p25 (AD)	Caveolin	Variable presentation	Elevated	Dystrophic changes, caveolin deficiency
Nebulin gene mutations	2q (AR)	Nebulin	Young adults; tibial and facial weakness	Normal	Some small nemaline rods

*This should be considered a myofibrillar myopathy.

AD, autosomal dominant; AR, autosomal recessive; HIBM, hereditary inclusion body myopathy; MyHC, myosin heavy chain; ZASP, Z-band alternatively spliced PDZ motif-containing protein.

Syndromic Congenital Muscular Dystrophies

A summary of the syndromic congenital muscular dystrophies (Fukuyama congenital muscular dystrophy, muscle-eye-brain disease, and Walker-Warburg syndrome) is shown in Table 19-1. These are three clinically defined CMDs with associated brain malformations. They involve the brain because the genes and protein products of these disorders are involved in glycosylation of both extracellular muscle and brain protein.

The treatment of CMDs is mostly symptomatic, and these approaches are discussed in Chapter 12. There is preclinical evidence that merosin-negative CMD can respond to costicosteroid treatment.[351] This has also been shown in patients with CMD 1A followed by one of the authors (DE). These patients clearly respond to prednisone at a dose similar to that used for DMD treatment, with increase in muscle strength and function sustained over many years. Thus, a trial of corticosteroid treatment in this form of CMD should be considered.

References

1. Emery AE: The muscular dystrophies, *Lancet* 359(9307):687–695, 2002.
2. Baumbach LL, Chamberlain JS, Ward PA, et al: Molecular and clinical correlations of deletions leading to Duchenne and Becker muscular dystrophies, *Neurology* 39(4):465–474, 1989.
3. Burmeister M, Lehrach H: Long-range restriction map around the Duchenne muscular dystrophy gene, *Nature* 324(6097):582–585, 1986.
4. Gillard EF, Chamberlain JS, Murphy EG, et al: Molecular and phenotypic analysis of patients with deletions within the deletion-rich region of the Duchenne muscular dystrophy (*DMD*) gene, *Am J Hum Genet* 45(4):507–520, 1989.
5. Hoffman EP, Fischbeck KH, Brown RH, et al: Characterization of dystrophin in muscle-biopsy specimens from patients with Duchenne's or Becker's muscular dystrophy, *N Engl J Med* 318(21):1363–1368, 1988.
6. Nicholson LV, Bushby KM, Johnson MA, et al: Predicted and observed sizes of dystrophin in some patients with gene deletions that disrupt the open reading frame, *J Med Genet* 29(12):892–896, 1992.
7. Patria SY, Alimsardjono H, Nishio H, et al: A case of Becker muscular dystrophy resulting from the skipping of four contiguous exons (71–74) of the dystrophin gene during mRNA maturation, *Proc Assoc Am Physicians* 108(4):308–314, 1996.
8. Arahata K, Beggs AH, Honda H, et al: Preservation of the C-terminus of dystrophin molecule in the skeletal muscle from Becker muscular dystrophy, *J Neurol Sci* 101(2):148–156, 1991.
9. Winnard AV, Mendell JR, Prior TW, et al: Frameshift deletions of exons 3–7 and revertant fibers in Duchenne muscular dystrophy: mechanisms of dystrophin production, *Am J Hum Genet* 56(1):158–166, 1995.
10. Arahata K, Hoffman EP, Kunkel LM, et al: Dystrophin diagnosis: comparison of dystrophin abnormalities by immunofluorescence and immunoblot analyses, *Proc Natl Acad Sci U S A* 86(18):7154–7158, 1989.
11. Koenig M, Beggs AH, Moyer M, et al: The molecular basis for Duchenne versus Becker muscular dystrophy: correlation of severity with type of deletion, *Am J Hum Genet* 45(4):498–506, 1989.
12. Malhotra SB, Hart KA, Klamut HJ, et al: Frame-shift deletions in patients with Duchenne and Becker muscular dystrophy, *Science* 242(4879):755–759, 1988.
13. Kunkel LM: Analysis of deletions in DNA from patients with Becker and Duchenne muscular dystrophy, *Nature* 322(6074):73–77, 1986.
14. den Dunnen JT, Bakker E, Breteler EG, et al: Direct detection of more than 50% of the Duchenne muscular dystrophy mutations by field inversion gels, *Nature* 329(6140):640–642, 1987.
15. Forrest SM, Cross GS, Speer A, et al: Preferential deletion of exons in Duchenne and Becker muscular dystrophies, *Nature* 329(6140):638–640, 1987.
16. Koenig M, Hoffman EP, Bertelson CJ, et al: Complete cloning of the Duchenne muscular dystrophy (DMD) cDNA and preliminary genomic organization of the *DMD* gene in normal and affected individuals, *Cell* 50(3):509–517, 1987.
17. Darras BT, Blattner P, Harper JF, et al: Intragenic deletions in 21 Duchenne muscular dystrophy (DMD)/Becker muscular dystrophy (BMD) families studied with the dystrophin cDNA: location of breakpoints on HindIII

and BglII exon-containing fragment maps, meiotic and mitotic origin of the mutations, *Am J Hum Genet* 43(5):620–629, 1988.

18. den Dunnen JT, Grootscholten PM, Bakker E, et al: Topography of the Duchenne muscular dystrophy (*DMD*) gene: FIGE and cDNA analysis of 194 cases reveals 115 deletions and 13 duplications, *Am J Hum Genet* 45(6):835–847, 1989.

19. Beggs AH, Koenig M, Boyce FM, et al: Detection of 98% of *DMD/BMD* gene deletions by polymerase chain reaction, *Hum Genet* 86:45–48, 1990.

20. Oudet C, Hanauer A, Clemens P, et al: Two hot spots of recombination in the DMD gene correlate with the deletion prone regions, *Hum Mol Genet* 1(8):599–603, 1992.

21. Nobile C, Galvagni F, Marchi J, et al: Genomic organization of the human dystrophin gene across the major deletion hot spot and the 3′ region, *Genomics* 28(1):97–100, 1995.

22. Jeppesen J, Green A, Steffensen BF, et al: The Duchenne muscular dystrophy population in Denmark, 1977–2001: prevalence, incidence and survival in relation to the introduction of ventilator use, *Neuromuscul Disord* 13 (10):804–812, 2003.

23. Brooks AP, Emery AE: The incidence of Duchenne muscular dystrophy in the South East of Scotland, *Clin Genet* 11(4):290–294, 1977.

24. Moser H: Duchenne muscular dystrophy: pathogenetic aspects and genetic prevention, *Hum Genet* 66:17–40, 1984.

25. Scheuerbrandt G, Lundin A, Lovgren T, et al: Screening for Duchenne muscular dystrophy: an improved screening test for creatine kinase and its application in an infant screening program, *Muscle Nerve* 9(1):11–23, 1986.

26. van Essen AJ, Busch HF, te Meerman GJ, et al: Birth and population prevalence of Duchenne muscular dystrophy in The Netherlands, *Hum Genet* 88:258–266, 1992.

27. Yoshioka M, Itagaki Y, Saida K, et al: Clinical and genetic studies of muscular dystrophy in young girls, *Clin Genet* 29(2):137–142, 1986.

28. Pena SD, Karpati G, Carpenter S, et al: The clinical consequences of X-chromosome inactivation: Duchenne muscular dystrophy in one of monozygotic twins, *J Neurol Sci* 79(3):337–344, 1987.

29. Kinoshita M, Ikeda K, Yoshimura M, et al: [Duchenne muscular dystrophy carrier presenting with mosaic X chromosome constitution and muscular symptoms—with analysis of the Barr bodies in the muscle], *Rinsho Shinkeigaku* 30(6):643–646, 1990.

30. Lesca G, Demarquay G, Llense S, et al: [Symptomatic carriers of dystrophinopathy with chromosome X inactivation bias], *Rev Neurol (Paris)* 159 (8–9):775–780, 2003.

31. Hoffman EP, Brown RH Jr, Kunkel LM: Dystrophin: the protein product of the Duchenne muscular dystrophy locus, *Cell* 51(6):919–928, 1987.

32. Hoffman EP, Knudson CM, Campbell KP, et al: Subcellular fractionation of dystrophin to the triads of skeletal muscle, *Nature* 330(6150):754–758, 1987.

33. Knudson CM, Hoffman EP, Kahl SD, et al: Evidence for the association of dystrophin with the transverse tubular system in skeletal muscle, *J Biol Chem* 263(17):8480–8484, 1988.

34. Rando TA: Role of nitric oxide in the pathogenesis of muscular dystrophies: a "two hit" hypothesis of the cause of muscle necrosis, *Microsc Res Tech* 55 (4):223–235, 2001.

35. Murphy ME, Kehrer JP: Free radicals: a potential pathogenic mechanism in inherited muscular dystrophy, *Life Sci* 39(24):2271–2278, 1986.

36. Baker MS, Austin L: The pathological damage in Duchenne muscular dystrophy may be due to increased intracellular oxy-radical generation caused by the absence of dystrophin and subsequent alterations in Ca^{2+} metabolism, *Med Hypotheses* 29(3):187–193, 1989.

37. Haycock JW, MacNeil S, Jones P, et al: Oxidative damage to muscle protein in Duchenne muscular dystrophy, *Neuroreport* 8(1):357–361, 1996.

38. Williams IA, Allen DG: The role of reactive oxygen species in the hearts of dystrophin-deficient *mdx* mice, *Am J Physiol Heart Circ Physiol* 293(3): H1969–H1977, 2007.

39. McDouall RM, Dunn MJ, Dubowitz V: Nature of the mononuclear infiltrate and the mechanism of muscle damage in juvenile dermatomyositis and Duchenne muscular dystrophy, *J Neurol Sci* 99(2–3):199–217, 1990.

40. Kissel JT, Lynn DJ, Rammohan KW, et al: Mononuclear cell analysis of muscle biopsies in prednisone- and azathioprine-treated Duchenne muscular dystrophy, *Neurology* 43(3 Pt 1):532–536, 1993.

41. Cai B, Spencer MJ, Nakamura G, et al: Eosinophilia of dystrophin-deficient muscle is promoted by perforin-mediated cytotoxicity by T cell effectors, *Am J Pathol* 156(5):1789–1796, 2000.

42. Spencer MJ, Tidball JG: Do immune cells promote the pathology of dystrophin-deficient myopathies? *Neuromuscul Disord* 11(6–7):556–564, 2001.

43. Lagrota-Candido J, Vasconcellos R, Cavalcanti M, et al: Resolution of skeletal muscle inflammation in *mdx* dystrophic mouse is accompanied by increased immunoglobulin and interferon-gamma production, *Int J Exp Pathol* 83(3):121–132, 2002.

44. Porter JD, Khanna S, Kaminski HJ, et al: A chronic inflammatory response dominates the skeletal muscle molecular signature in dystrophin-deficient *mdx* mice, *Hum Mol Genet* 11(3):263–272, 2002.

45. Li H, Mittal A, Makonchuk DY, et al: Matrix metalloproteinase-9 inhibition ameliorates pathogenesis and improves skeletal muscle regeneration in muscular dystrophy, *Hum Mol Genet* 18(14):2584–2598, 2009.

46. Wrogemann K, Pena SD: Mitochondrial calcium overload: a general mechanism for cell-necrosis in muscle diseases, *Lancet* 1(7961):672–674, 1976.

47. Yeung EW, Allen DG: Stretch-activated channels in stretch-induced muscle damage: role in muscular dystrophy, *Clin Exp Pharmacol Physiol* 31(8):551–556, 2004.

48. Suchyna TM, Sachs F: Mechanosensitive channel properties and membrane mechanics in mouse dystrophic myotubes, *J Physiol* 581(1):369–387, 2007.

49. Gervásio OL, Whitehead NP, Yeung EW, et al: TRPC1 binds to caveolin-3 and is regulated by Src kinase—role in Duchenne muscular dystrophy, *J Cell Sci* 121(13):2246–2255, 2008.

50. Iwata Y, Katanosaka Y, Arai Y, et al: Dominant-negative inhibition of Ca^{2+} influx via TRPV2 ameliorates muscular dystrophy in animal models, *Hum Mol Genet* 18(5):824–834, 2009.

51. Tindall RS, Rollins JA, Phillips JT, et al: Preliminary results of a double-blind, randomized, placebo-controlled trial of cyclosporine in myasthenia gravis, *N Engl J Med* 316(12):719–724, 1987.

52. Sandri M, Carraro U, Podhorska-Okolov M, et al: Apoptosis, DNA damage and ubiquitin expression in normal and *mdx* muscle fibers after exercise, *FEBS Lett* 373(3):291–295, 1995.

53. Spencer MJ, Walsh CM, Dorshkind KA, et al: Myonuclear apoptosis in dystrophic *mdx* muscle occurs by perforin-mediated cytotoxicity, *J Clin Invest* 99(11):2745–2751, 1997.

54. Smith J, Goldsmith C, Ward A, et al: IGF-II ameliorates the dystrophic phenotype and coordinately down-regulates programmed cell death, *Cell Death Differ* 7(11):1109–1118, 2000.

55. Adams V, Gielen S, Hambrecht R, et al: Apoptosis in skeletal muscle, *Front Biosci* 6:D1–D11, 2001.

56. Sandri M, El Meslemani AH, Sandri C, et al: Caspase 3 expression correlates with skeletal muscle apoptosis in Duchenne and facioscapulohumeral muscular dystrophy. A potential target for pharmacological treatment, *J Neuropathol Exp Neurol* 60(3):302–312, 2001.

57. Tews DS: Apoptosis and muscle fibre loss in neuromuscular disorders, *Neuromuscul Disord* 2(7–8):613–622, 2002.

58. D'Amore PA, Brown RH Jr, Ku PT, et al: Elevated basic fibroblast growth factor in the serum of patients with Duchenne muscular dystrophy, *Ann Neurol* 35(3):362–365, 1994.

59. Bernasconi P, Torchiana E, Confalonieri P, et al: Expression of transforming growth factor-beta 1 in dystrophic patient muscles correlates with fibrosis. Pathogenetic role of a fibrogenic cytokine, *J Clin Invest* 96(2):1137–1144, 1995.

60. Iannaccone S, Quattrini A, Smirne S, et al: Connective tissue proliferation and growth factors in animal models of Duchenne muscular dystrophy, *J Neurol Sci* 128(1):36–44, 1995.

61. Melone MA, Peluso G, Galderisi U, et al: Increased expression of IGF-binding protein-5 in Duchenne muscular dystrophy (DMD) fibroblasts correlates with the fibroblast-induced downregulation of DMD myoblast growth: an in vitro analysis, *J Cell Physiol* 185(1):143–153, 2000.

62. Yamazaki M, Minota S, Sakurai H, et al: Expression of transforming growth factor-beta 1 and its relation to endomysial fibrosis in progressive muscular dystrophy, *Am J Pathol* 144(2):221–226, 1994.

63. Luz MA, Marques MJ, Santo Neto H: Impaired regeneration of dystrophin-deficient muscle fibers is caused by exhaustion of myogenic cells, *Braz J Med Biol Res* 35(6):691–695, 2002.

64. Passerini L, Bernasconi P, Baggi F, et al: Fibrogenic cytokines and extent of fibrosis in muscle of dogs with X-linked golden retriever muscular dystrophy, *Neuromuscul Disord* 12(9):828–835, 2002.

65. Spurney CF, Knoblach S, Pistilli EE, et al: Dystrophin-deficient cardiomyopathy in mouse: expression of Nox4 and Lox are associated with fibrosis and altered functional parameters in the heart, *Neuromuscul Disord* 18 (5):371–381, 2008.

66. Wehling-Henricks M, Sokolow S, Lee JJ, et al: Major basic protein-1 promotes fibrosis of dystrophic muscle and attenuates the cellular immune response in muscular dystrophy, *Hum Mol Genet* 17(15):2280–2292, 2008.

67. Arahata K, Ishiura S, Ishiguro T, et al: Immunostaining of skeletal and cardiac muscle surface membrane with antibody against Duchenne muscular dystrophy peptide, *Nature* 333(6176):861–863, 1988.

68. Bonilla E, Samitt CE, Miranda AF, et al: Duchenne muscular dystrophy: deficiency of dystrophin at the muscle cell surface, *Cell* 54(4):447–452, 1988.

69. Watkins SC, Hoffman EP, Slayter HS, et al: Immunoelectron microscopic localization of dystrophin in myofibres, *Nature* 333(6176):863–866, 1988.

70. Zubrzycka-Gaarn EE, Bulman DE, Karpati G, et al: The Duchenne muscular dystrophy gene product is localized in sarcolemma of human skeletal muscle, *Nature* 333(6172):466–469, 1988.

71. Jung D, Yang B, Meyer J, et al: Identification and characterization of the dystrophin anchoring site on beta-dystroglycan, *J Biol Chem* 270(45):27305–27310, 1995.

72. Ervasti JM, Campbell KP: Membrane organization of the dystrophin-glycoprotein complex, *Cell* 66(6):1121–1131, 1991.

73. Vandebrouck C, Martin D, Colson-Van Schoor M, et al: Involvement of TRPC in the abnormal calcium influx observed in dystrophic (*mdx*) mouse skeletal muscle fibers, *J Cell Biol* 158(6):1089–1096, 2002.

74. Doran P, Dowling P, Lohan J, et al: Subproteomics analysis of Ca^+-binding proteins demonstrates decreased calsequestrin expression in dystrophic mouse skeletal muscle, *Eur J Biochem* 271(19):3943–3952, 2004.

75. Dowling P, Doran P, Ohlendieck K: Drastic reduction of sarcalumenin in Dp427 (dystrophin of 427 kDa)-deficient fibres indicates that abnormal calcium handling plays a key role in muscular dystrophy, *Biochem J* 79(Pt 2):479–488, 2004.

76. Woods CE, Novo D, DiFranco M, et al: The action potential-evoked sarcoplasmic reticulum calcium release is impaired in *mdx* mouse muscle fibres, *J Physiol* 557(Pt 1):59–75, 2004.

77. Clapham DE: TRP channels as cellular sensors, *Nature* 426(6966):517–524, 2003.

78. Mallouk N, Allard B: Stretch-induced activation of Ca^{2+}-activated K^+ channels in mouse skeletal muscle fibers, *Am J Physiol Cell Physiol* 278(3): C473–C479, 2000.

79. Vandebrouck C, Duport G, Raymond G, et al: Hypotonic medium increases calcium permeant channels activity in human normal and dystrophic myotubes, *Neurosci Lett* 323(3):239–243, 2002a.

80. Turner PR, Schultz R, Ganguly B, et al: Proteolysis results in altered leak channel kinetics and elevated free calcium in *mdx* muscle, *J Membr Biol* 133 (3):243–251, 1993.

81. Fraysse B, Liantonio A, Cetrone M, et al: The alteration of calcium homeostasis in adult dystrophic *mdx* muscle fibers is worsened by a chronic exercise in vivo, *Neurobiol Dis* 17(2):144–154, 2004.

82. Ansved T: Muscular dystrophies: influence of physical conditioning on the disease evolution, *Curr Opin Clin Nutr Metab Care* 6(4):435–439, 2003.

83. Allen DG: Skeletal muscle function: role of ionic changes in fatigue, damage and disease, *Clin Exp Pharmacol Physiol* 31(8):485–493, 2004.

84. Kumar A, Boriek AM: Mechanical stress activates the nuclear factor-κB pathway in skeletal muscle fibers: a possible role in Duchenne muscular dystrophy, *FASEB J* 17(3):386–396, 2003.

85. Rando TA: The dystrophin-glycoprotein complex, cellular signaling, and the regulation of cell survival in the muscular dystrophies, *Muscle Nerve* 24(12):1575–1594, 2001.

86. Ragusa RJ, Chow CK, Porter JD: Oxidative stress as a potential pathogenic mechanism in an animal model of Duchenne muscular dystrophy, *Neuromuscul Disord* 7(6–7):379–386, 1997.

87. Rando TA: Oxidative stress and the pathogenesis of muscular dystrophies, *Am J Phys Med Rehabil* 81(11 Suppl):S175–S186, 2002.

88. Spencer MJ, Montecino-Rodriguez E, Dorshkind K, et al: Helper ($CD4^+$) and cytotoxic ($CD8^+$) T cells promote the pathology of dystrophin-deficient muscle, *Clin Immunol* 98(2):235–243, 2001.

89. Thomas GD, Shaul PW, Yuhanna IS, et al: Vasomodulation by skeletal muscle-derived nitric oxide requires alpha-syntrophin-mediated sarcolemmal localization of neuronal nitric oxide synthase, *Circ Res* 92(5):554–560, 2003.

90. Sander M, Chavoshan B, Harris SA, et al: Functional muscle ischemia in neuronal nitric oxide synthase-deficient skeletal muscle of children with Duchenne muscular dystrophy, *Proc Natl Acad Sci U S A* 97(25): 13818–13823, 2000.

91. von Moers A, Zwirner A, Reinhold A, et al: Increased mRNA expression of tissue inhibitors of metalloproteinase-1 and -2 in Duchenne muscular dystrophy, *Acta Neuropathol (Berl)* 109(3):285–293, 2004.

92. Bernasconi P, Di Blasi C, Mora M, et al: Transforming growth factor-β1 and fibrosis in congenital muscular dystrophies, *Neuromuscul Disord* 9 (1):28–33, 1999.

93. Bertorini TE, Cornelio F, Bhattacharya SK, et al: Calcium and magnesium content in fetuses at risk and prenecrotic Duchenne muscular dystrophy, *Neurology* 34(11):1436–1440, 1986.

94. Gozal D: Pulmonary manifestations of neuromuscular disease with special reference to Duchenne muscular dystrophy and spinal muscular atrophy, *Pediatr Pulmonol* 29(2):141–150, 2000.

95. Nigro G, Politano L, Nigro V, et al: Mutation of dystrophin gene and cardiomyopathy, *Neuromuscul Disord* 4(4):371–379, 1994.

96. Melacini P, Vianello A, Villanova C, et al: Cardiac and respiratory involvement in advanced stage Duchenne muscular dystrophy, *Neuromuscul Disord* 6(5):367–376, 1996.

97. Wahi PL, Bhargava KC, Mohindra S: Cardiorespiratory changes in progressive muscular dystrophy, *Br Heart J* 33(4):533–537, 1971.

98. Leth A, Wulff K: Myocardiopathy in Duchenne progressive muscular dystrophy, *Acta Paediatr Scand* 65(1):28–32, 1976.

99. Ogasawara A: Downward shift in IQ in persons with Duchenne muscular dystrophy compared to those with spinal muscular atrophy, *Am J Ment Retard* 93(5):544–547, 1989.

100. Bushby KM, Appleton R, Anderson LV, et al: Deletion status and intellectual impairment in Duchenne muscular dystrophy, *Dev Med Child Neurol* 37(3):260–269, 1995.

101. Felisari G, Martinelli Boneschi F, Bardoni A, et al: Loss of Dp140 dystrophin isoform and intellectual impairment in Duchenne dystrophy, *Neurology* 55(4):559–564, 2000.

102. Hinton VJ, De Vivo DC, Nereo NE, et al: Poor verbal working memory across intellectual level in boys with Duchenne dystrophy, *Neurology* 54(11): 2127–2132, 2000.

103. Roccella M, Pace R, De Gregorio MT: Psychopathological assessment in children affected by Duchenne de Boulogne muscular dystrophy, *Minerva Pediatr* 55(3):267–276, 2003.

104. Borrelli O, Salvia G, Mancini V, et al: Evolution of gastric electrical features and gastric emptying in children with Duchenne and Becker muscular dystrophy, *Am J Gastroenterol* 10:695–702, 2005.

105. Gardner-Medwin D: Mutation rate in Duchenne type of muscular dystrophy, *J Med Genet* 7(4):334–337, 1970.

106. Francke U, Ochs HD, de Martinville B, et al: Minor Xp21 chromosome deletion in a male associated with expression of Duchenne muscular dystrophy, chronic granulomatous disease, retinitis pigmentosa, and McLeod syndrome, *Am J Hum Genet* 37(2):250–267, 1985.

107. Hoffman EP, Arahata K, Minetti C, et al: Dystrophinopathy in isolated cases of myopathy in females, *Neurology* 42(5):967–975, 1992.

108. Hoogerwaard EM, Bakker E, Ippel PF, et al: Signs and symptoms of Duchenne muscular dystrophy and Becker muscular dystrophy among carriers in The Netherlands: a cohort study, *Lancet* 353(9170):2116–2119, 1999.

109. Hoffman EP: Clinical and histopathological features of abnormalities of the dystrophin-based membrane cytoskeleton, *Brain Pathol* 6(1):49–61, 1996.

110. Hoogerwaard EM, van der Wouw PA, Wilde AA, et al: Cardiac involvement in carriers of Duchenne and Becker muscular dystrophy, *Neuromuscul Disord* 9(5):347–351, 1999.

111. Grain L, Cortina-Borja M, Forfar C, et al: Cardiac abnormalities and skeletal muscle weakness in carriers of Duchenne and Becker muscular dystrophies and controls, *Neuromuscul Disord* 11(2):186–191, 2001.

112. Nolan MA, Jones OD, Pedersen RL, et al: Cardiac assessment in childhood carriers of Duchenne and Becker muscular dystrophies, *Neuromuscul Disord* 13(2):129–132, 2003.

112a. Gualandi F, Rimessi P, Trabanelli C, et al: Intronic breakpoint definition and transcription analysis in DMD/BMD patients with deletion/duplication at the 5′ mutation hot spot of the dystrophin gene, *Gene* 370:26–33, 2006.

113. Abbs S, Bobrow M: Analysis of quantitative PCR for the diagnosis of deletion and duplication carriers in the dystrophin gene, *J Med Genet* 29(3):191–196, 1992.

114. Yau SC, Bobrow M, Mathew CG, et al: Accurate diagnosis of carriers of deletions and duplications in Duchenne/Becker muscular dystrophy by fluorescent dosage analysis, *J Med Genet* 33(7):550–558, 1996.

115. White S, Kalf M, Liu Q, et al: Comprehensive detection of genomic duplications and deletions in the *DMD* gene, by use of multiplex amplifiable probe hybridization, *Am J Hum Genet* 1(2):365–374, 2002.

116. Jay V, Becker LE, Ackerley C, et al: Dystrophin analysis in the diagnosis of childhood muscular dystrophy: an immunohistochemical study of 75 cases, *Pediatr Pathol* 13(5):635–657, 1993.

117. Drachman DB, Toyka KV, Myer E: Prednisone in Duchenne muscular dystrophy, *Lancet* 2(7894):1409–1412, 1974.

118. Brooke MH, Fenichel GM, Griggs RC, et al: Clinical investigation of Duchenne muscular dystrophy. Interesting results in a trial of prednisone, *Arch Neurol* 44(8):812–817, 1987.

119. DeSilva S, Drachman DB, Mellits D, et al: Prednisone treatment in Duchenne muscular dystrophy. Long-term benefit, *Arch Neurol* 44(8): 818–822, 1987.

120. Mendell JR, Moxley RT, Griggs RC, et al: Randomized, double-blind 6-month trial of prednisone in Duchenne's muscular dystrophy, *N Engl J Med* 320(24):1592–1597, 1989.

121. Fenichel GM, Florence JM, Pestronk A, et al: Long-term benefit from prednisone therapy in Duchenne muscular dystrophy, *Neurology* 41(12):1874–1877, 1991.

122. Griggs RC, Moxley RTD, Mendell JR, et al: Duchenne dystrophy: randomized, controlled trial of prednisone (18 months) and azathioprine (12 months), *Neurology* 43(3 Pt 1):520–527, 1993.

123. Griggs RC, Moxley RTD, Mendell JR, et al: Prednisone in Duchenne dystrophy. A randomized, controlled trial defining the time course and dose response. Clinical Investigation of Duchenne Dystrophy Group, *Arch Neurol* 48(4):383–388, 1991.

124. Alman BA, Raza SN, Biggar WD: Steroid treatment and the development of scoliosis in males with Duchenne muscular dystrophy, *J Bone Joint Surg Am* 86-A(3):519–524, 2004.

125. Biggar WD, Politano L, Harris VA, et al: Deflazacort in Duchenne muscular dystrophy: a comparison of two different protocols, *Neuromuscul Disord* 14(8–9):476–482, 2004.

126. Yilmaz O, Karaduman A, Topaloglu H: Prednisolone therapy in Duchenne muscular dystrophy prolongs ambulation and prevents scoliosis, *Eur J Neurol* 11(8):541–544, 2004.

127. Angelini C, Pegoraro E, Turella E, et al: Deflazacort in Duchenne dystrophy: study of long-term effect [published erratum appears in *Muscle Nerve* 17(7):833, 1994]. *Muscle Nerve* 17(4):386–391, 1994.

128. Campbell C, Jacob P: Deflazacort for the treatment of Duchenne dystrophy: a systematic review, *BMC Neurol* 3(1):7, 2003.

129. Merlini L, Cicognani A, Malaspina E, et al: Early prednisone treatment in Duchenne muscular dystrophy, *Muscle Nerve* 27(2):222–227, 2003.

130. Moxley RT, Ashwal S, Pandya S, et al: Practice parameter: corticosteroid treatment of Duchenne dystrophy: report of the Quality Standards Subcommittee of the American Academy of Neurology and the Practice Committee of the Child Neurology Society, *Neurology* 64(1):13–20, 2005.

131. Larson CM, Henderson RC: Bone mineral density and fractures in boys with Duchenne muscular dystrophy, *J Pediatr Orthop* 20(1):71–74, 2000.

132. Aparicio LF, Jurkovic M, DeLullo J: Decreased bone density in ambulatory patients with Duchenne muscular dystrophy, *J Pediatr Orthop* 22(2):179–181, 2002.

133. Bianchi ML, Mazzanti A, Galbiati E, et al: Bone mineral density and bone metabolism in Duchenne muscular dystrophy, *Osteoporos Int* 14(9): 761–767, 2003.

134. Mesa LE, Dubrovsky AL, Corderi J, et al: Steroids in Duchenne muscular dystrophy—deflazacort trial, *Neuromuscul Disord* 1(4):261–266, 1991.

135. Bonifati MD, Ruzza G, Bonometto P, et al: A multicenter, double-blind, randomized trial of deflazacort versus prednisone in Duchenne muscular dystrophy, *Muscle Nerve* 23(9):1344–1347, 2000.

136. Biggar WD, Gingras M, Fehlings DL, et al: Deflazacort treatment of Duchenne muscular dystrophy, *J Pediatr* 138(1):45–50, 2001.

137. Sansome A, Royston P, Dubowitz V: Steroids in Duchenne muscular dystrophy: pilot study of a new low-dosage schedule, *Neuromuscul Disord* 3(5–6): 567–569, 1993.

138. Dubowitz V, Kinali M, Main M, et al: Remission of clinical signs in early Duchenne muscular dystrophy on intermittent low-dosage prednisolone therapy, *Eur J Paediatr Neurol* 6(3):153–159, 2002.

139. Kinali M, Mercuri E, Main M, et al: An effective, low-dosage, intermittent schedule of prednisolone in the long-term treatment of early cases of Duchenne dystrophy, *Neuromuscul Disord* 12(Suppl 1):S169–S174, 2002.

140. Connolly A, Schierbecker J, Renna R, et al: High dose weekly oral prednisone improves strength in boys with Duchenne muscular dystrophy, *Neuromuscul Disord* 12(10):917–925, 2002.

141. Zanardi MC, Tagliabue A, Orcesi S, et al: Body composition and energy expenditure in Duchenne muscular dystrophy, *Eur J Clin Nutr* 57(2): 273–278, 2003.

142. Sharma KR, Mynhier MA, Miller RG: Cyclosporine increases muscular force generation in Duchenne muscular dystrophy, *Neurology* 43(3 Pt 1):527–532, 1993.

143. Mendell JR, Kissel JT, Amato AA, et al: Myoblast transfer in the treatment of Duchenne's muscular dystrophy, *N Engl J Med* 333(13): 832–838, 1995.

144. Escolar DM, Buyse G, Henricson E, et al: CINRG randomized controlled trial of creatine and glutamine in Duchenne muscular dystrophy, *Ann Neurol* 58(1):151–155, 2005.

145. Walter MC, Lochmuller H, Reilich P, et al: Creatine monohydrate in muscular dystrophies: a double-blind, placebo-controlled clinical study, *Neurology* 54 (9):1848–1850, 2000.

146. Tarnopolsky MA, Mahoney DJ, Vajsar J, et al: Creatine monohydrate enhances strength and body composition in Duchenne muscular dystrophy, *Neurology* 62(10):1771–1777, 2004.

147. Straathof CS, Overweg-Plandsoen WC, van den Burg GJ, et al: Prednisone 10 days on/10 days off in patients with Duchenne muscular dystrophy, *J Neurol* 256(5):768–773, 2009.

148. Barton-Davis ER, Cordier L, Shoturma DI, et al: Aminoglycoside antibiotics restore dystrophin function to skeletal muscles of *mdx* mice, *J Clin Invest* 104(4):375–381, 1999.

149. Wagner KR, Hamed S, Hadley DW, et al: Gentamicin treatment of Duchenne and Becker muscular dystrophy due to nonsense mutations, *Ann Neurol* 49(6):706–711, 2001.

150. Welch EM, Barton ER, Zhuo J, et al: PTC124 targets genetic disorders caused by nonsense mutations, *Nature* 447(7140):87–91, 2007.

151. Rando TA, Disatnik MH, Zhou LZ: Rescue of dystrophin expression in *mdx* mouse muscle by RNA/DNA oligonucleotides, *Proc Natl Acad Sci U S A* 97(10):5363–5368, 2000.

152. Gebski BL, Mann CJ, Fletcher S, et al: Morpholino antisense oligonucleotide induced dystrophin exon 23 skipping in *mdx* mouse muscle, *Hum Mol Genet* 12(15):1801–1811, 2003.

153. Wells KE, Fletcher S, Mann CJ, et al: Enhanced in vivo delivery of antisense oligonucleotides to restore dystrophin expression in adult *mdx* mouse muscle, *FEBS Lett* 552(2–3):145–149, 2003.

154. Lu QL, Mann CJ, Lou F, et al: Functional amounts of dystrophin produced by skipping the mutated exon in the *mdx* dystrophic mouse, *Nat Med* 9(8):1009–1014, 2003.

155. Errington SJ, Mann CJ, Fletcher S, et al: Target selection for antisense oligonucleotide induced exon skipping in the dystrophin gene, *J Gene Med* 5(6):518–527, 2003.

156. Mann CJ, Honeyman K, Cheng AJ, et al: Antisense-induced exon skipping and synthesis of dystrophin in the mdx mouse, *Proc Natl Acad Sci U S A* 98(1):42–47, 2001.

157. van Deutekom JC, Janson AA, Ginjaar IB, et al: Local dystrophin restoration with antisense oligonucleotide PRO051, *N Engl J Med* 357(26):2677–2686, 2007.

158. Laws N, Cornford-Nairn RA, Irwin N, et al: Long-term administration of antisense oligonucleotides into the paraspinal muscles of *mdx* mice reduces kyphosis, *J Appl Physiol* 105(2):662–668, 2008.

159. Yokota T, Lu QL, Partridge T, et al: Efficacy of systemic morpholino exon-skipping in Duchenne dystrophy dogs, *Ann Neurol* 65(6):667–676, 2009.

159a. Kinali M, Arechavala-Gomeza V, Feng L, Cirak S, Hunt D, et al: Local restoration of dystrophin expression with the morpholino oligomer AVI-4658 in Duchenne muscular dystrophy: a single-blind, placebo-controlled, dose-escalation, proof-of-concept study, *Lancet Neurol* 8(10):918–928, 2009. Epub 25, 2009 Aug.

160. Wang B, Li J, Xiao X: Adeno-associated virus vector carrying human minidystrophin genes effectively ameliorates muscular dystrophy in *mdx* mouse model, *Proc Natl Acad Sci U S A* 97(25):13714–13719, 2000.

161. Hartigan-O'Connor D, Kirk CJ, Crawford R, et al: Immune evasion by muscle-specific gene expression in dystrophic muscle, *Mol Ther* 4(6):525–533, 2001.

162. DelloRusso C, Scott JM, Hartigan-O'Connor D, et al: Functional correction of adult *mdx* mouse muscle using gutted adenoviral vectors expressing full-length dystrophin, *Proc Nat Acad Sci U S A* 99(20):12979–12984, 2002.

163. Scott JM, Li S, Harper SQ, et al: Viral vectors for gene transfer of micro-, mini-, or full-length dystrophin, *Neuromuscul Disord* 12(Suppl 1):S23–S29, 2002.

164. Gregorevic P, Blankinship MJ, Allen JM, et al: Systemic delivery of genes to striated muscles using adeno-associated viral vectors, *Nat Med* 10(8):828–834, 2004.

165. Wang B, Li J, Qiao C, et al: A canine minidystrophin is functional and therapeutic in *mdx* mice, *Gene Ther* 15(15):1099–1106, 2008.

166. Partridge T: Myoblast transplantation, *Neuromuscul Disord* 12(Suppl 1):S3–S6, 2002.

167. Munsat TL: Clinical trials in neuromuscular disease, *Muscle Nerve* 13(Suppl):S3–S6, 1990.

168. Miller RG, Sharma KR, Pavlath GK, et al: Myoblast implantation in Duchenne muscular dystrophy: the San Francisco study, *Muscle Nerve* 20(4):469–478, 1997.

169. Neumeyer AM, Cros D, McKenna-Yasek D, et al: Pilot study of myoblast transfer in the treatment of Becker muscular dystrophy, *Neurology* 51(2):589–592, 1998.

170. Huard J, Acsadi G, Jani A, et al: Gene transfer into skeletal muscles by isogenic myoblasts, *Hum Gene Ther* 5(8):949–958, 1994.

171. Tanaka KK, Hall JK, Troy AA, et al: Syndecan-4-expressing muscle progenitor cells in the SP engraft as satellite cells during muscle regeneration, *Cell Stem Cell* 4(3):217–225, 2009.

172. Tinsley JM, Potter AC, Phelps SR, et al: Amelioration of the dystrophic phenotype of *mdx* mice using a truncated utrophin transgene, *Nature* 384(6607):349–353, 1996.

173. Tinsley J, Deconinck N, Fisher R, et al: Expression of full-length utrophin prevents muscular dystrophy in *mdx* mice, *Nat Med* 4(12):1441–1444, 1998.

174. Deconinck N, Tinsley J, De Backer F, et al: Expression of truncated utrophin leads to major functional improvements in dystrophin-deficient muscles of mice, *Nat Med* 3(11):1216–1221, 1997.

175. Barton ER, Morris L, Kawana M, et al: Systemic administration of L-arginine benefits *mdx* skeletal muscle function, *Muscle Nerve* 32(6):751–760, 2005.

176. Burkin DJ, Wallace GQ, Nicol KJ, et al: Enhanced expression of the α7β1 integrin reduces muscular dystrophy and restores viability in dystrophic mice, *J Cell Biol* 152(6):1207–1218, 2001.

177. Maskarinec SA, Wu G, Lee KY: Membrane sealing by polymers, *Ann N Y Acad Sci* 1066:310–320, 2006.

178. Yasuda S, Townsend D, Michele DE, et al: Dystrophic heart failure blocked by membrane sealant poloxamer, *Nature* 436(7053):1025–1029, 2005.

179. Quinlan JG, Wong BL, Niemeier RT, et al: Poloxamer 188 failed to prevent exercise-induced membrane breakdown in *mdx* skeletal muscle fibers, *Neuromuscul Disord* 16(12):855–864, 2006.

180. Bogdanovich S, Krag TO, Barton ER, et al: Functional improvement of dystrophic muscle by myostatin blockade, *Nature* 420(6914):418–421, 2002.

181. Wagner KR, Fleckenstein JL, Amato AA, et al: A phase I/II trial of MYO-029 in adult subjects with muscular dystrophy, *Ann Neurol* 63(5):561–571, 2008.

182. Nakatani M, Takehara Y, Sugino H, et al: Transgenic expression of a myostatin inhibitor derived from follistatin increases skeletal muscle mass and ameliorates dystrophic pathology in *mdx* mice, *FASEB J* 22(2):477–487, 2008.

183. Alderton JM, Steinhardt RA: How calcium influx through calcium leak channels is responsible for the elevated levels of calcium-dependent proteolysis in dystrophic myotubes, *Trends Cardiovasc Med* 10(6):268–272, 2000.

184. Spencer MJ, Mellgren RL: Overexpression of a calpastatin transgene in *mdx* muscle reduces dystrophic pathology, *Hum Mol Genet* 11(21):2645–2655, 2002.

185. Wehling M, Spencer MJ, Tidball JG: A nitric oxide synthase transgene ameliorates muscular dystrophy in *mdx* mice, *J Cell Biol* 155(1):123–131, 2001.

186. Matsumura CY, Pertille A, Albuquerque TC, et al: Diltiazem and verapamil protect dystrophin-deficient muscle fibers of *MDX* mice from degeneration: a potential role in calcium buffering and sarcolemmal stability, *Muscle Nerve* 39(2):167–176, 2009.

187. Phillips MF, Quinlivan R: Calcium antagonists for Duchenne muscular dystrophy, *Cochrane Database Syst Rev* (4):CD004571, 2008.

188. Yeung EW, Head SI, Allen DG: Gadolinium reduces short-term stretch-induced muscle damage in isolated *mdx* mouse muscle fibres, *J Physiol* 552(Pt 2):449–458, 2003.

189. Yeung EW, Whitehead NP, Suchyna TM, et al: Effects of stretch-activated channel blockers on [Ca^{2+}]i and muscle damage in the *mdx* mouse, *J Physiol* 562(Pt 2):367–380, 2005.

190. Rolland JF, De Luca A, Burdi R, et al: Overactivity of exercise-sensitive cation channels and their impaired modulation by IGF-1 in *mdx* native muscle fibers: beneficial effect of pentoxifylline, *Neurobiol Dis* 24(3):466–474, 2006.

191. Bertorini TE, Palmieri GM, Griffin J, et al: Effect of dantrolene in Duchenne muscular dystrophy, *Muscle Nerve* 14(6):503–507, 1991.

192. Acharyya S, Villalta SA, Bakkar N, et al: Interplay of IKK/NF-κB signaling in macrophages and myofibers promotes muscle degeneration in Duchenne muscular dystrophy, *J Clin Invest* 117(4):889–901, 2007.

193. Radley HG, Davies MJ, Grounds MD: Reduced muscle necrosis and long-term benefits in dystrophic *mdx* mice after cV1q (blockade of TNF) treatment, *Neuromuscul Disord* 18(3):227–238, 2008.

194. Buyse GM, Van der Mieren G, Erb M, et al: Long-term blinded placebo-controlled study of SNT-MC17/idebenone in the dystrophin deficient *mdx* mouse: cardiac protection and improved exercise performance, *Eur Heart J* 30(1):116–124, 2009.

195. Brunelli S, Sciorati C, D'Antona G, et al: Nitric oxide release combined with nonsteroidal anti-inflammatory activity prevents muscular dystrophy pathology and enhances stem cell therapy, *Proc Natl Acad Sci U S A* 104(1):264–269, 2007.

196. Colussi C, Mozzetta C, Gurtner A, et al: HDAC2 blockade by nitric oxide and histone deacetylase inhibitors reveals a common target in Duchenne muscular dystrophy treatment, *Proc Natl Acad Sci U S A* 105(49):19183–19187, 2008. Erratum in *Proc Natl Acad Sci U S A* 106(5):1679, 2009.

197. Huebner KD, Jassal DS, Halevy O, et al: Functional resolution of fibrosis in *mdx* mouse dystrophic heart and skeletal muscle by halofuginone, *Am J Physiol Heart Circ Physiol* 294(4):H1550–H1561, 2008.

198. Minetti GC, Colussi C, Adami R, et al: Functional and morphological recovery of dystrophic muscles in mice treated with deacetylase inhibitors, *Nat Med* 12(10):1147–1150, 2006.

199. Cohn RD, van Erp C, Habashi JP, et al: Angiotensin II type 1 receptor blockade attenuates TGF-β-induced failure of muscle regeneration in multiple myopathic states, *Nat Med* 13(2):204–210, 2007.

200. Gibson B: Long-term ventilation for patients with Duchenne muscular dystrophy: physicians' beliefs and practices, *Chest* 119(3):940–946, 2001.

201. Do T: Orthopedic management of the muscular dystrophies, *Curr Opin Pediatr* 14(1):50–53, 2002.

202. Corrado G, Lissoni A, Beretta S, et al: Prognostic value of electrocardiograms, ventricular late potentials, ventricular arrhythmias, and left ventricular systolic dysfunction in patients with Duchenne muscular dystrophy, *Am J Cardiol* 89(7):838–841, 2002.

203. Bushby K, Muntoni F, Bourke JP: 107th ENMC International Workshop: the management of cardiac involvement in muscular dystrophy and

myotonic dystrophy. 7th–9th June 2002, Naarden, The Netherlands, *Neuromuscul Disord* 13(2):166–172, 2003.

204. Finsterer J, Stollberger C: The heart in human dystrophinopathies, *Cardiology* 99(1):1–19, 2003.

205. Griggs RC, Mendell JR, Brooke MH, et al: Clinical investigation in Duchenne dystrophy: V. Use of creatine kinase and pyruvate kinase in carrier detection, *Muscle Nerve* 8(1):60–67, 1985.

206. Milhorat AT, Goldstone L: The carrier state in muscular dystrophy of the Duchenne type, *JAMA* 194(2):130–134, 1965.

207. Maunder-Sewry CA, Dubowitz V: Needle muscle biopsy for carrier detection in Duchenne muscular dystrophy. Part 1. Light microscopy—histology, histochemistry and quantitation, *J Neurol Sci* 49(2):305–324, 1981.

208. Ionasescu V, Zellweger H, Conway TW: A new approach for carrier detection in Duchenne muscular dystrophy. Protein synthesis of muscle polyribosomes in vitro, *Neurology* 21(7):703–709, 1971.

209. Ionasescu V, Zellweger H, Conway TW: Ribosomal protein synthesis in Duchenne muscular dystrophy, *Arch Biochem Biophys* 144(1):51–58, 1971.

210. Ionasescu V, Burmeister L, Hanson J: Discriminant analysis of ribosomal protein synthesis findings in carrier detection of Duchenne muscular dystrophy, *Am J Med Genet* 5(1):5–12, 1980.

211. Kuller JA, Hoffman EP, Fries MH, et al: Prenatal diagnosis of Duchenne muscular dystrophy by fetal muscle biopsy, *Hum Genet* 90(1–2):34–40, 1992.

212. Vassilopoulos D, Emery AE: Muscle nuclear changes in fetuses at risk for Duchenne muscular dystrophy, *J Med Genet* 14(1):13–15, 1977.

213. Heiman-Patterson TD, Natter HM, Rosenberg HR, et al: Malignant hyperthermia susceptibility in X-linked muscle dystrophies, *Pediatr Neurol* 2(6):356–358, 1986.

214. Smith CL, Bush GH: Anaesthesia and progressive muscular dystrophy, *Br J Anaesth* 57(11):1113–1138, 1985.

215. Witte RA: The psychosocial impact of a progressive physical handicap and terminal illness (Duchenne muscular dystrophy) on adolescents and their families, *Br J Med Psychol* 58(Pt 2):179–187, 1985.

216. Fitzpatrick C, Barry C, Garvey C: Psychiatric disorder among boys with Duchenne muscular dystrophy, *Dev Med Child Neurol* 28(5):589–595, 1986.

217. Song KS, Scherer PE, Tang Z, et al: Expression of caveolin-3 in skeletal, cardiac, and smooth muscle cells. Caveolin-3 is a component of the sarcolemma and co-fractionates with dystrophin and dystrophin-associated glycoproteins, *J Biol Chem* 271(25):15160–15165, 1996.

218. Tang Z, Scherer PE, Okamoto T, et al: Molecular cloning of caveolin-3, a novel member of the caveolin gene family expressed predominantly in muscle, *J Biol Chem* 271(4):2255–2261, 1996.

219. Dincer P, Leturcq F, Richard I, et al: A biochemical, genetic, and clinical survey of autosomal recessive limb-girdle muscular dystrophies in Turkey, *Ann Neurol* 42(2):222–229, 1997.

220. Richard I, Brenguier L, Dincer P, et al: Multiple independent molecular etiology for limb-girdle muscular dystrophy type 2A patients from various geographical origins, *Am J Hum Genet* 60(5):1128–1138, 1997.

221. Topaloglu H, Dincer P, Richard I, et al: Calpain-3 deficiency causes a mild muscular dystrophy in childhood, *Neuropediatrics* 28(4):212–216, 1997.

222. Chae J, Minami N, Jin Y, et al: Calpain 3 gene mutations: genetic and clinico-pathologic findings in limb-girdle muscular dystrophy, *Neuromuscul Disord* 11(6–7):547–555, 2001.

223. Johnson P: Calpains (intracellular calcium-activated cysteine proteinases): structure-activity relationships and involvement in normal and abnormal cellular metabolism, *Int J Biochem* 22(8):811–822, 1990.

224. Chiannilkulchai N, Pasturaud P, Richard I, et al: A primary expression map of the chromosome 15q15 region containing the recessive form of limb-girdle muscular dystrophy (LGMD2A) gene, *Hum Mol Genet* 4(4):717–725, 1995.

225. Richard I, Broux O, Allamand V, et al: Mutations in the proteolytic enzyme calpain 3 cause limb-girdle muscular dystrophy type 2A, *Cell* 81(1):27–40, 1995.

226. Saenz A, Leturcq F, Cobo AM, et al: LGMD2A: genotype-phenotype correlations based on a large mutational survey on the calpain 3 gene, *Brain* 128(4):732–742, 2005.

227. Spencer MJ, Guyon JR, Sorimachi H, et al: Stable expression of calpain 3 from a muscle transgene in vivo: immature muscle in transgenic mice suggests a role for calpain 3 in muscle maturation, *Proc Natl Acad Sci U S A* 99(13):8874–8879, 2002.

228. Zatz M, de Paula F, Starling A, et al: The 10 autosomal recessive limb-girdle muscular dystrophies, *Neuromuscul Disord* 13(7–8):532–544, 2003.

229. Baghdiguian S, Martin M, Richard I, et al: Calpain 3 deficiency is associated with myonuclear apoptosis and profound perturbation of the IκBα/NF-κB pathway in limb-girdle muscular dystrophy type 2A, *Nat Med* 5(5):503–511, 1999.

230. Taveau M, Bourg N, Sillon G, et al: Calpain 3 is activated through autolysis within the active site and lyses sarcomeric and sarcolemmal components, *Mol Cell Biol* 23(24):9127–9135, 2003.

231. Rey MA, Davies PL: The protease core of the muscle-specific calpain, p94, undergoes Ca^{2+}-dependent intramolecular autolysis, *FEBS Lett* 532(3):401–406, 2002.

232. Beckmann JS, Bushby KM: Advances in the molecular genetics of the limb-girdle type of autosomal recessive progressive muscular dystrophy, *Curr Opin Neurol* 9(5):389–393, 1996.

233. Fanin M, Nascimbeni AC, Fulizio L, et al: Loss of calpain-3 autocatalytic activity in LGMD2A patients with normal protein expression, *Am J Pathol* 163(5):1929–1936, 2003.

234. Bansal D, Miyake K, Vogel SS, et al: Defective membrane repair in dysferlin-deficient muscular dystrophy, *Nature* 423(6936):168–172, 2003.

235. Matsuda C, Aoki M, Hayashi YK, et al: Dysferlin is a surface membrane-associated protein that is absent in Miyoshi myopathy, *Neurology* 53(5):1119–1122, 1999.

236. Gallardo E, Rojas-Garcia R, de Luna N, et al: Inflammation in dysferlin myopathy: immunohistochemical characterization of 13 patients, *Neurology* 57(11):2136–2138, 2001.

237. Takahashi T, Aoki M, Tateyama M, et al: Dysferlin mutations in Japanese Miyoshi myopathy: relationship to phenotype, *Neurology* 60(11):1799–1804, 2003.

238. Ueyama H, Kumamoto T, Horinouchi H, et al: Clinical heterogeneity in dysferlinopathy, *Intern Med* 41(7):532–536, 2002.

239. Mahjneh I, Marconi G, Bushby K, et al: Dysferlinopathy (LGMD2B): a 23-year follow-up study of 10 patients homozygous for the same frameshifting dysferlin mutations, *Neuromuscul Disord* 11(1):20–26, 2001.

240. Ho M, Gallardo E, McKenna-Yasek D, et al: A novel, blood-based diagnostic assay for limb-girdle muscular dystrophy 2B and Miyoshi myopathy, *Ann Neurol* 51(1):129–133, 2002.

241. Nigro V, Piluso G, Belsito A, et al: Identification of a novel sarcoglycan gene at 5q33 encoding a sarcolemmal 35kDa glycoprotein, *Hum Mol Genet* 5(8):1179–1186, 1996.

242. Zatz M, Passos-Bueno MR, Rapaport D: Estimate of the proportion of Duchenne muscular dystrophy with autosomal recessive inheritance, *Am J Med Genet* 32(3):407–410, 1989.

243. Matsumura K, Tome FM, Collin H, et al: Deficiency of the 50K dystrophin-associated glycoprotein in severe childhood autosomal recessive muscular dystrophy, *Nature* 359(6393):320–322, 1992.

244. Azibi K, Bachner L, Beckmann JS, et al: Severe childhood autosomal recessive muscular dystrophy with the deficiency of the 50 kDa dystrophin-associated glycoprotein maps to chromosome 13q12, *Hum Mol Genet* 2(9):1423–1428, 1993.

245. Mizuno Y, Noguchi S, Yamamoto H, et al: Selective defect of sarcoglycan complex in severe childhood autosomal recessive muscular dystrophy muscle, *Biochem Biophys Res Commun* 203(2):979–983, 1994.

246. Hoffman EP, Clemens PR: HyperCKemic, proximal muscular dystrophies and the dystrophin membrane cytoskeleton, including dystrophinopathies, sarcoglycanopathies, and merosinopathies, *Curr Opin Rheumatol* 8(6):528–538, 1996.

247. Krasnianski M, Neudecker S, Deschauer M, et al: [The clinical spectrum of limb-girdle muscular dystrophies type 2I in cases of a mutation in the fukutin-related protein gene], *Nervenarzt* 75(8):770–775, 2004.

248. Walter MC, Petersen JA, Stucka R, et al: FKRP (826C>A) frequently causes limb-girdle muscular dystrophy in German patients, *J Med Genet* 41(4):e50, 2004.

249. Brockington M, Blake DJ, Prandini P, et al: Mutations in the fukutin-related protein gene (FKRP) cause a form of congenital muscular dystrophy

with secondary laminin α2 deficiency and abnormal glycosylation of alpha-dystroglycan, *Am J Hum Genet* 69(6):1198–1209, 2001.

250. Brockington M, Yuva Y, Prandini P, et al: Mutations in the fukutin-related protein gene (*FKRP*) identify limb-girdle muscular dystrophy 2I as a milder allelic variant of congenital muscular dystrophy MDC1C, *Hum Mol Genet* 10(25):2851–2859, 2001.

251. Mercuri E, Brockington M, Straub V, et al: Phenotypic spectrum associated with mutations in the fukutin-related protein gene, *Ann Neurol* 53(4):537–542, 2003.

252. Poppe M, Cree L, Bourke J, et al: The phenotype of limb-girdle muscular dystrophy type 2I, *Neurology* 60(8):1246–1251, 2003.

253. Schneiderman LJ, Sampson WI, Schoene WC, et al: Genetic studies of a family with two unusual autosomal dominant conditions: muscular dystrophy and Pelger-Huet anomaly. Clinical, pathologic and linkage considerations, *Am J Med* 46(3):380–393, 1969.

254. Gilchrist JM, Pericak-Vance M, Silverman L, et al: Clinical and genetic investigation in autosomal dominant limb-girdle muscular dystrophy, *Neurology* 38(1):5–9, 1988.

255. Yamaoka LH, Westbrook CA, Speer MC, et al: Development of a microsatellite genetic map spanning 5q31-q33 and subsequent placement of the LGMD1A locus between D5S178 and IL9, *Neuromuscul Disord* 4(5–6):471–475, 1994.

256. Hauser MA, Conde CB, Kowaljow V, et al: Myotilin mutation found in second pedigree with LGMD1A, *Am J Hum Genet* 71(6):1428–1432, 2002.

257. Selcen D, Engel AG: Mutations in myotilin cause myofibrillar myopathy, *Neurology* 62(8):1363–1371, 2004.

258. Selcen D, Ohno K, Engel AG: Myofibrillar myopathy: clinical, morphological and genetic studies in 63 patients, *Brain* 127(Pt 2):439–451, 2004.

259. Schroder R, Reimann J, Salmikangas P, et al: Beyond LGMD1A: myotilin is a component of central core lesions and nemaline rods, *Neuromuscul Disord* 13(6):451–455, 2003.

260. Valle G, Faulkner G, De Antoni A, et al: Telethonin, a novel sarcomeric protein of heart and skeletal muscle, *FEBS Lett* 415(2):163–168, 1997.

261. Moreira ES, Vainzof M, Marie SK, et al: The seventh form of autosomal recessive limb-girdle muscular dystrophy is mapped to 17q11–12, *Am J Hum Genet* 61(1):151–159, 1997.

262. Granzier HL, Labeit S: The giant protein titin: a major player in myocardial mechanics, signaling, and disease, *Circ Res* 94(3):284–295, 2004.

263. McElhinny AS, Perry CN, Witt CC, et al: Muscle-specific RING finger-2 (*MURF-2*) is important for microtubule, intermediate filament and sarcomeric M-line maintenance in striated muscle development, *J Cell Sci* 117(Pt 15):3175–3188, 2004.

264. Hackman P, Vihola A, Haravuori H, et al: Tibial muscular dystrophy is a titinopathy caused by mutations in *TTN*, the gene encoding the giant skeletal-muscle protein titin, *Am J Hum Genet* 71(3):492–500, 2002.

265. Bione S, Maestrini E, Rivella S, et al: Identification of a novel X-linked gene responsible for Emery-Dreifuss muscular dystrophy, *Nat Genet* 8(4):323–327, 1994.

266. Bonne G, Di Barletta MR, Varnous S, et al: Mutations in the gene encoding lamin A/C cause autosomal dominant Emery-Dreifuss muscular dystrophy, *Nat Genet* 21(3):285–288, 1999.

267. Gruenbaum Y, Goldman RD, Meyuhas R, et al: The nuclear lamina and its functions in the nucleus, *Int Rev Cytol* 226:1–62, 2003.

268. Emery AE: Emery-Dreifuss muscular dystrophy—a 40 year retrospective, *Neuromuscul Disord* 10(4–5):228–232, 2000.

269. Bonne G, Mercuri E, Muchir A, et al: Clinical and molecular genetic spectrum of autosomal dominant Emery-Dreifuss muscular dystrophy due to mutations of the lamin A/C gene, *Ann Neurol* 48(2):170–180, 2000.

270. Brown CA, Lanning RW, McKinney KQ, et al: Novel and recurrent mutations in lamin A/C in patients with Emery-Dreifuss muscular dystrophy, *Am J Med Genet* 102(4):359–367, 2001.

271. Bonne G: The laminopathy saga, *Rev Neurol* 37(8):772–774, 2003.

271a. Zhang Q, Bethmann C, Worth NF, Davies JD, et al: Nesprin-1 and -2 are involved in the pathogenesis of Emery Dreifuss muscular dystrophy and are critical for nuclear envelope integrity, *Hum Mol Genet* 16(23):2816–2833, 2007.

271b. Quinzii CM, Vu TH, Min KC, et al: X-linked dominant scapuloperoneal myopathy is due to a mutation in the gene encoding four-and-a-half-LIM protein 1, *Am J Hum Genet* 82(1):208–213, 2008.

272. Muntoni F, Lichtarowicz-Krynska EJ, Sewry CA, et al: Early presentation of X-linked Emery-Dreifuss muscular dystrophy resembling limb-girdle muscular dystrophy, *Neuromuscul Disord* 8(2):72–76, 1998.

273. Fujimoto S, Ishikawa T, Saito M, et al: Early onset of X-linked Emery-Dreifuss muscular dystrophy in a boy with emerin gene deletion, *Neuropediatrics* 30(3):161–163, 1999.

274. Emery AE: Emery-Dreifuss syndrome, *J Med Genet* 26(10):637–641, 1989.

275. Becane HM, Bonne G, Varnous S, et al: High incidence of sudden death with conduction system and myocardial disease due to lamins A and C gene mutation, *Pacing Clin Electrophysiol* 23(11 Pt 1):1661–1666, 2000.

276. Bonne G, Yaou RB, Beroud C, et al: 108th ENMC International Workshop, 3rd Workshop of the MYO-CLUSTER project: EUROMEN, 7th International Emery-Dreifuss Muscular Dystrophy (EDMD) Workshop, 13–15 September 2002, Naarden, The Netherlands, *Neuromuscul Disord* 13(6):508–515, 2003.

277. Danièle N, Richard I, Bartoli M: Ins and outs of therapy in limb girdle muscular dystrophies, *Int J Biochem Cell Biol* 39(9):1608–1624, 2007.

277a. Mendell RJ, Rodino-Klapac LR, Rosales-Quinteros X, et al: Limb-girdle muscular dystrophy type 2D gene therapy restores alpha-sarcoglycan and associated proteins, *Ann Neurol* 66:267–270, 2009.

278. Angelini C, Fanin M, Menegazzo E, et al: Homozygous alpha-sarcoglycan mutation in two siblings: one asymptomatic and one steroid-responsive mild limb-girdle muscular dystrophy patient, *Muscle Nerve* 21(6):769–775, 1998.

279. Connolly AM, Pestronk A, Mehta S, et al: Primary alpha-sarcoglycan deficiency responsive to immunosuppression over 3 years, *Muscle Nerve* 21(11):1549–1553, 1998.

280. Zatz M, Marie SK, Passos-Bueno MR, et al: High proportion of new mutations and possible anticipation in Brazilian facioscapulohumeral muscular dystrophy families, *Am J Hum Genet* 56(1):99–105, 1995.

281. Wijmenga C, Frants RR, Hewitt JE, et al: Molecular genetics of facioscapulohumeral muscular dystrophy, *Neuromuscul Disord* 3(5–6):487–491, 1993.

282. Tawil R: Facioscapulohumeral muscular dystrophy, *Neurotherapeutics* 5(4):60–66, 2008.

283. Brouwer OF, Padberg GW, Bakker E, et al: Early onset facioscapulohumeral muscular dystrophy, *Muscle Nerve* 2:S67–S72, 1995.

284. Brouwer OF, Padberg GW, Wijmenga C, et al: Facioscapulohumeral muscular dystrophy in early childhood, *Arch Neurol* 51(4):387–394, 1994.

285. Yamanaka G, Goto K, Ishihara T, et al: FSHD-like patients without 4q35 deletion, *J Neurol Sci* 219(1–2):89–93, 2004.

286. Tawil R, Figlewicz DA, Griggs RC, et al: Facioscapulohumeral dystrophy: a distinct regional myopathy with a novel molecular pathogenesis. FSH Consortium, *Ann Neurol* 43(3):279–282, 1998.

287. Small RG: Coats' disease and muscular dystrophy, *Trans Am Acad Ophthalmol Otolaryngol* 72(2):225–231, 1968.

288. Taylor DA, Carroll JE, Smith ME, et al: Facioscapulohumeral dystrophy associated with hearing loss and Coats syndrome, *Ann Neurol* 12(4):395–398, 1982.

289. Fitzsimons RB, Gurwin EB, Bird AC: Retinal vascular abnormalities in facioscapulohumeral muscular dystrophy. A general association with genetic and therapeutic implications, *Brain* 110(Pt 3):631–648, 1987.

290. Rothstein TL, Carlson CB, Sumi SM: Polymyositis with facioscapulohumeral distribution, *Arch Neurol* 25(4):313–319, 1971.

291. Bunch WH, Siegel IM: Scapulothoracic arthrodesis in facioscapulohumeral muscular dystrophy. Review of 17 procedures with 3- to 21-year follow-up, *J Bone Joint Surg Am* 75(3):372–376, 1993.

292. Twyman RS, Harper GD, Edgar MA: Thoracoscapular fusion in facioscapulohumeral dystrophy: clinical review of a new surgical method, *J Shoulder Elbow Surg* 5(3):201–205, 1996.

293. McCartney N, Moroz D, Garner SH, et al: The effects of strength training in patients with selected neuromuscular disorders, *Arch Phys Med Rehabil* 20:362–368, 1998.

294. Olsen DB, Ørngreen MC, Vissing J: Aerobic training improves exercise performance in facioscapulohumeral muscular dystrophy, *Neurology* 64(6):1064–1066, 2005.

295. Kissel JT, McDermott MP, Mendell JR, et al: Randomized, double-blind, placebo-controlled trial of albuterol in facioscapulohumeral dystrophy, *Neurology* 57(8):1434–1440, 2001.

296. van der Kooi EL, Vogels OJ, van Asseldonk RJ, et al: Strength training and albuterol in facioscapulohumeral muscular dystrophy, *Neurology* 63(4):702–708, 2004.

297. Rose MR, Tawil R: Drug treatment for facioscapulohumeral muscular dystrophy, *Cochrane Database Syst Rev* (2):CD002276, 2004.

298. van der Kooi EL, de Greef JC, Wohlgemuth M, et al: No effect of folic acid and methionine supplementation on D4Z4 methylation in patients with facioscapulohumeral muscular dystrophy, *Neuromuscul Disord* 6(11):766–769, 2006.

299. Redman JB, Fenwick RG Jr, Fu YH, et al: Relationship between parental trinucleotide GCT repeat length and severity of myotonic dystrophy in offspring, *JAMA* 269(15):1960–1965, 1993.

300. De Temmerman N, Sermon K, Seneca S, et al: Intergenerational instability of the expanded CTG repeat in the *DMPK* gene: studies in human gametes and preimplantation embryos, *Am J Hum Genet* 75(2):325–329, 2004.

301. Cho DH, Tapscott SJ: Myotonic dystrophy: emerging mechanisms for DM1 and DM2, *Biochim Biophys Acta* 1772(2):195–204, 2007.

302. Cooper TA: A reversal of misfortune for myotonic dystrophy? *N Engl J Med* 355(17):1825–1827, 2006.

303. Philips AV, Timchenko LT, Cooper TA: Disruption of splicing regulated by a CUG-binding protein in myotonic dystrophy, *Science* 280:737–741, 1998.

304. Savkur RS, Philips AV, Cooper TA: Aberrant regulation of insulin receptor alternative splicing is associated with insulin resistance in myotonic dystrophy, *Nat Genet* 29(1):40–47, 2001.

305. Savkur RS, Philips AV, Cooper TA, et al: Insulin receptor splicing alteration in myotonic dystrophy type 2, *Am J Hum Genet* 74(6):1309–1313, 2004.

306. Mankodi A, Takahashi MP, Jiang H, et al: Expanded CUG repeats trigger aberrant splicing of ClC-1 chloride channel pre-mRNA and hyperexcitability of skeletal muscle in myotonic dystrophy, *Mol Cell* 10(1):35–44, 2002.

307. Yadava RS, Frenzel-McCardell CD, Yu Q, et al: RNA toxicity in myotonic muscular dystrophy induces NKX2-5 expression, *Nat Genet* 40(1):61–68, 2008.

308. Hawley RJ, Milner MR, Gottdiener JS, et al: Myotonic heart disease: a clinical follow-up, *Neurology* 41(2[Pt 1]):259–262, 1991.

309. Hudson AJ, Huff MW, Wright CG, et al: The role of insulin resistance in the pathogenesis of myotonic muscular dystrophy, *Brain* 110(Pt 2):469–488, 1987.

310. Rubinsztein JS, Rubinsztein DC, Goodburn S, et al: Apathy and hypersomnia are common features of myotonic dystrophy, *J Neurol Neurosurg Psychiatry* 64(4):510–515, 1998.

311. Webb D, Muir I, Faulkner J, et al: Myotonia dystrophica: obstetric complications, *Am J Obstet Gynecol* 132(3):265–270, 1978.

312. Thornton CA, Griggs RC, Moxley RT III: Myotonic dystrophy with no trinucleotide repeat expansion, *Ann Neurol* 35(3):269–272, 1994.

313. Ricker K, Koch MC, Lehmann-Horn F, et al: Proximal myotonic myopathy: a new dominant disorder with myotonia, muscle weakness, and cataracts, *Neurology* 44(8):1448–1452, 1994.

314. Ricker K, Koch MC, Lehmann-Horn F, et al: Proximal myotonic myopathy. Clinical features of a multisystem disorder similar to myotonic dystrophy, *Arch Neurol* 52(1):25–31, 1995.

315. Ranum LP, Rasmussen PF, Benzow KA, et al: Genetic mapping of a second myotonic dystrophy locus, *Nat Genet* 19(2):196–198, 1998.

316. Liquori CL, Ricker K, Moseley ML, et al: Myotonic dystrophy type 2 caused by a CCTG expansion in intron 1 of ZNF9, *Science* 293(5531):864–867, 2001.

317. Day JW, Ricker K, Jacobsen JF, et al: Myotonic dystrophy type 2: molecular, diagnostic and clinical spectrum, *Neurology* 60(4):657–664, 2003.

318. Day JW, Ranum LP: RNA pathogenesis of the myotonic dystrophies, *Neuromuscul Disord* 15(1):5–16, 2005.

319. Trip J, Drost G, van Engelen BG, et al: Drug treatment for myotonia, *Cochrane Database Syst Rev* (1):CD004762, 2006.

320. Furling D, Doucet G, Langlois MA, et al: Viral vector producing antisense RNA restores myotonic dystrophy myoblast functions, *Gene Ther* 10(9):795–802, 2003.

321. Langlois MA, Lee NS, Rossi JJ, et al: Hammerhead ribozyme-mediated destruction of nuclear foci in myotonic dystrophy myoblasts, *Mol Ther* 7 (5[Pt 1]): 670–680, 2003.

322. Wheeler TM, Lueck JD, Swanson MS, et al: Correction of ClC-1 splicing eliminates chloride channelopathy and myotonia in mouse models of myotonic dystrophy, *J Clin Invest* 117(12):3952–3957, 2007.

323. Wheeler TM: Myotonic dystrophy: therapeutic strategies for the future, *Neurotherapeutics* 5(4):592–600, 2008.

324. Halliday D, Ford GC, Edwards RH, et al: In vivo estimation of muscle protein synthesis in myotonic dystrophy, *Ann Neurol* 17(1):65–69, 1985.

325. Griggs RC, Jozefowicz R, Kingston W, et al: Mechanism of muscle wasting in myotonic dystrophy, *Ann Neurol* 27(5):505–512, 1990.

326. Griggs RC, Pandya S, Florence JM, et al: Randomized controlled trial of testosterone in myotonic dystrophy, *Neurology* 39(2[Pt 1]):219–222, 1989.

327. Walter MC, Reilich P, Lochmüller H, et al: Creatine monohydrate in myotonic dystrophy: a double-blind, placebo-controlled clinical study, *J Neurol* 249(12):1717–1722, 2002.

328. Schneider-Gold C, Beck M, Wessig C, et al: Creatine monohydrate in DM2/PROMM: a double-blind placebo-controlled clinical study. Proximal myotonic myopathy, *Neurology* 60(3):500–502, 2003.

329. Sugino M, Ohsawa N, Ito T, et al: A pilot study of dehydroepiandrosterone sulfate in myotonic dystrophy, *Neurology* 51(2):586–589, 1998.

330. Abu-Baker A, Rouleau GA: Oculopharyngeal muscular dystrophy: recent advances in the understanding of the molecular pathogenic mechanisms and treatment strategies, *Biochim Biophys Acta* 1772(2):173–185, 2007.

331. Brais B, Xie YG, Sanson M, et al: The oculopharyngeal muscular dystrophy locus maps to the region of the cardiac alpha and beta myosin heavy chain genes on chromosome 14q11.2-q13, *Hum Mol Genet* 4(3):429–434, 1995.

332. Barbeau A: Ocular myopathy in French Canada. A preliminary study, *J Genet Hum* 15(Suppl):49–55, 1966.

333. Rose MR, Landon DN, Papadimitriou A, et al: A rapidly progressive adolescent-onset oculopharyngeal somatic syndrome with rimmed vacuoles in two siblings, *Ann Neurol* 41(1):25–31, 1997.

334. Amato AA, Jackson CE, Ridings LW, et al: Childhood-onset oculopharyngodistal myopathy with chronic intestinal pseudo-obstruction, *Muscle Nerve* 18(8):842–847, 1995.

335. Davies JE, Sarkar S, Rubinsztein DC: Trehalose reduces aggregate formation and delays pathology in a transgenic mouse model of oculopharyngeal muscular dystrophy, *Hum Mol Genet* 15(1):23–31, 2006.

336. Verheesen P, de Kluijver A, van Koningsbruggen S, et al: Prevention of oculopharyngeal muscular dystrophy-associated aggregation of nuclear polyA-binding protein with a single-domain intracellular antibody, *Hum Mol Genet* 15(1):105–111, 2006.

337. Davies JE, Wang L, Garcia-Oroz L, et al: Doxycycline attenuates and delays toxicity of the oculopharyngeal muscular dystrophy mutation in transgenic mice, *Nat Med* 11(6):672–677, 2005.

338. Mouly V, Aamiri A, Périé S, et al: Myoblast transfer therapy: is there any light at the end of the tunnel? *Acta Myol* 24(2):128–133, 2005.

339. Mostacciuolo ML, Miorin M, Martinello F, et al: Genetic epidemiology of congenital muscular dystrophy in a sample from north-east Italy, *Hum Genet* 97(3):277–279, 1996.

340. Vachon PH, Loechel F, Xu H, et al: Merosin and laminin in myogenesis; specific requirement for merosin in myotube stability and survival, *J Cell Biol* 134(6):1483–1497, 1996.

341. Caro PA, Scavina M, Hoffman E, et al: MR imaging findings in children with merosin-deficient congenital muscular dystrophy, *AJNR Am J Neuroradiol* 20(2):324–326, 1999.

342. Pegoraro E, Marks H, Garcia CA, et al: Laminin α2 muscular dystrophy: genotype/phenotype studies of 22 patients, *Neurology* 51(1):101–110, 1998.

343. Hayashi YK, Chou FL, Engvall E, et al: Mutations in the integrin alpha7 gene cause congenital myopathy, *Nat Genet* 19(1):94–97, 1998.

344. Moghadaszadeh B, Petit N, Jaillard C, et al: Mutations in *SEPN1* cause congenital muscular dystrophy with spinal rigidity and restrictive respiratory syndrome, *Nat Genet* 29(1):17–18, 2001.

345. Flanigan KM, Kerr L, Bromberg MB, et al: Congenital muscular dystrophy with rigid spine syndrome: a clinical, pathological, radiological, and genetic study, *Ann Neurol* 47(2):152–161, 2000.

346. Vanegas OC, Zhang RZ, Sabatelli P, et al: Novel *COL6A1* splicing mutation in a family affected by mild Bethlem myopathy, *Muscle Nerve* 25(4): 513–519, 2002.

347. Zhang RZ, Sabatelli P, Pan TC, et al: Effects on collagen VI mRNA stability and microfibrillar assembly of three *COL6A2* mutations in two families with Ullrich congenital muscular dystrophy, *J Biol Chem* 277(46):43557–43564, 2002.

348. Furukawa T, Toyokura Y: Congenital, hypotonic-sclerotic muscular dystrophy, *J Med Genet* 14(6):426–429, 1977.

349. Higuchi I, Horikiri T, Niiyama T, et al: Pathological characteristics of skeletal muscle in Ullrich's disease with collagen VI deficiency, *Neuromuscul Disord* 13(4):310–316, 2003.

350. Bethlem J, Wijngaarden GK: Benign myopathy, with autosomal dominant inheritance. A report on three pedigrees, *Brain* 99(1):91–100, 1976.

351. Connolly AM, Keeling RM, Streif EM, et al: Complement 3 deficiency and oral prednisolone improve strength and prolong survival of laminin alpha2-deficient mice, *J Neuroimmunol* 127(1–2):80–87, 2002.

Bassam A. Bassam, MD
Tulio E. Bertorini, MD

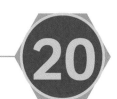

Neuromuscular Manifestations of Acquired Metabolic, Endocrine, and Nutritional Disorders

Endocrine Disorders

Diabetes Mellitus; Diabetic Neuropathies

Diabetic neuropathy (DN) is one of the most common complications of diabetes mellitus (DM), and its prevalence is increasing with the growing number of patients with DM. The reported prevalence of DN varies with the type and the criteria by which it is defined. Using criteria that include clinical symptoms, supported by examination and electrodiagnostic studies, reveals a prevalence of 6% to 15% at the time of diagnosis and more than 50% after 25 years of disease (Fig. 20-1).[1,2] Risk factors for the development of DN include the severity and duration of DM, smoking, and the presence of other complications, such as retinopathy and nephropathy.[3]

The precise etiology of DN remains unknown, and it is likely that DM affects the peripheral nerves by several mechanisms. Two main hypotheses, the microvascular and the metabolic, have been postulated for the development of DN. At one end of the spectrum, it appears that microangiopathy and arteriosclerosis affecting the vasa nervorum inflict ischemic insult to neurons and axons.[4,5] At the other end, oxidative stress with excessive accumulation of glycoproteins and polyol flux induce axonal degeneration.[6,7] Several investigators have provided evidence that oxidative stress damages axons, Schwann cells, and probably neurons.[8,9] Increased activation of the polyol pathway, which converts glucose to sorbitol, results in increased tissue accumulation of sorbitol and depletion of myoinositol, causing a reduction in Na^+/K^+-ATPase and subsequent slowing of nerve conduction.[10]

DM is associated with a wide spectrum of neuropathy syndromes, ranging from mild asymptomatic distal sensory polyneuropathy (PN) or sensorimotor neuropathy to a severe disabling neuropathy of variable symmetric or asymmetric presentation (Box 20-1); these disorders often co-exist.

Distal Sensorimotor Polyneuropathy

Distal sensory predominant or sensorimotor PN is the most common neuropathy in patients with DM. This usually develops when DM has been present for several years, although nerve conduction study abnormalities are demonstrated in 10% to 18% of patients at the time of diagnosis of DM.[11]

Clinically, symmetric sensory symptoms typically predominate; these may include positive symptoms (prickling, tingling, pins and needles, burning, crawling, itching, or pain) or negative symptoms (numbness, decreased sensibility, painless injuries) in the toes and feet. These symptoms progress slowly and extend up to the ankles and legs, and later to the fingers and hands. Neuropathic pain can be severe, is more prominent at night, and may compromise quality of life. Painless repetitive foot injury secondary to loss of protective sensory input contributes to the development of foot ulceration, which is a common medical cause of eventual amputation.[12] Autonomic symptoms are variably encountered. Weakness usually is absent or minimal, especially in the early years of symptom onset, but in severe cases distal weakness and atrophy of the intrinsic muscles of the feet may be present. Coexisting upper limb mononeuropathies (median nerve at the wrist or ulnar nerve at the elbow) are relatively common.[13]

Examination demonstrates distal symmetric sensory loss or deficit in a stocking-glove pattern, diminished or absent ankle tendon reflexes, and, in more severe cases, loss of knee reflexes or upper-limb tendon reflexes. Weakness of toe and foot dorsiflexion and atrophy of the intrinsic muscles of the feet usually are noted later in the course of the disease.

Autonomic Neuropathy

Diabetic autonomic neuropathy usually coexists with sensorimotor polyneuropathy from involvement of small autonomic nerve fibers, and autonomic symptoms usually become prominent with increased duration and severity of the neuropathy. Impotence is among the most common manifestations of autonomic neuropathy. Sweating abnormalities, including distal anhidrosis and truncal and gustatory sweating, are relatively common. Other manifestations include constipation alternating with diarrhea, gastroparesis and bloating, orthostatic light-headedness, postural hypotension, and bowel or urinary disturbances. Cardiac arrhythmia secondary to parasympathetic denervation contributes to increased cardiac morbidity and mortality. Diabetic patients who suffer an acute myocardial infarction are

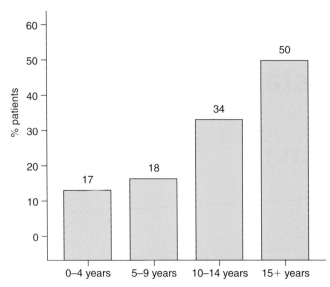

Figure 20-1 Prevalence of distal polyneuropathy by duration of noninsulin-dependent diabetes mellitus.

Box 20-1 Clinical Classification of Diabetic Neuropathies

Symmetric

Distal sensorimotor polyneuropathy
Autonomic neuropathy
Acute painful neuropathy (insulin neuritis, neuropathic cachexia)

Asymmetric

Diabetic lumbosacral plexopathy
Compression mononeuropathies
Cranial neuropathies
Isolated thoracic radiculopathies

twice as likely to die as matched controls because of a combination of accelerated coronary artery atherosclerosis, hypertension, and autonomic neuropathy.[14,15] These manifestations and their treatment are covered in detail in Chapter 5.

Acute Painful Neuropathy

A variant of acute or subacute severe painful neuropathy has been described in diabetic patients with rapid unwanted weight loss and poor glycemic control. It is characterized by intense diffuse neuropathic pain and has a monophasic course[16]; patients appear acutely ill. Typically, it manifests in two settings: one form, which occurs after the initiation of improved glycemic control, is called *insulin neuritis*; the other form occurs in poorly controlled non–insulin-dependent diabetes mellitus (NIDDM) and is called *diabetic neuropathic cachexia.*

Insulin neuritis was first described by Caravati in 1933.[17] It is an uncommon and highly unpleasant entity that typically appears after the initiation of aggressive insulin therapy or oral agents. Patients develop intense burning pain in the feet and legs, often requiring narcotics. Objective findings on neurologic examination and electrodiagnostic studies are mild. The pain generally resolves in a few months, although the underlying polyneuropathy often remains. Nutritional supplements and blood glucose level monitoring are helpful.

Diabetic neuropathic cachexia occurs in males with poorly controlled NIDDM. It is characterized by anorexia, severe weight loss, and intense pain that requires narcotic analgesics. The neurologic

examination and nerve conduction studies are unrevealing or show only mild abnormalities. Weight gain after glycemic control is usually followed by slow improvement over months.[18]

Diabetic Lumbosacral Plexopathy

Diabetic lumbosacral plexopathy (DLSP) is also known as *diabetic radiculoplexus neuropathy, diabetic amyotrophy, Bruns-Garland syndrome,* or *asymmetric proximal diabetic neuropathy.* It is an uncommon debilitating neuropathy seen in 1% of patients with NIDDM.[11] This syndrome usually involves the lumbosacral plexus and much less commonly the thoracic and cervical roots, plexus, or nerves. The condition usually occurs in patients with NIDDM who are older than age 50 years and is more common in males. It presents with sudden-onset unilateral anterior thigh pain, followed by weakness and muscle atrophy. The pain is severe, sharp, burning, or aching and often subsides in a few weeks. The weakness and muscle atrophy affect the involved segments (anterior thigh muscles) and often are so severe and debilitating that the patient may require walking aids. Sensory loss usually is minimal, and knee tendon reflex is diminished or absent. The syndrome usually is monophasic, and spontaneous slow recovery occurs over several months. The pathophysiology of DLSP is mostly microvasculopathy and inflammatory changes; secondary immune response is suspected.[19,20] Variations of DLSP include spreading to the contralateral side or symmetric bilateral involvement, foot drop, upper limb involvement, and thoracic radiculopathy.

Compression Neuropathies

As mentioned before, compression neuropathies are more common in diabetic patients, particularly those with associated polyneuropathy. It is unclear why diabetic patients have an increased risk of developing these neuropathies, although an increased obesity rate may be a factor.

Median neuropathy at the wrist, widely known as *carpal tunnel syndrome* (CTS), is the most common, and its prevalence increases with a longer duration of DM. Nerve conduction studies demonstrate CTS in nearly 30% of diabetic patients, of whom 6% to 10% are symptomatic.[2] Thus, CTS should be suspected in any diabetic patient who complains of pain, paresthesia, and numbness in the hands, worsening at night or on awakening. Weakness of the thenar muscles is rare except in long-standing severe cases. The diagnosis is best made by nerve conduction studies; however, coexistent polyneuropathy may impose a diagnostic challenge, best assessed by testing other nerves in the upper limb not subject to compression.

Other compression neuropathies include ulnar neuropathy at the elbow and possibly peroneal neuropathy at the fibular head. Radial neuropathy and lateral femoral cutaneous neuropathy (meralgia paresthetica) have been rarely described in diabetic patients and are indistinguishable from similar neuropathies in nondiabetic patients.[21]

Ulnar neuropathy at the elbow occurs less frequently than CTS and has been reported in 2% of diabetic patients. Clinically, ulnar neuropathy causes sensory symptoms in the ring and small fingers.[2] More severe ulnar neuropathy at the elbow is associated with progressive weakness and atrophy of the ulnar-innervated hand muscles and may have significant impact on hand function. Asymptomatic mild slowing of ulnar motor conduction across the elbow is common in diabetic patients.

Diabetic focal limb mononeuropathies not at common nerve entrapment sites are rare and coincidental, and other common causes should be considered. Lateral femorocutaneous neuropathy or meralgia paresthetica appears to be more common in obese patients with NIDDM. Likewise, mononeuritis multiplex is not among the encountered complications of diabetes mellitus.

Cranial Mononeuropathies

Oculomotor neuropathy with pupillary sparing is characteristic of diabetic third cranial nerve palsy. The onset usually is acute and is associated with severe headache, diplopia, and ptosis. Recovery often is complete or near-complete over a few weeks to a few months.

Other cranial nerve palsies associated with diabetes include abducens, trochlear, and facial neuropathy. Facial neuropathy is more common in older diabetic patients, usually is unilateral, and has a clinical course similar to that of idiopathic facial palsy (Bell palsy).

The overall incidence of cranial neuropathies in diabetic patients is relatively low, in the range of 2% to 5%; however, a higher incidence of facial nerve palsy (6% to 10%) has been reported. This is even higher if individuals with abnormal glucose tolerance tests are included.[22,23] Pain often is present and is associated with upper and lower facial weakness and infrequently with loss of taste and hyperacusis.

Isolated Thoracic Radiculopathy

Isolated thoracic radiculopathy, also termed *truncal radiculo-neuropathy* or *diabetic thoracoabdominal neuropathy*, is a distinctive disorder that often suggests DM. It is uncommon and usually occurs in older patients, often associated with weight loss and poor glycemic control. Patients develop segmental chest or abdominal pain, cutaneous hypersensitivity or allodynia, and sensory loss. The pain usually is intense and of a burning or aching quality and may not follow a classic dermatomal distribution. Likewise, the sensory deficit may not follow a typical dermatomal pattern. The pain presentation may mimic chest or abdominal medical or surgical emergencies. The diagnosis of isolated thoracic radiculopathy is clinical, and needle electromyographic (EMG) examination may show denervation potentials in the intercostal, abdominal, or thoracic paraspinal muscles.[24] The pathogenesis of this disorder remains uncertain but probably is similar to that of proximal diabetic neuropathy. The site of the lesion is not firmly established, but it is likely to be at the thoracic roots, posterior rami, or both.

Diagnosis and Evaluation

Assessment of DN is mostly noninvasive; however, rarely invasive studies are needed (Box 20-2). Nerve conduction studies remain the gold standard in evaluation. They are widely available and are used in both clinical practice and clinical trials. The distal symmetric PN is sensory and predominantly axonal; a decline in the sensory nerve action potential (SNAP) amplitude is typically the earliest sensitive finding of PN. The most commonly used nerve conduction study is measurement of the sural SNAP amplitude behind the ankle. A decline of the sural SNAP amplitude below 6 to 8 mV baseline to peak, with a surface skin temperature of 31° Celsius, is considered abnormal.[25] Mild conduction slowing of the sural sensory

---

Box 20-2 Assessment of Diabetic Neuropathy

Noninvasive

Nerve conduction velocity/EMG
Quantitative sensory testing
Autonomic function tests

Invasive

Punch cutaneous biopsy
Sural nerve biopsy
Lumbar puncture

---

conduction velocity or peroneal motor conduction velocity and prolonged F-waves often are noted and indicate mild demyelination. Demyelinating features out of proportion to axonal loss are rare and raise suspicion of a superimposed focal neuropathy or an autoimmune demyelinating neuropathy. Superficial radial SNAP recorded at the base of the thumb is a useful index when the sural SNAP is unobtainable. Compound muscle action potential (CMAP) amplitudes usually are preserved early in the disease course; however, reduced CMAP amplitudes, especially of the foot muscles, often are seen as the disease progresses. An associated increased conduction time across the carpal tunnel or other common entrapment sites in asymptomatic patients may be encountered. Needle EMG examination of distal leg or foot muscles often shows fibrillation potentials, an increased number of large motor unit potentials, and reduced recruitment, indicating chronic mild motor axonal loss and compensatory reinnervation, particularly in chronic cases. Nonetheless, in early small-fiber sensory neuropathy, nerve conduction studies can be normal and other diagnostic tools, such as skin biopsy to assess intraepidermal nerve fiber density or autonomic testing, often are more useful.

Autonomic testing is most useful in evaluation of suspected selective autonomic neuropathy or autonomic manifestations associated with diabetic PN; they are, however, not widely used. Sympathetic skin response is easily tested, but this usually is unrevealing except in severe autonomic neuropathy. Evaluation of heart rate variability and blood pressure changes with deep inspiration-expiration, Valsalva maneuver, and changes in posture are more informative tests and can be used to confirm autonomic neuropathy.[26] Decreased heart rate variability for matched age is a common autonomic dysfunction in diabetic patients and appears earlier than other autonomic manifestations.[27] Tests of sudomotor function evaluate the sympathetic efferent to sweat glands, but they are somewhat cumbersome and usually performed at specialized laboratories. These are discussed in detail in Chapter 5.

Quantitative sensory testing for vibration perception threshold, warm and cold detection thresholds, and heat pain detection threshold modalities using computers have been useful in clinical trials, but their use and reproducibility in clinical practice are limited.[28]

Electrodiagnostic studies in lumbosacral plexopathy demonstrate active denervation in affected muscles and often bilaterally despite unilateral symptoms, with only mild conduction slowing, consistent with axonal loss. Magnetic resonance imaging (MRI) should be obtained to exclude structural lesions.

Focal and isolated mononeuropathies such as CTS, ulnar neuropathy, or peroneal neuropathy are best diagnosed by nerve conduction studies. Sural nerve biopsy is used on a limited scale in the diagnosis of diabetic peripheral neuropathy and is rarely needed.

Differential Diagnosis

Other causes of PN must be considered or excluded in diabetic patients. In patients with distal symmetric polyneuropathy, screening laboratory studies for other metabolic, toxic, drug-induced, nutritional, neoplasm-related, or infectious causes are recommended. Typically blood count, thyroid studies (thyrotropin or thyroxine [T_4]), serum protein, and serum immunoelectrophoresis are necessary. Human immunodeficiency virus (HIV) antibody and urine and blood heavy metal screens are requested if indicated. Sjögren syndrome antibodies, vitamin B_6 and vitamin E levels, and screening for malignancy and measurement of Hu antibody and MAG antibodies can be considered in patients with large-fiber sensory polyneuropathy. Screening for amyloidosis, porphyria, and paraneoplastic or hereditary causes also is indicated in neuropathy with prominent autonomic symptoms. A detailed family history and, at times, nerve conduction studies of suspected family members and DNA testing are essential if a hereditary neuropathy is strongly suspected.

In those whose PN has prominent demyelinating features on nerve conduction studies, screening for hepatitis and infectious mononucleosis, serum immunoelectrophoresis, and cerebrospinal fluid studies are indicated. Recommended diagnostic considerations in diabetic mononeuropathy or multiple mononeuropathy include testing for vasculitis, connective tissue disease, and infiltrative processes such as neoplasia or sarcoidosis.

Treatment and Management

Clinical trials include several therapeutic trials for diabetic neuropathy addressing the proposed pathophysiology. These trials showed only modest stabilization (Box 20-3). Clinical trials have examined aldose reductase inhibitors, alpha-linolenic acid, alpha-lipoic acid, myoinositol substitution, angiotensin-converting enzyme inhibitors, and neurotrophic nerve growth factors.[29] The aldose reductase inhibitors (sorbinil, tolrestat, ponalrestat, and epalrestat) have been used in a number of trials since 1980 and aimed to prevent excessive sorbitol flux in peripheral nerves.[30] These trials, however, have been confounded by side effects, poor trial design, and lack of convincing, clinically meaningful effects. More recently, trial of the aldose reductase inhibitors ranirestat and fidarestat showed modest improvement in nerve conduction and quantitative sensory testing.[31,32] Other clinical trials of DN treatment using dietary supplementation with myoinositol, two antioxidants—gamma-linoleic acid (evening primrose oil) and alpha-lipoic acid—showed no convincing effectiveness, although some benefit was observed.[33,34] Protein kinase C-β inhibitors showed some benefit in animal studies, and in small human studies amelioration of sensory nerve dysfunction by C-peptide in patients with insulin-dependent DM (IDDM) was reported.[35,36] Nerve growth factor (NGF) is a neurotrophic factor that promotes survival, differentiation, and maintenance of small sensory fibers and sympathetic neurons in the peripheral nervous system. Skin biopsy specimens from patients with PN showed reduced NGF and impaired retrograde axonal transport. A 6-month phase II controlled trial of NGF in diabetic neuropathy showed a statistical trend toward improvement; however, a large phase III multicenter trial over 1 year was not able to confirm any beneficial effects.[37,38] Treatment using gene therapy by intramuscular administration of vascular endothelial growth factor in animal models, tested for its ability to increase blood flow in DN, showed improvement in nerve conduction and histologic changes; however, no human studies have been conducted.

Although an immune or inflammatory response may play a primary role or accelerate some forms of neuropathy initiated by a metabolic or vascular injury, there is not an established role for immunosuppression or intravenous immunoglobulin (IVIg) therapy in clinical DN. Nonetheless, Stewart et al described diabetic patients with symmetric distal and proximal progressive neuropathy meeting the clinical and electrodiagnostic criteria for chronic inflammatory demyelinating polyradiculoneuropathy (CIDP) that responded to CIDP treatment.[39] This should be considered in patients with prominent demyelinating features.

Distal symmetric sensorimotor polyneuropathy is generally slowly progressive, but early detection of neuropathy and implementation of close diabetic control are essential and seemingly prevent or delay the progression of neuropathy, retinopathy, and nephropathy. Maintaining strict blood glucose control has been demonstrated to stabilize, improve, and reduce the occurrence of diabetic neuropathy and other diabetic complications in large clinical trials, such as the Diabetic Control and Complications Trial (DCCT). This study followed a large number of patients with IDDM for 3.5 to 9 years to compare strict glycemic control by means of intensive insulin pump or multiple injections to routine diabetic control. In this trial, intensive insulin therapy reduced the occurrence of neuropathy at 5 years by 64% compared with conventional therapy.[40,41] However, this degree of glycemic control is practically difficult and is associated with a higher risk of hypoglycemic reactions. Additionally, 25% of patients with intensive glycemic control develop neuropathy over 6 to 9 years. Similar protective effects are yet to be documented in patients with NIDDM. The United Kingdom Prospective Diabetes Study Research Group (UKPDS), in a large number of patients with NIDDM followed for an average of 10 years, showed a 25% reduction in the risk of neuropathy and microvascular complications with glycemic control (HbA_{1c}, 7%) when compared with the standard treatment group (HbA_{1c}, 7.9%).[42] Pancreatic transplant was shown to halt the progression and improve the symptoms of diabetic neuropathy better than intensive glycemic control with insulin in patients followed for up to 10 years. Transplant patients showed marked improvement in nerve conduction indices and slight improvement on clinical examination, whereas the control group steadily worsened in all study outcomes.[43] Nonetheless, pancreatic transplantation is effective for DN only early in the disease, before axonal loss is extensive, and the effect was not sustained in long-term follow-up.

Diabetic lumbosacral plexopathy or proximal diabetic neuropathy has no currently effective therapy, despite reported improvement with intravenous methylprednisolone in a controlled clinical trial.[44] High-dose corticosteroids may compromise diabetes control. Likewise, the role of corticosteroids or IVIg in isolated thoracic radiculopathy is uncertain.

Proximal diabetic neuropathy initially progresses rapidly, followed by slow, varying degrees of improvement. Most patients achieve good recovery and pain usually improves, but in a small number of patients variable degrees of residual disabling weakness persist.[45,46] Immunotherapy can be considered in those with progressive or disabling symptoms. The pain in proximal diabetic neuropathy or thoracic radiculopathy can be intense and difficult to treat and may require narcotic analgesics.

Physical therapy is important, and protein-caloric supplements may be useful for those with associated significant weight loss.

Compression neuropathies, including CTS and ulnar neuropathy, should be treated in the same way as the idiopathic forms. Surgical decompression in symptomatic CTS is a widely used treatment, although there are no comparative outcome studies for carpal tunnel release in diabetic and nondiabetic patients. Nocturnal pain and hand paresthesia are expected to improve after surgical carpal tunnel release; however, symptoms related to the underlying polyneuropathy will not change. Ulnar neuropathy at the elbow may improve with conservative treatment, including avoidance of ulnar compression and the use of soft pads at the elbow. Surgical decompression should be considered for progressive hand weakness

---

Box 20-3 Treatment Rationale Based on Metabolic Hypothesis

Polyol pathway activation → Aldose reductase inhibitors
Reduction of myoinositol → Myoinositol substitution
Reduced nerve growth factor (NGF) → Human recombinant NGF
Alteration in fatty acid metabolism → Gamma-linolenic acid (primrose oil)
Acetyl-L-carnitine depletion → Substitution of acetyl-L-carnitine
Free radical–mediated oxidative stress → Antioxidants (alpha-lipoic acid)

and muscle atrophy, although the outcome is not always successful. Multiple surgical decompressions in DN are not beneficial and should be discouraged.[47,48]

Cranial mononeuropathies, including diabetic ocular mononeuropathy, have no specific treatment; however, most patients have a spontaneous complete recovery over several weeks. The recovery of facial nerve palsy depends on the degree of axonal loss, estimated by measuring the amplitude of the facial CMAP at least 1 week after the onset of weakness.[49] Physical therapy is needed, as well as the use of eye patches for corneal protection. The treatment is otherwise the same as for the idiopathic form.

The pharmacologic management of DM, particularly IDDM, is with the use of insulin. Intensive insulin therapy should be done by a specialist. Barriers to intensive therapy may include the need for the patients to adhere to the recommended diet, avoidance of hypoglycemia, and the cost. Insulin usually is given using a combination of regular insulin or a rapid analog with meals and intermediate insulin twice a day or a long-acting insulin analog once a day. The recommended starting dosage of insulin is 0.3 to 0.6 units/kg of body weight/day, increasing as needed. Most patients require about 0.6 to 0.7 units/kg/day.[50]

Insulin pumps using short-acting analogue insulin improve lifestyle and help achieve an HbA1C below 7%.

In patients with type 2 DM (NIDDM), the initial treatment should be aimed at lifestyle changes, including diet, weight loss, and exercise. If there are no contraindications, metformin should be part of the initial therapy at diagnosis (Fig. 20-2). The initial dose is 500 mg twice daily to avoid gastrointestinal symptoms, titrated up to 2500 mg/day if necessary over a 2–3 month period. Metformin does not usually produce hypoglycemia but can be associated with lactic acidosis in patients with kidney disease or infection and in those undergoing surgery or receiving contrast radiologic agents. If contraindications to metformin exist, sulfonylureas such as glipizide or thiazolidinediones such as pioglitazone should be used.[51,52] Meglitinides could be used if the patient has an allergy to sulfonylureas; unfortunately, these are more expensive. Insulin could be the first-line agent in patients with HbA1C above 10%, fasting glucose over 250 mg/dL, or random glucose over 300 mg/dL, or when it is difficult to distinguish between type 1 and type 2 DM.

If proper glycemic control is not achieved (HbA1C > 7%) after 3 months, a second-line agent should be started. The American Diabetes Association (ADA) and the European Association for the study of Diabetes (EASD) consensus guideline suggests either a basal insulin such as glargine (Lantus) or detemir (Levemir) or a sulfonylurea such as glipizide (Glucotrol) as well-validated core therapies.[53,54] If target HbA1C is not achieved with a second-line agent, the ADA/EASD suggest starting or intensifying insulin therapy. Other less well-validated second- and third-line agents are pioglitazone (Actos), GLP-1 agonist such as exenatide (Byetta) or liraglutide (Victosa), DDP4 inhibitors such as sitagliptin (Januvia) or saxagliptin (Onglyza), alpha glucosidase inhibitors such as acarbose (Precose) or miglitol (Glyset). Synthetic analogues of amylin such as pramlintide (Symlin) can be used in conjunction with insulin for patients who are overweight and are inadequately controlled on insulin.

Symptomatic Treatment of Diabetes Mellitus

Neuropathic pain is common in patients with diabetic neuropathy. Nearly one third of patients with diabetic neuropathy develop neuropathic pain, which may compromise the quality of daily life and requires specific therapy. The pain can be spontaneous (lancinating, burning, paroxysmal, cramping) or evoked (allodynia, hyperalgesia, or hyperpathia). Clinical trials of pharmacologic management of

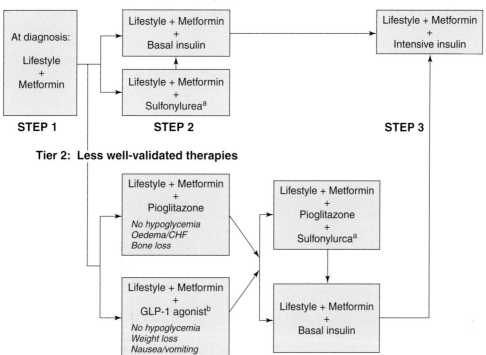

Figure 20-2 Algorithm for the metabolic management of type 2 diabetes. Reinforce lifestyle interventions at every visit and check A1C every 3 months until A1C is <7% and then at least every 6 months. The interventions should be changed if A1C is ≥7%. [a]Sulfonylureas other than glybenclamide (glyburide) or chlorpropamide. [b]Insufficient clinical use to be confident regarding safety. (Reproduced with permission from Nathan DM, Buse JB, Dausou MD, et al: Initiation and adjustment of therapy: a consensus statement of the American Diabetes Association and the European Association for the Study of Diabetes, *Diabetes Care* 32:193–203, 2009.)

painful diabetic neuropathy have included several drugs, such as anti-depressants, anticonvulsants, topical formulations, narcotic analgesics, and others[55–62]; these are discussed in detail in Chapter 6.

Treatment of Autonomic Neuropathy

Autonomic symptoms are important and should be managed with proper therapy. Diabetic cardiac autonomic neuropathy is associated with increased arrhythmias, silent myocardial infarction, and a high mortality rate.[63] Patients should be evaluated for cardiovascular auto-nomic dysfunction, and preventive measurements should be taken, including the treatment of arrhythmia and the prevention of myocardial infarcts. An exercise stress test is recommended before patients with autonomic neuropathy begin an exercise program. Orthostatic hypo-tension should be treated with hydration, elastic stockings, increased salt intake, or, rarely, with short-acting pressor agents.

Erectile dysfunction is among the most common complaints in patients with autonomic DN. This could be confounded by a psy-chogenic component, and a decreased testosterone level should be ruled out or treated. Moderately effective treatments include silden-afil, penile injection of erectogenic agents, and vacuum devices.[64]

Gastrointestinal manifestations include anorexia, early satiety, gastroparesis, bloating, constipation, and diarrhea. These man-ifestations and their treatment, as well as the treatment of bladder dysfunction, are discussed in detail in Chapter 5.

Hyperthyroidism

Hyperthyroidism caused by Graves' disease is defined as the over-production of thyroid hormone caused by antibodies against thyro-tropin receptors in the thyroid gland, also resulting in its enlargement.[65] This is an autoimmune disorder most frequently seen in women and is associated with certain human leukocyte antigen titers. Hyperthyroidism can occur alone or in conjunction with other immune conditions[66]; it also can be caused by drugs, adenomas, and rarely by disorders of the pituitary gland.[65,66]

Diagnosis and Evaluation

Patients with hyperthyroidism generally appear thin, anxious, and irri-table; they have hand tremors and insomnia. They may have auto-nomic symptoms from tachycardia and sometimes cardiac arrhythmia. The enlargement of the thyroid gland is sometimes accompanied by a bruit in the area. Patients also frequently have a var-iable degree of thyroid ophthalmopathy characterized by proptosis, with eyelid retraction and diplopia caused by ophthalmoparesis,[66–69] with swelling of the orbits and the extraorbital tissue.

The disorder can be associated with myasthenia gravis, and 3% of patients with myasthenia gravis have hyperthyroidism.[65,69–71] Myas-thenia should be suspected in patients with ophthalmopathy with extraocular muscle weakness that exceeds the proptosis. In these patients, proper measurement of acetylcholine receptor antibodies, edrophonium (tensilon) test, and electrophysiologic studies are necessary.[65] The forced duction test also helps in the diagnosis.

Hyperthyroidism also may cause a polyneuropathy,[72,73] diffuse muscle weakness, and fatigue. Some patients also show focal pretibial myxedema and acropachy, characterized by swelling and clubbing of the distal phalanges of the fingers and toes.[73]

Hyperthyroidism rarely causes attacks of periodic paralysis, which occur particularly, but not always, in those of Asian ethnicity.[74,75] This should be suspected in patients with an acute onset of weakness.

Measurement of thyrotropin is important in making the diagno-sis, and thyroxine is always low or undetectable. Evaluation also should include measurement of T_4 and particularly free T_4 and triiodothyronine (T_3) level, which should be elevated.[65,76,77] An elevated level of thyroid globulin-binding antibodies confirms the presence of autoimmunity.[78]

Thyroid ultrasound helps in the diagnosis, particularly to detect not only an enlarged gland, but also thyroid nodular disorders. Radioiodine uptake is not always required, but can be used to rule out silent subacute thyroiditis and to diagnose factitious and drug-induced thyrotoxicosis. Serum creatine kinase (CK) and electrolytes should be measured in patients with acute paralysis.

Treatment and Management

The treatment of hyperthyroidism consists of pharmacologic sup-pression of hormonal secretion, radioactive iodine, or surgery.[79] Treatment choice is based on the patient's age, response to drug therapy, and the size of the gland.

Pharmacologic management includes the use of thionamides such as methimazole and prophylthiouracyl (PTU). These agents block the synthesis of thyroid hormone. Because methimazole is 10 times more potent than PTU, its dosage is 20 to 40 mg/day compared to 200 to 400 mg/day for PTU, aiming to maintain the euthyroid state with the minimal dose.[65] Higher doses in addition to levothyroxine supplements are recommended by some.[80] This treatment should be used for 2 years; lack of response or relapse is an indication for radi-ation or thyroidectomy. Inorganic iodine can be given for a short period in preparation for surgery.

In older patients, radioactive isotopes are used to destroy the gland, using dosages of 80 to 100 μCi/g; supplemental levothyroxine may be required.

Patients with severe hyperthyroidism can be treated acutely with beta blockers, which suppress the autonomic dysfunction, or with corticosteroids, which block the conversion of T_4 to T_3 and decrease T_4 secretion.

Thyroid ophthalmopathy is treated with 30 to 40 mg of predni-sone daily for a short period; in severe cases decompression or radi-ation treatment is necessary. Immunosuppressant therapy also can be used.[67]

Myasthenia gravis should be treated with anticholinesterase drugs and with corticosteroids or immunosuppressants as necessary.

Attacks of thyrotoxic periodic paralysis are treated with potas-sium supplements; patients should then follow low-sodium, low-carbohydrate diets with potassium supplementation. Propranolol can be used in acute attacks.[74,75]

Hypothyroidism

Thyroid hormone is important in neuromuscular function because it binds to intracellular and other adrenergic receptors, regulating gly-cogenolysis and mitochondrial oxidation.[81] It regulates the activity of calcium ATPase, and in hypothyroidism there is an increase in the ratio of inorganic phosphate to ATP in resting muscle and a decrease in phosphocreatine in working muscle.[82] The hormone also participates in the mobilization of mucopolysaccharides; in hypothy-roidism, thickening of the skin is caused by deposits of these substances in the subcutaneous tissue, which might be associated with nerve entrapment such as CTS.[83]

The most common cause of hypothyroidism is dysfunction of the gland from a chronic thyroiditis, but it also can occur after thyroid surgery, radiation, infiltrations, iodine deficiency, or the use of some drugs, such as lithium and amiodarone.[84] Secondary hypothyroidism is caused by decreased production of thyrotropin by the pituitary gland, for example, from tumors or rarely by decreased secretion of thyroid hormone–releasing hormone by the hypothalamus.

Diagnosis and Evaluation

The clinical manifestations of hypothyroidism include slowness of movements; tough, thick skin; increased weight; cold intolerance; and constipation.

Neurologic complications include encephalopathy, ataxia, and sometimes even coma. Cranial nerve dysfunction can cause hoarseness and rarely diaphragmatic paralysis.[85] Patients may exhibit bradycardia, myoedema, and delayed relaxation of the ankle reflex.

Neuromuscular complications include sensorimotor polyneuropathy[86,87] and entrapment neuropathies, particularly CTS.[87] Some patients also have diffuse muscle weakness and fatigue,[88–91] which can be accompanied by stiffness. Rare cases of rhabdomyolysis have been reported.[92–95]

Muscle enlargement accompanied by pain in adults with hypothyroidism is called *Hoffmann syndrome*[96,97]; in children this also manifests with dysmorphic features and muscle swelling, but without pain, and is called Kocher-Debré-Semelaigne syndrome.[98] (For neuromuscular complications caused by hypothyroidism and other endocrine disorders, see Table 20-1.)

Serum cholesterol, triglycerides, and serum CK levels frequently are elevated,[99] likely because of decreased secretion of the enzyme.[100] CK levels may be elevated in subclinical cases misdiagnosed with "idiopathic hyperCKemia." Thyroid hormone levels should be measured in these patients, particularly those with hyperlipidemia, before placing them on cholesterol-lowering drugs.

The evaluation of hypothyroidism includes measurement of serum T_4, particularly free thyroxine, T_3, and particularly thyrotropin, which is elevated in the primary form. Measurement of thyroid peroxidase antibodies is used to diagnose chronic autoimmune thyroiditis.[84] Thyroid ultrasound and thyroid scans can be used in those with enlargement of the gland.

Treatment and Management

The treatment of hypothyroidism consists of eliminating possible causes, such as medications, and treating the iodine deficiency, but the most important therapy consists of hormonal replacement with oral levothyroxine, initially in a dosage of 1.3 μg/kg/day orally and later with a maintenance dose of about 125 μg daily; this dosage varies between 50 and 200 μg daily with proper monitoring of thyrotropin levels. The dosage should be adjusted according to the effects of diet, medications, and particularly weight. The combination of levothyroxine and levothyronine at a ratio of 4:1 also is used by some.[84]

Management also includes surgery for CTS, exercise, and physical therapy.

Hyperparathyroidism

Primary hyperparathyroidism is caused by an excessive release of parathyroid hormone (PTH) by adenomas or hyperplasia of the glands and rarely by parathyroid cancer.[101] These tumors may be a manifestation of familial multiple endocrine neoplasms.[102]

Normally, PTH acts in the kidneys by increasing calcium reabsorption and converting 25-hydroxy vitamin D_3 to the more potent metabolite 1,25-dihydroxy vitamin D.[103] This action is exaggerated in primary hyperparathyroidism.

In renal disease, failure to convert 25-hydroxy vitamin D to 1,25-dihydroxy vitamin D decreases calcium reabsorption and causes hypocalcemia, which increases PTH production (secondary hyperparathyroidism). In these patients, hypocalcemia and vitamin D deficiency are accompanied by hyperphosphatemia. Tertiary hyperparathyroidism refers to an autonomous production of PTH even with normal or elevated serum calcium levels.[101,104]

The mechanism by which hyperparathyroidism causes neuromuscular disease is unclear, but elevated levels of PTH with hypercalcemia and hypophosphatemia impair muscle function.[105–107] The proximal muscle weakness that occurs in vitamin D deficiency and osteomalacia suggests a link between abnormal vitamin D metabolism and neuromuscular disease.

Diagnosis and Evaluation

Primary hyperparathyroidism is frequently diagnosed during routine laboratory studies in asymptomatic individuals by the presence of hypercalcemia.[108] The disease can manifest clinically as bone disease (osteitis fibrosa cystica), kidney stones, peptic ulcers, and psychiatric symptoms.[109]

Neuromuscular manifestations include fatigability and prominent proximal muscle weakness, with atrophy mainly in the leg muscles (hyperparathyroid myopathy). Serum CK levels are normal.[109] This presentation occurs in both primary and secondary hyperparathyroidism.[111]

Unusual symptoms include diplopia, myotonia, and severe hypotonia. An acute necrotizing myopathy has been reported.[112] Rarely, symptoms resemble those of amyotrophic lateral sclerosis,[110] and "dropped head syndrome" can also occur.[113]

Short-duration polyphasic motor unit action potentials can be seen on EMG and increased neuromuscular jitter on single-fiber EMG, indicating a disorder of the neuromuscular junction.[114] Type II muscle fiber atrophy is demonstrated on muscle biopsy, which also may show scattered esterase-positive atrophic denervated muscle fibers. Another important finding is the presence of calcium deposits in vessel walls[115]; this vasculopathy in other tissues could play a role in the cardiovascular complications of hyperparathyroidism.

The laboratory diagnosis of hyperparathyroidism is based on the presence of hypercalcemia and elevated levels of PTH. However, hypercalcemia can also occur with malignancy, excessive vitamin D and A intake, and other endocrine disorders, such as thyrotoxicosis and Addison disease. In all of these, PTH levels are suppressed except for rare cases of ectopic PTH secretion in malignancy. Hypercalcemia also occurs in patients receiving lithium and thiazides and in the hypercalcemic hypocalciuric syndrome.[101,104]

Serum phosphate may be normal in primary hyperparathyroidism, but it is elevated in secondary hyperparathyroidism. Radiographs and densitometry occasionally provide valuable diagnostic clues.

Once the diagnosis is made, there are several methods for localization of the adenoma, including MRI, computed tomography (CT), and ultrasound. The most sensitive method is Tc-99 sestamibi uptake, especially when combined with initial single-photon emission CT scan.

Treatment and Management

The treatment of primary hyperparathyroidism consists of surgical removal of the adenoma.[101,116,117] In patients who cannot tolerate surgery, medical therapies include oral phosphate, which can cause gastrointestinal symptoms. Subcutaneous bisphosphonates are used for control of osteitis fibrosa, reducing bone turnover without affecting PTH secretion. Of the bisphosphonates, alendronate has been shown to increase bone density in hyperparathyroidism.[118] Estrogen replacement can be used in postmenopausal women, but this can be associated with deleterious effects. Inhibition of PTH synthesis can be obtained by drugs such as cinacalcet that act in the calcium-sensing receptor in parathyroid cells.[101]

Treatment of secondary hyperparathyroidism consists of low-phosphate diets and vitamin D replacement. Aluminum-containing

Table 20-1 Neuromuscular Manifestation of Endocrine Disorders

Disorder	Symptoms	Laboratory Test Results	EMG	Biopsy	Treatment
Acromegaly	Proximal weakness, CTS, neuropathy, muscle atrophy	Normal CK (may be elevated), elevated growth hormone, IGF-1, TSH	Normal or myopathic	Nonspecific; some fiber necrosis may be seen	Removal of tumor
Hypopituitarism	Weakness (may be severe); muscle fatigue	Normal CK; multiple hormone deficiencies	Not defined	Not defined	Hormone replacement
Adrenal insufficiency, Addison disease	Proximal weakness, cramps, fatigue	Elevated potassium, reduced cortisol levels, abnormally high corticotropin, normal CK	Normal	N/A	Mineralocorticoids, glucocorticoids, fluid and electrolyte replacement
Thyrotoxic periodic paralysis	Weakness with hypokalemia, usually after high-carbohydrate meals (occurs mainly in Asians, more common in men)	Elevated CK during attacks	Normal except for decreased CMAP during attacks, after exercise	Nonspecific; may show vacuolated fibers	Beta blockers, potassium supplement, PTU, methimazole, surgery
Hypothyroidism (adult: Hoffmann syndrome; children: Kocher-Debré-Semelaigne)	Proximal weakness, muscle spasms, pain (adults); myoedema, delayed relaxation of reflexes; peripheral neuropathy, entrapment neuropathies, CTS	Elevated CK, elevated thyrotropin or low T_4	Nonspecific	Nonspecific	Thyroid replacement
Hyperthyroidism or thyrotoxic myopathy	Proximal weakness with little atrophy, more common in women; distal weakness in 20%, some bulbar involvement; Graves ophthalmopathy can occur, myasthenia gravis and periodic paralysis may occur; fasciculations and myokymia; peripheral neuropathy	Normal CK, high T_4 and T_3, reduced thyrotropin	Myopathy, with fibrillations and fasciculations	Normal or nonspecific	Beta blockers, surgery, radioactive iodine
Diabetes	Peripheral polyneuropathy, focal neuropathy; myopathy unusual; muscle infarcts causing unilateral weakness, swelling; proximal muscle weakness (diabetic amyotrophy)	Elevated CK	Motor unit action potentials		
Cushing disease (primary or drug-induced)	Proximal weakness, myalgia, truncal adipose tissue accumulation, moon face	Normal CK, low potassium, elevated plasma cortisol	May show myopathic motor unit action potentials	Atrophy of type II fibers, mainly IIB	Reduction of steroids, removal of tumor
Hyperparathyroidism, primary or secondary from renal disease	Proximal weakness and atrophy, muscle cramps, possible hypotonia	Elevated calcium levels, usually low phosphate and high alkaline phosphatase, normal or mildly elevated CK, elevated PTH and vitamin D levels	Small polyphasic motor units or potentials	Type II fiber atrophy, angular atrophic fibers, increased calcium in capillaries	Removal of the adenoma, bisphosphonates, cinacalcet, vitamin D supplementation (secondary hyperparathyroidism), calcitriol
Hypoparathyroidism	Hypocalcemia-induced tetany (Chvostek, Trousseau signs), cramps	Mildly elevated CK, hypocalcemia, hypomagnesemia	Multiplex discharges	?	Calcium and vitamin D

CK, creatine kinase; CMAP, compound muscle action potential; CTS, carpal tunnel syndrome; EMG, electromyography; IGF-1, insulin-like growth factor-1; PTH, parathyroid hormone; PTU, propylthiouracil.

Modified with permission from Bertorini TE: *Neuromuscular Case Studies*, Philadelphia, 2008, Butterworth-Heinemann.

phosphate-binding agents also can be used, but these can increase aluminum levels, which could cause weakness and encephalopathy and occasionally hypercalcemia. Currently, calcium carbonate is used in dosages not exceeding 2 g/day. Calcitriol or its analogs also can be used to inhibit PTH production. Alpha calcitriol has similar effects. Treatment also should include proper dialysis and ideally kidney transplantation.

Hypoparathyroidism

Hypoparathyroidism is defined as the decreased production of PTH; a lack of response of the target tissue to the PTH is called *pseudohypoparathyroidism*.[119] Both disorders result in hypocalcemia and hyperphosphatemia.

Decreased production of PTH is more often the result of unintentional damage to the parathyroid glands during neck surgery for cancer or adenomas and for hyperthyroidism, and less frequently by radiation,[120] infiltrations such as iron overload in hemochromatosis and multiple transfusions,[119] and Wilson disease.[121] Idiopathic hypoparathyroidism represents a heterogeneous group of rare diseases, such as autoimmune familial hypoparathyroidism associated with multiglandular syndrome[122] and congenital disorders such as DiGeorge syndrome.[123] Chronic hypermagnesemia may cause decreased production of PTH,[124] as in Kearns-Sayre syndrome, a mitochondrial disorder.[125] Hypermagnesemia also can cause decreased secretion of PTH, such as occurs, for example, with high doses of intravenous magnesium used to treat toxemia.[119]

PTH regulates calcium concentrations in the extracellular space. About 50% is protein bound, and the rest is ionized calcium. The hormone increases calcium mobilization from bone and reabsorption from the kidneys, and its deficiency results in hypocalcemia. Hyperphosphatemia is caused by diminished phosphate clearance by the kidneys.

Pseudohypoparathryoidism occurs in a group of disorders in which there is hypocalcemia with hyperphosphatemia and is associated with increased PTH production but a reduced response to the biologic action of the hormone.[126]

Vitamin D deficiency also can cause hypocalcemia by decreasing intestinal calcium absorption, which enhances PTH production (secondary hyperparathyroidism).

Diagnosis and Evaluation

Hypocalcemia may be asymptomatic or may cause neuromuscular irritability in acute cases, presenting as seizures and syncope or choreoatetosis, particularly in children with rickets.[127] In adults, osteomalacia is most often caused by vitamin D deficiency. Chronic hypocalcemia in hypoparathyroidism causes muscle pains, weakness, coarse hair, dry skin, and bone disease.[128,129] Muscle weakness is accompanied by normal serum CK levels and nonspecific muscle biopsy findings.[130] Statin-induced myalgia in vitamin D–deficient patients have been reported to improve with vitamin D supplementation[131]; thus, its deficiency may play a role in this complication.

Acute hypoparathyroidism presents clinically as neuromuscular irritability with carpopedal spasms, sometimes with opisthotonic posture, and positive Trousseau and Chvostek signs on examination.[132]

Laboratory findings consist of a reduction of serum calcium and PTH; phosphate levels may be normal or elevated. In vitamin D deficiency, however, PTH levels are elevated and are accompanied by high levels of phosphate and alkaline phosphatase and decreased vitamin D. Also, when evaluating patients with neuromuscular irritability, it is important to measure magnesium levels, because hypomagnesemia could have a similar presentation.[133]

Electrophysiologic tests show normal nerve conduction velocities, and the needle EMG test demonstrates the characteristic "multiplets" motor action potentials. In acute hypoparathyroidism, electroencephalography shows no specific abnormalities, and electrocardiography may show prolongation of the QT interval.

Basal ganglia calcifications may be seen on CT scans in chronic hypoparathyroidism.[134,135]

Treatment and Management

Acute hypocalcemia is treated with intravenous infusions of calcium gluconate in doses of 1 to 3 g in 10 to 30 mL (10%) for 10 minutes, followed by 5% dextrose in 100 mL of calcium gluconate (10%). Oral calcium gluconate should then be given in doses of 1 to 3 g/day.[119]

Patients with osteomalacia and rickets should receive vitamin D and calcium supplementation.

Long-term treatment of hypocalcemia in patients with hypoparathyroidism requires administration of oral calcium and vitamin D. Older patients require vitamin D analogs in addition to calcium. Calcitriol, which is the active form of vitamin D, is the treatment of choice. Patients can be effectively treated with dosages of 0.25 μg twice a day to 0.5 μg four times a day.[119] Ergocalciferol (vitamin D_2) and cholecalciferol (vitamin D_3) also are frequently used in long-term management, and their cost is significantly lower than that of calcitriol.

Because thiazide diuretics increase calcium reabsorption and glucocorticoids influence vitamin D metabolism, these agents should be given with caution and frequent monitoring of the serum calcium and phosphorus levels.[136]

Cushing Syndrome

Cushing syndrome (CS) is a metabolic disorder associated with elevated levels of cortisol affecting carbohydrate, protein, and lipid metabolism. Clinical manifestations include hypertension, obesity, osteoporosis, and hyperglycemia. The most common cause of CS is the exogenous administration of corticosteroids for therapeutic purposes.[137] Endogenous CS is caused by excessive cortisol secretion, and the syndrome may be adrenocorticotropin hormone (ACTH)-dependent or independent. ACTH-dependent CS is caused by secondary adrenal hyperplasia from pituitary adenomas (Cushing disease) and more rarely by ectopic corticotropin-releasing factor secretion, which can be caused by tumors such as small cell carcinoma of the lung. Corticotropin-independent CS occurs in 15% to 20% of cases and is caused by adrenal adenomas, carcinomas, or micronodular hyperplasia.[138,139]

Diagnosis and Evaluation

The neurologic manifestations of CS are multiple and are discussed in Chapter 7 where the complications of corticosteroid treatment in neuromuscular diseases are covered. These include neuropsychiatric symptoms such as mania and depression, back pain due to compression fractures, and cranial nerve palsies caused mostly by mechanical compression from the pituitary masses. Some patients also develop symmetric muscle weakness and wasting, predominantly in the legs, sometimes accompanied by myalgia. In these patients, serum CK usually is normal.[138,139,142] Those receiving corticosteroids and paralyzing agents in the intensive care unit might also develop critical illness myopathy, which is discussed in Chapter 10.

Nerve conduction tests are normal in steroid-induced weakness, and the needle EMG examination shows small motor unit action potentials without spontaneous potentials. Histologically, selective type II muscle fiber atrophy, particularly of type IIB fibers, is present.

The differential diagnoses are multiple, including inflammatory myopathies, which could be an important challenge in those treated with corticosteroids that get weaker during therapy, because this could be caused by the effects of treatment or the primary disease.

When Cushing disease is suspected, initial tests should include measurements of sugar, electrolytes, and serum CK. Bone density testing is important to assess for osteoporosis. The first steps in the diagnose of endogenous CS are the demonstration of elevated levels of free cortisol in urine and the late evening salivary cortisol[140] and the demonstration of an inadequate suppression of cortisol secretion during the dexamethasone suppression test.[141] Once the diagnosis is established, the second step is to determine if CS is corticotropin-dependent or -independent.[139] Plasma cortisol levels of more than 15 pg/dL and corticotropin concentrations less than 5 pg/mL are diagnostic of cortisol secretion and corticotropin-independent CS; corticotropin concentrations of more than 15 pg/mL are diagnostic of corticotropin-dependent CS.[138,139]

Treatment and Management

Adrenalectomy can be done in patients with adrenal hyperplasia. In those with Cushing disease caused by pituitary adenomas, treatment consists of transphenoidal microadenomectomy.[138] The treatment of exogenous CS consists in tapering of the corticosteroid dosage and using other drugs as steroid-sparing agents if necessary.

Proper management of complications is important, such as control of hyperglycemia, hypokalemia, hypertension, and osteopenia. Physical therapy and gentle aerobic activity are recommended.

Hyperaldosteronism

Hyperaldosteronism is defined as a selective increase of mineralocorticoids caused by a disorder of the zona glomerulosa of the adrenal gland, resulting in hypertension, hypokalemia, and metabolic alkalosis. This may be accompanied by muscle weakness and fatigue related to the hypokalemia.[138] Patients also may complain of paresthesias and may develop periodic paralysis or persistent myopathy.

Hyperaldosteronism can be primary, from adenomas or inflammation of the gland, or secondary to an alteration of the renin-angiotensin system, such as in renovascular hypertension, estrogen administration, and renin-secreting tumors. Bartter syndrome is a congenital metabolic disorder manifesting as hypokalemia and alkalosis with hyperreninemia and hyperaldosteronism.[138] Patients with Kearns-Sayre syndrome, which causes muscle weakness, deafness, cardiac arrhythmia, and short stature, can also develop hyperaldosteronism with symptoms similar to those of Bartter syndrome.[143]

Diagnosis and Evaluation

The diagnosis should be considered in patients who present with muscle weakness associated with hypokalemia, regardless of the degree of hypertension,[144,145] and also in those with severe hypertension. Other neurologic manifestations of hyperaldosteronism include tremors, encephalopathy, and syncope, as well as tetany from metabolic alkalosis.[146]

The laboratory diagnosis is made by measurements of electrolytes, aldosterone, and plasma renin in the early morning hours. A serum aldosterone-to-renin ratio of more than 30 suggests a diagnosis (assuming the aldosterone level is reported in nanograms per deciliter and the renin level in nanograms per milliliter per hour). Localization of the adenoma with imaging is then necessary.

Treatment and Management

In hyperaldosteronism, electrolyte balance and treatment of hypertension are mandatory. The specific therapy consists of correction of the cause; for example, those with renovascular hypertension may require angioplasty, and those with tumors such as adenomas may require a laparoscopic adrenalectomy.[147]

Adrenal Insufficiency

Adrenal insufficiency (AI) results from inadequate secretion of corticotropin caused by pituitary adenomas or a hypothalamic disease, both of which are considered secondary AI. AI usually is associated with an intact renin-angiotensin-aldosterone system and can be caused by withdrawal of glucocorticoid therapy or by surgical removal of pituitary tumors or hypopituitarism. Less common causes include infections, radiation, pituitary apoplexy, Sheehan syndrome, lymphocytic hypophysitis, and tumors.[148,149]

Primary AI or Addison disease is caused by a disorder of the adrenal gland, which often is autoimmune or caused by infections such as tuberculosis, histoplasmosis, cysticercosis, cytomegalovirus,[148] or human immunodeficiency virus[150]; amyloidosis, hemorrhage, surgical removal of the gland, or metastasis. Other causes of AI are adrenoleukodystrophy and adrenomyeloneuropathy.[138,148] These are X-linked inherited disorders related to a defect in chromosome Xq20a that causes a deficiency of the enzyme acyl-coenzyme A synthetase, resulting in the inability to degrade very long chain fatty acids in peroxisomes, leading to accumulation and the formation of cytoplasmic inclusions.[151] Adrenoleukodystrophy is characterized by a primary adrenal insufficiency with a progressive demyelinating process of the cerebral hemispheres.[151,152] The classic form occurs in childhood and is rapidly progressive. Adrenomyeloneuropathy is a variant that affects the central and peripheral nervous systems. These disorders are discussed in detail in Chapter 13.

Diagnosis and Evaluation

The clinical symptoms of adrenal insufficiency include nausea, vomiting, weakness and fatigue, depression, malaise, weight loss, and orthostatic hypotension. It also may manifest as hyperkalemia and severe weakness. In primary AI, hyperpigmentation of the skin and loss of the axillary hair also are present. Secondary AI may occur in association with other hormonal deficiencies.

Adrenal insufficiency can present acutely as hyperkalemia and alkalosis, and patients may develop an Addisonian crisis with severe weakness and hypotension.

The laboratory tests used in evaluation include electrolyte measurements and the demonstration of reduced plasma cortisol levels. Imaging of the adrenal or the pituitary glands also helps establish the diagnosis. Cortisol concentration should be measured between 6:30 and 8:00 AM, and levels below 3 µg/dL indicate adrenal insufficiency, whereas levels of 19 µg/dL or more rule out this disorder. In primary AI, corticotropin concentration usually is above 100 pg/mL, whereas aldosterone levels are low. Corticotropin levels sometimes are normal. The corticotropin stimulation test is a more specific test for the diagnosis of primary AI. Results are considered normal if plasma cortisol levels are more than 18 µg/dL after a synthetic corticotropin (Cosyntropin) 25 µg is given intravenously.[138,153]

Treatment and Management

Treatment of AI consists in replacement of glucocorticoids and mineralocorticoids in conjunction with fluid and electrolyte replacement. Patients should receive hydrocortisone or cortisone. The oral dosage of hydrocortisone is 25 mg a day (15 mg in the morning and 10 mg at night). Cortisone could be given in dosages of 25 mg in the morning and 12.5 mg in the evening.[138,148] For mineralocorticoid replacement in primary adrenal insufficiency, oral fludrocortisone is given in doses of 0.05 to 2 mg daily.

During times of stress and when surgery is performed, the dosage of hydrocortisone should be doubled or tripled. In an Addisonian crisis, patients should receive hydrocortisone intravenously in a dosage of 100 mg every 8 hours.

Patients with adrenal insufficiency should be advised regarding the risk of an Addisonian crisis, particularly during times of stress or during surgery. Patients and families should receive genetic counseling. Physical therapy and gait training are most important.

Neuromuscular Complications of Uremia

Patients with chronic renal failure can develop multiple neurologic complications, including peripheral neuropathy and focal neuropathies, such as CTS or other entrapment syndromes. They may also develop shunt-related neuropathies, vascular steal syndromes, or myopathy, all of which can have multiple etiologies[154] (Table 20-2 and Box 20-4).

Table 20-2 Uremic Neuropathies

Type	Etiology
Polyneuropathy	Middle molecule toxins Miscellaneous (vitamin deficiency, malnutrition, secondary hyperparathyroidism, abnormal carbohydrate metabolism)
Mononeuropathy	Ischemic monomelic Acute ischemia ± underlying diabetes mellitus with neuropathy, peripheral neuropathy, and atherosclerotic vascular disease
Steal syndrome	Reversal of arterial blood flow from shunt
Carpal tunnel syndrome	Dialysis amyloid (β_2-microglobulin) accumulation
Compressive neuropathies	Nerve compression (cachetic bedridden patients)
Traumatic	Self-retaining retractors (kidney transplant or surgical positioning)

Box 20-4 Causes of Uremia-associated Myopathy*

Secondary hyperparathyroidism
Aluminum intoxication
Iron overload
β_2-microglobulin-associated amyloidosis
Vitamin D deficiency
Chronic phosphate depletion
Hypokalemia
Hyperkalemia
Hyercalcemia
Carnitine deficiency
Azotemic vasculopathy (necrotizing myopathy)
Disuse atrophy (type II muscle fiber)
Associated vasculitides
Connective tissue disease
Myopathy in dialysis-associated systemic fibrosis
Idiopathic

*Weakness could also occur, particularly in those receiving drugs that affect neuromuscular transmission.

Polyneuropathy

Uremic PN is an axonal neuropathy with secondary demyelination that causes sensory loss and later weakness.[154-156] This has multiple etiologies, including the accumulation of middle molecular weight molecules,[157-159] multiple vitamin deficiencies and malnourishment, secondary hyperparathyroidism with low vitamin D,[160] and a hyperkalemia-induced hyperpolarizing state[155] (Fig. 20-3).

Diagnosis and Evaluation

Patients with uremia usually complain of burning paresthesia and numbness and may have restless leg syndrome. They also may develop dysautonomia with significant orthostatic hypotension.

The neurologic examination demonstrates signs of a sensorimotor PN with stocking-glove sensory deficits, absent distal reflexes, and later weakness. A drop in blood pressure also may be demonstrated clinically or with a tilt-table test.

Electrophysiologic studies document the presence of an axonopathy and secondary demyelination with low-amplitude CMAPs and SNAPs and some slowing of nerve conduction with prolonged distal latencies. The needle EMG may show signs of denervation with large motor unit action potentials.

During the evaluation clinicians should be aware of other superimposed or associated causes of neuropathy and entrapment, which should be ruled out.

Treatment and Management

The treatment consists of proper vitamin supplementation, particularly vitamins D, B_6, and calcium; physical activity; pain modulators[161]; and particularly hemodialysis.[154] The best result is obtained with kidney transplantation, which markedly improves the neuropathy.[162]

Focal Uremic Neuropathies

Focal uremic neuropathies include CTS and other entrapment syndromes, damage of nerves such as the lateral femoral cutaneous nerve from compression during transplantation, and peroneal and ulnar nerve palsies, as well as shunt-related neuropathies.

CTS is common in patients with uremic neuropathy, particularly in those receiving prolonged hemodialysis. This is caused by accumulation of β_2-microglobulin in the carpal tunnel, compressing the median nerve.[163-165]

Ischemic monomelic neuropathy is an acute ischemic neuropathy caused by shunt occlusion after placement or by infections, manifesting as a distal axonal neuropathy in the affected limb.[166] The symptoms develop abruptly without muscle necrosis. This is more common in diabetic patients.

Vascular steal syndrome is an insidious neuropathy that manifests days to months after shunt placement, causing neurologic deficits in the affected limbs, as well as ischemic changes in the skin. The syndrome is thought to be caused by reversal of the arterial blood flow away from the digits.[167-169]

Shunt-related entrapment neuropathies occur frequently after placement of an arterial venous shunt and cause ulnar and median nerve entrapments, particularly in women with high fistular flows.[170]

Diagnosis and Evaluation

The diagnosis of CTS should be suspected in patients with uremic polyneuropathy who have more prominent symptoms in the median nerve distribution and swelling of the wrist. Electrophysiologic studies demonstrate prolongation of the median nerve CMAP and SNAP distal latencies.

Patients with ischemic monomelic neuropathy have impairment of all sensory modalities distally in the affected limbs, which is more

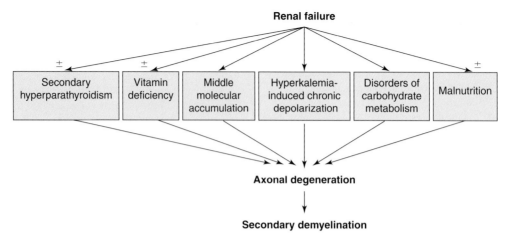

Figure 20-3 Possible pathogenesis of uremic polyneuropathy.

prominent than the weakness. Usually there are no signs of vascular insufficiency. Electrophysiologic tests show evidence of axonal loss with low-amplitude SNAPs and to a lesser extent CMAPs.[171] Conduction block also may be evident.[172,173]

Patients with vascular steal syndrome have painful paresthesias with pallor and ischemic changes in the skin that can progress to gangrene and sensory deficits in the median and ulnar nerve distributions. Nerve conduction studies document low-amplitude SNAPs and later CMAPs. Ultrasonography reveals reversal of the shunt flow, although some patients with retrograde flow in the shunt may be asymptomatic.[154,169] Fistulography may be necessary. Digital oximetry shows decreased oxygen saturation.[154,169]

The examination of patients with shunt-related entrapment syndromes demonstrates sensory and motor deficits in the hands and often deficits and swelling of the affected limbs.[174]

Treatment and Management
The treatment of CTS is conservative, but decompression of the carpal tunnel is frequently necessary. During surgery there is evidence of an accumulation of a mucinous material, which represents β_2-microglobulin.[164,165]

The treatment of ischemic monomelic neuropathy consists of immediate ligation of the arteriovenous graft, and its removal might be required to preserve neurologic function. The shunt should then be placed at another site.[167] Antibiotic therapy and pain management are necessary.

Vascular steal syndrome is treated with fistular banding, but removal of the shunt might be required.[169,170]

For shunt-related entrapment syndromes, treatment depends on the severity of the symptoms. Nerve decompression can produce marked relief. Removal of the shunt also may be necessary.

Uremic Myopathy
Patients with uremia can develop insidious proximal muscle weakness related to end-stage renal disease or complications of therapy.[175–179] The causes of uremic myopathy are multiple and include secondary hyperparathyroidism,[178,179] aluminum intoxication,[180] iron overload,[181] electrolyte imbalance, and carnitine deficiency.[182] β_2-Microglobulin deposits also have been associated with weakness[154] (see Box 20-4).

Some patients may develop nephrogenic fibrosing dermopathy, particularly those who receive gadolinium contrast for imaging. Symptoms include systemic fibrosis with joint contractures and weakness.[183,184]

Patients with uremia also rarely develop increased muscle fatigue during daily activities secondary to a defect of neuromuscular transmission. In those receiving carnitine, the defect is believed to be related to the similarity of carnitine and acetylcholine.[185] Impairment of neuromuscular transmission also can be secondary to neuropathy, which might be aggravated by some drugs that affect neuromuscular transmission.[186]

Diagnosis and Evaluation
Patients with uremic myopathy have proximal weakness out of proportion to the distal peripheral neuropathy, and EMG studies may show evidence of "myopathic" motor unit action potentials and sometimes denervation potentials.

The evaluation should include measurement of vitamin D, calcium, phosphate, electrolytes, and CK, and, if necessary, measurement of serum carnitine. Measurements of serum aluminum levels and muscle biopsy also may help to demonstrate the deposits of iron or β_2-microglobulin or iron accumulation in muscle.

The diagnosis of a superimposed disorder of neuromuscular transmission depends on proper clinical assessment, and the repetitive stimulation test is necessary to document a decrement of the CMAP area. If myasthenia gravis is a clinical consideration, acetylcholine receptor antibodies should be measured.

Treatment and Management
Those with carnitine deficiency require its replacement,[181] and chelation therapy may benefit those with aluminum and iron overload.[180,181] Systemic fibrosis is treated conservatively. The anemia in renal disease should be corrected, and patients should receive vitamin D[179] and other vitamin replacements. Physical therapy and increased muscle activity are important. The best treatment of most of these complications is kidney transplantation. The treatment of those with a disorder of neuromuscular transmission is removal of the cause, particularly drugs that might impair neuromuscular transmission, or discontinuation of carnitine suppression.

Malnutrition and Vitamin Deficiencies

Malnutrition is seen commonly in poor countries where people have low protein and vitamin intake, but it also occurs in patients with malabsorption syndrome from infections, celiac disease, parenteral nutrition, or gastrointestinal surgery. This also is frequently seen in alcoholics.[187,188] Only the most important neuromuscular manifestations of malnutrition and vitamin deficiencies are discussed here.

Vitamin A

Vitamin A is a fat-soluble vitamin that includes the preformed compounds retinol and retinal, which are contained in animal foods. The provitamin A is beta-carotene. This and other carotenoids are converted in the body to retinal.[189,190] Retinal and carotene are converted to retinyl palmitate, which is stored in the liver.[190]

Most complications of vitamin A deficiency are ophthalmalogic, but some patients also develop bulbar weakness, ataxia, and sometimes generalized weakness.

Diagnosis and Evaluation

Patients with this deficiency usually present with night blindness, exophthalmia, dry eyes, keratitis, and rarely ataxia. Vitamin A deficiency should be suspected in patients with these symptoms, and its levels should be measured in those with malabsorption and ocular manifestations.

Treatment and Management

The recommended daily allowance of vitamin A is 1,000 mcg for men and 800 mcg for women. The daily allowance for children younger than age 1 year is 375 μg and for those between ages 1 and 3 years of age, 400 μg; from age 4 to 10 years, this increases to 500 μg.

Patients with severe vitamin A deficiency should receive up to 500,000 units/day for 3 days and then 50,000 units/day for 14 days followed by 10,000 to 20,000 units/day for 2 months. If oral administration is not possible, 10,000 to 50,000 units/day should be given parenterally. The maintenance dose is 400 to 500 units/day orally, increasing to 10,000 units in patients with malabsorption. Vitamin A levels should be monitored because overdoses can cause complications such as increased intracranial pressure. Normal vitamin A levels in serum are 38 to 100 μg/dL, and the normal levels of carotene are 70 to 300 μg/mL.

Vitamin B₁ (Thiamine)

Thiamine is a water-soluble vitamin contained in cereals and grains, particularly in those that maintain their outer layers. The recommended daily allowance of vitamin B_1 is 0.5 mg/1,000 kcal or a daily intake of 1.2 mg, increasing to 1.4 mg during pregnancy and lactation. Requirements might be increased during dialysis, thyrotoxicosis, and diuretic therapy[191] and are particularly during periods of high metabolic demands and high carbohydrate, particularly glucose, intake. The active form of vitamin B_1 is thiamine pyrophosphate (TPP), which participates in the intermediate metabolism of carbohydrates.[188,192]

Decreased levels of TPP cause elevated levels of pyruvate and sometimes lactate and reduce red blood cell (RBC) activity of transketolase, with reduction of oxygen uptake and transketolase activity in the brain stem.[191,192]

Thiamine deficiency causes a sensorimotor polyneuropathy and can cause cardiomyopathy and Wernicke-Korsakoff syndrome.[191]

Diagnosis and Evaluation

The early symptoms of the polyneuropathy include dysesthesia and numbness, predominantly in the lower extremities. Physical examination reveals weakness and wasting in the distal muscles of the legs with areflexia. Rarely, patients have involvement of the recurrent laryngeal nerve, causing hoarseness.[193] Electrophysiologic studies demonstrate an axonal, predominantly sensory neuropathy.

Normal thiamine levels in serum are 1.1 to1.6 mg/dL, but its measurement has a limited value; measurement of serum pyruvate and lactate levels may be helpful.[191] More reliable tests include the measurement of RBC transketolase activity[194] and TPP stimulation of RBC transkelotase levels.[195] The measurement of 24-hour excretion of thiamine is also useful.

Treatment and Management

Treatment of vitamin B_1 deficiency includes a well-balanced diet with supplements of this and other vitamins. In symptomatic deficiencies, the initial replacement is given parenterally in a dosage of 50 to 100 mg/day for 3 to 5 days and then the same dosage orally.

Alcoholics and malnourished patients should receive intravenous thiamine before receiving intravenous glucose to avoid the development of Wernicke encephalopathy. Patients receiving parenteral nutrition should receive supplementation in a dosage of 6 mg/day, increasing to 25 to 50 mg in those with a history of alcohol intake. In symptomatic children, the dosage is 10 to 25 mg/day either orally or parenterally. The dosage for infants is 0.2 mg/day, and for those age 7 to 12 years the dosage is 0.3 mg/day.

Vitamin B₃ (Niacin)

Niacin is a vitamin that includes both nicotinamide and nicotinic acid. Niacin is formed in the body from tryptophan. Its deficiency is prevented by exogenous intake in cereals, beef liver, and fish.

Nicotinic acid and nicotinamide form nicotinamide adenine dinucleotide (NAD) and NAD phosphate; many important enzymes of energy metabolism depend on these.

Niacin is contained in legumes, peanuts, coffee, tea, meat, and fruit. Niacin deficiency is seen in people whose diet consists mainly of some cereals such as maize, which contain solid forms of the vitamin that are not nutritionally available. Niacin deficiency also occurs in alcoholics and those receiving isoniazid. The recommended daily allowance of the vitamin is 15 to 19 mg/day.

Diagnosis and Evaluation

The clinical presentation of vitamin B_3 deficiency is called *pellagra* and is characterized by the triad of dermatitis, dementia, and diarrhea.

A selective deficiency of niacin is seldom seen except in very poor countries. The clinical presentation includes diarrhea with dermatitis and central nervous system disorders. Patients exhibit irritability, confusion, and dementia and may have ataxia, extrapyramidal symptoms, and occasionally a peripheral neuropathy[196] or myelopathy.[189,191]

Treatment and Management

Pellagra should be treated with 25 mg of niacin intravenously two or three times a day in addition to other vitamins, particularly thiamine. Oral nicotinic acid is then given in a dosage of 50 to 100 mg three times a day until symptoms disappear. A maintenance dosage of 50 mg/day is recommended.[191,197]

Vitamin B₆ (Pyridoxine)

Pyridoxine is another water-soluble vitamin for which the recommended daily allowance is 2 mg orally in adults and 0.9 to 1.6 mg in children. This vitamin is included in most foods, particularly enriched breads, cereals, grain, chicken, and fruits. Pyridoxine deficiency is uncommon but can occur with malnutrition or alcoholism and in infants from deficient mothers. Vitamin B_6 deficiency also occurs in patients receiving medications that are considered its antagonists, such as isoniazid, hydralazine, and D-penicillamine.

The active form of pyridoxine is pyridoxal phosphate, which is a coenzyme of amino acid metabolism, particularly methionine and tryptophan. Pyridoxal phosphate also is required in the production of niacin; thus, pyridoxine deficiency can produce a secondary deficiency of vitamin B_3. Pyridoxine also is involved in the synthesis of neurotransmitters such as GABA, dopamine, other catecholamines, and serotonin.[191]

Diagnosis and Evaluation

Vitamin B_6 deficiency produces a mixed symmetric sensorimotor polyneuropathy characterized by numbness and pain and later atrophy and weakness. Distal reflexes are absent, and there is sensory loss to all modalities. Electrophysiologic studies demonstrate a predominantly axonal polyneuropathy.

Pyridoxine levels can be measured in the plasma (normal levels are 5 to 30 ng/mL).

Treatment and Management

The recommended daily dosage of vitamin B_6 is 100 to 450 mg/day, and this dosage should be used to prevent the development of neuropathy in patients receiving medications such as isoniazid. For prophylaxis in those at risk, the recommended dosage is 25 mg to 100 mg/day of the oral supplement.

An important consideration is that the usage of megadoses of pyridoxine as large as 2 g/day could produce a predominantly sensory ataxic polyneuropathy,[198] but this has also been reported in patients receiving lower dosages.[199]

Vitamin B_{12} (Cobalamin)

Cobalamin is a compound that participates in the conversion of methylmalonic coenzyme A (CoA) from methylmalonic acid to form succinyl CoA, an important enzyme of the intermediate metabolism. It also participates in the synthesis of methionine from homocysteine and tetrahydrofolate from folic acid. Methionine and tetrahydrofolate are used in DNA synthesis and methylation reactions in the nervous system (Figs. 20-4 and 20-5).

Cobalamin is an essential vitamin that is not synthesized in the body and requires proper supplementation from meats and dairy products. Cobalamin is liberated in the stomach by the action of gastric acid, where it binds to haptocorrins (R-binders). It is liberated by tripsin in the duodenum, where it binds to an intrinsic factor produced by the parietal cells of the stomach; ultimately the vitamin is absorbed in the ileum (Table 20-3).

Vitamin B_{12} deficiency is caused by a lack of the intrinsic factor, as in pernicious anemia, gastric surgery, and excessive use of proton pump inhibitors. It also occurs in patients with pancreatic

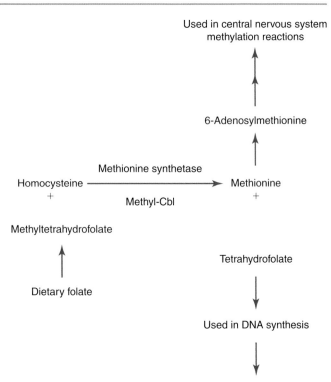

Figure 20-5 Synthesis of methionine from homocysteine and methylcobalamin (Cbl). (Reprinted with permission from Snow CF: Laboratory diagnosis of vitamin B_{12} and folate deficiency, *Arch Intern Med* 159:1289-1298,1999.)

insufficiency and malabsorption or bacterial overgrowth and from deficiencies of transcobalamin II, a protein that binds cobalamin after absorption. Vitamin B_{12} deficiency also can be caused by chronic exposure to nitrous oxide because this inhibits the formation of methionine[200,201] (Box 20-5).

Diagnosis and Evaluation

Patients with vitamin B_{12} deficiency present with numbness in the feet and hands, and there could be evidence of a distal predominantly sensory neuropathy.[202,203] Patients also may develop confusion, dementia, and combined degeneration of the spinal cord with spasticity, hyperreflexia, and a positive Babinski sign. Some patients, however, are hyporeflexic.[204]

MRI studies show lesions with an increased signal on T2-weighted images of the cervical cord. Somatosensory evoked responses show abnormalities of conduction in the central sensory pathways.[205] EMG studies document the presence of a predominantly sensory neuropathy.

Blood tests show a macrocytic anemia with hypersegmented white cells; vitamin B_{12} levels should always be measured in patients with these findings. Because neurologic disorders can be seen in patients with "normal" vitamin B_{12} levels, homocysteine and methylmalonic acid should be measured; both are elevated in vitamin B_{12} deficiency. Misleading abnormal levels can be seen in several conditions (Box 20-6).

Although still useful, the Schilling test is not routinely done. When malabsorption is suspected, stage 3 of the test is useful. This stage of the test is repeated after antibiotic therapy (Table 20-4). Evaluation of the gastrointestinal tract and measurement of parietal cell antibodies can be valuable.[201] Those suspected of having a malabsorption syndrome should be evaluated for its causes, such as parasites in the stools.

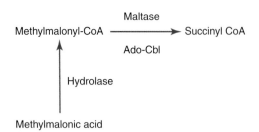

Figure 20-4 Conversion of methylmalonyl coenzyme A (CoA) to succinyl CoA. Ado-Cbl, adenosyl cobalamin; Cbl, cobalamin. (Reprinted with permission from Snow CF: Laboratory diagnosis of vitamin B_{12} and folate deficiency, *Arch Intern Med* 159:1289-1298,1999.)

Table 20-3 Cobalamin Absorption and Transport

Step	Clinical Significance
In many foods, Cbl is bound to proteins. When food enters the stomach, acid facilitates the even release of Cbl. The presence of food also stimulates the secretion of IF, a glycoprotein produced by gastric parietal cells. However, in conditions of low pH, unbound Cbl preferentially attaches to salivary haptocorrin (formerly referred to as R-binder) rather than to IF.	If gastric production of acid is reduced, Cbl absorption from food may be impaired, even when IF is present. However, unbound Cbl supplemental vitamin preparations will still be absorbed normally. A decrease in serum Cbl levels has been demonstrated after 3 to 4 years of omeprazole therapy, and it has been suggested that serum Cbl levels be measured in patients undergoing prolonged treatment with proton pump inhibitors.
In the neutral pH of the duodenum, IF displaces the salivary haptocorrin with the aid of pancreatic enzymes.	Patients with pancreatic insufficiency may have reduced Cbl absorption, although they rarely become Cbl deficient.
The IF-Cbl complex passes through the small intestine and is taken up by receptor-mediated endocytosis in the terminal ileum.	Bacterial overgrown of fish tapeworm infestation may cause Cbl deficiency because of competition for Cbl in the intestine before the IF-Cbl complex reaches the terminal ileum.
Cbl is released from the complex and binds either to the TC II protein or to serum haptocorrins despite normal serum Cbl levels. In some patients with myeloproliferative disorders or liver disease, levels of serum haptocorrins may increase, leading to increases in the measured serum Cbl level.	Congenital TC II deficiency may cause megaloblastic anemia (formerly referred to as TC I and TC III). TC II, which accounts for only 10% to 30% of the measurable serum Cbl level, is the physiologically important transport protein.
An active enterohepatic circulation conserves the vitamin. Once Cbl reenters the gut in the bile, IF is again necessary for reabsorption.	Compared with patients with pernicious anemia, strict vegetarians (who produce IF normally) retain more Cbl from the enterohepatic circulation and therefore take much longer (10 to 20 years) to become Cbl deficient.

Cbl, cobalamin; IF, intrinsic factor; TC, transcobalamin.
Reprinted with permission from Snow CD: Laboratory diagnosis of vitamin B$_{12}$ and folate deficiency. *Arch Intern Med* 159:1294, 1999.

Box 20-5 Causes of Cobalamin Deficiency

Malabsorption: pernicious anemia, gastrectomy or gastric bypass, protein-bound cobalamin malabsorption, ileal disease or resection, pancreatic insufficiency, abuse of nitrous oxide, drug-induced (colchicine, neomycin, aspirin, or omeprazole), congenital absence or dysfunction of intrinsic factor
Biologic competition for dietary cobalamin, bacterial overgrowth syndromes, fish tapeworm infestation
Dietary lack: strict vegetarians
Impaired utilization: congenital transcobalamin II deficiency

Modified with permission from Snow CF: Laboratory diagnosis of vitamin B$_{12}$ and folate deficiency, *Arch Intern Med* 159:1291, 1999.

Treatment and Management

The treatment of vitamin B$_{12}$ deficiency consists initially of replacement therapy with intramuscular injections of 1000 µg/week for 4 weeks and then 1000 µg monthly. Periodic monitoring every 3 to 6 months is recommended. Some nasal preparations are

Box 20-6 Causes of Misleading Serum Cobalamin Levels

Falsely Normal

Myeloproliferative disorders: polycythemia vera, chronic myelogenous leukemia, others
Liver disease
Antecedent administration of cobalamin

Falsely Low

Folate deficiency
Pregnancy
Use of oral contraceptives
Congenital deficiency of serum haptocorrins
Multiple myeloma

Modified with permission from Snow CF: Laboratory diagnosis of vitamin B$_{12}$ and folate deficiency, *Arch Intern Med* 159;1289–1298, 1999.

Table 20-4 Interpretation of Schilling Test Results in Cobalamin-deficient Patients

Stage, Result	Possible Interpretations
1, normal	Dietary deficiency, protein-bound Cbl malabsorption, hypochlorhydria, partial gastrectomy, congenital transcobalamin II deficiency
1, abnormal; 2, normal	Pernicious anemia, previous gastrectomy or gastric bypass, congenital absence or dysfunction of intrinsic factor, inadequate urine collection in stage 1.
1 and 2, both abnormal	Ileal disease or resection, pernicious anemia with ileal dysfunction secondary to prolonged Cbl deficiency, pernicious anemia with inadequate urine collection in stage 2; renal insufficiency, inadequate urine collection in both stages 1 and 2; bacterial overgrowth syndromes, fish, tapeworm infestation, pancreatic insufficiency.

Cbl, cobalmin.
Reprinted with permission from Snow CD: Laboratory diagnosis of vitamin B$_{12}$ and folate deficiency. *Arch Intern Med* 159:1294, 1999.

available and can be used to avoid intramuscular injections. Vitamin B$_{12}$ supplementation should be given orally in vegetarians.

Patients should undergo physical therapy, rehabilitation, and management of the symptomatic neuropathy.

Folic Acid

Folic acid is an important vitamin used in nervous system metabolism in all age groups, and its deficiency has been associated with several congenital malformations, particularly in newborns from mothers who do not receive adequate amounts during pregnancy.[206]

Folic acid is present in foods such as leafy vegetables and fruits. The deficiency occurs in alcoholics, those with malabsorption syndromes, and those with vitamin B$_{12}$ deficiency.[207]

Deficiency of folic acid causes hyperhomocysteinemia, which could increase the risk of stroke and peripheral neuropathy. Folic acid deficiency also may cause a combined degeneration of the spinal cord similar to that seen in pernicious anemia.

Diagnosis and Evaluation

Folic acid deficiency should be suspected in patients with macrocytic anemia, depression, or dementia, particularly when vitamin B_{12} deficiency has been ruled out as a cause. Electrophysiologic tests, imaging, and somatosensory evoked responses may be useful.

Normal serum folate levels are 2.5 to 20 µg/mL. Normal RBC folate levels are 40 mg or above. During evaluation, vitamin B_{12}, homocysteine, and methylmalonic acid should be measured because methylmalonic acid levels are elevated in vitamin B_{12} deficiency but usually are normal in folate deficiency.

Treatment and Management

There are no clear guidelines on treatment, but patients should receive about 1 to 5 mg of folate a day to reverse the clinical manifestations and allow metabolic recovery.

Vitamin D

The name vitamin D is applied to fat-soluble substances, called cholecalciferol or D3 and calciferol or D2 (what is called vitamin D1 is in reality a mixture of substances with antirachitic activity). The principal provitamin is 7-dehydrocholesterol, which is converted to cholecalciferol by ultraviolet light and by a thermal reaction. This is then hydrolyzed in the liver to 25-hydroxy vitamin D, and in the kidney this forms 1,25-dihydroxy vitamin D, the biologically active form of the vitamin,[189] which is important in the metabolism of calcium and phosphorus. The clinical manifestations of vitamin D deficiency are related to its effects on bone and muscle.

Diagnosis and Evaluation

Infants and children with vitamin D deficiency exhibit rickets, which may be associated with bone disease and hypotonia. Adults have characteristic osteomalatic bone disease accompanied by generalized weakness and muscle pain.

Electromyographic studies may demonstrate the presence of a sensorimotor polyneuropathy, but myopathic motor unit action potentials may be seen on needle EMG. Muscle biopsy shows type II muscle fiber atrophy.

Treatment and Management

Vitamin D supplementation is necessary in patients at risk, such as those with fat malabsorption, decreased fat absorption, or kidney disease; those receiving certain medications; and those with decreased exposure to sunlight. Levels should be maintained between 30 and 50 mg/mL, and oral supplements of vitamin D_2 should be given in the form of 50,000 units weekly with close monitoring of levels. Patients should be reevaluated after 8 weeks and periodically thereafter.

Vitamin E

Vitamin E is a fat-soluble vitamin present in vegetable oils and wheat. It is absorbed in the intestine in the form of alpha-tocopherol, which is converted in the liver to the active form of the vitamin. The daily allowance is 15 mg, increasing to 19 mg during lactation.[207]

Vitamin E is an antioxidant and free-radical scavenger, and its deficiency is seen particularly in patients with malabsorption, those receiving parenteral nutrition, and in children with cystic fibrosis,

but it also can occur in some genetic disorders, particularly in the autosomal recessive disease caused by mutation of the *aTTP* gene on chromosome 8q13.[208]

The neurologic manifestation of vitamin E deficiency is related to its antioxidant and free-radical scavenger functions.

Diagnosis and Evaluation

Patients with vitamin E deficiency usually have weakness, ataxia, dysarthria, and areflexia and may exhibit a myelopathy similar to Freidreich ataxia, with retinitis pigmentosa and cardiomyopathy.[189,209,210]

Alpha-tocopherol can be measured in serum, and normal levels are 5 µg/mL or greater in adults. In children older than age 12 years, normal levels are 3 to 4 µg/mL. Because vitamin E may appear normal in hyperlipemic states, the ratio of vitamin E to total lipids should be measured in those patients. The normal ratio in children is 0.6 mg/g and in adults 0.8 mg/g or less.[189]

Electrophysiologic studies document a predominantly sensory neuropathy. The assessment also may require somatosensory evoked responses and MRI of the cervical spine and brain to rule out other causes.

Treatment and Management

Vitamin E replacement may halt the progression of neurologic symptoms when used in dosage of 1 to 4 g/day of oral supplementation. In children with cystic fibrosis, it should be given orally in a dosage of 5 to 10 mg/kg. This is adjusted according to alpha-tocopherol levels.

Copper

Copper is a trace mineral that is incorporated in many enzymes in the body, such as ceruloplasmin and superoxide dismutase. Its deficiency can be associated with abnormalities of mitochondrial function and oxidative metabolism.

The dietary requirements for copper are low because this metal is commonly found in nature; a deficiency, however, can occur in patients who undergo gastric surgery or have malabsorption syndromes. Copper is absorbed in the stomach and the proximal bowel, and this absorption is impaired by excessive intake of zinc, iron, phosphate, and calcium. Vitamin C can also reduce copper from its cupric state to its less bioavailable cuprous state. In some cases the exact cause of copper deficiency is unknown.[211]

Patients with copper deficiency may develop ataxic syndrome and have manifestations of combined degeneration of the spinal cord similar to those in patients with vitamin B_{12} deficiency.[212,213] They also may develop neuropathy or polyneuropathy. Swayback is a neurologic dysfunction seen in copper-deficient animals, particularly rodents, in which pathologic studies demonstrate prominent demyelination and axonal degeneration.[211]

Diagnosis and Evaluation

Patients present with gait difficulty and have paresthesia with clinical evidence of sensory ataxia, spasticity, and hyperreflexia with Babinski signs or hyporeflexia.[213]

Copper levels and particularly zinc levels should be measured; zinc levels have been found to be elevated in copper deficiency, sometimes even in patients not receiving zinc supplements.[214,215]

Somatosensory evoked responses document conduction abnormalities of the spinal cord and MRI shows lesions of the posterior columns in T2-weighted images.

Electromyographic studies demonstrate the presence of a predominantly sensory neuropathy.[216,217]

Treatment and Management

The initial treatment consists of 6 mg/day in three divided doses for a week, tapered to 4 mg/day for another week, and then maintained at 2 mg/day with proper frequent monitoring.[211] Removal of the cause, such as excessive intake of zinc, is important. Patients should receive physical therapy and gait training when necessary.

Strachan Syndrome

This syndrome, which is likely caused by multiple vitamin deficiencies, was described initially in Jamaican sugar cane workers who presented with a sensorimotor polyneuropathy that was called *peripheral neuritis of Jamaica*. The neuropathy is accompanied by other neurologic dysfunctions and optic neuropathy.[218,219] The same disorder apparently occurred in Canadian prisoners of war during World War II[218–220] and more recently in Cuba when patients developed myeloneuropathy and optic neuropathy.[220–222]

Diagnosis and Evaluation

The most common manifestation is a peripheral and sensory motor polyneuropathy with visual loss from central or cecocentral scotomas, gingival lesions, and sensory nerve hearing loss.

The diagnosis is made by the neurologic manifestations, which are usually accompanied by other signs of malnutrition, although they might not be present. Measurements of vitamins, particularly the B vitamins, folate, and vitamin B_{12}, is important.

Nerve conduction tests and visual evoked responses are useful.

Treatment and Management

Treatment consists of supplementation of all deficient vitamins, particularly the B group, and proper nutrition with adequate caloric and protein intake, which could reverse the neurologic symptoms.[191]

Acknowledgment

The authors thank Drs. Genero Palmieri, Abbas Kitabchi, and Cesar Magsino for their insightful comments.

References

1. Pirart J: Diabetes mellitus and its degenerative complications: a prospective study of 4,400 patients observed between 1947 and 1973 (3rd and last part), *Diabetes Care* 3:245–256, 1977.
2. Dyck PJ, Kratz KM, Karnes JL, et al: The prevalence by staged severity of various types of diabetic neuropathy, retinopathy and nephropathy in population-based cohort: the Rochester Diabetic Neuropathy Study, *Neurology* 43:817–824, 1993.
3. Dyck PJ, Davies JL, Wilson DM, et al: Risk factors for severity of diabetic polyneuropathy: intensive longitudinal assessment of the Rochester Diabetic Neuropathy Study cohort, *Diabetes Care* 22:1479–1486, 1999.
4. Dyck PJ, Karnes JL, O'Brien P, et al: The spatial distribution of fiber loss in diabetic polyneuropathy suggests ischemia, *Ann Neurol* 19:440–449, 1986.
5. Malik RA, Tesfaye S, Thompson SD, et al: Endoneurial localization of microvascular damage in human diabetic neuropathy, *Diabetologia* 36:454–459, 1993.
6. Greene DA, Lattimer SA, Sima AA: Sorbitol, phosphoionositides, and sodium-potassium ATPase in the pathogenesis of diabetic complications, *N Engl J Med* 316:599–606, 1987.
7. Mizisin AP, Li L, Calcutt NA: Sorbitol accumulation and transmembrane efflux in osmotically stressed JSI schwannoma cells, *Neurosci Lett* 229:53–56, 1977.
8. Mizisin AP, Powell HC: Schwann cell changes induced as early as one week after galactose intoxication, *Acta Neuropathol* 93:611–618, 1997.
9. Low PA, Nickander KK, Tritschler HJ: The roles of oxidative stress and antioxidant treatment in experimental diabetic neuropathy, *Diabetes* 46: S38–S42, 1997.
10. Stevens MJ, Dananberg J, Feldman E, et al: The linked roles of nitric oxide, aldose reductase and (Na^+, K^+)-ATPase in the slowing of nerve conduction in the streptozotocin diabetic rat, *J Clin Invest* 94:853–859, 1994.
11. Lehtinen JM, Uuistupa M, Sutonene O, et al: Prevalence of neuropathy in newly diagnosed NIDDM and nondiabetic control subjects, *Diabetes* 38:1308–1313, 1989.
12. Abbott CA, Carrington AL, Ashe H, et al: The North-West Diabetes Foot Care Study: incidence of, and risk factors for, new diabetic foot ulceration in a community-based patient cohort, *Diabetes Med* 19:377–384, 2002.
13. Dyck JB, Dyck PJ: Paresthesia, pain and weakness in hands of diabetic patients is attributable to mononeuropathies or radiculopathy not polyneuropathy: The Rochester (RDNS) and Pancreas Renal Transplant (MC-PRT) Studies, *Neurology* 50:A333, 1998.
14. Hilsted J, Low PA: Diabetic autonomic neuropathy. In Low PA, editor: *Clinical Autonomic Disorders*, Philadelphia, 1997, Lippincott-Raven, pp 487–507.
15. Benvenuti F, Boncinelli L, Vignoli GC: Male sexual impotence in diabetes mellitus: vasculogenic versus neurogenic factors, *Neurourol Urodyn* 12:145–151, 1993.
16. Archer A, Watkins PJ, Thomas PK: The natural history of acute painful neuropathy in diabetes mellitus, *J Neurol Neurosurg Psychiatry* 46:491–497, 1983.
17. Caravati CM: Insulin neuritis: a case report, *Va Med* 59:745–746, 1933.
18. Ellenberg M: Diabetic neuropathic cachexia, *Diabetes* 23:418–423, 1974.
19. Dyck PJB, Windebank AJ: Diabetic and non-diabetic lumbosacral radiculoplexus neuropathies: New insights into pathophysiology and treatment, *Muscle Nerve* 25:477–491, 2002.
20. Said G, Elgrably F, Lacroix C, et al: Painful proximal diabetic neuropathy: inflammatory nerve lesions and spontaneous favorable outcome, *Ann Neurol* 41:762–770, 1997.
21. Wilbourn AJ: Diabetic entrapment and compression neuropathies. In Dyck PJ, Thomas PK, editors: *Diabetic Neuropathy*, Philadelphia, 1999, Saunders, pp 481–508.
22. Smith BE: Cranial neuropathy in diabetes mellitus. In Dyck PJ, Thomas PK, editors: *Diabetic Neuropathy*, Philadelphia, 1999, Saunders, pp 457–467.
23. Aminoff MJ, Miller AL: The prevalence of diabetes mellitus in patients with Bell's palsy, *Acta Neurol Scand* 48(3):381–384, 1972.
24. Sun SF, Streib EW: Diabetic thoracoabdominal neuropathy: clinical and electrodiagnostic features, *Ann Neurol* 9:75–79, 1981.
25. Bril V: Electrophysiological testing. In Gries FA, Cameron NE, Low PA, editors: *Textbook of Diabetic Neuropathy*, New York, 2003, Thieme, pp 177–184.
26. Low PA: Autonomic nervous system function, *J Clin Neurophys* 10:14–27, 1993.
27. Zeigler D, Dannehl K, Muhlen H, et al: Prevalence of cardiovascular autonomic dysfunction assessed by spectral analysis, vector analysis and standard test of HR variation and blood pressure responses at various stages of diabetic neuropathy, *Diabetes Med* 2:806–814, 1992.
28. Shy ME, Frohman EM, So YT, et al: Quantitative sensory testing: report of the Therapeutics and Technology Assessment Subcommittee of the American Academy of Neurology, *Neurology* 60:898–904, 2003.
29. Pfeifer M, Schumer M: Clinical trials of diabetic neuropathy: past present and future, *Diabetes* 44:1355–1361, 1995.
30. Pfeifer M, Schumer M, Gelber D: Aldose reductase inhibitors: the end of an era or the need for different trial designs? *Diabetes* 46:82–89, 1997.
31. Bril V, Buchanan RA: Long-term effects of ranirestat (AS-3201) on peripheral nerve function in patients with diabetic sensorimotor polyneuropathy, *Diabetes Care* 29:68–72, 2006.
32. Hotta N, Toyota T, Matsuoka K, et al: Clinical efficacy of fidarestat, a novel aldose reductase inhibitor, for diabetic peripheral neuropathy: a 52-week multicenter placebo-controlled double-blind parallel group study, *Diabetes Care* 24:776–782, 2001.
33. Keen H, Payan J, Allawi J, et al: Treatment of diabetic neuropathy with gamma-linolenic acid, The T-Linolenic Acid Multicenter Trial Group, *Diabetes Care* 16:8–15, 1993.

34. Ziegler D, Nowak H, Kempler P, et al: Treatment of symptomatic diabetic polyneuropathy with the antioxidant alpha-lipoic acid: a meta-analysis, *Diabetes Med* 21:114–121, 2004.

35. Ahlgren SC, Levine JD: Protein kinase C inhibitors decrease hyperalgesia and C-fiber hyperexcitability in the streptozotocin-diabetic rat, *J Neurophysiol* 72:684–692, 1994.

36. Ekberg K, Brismar T, Johansson BL, et al: Amelioration of sensory nerve dysfunction by C-peptide in patients with type I diabetes, *Diabetes* 52:536–541, 2003.

37. Wellmer A, Misra VP, Sharief MK, et al: A double-blind placebo-controlled clinical trial of recombinant human brain-derived neurotrophic factor (rhBDNF) in diabetic polyneuropathy, *J Peripher Nerv Syst* 6:204–210, 2001.

38. Apfel SC, Schwartz S, Adornato BT, et al: Efficacy and safety of recombinant human nerve growth factor in patients with diabetic polyneuropathy: a randomized controlled trial. rhNGF Clinical Investigator Group, *JAMA* 284:215–2221, 2000.

39. Stewart JD, McKelvey R, Durcan L, et al: Chronic inflammatory demyelinating polyneuropathy (CIDP) in diabetes, *J Neurol Sci* 142:59–64, 1996.

40. Dyck JB, Windebank AJ: Diabetic and nondiabetic lumbosacral radiculoplexus neuropathies: new insights into pathophysiology and treatment, *Muscle Nerve* 25:477–491, 2002.

41. Mondelli M, Aretini A, Rossi S: Ulnar neuropathy at the elbow in diabetes, *Am J Phys Med Rehabil* 88:1–7, 2009.

42. Chaudhry V, Stevens JC, Kincaid J, et al: Practice advisory: utility of surgical decompression for treatment of diabetic neuropathy: report of the Therapeutics and Technology Assessment Subcommittee of the American Academy of Neurology, *Neurology* 66:1805–1808, 2006.

43. The Diabetes Control and Complications Research Group: The effect of intensive treatment of diabetes on the development and progression of long-term complications in insulin-dependent diabetes mellitus, *N Engl J Med* 329:977–986, 1993.

44. The Diabetes Control and Complications Trial Research Group: The effect of intensive diabetes therapy on the development and progression of neuropathy, *Ann Intern Med* 122:561–568, 1995.

45. UK Prospective Diabetes Study Group: Prospective diabetes study 33: intensive blood-glucose control with sulfonylureas or insulin compared with conventional treatment and risk complication in patients with type II diabetes, *Lancet* 352:837–853, 1998.

46. Navaro X, Sutherland D, Kennedy W: Long-term effects of pancreatic transplantation on diabetic neuropathy, *Ann Neurol* 42:727–736, 1997.

47. Pascoe MK, Low PA, Windebank AJ, et al: Subacute diabetic proximal neuropathy, *Mayo Clin Proc* 72:1123–1132, 1997.

48. Chokrovertz S, Reyer MS, Rubino FA, et al: The syndrome of diabetic amyotrophy, *Ann Neurol* 2:181–194, 1977.

49. Thomander L, Stalberg E: Electroneuronography in the prognostication of Bell's palsy, *Acta Laryngol* 92:221–228, 1981.

50. McCulloch DK: Insulin therapy in type 2 diabetes mellitus, *UpToDate* 1–25, 2008.

51. McCulloch DK: Initial management of blood glucose in type 2 diabetes mellitus, *UpToDate* 1–20, 2008.

52. McCulloch DK: Sulfonylureas and meglitidines in the treatment of diabetes mellitus, *UpToDate* 1–7, 2008.

53. Nathan D, Buse J, Davidson M, et al: Management of hyperglycemia in type 2 diabetes: A consensus algorithm for the initiation and adjustment of therapy: a consensus statement from the American Diabetes Association and the European Association for the Study of Diabetes, *Diabetes Care* 29:1963–1972, 2006.

54. Nathan DM, Buse JB, Dausou MD, et al: Initiation and adjustment of therapy: a consensus statement of the American Diabetes Association and the European Association for the Study of Diabetes, *Diabetes Care* 32:193–203, 2009.

55. Max MB, Lynch SA, Muir J, et al: Effects of desipramine, amitriptyline, and fluoxetine on pain in diabetic neuropathy, *N Engl J Med* 326:1250–1256, 1992.

56. Oskarsson P, Ljunggren JC, Lins PE: Efficacy and safety of mexiletine in the treatment of painful diabetic neuropathy. The Mexiletine Study Group, *Diabetes Care* 20:1594–1597, 1997.

57. Beydoun A, Shaibani A, Hopwood M, et al: Oxcarbazepine in painful diabetic neuropathy: results of a dose-ranging study, *Acta Neurol Scand* 113:395–404, 2006.

58. Backonja MM: Gabapentin monotherapy for the symptomatic treatment of painful neuropathy: a multicenter, double-blind, placebo-controlled trial in patients with diabetes mellitus, *Epilepsia* 40(Suppl 6):S57–S59, 1999.

59. McQuay H, Carroll D, Jadad AR, et al: Anticonvulsant drugs for management of pain: a systematic review, *BMJ* 311:1047–1052, 1995.

60. Harati Y, Gooch C, Swenson M, et al: Double-blind randomized trial of tramadol for the treatment of the pain of diabetic neuropathy, *Neurology* 50:1842–1846, 1998.

61. Gimbel JS, Richards P, Portenoy RK: Controlled-release oxycodone for pain in diabetic neuropathy: a randomized controlled trial, *Neurology* 60:927–934, 2003.

62. Goldstein DJ, Lu Y, Detke MJ, et al: Duloxetine vs placebo inpatients with painful diabetic neuropathy, *Pain* 116:109–118, 2005.

63. Aronson D, Rayfield EJ, Chesebro JH: Mechanisms determining course and outcome of diabetic patients who have had acute myocardial infarction, *Ann Intern Med* 126:296–306, 1997.

64. Dunsmuir WD, Holmes SA: The etiology and management of erectile, ejaculatory, and fertility problems in men with diabetes mellitus, *Diabetes Med* 13:700–708, 1996.

65. Marino M, Chiovato L, Pinchera A: Graves' disease. In DeGrott LJ, Jameson LJ, editors: *Endocrinology*, 5th ed, Philadelphia, 2008, Saunders, pp 1995–2028.

66. Kattah J: Thyroid dysfunction. In Biller J, editor: *Interface of Neurology and Internal Medicine*, Philadelphia, 2008, Lippincott Williams and Wilkins, pp 471–475.

67. Merchant MP, Ahmad A: Orbital disease. In Biller J, editor: *The Interface of Neurology and Internal Medicine*, Philadelphia, 2008, Lippincott Williams and Wilkins, pp 819–822.

68. Burch HB, Bahn RS: Graves ophthalmology. In DeGrott LJ, Jameson LJ, editors: *Endocrinology*, 5th ed, Philadelphia, 2008, Saunders, pp 2029–2042.

69. Bahn R: Graves' opthalmopathy, *N Engl J Med* 362:726–738, 2010.

70. Ohno M, Hamada N, Yamikawa J, et al: Myasthenia gravis associated with Graves' disease in Japan, *Jpn J Med* 26:2–6, 1987.

71. Marino M, Ricciardi R, Pinchera A, et al: Mild clinical expression of myasthenia gravis associated with autoimmune thyroid diseases, *J Clin Endocrinol Metab* 82:438–443, 1997.

72. Feibel JH, Campa JF: Thyrotoxic neuropathy (Basedow's paraplegia), *J Neurol Neurosurg Psychiatry* 39:419–497, 1976.

73. Pandit L, Shankar SK, Gaythri N, et al: Acute thyrotoxic neuropathy: Basedow's paraplegia revisited, *J Neurol Sci* 155:211–214, 1998.

74. Bertorini TE: An African American man with hyperthyroidism and acute paralysis, Case 73B. In Bertorini TE, editor: *Neuromuscular Case Studies*, Philadelphia, 2008, Butterworth-Heinemann, pp 470–471.

75. Pichon B, Lidove O, Delbott T, et al: Thyrotoxic periodic paralysis in Caucasian patients. A diagnostic challenge, *Eur J Intern Med* 16(5):372–374, 2005.

76. Bartalena L, Bogazzi F, Brogioni S, et al: Measurement of serum free thyroid hormone concentrations, An essential tool for the diagnosis of thyroid dysfunction, *Horm Res* 45:142–147, 1996.

77. Sterling K, Refetoff S, Selenkow HA: 53 thyrotoxicosis: thyrotoxicosis due to elevated serum triiodothyronine levels, *JAMA* 313:571–575, 1970.

78. Schwartz-Lauer L, Chazenbalk GD, Mclachlan SM, et al: Evidence for a simplified view of autoantibody interactions with the thyrotropin receptor, *Thyroid* 12:115–120, 2002.

79. Sugino K, Mimura T, Toshima K, et al: Follow-up evaluation of patients with Graves' disease treated by subtotal thyroidectomy and risk factor analysis for post-operative thyroid dysfunction, *J Endocrinol Invest* 16:195–199, 1993.

80. Rittmaster RS, Abbott EC, Douglas R, et al: Effect of methimazole, with our without L-thyroxine on remission rates in Graves' disease, *J Clin Endocrinol Metab* 83:814–818, 1998.

81. Kaminski P, Robin-Lherbier B, Brunotte F, et al: Energetic metabolism in hypothyroid skeletal muscle, as studied by phosphorus magnetic resonance spectroscopy, *J Clin Endocrinol Metab* 74:124–129, 1992.

82. Monzani F, Caraccio N, Siciliano G, et al: Clinical and biochemical features of muscle dysfunction in subclinical hypothyroidism, *J Clin Endocrinol Metab* 82:3315–3318, 1997.

83. Cakir M, Samanci N, Balci N, et al: Musculoskeletal manifestations in patients with thyroid disease, *Clin Endocrinol* 59:162–167, 2003.

84. Wiersinga WM: Hypothyroidism and myxedema coma. In DeGroot LJ, Jameson LJ, editors: *Endocrinology*, 5th ed, Philadelphia, 2006, Saunders, pp 2081–2099.

85. Crum BA, Bolton CF: Peripheral neuropathy in systemic disease. In Brown WF, Bolton CF, Aminoff MJ, editors: *Neuromuscular Function and Disease*, Philadelphia, 2002, Saunders, pp 1081–1108.

86. Dyck PJ, Lambert EH: Polyneuropathy associated with hypothyroidism, *J Neuropathol Exp Neurol* 29:631–658, 1970.

87. Shirabe T, Tawara S, Terao A, et al: Myxedematous polyneuropathy: a light and electron microscopic study of the peripheral nerve and muscle, *J Neurol Neurosurg Psychiatry* 38:241–247, 1975.

88. Al-Shekhlee A, Kaminiski HJ, Ruff RL: Endocrine myopathies and muscle disorders related to electrolyte disturbance. In Katirgi B, Kaminski HT, Preston DC, et al, editors: *Neuromuscular Disorders in Clinical Practice*, Boston, 2002, Butterworth-Heinemann, pp 1187–1204.

89. Madariaga M: Polymyositis-like syndrome in hypothyroidism: review of case reports over the past 25 years, *Thyroid* 12:331–336, 2002.

90. Duyff RF, Van den Bosch J, Laman DM, et al: Neuromuscular findings in thyroid dysfunction: a prospective clinical and electrodiagnostic study, *J Neurol Neurosurg Psychiatry* 68:750–755, 2000.

91. Tornero Estebanez C: Myopathy in hypothyroidism, *Ann Med Intern* 18(6):345–346, 2001.

92. Kisakol G, Tune R, Kaya A: Rhabdomyolysis in a patient with hypothyroidism, *Endocr J* 50(2):221–223, 2003.

93. Kar PM, Hirani A, Allen MJ: Acute renal failure in a hypothyroid patient with rhabdomyolysis, *Clin Nephrol* 60(6):428–429, 2003.

94. Barahona MJ, Mauri A, Sucunza N, et al: Hypothyroidism as a cause of rhabdomyolysis, *Endocr J* 49(6):621–623, 2002.

95. Scott KR, Simmons Z, Boyer PJ: Hypothyroid myopathy with a strikingly elevated serum creatine kinase level, *Muscle Nerve* 26(1):141–144, 2002.

96. Benito-Leon J, Marin E, Mendez M, et al: Muscle pseudo-hypertrophy associated with hypothyroidism (Hoffman's syndrome), *Rev Neurol* 32(10):998–999, 2001.

97. Mastropasqua M, Spagna G, Baldini V, et al: Hoffman's syndrome: muscle stiffness, pseudo hypertrophy and hypothyroidism, *Horm Res* 59(2):105–108, 2003.

98. Rullu MS, Udgirkar VS, Maranjan MN, et al: Kocher-Debro-Semelaigne syndrome: hypothyroidism with muscle pseudo hypertrophy, *Indian J Pediatr* 70(8):671–673, 2003.

99. Bertorini T: A woman with weakness, elevated cholesterol and serum creatine kinase, Case 87. In Bertorini TE, editor: *Neuromuscular Disorder Case Studies*, Philadelphia, 2008, Butterworth-Heinemann, pp 550–553.

100. Karlsberg RD, Roberts R: Effect of altered thyroid function on plasma creatine kinase clearance in the dog, *Am J Physiol* 235:E614–E618, 1978.

101. Silverberg Shonni J, Bilezikian JP: Primary hyperparathyroidism. In DeGroot LJ, Jameson JL, editors: *Endocrinology*, 5th ed, Philadelphia, 2006, Saunders, pp 1533–1554.

102. Attie JN, Bock G, Auguste L: Multiple parathyroid adenomas: report of 33 cases, *Surgery* 108:1014–1019, 1980.

103. Feldman D: Vitamin D, parathyroid hormone and calcium: a complex regulatory network, *Am J Med* 107:637–639, 1999.

104. Sirdofsky Michael D, Kroges L: Neurological complications of parathyroid gland disorders: hypoparathyroidism and hyperparathyroidism. In Biller J, editor: *The Interface of Neurology and Internal Medicine*, Philadelphia, 2008, Lippincott Williams and Wilkins, pp 476–481.

105. Baczynski R, Massry SG, Magott M, et al: Effect of parathyroid hormone on energy metabolism of skeletal muscle, *Kidney Int* 28(5):722–7272, 1985.

106. Garber AJ: Effects of parathyroid hormone on skeletal muscle protein and amino acid metabolism in the rat, *J Clin Invest* 71(6):1806–1821, 1983.

107. Wrogemann K, Pena SD: Mitochondrial calcium overload. A general mechanism for cell necrosis in muscle disease, *Lancet* 1:672–674, 1976.

108. Scholz DA, Purnell DC: Asymptomatic primary hyperparathyroidism, *Mayo Clin Proc* 56:473–478, 1981.

109. Joborn C, Hetta J, Johansson H, et al: Psychiatric morbidity in primary hyperparathyroidism, *World J Surg* 1:476–481, 1998.

110. Pattern BM, Bilezikian JP, Mallette LE, et al: The neuromuscular disease of primary hyperthyroidism, *Ann Intern Med* 80:182–194, 1974.

111. Mallette LE, Patten BM, Engel WK: Neuromuscular disease in secondary hyperparathyroidism, *Ann Intern Med* 82:474–483, 1975.

112. Bertorini TE: Histologic studies in muscle of hyperparathyroidism. In Massry SG, Fujita T, editors: *New Actions of Parathyroid Hormone*, New York, 1989, Plenum Press, pp 173–182.

113. Rymanowski JV, Twydell PT: Treatable dropped head syndrome in hyperparathyroidism, *Muscle Nerve* 3:409–410, 2009.

114. Frame B, Heinze EG, Block MA, et al: Myopathy in primary hyperparathyroidism: observations in three patients, *Ann Intern Med* 68:1022–1027, 1968.

115. Kaplan PE, Hines JR, Leestma JE, et al: Neuromuscular junction transmission deficit in a patient with primary hyperparathyroidism, *Electromyograph Clin Neurophysiol* 20:359–367, 1980.

116. Wersall-Robertson E, Hamberger B, Ehren H, et al: Increase in muscular strength following surgery for primary hyperparathyroidism, *Acta Med Scand* 220:233–235, 1986.

117. Delbridge L, Marshman D, Reeve T, et al: Neuromuscular symptoms in elderly patients with hyperparathyroidism: improvement with parathyroid surgery, *Med J Aust* 149:74–76, 1988.

118. Hassani S, Braunstein GD, Seibel MJ, et al: Alendronate therapy of primary hyperparathyroidism, *Endocrinologist* 11:459–464, 2001.

119. Levine MA: Hypoparathyroidism and pseudohypoparathyroidism. In DeGroot LJ, Jameson JL, editors: *Endocrinology*, Philadelphia, 2006, Saunders, pp 1611–1636.

120. Edis AJ: Prevention and management of complications associated with thyroid and parathyroid surgery, *Surg Clin North Am* 59:83–92, 1979.

121. Carpenter TO, Carnes DL Jr, Anast CS: Hypoparathyroidism in Wilson's disease, *N Engl J Med* 309:873–877, 1983.

122. Obermayer-Straub P, Manns MP: Autoimmune polyglandular syndromes, *Baillieres Clin Gastroenterol* 12:293–315, 1998.

123. Baldini A: DiGeorge syndrome: an update, *Curr Opin Cardiol* 19:201–204, 2004.

124. Fatemi S, Ryzen E, Flores J, et al: Effect of experimental human magnesium depletion on parathyroid hormone secretion and 1, 25 dihydroxyvitamin D metabolism, *J Clin Endocrinol Metab* 73:1067–1072, 1991.

125. Katsanos KH, Elisaf M, Bairaktari E, et al: Severe hypomagnesemia and hypoparathyroidism in Kearns-Sayre syndrome, *Am J Nephrol* 21:150–153, 2001.

126. Breslau NA: Pseudohypoparathyroidism: current concepts, *Am J Med Sci* 298:130–140, 1989.

127. Schutt-Aine JC, Young MA, Pescovitz DH, et al: Hypoparathyroidism: a possible cause of ricketts, *J Pediatr* 106:255–259, 1985.

128. Erkal MZ, Wilde J, Bilgin Y, et al: High prevalence of vitamin D deficiency, secondary hyperparathyroidism and generalized bone pain in Turkish immigrants in Germany: identification of risk factors, *Osteoporos Int* 17:1133–1140, 2006.

129. Bischoff-Ferrari HA, Dietrich T, Orav EJ, et al: Higher 25-hydroxy vitamin D concentrations are associated with better lower-extremity function in both active and inactive persons aged ≥ 60 y, *Am J Clin Nutr* 80:752–758, 2004.

130. Ziambaras K, Dagogo-Jack S: Reversible muscle weakness in patients with vitamin D deficiency, *West J Med* 167:435–439, 1997.

131. Ahmed W, Khan N, Glueck CJ, et al: Low serum 25 (OH) vitamin D levels (<32 ng/mL) are associated with reversible myositis-myalgia in statin-treated patients, *Transl Res* 153:11–16, 2009.

132. Hoffman E: The Chvostek sign: a clinical study, *Am J Surg* 96:33, 1958.

133. Abbott LG, Rude RK: Clinical manifestations of magnesium deficiency, *Miner Electrolyte Metab* 19:314–322, 1993.

134. Illum F, Dupont E: Prevalences of CT-detected calcification of the basal ganglia in idiopathic hypoparathyroidism, *Neuroradiology* 27:32–37, 1985.

135. Knowdley KV, Coull BM, Orwoll ES: Cognitive impairment and intracranial calcification in chronic hypoparathyroidism, *Am J Med Sci* 317:273–277, 1999.

136. Parfitt AM: The interactions of thiazide diuretics with parathyroid hormone and vitamin D: studies in patients with hypoparathyroidism, *J Clin Invest* 51:1879–1888, 1972.

137. David N: Cushing's syndrome, *N Engl J Med* 332:791–803, 1995.

138. Bertorini TE, Perez AS, Tamara M: Disorders of the adrenal glands and neuroendocrine tumors. In Biller J, editor: *The Interface of Neurology and Internal Medicine*, Philadelphia, 2008, Lippincott Williams and Wilkins, pp 482–496.

139. Nieman LK: *Establishing the diagnosis of Cushing's Syndrome*, UpToDate, Waltham MA, 2007.

140. Gilbert R, Lim EM: The diagnosis of Cushing's syndrome: an Endocrine Society Clinical Practice Guideline, *Clin Brioche Rev* 29(3):103–106, 2008.

141. Fondling JW, Raff H, Aaron DC: The low-dose dexamethasone suppression test: a reevaluation in patients with Cushing's syndrome, *J Clin Endocrinol Metab* 89:1222–1226, 2004.

142. McDougall D, Bhibhatbhan A, Toth C: Adverse effects of corticosteroid therapy in neuromuscular diseased patients are common and receive insufficient prophylaxis, *Acta Neurol Scan* 120:364–367, 2009.

143. Emma F, Pizzini C, Tessa A, et al: "Bartter-like" phenotype in Kearnes-Sayre syndrome, *Pediatr Nephrol* 21:355–360, 2006.

144. Bautista J, Gil-Neciga E, Gil-Peralta A: Hypokalemic periodic paralysis in primary hyperaldosteronism: subclinical myopathy with atrophy of the 2A muscle fibers as the most pronounced alteration, *Eur Neurol* 18(6): 415–420, 1979.

145. Talib B, Mahmood K, Yamagudin, et al: Hypokalemic quadriparesis with normotensive primary hyperdaldosteronism, *J Coll Physicians Surg Pak* 14: 492–493, 2004.

146. Fujihara K, Miyoshi T, Yamagunchi Y, et al: Tetany as a sole manifestation in a patient with Barrter's syndrome and a successful treatment with indomethacin, *Rinsho Shinkeigaku* 30:529–532, 1990.

147. Duncan JL 3rd, Fuhrmang GM, Bolton JS, et al: Laparoscopic adrenalectomy in subjects to an open approach h to treat primary hyperaldosteronism, *Am Surg* 66:932–935, 2000.

148. Wolfgand O: Adrenal insufficiency, *N Engl J Med* 335:1206–1212, 1996.

149. Carey R: The changing clinical spectrum of adrenal insufficiency, *Ann Intern Med* 127:1103–1105, 1997.

150. Piedrola G, Casado JL, Lopez E, et al: Clinical features of adrenal insufficiency in patients with acquired immunodeficiency syndrome, *Clin Endocrinol (Oxf)* 45:97–101, 1996.

151. Moser HW, Raymond GV, Lu SE, et al: Follow-up of 89 asymptomatic patients with adrenoleukodystrophy treated with Lorenzo's oil, *Arch Neurol* 62:1073–1080, 2005.

152. Mukherjee S, Newby E, Harvey J: Adrenomyeloneuropathy in patients with Addison's disease: genetic case analysis, *J R Soc Med* 99:245–249, 2006.

153. Grinspook SK, Biller BM: Laboratory assessment of adrenal insufficiency, *J Clin Endocrinol Metab* 79:923–931, 1997.

154. Al-Hayk K, Bertorini TE: Neuromuscular complications in uremics: a review, *Neurologist* 13:188–196, 2007.

155. Krishnan AV, Kiernan MC: Uremic neuropathy: clinical features and new pathphysiological insights, *Muscle Nerve* 35:273–290, 2007.

156. Dyck PJ, Johnson WJ, Lambert EH, et al: Segmental demyelination secondary to axonal degeneration in uremic neuropathy, *Mayo Clin Proc* 46:400–431, 1971.

157. Babb AL, Ahmad S, Bergstrom J, et al: The middle molecule hypothesis in perspective, *Am J Kidney Dis* 1:46–50, 1981.

158. Man NK, Terlain B, Paris J, et al: An approach to "middle molecules" identification in artificial kidney dialysate, with reference to neuropathy prevention, *Trans Am Soc Artif Intern Organs* 19:320–324, 1973.

159. Milutinovic J, Babb AL, Eschbach JW, et al: Uremic neuropathy: evidence of middle molecule toxicity, *Artif Organs* 2(1):45–51, 1978.

160. DiGiulio S, Chkoff N, Lhoste F, et al: Parathormone as a nerve poison in uremia, *N Engl J Med* 299:1134–1135, 1978.

161. Mendell JR, Sahenk Z: Clinical practice: painful sensory neuropathy, *N Engl J Med* 348:1243–1255, 2003.

162. Bolton CF: Electrophysiologic changes in uremic neuropathy after successful renal transplantation, *Neurology* 26:152–161, 1976.

163. Gilbert MS, Robinson A, Baez A, et al: Carpal tunnel syndrome in patients who are receiving long term renal hemodialysis, *J Bone Joint Surg Am* 70:1145–1153, 1988.

164. Ritz E, Bomer J: Beta-2 microglobulin-derived amyloid-problems and perspectives, *Blood Purif* 6:61–68, 1988.

165. Schwarz A, Keller F, Seyfert S, et al: Carpal tunnel syndrome: a major complication in long-term hemodialysis patients, *Clin Nephrol* 22:133–137, 1984.

166. Wilbourn AJ, Furlan AJ, Hulley W, et al: Ischemic monomelic neuropathy, *Neurology* 33:447–451, 1983.

167. Hebl JR, Horlocker TT: Brachial neuropathy after hemodialysis shunt placement under axillary blockade, *Anesth Analg* 89:1025–1026, 1999.

168. Miles AM: Vascular steal syndrome and ischemic monomelic neuropathy: two variants of upper limb ischemia after hemodialysis vascular access surgery, *Nephrol Dial Transplant* 14:297–300, 1999.

169. Miles AM: Upper limb ischemia after vascular access surgery: differential diagnosis and management, *Semin Dial* 13:312–315, 2000.

170. Padbert FT Jr, Calligaro KD, Sidawy AN: Complications of arteriovenous hemodialysis access: recognition and management, *J Vasc Surg* 48:55S–80S, 2008.

171. Bolton CF, Driedger AA, Lindsay RM: Ischemic neuropathy in uremic patients caused by bovine arteriovenous shunt, *J Neurol Neurosurg Psychiatry* 42:810–814, 1979.

172. Kaku DA, Malamut RI, Frey DJ, et al: Conduction block as an early sign of reversible injury in ischemic monomelic neuropathy, *Neurology* 43:1126–1130, 1993.

173. Goldstein LJ, Helfend LK, Kordestani RK: Postoperative edema after vascular access causing nerve compression secondary to the presence of a perineuronal lipoma: case report, *Neurosurgery* 50:412–413, 2002.

174. Delmez JA, Holmann B, Sivard SA, et al: Peripheral nerve entrapment syndromes in chronic hemodialysis patients, *Nephron* 30:118–123, 1982.

175. Lazaro RP, Kirshner HS: Proximal muscle weakness in uremia: case reports and review of the literature, *Arch Neurol* 37:555–558, 1980.

176. Floyd M, Ayyar DR, Barwick DD, et al: Myopathy in chronic renal failure, *Q J Med* 43:509–524, 1974.

177. Quintanilla AP, Sahgal V: Uremic myopathy, *Int J Artif Organs* 7:239–242, 1984.

178. Campistol JM: Uremic myopathy, *Kidney Int* 62:1901–1913, 2002.

179. Wanic-Kossowska M, Grzegorzewska A, Plotast H, et al: Does calcitriol therapy improve muscle function in uremic patients? *Perit Dial Int* 16(Suppl 1): S305–S308, 1996.

180. Marsden SN, Parkinson IS, Ward MK, et al: Evidence for aluminum accumulation in renal failure, *Proc Eur Dial Transplant Assoc* 16:588–596, 1979.

181. Bregman H, Gelfand MC, Winchester JF, et al: HLA-linked iron overload and myopathy in maintenance hemodialysis patients, *Trans Am Soc Artif Intern Organs* 26:366–368, 1980.

182. Thompson CH, Irish AB, Kemp GJ, et al: The effect of propionyl L-carnitine on skeletal muscle metabolism in renal failure, *Clin Nephrol* 47:372–378, 1977.

183. Levine JM, Taylor RA, Elman LB, et al: Involvement of skeletal muscle in dialysis-associated systemic fibrosis (nephrogenic fibrosing dermopathy), *Muscle Nerve* 30:569–577, 2004.

184. Cowper SE: Nephrogenic fibrosing dermopathy: the first 6 years, *Curr Opin Rheumatol* 15:786–790, 2003.

185. DeGrandis D, Mezzina C, Fiaschi A, et al: Myasthenia due to carnitine treatment, *J Neurol Sci* 46:365–371, 1980.

186. Niakan E, Bertorini TE, Acchiardo SR, et al: Procainamide-induced myasthenia-like weakness in a patient with peripheral neuropathy, *Arch Neurol* 38:378–379, 1981.

187. Denny-Brown DE: Neurological conditions resulting from prolonged and severe dietary restriction, *Medicine (Baltimore)* 26:41–113, 1947.

188. Windebank AJ: Polyneuropathy due to nutritional deficiency and alcoholism. In Dick PJ, Thomas PK, Griffin JW, et al, editors: *Peripheral Neuropathy*, 3rd ed, Philadelphia, 1993, Saunders, pp 1310–1321.

189. Hammond N, Wang Y: Fat soluble vitamins. In Biller J, editor: *The Interface of Neurology and Internal Medicine*, Philadelphia, 2008, Lippincott Williams and Wilkins, pp 449–458.

190. Blomhoff R: Vitamin A metabolism. New perspective on absorption, transport and storage, *Physiol Rev* 71:951–990, 1991.

191. Pingrade NA: Hydrosoluble vitamins (except B_{12} and folate). In Biller J, editor: *The Interface of Neurology and Internal Medicine*, Philadelphia, 2008, Lippincott Williams and Wilkins, pp 443–452.

192. Jukes TH: The prevention and conquest of scurvy, beri-beri and pellagra, *Prevent Med* 18:877–883, 1989.
193. Zak J, Burns D, Lingenfelser T, et al: Dry beriberi: unusual complication of prolonged parenteral nutrition, *JPEN J Parenter Enteral Nutr* 15:200–201, 1991.
194. Brin M: Erythrocyte transketolase in early thiamine deficiency, *Ann N Y Acad Sci* 98:528–541, 1962.
195. Jeyasingham MD, Pratt OE, Burns A, et al: The activation of red blood cell transketolase in groups of patients especially at risk for thiamine deficiency, *Psychol Med* 17:311–318, 1987.
196. Lewy FH, Spies TD, Aring CD: The incidence of neuropathy in pellagra: the effect of cocarboxylase upon its neurologic signs, *Am J Med Sci* 199: 840–849, 1940.
197. Ruffin JM, Smith DT: Treatment of pellagra with special reference to the use of nicotinic acid, *South Med J* 32:40–47, 1939.
198. Albin RL, Albers JW: Long-term follow-up of pyridoxine-induced acute sensory neuropathy-neuronopathy, *Neurology* 40:1319, 1990.
199. Parry GJ, Bredesen DE: Sensory neuropathy with low-dose pyridoxine, *Neurology* 35:1466–1468, 1985.
200. Wang Y, Aamodt C, Barohn R: Cobalamine (B_{12}) deficiency. In Biller J, editor: *The Interface of Neurology and Internal Medicine*, Philadelphia, 2008, Lippincott Williams and Wilkins, pp 453–455.
201. Snow CF: Laboratory diagnosis of vitamin B_{12} and folate deficiency. A guide for the primary care physician, *Arch Intern Med* 159:1289–1298, 1999.
202. Cox-Klazinga M, Endtz LJ: Peripheral nerve involvement of pernicious anemia, *J Neurol Sci* 45:367–371, 1980.
203. Healton EB, Savage DG, Brust JCM, et al: Neurologic aspects of cobalamine deficiency, *Neurology* 45:1435–1440, 1995.
204. Victor M, Lear AA: Subacute combined degeneration of the spinal cord: current concepts of the disease process: value of serum B_{12} determinations in clarifying some of the common clinical problems, *Am J Med* 20: 896–911, 1956.
205. Fine EJ, Sovia E, Paroski MW, et al: The neurophysiological profile of vitamin B_{12} deficiency, *Muscle Nerve* 13:158–164, 1990.
206. Aurora TK, Suri P: Folic acid deficiency. In Biller J, editor: *The Interface of Neurology and Internal Medicine*, Philadelphia, 2008, Lippincott Williams and Wilkins, pp 456–458.

207. Evans HM, Burr GO: Development of paralysis in the suckling young of mothers deprived of vitamin E, *J Biol Chem* 76:273–297, 1928.
208. Amato JCE, AA BRJ: Isolated vitamin E deficiency, *Muscle Nerve* 19:1161–1165, 1996.
209. Sokol RJ: Vitamin E and neurologic deficits, *Adv Pediatr* 37:119–148, 1990.
210. Binder HJ, Solitare GB, Spiro HM: Neuromuscular disease in patients with steatorrhea, *Gut* 8:605–611, 1967.
211. Kumar N: Copper deficiency myelopathy (human swayback), *Mayo Clin Proc* 81(10):1371–1384, 2006.
212. Kumar N, Gross JB Jr, Ahlskog JE: Myelopathy due to copper deficiency, *Neurology* 61:272–274, 2003.
213. Kumar N, Crum B, Petersen RC, et al: Copper deficiency myelopathy, *Arch Neurol* 61:762–766, 2004.
214. Steinberg SAL, FU GJG: Morphologic findings in bone marrow precursor cells in zinc-induced copper deficiency anemia, *Am J Clin Pathol* 97: 665–668, 1991.
215. Willis MS, Monaghan SA, Miller ML, et al: Zinc-induced copper deficiency: a report of three cases initially recognized on bone marrow examination, *Am J Clin Pathol* 123:125–131, 2005.
216. Crum BA, Kumar N: Electrophysiologic findings in copper deficiency myeloneuropathy [abstract], *Neurology* 64(6 Suppl 1):A123, 2005 Abstract P02.161.
217. Chai Y, Bertorini TE: A female with progressive four-limb paresthesias, *J Clin Neuromuscul Dis* 11(4):191–197, 2010.
218. Strachan H: Malarial multiple peripheral neuritis, *Annu Univers Med Sci* 1:139–142, 1888.
219. Strachan H: On a form of multiple neuritis prevalent in the West Indies, *Practitioner* 59:477–484, 1897.
220. Scott HH: An investigation into an acute outbreak of "central neuritis," *Ann Trop Med Parasitol* 12:109–196, 1918.
221. Fisher CM: Residual neuropathological changes in Canadians held prisoners of war by the Japanese, *Can Serv Med J* 11:157–199, 1955.
222. Borrajero I, Perez JL, Dominguez C, et al: Epidemic neuropathy in Cuba: morphological characterization of peripheral nerve lesions in sural nerve biopsies, *J Neurol Sci* 127:68–76, 1994.

Marinos C. Dalakas, MD

Treatment and Management of Autoimmune Myopathies

21

The autoimmune inflammatory myopathies comprise three major and distinct subsets: *polymyositis* (PM), *dermatomyositis* (DM), and *inclusion body myositis* (IBM). Although the presence of moderate to severe muscle weakness, endomysial inflammation, and variable creatine kinase (CK) elevation are common features in all these conditions, unique clinical, immunopathologic, and histologic criteria characterize each subset.[1–10] A rare form of myositis, the *acute necrotizing myopathy*, has emerged as a distinct subset that needs to be distinguished from the other three because of generally incomplete response to therapies. Fasciitis, another autoimmune condition in which the pathologic picture consists of inflammation of the fascia and perimysium, is also briefly described here.

Dermatomyositis

Dermatomyositis occurs in both children and adults. It is a distinct clinical entity because of a characteristic rash that accompanies or, more often, precedes muscle weakness. The skin manifestations include a heliotrope rash (blue-purple discoloration) with edema on the upper eyelids, a flat red rash on the face and upper trunk, and erythema of the knuckles with a raised violaceous scaly eruption (Gottron rash) (Fig. 21-1).[1,7,8] The erythematous rash can also occur on other body surfaces, including the knees, elbows, malleoli, neck and anterior chest (often in a V sign), and back and shoulders (shawl sign) and may be exacerbated after exposure to the sun. The initial erythematous lesions may result in scaling of the skin accompanied by pigmentation and depigmentation, giving a shiny appearance at times. Dilated capillary loops at the base of the fingernails are also characteristic of dermatomyositis. The cuticles may be irregular, thickened, and distorted, and the lateral and palmar areas of the fingers may become rough and cracked, with irregular, "dirty" horizontal lines, resembling "mechanic's hands." Dermatomyositis in children resembles the adult disease. An early abnormality in children is "misery," defined as an irritable child that feels uncomfortable, has a red flush on the face, is fatigued, does not feel like socializing, and has a varying degree of muscle weakness.[7] A tiptoe gait due to flexion contracture of the ankles is not unusual. In DM, the affected muscles are predominantly proximal but the degree of weakness varies. It can be mild, moderate, or severe, leading to quadriparesis. In advanced cases, atrophy of the affected muscles takes place. Ocular and facial muscles remain normal even

in advanced cases, and if these muscles are affected, the diagnosis of inflammatory myopathy should be in doubt. The pharyngeal and neck extensor muscles can be involved, causing dysphagia and difficulty holding up the head. The tendon reflexes are preserved but may be absent in severely weakened or atrophied muscles. The respiratory muscles are rarely affected but respiratory symptoms may not be uncommon due to interstitial lung disease. Myalgia and muscle tenderness may occur early in the disease, especially when DM occurs in the setting of a connective tissue disorder. In patients with DM who have severe muscle pain, involvement of the fascia should be suspected.

Some patients with the classic skin lesions may have clinically normal strength, even 3 to 5 years after onset. This form of DM, referred to as *dermatomyositis sine myositis* or *amyopathic dermatomyositis,*[8] has a better overall prognosis. Although in these cases the disease appears limited to the skin, the muscle biopsy shows significant perivascular and perimysial inflammation with immunopathologic features identical to those seen in classic dermatomyositis, suggesting that the amyopathic and myopathic forms are part of the range of dermatomyositis affecting skin and muscle to a varying degree.[7]

Dermatomyositis usually occurs alone, but it may overlap with scleroderma and mixed connective tissue disease. Fasciitis and skin changes similar to those found in dermatomyositis have occurred in patients with eosinophilia-myalgia syndrome caused by the ingestion of contaminated L-tryptophan and in patients with eosinophilic fasciitis or macrophagic myofasciitis. In up to 15% of adult patients, the DM has a paraneoplastic association. Ovarian cancer is most frequent, followed by intestinal, breast, lung, and liver cancer. In Asian populations, nasopharyngeal cancer is more common.[8] Because tumors are often uncovered at autopsy or on the basis of abnormal findings on medical history and physical examination, blind radiologic searches are rarely fruitful. A complete annual physical examination with breast, pelvic, and rectal examinations (including colonoscopy in high-risk patients), urinalysis, complete blood cell count, blood chemistry tests, and chest radiograph, is usually sufficient and is highly recommended, especially for the first 3 years.

Extramuscular manifestations may also be prominent in some patients with dermatomyositis and include (1) dysphagia; (2) subcutaneous calcifications (Fig. 21-2), sometimes opening onto the skin and causing ulcerations and infections, especially in children[7]; (3) contractures of the joints, especially in the childhood form; (4) pulmonary involvement due to interstitial lung disease, especially in

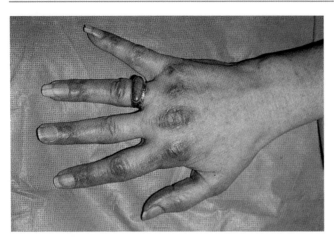

Figure 21-1 The characteristic Gottron rash seen in a patient with dermatomyositis.

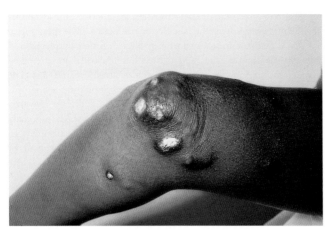

Figure 21-2 Subcutaneous calcifications in the elbow of a patient with dermatomyositis.

patients who have anti-Jo-1 antibodies, as discussed later; (5) gastrointestinal ulcerations, due to vasculitis or infections; (6) general systemic disturbances, such as fever, malaise, weight loss, arthralgia; and (7) Raynaud phenomenon, especially when dermatomyositis is associated with a connective tissue disorder.

Polymyositis

Polymyositis has no unique clinical features, and it is often a diagnosis of exclusion.[1,7,9,10] This disease is best defined as an inflammatory myopathy of subacute onset (weeks to months) and steady progression that occurs in adults who do not have rash on the face, trunk, or fingers, as seen in dermatomyositis; involvement of eye and facial muscles; family history of a neuromuscular disease; endocrinopathy; history of exposure to myotoxic drugs or toxins; and another myopathy such as dystrophy, metabolic myopathy, or inclusion body myositis. Unlike dermatomyositis, in which the rash secures early recognition, the actual onset of polymyositis cannot be easily determined and the disease may exist for several months before the patient seeks medical advice.

Patients with polymyositis commonly present with proximal and often symmetrical muscle weakness that develops over weeks to months, and rarely acutely. An acute onset should raise the suspicion

of a necrotizing myopathy. Fine-motor movements that depend on the strength of distal muscles are affected only late in the disease. If these muscles are affected from the outset or early in the course of the disease, the diagnosis of inclusion body myositis should be suspected. In advanced cases, atrophy of the affected muscles takes place. Ocular muscles remain normal even in advanced cases, and if these muscles are affected, the diagnosis of inflammatory myopathy should be in doubt. In contrast with IBM, in which the facial muscles are affected in the majority of patients, in PM, the strength of the facial muscles remains normal except for in rare advanced cases. The pharyngeal and neck extensor muscles can be involved, causing dysphagia and difficulty holding up the head. The tendon reflexes are preserved but may be absent in severely weakened or atrophied muscles. The respiratory muscles are rarely affected, but respiratory symptoms are not uncommon owing to interstitial lung disease, especially in patients with anti-Jo-1 antibodies or antibodies to various ribonucleoproteins.[1,7,9-11] Although myalgia may occur early in the disease, most often in the setting of a coexisting connective tissue disorder, severe muscle pain should raise the suspicion of fasciitis even if there are no overt signs of skin induration and thickness.

Polymyositis is extremely rare in childhood, and if a diagnosis is made in patients younger than age 16 years, a careful review is needed to exclude another disease, especially one of the inflammatory dystrophies.

Polymyositis appears to be a syndrome of diverse causes. As a stand-alone clinical entity, it is rather uncommon. It is more frequently seen in association with connective tissue disorders, systemic autoimmune diseases, or viral infections, such as Sjögren syndrome, rheumatoid arthritis, Crohn disease, vasculitis, sarcoidosis, primary biliary cirrhosis, adult celiac disease, chronic graft-versus-host disease, discoid lupus, ankylosing spondylitis, Behçet disease, myasthenia gravis, acne fulminans, dermatitis herpetiformis, psoriasis, Hashimoto disease, granulomatous diseases, agammaglobulinemia, hypereosinophilic syndrome, Lyme disease, Kawasaki disease, autoimmune thrombocytopenia, hypergammaglobulinemic purpura, hereditary complement deficiency, IgA deficiency, and acquired immunodeficiency syndrome (AIDS). Among viruses, human immunodeficiency virus (HIV) and human T-lymphotrophic virus type I (HTLV-I) are the only viruses convincingly associated with polymyositis. Claims that other viruses, such as enteroviruses, can be causally connected with polymyositis are unproved. In contrast to dermatomyositis, polymyositis is not more frequently associated with cancer compared to other chronic autoimmune disorders treated with immunosuppressants.

Several animal parasites, such as protozoa (*Toxoplasma, Trypanosoma*), cestodes (*cysticerci*), and nematodes (*trichinae*), may produce a focal or diffuse inflammatory myopathy known as "parasitic polymyositis."[1] In the tropics, a suppurative myositis known as "tropical polymyositis" or "pyomyositis" may be produced by *Staphylococcus aureus*, *Yersinia*, *Streptococcus*, or other anaerobes. Pyomyositis, previously rare in the West, can now be seen in patients with AIDS. Certain bacteria, such as *Borrelia burgdorferi* of Lyme disease and *Legionella pneumophila* of legionnaires' disease may infrequently be the cause of polymyositis.

Drugs do not cause PM. The only drug that could change immunoregulation and trigger PM is D-penicillamine and occasionally statins.[11,12] Zidovudine and the cholesterol-lowering drugs can be myototoxic, but they cause a mitochondrial or a necrotizing myopathy that lacks the features of primary endomysial inflammation as seen in polymyositis. In these cases, the muscle fibers demonstrate prominent mitochondrial or necrotic features.

Inclusion Body Myositis

IBM is the most common of the inflammatory myopathies. It affects men more often than women and is the most commonly acquired myopathy in men older than 50 years. Although IBM may be suspected when a patient with presumed polymyositis does not respond to therapy, involvement of distal muscles, especially foot extensors and deep finger flexors in almost all cases (Fig. 21-3), should be a clue to an early clinical diagnosis.[1,13-21] Some patients present with falls because their knees collapse owing to early weakness of the quadriceps muscles. Others present with weakness in the small muscles of the hands, especially the long finger flexors, and complain of inability to hold certain objects such as golf clubs, play the guitar, turn a key, or tie a knot. The weakness and the accompanying atrophy can be asymmetrical, with preferential involvement of the quadriceps (Fig. 21-3A–C), iliopsoas, triceps, biceps, and finger flexors in the forearm. This involvement is in contrast to the hereditary or familial quadriceps-sparing IBM,[22-24] in which the quadriceps remains strong in spite of the weakness in the other muscles. The selective involvement of the flexor digitorum profundus has been confirmed with magnetic resonance imaging (MRI).[25] Dysphagia is quite common, occurring in up to 60% of the patients, especially late in the disease. Because of the distal and at times asymmetrical weakness and atrophy and the early loss of the patellar reflex, a lower motor neuron disease is occasionally suspected, especially since serum CK activity is either not elevated or only moderately increased.[1] Sensory examination is generally normal except for a mildly diminished vibratory sensation at the ankles, presumably related to the patient's age. Contrary to early suggestions, the distal weakness does not represent neurogenic involvement but is part of the distal myopathic process, as confirmed

with macro-electromyography (EMG).[26] In contrast to PM and DM, in which facial muscles are spared, mild facial muscle weakness is very common and is noted in more than 60% of IBM patients.[16]

Sporadic IBM (s-IBM) can be associated with systemic autoimmune or connective tissue diseases in up to 33% of affected patients.[27,28] An increased frequency of DRb10301 and DQb10201 alleles associated with DR and DQ phenotypes has been documented in up to 75% of patients.[29] A frequent association with HLA-B8-DR3 haplotype has been also observed.[28] Familial aggregation of IBM with the typical clinical phenotype of s-IBM, and with histologic and immunopathologic features identical to the sporadic form, can also occur, as seen in other autoimmune disorders.[30] Our group has designated this as *familial inflammatory IBM* and emphasized that it should be distinguished from hereditary inclusion body myopathy (h-IBM), a noninflammatory vacuolar myopathy that spares the quadriceps[22,31] and occurs mostly in Iranian Jews but also in other ethnic groups.[22,31] This disorder results from mutations in the uridine diphosphate-N-acetylglucosamine 2-epimerase/N-acetylmannosamine kinase (GNE) gene.[32]

Progression of s-IBM is slow but steady. Data from 86 patients studied consecutively by the author's group revealed that progression is faster when the disease begins later in life. Patients whose disease began in their 60s required an assistive device many years later compared with those whose disease began in their 70s, presumably because of lesser reserves.[33]

Eosinophilic Syndromes and Fasciitis

Prominent presence of eosinophilic polymorphonuclear leukocytes in muscle (or fascia) can occur in isolation or with systemic eosinophilia and is due to parasitic infection, vasculitis, hypereosinophilic syndrome, or toxic factors. In eosinophilic polymyositis,[34,35] muscle involvement is part of a systemic hypereosinophilic syndrome. A marked systemic eosinophilia is present. Proximal limb muscles show stiffness, pain, and variable weakness. Serum CK activity is moderately elevated. The pathologic picture is similar to that of idiopathic PM, except that there is a conspicuous presence of eosinophilic polymorphonuclear leukocytes in the inflammatory infiltrates. Recent evidence suggests that certain patients with genetically defined calpain-gene mutations have eosinophilic infections in their muscle.[36] The frequency of this phenomenon and the role of eosinophils in myopathy remain unclear.

In eosinophilic fasciitis, the inflammatory reaction is restricted to the fascia and is best shown by a biopsy of the fascia lata. The eosinophilia-myalgia syndrome is caused by prolonged oral intake of large doses of a contaminated L-tryptophan preparation as a therapeutic agent, mainly for insomnia.[37] There was marked systemic eosinophilia with generalized myalgia and moderate muscle weakness.[37] Another important feature is thickening of the skin, mimicking scleroderma. In severe disease, myocarditis and other visceral involvements can supervene. The lymphocytic inflammatory infiltrates (CD8+ cytotoxic cells) also include either abundant or few eosinophilic polymorphonuclear leukocytes, mainly in the perimysial region, and less often in the interstitial space of muscle.[38,39] Muscle fiber necrosis was rare and serum CK activity did not rise significantly. Coexisting peripheral neuropathy may cause denervation atrophy. In some cases, the muscle biopsy shows no abnormality, despite clinical symptoms. The pathogenic factor appears to be a contamination of L-tryptophan with an acetaldehyde ditryptophan derivative, which seems to induce an autosensitization. The disease usually subsides after cessation of

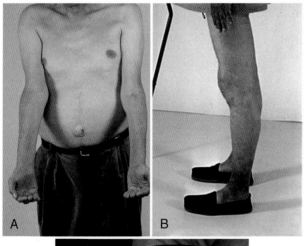

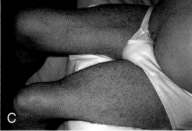

Figure 21-3 Notice the following in a patient with inclusion body myositis: wasting of the forearm muscles with difficulty making a grip (**A**); quadriceps atrophy (**B, C**), and "locking up" of the knee to avoid falls (**B**). (**B**); and atrophy of the quadriceps and overextension of the knee (**C**).

exposure, but resolution may be slow. Corticosteroid therapy may help to accelerate recovery.

A distinctive inflammatory muscle disorder was also identified in up to 80 French patients who presented with myalgias, fatigue, and mild muscle weakness.[40] Muscle biopsy revealed pronounced infiltration of the connective tissue around the muscle (epimysium, perimysium, and perifascicular endomysium) by sheets of periodic acid–Schiff base-positive macrophages and occasional CD8+ T cells. The serum CK or erythrocyte sedimentation rate may at times be elevated. Most patients respond to glucocorticoid therapy, and the overall prognosis is favorable. The pathologic change is almost always seen at the sites of previous vaccinations, even several months later, and has been linked to a type of aluminum component used as a substrate for preparation of the vaccines. Macrophagic myofasciitis has been reported exclusively from France.

Diagnosis and Evaluation

The diagnosis of these disorders is based on the combination of clinical history, serum muscle enzymes, electromyography (EMG), and muscle biopsy. The CK is elevated in all three subsets, but it can be normal or only slightly elevated in DM and IBM. The EMG is myopathic in all three and, although useful to exclude neurogenic disorders, it is insensitive to differentiate an inflammatory myopathy from other toxic or dystrophic myopathic processes. The muscle biopsy shows inflammatory features distinct for each subset and remains the most sensitive diagnostic tool. In DM, the inflammation is perivascular or at the periphery of the fascicle and is often associated with perifascicular atrophy (Fig. 21-4); in PM and IBM the inflammation is in multiple foci within the endomysial parenchyma (Fig. 21-5) and consists predominantly of CD8+ T cells that invade healthy muscle fibers expressing the major histocompatibility complex class I (MHC-I) antigen.[41] The MHC/CD8 complex is characteristic and useful for the diagnosis of PM and IBM.[1,6,7] Plasma cells and dendritic cells are frequent among the infiltrates in all three disorders.[42] An additional feature in IBM is the presence of vacuoles containing 12 to 16 nm tubulofilaments with tiny deposits of amyloid and amyloid-related proteins (Fig. 21-6).[43,44] In IBM, the presence of 15- to 18-nm tubular filamentous masses in nuclei or cytoplasm of muscle fibers can be demonstrated with extensive ultrastructural scrutiny.[45] These filamentous masses are not disease-specific but have been reported to be identical to the paired helical

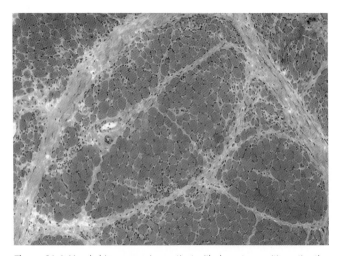

Figure 21-4 Muscle biopsy seen in a patient with dermatomyositis, notice the characteristic perifascicular muscle atrophy and necrosis. (H&E stain ×100.)

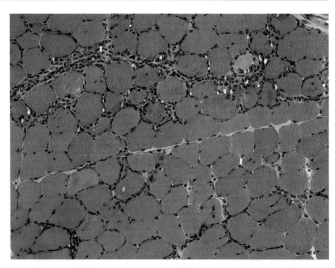

Figure 21-5 Interstitial inflammation in polymyositis and some regenerating muscle fibers. (H&E stain ×200.)

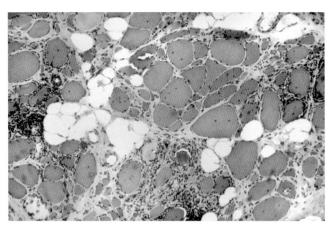

Figure 21-6 Muscle biopsy of a patient with inclusion body myositis. Notice fiber atrophy, internalized nuclei, interstitial inflammatory infiltrates, and rimmed vacuoles. There is also proliferation of endomysial connective tissue and fat. (H&E stain ×200.)

filaments found in neurons in Alzheimer disease.[46] The blue granules, located in or along the wall of the vacuoles, correspond to whorls of cytomembranes or myelin figures, detectable by electron microscopy.[9] Most important, congophilic material, best visualized by Texas-red fluorescent optics, can be found in a variable number of fibers usually in or near rimmed vacuoles.[47–49] Other degeneration-associated molecules such as beta-amyloid and its precursor protein, alpha-chymotrypsin, tau proteins, ubiquitin, apolipoprotein E, prion protein, and others are also found in a small percentage of fibers.[50,51] Although they help toward confirming the histologic diagnosis of IBM, they are not specific because they have been found in other myopathies[52] or even in chronic neurogenic conditions such as the postpolio syndrome.[53] In IBM, the beta-amyloid appears targeted for lysosomal degradation via macroautophagy, as recent studies indicate.[54] The contention that the rimmed vacuoles are a consequence of the myonuclear breakdown, based partly on the observation that they express myonuclear molecules,[55] remains theoretical, if not unrealistic. Ragged red, cytochrome oxidase–negative muscle fibers with mitochondrial excess and multiple mitochondrial DNA deletions have been demonstrated in most examined cases.[56] Uniform expression of class I MHC products at the surface of most muscle fibers is characteristic of PM and IBM, whereas in DM this phenomenon may be evident only in the perifascicular or other random regions.[41,57] Ubiquitous expression of MHC class I does not occur in limb girdle dystrophy, denervating diseases, or metabolic myopathies (except in regenerating fibers or in fiber invaded by macrophages and lymphoid cells), which makes MHC immunostaining a very helpful diagnostic tool for PM and IBM.[58]

Causes of Misdiagnosis

A relatively common erroneous practice that has an impact on investigative and therapeutic decisions is the failure to distinguish IBM from PM and PM from "inflammatory dystrophies" (muscular dystrophies with prominent inflammation seen on histologic examination).[59] The most common cause of a clinical misdiagnosis is an erroneous pathologic interpretation of the biopsy based on the following errors[9,60]:

1. Failure to distinguish the muscle fiber necrosis due to invasion of muscle fibers by cytotoxic lymphocytes, as seen in PM and IBM, from the invasion of muscle fibers by macrophages, as seen in inflammatory dystrophies. In some of these dystrophies (i.e., Duchenne muscular dystrophy, dysferlinopathy, calpainopathy, merosin-deficient sarcoglycanopathy), endomysial infiltration by lymphocytes may also occur but these cells lack the MHC/CD8 complex typical of PM and IBM, as discussed later.[60]

2. Failure to recognize that the pathologic involvement may be spotty and a given biopsy may not contain convincing pathologic changes ("skip areas") requiring repeat biopsy.

3. Being unaware that in DM, changes typical of perifascicular atrophy are diagnostic, even if there is the lack of inflammatory cell infiltrates.

4. Failure to recognize that up to 15% of biopsies from patients with typical clinical features of IBM demonstrate inflammation like that seen in PM but without the classic vacuoles. These patients recently have been labeled as having PM/IBM.[61] A careful view of these biopsies, however, shows a large number of COX-negative fibers and signs of chronicity (large fibers, splitting, increased connective tissue) that denote probable IBM.[58]

These errors can be avoided by a combined evaluation of the clinical picture with the histologic and immunopathologic findings.[61]

Immunopathology

The cause of PM, DM, and IBM is unknown, but an autoimmune pathogenesis is strongly implicated.

Immunopathology of Dermatomyositis
In DM, there is evidence of a humoral-mediated process based on immunopathologic studies performed on muscle biopsy specimens. The primary antigenic targets appear to be components of the endothelium of the blood vessels in the endomysium and probably the skin. Alterations in the endothelial cells consisting of pale and swollen cytoplasm with microvacuoles and tubuloreticular aggregates appear early in the disease. These changes are caused by immune complexes immunolocalized in the endomysial blood vessels along with the C5b-9 membranolytic attack complex, the lytic component of the complement pathway. The membranolytic attack complex and the early complement components C3b and C4b are deposited on the capillaries early in the disease and precede the signs of inflammation or structural changes in the muscle fibers.[1,2,7,59] These

complement fragments are also detected in the serum and correlate with disease activity. The disease probably begins when putative antibodies or other factors activate complement C3, C3b, and C4b fragments that lead to formation of membranolytic attack complex, which is deposited in the endomysial microvasculature and leads to osmotic lysis of the endothelial cells and capillary necrosis.[1,2,4,7,9] As a result, there is reduction in the number of capillaries per muscle fiber, impaired perfusion, and dilatation of the loop of the remaining capillaries in an effort to compensate for the ischemic process. Larger intramuscular blood vessels are also affected in the same pattern, leading to muscle fiber destruction (often resembling microinfarcts) and inflammation. The perifascicular atrophy often seen in more chronic stages is probably a reflection of the endofascicular hypoperfusion that is prominent distally.

The activation of complement induces the release of cytokines and chemokines such as interleukins (IL-1, IL-6) and tumor necrosis factor (TNF), which, in turn, upregulate the expression of VCAM-1 (vascular cell adhesion molecule-1) and ICAM-1 (intercellular adhesion molecule-1) on the endothelial cells and facilitate the transmigration of activated T cells to the perimysial and endomysial spaces. Immunophenotypic analysis of the lymphocytic infiltrates demonstrates B cells, CD4+ cells, and plasmacytoid dendritic cells in the perimysial and perivascular regions, supporting the view that a humoral-mediated mechanism plays the major role in the disease. In the perifascicular regions, there is also upregulation of various molecules such as cathepsins and signal transduction and activation of transducer molecules, probably triggered by interferon-γ, TGF-β (transforming growth factor-beta), and myxovirus resistance protein MxA induced by α/β interferon, which is probably secreted by the large number of plasmacytoid dendritic cells.[42] Based on gene arrays, a number of adhesion molecules, cytokines, and chemokine genes are also upregulated in the muscles of DM patients. Most notable among those genes are the X-linked Kallmann syndrome-1 protein (KAL-1) adhesion molecule,[62] and genes induced by α/β interferon.[42] The KAL-1 is upregulated by TGF-β and may have a deleterious role in DM by inducing fibrosis. Of interest, KAL-1, along with TGF-β, is downregulated in the muscles of DM patients who improved after therapy, and it is most clinically relevant.[63] A summary of the immunopathology of DM is shown in Figure 21-7.

Autoantibodies against nuclear (antinuclear antibodies) and cytoplasmic antigens directed against ribonucleoproteins involved in translation and protein synthesis are also found in up to 20% of DM and PM patients. The antibody directed against the histidyl-transfer RNA synthetase, called *anti-Jo-1*, accounts for 75% of all the antisynthetases and is clinically useful because up to 80% of dermatomyositis patients with anti-Jo-1 antibodies develop interstitial lung disease. These antibodies are not pathogenic, however, and may also occur in patients who have only interstitial lung disease without myositis. Patients with the overlap syndrome of dermatomyositis and systemic sclerosis may also have autoantibodies of unclear significance, including the anti-polymyositis/Scl, directed against a nucleolar protein complex, anti-Ku, and others.

Immunopathology of Polymyositis and Inclusion Body Myositis
Polymyositis and IBM may be some of the best studied or prototypic T cell–mediated disorders in which cytotoxic T cells directed against heretofore unidentified muscle antigens form an immunologic synapse with the MHC class I antigen expressed on the surface of muscle fibers. The cytotoxicity of the autoinvasive T cells has been supported by the presence of perforin granules that are directed toward the surface of the muscle fiber and lead to muscle fiber necrosis on release. The specificity of the T cells has been further

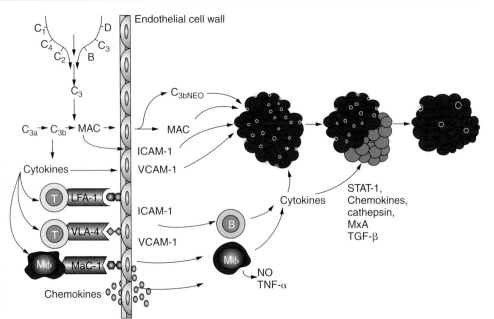

Figure 21-7 Proposed mechanisms in the immunopathogenesis of dermatomyosis. C3bNEO, complement component 3b neoantigen; ICAM-1, intercellular adhesion molecule-1; LFA-1, lymphocyte function–associated antigen 1; MAC, membrane attack complex; MaC-1, macrophage 1 antigen; MxA, myxovirus (influenzavirus) resistance protein 1; NO, nitrous oxide; STAT-1, signal transducer and activator of transcription protein 1; TGF-ß, transforming growth factor-beta; TNF-α, tumor necrosis factor-alpha; VCAM-1, vascular cell adhesion molecule-1; VLA-1, very late antigen-1.

examined by studying the gene rearrangement of the T-cell receptors (TCR) of the autoinvasive T cells.[64,65] In patients with polymyositis, as well as inclusion body myositis, only certain T cells of specific T-cell receptor alpha and T-cell receptor beta families are recruited to the muscle from the circulation. Cloning and sequencing of the amplified endomysial T-cell receptor gene families has demonstrated a restricted use of the *J-beta* gene with conserved amino acid sequence in the CDR3 region, the antigen-binding region of the TCR, indicating that CD8+ cells are specifically selected and clonally expanded in situ by muscle-specific autoantigens. Studies combining laser microdissection, immunocytochemistry, polymerase chain reaction (PCR), and sequencing of the most prominent T-cell receptor families have shown that only the autoinvasive, not the perivascular, endomysial CD8+ cells are clonally expanded. Comparison of the T-cell receptor repertoire between polymyositis and dermatomyosis with spectratyping has confirmed that perturbations of the T-cell receptor families occur only in polymyositis but not dermatomyosis. Further, among the circulating T cells, clonal expansion occurs only in the cytotoxic CD8+ cells that express genes for perforin and infiltrate the MHC-I–expressing muscle fibers (Fig. 21-8).

The clonally expanded CD8+ T cells form immunologic synapses with the muscle fibers they invade, as supported by the co-expression of costimulatory molecules B7-1, B7-2, BB1, CD40, or inducible costimulator (ICOS) ligand (ICOS-L) on the muscle fibers and the respective counter-receptors CD28, cytotoxic T-lymphocyte antigen-4 (CTLA-4), CD40 ligand (CD40L), or ICOS on autoinvasive T cells.[64–66] Cytokines, chemokines, and metalloproteinases (fundamental molecules for T-cell activation, trafficking, antigen recognition, and T-cell attachment) are also upregulated in the muscle tissue. Some of these cytokines, such as interferon-γ, IL-1β, and TNF may exert a direct cytotoxic effect on the muscle tissue. Unique to the muscle is the observation that the various cytokines and chemokines can also stimulate the muscle fibers to endogenously produce certain proinflammatory cytokines, such as interferon-γ, which enhances and perpetuates the immune response.

In PM, MHC-I is expressed in all fibers, even in those not invaded by T cells, often throughout the course of the disease. Such a chronic MHC-I upregulation may be exerting a deleterious stress effect to the endoplasmic reticulum (ER) of the myofiber, independent of T cell–mediated cytotoxicity, as discussed next.

The factors triggering the T cell–mediated process in polymyositis and IBM remain unclear. Viruses may be responsible for breaking tolerance and several of the common viruses, including coxsackievirus, influenza virus, paramyxoviruses, cytomegalovirus, and Epstein-Barr virus, have been directly associated with chronic and acute myositis.[67] Very sensitive PCR studies, however, have repeatedly failed to confirm the presence of such viruses in these patients' muscle biopsies.[68,69]

The best evidence of possible viral connection in PM and IBM is with the retroviruses. Monkeys infected with the simian immunodeficiency virus and humans infected with HIV and HTLV-I develop PM or IBM. In humans infected with HIV or HTLV-I, an isolated inflammatory myopathy may occur as the initial manifestation of the retroviral infection or myositis may develop later in the disease course.[70–81] The association of retroviruses with s-IBM is more than a coincidence because more than 30 cases of HIV/HTLV-I positive patients with IBM have been reported or known to us.[74,75,79,80,81] In these seropositive patients, the disease appears before the age of 50 but several years after the first manifestations of the retroviral infection, suggesting that in HIV-positive patients who live longer and harbor the virus for several years, the disease is more frequently recognized. The clinical phenotype and muscle histologic findings in HIV-IBM patients are identical to the retroviral-negative IBM.[74,81] Using in situ hybridization, PCR, immunocytochemisty, and electron microscopy, viral antigens could not be detected within the muscle fibers but only in occasional endomysial macrophages.[74–81] Molecular immunologic studies using tetramers have shown that retrovirus-specific cytotoxic T cells, whose T-cell receptor contains amino acid residues for specific HLA/viral peptides, are recruited within the clonally expanded T cells and invade muscle fibers.[80,81] We have interpreted these observations to suggest that in HIV- and HTLV-I IBM, there is no evidence of persistent infection of the muscle fibers with the virus or viral replication within the muscle but rather that the chronic retroviral infection, in genetically susceptible individuals, triggers a persistent inflammatory process that leads to s-IBM.[90,91]

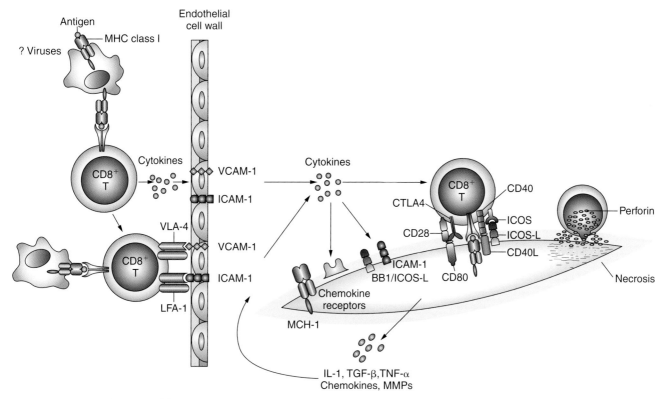

Figure 21-8 Immunopathogenesis of dermatomyositis. BB1/ICOS-L, BB1-costimulatory molecule ligand; CD40L, CD40 ligand; CTLA-4, cytotoxic T-lymphocyte antigen-4; ICAM-1, intercellular adhesion molecule-1; ICOS, inducible costimulator; IL-1, interleukin 1; LFA-1, lymphocyte function–associated antigen 1; MHC, major histocompatibility complex; MCH-1, major histocompatibility complex I; MMPs, matrix metalloproteinases; TGF-ß, transforming growth factor-beta; TNF-α, tumor necrosis factor-alpha; VCAM-1, vascular cell adhesion molecule-1; VLA-4, very late antigen-4.

Nonimmune Features in the Muscles of Inclusion Body Myositis: Reconciling the Roles of Inflammation and "Degeneration"

IBM is a more complex disease because in addition to the primary autoimmune and inflammatory features discussed previously, there are concomitant features of cell stress and degeneration molecules highlighted by the presence of rimmed vacuoles (almost always in fibers not invaded by T cells), intracellular deposition of Congo red–positive amyloid, and accumulation of amyloid-related molecules, including β-APP, phosphorylated tau, presenilin-1, apolipoprotein E, γ-tubulin, clusterin, α-synuclein, and gelsolin. These accumulations are not, however, unique to s-IBM, because they are also observed to a similar extent in other vacuolar myopathies and most of the the myofibrillar ones. What appears unique to IBM, however, compared to other chronic vacuolar myopathies, is the strong presence of primary inflammation and the overexpression of MHC-I molecule on most, if not all, of the fibers. It has been proposed that in muscle fibers overloaded by MHC molecules the presented antigenic peptides cannot undergo proper conformational change to bind to MHC-I complex, leading to endoplasmic reticulum (ER) stress and protein misfolding.[58,68,82] This model is supported by the noted enhanced immunoproteasome activity, enhanced MHC class I protein assembly, misfolding of accumulated glycoproteins, and signs of a cell stress response, with upstream upregulation of αB-crystallin in intact and MHC-I–positive muscle fibers.[83–87] Such stressor effects are also seen in transgenic mice that overexpress MHC class I, indicating that chronic overexpression of MHC class I alone might be sufficient to induce ER stress to myofiber.[82]

Although the factors triggering immune and protein dysregulation or vacuolar formation remain unknown, our group favors a primary inflammatory process that leads to degeneration[58,63,86,88] because (1) IBM is frequently seen with autoimmune disorders and increasingly with HIV and HTLV-I infection, (2) T cell invasion of non-necrotic fibers is found early and in higher frequency than the Congo red–positive fibers,[89] (3) the cytotoxic T cells at the immunologic synapses do not recognize amyloid-related proteins as antigens, and (4) the cytokine-induced upregulation of MHC-I occurs early and is capable of triggering cell stress and degeneration.[88] Most important, endomysial inflammation alone can cause muscle destruction and clinical weakness, as seen in polymyositis; whether the tiny amyloid deposits are sufficient alone to trigger muscle degeneration in humans remains unclear, especially because the same molecules accumulate in various vacuolar myopathies and muscular dystrophies caused by genetic mutations, but in other conditions these deposits appear innocuous.

The possibility that "degenerative" changes are the primary events while the inflammatory features are secondary is another view. In this scenario, accumulation of altered elements of muscle fibers may not only be toxic but also represent neoantigens as a result of transcriptional dysregulation of certain molecules, triggering cytotoxic lymphocytic attack on muscle fiber.[91] Our group views this possibility unlikely, however, because there has not been any evidence supporting it.

Regardless of whether the primary event is a dysimmune or protein dysregulation process, there is now strong evidence that in IBM, proinflammatory cytokines not only correlate with the intramuscular accumulation of amyloid, phosphorylated tau, ubiquitin, and αB-crystallin but that inflammatory mediators such as IL-1 can enhance the production and intracellular accumulation of amyloid and stressor proteins such as αB-crystallin.[86,88] Cytokines also stimulate myofibers to produce inflammatory mediators in an autoamplificatory mechanism, further enhancing the chronicity of inflammation, amyloid formation, and cell stress.[86,88] Theoretically, successful inhibition of inflammatory molecules can halt the degenerative process and stop the disease progression.[88]

Treatment and Management of Inflammatory Myopathies

Goals of Therapy

The goal of therapy in inflammatory myopathies is to improve muscle strength and activities of daily living. Although when the strength improves the serum CK falls concurrently, the reverse is not always true because most of the immunosuppressive therapies can result in a decrease of serum muscle enzymes without necessarily improving muscle strength.[60,90] Unfortunately, this is commonly interpreted as a positive sign and, when associated with a patient's subjective sense of feeling better (but not stronger), gives the erroneous impression of improvement and forms the basis for the common habit of "chasing" or "treating" the CK level instead of the muscle weakness. It is essential, therefore, to discontinue the applied therapies if an adequate trial has led only to a reduction in CK and not to an objective improvement in muscle strength. The level of CK is helpful only as an auxiliary measure and not as a guide to start or monitor therapy.

On assessing strength, in addition to using routine Medical Record Council (MRC) scales, it is essential to ask the patients specific questions about changes in performing routine physical tasks at home or work and activities of daily living. The patients also need to be informed from the onset that these are chronic disorders and long-term therapy is anticipated. The potential long-term side effects of the drugs need to be explained and the patient's cooperation should be sought from the outset. This is especially useful when steroids are used and the patients need to adhere to a strict dietetic regimen.

Treatment of Dermatomyositis and Polymyositis

In spite of the progress in elucidating the specificity of the immune response, a number of fundamental issues remain unanswered, hindering the prospects of specific immunotherapy. Accordingly, none of the available therapies are selective or antigen-specific but rather attack indiscriminately the various T-cell or B-cell functions.[91,92–94]

Starting Therapy: The Role of Corticosteroids

Prednisone is the first drug of choice, based on experience but not on controlled trials. Because the effectiveness and relative safety of prednisone therapy[60,90,92–96] determines the future need for stronger immunosuppressive drugs, our preference has been to start with a high-dose prednisone beginning early in the disease. A high dose, at least 1 mg/kg or 60 to 80 mg/day, as a single daily morning dose (after breakfast) for an initial period of 3 to 4 weeks is preferable. In patients with severe PM or DM and systemic manifestations, I prefer to start treatment with IV methylprednisolone 1 g/day for 3 to 5 days and then continue with the oral prednisone regimen, as mentioned above. After 1 month of high-dose, oral, daily prednisone, I switch to an alternate-day dose. This is accomplished by gradually

reducing the alternate, "off-day" dose by 5 to 10 mg per 1 or 2 weeks, or faster if necessitated by side effects. When reaching the every other day regimen without serious adverse effects, the dosage is reduced gradually by 5 to 10 mg every 3 to 4 weeks until the lowest possible dose that controls the disease is reached. The single-dose, alternate-day program minimizes adverse effects while adequately maintaining control of the underlying disease. It has been my preference to give the prednisone as a single dose in the morning because it is less likely to suppress the evening secretion of adrenocorticotropic hormone (ACTH) and more likely to secure a normal endogenous cortisol secretion the next morning (corticosteroids and other immunosuppressant drugs are discussed in detail in Chapter 7).

The ultimate goal in a patient who responds to steroid therapy is to find the lowest dose that controls the disease with the fewest adverse effects. This is often accomplished by adding a steroid-sparing drug, while lowering the amount of steroid, without a breakthrough of disease. We do not advocate a concurrent use of steroids with another immunosuppressant from the outset of treatment except if the disease has a very aggressive course and the patient is rapidly worsening. Conversely, if by the time the steroid dosage has been reduced to 60 to 80 mg every other day (approximately 14 weeks after initiating therapy), there is no objective benefit (defined as increased muscle strength and not as lowering of the CK or a subjective feeling of increased energy), the patient may be considered unresponsive to prednisone, and tapering is accelerated while the next mode of therapy is started.

To minimize side effects, every patient should be requested from the beginning of steroid therapy to start a strict low-carbohydrate, low-salt, high-protein diet. Antacids or one of the histamine H_2-receptor antagonists may be used if patients experience stomach upset. Co-administration of calcium supplement (1 g/day) and vitamin D (50,000 units per week) may be useful for long-term steroid administration. In postmenopausal women, when long-term therapy is required, I consider adding Fosamax once weekly based on its proven efficacy in the prophylaxis of steroid-related osteoporosis. Monitoring for osteoporosis with dual-energy x-ray absorptiometry (DEXA) scan may be helpful.

Steroid Myopathy versus Disease Activity

The long-term use of prednisone may theoretically cause worsening of muscle strength associated with a normal or unchanged CK level, referred to as *steroid myopathy*. The term *steroid myopathy* is a misnomer because steroids do not cause histologic signs of myopathy but, rather, selective atrophy of type II muscle fibers. Contrary to what is believed, the condition is not common. Rarely, it may be difficult to distinguish a developing steroid-induced myopathic weakness from the increased weakness related to disease activity or to other factors such as decreased mobility, infections, or a concomitant systemic illness. The decision to adjust the prednisone dosage in a patient with myositis who has previously responded to treatment may be influenced by reviewing the past 1 to 2 months' history of strength, mobility, serum CK, medication changes, and associated medical conditions.[4,98] For example, in a patient who for the past 1 to 2 months has had increased CK levels, no new overt signs of steroid toxicity with reduced or unchanged dosage of steroids, and no evidence of a systemic illness or infection, increasing muscle weakness is most likely due to worsening of the disease that either may require more prednisone or has become steroid-resistant, requiring another drug. When these signs are not clear, one may arbitrarily raise the prednisone dosage and wait for the answer, which can be evident in about 2 to 8 weeks, according to the change in the patient's strength. A clinical sign that I have found to be of some help in a few patients is the strength of neck extensor muscles, which usually worsens with exacerbation of the disease but remains unchanged with steroid-induced muscle intoxication. Electromyography, when it shows increased spontaneous activity, is also useful to explore evidence of active disease.

Relapses While on Maintenance Steroid Therapy

Relapses may occur while the steroid dose is decreased below a critical level for a given patient or in patients who are seemingly stable but decompensate after a viral illness, during a concurrent infection, or because of disease worsening. Many such patients can be controlled if the dose of prednisone is increased to a high single daily dose (as high as the initial), or to a high alternate-day dose (if the relapse is mild), for a month followed by a slow taper. More often, however, relapses require more aggressive strategies, such as intravenous immunoglobulin (IVIG) or addition of an immunosuppressant, as described later.

Use of Steroid-Sparing Regimens in Steroid-Responsive Patients

The decision to start an immunosuppressive drug is based on its "steroid-sparing" effect when, in spite of steroid responsiveness, the patient has developed significant complications or when attempts to lower a high steroid dosage have resulted in worsening of muscle strength. The preference for selecting an immunosuppressive drug for these circumstances is empirical because control studies have not been conducted. The choice is usually based on our prejudices or personal experience with each drug, and our own assessment of the relative efficacy/safety ratio. My preference depends on disease severity, clinical setting, and other conditions. The following immunosuppressive drugs are used.[91,92,97]

Azathioprine

Although lower doses (1.5–2.0 mg/kg) are commonly used, I prefer higher doses up to 3 mg/kg for effective immunosuppression. Because azathioprine is usually effective after 6 months of treatment, patience is required before it is concluded that the drug is ineffective. The major toxicity of azathioprine includes thrombocytopenia, anemia, leukopenia, pancytopenia, drug fever, nausea, and liver toxicity. An elevation of liver enzymes, if slight, needs only observation. Azathioprine, which is metabolized by xanthine oxidase, if given concurrently with allopurinol, can be severely toxic to the liver or bone marrow and combined use of these two drugs is not recommended. The susceptibility to toxicity is genetically dependent on interindividual variations in thiopurine S-methyl transferase (TPMT) enzyme activity based on the genetic polymorphism of high- versus low-metabolizing alleles. Patients with low enzyme activity concentrations have an increased risk of bone marrow suppression. Because of these side effects, I prefer to use mycophenolate mofetil (Cellcept), which also acts faster.

Mycophenolate Mofetil

This drug is a morpholinoethylester of mycophenolic acid that blocks de novo purine synthesis and acts on both B and T cells. It is an antipurine antimetabolite, like azathioprine, but it does not cause significant bone marrow suppression or hepatotoxicity. It is a well-tolerated drug when used at doses up to 3 g/day. It does not work as fast as initially thought, and it may take up to 2 or 3 months to see any clinical benefit. In organ rejection, Cellcept works fast because it inhibits the production of new B and T cells; in autoimmune diseases, however, the initial goal is to affect the autoreactive, existing lymphocytes, which is accomplished with other

drugs, such as prednisone, while waiting for Cellcept to act later by inhibiting the new B or T cells.

Methotrexate

An antagonist of folate metabolism, methotrexate is a useful drug. I prefer the oral route starting at 7.5 mg weekly for the first 3 weeks (given in a total of three doses, 2.5 mg every 12 hours), increasing it gradually by 2.5 mg per week up to a total of 25 mg weekly. A rarely reported side effect (but admittedly never seen by this author) is methotrexate pneumonitis, which can be difficult to distinguish from the interstitial lung disease seen in some patients with inflammatory myopathies. Other adverse effects include stomatitis, gastrointestinal symptoms, leukopenia, thrombocytopenia, renal toxicity, hepatotoxicity, and malignancies. Because it acts faster than azathioprine it might be preferable to use as a steroid-sparing agent.

Cyclosporine

Cyclosporine affects T cell–mediated immunity by inhibiting transcription of certain genes, mostly the IL-2 gene, resulting in reduced IL-2 and other cytokines. At doses of 150 mg twice a day (not more than 5 mg/kg/day) and frequent monitoring of the optimal trough serum level (100–200 ng/mL), this drug can be given without major complications. The kidney function should be closely monitored and nonsteroidal anti-inflammatory drugs (e.g., ibuprofen) are avoided. When creatinine increases more than 30%, the drug should be discontinued. The concomitant use of ketoconazole (which inhibits the P480 cytochromal enzyme in the liver) allows for a lower (up to 80%) dose with less toxicity. The advantage of cyclosporine compared to azathioprine is that it acts faster.

When Steroids Are Inadequate: The Use of High-Dose Intravenous Immunoglobulin

In my experience, when corticosteroids have failed to induce remission, or in rapidly progressive cases with evolving severe weakness, the aforementioned immunosuppressive agents, used only for "steroid-sparing" toxicity, are inadequate to substantially increase strength. In these circumstances, the choice is IVIG.

IVIG has multiple mechanisms of actions, most of which include inhibition of cytokines, competition with autoantibodies, inhibition of complement deposition, interference with Fc receptor binding on macrophages or the immunoglobulins on B cells, blocking the Fc receptors on target antigens, interaction with sialic acid–specific receptors on regulatory macrophages exerting an anti-inflammatory effect, or interference with antigen recognition by sensitized T cells. More than one of these actions is probably responsible for the observed benefit.[98] The dose is 2 g/kg, given in two to five divided daily doses, every 5 to 8 weeks, as clinically required. In a double-blind study conducted in patients with refractory dermatomyositis, IVIG significantly improved the patients' strength compared to placebo.[99] The improvement becomes noticeable about 15 days after the first IVIG infusion, and it is clear and definitive after the second infusion. Marked improvement is also noticed in the active violaceous rash or the chronic scaly eruptions on the knuckles. Repeated infusions may be required every 6 to 12 weeks to maintain improvement. In several patients we have been able to lower the prednisone dose and keep only a low maintenance dose. Some patients with DM who had become unresponsive to steroids may respond again to prednisone after a few IVIG infusions.

Because DM responds to steroids, IVIG therapy is best reserved for steroid-resistant patients, either as a second-line therapy or as a third-line add-on therapy in patients who are not adequately controlled with combination of steroids and methotrexate or azathioprine and for patients who are immunodeficient or in whom immunosuppressants are contraindicated. In children and in older patients, it can be used as a first-line therapy after a short course of steroids.

The beneficial effect of IVIg in PM has been documented only in open-label trials. A controlled study started by this group 15 years ago was never completed. It is common experience, however, that IVIg is effective in the majority of patients with PM.

If Steroids and IVIg are Ineffective or Inadequate to Induce Remission

In most of these cases, it is prudent to evaluate the patient's diagnosis. If the diagnosis is secured (based on the unique clinical features, as in DM, or with new muscle biopsy, as in PM) or the patient had clearly responded to steroid and IVIg early in the disease course, the following can be used.

Rituximab

This drug is a monoclonal antibody against CD20+ B cells resulting in B-cell depletion that lasts for at least 6 months. There is evidence based on number of reports that rituximab at 375 $\mu g/m^2$ once a week for 4 weeks or 2 g (divided in two biweekly infusions) can be beneficial to patients with DM and PM resistant to therapies.[101,102,102a] A NIH-sponsored multicenter trial is in progress.

Cyclophosphamide

In patients who have interstitial lung disease and severe clinical myopathy unresponsive to other agents, this drug can be used at doses of 0.5 to 1 g/m^2 intravenously per month. Adequate hydration the day before and antiemetics are helpful. Adverse reactions include nausea, vomiting, alopecia, hemorrhagic cystitis, bone marrow suppression, secondary malignancies, and sterility. Contraceptives are recommended for women and sperm preservation for men. It is critical to monitor the neutrophil count (no less than 1500–2000) and the lymphocyte count (no less than 1000) at 7, 10, 14, and 21 days and perform frequent urinalysis even after the drug was stopped.

Tacrolimus

Formerly known as FK 506, tacrolimus is structurally different from cyclosporine, although they share the ability to selectively inhibit the transcription of cytokines, specifically IL-2. There is evidence that tacrolimus is effective in some difficult cases of polymyositis, especially when there is interstitial lung disease.[103–105]

Other, Newer Agents

In difficult cases, other agents have been used with limited success. These include anti-TNF-α agents such as etanercep (Embrel) and infliximab, sirolimus, and Campath.[106–108]

Step-by-Step Approach

In the absence of evidence-based studies, an algorithm in the management of these diseases remains empirical and somewhat biased. In my experience, the excellent effect of IVIg in many DM and PM patients and the limited beneficial effect achieved by the other immunosuppressants have changed the order in which I use these agents. If steroids are inadequate, I go directly to IVIg, followed by the addition of one of the aforementioned immunosuppressants. A personal step-by-step approach to the treatment of DM and PM is as follows:

Step 1. Prednisone (in aggressive cases, combination with another agent listed in steps 2 and 3 is preferred by some practitioners).

Step 2. IVIg (the use of IVIg as a second-line therapy is justified based on the observation that the immunosuppressants listed in step 3 have a mild effect alone and mostly a steroid-sparing effect).

Step 3. Immunosuppressants, such as azathioprine, methotrexate, mycophenolate, or cyclosporine, only as steroid-sparing agents. These drugs are usually ineffective in steroid-resistant cases.

Step 4. Newer agents: rituximab, tacrolimus, rapamycin, Campath.

Treatment of Inclusion Body Myositis

In spite of immunopathologic features identical with PM, IBM patients are difficult to treat. Although a number of patients may transiently respond to steroids, the majority do not. Methotrexate in a controlled study was not better than placebo. Cyclosporine, azathioprine, and Cellcept are mostly ineffective although some patients may initially respond to some degree. IVIg may provide some benefit to a small number of patients for a period of time, especially in dysphagia, as demonstrated with controlled studies.[109–111] Although no statistically significant differences were noted overall, regional difference in certain muscle groups, especially the muscles of swallowing, were observed.[109] Dysphagia appears to be the main symptom that improves consistently, as documented on subsequent open-label trials.[111] Because dysphagia is life-threatening, IVIG can be considered in patients with significant swallowing difficulties and choking episodes.[4,98,107] Cricopharyngeal myotomy may be another option,[112] although in our experience it does not always work. Collectively, my approach to the treatment of patients with IBM is sequentially as follows:

1. Inform the patient that there is no proven effective therapy. I prescribe coenzyme Q_{10}, even though there is no demonstrable benefit, as a means to enhance endurance, given the mitochondrial changes in the biopsy. I also advocate a systematic nonfatiguing exercise program that has shown to be of benefit.[113]

2. Administer low-dose, every-other-day prednisone combined with mycophenolate in some patients hoping for disease stability with a clear explanation that the benefit from this regimen is anecdotal and short-lived and is not based on controlled studies.

3. Begin a trial with IVIg if there is significant worsening of muscle strength or life-threatening dysphagia.

4. Encourage patients to participate in one of the experimental trials. Our recently completed anecdotal and small trial with Campath has been encouraging in inducing some short-term stability.[114]

Supportive Therapy

We recommend physical therapy early in the disease to preserve existing muscle function, avoid disuse atrophy of the weak muscles, and prevent joint contractures. Evaluation of swallowing function is also recommended because dysphagia is common, especially in IBM. Speech pathologists provide practical tips on how to prevent choking episodes and diminish the anxiety of an impending aspiration not only for the patient but also for the immediate family.

Occupational and rehabilitation therapists help the patients with their ambulation by providing canes, braces, or wheelchairs according to the stage of their disease or by teaching them how to walk without falling (by "locking" on the knees or by using light braces), and how to perform easier fine motor tasks. Proper emotional support to accept these aids is essential; the patients and their families should be convinced that these means are not demoralizing but realistic approaches to improve transportation and socialization.

Emotional support is also fundamental, especially for young patients with DM who are discouraged by a disfiguring rash, calcifications, and steroid side effects. Reassurance that these symptoms improve with aggressive therapies and many steroid side effects are short-lived is important.

Practical Therapeutic Considerations

In light of the information presented earlier regarding the efficacy of these therapies, the following observations and practical tips may be useful:

- Patients with bona fide PM and DM should almost always respond to prednisone to a certain degree and for some period of time.

- A patient with presumed PM who has not responded to any form of immunotherapy most likely has IBM or an "inflammatory dystrophy." In these cases, a repeat muscle biopsy and a more vigorous search for the other disease are recommended.

- Calcinosis, a manifestation of DM, does not resolve with immunotherapies. New calcium deposits may be prevented if the primary disease responds to the available therapies. Diphosphonates, aluminum hydroxide, probenecid, colchicines, low doses of warfarin, and surgical excision have all been tried without success. Diltiazem may also be of benefit.[115]

- If prednisone or the other immunosuppressive therapies have not helped or have become ineffective in improving the patient's strength, they should be discontinued to avoid severe, irreversible adverse effects because, contrary to common belief, there is no evidence that their continuation maintains stability or prevents further disease progression.

- In patients with cancer-associated myositis, the treatment should be aggressive to treat the cancer. Searches for possible cancer in DM patients should be a consideration during the first 3 years.

- Patients with interstitial lung disease may have a high mortality rate and require aggressive treatment with cyclophosphamide, cyclosporine, or tacrolimus.

- Physical therapy to preserve existing muscle function, avoid disuse atrophy of the weak muscles, and prevent joint contractures should start early in the disease.

- When treatment of PM is unsuccessful, the patient should be reevaluated and the muscle biopsy reexamined. A new biopsy might be considered to make sure that the diagnosis is correct and that IBM or one of the inflammatory dystrophies has not been overlooked. The disorders most commonly mistaken for PM are IBM, an inflammatory sporadic limb girdle dystrophy with endomysial inflammation resembling polymyositis (such as dysferlinopathies, calpainopathy, caveolinopathy, sarcoglyconopathy), metabolic myopathy (such as phosphorylase or acid maltase deficiency), endocrinopathy, drug-induced myopathies with some secondary inflammatory features (such as the one due to statins), and neurogenic muscular atrophies.

The major pitfalls leading to failure of steroid or immunosuppressive treatment include the following:

- Inadequate initial dose of prednisone or cytotoxic drugs
- Short duration of therapy or quick tapering
- Early discontinuation of prednisone without keeping a "maintenance" low-dose therapy
- Early development of preventable side effects necessitating early discontinuation of prednisone
- Wrong diagnosis

Outcome

DM responds more favorably to therapy than PM. Overall, most patients improve, and many of them make a full functional recovery, which is sustained with maintenance therapy.[96] However, up to 30% of the patients may be left with residual muscle weakness or calcifications. The 5-year survival rate for treated patients with PM and DM is now approaching 80%. On the other hand, IBM is predictably disabling. Most of these patients will require use of an assistive device such as a cane, walker, or wheelchair. The older the age at onset, the more rapidly progressive the course of IBM appears to be.

References

1. Dalakas MC: Polymyositis, dermatomyositis and inclusion body myositis, *N Engl J Med* 325:1487–1498, 1991.
2. Engel AG, Hohlfeld R: The polymyositis and dermatomyositis syndromes. In Engel AG, Franzini-Armstrong C, editors: *Myology*, 3rd ed, New York, 2004, McGraw-Hill, pp 1321–1366.
3. Mastaglia FL, Phillips BA: Idiopathic inflammatory myopathies: epidemiology, classification and diagnostic criteria, *Rheum Dis Clin North Am* 28:723–741, 2002.
4. Dalakas MC: Immunopathogenesis of inflammatory myopathies, *Ann Neurol* 37:74–86, 1995.
5. Dalakas MC: Inflammatory disorders of muscle: progress in polymyositis, dermatomyositis and inclusion body myositis, *Curr Opin Neurol* 17:561–567, 2004.
6. Dalakas MC, Hohlfeld R: Diagnostic criteria for polymyositis and dermatomyositis, *Lancet* 362:1762–1763, 2003.
7. Dalakas MC, Hohlfeld R: Polymyositis and dermatomyositis, *Lancet* 362:971–982, 2003.
8. Callen JP: Dermatomyositis, *Lancet* 355(9197):53–57, 2000.
9. Dalakas MC, Karpati G: The inflammatory myopathies. In Karpati G, David Hilton-Jones D, Griggs RC, editors: *Disorders of Voluntary Muscle*, 8th ed, Cambridge, 2010, Cambridge University Press, pp 427–452.
10. Mastaglia FL: Neuromuscular disorders: molecular and therapeutic insights, *Lancet Neurol* 4(1):6–7, 2005.
11. Dalakas MC: Toxic and drug-induced myopathies, *J Neurol Neurosurg Psychiatry* 80:832–838, 2009.
12. Dalakas MC: Inflammatory and toxic myopathies, *Curr Opin Neurol Neurosurg* 5(5):645–654, 1992.
13. Hohlfeld R, Goebels N, Engel AG: Cellular mechanisms in inflammatory myopathies, *Baillieres Clin Neurol* 2(3):617–635, 1993.
14. Karpati G, Carpenter S: Pathology of the inflammatory myopathies, *Baillières Clin Neurol* 2:527–556, 1993.
15. Needham M, Mastaglia FL: Inclusion body myositis: current pathogenetic concepts and diagnostic and therapeutic approaches, *Lancet Neurol* 6(7):620–631, 2007. Review.
16. Sekul EA, Dalakas MC: Inclusion body myositis: new concepts, *Semin Neurol* 13:256–263, 1993.
17. Engel AG, Arahata K: Monoclonal antibody analysis of mononuclear cells in myopathies. II: phenotypes of autoinvasive cells in polymyositis and inclusion body myositis, *Ann Neurol* 16:209–215, 1984.
18. Griggs RC, Askanas V, DiMauro S, et al: Inclusion body myositis and myopathies, *Ann Neurol* 38:705–713, 1995.
19. Carpenter S: Inclusion body myositis, a review, *J Neuropathol Exp Neurol* 55(11):1105–1114, 1996.
20. Karpati G: Inclusion body myositis—status, *Neurologist* 3:201–208, 1997.
21. Dalakas MC: Inflammatory, immune, and viral aspects of inclusion-body myositis, *Neurology* 66(2 Suppl 1):S33–S38, 2006.
22. Sivakumar K, Dalakas MC: The spectrum of familial inclusion body myopathies in 13 families and description of a quadriceps sparing phenotype in non-Iranian Jews, *Neurology* 47:977–984, 1996.
23. Sivakumar K, Dalakas MC: Inclusion body myositis and myopathies, *Curr Opin Neurol* 10:413–420, 1997.
24. Argov Z, Yarom R: 'Rimmed vacuole myopathy' sparing the quadriceps: a unique disorder in Iranian Jews, *J Neurol Sci* 64:33–43, 1984.

25. Sekul EA, Chow C, Dalakas MC: Magnetic resonance imaging of the forearm as a diagnostic aid in patients with inclusion body myositis, *Neurology* 48:863–866, 1997.

26. Luciano CA, Dalakas MC: A macro-EMG study in inclusion-body myositis: no evidence for a neurogenic component, *Neurology* 48:29–33, 1997.

27. Koffman BM, Rugiero M, Dalakas MC: Autoimmune diseases and autoantibodies associated with sporadic inclusion body myositis, *Muscle Nerve* 21:115–117, 1998.

28. Badrising UA, Schreuder GM, Giphart MJ, et al: Associations with autoimmune disorders and HLA class I and II antigens in inclusion body myositis, *Neurology* 63(12):2396–2398, 2004.

29. Koffman BM, Sivakumar K, Simonis T, et al: HLA allele distribution distinguishes sporadic inclusion body myositis from hereditary inclusion body myopathies, *J Neuroimmunol* 84:139–142, 1998.

30. Sivakumar K, Semino-Mora C, Dalakas MC: An inflammatory, familial, inclusion body myositis with autoimmune features and a phenotype identical to sporadic inclusion body myositis: studies in 3 families, *Brain* 120:653–661, 1997.

31. Argov Z, Tiram E, Eisenberg I, et al: Various types of hereditary inclusion body myopathies map to chromosome 9p1–q1, *Ann Neurol* 41(4):548–551, 1997.

32. Rosenbaum ML, Silverberg NB: Amyopathic dermatomyositis associated with familial polyposis coli, *Pediatr Dermatol* 21(1):91–92, 2004.

33. Peng A, Koffman BM, Malley JD, et al: Disease progression in sporadic inclusion body myositis (s-IBM): observations in 78 patients, *Neurology* 55:296–298, 2000.

34. Layzer RB, Shearn MA, Satya-Murti S: Eosinophilic polymyositis, *Ann Neurol* 1:65–71, 1977.

35. Lakhanpal S, Duffy J, Engel AG: Eosinophilia associated with perimyositis and pneumonitis, *Mayo Clin Proc* 63(1):37–41, 1988.

36. Krahn M, Lopez de Munain A, Streichenberger N, et al: CAPN3 mutations in patients with idiopathic eosinophilic myositis, *Ann Neurol* 59:905–911, 2006.

37. Hertzman PA, Blevins WL, Mayer J, et al: Association of the eosinophilia-myalgia syndrome with the ingestion of tryptophan, *N Engl J Med* 322:869–873, 1990.

38. Seidman RJ, Kaufman LD, Sokoloff L, et al: The neuromuscular pathology of the eosinophilia-myalgia syndrome, *J Neuropathol Exp Neurol* 50(1):49–62, 1991.

39. Illa I, Dinsmore S, Dalakas MC: Immune-mediated mechanisms and immune activation of fibroblasts in the pathogenesis of eosinophilia-myalgia syndrome induced by L-tryptophan, *Hum Pathol* 24:702–709, 1993.

40. Gherardi RK, Coquet M, Cherin P, et al: Macrophagic myofasciitis: an emerging entity. Groupe d'Etudes et Recherche sur les Maladies Musculaires Acquises et Dysimmunitaires (GERMMAD) de l'Association Francaise contre les Myopathies (AFM), *Lancet* 352(9125):347–352, 1998.

41. Karpati G, Pouliot Y, Carpenter S: Expression of immunoreactive major histocompatibility complex products in human skeletal muscles, *Ann Neurol* 23:64–72, 1988.

42. Greenberg SA: Proposed immunologic models of inflammatory myopathies and potential therapeutic implications, *Neurology* 69:2008–2019, 2007.

43. Askanas V: Engel WK Sporadic inclusion-body myositis and hereditary inclusion-body myopathies: current concepts of diagnosis and pathogenesis, *Curr Opin Rheumatol* 10:530–542, 1998.

44. Mendell JR, Sahenk Z, Gales T, et al: Amyloid filaments in inclusion body myositis, *Arch Neurol* 48:1229–1234, 1991.

45. Lotz BP, Engel AG, Nishino H, et al: Inclusion body myositis. Observations in 40 patients, *Brain* 112:727–747, 1989.

46. Askanas V, Engel WK, Bilak M, et al: Twisted tubulofilaments of inclusion body myositis muscle resemble paired helical filaments of Alzheimer brain containing hyperphosphorylated tau, *Am J Pathol* 144:177–187, 1994.

47. Askanas V, Serdaroglu P, Engel WK, et al: Immunocytochemical localization of ubiquitin in inclusion body myositis allows its light-microscopic distinction from polymyositis, *Neurology* 42:460–461, 1992.

48. Askanas V, Engel WK, Alvarez RB, et al: 4-Amyloid protein immunoreactivity in muscle of patients with inclusion-body myositis, *Lancet* 339:560–561, 1992.

49. Askanas V, Engel WK, Alvarez RB: Enhanced detection of Congo-red-positive amyloid deposits in muscle fibers of inclusion body myositis

50. Mendel JR, Sahenk Z, Gales L, Paul L: Amyloid filaments in inclusion body myositis. Novel findings provide insight into nature of filaments, *Arch Neurol* 48:1229–1234, 1991.

51. Askanas V, Engel WK: Inclusion-body myositis: a myodegenerative conformational disorder associated with Abeta, protein misfolding, and proteasome inhibition, *Neurology* 66(2 Suppl 1):S39–S48, 2006.

52. De Bleecker JL, Ertl BB, Engel AG: Patterns of abnormal protein expression in target formations and unstructured cores, *Neuromuscul Disord* 6:339–349, 1996.

53. Semino-Mora C, Dalakas MC: Rimmed vacuoles with β-amyloid and ubiquitinated filamentous deposits in the muscles of patients with long-standing denervation (post-poliomyelitis muscular atrophy): similarities with inclusion body myositis, *Hum Pathol* 29:1128–1133, 1998.

54. Lünemann JD, Schmidt J, Schmid D, et al: Beta-amyloid is a substrate of autophagy in sporadic inclusion body myositis, *Ann Neurol* 61(5):476–483, 2007.

55. Greenberg SA, Watts GD, Kimonis VE, et al: Nuclear localization of valosin-containing protein in normal muscle and muscle affected by inclusion-body myositis, *Muscle Nerve* 36(4):447–454, 2007.

56. Horvath R, Fu K, Genge A, et al: Characterization of the mitochondrial DNA abnormalities in the skeletal muscle of patients with inclusion body myositis, *J Neuropath Exp Neurol* 57:396–403, 1998.

57. Emslie-Smith AM, Arahata K, Engel AG: Major histocompatibility complex class I antigen expression, immunologicalization of interferon subtypes, and T cell–mediated cytotoxicity in myopathies, *Hum Pathol* 20:224–231, 1989.

58. Dalakas MC: Sporadic inclusion body myositis—diagnosis, pathogenesis and therapeutic strategies, *Nat Clin Pract Neurol* 2(8):437–447, 2006.

59. Kissel JT, Burrow KL, Rammohan KW, for the CIDD Group. Mononuclear cell analysis of muscle biopsies in prednisone-treated and untreated Duchenne muscular dystrophy, *Neurology* 41:667–672, 1991.

60. Dalakas MC: Advances in the treatment of Myositis, *Nature Review Rheumatol* 129–137, 2010.

61. Chahin N, Engel AG: Correlation of muscle biopsy, clinical course, and outcome in PM and sporadic IBM, *Neurology* 70(6):418–424, 2008.

62. Raju R, Dalakas MC: Gene expression profile in the muscles of patients with inflammatory myopathies: effect of therapy with IVIG and biological validation of clinically relevant genes, *Brain* 128(Pt 8):1887–1896, 2005.

63. Dalakas MC: Inflammatory muscle diseases: a critical review on pathogenesis and therapies, *Curr Opin Pharmacol* 2010 (in press).

64. Hohlfeld R, Engel AG: The immunobiology of muscle, *Immunol Today* 15(6):269–274, 1994.

65. Wiendl H, Hohlfeld R, Kieseier BC: Immunobiology of muscle: advances in understanding an immunological microenvironment, *Trends Immunol* 26(7):373–380, 2005.

66. Dalakas MC: Treatment of polymyositis and dermatomyositis. Signaling pathways and immunobiology of inflammatory myopathies, *Nat Clin Pract Rheumatol* 2:219–227, 2006.

67. Dalakas MC: Viral myopathies. In Engel AG, Franzini-Armstrong C, editors: *Myology*, vol II, New York, 2006, McGraw-Hill, pp 1419–1437.

68. Nishino H, Engel AG, Rima BK: Inclusion body myositis: the mumps virus hypothesis, *Ann Neurol* 25:260–264, 1989.

69. Leff RL, Love LA, Miller FW, et al: Viruses in the idiopathic inflammatory myopathies: absence of candidate viral genomes in muscle, *Lancet* 339:1192–1195, 1992.

70. Dalakas MC, Pezeshkpour GH, Gravell M, et al: Polymyositis in patients with AIDS, *JAMA* 256:2381–2383, 1986.

71. Dalakas MC, London WT, Gravell M, et al: Polymyositis in an immunodeficiency disease in monkeys induced by a type D retrovirus, *Neurology* 36:569–572, 1986.

72. Dalakas MC, Pezeshkpour GH: Neuromuscular diseases associated with human immunodeficiency virus infection, *Ann Neurol* 23(Suppl):38–48, 1988.

73. Morgan O St C, Rodgers-Johnson P, Mora C, et al: HTLV-1 and polymyositis in Jamaica, *Lancet* 2:1184–1187, 1989.

74. Cupler EJ, Leon-Monzon M, Miller J, et al: Inclusion body myositis in HIV-I and HTLV-I infected patients, *Brain* 19:1887–1893, 1996.

and brain of Alzheimer disease using fluorescence technique, *Neurology* 43:1265–1267, 1993.

75. Ozden S, Gessain A, Gout O, et al: Sporadic inclusion body myositis in a patient with human T cell leukemia virus type 1–associated myelopathy, *Clin Infect Dis* 32(3):510–514, 2001.

76. Illa I, Nath A, Dalakas MC: Immunocytochemical and virological characteristics of HIV-associated inflammatory myopathies: similarities with seronegative polymyositis, *Ann Neurol* 29:474–481, 1991.

77. Leon-Monzon M, Lamperth L, Dalakas MC: Search for HIV proviral DNA and amplified sequences in the muscle biopsies of patients with HIV-polymyositis, *Muscle Nerve* 16:408–413, 1993.

78. Leon-Monzon M, Illa I, Dalakas MC: Polymyositis in patients infected with HTLV-1: the role of the virus in the cause of the disease, *Ann Neurol* 36:643–649, 1994.

79. Saito M, Higuchi I, Saito A, et al: Molecular analysis of T cell clonotypes in muscle-infiltrating lymphocytes from patients with human T lymphotropic virus type 1 polymyositis, *J Infect Dis* 186(9):1231–1241, 2002.

80. Ozden S, Cochet M, Mikol J, et al: Direct evidence for a chronic CD8$^+$-T-cell-mediated immune reaction to tax within the muscle of a human T-cell leukemia/lymphoma virus type 1-infected patient with sporadic inclusion body myositis, *J Virol* 78(19):10320–10327, 2004.

81. Dalakas MC, Rakocevic G, Shatunov A, et al: Inclusion body myositis with human immunodeficiency virus infection: four cases with clonal expansion of viral-specific T cells, *Ann Neurol* 61(5):466–475, 2007.

82. Nagaraju K, Casciola-Rosen L, Lundberg I, et al: Activation of the endoplasmic reticulum stress response in autoimmune myositis: potential role in muscle fiber damage and dysfunction, *Arthritis Rheum* 52(6):1824–1835, 2005.

83. Ferrer I, Martín B, Castaño JG, et al: Proteasomal expression, induction of immunoproteasome subunits, and local MHC class I presentation in myofibrillar myopathy and inclusion body myositis, *J Neuropathol Exp Neurol* 63(5):484–498, 2004.

84. Vattemi G, Engel WK, McFerrin J, et al: Endoplasmic reticulum stress and unfolded protein response in inclusion body myositis muscle, *Am J Pathol* 164(1):1–7, 2004.

85. Askanas V, Engel WK: Proposed pathogenetic cascade of inclusion-body myositis: importance of amyloid-beta, misfolded proteins, predisposing genes, and aging, *Curr Opin Rheumatol* 15(6):737–744, 2003.

86. Schmidt J, Barthel K, Wrede A, et al: Interrelation of inflammation and APP in sIBM: IL-1β induces accumulation of β-amyloid in skeletal muscle, *Brain* 131:1228–1240, 2008.

87. Banwell BL, Engel AG: AlphaB-crystallin immunolocalization yields new insights into inclusion body myositis, *Neurology* 54(5):1020–1021, 2000.

88. Dalakas MC: Interplay between inflammation and degeneration: using inclusion body myositis to study "neuroinflammation," *Ann Neurol* 64(1):1–3, 2008.

89. Pruitt JN 2nd, Showalter CJ, Engel AG: Sporadic inclusion body myositis: counts of different types of abnormal fibers, *Ann Neurol* 39(1):139–143, 1996.

90. Dalakas MC: Therapeutic approaches in patients with inflammatory myopathies, *Semin Neurol* 23(2):199–206, 2003.

91. Gold R, Dalakas MC, Toyka KV: Immunotherapy in autoimmune neuromuscular disorders, *Lancet Neurol* 2:22–32, 2003.

92. Hohlfeld R, Dalakas MC: Basic principles of immunotherapy in neurological diseases, *Semin Neurol* 23:121–132, 2003.

93. Mastaglia FL, Phillips BA, Zilko PJ: Treatment of inflammatory myopathies, *Muscle Nerve* 20:651–664, 1997.

94. Mastaglia FL: Treatment of autoimmune inflammatory myopathies, *Curr Opin Neurol* 13:507–509, 2000.

95. Dalakas MC: Therapy for immune-mediated inflammatory myopathies. In Johnson RT, Griffin JW, McArthur JC, editors: *Current Therapy in Neurologic Disease*, vol 7, Philadelphia, 2005, Mosby.

96. Dalakas MC: Polymyositis, dermatomyositis and inclusion body myositis. In Braunwald E, Fauci AS, Kasper DL, Hauser SL, Longo DL, Jameson JL, editors: *Harrison's Principles of Internal Medicine*, 15th ed, New York, 2001, McGraw-Hill, pp 2524–2529.

97. Dalakas MC: Advances in the immunobiology and treatment of inflammatory myopathies, *Curr Rheumatol Rep* 9(4):291–297, 2007.

98. Dalakas MC: Therapeutic targets in patients with inflammatory myopathies: present approaches and a look to the future, *Neuromuscul Disord* 16:223–236, 2006.

99. Dalakas MC: The use of intravenous immunoglobulin in the treatment of autoimmune neurological disorders: evidence-based indications and safety profile, *Pharmacol Ther* 102:177–193, 2004.

100. Dalakas MC, Illa I, Dambrosia JM, et al: A controlled trial of high-dose intravenous immunoglobulin infusions as treatment for dermatomyositis, *N Engl J Med* 329:1993–2000, 1993.

101. Levine TD: Rituximab in the treatment of dermatomyositis: an open-label pilot study, *Arthritis Rheum* 52:601–607, 2005.

102. Chung L, Genovese MC, Fiorentino DF: A pilot trial of rituximab in the treatment of patients with dermatomyositis, *Arch Dermatol* 143(6):763–767, 2007.

102a. Valiyil R, Casciola-Rosen L, Hong G, et al: Rituximab therapy for myopathy associated with anti-signal recognition particle antibodies: a case series, *Arthritis Care Res*, in press.

103. Oddis CV, Sciurba FC, Elmagd KA, et al: Tacrolimus in refractory polymyositis with interstitial lung disease, *Lancet* 353:1762–1763, 1999.

104. Shimojima Y, Gono T, Yamamoto K, et al: (Efficacy of tacrolimus in treatment of polymyositis associated with myasthenia gravis), *Clin Rheumatol* 23:262–265, 2004.

105. Yamada A, Ohshima Y, Omata N, et al: Steroid-sparing effect of tacrolimus in a patient with juvenile dermatomyositis presenting poorbioavailability of cyclosporine A, *Eur J Pediatr* 163:561–562, 2004.

106. Hengstman GJ, van den Hoogen FH, Barrera P, et al: Successful treatment of dermatomyositis and polymyositis with anti-tumor necrosis factor-alpha: preliminary observations, *Eur Neurol* 50:10–15, 2003.

107. Labioche I, Liozon E, Weschler B, et al: Refractory polymyositis responding to infliximab: extended follow-up, *Rheumatology (Oxford)* 43:531–532, 2004.

108. Nadiminti U, Arbiser JL: Rapamycin (sirolimus) as a steroid-sparing agent in dermatomyositis, *J Am Acad Dermatol* 52:17–19, 2005.

109. Dalakas MC, Sonies B, Dambrosia J, et al: Treatment of inclusion body myositis with IVIG: a double-blind, placebo-control study, *Neurology* 48:712–716, 1997.

110. Walter MC, Lochmuller H, Toepfer M, et al: High-dose immunoglobulin therapy in sporadic inclusion body myositis: a double-blind, placebo-controlled study, *J Neurol* 247:22–28, 2000.

111. Cherin P, Pelletier S, Teixeira A, et al: Intravenous immunoglobulin for dysphagia of inclusion body myositis, *Neurology* 58:326, 2002.

112. Verma A, Bradley W, Adesina AM, et al: Inclusion body myositis with cricopharyngeus muscle involvement and severe dysphagia, *Muscle Nerve* 14:470–473, 1991.

113. Spector SA, Lemmer MS, Koffman BM, et al: Safety and efficacy of strength training in patients with sporadic inclusion body myositis, *Muscle Nerve* 20:1242–1248, 1997.

114. Dalakas MC, Rakocevic G, Schmidt J, et al: Effect of alemtuzumab (Campath 1-H), in patient with inclusion body myositis, *Brain* 132(Pt 6):1536–1544, 2009.

115. Bertorini TE, Sebes JI, Palmieri GM, et al: Dialtiazem in the treatment of calcinosis in juvenile dermatomyositis, *J Clin Neuromuscul Dis* 2:191–193, 2001.

Matthias Vorgerd, MD
Marcus Deschauer, MD

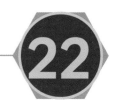

Treatment and Management of Hereditary Metabolic Myopathies

Hereditary metabolic myopathies are a group of muscle disorders that result from a shortage of energy producton (i.e., deficiency of adenosine triphosphate [ATP]). In muscle, ATP is produced by aerobic glycogenesis or glycogenolysis and glycolysis, using the respiratory chain, or by anaerobic glycolysis, resulting in lactate production. For sustained work, muscle switches its energy source to fatty acid oxidation. Important pathways in muscle metabolism are shown in Figure 22-1. Therefore, metabolic myopathies typically present with exercise-induced symptoms, including myalgia, cramps, muscle weakness, and rhabdomyolysis resulting in myoglobinuria. In glycogenoses symptoms typically emerge after short exercise, whereas myopathies of lipid metabolism manifest after prolonged exercise. However, these typical signs are not present in all metabolic myopathies. In some disorders there is permanent, predominantly proximal muscle weakness that resembles limb girdle muscular dystrophies.

Many different enzyme defects are known to cause metabolic myopathies. They are classified as glycogenoses, myopathies of lipid metabolism, and mitochondrial myopathies. Some of them are very rare, but a few disorders are rather common. Myophosphorylase deficiency (McArdle disease) and acid α-glucosidase deficiency (Pompe disease) are common glycogenoses. Carnitine palmitoyltransferase II (CPT II) deficiency is a common disorder of lipid metabolism and a frequent cause of hereditary myoglobinuria. Chronic progressive external ophthalmoplegia (CPEO) is a common mitochondrial disorder. These conditions are discussed in some detail in this chapter. Additionally, this chapter also covers the evaluation and management of myoglobinuria.

Muscle Disorders of Glycogen Metabolism

Disorders of glycogen metabolism, termed *glycogenoses* or *glycogen storage diseases* (GSD), are caused by genetic deficiencies of various enzymes or transporters, involved either directly in the synthesis or breakdown of glycogen or in the utilization of its catabolite, glucose-1-phosphate (Fig. 22-2). Glycogenoses can be multisystemic disorders or can preferentially affect only certain tissues, often but not always reflecting the tissue specificity of expression of the mutant gene. Liver and muscle are the tissues in which glycogen is most abundant and in which it plays its most prominent physiologic roles: as a reservoir for systemic glucose homeostasis in liver, and for local glycolytic energy production in exercising muscle. Therefore, most glycogenoses manifest primarily in liver, in muscle,

or in both, although in some forms the kidney, heart, nervous system, or erythrocytes can also be affected.

Here we present in more detail the glycogenoses that predominantly affect skeletal muscle metabolism, causing neuromuscular symptoms (Table 22-1). The two main syndromes of muscle glycogenoses can be defined as exercise intolerance with myalgia, early fatigue, and painful cramps or permanent muscle atrophy and weakness. In some GSD patients, these syndromes may overlap from the beginning or muscle weakness may appear years after symptoms of exercise intolerance begin.

Clinical Presentation of Myopathies Caused by Enzyme Defects of Glycogen Metabolism

GSD II (Pompe Disease)

Glycogen storage disease type II (Pompe disease) is an autosomal recessive disorder caused by a lack of the lysosomal enzyme acid α-glucosidase, also called *acid maltase*. Acid α-glucosidase catalyzes the hydrolysis of glycogen to glucose within the acidic milieu of lysosomes. In acid α-glucosidase deficiency, the pool of glycogen that enters the lysosomes via autophagy is poorly degraded and overloads the lysosomal system. This leads to a progressive and irreversible cellular damage, mostly of the skeletal and cardiac muscle fibers.

The number of individuals born with GSD II is estimated to be 1 in 40,000. GSD II patients present with a continuous spectrum of phenotypes, with variable age at onset, variable severity, and variable rate of progression. Although there is a wide continuum, three forms have been described in more detail in the literature: (1) infantile GSD II ("classic" Pompe disease) presents in the first few months of life, and most infants die within 12 months from cardiorespiratory insufficiency, (2) "nonclassic" GSD II begins between ages 1 and 2 years, and (3) late-onset GSD has the onset of symptoms at any time after age 2 years, including GSD II presenting in childhood, adolescence, and adulthood (Fig. 22-3). The natural course of late-onset GSD II was studied in detail in 54 Dutch patients from 45 families. In this large group of patients, the first complaints started at a mean age of 28 ± 14.3 years and were mostly related to mobility problems and limb-girdle weakness. Problems in running and playing sports were reported in approximately 70%, climbing stairs in about 30%, rising from an armchair in 20%, walking in 17%, and rising from a lying position in about 10% of the patients. Fatigue and muscle cramps were frequent first complaints. Approximately 60% of the adult patients had mild muscular symptoms

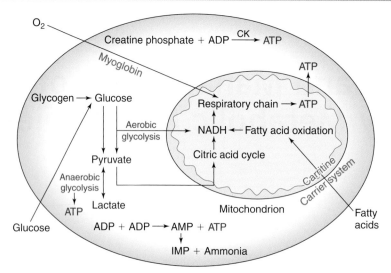

Figure 22-1 Schematic presentation of important energy pathways in muscle metabolism. ADP, adenosine diphosphate; AMP, adenosine monophosphate; ATP, adenosine triphosphate; CK, creatine kinase; IMP, inosine 5′-phosphate; NADH, reduced nicotinamide adenine dinucleotide.

during childhood, such as running more slowly than other children, being unable to keep up with other children during physical exercise or when playing games, as well as frequent falls or gait disturbance. In 28% of the patients, the final diagnosis was made more than 5 years after the first visit to a physician for disease-related symptoms. Some patients were initially diagnosed as having spinal muscular atrophy, Duchenne muscular dystrophy, or Becker muscular dystrophy. Nearly all patients experienced problems walking, varying from imbalance or a waddling gait to a complete inability to walk. About 50% of the group used a wheelchair, and the mean age at which patients started using a wheelchair was 46.1 ± 12.4 years. Approximately 40% required artificial ventilation at the time of investigation, either noninvasively by nose hood or facemask or invasively by trachea cannula. The mean age at the start of artificial ventilation was 48.6 ± 16.3 years. The course of the late-onset GSD II form was shown to be quite variable between patients with respect to age at onset and rate of disease progression. There was also variability regarding the time at which patients first needed wheelchairs or artificial ventilation.

More than 200 different mutations within the *GAA* gene have been identified so far (www.pompecenter.nl). Approximately 63% of these lead to total loss of acid α-glucosidase, 12% to partial deficiency, and 25% are nonpathogenic. In general, there is good correlation between the nature of the mutation, the degree of residual enzyme activity, and the severity of the clinical presentation. Many patients with the late-onset form carry the c.-32-13T>G mutation on one allele with another *GAA* mutation on the second allele. Some of the mutations are found more frequently in different ethnic groups.[1] In the Netherlands, where extended molecular studies have been undertaken, a deletion at nucleotide 525 in exon 2 (del525T) leading to a frameshift (p.Glu176fsX45) and a large deletion of exon 18 (c.2481+102_2646+31del) are frequent. The p.R854X (c.2560C>T) mutation was frequently found among African Americans, and the p.D645E (c.1935C>A) mutation among Asians.

GSD III
Glycogen-debranching enzyme plays an important role in the degradation of glycogen and has two independent catalytic activities, oligo-1,4→1,4-glucanotransferase and amylo-1,6-glucosidase, on a single 160-kDa protein. Both activities and glycogen binding are required for complete function. In GSD III, debrancher activities are virtually

absent in affected organs; the deficiency causes excessive accumulation of abnormal glycogen with truncated outer chains. Most patients (GSD IIIa) have liver and muscle involvement of variable severity and clinical onset. Typical symptoms include fasting hypoglycemia, hepatomegaly, growth retardation, progressive myopathy, and cardiomyopathy. Some patients have only liver involvement without evidence of a myopathy (GSD IIIb).

GSD IV (Andersen Disease)
Andersen disease (GSD IV, or amylopectinosis) is an autosomal recessive disease caused by mutations in the glycogen branching enzyme 1 (*GBE1*) gene, resulting in deficiency of the glycogen branching enzyme (GBE). GBE participates with glycogen synthase in the synthesis of glycogen by transferring a minimum of six α-1,4-linked glycosyl units into an α-1,6 position. The human *GBE1* gene is located on chromosome 3p12.3, and has a coding sequence of 2.106 bp with 16 exons encoding a 702–amino acid GBE protein, which is ubiquitously expressed.

Deficiency of GBE results in the accumulation of abnormal, amylopectin-like polysaccharide with fewer branching points, more 1,4-linked units, and longer outer branches than normal glycogen. These are called *polyglucosans*, and they accumulate in all tissues to various degrees. The typical clinical phenotype of GSD IV as originally described is characterized by failure to thrive, hepatosplenomegaly, and progressive liver cirrhosis leading to death in early childhood. The neuromuscular presentation of GSD IV is remarkably heterogeneous with four main variants. The perinatal form presents as fetal akinesia deformation sequence and is characterized by multiple congenital contractures (arthrogryposis multiplex congenita), hydrops fetalis, and perinatal death. The congenital form includes hypotonia, muscle wasting, neuronal involvement, inconsistent cardiomyopathy, and death in early infancy. The childhood form is dominated by myopathy, a neuromuscular form, or by cardiomyopathy. The adult form can present as an isolated myopathy or as a multisystem disorder with central and peripheral nervous system involvement (adult polyglucosan body disease).

GSD V (McArdle Disease)
Glycogenosis type V (GSD V), also known as myophosphorylase deficiency or McArdle disease, is the most common disorder of

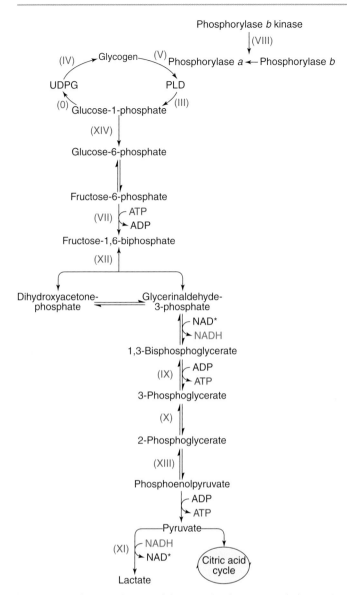

Phosphorylase *b* kinase

$|$(VIII)

(IV) → Glycogen — (V) Phosphorylase *a* ← Phosphorylase *b*

UDPG   PLD

(0) Glucose-1-phosphate   (III)

(XIV)

Glucose-6-phosphate

Fructose-6-phosphate

(VII) ⌐ ATP
      ⌊→ ADP

Fructose-1,6-biphosphate

(XII)

Dihydroxyacetone-   Glycerinaldehyde-
phosphate   3-phosphate

⌐ NAD*
⌊→ NADH

1,3-Bisphosphoglycerate

(IX) ⌐ ADP
     ⌊→ ATP

3-Phosphoglycerate

(X)

2-Phosphoglycerate

(XIII)

Phosphoenolpyruvate

⌐ ADP
⌊→ ATP

Pyruvate

(XI) ⌐ NADH   Citric acid
     ⌊→ NAD*   cycle

Lactate

Figure 22-2 Schematic diagram of the cytosolic glycogen metabolism and glycolysis. Roman numerals indicate the enzymes that are deficient in muscle glycogenoses: III, debranching enzyme; IV, branching enzyme; V, myophosphorylase; VII, phosphofructokinase; VIII, phosphorylase kinase; IX, phosphoglycerate kinase; X, phosphoglycerate mutase; XI, lactate dehydrogenase; XII, aldolase A; XIII, β-enolase; XIV, phosphoglucomutase 1; UDPG, uridine diphosphate glucose; PLD, phosphorylase-limit dextrin. Glycogen storage disease II is caused by a defect of acid maltase, which is located within the lysosomes (not shown in the figure). ADP, adenosine diphosphate; ATP, adenosine triphosphate; NAD, nicotinamide adenine dinucleotide; NADH, reduced nicotinamide adenine dinucleotide. (Modified from DiMauro S, Lamperti C: Muscle glycogenoses, *Muscle Nerve* 24: 984–999, 2001.)

skeletal muscle carbohydrate metabolism. GSD V is inherited in an autosomal recessive manner; patients have mutations in both alleles of the *PYGM* gene, which encodes myophosphorylase, the skeletal muscle isoform of glycogen phosphorylase. Myophosphorylase initiates the breakdown of muscle glycogen by removing α-1,4-linked glycosyl units from the outer branches of glycogen, which leads to the liberation of glucose-1-phosphate. Glucose-1-phosphate is normally converted to glucose-6-phosphate, which subsequently undergoes glycolysis, resulting in pyruvate production. Muscle

pyruvate can be converted to lactate in anaerobic conditions, which is then released to the blood. Most of the pyruvate crosses the mitochondrial membrane, where it is converted to acetyl coenzyme A (acetyl-CoA) and further metabolized in the citric acid cycle. GSD V patients have absent myophosphorylase activity and are unable to mobilize muscle glycogen stores during exercise. However, they can take up glucose from the blood, which is converted to glucose-6-phosphate and metabolized via the intact glycolytic pathway.

Glycogen storage disease V typically presents with symptoms of exercise intolerance, such as myalgia, painful cramps, muscle contractures, premature fatigue, and episodic myoglobinuria during static or dynamic exercise. In most patients, a few minutes of rest relieves these symptoms. The onset of exercise intolerance usually occurs in childhood; fixed weakness may occur with increasing age.

We examined the muscle pain characteristics in 24 German patients with McArdle disease using detailed pain questionnaires[2]; 23 patients complained of intermittent pain, and it was exercise-induced in 15. Eight patients reported a more permanent muscle pain, and 7 of those had superimposed exercise-induced myalgia. The patients with permanent pain were more often female, and they experienced more problems during higher impact general activities, resulting in decreased sleep and more fatigue. This study showed that a substantial number of McArdle disease patients have permanent pain as a major complaint. Because this permanent pain is not related to age or disease duration, it might represent a clinically relevant subgroup of McArdle disease, differing from those with "pure" exercise-induced symptoms.

A specific feature of GSD V is the "second-wind" phenomenon, which denotes a sudden improvement in exercise capacity after a few minutes of sustained exercise or when resuming exercise after a brief rest. This second wind is produced by an exercise-related increase in the capacity for muscle oxidative phosphorylation, which correlates with increased availability of blood-borne fuels such as glucose and free fatty acids. It was recently shown that fat oxidation is augmented with the onset of second wind in GSD V patients during a prolonged, low-intensity exercise of 50% to 60% of maximal oxygen uptake capacity.[3] These results support the theory that the energy deficit in GSD V may be compensated by trials of moderate aerobic exercise to enhance fat oxidation.

In rare cases, GSD V may present with a severe generalized weakness at birth and death in childhood or with late-onset permanent muscle atrophy and weakness not preceded by symptoms of exercise intolerance.

Heterozygous individuals carrying one mutation in the *PYGM* gene may develop muscle symptoms that are considered to be caused by a critically low residual level (30%–40%) of myophosphorylase activity in muscle. A few GSD V families with an apparent autosomal dominant transmission have been reported. Molecular genetic analysis in such "pseudo-dominant" families identified either symptomatic heterozygous carriers in one parent or "true" recessive GSD V in one parent and heterozygosity in the other.

The most common mutation in European and North American GSD V patients is the nonsense mutation at R50X (previously referred to as R49X). More than 60 different mutations located throughout the entire *PYGM* gene on chromosome 11q13 have been reported. We performed molecular genetic analysis in a large cohort of 56 GSD V patients from Germany, the United Kingdom, and several other European countries. Allele frequency of the R50X mutation was 58%, and 71% of the McArdle disease patients carried this mutation on at least one allele. This study also detected 26 other less common mutations, with no clear genotype-phenotype correlation with respect to age of onset or severity.[4]

Table 22-1 Clinical Symptoms and Classification of Muscle Glycogen Storage Diseases

GSD	Enzymatic Defect	Chromosome	Clinical Syndrome(s)	Characteristic Features on Muscle Biopsy
Defects in Glycogen Metabolism				
I	Muscle glycogen synthase	19q13	Cardiomyopathy, exercise intolerance	Lack of glycogen
II (Pompe)	Lysosomal α-1,4-1,6-glucosidase (acid maltase)	17q25	Infantile "classic" form: multiorgan involvement (heart, muscle, liver) Late-onset form: myopathy with atrophy and weakness, respiratory insufficiency	PAS-positive vacuoles; secondary changes: increased acid phosphatase reaction, mitochondrial alterations, autophagic vacuoles, neurogenic-like changes
III (Cori-Forbes)	Debranching enzyme (oligo-1,4-1,4-glucanotransferase, amylo-1,6-glucosidase)	1p21	IIIa: liver (hepatomegaly, growth retardation, fasting hypoglycemia), myopathy with atrophy and weakness or exercise intolerance IIIb: only liver involvement	PAS-positive vacuoles
IV (Andersen)	Branching enzyme (amylo-1,4-1,6-transglucosidase)	3p12	Congenital form: myopathy, cardiomyopathy, neuronal involvement Childhood form: myopathy, cardiomyopathy Adult form: myopathy or APBD	Diastase-resistant PAS-positive deposits; polyglucosan bodies
V (McArdle)	Myophosphorylase	11q13	Exercise intolerance, myopathy with atrophy and weakness (during late disease course),infantile form	PAS-positive deposits; negative phosphorylase staining
VIII	Phosphorylase kinase α (muscle) subunit or β-subunit	Xq13 16q13	Exercise intolerance, muscle weakness Liver and muscle involvement	PAS-positive deposits
XIV	Phosphoglucomutase 1	1p31	Exercise intolerance	PAS-positive vacuoles
Defects of Glycolytic Metabolism				
VII (Tarui)	Phosphofructokinase (muscle isoform)	12q13.3	Exercise intolerance, chronic hemolysis, infantile form (rare)	PAS-positive deposits; negative PFK staining; polyglucosan bodies
IX	Phosphoglycerate kinase	Xq13	Exercise intolerance, chronic hemolysis; rare form with CNS involvement (oligophrenia, delayed motor development, epilepsy)	PAS-positive deposits
X	Phosphoglycerate mutase (muscle isoform)	7p12	Exercise intolerance	PAS-positive deposits
XI	Lactate dehydrogenase (muscle isoform)	11p15	Exercise intolerance, dermatologic symptoms	Normal
XII	Aldolase A	16q22-q24	Exercise intolerance, chronic hemolysis	Normal
XIII	β-Enolase	17pter-p12	Exercise intolerance	PAS-positive deposits
	Triosephosphate isomerase		Myopathy with atrophy and weakness, chronic hemolysis	PAS-positive deposits; secondary changes; mitochondrial alterations

APBD, adult polyglucosan body disease (motor neuron involvement, polyneuropathy, dementia, urinary incontinence); CNS, central nervous system; GSD, glycogen storage disease; PAS, periodic acid-Schiff; PFK, phosphofructokinase.

GSD VII (*Tarui Disease*)

Tarui disease (GSD VII) is caused by an inherited deficiency of muscle phosphofructokinase (PFK) and manifests with the combination of myopathy and hemolysis. Typically, GSD VII begins in early childhood and causes painful cramps or contractures on exercise, limitation of vigorous activity, hyperuricemia, a compensated hemolytic anemia, and, less frequently, myoglobinuria. The disease seems to be prevalent among people of Jewish-Russian ancestry, and the transmission is autosomal recessive. The clinical phenotype of GSD VII is similar to that of McArdle disease, so definitive diagnosis requires biochemical demonstration of the enzyme defect.

GSD VIII

Phosphorylase kinase (Phk) is a regulatory protein kinase that stimulates glycogen breakdown. It receives input from hormonal and neuronal signals transmitted through the second messengers Ca^{2+} and adenosine 3′,5′-cyclic monophosphate (cAMP) and responds by phosphorylating and thus activating glycogen phosphorylase. Phk deficiency alone accounts for approximately 25% of all cases of glycogen storage diseases. Phk consists of four subunits in a hexadecameric complex $(\alpha\beta\gamma\delta)_4$, and each of these subunits has isoforms or splice variants differentially expressed in different tissues. Consequently, Phk deficiency occurs in several subtypes that differ in mode of inheritance and tissue involvement.

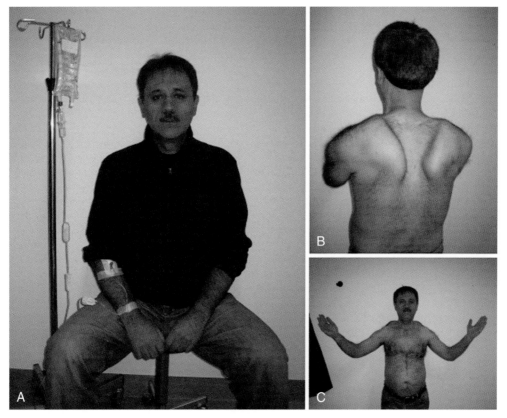

Figure 22-3 A, Patient with late-onset glycogen storage disease II on intravenous enzyme replacement therapy. **B** and **C,** He presents with scapula alata and proximal muscle weakness.

Muscle-specific glycogenosis due to Phk deficiency can manifest in three different clinical forms. Frequently, the disorder becomes clinically apparent at a juvenile or early adult age, presenting with exercise intolerance, which includes pain, cramps, early fatigue, and sometimes myoglobinuria, resembling GSD V. A late-adult onset form, manifesting with slowly progressive atrophy and weakness, as well as a neonatal form with generalized muscle hypotonia and respiratory insufficiency have also been described. Most patients with muscle-specific Phk deficiency are male, and mutations in the X-chromosomal gene of the muscle isoform of the Phkα subunit (*PHKA1*) have been identified in a mouse mutant and in two male human patients.[5]

Other Muscle Glycogenoses
Recently, a family with cardiomyopathy and exercise intolerance caused by mutations in the muscle glycogen synthase gene (*GYS1*) was reported by Kollberg et al.[6] Glycogen synthase catalyzes the addition of glucose monomers to the growing glycogen molecule through the formation of α-1,4-glycoside linkages (see Fig. 22-2). Although this autosomal recessive metabolic myopathy showed a lack of glycogen deposition in muscle biopsy specimens, it has been classified as muscle glycogen storage disease type 0 (GSD 0) because of its enzyme defect within the first step of muscle glycogen synthesis.

Phosphoglycerate kinase deficiency (GSD IX), phosphoglycerate mutase deficiency (GSD X), lactate dehydrogenase (LDH) deficiency (GSD XI), and β-enolase deficiency (GSD XIII) are rare disorders that present mainly with symptoms of exercise intolerance. In addition to muscle symptoms, most of the glycolytic defects may produce signs of chronic hemolytic anemia. GSD IX and a subform of GSD VIII are inherited in an X-chromosomal recessive manner and only males are reported to be affected, whereas the other muscle GSDs are autosomal recessive disorders. In aldolase A deficiency (GSD XII), muscle atrophy and weakness were associated with symptoms of exercise intolerance. Triosephosphate isomerase deficiency was described in a young girl with chronic hemolytic anemia and myopathy, and her muscle biopsy revealed elevated glycogen and mitochondrial alterations.[7]

An additional group of patients present with neuromuscular symptoms and periodic acid-Schiff (PAS)–positive vacuolar changes on muscle biopsy with increased glycogen concentration and without a definite enzymatic defect. These patients should be classified as having a *muscle GSD with an unclear primary defect* and should be further studied on a molecular level when we have more knowledge of the complex regulation and fine-tuning of glycogen metabolism in muscle.

Diagnosis and Evaluation

Increased levels of serum creatine kinase (CK) at rest are typical in muscle GSD and may reach the highest levels in rhabdomyolysis as a severe complication of the disease. The degree of CK elevation, however, is not specific for any of the GSD forms and may vary significantly during the disease course. Serum CK can even be normal in some GSD patients, so that normal values do not exclude the diagnosis of GSD.

The ischemic ("anaerobic") forearm test is a simple, widely used test to screen for disorders of muscle glycogen metabolism. It involves measuring plasma ammonia and lactate levels after a short period of isometric contraction of the forearm muscles under ischemic conditions. This test is useful to screen patients before more invasive or expensive investigations, such as muscle biopsy, genetic analysis, or enzymatic analyses, are performed. It shows a characteristic flat lactate response and enhanced ammonia production in most muscle glycogenoses, but may produce false-negative results in weak or less-motivated patients. In GSD II and IV patients, the forearm test is normal because the cytoplasmic glycogen degradation and glycolytic production of pyruvate are not primarily affected. Compartment syndrome has been described as a severe complication of the ischemic forearm test, so a modified, less unpleasant, and less traumatic aerobic version of the noninvasive test has been developed. This does not require restriction of blood circulation; thus it is better tolerated and is as sensitive as the classic ischemic test.[8]

If, during the exercise test there is a lasting lack of raised lactate, the procedure should be repeated including measurement of pyruvate to detect a possible LDH defect. In LDH deficiency an excessive increase of pyruvate is seen, in contrast to other defects of glycolysis, in which no rise of pyruvate occurs because the metabolic block is located "above" the level of LDH (see Fig. 22-2).

Myoadenylate deaminase (MAD) catalyzes the deamination of AMP to inosine monophosphate in skeletal muscle and plays an important role in the purine nucleotide cycle. In primary MAD deficiency, a flat response of ammonia and a normal increase of lactate can be documented with the forearm test. Thus, this simple test is a useful screening test not only for muscle GSD, but also for the more common MAD defect. MAD deficiency presents in approximately 3% of the normal population, and the pathogenic relevance of this enzyme defect is doubtful.[9]

The diagnostic gold standard in muscle glycogenoses is the skeletal muscle biopsy and demonstration of the primary enzyme defect. Histochemical examination of muscle biopsies typically shows vacuoles filled with PAS-positive glycogen in most patients (Fig. 22-4). Diastase can degrade glycogen in skeletal muscle; thus PAS-positive staining disappears with diastase preincubation, but not in atypical glycogen storage, as in polyglucosan storage disease (GSD IV). PAS-positive deposits of glycogen may be very subtle and only present under the sarcolemma in some muscle fibers. Some GSDs with glycolytic defects may not show increased glycogen with PAS staining. In GSD 0, there is a lack of glycogen in skeletal muscle. Acid phosphatase staining of muscle biopsy in GSD II patients often shows an increased lysosomal activity within cytoplasmic vacuoles (see Fig. 22-4). In GSD V and GSD VII, absent histochemical staining for myophosphorylase or PFK leads to the diagnosis (Fig. 22-5). In GSD X, tubular aggregates in addition to glycogen storage are characteristic.

Enzymatic testing can provide a definitive diagnosis of GSD. In GSD II, GSD III, GSD IV, and GSD VII, the enzymatic tests can be performed not only on skeletal muscle tissue, but also on leukocytes, because the enzymes primarily involved in these disorders are also expressed in blood cells. In most types of GSD, the enzymatic assays show either absent activity or some residual activity of the defective enzyme, usually with variable and unspecific increase in glycogen concentration.

Molecular genetic analysis is performed mostly to confirm the diagnosis. In GSD families with a known mutation, it is the method of choice in symptomatic members suspected to have the disease.

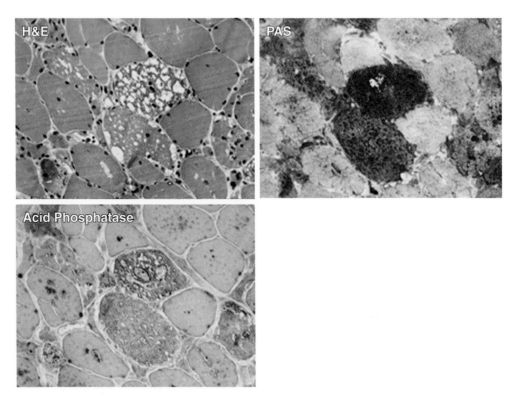

Figure 22-4 Vacuolar myopathy in late-onset glycogen storage disease II (Pompe disease). Muscle fibers harbor vacuoles in frozen sections stained with hematoxylin and eosin (H&E). Many fibers are reactive for acid phosphatase, and most vacuoles are filled with periodic acid-Schiff (PAS)–positive material.

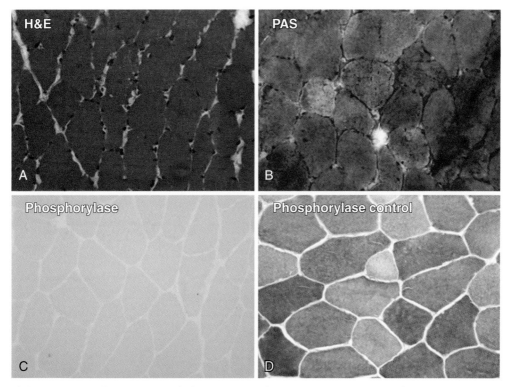

Figure 22-5 A, Muscle biopsy specimen from a patient with glycogen storage disease V (myophosphorylase deficiency). Hematoxylin and eosin (H&E) stain shows subsarcolemmal vacuoles. Some fibers harbor periodic acid-Schiff (PAS)–positive deposits of glycogen (*darkly stained*) under the sarcolemma (**B**). All fibers show absent histochemical reaction for phosphorylase (**C**), whereas phosphorylase reaction is normal in a control patient (**D**).

In such cases, muscle biopsy and enzymatic testing can be avoided. Mutation analysis should also be considered in patients in whom a definite diagnosis cannot be achieved on the basis of clinical, laboratory, and enzymatic studies alone.

We have used phosphorus-31 magnetic resonance spectroscopy (^{31}P-MRS) to measure muscle energy metabolism noninvasively in various muscle GSDs. In GSD V patients, 3 minutes of isometric exercise at 30% to 40% of maximal voluntary contraction results in a strong H^+ consumption and an increase in pH by about 0.3 units. In contrast, H^+ consumption assessed by phosphocreatine (PCr) breakdown is typically overwhelmed by lactic acidosis in healthy subjects, resulting in moderate acidosis. GSD V patients typically consume more PCr for a given workload, and in most patients ATP levels decrease because CK reaction and oxidative phosphorylation cannot compensate for the ATP consumption (Fig. 22-6). In GSD VII, muscle exercise additionally results in an impressive increase in the phosphomonoester peak, representing a massive sugar phosphate accumulation "above" the enzymatic block of PFK (Fig. 22-7). Taking these findings to the bedside, we use ^{31}P-MRS to screen patients with symptoms of exercise intolerance suspected to have GSD V or GSD VII. If they show such typical MRS findings, we go forward with mutational studies to reach a definite diagnosis and avoid a muscle biopsy. This method is available in only a few centers and is not done routinely.

Treatment

GSD II

Enzyme replacement therapy (ERT) with recombinant alglucosidase alfa (Myozyme, Genzyme Corp., Framingham, MA) became available in 2006 for all forms of GSD II; this represents the first effective, disease-specific treatment for Pompe disease patients. It has

been demonstrated that ERT reverses pathology in cardiac muscle and extends life expectancy in infantile GSD II patients.[10–16] Two large clinical trials in late-onset GSD II indicate that ERT improves walking and pulmonary outcomes, but the results have not yet been published. Evidence on the effects of alglucosidase alfa on skeletal muscles is still inconclusive, particularly in adult GSD II patients. It is important to learn whether ERT stably increases α-glucosidase activity in skeletal muscle and also improves skeletal muscle function for a long time; this should be studied in more detail.

Current data supports initiating ERT early to improve the chances of effectiveness. ERT is expensive; patients receiving this treatment must have a definite diagnosis based on enzymatic or genetic data. The commonly used treatment protocol consists of alglucosidase alfa 20 mg/kg body weight infusion every other week, although doses as high as 40 mg/kg per infusion have been used in individual patients. We perform regular 6-minute walking tests and forced vital capacity to follow the individual disease course and evaluate the treatment effects in adult Pompe disease patients receiving ERT.

GSD V

In contrast to GSD II, no ERT or effective gene therapy is available for the other muscle GSDs. In these disorders, treatment is mainly symptom-oriented.[17] Creatine is an amino acid formed from arginine, glycine, and methionine in a two-step reaction that takes place in the kidneys and liver. After this, creatine incorporates in skeletal muscle, where it is transported across the cell membrane via a sodium-dependent creatine membrane transporter.[18] Due to the equilibrium reaction of CK, it is expected that an uptake of creatine by muscle fibers results in an elevation of intracellular PCr levels. Transphosphorylation of ATP on creatine and subsequent rephosphorylation of ADP by oxidative phosphorylation should

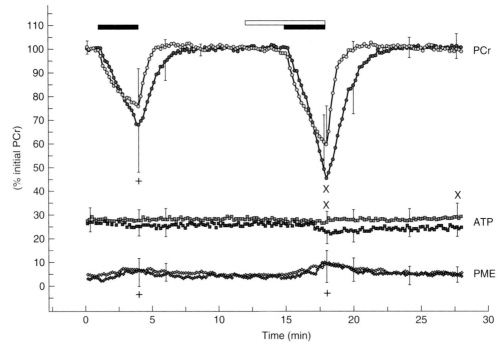

Figure 22-6 Phosphorus-31 magnetic resonance spectroscopy in the calf muscle of patients with glycogen storage disease V (GSD V; McArdle disease) (*dark circles*) and healthy controls (*open circles*). During aerobic (*filled bar*) and muscle contraction with arterial occlusion (*open bar*), moderate acidosis and moderate phosphocreatine (PCr) consumption is found in healthy controls, while adenosine triphosphate (ATP) is kept on constant levels. In patients with GSD V, however, the test contractions always result in a large alkalinization. Alkalinization is caused by the significantly larger PCr consumption than in controls and the absent increase of H$^+$ by lactic acid formation. In most GSD V patients, a distinct drop in ATP levels is found, which on average resulted in significantly lower ATP concentrations at the end of contraction compared to the previous state at rest and to corresponding values of healthy controls. The decrease in ATP is mirrored by an increase in the phosphomonoester (PME) signal, most likely indicating an increase in inosine monophosphate by the degradation of the total adenosine phosphate pool. (From Zange J, Grehl T, Disselhorst-Klug C: Breakdown of adenine nucleotide pool in fatiguing skeletal muscle in McArdle disease: a noninvasive 31P-MRS and EMG study, *Muscle Nerve* 27:728–736, 2003.)

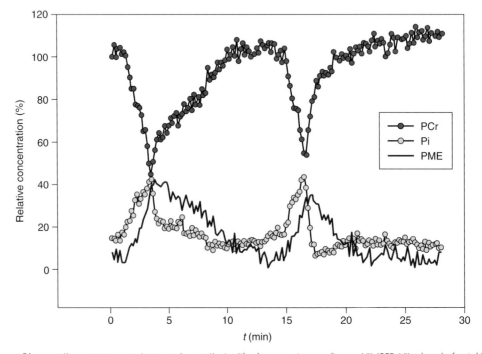

Figure 22-7 Phosphorus-31 magnetic resonance spectroscopy in a patient with glycogen storage disease VII (GSD VII: phosphofructokinase deficiency). The absence of glycolytic adenosine triphosphate production results in a linear time course of phosphocreatine (PCr) breakdown during aerobic (first 3 minutes) and ischemic submaximal contraction of calf muscle. The level of phosphomonoesters (PME) shows a drastic increase during aerobic and ischemic muscle contraction, indicating an excessive accumulation of hexose phosphates (e.g., glucose-6- and fructose-6-phosphate) during submaximal exercise. Pi, inorganic phosphate. (From Grehl T, Müller K, Vorgerd M, et al: Impaired aerobic glycolysis in muscle phosphofructokinase deficiency results in biphasic post-exercise phosphocreatine recovery in 31P magnetic resonance spectroscopy, *Neuromuscul Disord* 8:408–488, 1998.)

result in detection of elevated PCr/ATP ratios in ^{31}P-MRS of muscle. However, in patients with McArdle disease, oral creatine supplementation at both high (150 mg/kg/day) and low (60 mg/kg/day) doses did not result in elevated PCr/ATP ratios. With low-dose creatine, working capacity during ischemic exercise improved; a higher consumption of PCr during aerobic and low-level ischemic low-level exercise was seen in McArdle disease patients.[19] However, high-dose creatine cannot be recommended because it worsened clinical symptoms of exercise intolerance; patients reported an increase in the number of pain episodes and an increase in the myalgia pain score.[20]

In a crossover open design, we compared the effects of a carbohydrate-rich (20% fat, 15% protein, 65% carbohydrate) versus a protein-rich (15% fat, 55% proteins, 30% carbohydrate) diet in GSD V patients. Exercise tolerance and maximal work capacity were tested on a cycle ergometer, using a constant workload for 15 minutes, followed by an incremental workload to exhaustion. The carbohydrate-rich diet improved the maximal work capacity and the exercise tolerance of submaximal workloads.[21]

Moderate aerobic exercise was tested in GSD V patients who pedaled a cycle ergometer for 30 to 40 minutes a day, 4 days a week, for 14 weeks, at an intensity corresponding to 60% to 70% of maximal heart rate. This exercise program increased average work capacity, oxygen uptake, cardiac output, and mitochondrial enzyme levels without causing pain or cramping or increasing serum CK. This study suggests that regular, submaximal aerobic exercise increases oxidative capacity and should be a consistent component of therapy in GSD V patients.[22]

In GSD V patients a genotype (D/D) associated with higher angiotensin-converting enzyme (ACE) activity showed a more severe phenotype of exercise intolerance.[23,24] It was suggested that modulation of ACE activity through the use of inhibitors such as ramipril could positively affect disease expression and increase exercise capacity. A controlled trial of 12 weeks of low-dose ramipril treatment (2.5 mg/day) in GSD V patients did not show changes in the primary outcome measures of exercise physiology, although it showed a possible benefit in patients with the D/D ACE genotype.[25]

Aminoglycosides may allow the potential to read through stop codons and thus may induce synthesis of a full-length protein. In most GSD V patients the primary genetic abnormality is a missense mutation R50X in the phosphorylase gene, leading to a premature stop codon. Daily intravenous gentamicin sulfate 8 mg/kg/day was given for 10 days in four R50X homozygous GSD V patients in an open study. This short-term aminoglyoside treatment appeared to have no effect on muscle energy metabolism as assessed by ^{31}P-MRS.[26] It is possible that the lack of benefit was due to the short treatment time or that the type of nonsense mutation was not amenable to the effects of the drug. This potential therapeutic strategy may be exploited in the future with new pharmacologic compounds with similar effects.

Sucrose, a disaccharide of glucose and fructose, is the most important sugar in plants. Six GSD V patients were tested after ingestion of either 75 g of sucrose 40 minutes before exercise or 37 g of sucrose 5 minutes before exercise.[27] Treatment effects were assessed by monitoring heart rate and perceived exertion during exercise. Both sucrose treatments improved exercise tolerance; the low-dose, 5-minute sucrose trial had a more sustained effect on exercise capacity than the 40-minute trial. The authors recommend low-dose sucrose ingestion immediately before episodes of more strenuous exercise. This provides a sustained elevation in plasma glucose during exercise, which partially rescues muscle oxidative metabolism early in exercise (Box 22-1).

Box 22-1 Treatment Options in McArdle Disease (GSD V)

High-carbohydrate and low-fat diet
Low-intensity aerobic exercise
Supplementation with oral creatine (60 mg/kg/day)
Sucrose before exercise

A ketogenic diet may bypass the enzyme defect of glycogen utilization and may be a feasible tool to improve GSD V symptoms; this has been demonstrated in one patient.[28] Another dietary approach is the ingestion of vitamin B6, which has shown beneficial effects in one GSD V patient.[29] Both approaches, however, require more systematic evaluation in a larger group of patients.

In summary, in the most severe infantile GSD II patients without ERT, death results from cardiac and respiratory failure within the first 1 or 2 years of life. In the milder late-onset forms, cardiac muscle is usually spared and a progressive skeletal muscle weakness is the main symptom. Weakness of respiratory muscle is the major cause of death in late-onset GSD II. The long-term effects of ERT on skeletal and pulmonary functions in GSD II remain to be systematically studied and will show whether ERT will stabilize or even improve the long-term clinical course.

In most cases, the natural course of GSD V and GSD VII appears nonprogressive, without significant limitations of life expectancy and without severe cardiorespiratory complications. Currently no systematic data is available on the natural disease course of the other muscle glycogenoses due to the extreme rarity of these conditions.

When subjected to surgery and anesthesia, GSD patients have the potential to develop perioperative complications, such as hypoglycemia, rhabdomyolysis, myoglobinuria, acute renal failure, postoperative fatigue, and possibly malignant hyperthermia. Because a small subset of GSD V patients were shown to have a positive in vitro contracture test, in all GSD patients simple prophylactic measures as with malignant hyperthermia must be recommended (also see Chapter 10).

Conclusion

Thus far, an effective causative therapy in glycogen storage myopathies is only available for the lysosomal GSD II (Pompe disease), underscoring the need for a definite and early diagnosis in this disease. All GSD patients reporting exercise intolerance must be advised to avoid trigger factors of rhabdomyolysis (e.g., static and dynamic muscle contractions at a high-intensity level) and should follow a high-carbohydrate diet. Nutritional supplementation with low-dose creatine or sucrose may help to reduce symptoms of exercise intolerance in GSD V and possibly the other GSDs with similar symptoms. There is an urgent need to further develop molecular-oriented therapeutic strategies in the future.

Muscle Disorders of Lipid Metabolism

Enzyme deficiencies that affect lipid metabolism, impairing the transport of fatty acids into the mitochondria (carnitine transporter system), beta-oxidation, and utilization of triglycerides can cause muscle disease. The frequently used term *lipid storage myopathies* for these disorders is accurate only for some forms, because several of these disorders do not show lipid accumulation on muscle biopsy.

Table 22-2 Defects of Lipid Metabolism Resulting in Myopathy

Biochemical Defect	Affected Gene(s)	Typical Muscle Phenotype	Characteristic Changes of Acyl-carnitine Spectrum in Blood	Muscle Histology
Carnitine palmitoyl-transferase II deficiency	CPT II	Attacks with myoglobinuria	C16:0 and C18:1 carnitine elevated	Often normal interictally
Multiple acyl-CoA dehydrogenase deficiency (glutaric aciduria type 2)	ETFDH, ETFA, or ETFB	Permanent muscle weakness	Multiple acyl-carnitines (C4–C18:1) elevated	Lipid storage
Medium-chain acyl-CoA dehydrogenase deficiency	MCAD	Attacks with myoglobinuria; permanent muscle weakness	C8 carnitine elevated	Lipid storage
Very long chain acyl-CoA dehydrogenase deficiency	ACADVL	Attacks with myoglobinuria	C14:1 carnitine elevated	Often normal interictally
Primary muscle carnitine deficiency	Unknown	Permanent muscle weakness	Carnitine rarely reduced	Lipid storage
Primary systemic carnitine deficiency (carnitine transporter defect)	SLC22A5 (OCTN2)	Hypotonia, cardiomyopathy	Carnitine reduced	Lipid storage
Trifunctional protein deficiency (deficiency of long-chain 3-hydroxyacyl-CoA dehydrogenase, long-chain 2-enoyl-CoA hydratase, and long-chain 3-ketoacyl-CoA thiolase)	HADHA and HADHB	Attacks with myoglobinuria	3-hydroxy C16 and C18 acyl-carnitine elevated (can be normal interictally)	Often normal interictally
Short-chain acyl-CoA dehydrogenase deficiency	ACADS	Hypotonia	C4 carnitine elevated	Sometimes lipid storage
Neutral lipid storage disease with ichthyosis	ABHD5 (GCI58)	Permanent muscle weakness	Normal	Abundant lipid storage
Neutral lipid storage disease without ichthyosis	PNPLA2 (ATGL)	Permanent muscle weakness	Normal	Abundant lipid storage

Thus, the term *myopathies of lipid metabolism* is more appropriate for this group of metabolic myopathies. All known enzyme defects of lipid metabolism follow an autosomal recessive mode of inheritance. Muscle is not the only tissue affected in these disorders; brain, heart, liver, and skin can also be involved. In children, myopathy is often overshadowed by encephalopathy or cardiomyopathy, but in adults muscle problems are usually the primary manifestation. At present, nine different enzyme defects are known to affect lipid metabolism of muscle (Table 22-2). Some of these have been described in only a few patients, whereas others are more common. However, data about the frequency of myopathies due to disorders of lipid metabolism is not available. CPT II deficiency seems to be the most frequent form.

Clinical Presentation

Disorders of lipid metabolism can present with a profound enzyme deficiency, resulting in severe early onset multisystemic disease. Typically, episodes of hypoketotic hypoglycemia and liver failure (Reye-like disease) occur. These children present with encephalopathy leading to lethargy and coma, muscle weakness, and cardiac arrhythmias. Milder phenotypes are restricted to muscle with onset not only in childhood, but also in adulthood. These show higher residual enzyme activities in regard to muscle involvement. Two clinical presentations can be distinguished. Some manifest with recurrent attacks of rhabdomyolysis triggered by long-lasting exercise, fasting, infections, or cold. Other disorders present with permanent muscle weakness.

Recurrent attacks of rhabdomyolysis occur in CPT II deficiency. The enzymes CPT I and II are part of the carnitine transporter system located in the outer (CPT I) and inner (CPT II) mitochondrial membranes to incorporate long-chain fatty acids from the cytosol into the mitochondrial matrix (Fig. 22-8). In the most common form of CPT II deficiency, symptoms are restricted to muscle. This form is a common cause of hereditary rhabdomyolysis and is also called the "adult" form of CPT II deficiency. Despite the common adult onset, first attacks can occur in early childhood. In contrast to McArdle disease (GSD V)—another rather frequent metabolic myopathy that causes rhabdomyolysis—patients with CPT II deficiency do not suffer from muscle cramps. In addition to the muscle form of CPT II deficiency, a multisystemic form is seen in infants, affecting the liver and heart and sometimes associated with muscle weakness. This type manifests mainly with lethargy and encephalopathy as consequences of hypoketotic hypoglycemia. Finally, there is a neonatal lethal form with congenital anomalies. However, these forms are much less common than the muscle form.[43]

Another disorder of the carnitine carrier system that involves muscle is primary carnitine deficiency, which results from a defect of the carnitine transporter. These patients excrete the filtered carnitine in the urine. There are two clinical manifestations of primary carnitine deficiency: systemic primary carnitine deficiency, which presents as a multisystemic infantile disease with metabolic crises, and primary muscle carnitine deficiency, with late-onset and permanent muscle weakness.[31] Secondary forms of carnitine deficiency are observed in several other muscle disorders, including acyl-CoA

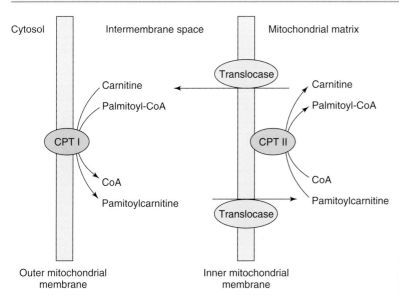

Figure 22-8 Carnitine shuttle system for import of long-chain fatty acids through the inner mitochondrial membrane. CoA, coenzyme A; CPT, carnitine palmitoyltransferase.

dehydrogenase deficiencies. Moreover, drugs such as valproate and zidovudine can also cause a secondary carnitine deficiency.

Different enzymes are necessary for beta-oxidation of fatty acids within the mitochondria depending on the length of the fatty acids that are metabolized (short, medium, long, and very long chain acyl-CoA). The different defects can result in late-onset metabolic myopathies or in infantile multisystemic diseases, including muscular hypotonia.

Clinical presentation of the late-onset myopathic form of very long chain acyl-CoA dehydrogenase (VLCAD) deficiency is similar to that of muscle CPT II deficiency. Patients present with attacks of rhabdomyolysis after long-lasting exercise or fasting.[32] In patients with infantile hepatic manifestations of VLCAD deficiency, the myopathic phenotype can present in later life.[33] Attacks of rhabdomyolysis are also observed in the late-onset form of trifunctional protein deficiency, frequently associated with peripheral neuropathy. However, in contrast to VLCAD and CPT II deficiencies, these were observed only in childhood.[34]

Multiple acyl-CoA dehydrogenase deficiency (MADD) is caused by defects in flavoproteins that are responsible for transfer of electrons from flavin adenine dinucleotide to the respiratory chain: electron transfer flavoprotein (ETF), encoded by two genes—*ETFA* (subunit A) and *ETFB* (subunit B), and electron transfer flavoprotein ubiquinone oxidoreductase (ETF:QO), encoded by the *ETFDH* gene. MADD affects not only multiple acyl-CoA dehydrogenases, but also the metabolism of amino acids and choline. The defect of amino acid metabolism results in glutaric aciduria; MADD is also called *glutaric aciduria type II*. MADD can manifest as a severe neonatal disorder, but later-onset cases are seen in children and adults, affecting muscle only and resulting in permanent weakness. Some patients with later onset can also have episodes of encephalopathy generally precipitated by an infection. Children typically suffer from recurrent episodes of vomiting.[35,36]

Medium-chain acyl-CoA dehydrogenase (MCAD) deficiency is a common disorder of fatty acid metabolism resulting in infantile metabolic decompensation, including hypotonia or rhabdomyolysis.[37] Late-onset disease with predominant muscle involvement is rare. Short-chain dehydrogenase deficiency typically manifests in childhood. Muscle weakness is seen in some patients as a manifestation

of a mild multisystemic presentation in which developmental delay is the leading feature. A juvenile late-onset form with muscle weakness is observed rarely.[38]

Finally, there are disorders affecting the utilization of stored triglycerides due to a defect of the triglyceride lipase. These are called *neutral lipid storage diseases*. Two different forms of neutral lipid storage disease are associated with different gene defects: neutral lipid storage disease with ichthyosis, also known as *Chanarin-Dorfman syndrome* (*ABHD5* gene), which manifests an ichthyosiform non-bullous erythroderma,[39] and *neutral lipid storage disease without ichthyosis* (*PNPLA2* gene).[40] The latter form can present not only with proximal, but also with distal muscle weakness.

Diagnosis and Evaluation

Analysis of the acyl-carnitine profile and carnitine level in blood by tandem mass spectrometry can provide insights about the underlying enzyme deficiency of lipid metabolism. This is a useful screening test in patients with unknown myopathy and can be performed before a muscle biopsy. It can also be used in newborn screening and can be done not only on serum samples, but also on dried blood spots (Guthrie card). In enzyme defects of lipid metabolism there is accumulation of certain fatty acids in blood. For example, in CPT II deficiency the long-chain fatty acids C16 and C18:1 are increased.[41] Typical profiles of different disorders of muscle lipid metabolism are listed in Table 22-2. The diagnostic yield is maximized if the specimens are obtained during a metabolic crisis or after fasting overnight. A normal acyl-carnitine spectrum does not exclude a myopathy of lipid metabolism because the acyl-carnitine profile can be normal between attacks.

Serum CK is often normal between attacks in muscle disorders of lipid metabolism that are characterized by episodes of rhabdomyolysis. A mild or moderate elevation of CK is typically observed in patients with permanent weakness. Creatinine levels should always be obtained to detect renal failure in patients with rhabdomyolysis. Myoglobin and ketones should be measured in blood and urine. In children with Reye-like symptoms mild hyperammonemia and elevated liver enzymes can be present. Analysis of organic acid profile in urine is important, especially to detect glutaric aciduria in MADD.

Histologic studies typically reveal clear lipid accumulation only in those with permanent weakness. In patients with attacks of myoglobinuria, muscle biopsies done during the acute phase can show only necrotic fibers, but these are frequently normal inter-ictally, and these forms may demonstrate little or no lipid accumulation. Muscle biopsies should not be taken during the phase of rhabdomyolysis, but several weeks later because necrosis can mask the characteristic features of metabolic myopathies. Lipid accumulation is frequently more pronounced in the oxidative type I fibers than in type II fibers, because normal muscle also contains more lipid in type I fibers. The most pronounced lipid accumulation is seen in neutral lipid storage disease. Lipid droplets can be stained by Oil Red O (Fig. 22-9) or by Sudan Black. VLCAD deficiency can be detected by immunohistochemistry.[42] In neutral lipid storage diseases peripheral blood smears typically show neutral lipid vacuoles in leukocytes (Jordan's anomaly).[39,40]

Further investigations of the enzyme molecular genetic defect are necessary to confirm the diagnosis of lipid myopathies. In late-onset cases, there is often considerable residual enzyme activity that makes diagnosis difficult. For example, in patients with muscle CPT II deficiency, there is normal activity of CPT under optimal assay conditions. However, abnormal regulation of the enzyme can be seen by abnormal inhibition by malonyl CoA.[43] Biochemical analysis of enzyme deficiencies in lipid metabolism of muscle is difficult, and these studies are performed only in specialized laboratories. Fibroblasts and lymphocytes are also tissues in which the enzymes can be measured. Fatty acid oxidation rates can be measured in fibroblasts by incubating cells with radiolabeled fatty acids of different chain length. This method can differentiate short-, medium-, or long-chain defects. Carnitine levels can be measured not only in blood, but also in muscle, bearing in mind that secondary carnitine deficiency is quite common. Secondary coenzyme Q (CoQ) deficiency in muscle can be measured in MADD due to a defect of ETF:QO.[41]

Molecular genetic testing is relatively simple for CPT II and MCAD deficiencies. Although more than 40 mutations are known in the *CPT2* gene, a missense mutation S113L in patients with muscle CPT II deficiency is found in approximately 60% of mutant alleles. More than 90% of the patients carry this mutation on at least one allele.[43] In patients with MCAD deficiency, there is a common point mutation 985A>G with similar frequency compared to the CPT II mutation S113L.[37] Such common mutations are not present in other genes affected in myopathies of lipid metabolism, and molecular genetic testing requires primary sequencing of the gene.

Treatment

Treatment strategies for myopathies caused by defects of lipid metabolism include avoidance of exacerbating factors, dietary regimens containing high amounts of carbohydrate, supplementation with fatty acids that bypass the enzyme defect, riboflavin or carnitine, and IV glucose.

Avoidance of exacerbating factors still plays a large role in the management of patients with attacks of rhabdomyolysis or metabolic crises. In children, fasting and infections are the major causes of metabolic decompensation and rhabdomyolysis. Thus, regular feedings are essential in children. In adults, exercise and cold temperatures are the major precipitants of rhabdomyolysis. Thus, avoidance of intense or prolonged exercise and protection from cold is necessary. Certain drugs, such as valproate, diazepam, and ibuprofen, can trigger attacks in patients with CPT II deficiency.

In general, the recommended dietary regimen for patients with disorders of lipid metabolism is a high-carbohydrate, low-fat diet with frequent and regularly scheduled meals. Slow-release carbohydrate intake should be increased during intercurrent illness or sustained exercise.

In patients with muscle CPT II deficiency it has been shown that ingestion of polysaccharides can improve exercise intolerance, whereas oral glucose ingestion does not.[44] This study also demonstrated that intravenous (IV) glucose infusions improve exercise intolerance in patients with CPT II deficiency (Box 22-2). IV glucose can be recommended in crises of infantile CPT II deficiency (including insulin that reduces mobilization of the stored lipids),[45] but is not generally given in patients with other disorders of lipid metabolism. A study in patients with VLCAD deficiency did not show a benefit of IV glucose[3] (Box 22-2).

Supplementation with medium-chain triglycerides (MCT) could be beneficial in disorders with long-chain fatty acid oxidation defects because medium-chain acyl-CoA esters can bypass the long-chain oxidation enzymes. Anecdotal evidence suggests that MCT is effective in cases of trifunctional protein deficiency, VLCAD, and CPT II deficiency. However, no effect of oral medium-chain triglycerides was observed in a study on patients with VLCAD deficiency.[3] MCT supplements are contraindicated in patients with medium- or short-chain beta-oxidation defects or MADD.

Oral intake of the triglyceride triheptanoin, which contains the odd-chain (C7) fatty acid hepanoate, can provide an alternative source to fill the citric cycle. This so-called *anaplerotic diet* was investigated for patients with VLCAD deficiency[46] and muscle CPT II deficiency.[47] In children with VLCAD deficiency, cardiomyopathy, hepatomegaly, and muscle weakness were improved.

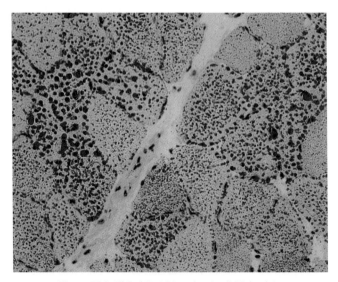

Figure 22-9 Oil Red O staining showing lipid droplets.

Box 22-2 Treatment Options in Carnitine Palmitoyltransferase II Deficiency

---

High-carbohydrate and low-fat diet with frequent and regularly scheduled meals
Increased intake of polysaccharides during sustained exercise
IV glucose in crisis
Supplementation with medium-chain triglycerides (MCT)
Oral intake of the triglyceride triheptanoin
Bezafibrate

In patients with CPT II deficiency, triheptanoin intake reduced muscle pain after exercise and might prevent attacks of rhabdomyolysis.

L-Carnitine substitution (100–400 mg/kg/day in children and 2–4 g/day in adults) is unequivocally beneficial in cases of primary carnitine deficiency.[31] The role of carnitine supplementation in other fatty acid oxidation disorders remains controversial. Secondary carnitine deficiency is common, caused either by acylcarnitine wastage or inhibition of the plasma membrane carnitine transporter by accumulating acylcarnitines.

Riboflavin (vitamin B$_2$) is the cofactor shared by ETF, ETFDH, and all acyl-CoA dehydrogenases. Many of the patients with MADD presenting with myopathy improve with riboflavin supplementation (100–400 mg/day). It has been shown that riboflavin-responsive myopathy with MADD is frequently caused by *ETFDH* mutations.[35,36] A secondary CoQ deficiency was observed in one study,[35] arguing that additional CoQ supplementation (150–500 mg/day) should be considered.

A future therapeutic option might consist of bezafibrate, which can induce up-regulation of different genes involved in lipid metabolism by activating the peroxisome proliferator-activated receptor α. In fibroblasts and myoblasts from patients with muscle CPT II deficiency and in fibroblasts of patients with VLCAD deficiency, bezafibrate improved the biochemical defect.[48,49]

Recently it was shown that administration of bezafibrate (600 mg/day for 6 months) in six patients with muscle CPT II deficiency resulted in an increased rate of palmitoylcarnitine oxidation in muscle mitochondria.[60] In this study, a self-assessment score for general health improved. Frequency of attacks with rhabdomyolysis and maximal CK levels were lower during treatment compared to a 6-month period before, but it was not shown that there was a statistically significant decrease. No adverse effects were reported,[60] an important finding because rhabdomyolysis is a potential side effect of bezafibrate. However, as long as no placebo-controlled, double-blind study has proven its efficacy, bezafibrate cannot be recommended, in general, for treatment of patients with muscle CPT II deficiency.

In conclusion, treatment of myopathies of lipid metabolism remains inadequate. Bezafibrate treatment offers promising results. However, dietary advice is the only therapeutic option as long as there are no therapeutic effects of specific drugs. Because many disorders of lipid metabolism are rare, clinical studies are difficult to perform. In the future, gene therapy might correct the metabolic defect.

Outcome

The outcome is usually much better in patients with myopathies of lipid metabolism that manifest late in life only with muscular symptoms than in those with infantile multisystemic manifestations. The most favorable disease course is seen in patients presenting with attacks of rhabdomyolysis, such as the muscle form of CPT II deficiency. At rest and except for episodes of myoglobinuria, muscle strength is normal. Patients usually have an excellent long-term prognosis. In many cases, attacks can be effectively prevented after the diagnosis is made by avoiding situations that can provoke rhabdomyolysis and by increasing carbohydrate intake during prolonged exercise or other situations that provoke attacks. Acute tubular necrosis as a result of massive myoglobinuria is the only life-threatening complication. Although renal failure has been documented in approximately 25% of patients, if it is promptly recognized and appropriately treated, a complete recovery should be expected in virtually all cases. Cardiac arrest can occur very rarely during an attack in the muscle form of CPT II deficiency. Only one case with a fatal outcome has been reported,[50] and respiratory failure from muscle weakness was reported in another patient.[51]

In patients with muscle disorders of lipid metabolism with persistent weakness, the disease is usually slowly progressive but can lead to significant disability over years. Typically, proximal weakness is present, but involvement of facial, bulbar, or respiratory muscles is rare. Cardiomyopathy can result in heart failure or in cerebral cardiac embolism.[40] Children with metabolic crises can progress into coma if they are not treated promptly with IV glucose. These children have a high risk of sudden death due to cardiac arrhythmia.

Mitochondrial Myopathies

The term *mitochondrial myopathy* is generally used only for defects of the respiratory chain. Myopathies with defects located elsewhere in the metabolic pathways within the mitochondria are generally not classified as mitochondrial myopathies (e.g., myopathies due to defects in the beta-oxidation of fatty acids are classified as myopathies of lipid metabolism). Mitochondrial disorders are frequently multisystemic diseases; the term *mitochondrial myopathy* is used for those with predominant muscle involvement.

From the genetic point of view, mitochondrial disorders are unique because mitochondria have their own genome, enabling intramitochondrial protein synthesis. However, only a very small proportion of mitochondrial proteins are encoded by the mitochondrial DNA. The majority are encoded by nuclear DNA, and these proteins are imported into the mitochondria. Therefore, mitochondrial disorders can follow both mendelian and maternal traits of inheritance.

Mitochondrial genetics differ from mendelian genetics in several aspects. Due to the polyploid nature of the mitochondrial genome, with several thousand copies per cell, a mixture of mutant and normal mtDNA is frequently observed. Called *heteroplasmy*, this has implications for molecular diagnostics because the mutant mtDNA may be absent or present only in very low levels in certain tissues. Moreover, the level of heteroplasmy influences the phenotype: a threshold of mutant mtDNA has to be reached before biochemical effects and phenotypical abnormalities occur.

Clinical Presentation

Chronic progressive external ophthalmoplegia (CPEO) is the most common form of mitochondrial myopathy; it can present as an isolated disorder or as the leading manifestation of a multisystemic syndrome. Ptosis is frequently the first symptom, and old photographs are helpful for establishing the age of onset. The disease typically manifests in the teenage years or early adulthood, but childhood or late adult onset also occurs. Ptosis may occur unilaterally at first, but will eventually become bilateral (Fig. 22-10).

Ophthalmoparesis develops over many years and may lead to complete ocular paralysis. Additionally, many patients have some weakness of the orbicularis muscle. Some patients seek medical attention only when ptosis covers the optic axis and leads to visual disturbance. Patients with CPEO use their frontalis muscles to lift their eyelids and show compensatory chin elevation. Together with the ptosis this is called *Hutchinson's triad*. Ophthalmoplegia is often symmetric and may not lead to complaints because patients simply turn their heads to compensate. Only a minority of patients suffer from diplopia. Muscle weakness is often not restricted to the extraocular muscles, and severe weakness of the facial muscles can present with the facies myopathica. Many patients also suffer from exercise intolerance. In most cases, neurologic examination shows limb weakness, most prominent in the proximal muscles of the lower extremities.

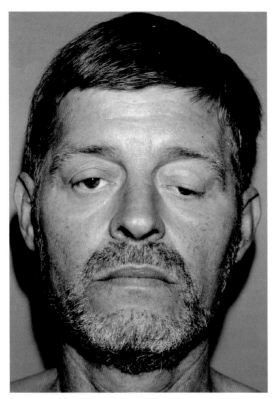

Figure 22-10 Patient with chronic progressive external ophthalmoplegia showing ptosis (left > right) and strabismus.

Important differential diagnoses of CPEO are oculopharyngeal muscular dystrophy (OPMD) and ocular myasthenia. OPMD typically manifests after age 40 years, whereas CPEO typically starts before that age. Ocular myasthenia symptoms fluctuate and, in both OPMD and ocular myasthenia, ptosis is more prominent than ophthalmoplegia throughout the disease course.

Additionally, involvement of systems other than muscle is possible in CPEO. The term *CPEO-plus* was established for these patients. Ocular manifestations include retinopathy (typically with a salt-and-pepper like appearance), optic atrophy, and, rarely, cataracts. Cardiac manifestations include cardiac conduction block and cardiomyopathy. Cerebral manifestations include epilepsy, cerebellar ataxia, and dementia. The peripheral nervous system can also be affected, typically with axonal sensory neuropathy. Endocrine involvement includes diabetes mellitus, hypothyroidism, hypoparathyroidism, and hypogonadism. Sensorineural hearing loss and gastrointestinal involvement are also possible. Typical multisystemic signs and symptoms of CPEO-plus are shown in Figure 22-11.

Some specific CPEO-plus syndromes have been defined; of these, Kearns-Sayre syndrome is a severe multisystemic phenotype with onset before age 20. This syndrome is characterized by CPEO with retinopathy, heart block, and cerebellar ataxia as well as elevated protein in cerebrospinal fluid (CSF).[52] Two other multisystemic mitochondrial syndromes associated with CPEO are SANDO (sensory ataxia, neuropathy, dysarthria and ophthalmoplegia)[53] and MNGIE (mitochondrial neurogastrointestinal encephalomyopathy). MNGIE is a rare disorder with prominent gastrointestinal symptoms leading to cachexia.[54] There is, however, a significant overlap between these syndromes and there are doubts as to whether they all represent specific disease entities, because most do not result from specific genetic defects.

Myopathy is also observed in other classical mitochondrial syndromes that predominantly affect the brain, such as MERRF (myoclonic epilepsy with ragged-red fibers) and MELAS (mitochondrial encephalomyopathy with lactic acidosis and strokelike episodes).[55] In children with Leigh syndrome or Leigh-like syndrome, hypotonia can be observed.

Although CPEO is the prominent feature of mitochondrial myopathies, patients with mitochondrial myopathies without CPEO or multisystemic involvement have been increasingly recognized. These patients can present with mild disease (exercise intolerance, muscle stiffness, and attacks of myoglobinuria) or with progressive severe proximal limb weakness resembling limb girdle muscular dystrophy.[56–59]

Another autosomally inherited mitochondrial myopathy is caused by CoQ deficiency. This is important because this disorder is treatable by oral supplementation. Patients genetically proven to have primary CoQ deficiency can manifest with a pure myopathy, but may also have multisystemic involvement, frequently presenting with cerebellar ataxia.[61] CPEO has not been described in patients with genetically proven CoQ deficiency, although a secondary CoQ deficiency is documented occasionally in CPEO.[62]

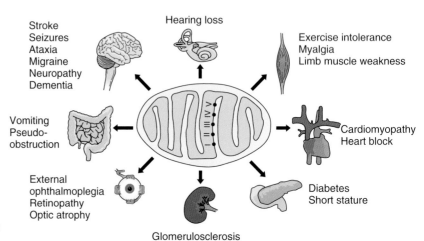

Figure 22-11 Possibilities of multisystemic involvement in mitochondrial disorders.

Diagnosis and Evaluation

Clinical Examinations

The diagnosis of mitochondrial myopathies requires a close collaboration between clinicians and laboratory investigators. Because of multisystemic involvement, patients should be examined by an ophthalmologist, cardiologist, and otorhinolaryngologist, in addition to a neurologist.

Knowledge of the patient's family history is extremely important. It is also helpful to perform a clinical examination of family members because oligosymptomatic patients are possible (e.g., with mild sensorineural hearing loss or ptosis).

Laboratory testing should include resting lactate which, when elevated, indicates impaired oxidative phosphorylation. A more sensitive test is to measure lactate after low-level cycling exercise (30 W for 15 min), showing an abnormal lactate increase (Fig. 22-12), with a sensitivity of 70%. One must keep in mind that moderate lactate elevations (not exceeding 4 mmol/L with the above-mentioned protocol) can be observed in patients with other myopathies. Specificity of the bicycle exercise test has been estimated at 90%.[63] In patients with mitochondrial disorders affecting the brain, lactate should also

be measured in CSF. In addition to an increased lactate level, pyruvate can also be elevated, resulting in a decreased ratio of lactate/pyruvate in blood and CSF, especially in patients with pyruvate dehydrogenase complex deficiency. In this childhood disorder, alanine can be increased in blood or urine because pyruvate is metabolized to alanine instead of acetyl-CoA. Mild elevation of CK is frequently seen in patients with mitochondrial myopathies. Measurement of glucose metabolism can disclose diabetes mellitus. Measurements of thyroid hormones, thyrotropin, corticotropin, cortisol, parathyroid hormone, growth hormone, estradiol, progesterone, and testosterone are also useful in some patients.

Audiograms may detect subclinical hearing impairment, and electrophysiologic examination of the peripheral nerves may reveal a subclinical neuropathy. Cardiac examination should include electrocardiography and echocardiography. Brain magnetic resonance imaging is necessary to detect cerebral involvement. Magnetic resonance imaging may detect a leukencephalopathy, strokelike lesions typically with occipital localization, or lesions within the basal ganglia, indicating Leigh syndrome. Analysis of CSF may show elevated protein.

Analysis of Muscle Biopsy

Clinical examination can suggest mitochondrial myopathy, but the diagnosis must be confirmed by histologic and biochemical analysis of muscle biopsy. Moreover, muscle is the best tissue to test for mutations in mtDNA.

Myohistologic analysis shows abnormal mitochondrial proliferation in modified Gomori's trichrome staining or in succinate dehydrogenase (SDH) staining. These fibers are called *ragged-red fibers* (Fig. 22-13A). Sometimes the classical ragged-red fibers are missing; some fibers show only subsarcolemmal accumulation of mitochondria without a ragged appearance. These fibers are called *ragged red–like fibers*. A more sensitive technique is sequential histochemical staining for cytochrome *c* oxidase (COX = complex IV) and SDH to detect COX-negative fibers (Fig. 22-13B). However, in patients with gene defects that do not affect COX, this staining is normal. Some patients with mitochondrial myopathy only show minor changes in histology (less than 5% abnormal fibers).[64] In such cases, only molecular genetic testing can confirm the diagnosis.

It is important to recognize that mitochondrial abnormalities in muscle biopsies are also seen in normal aging and in other muscle diseases (e.g., myositis). Electronmicroscopy typically shows enlarged and irregularly shaped mitochondria with paracrystalline inclusions. In general, however, electronmicroscopy is not mandatory for

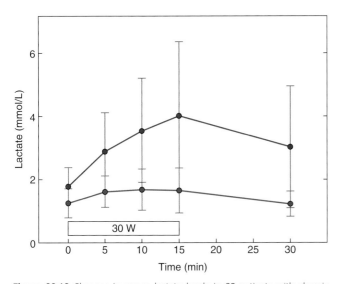

Figure 22-12 Changes in serum lactate levels in 22 patients with chronic progressive external ophthalmoplegia after bicycle exercise shown in *red* compared to normal controls shown in *blue*. Error *bars* show one standard deviation, *circles* show mean values.

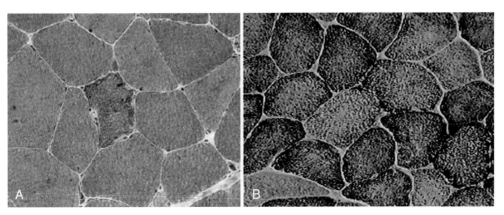

Figure 22-13 A, Modified Gomori-trichrome staining showing a ragged-red fiber. **B,** Sequential cytochrome *c* oxidase/succinate dehydrogenase staining showing cytochrome *c* oxidase–negative fibers in *blue*.

diagnosis. Abnormal mitochondria can be seen with electron-microscopy in many other myopathies, indicating only secondary alterations.

Biochemistry

Biochemistry of muscle biopsy samples can show decreased activity of respiratory chain complexes. Frequently there is a combined defect in the complexes because the underlying genetic defect of the mtDNA (large-scale deletions or tRNA mutations) affects several subunits of different complexes.[65] If there is an isolated deficiency of one complex, a genetic defect in one subunit can be assumed. This is more frequent in children with mitochondrial disorders. Additionally, mitochondrial enzymes that are not encoded by mtDNA, such as citrate synthase or SDH, can be increased, indicating mitochondrial proliferation. Generally, biochemistry is not as important as histology for the diagnosis. The enzyme testing is complex and is available only in specialized laboratories. However, it is important to measure CoQ levels in muscle if histology shows lipid accumulation in addition to mitochondrial proliferation, because these findings can be present in treatable CoQ deficiency.

Molecular Genetic Investigations

Genetic analysis is important not only to confirm the diagnosis, but also to allow for genetic counseling. Patients with CPEO have different underlying genetic defects. Approximately 50% of those with CPEO carry large-scale single deletions of mtDNA. These single deletions are heteroplasmic with a length between 1 and 9 kb and are commonly located within the major arc of mtDNA between both origins of replication (origin of heavy-strand replication O_H and light-strand replication O_L) (Fig. 22-14). There is one common deletion with a length of 5 kb. The deletion break points are typically characterized by direct repeats. Most cases of CPEO with single deletions are sporadic. It is postulated that deletions occur in the

oocyte, and mitotic segregation during embryogenesis results in high levels of deleted mtDNA in certain tissues like muscle, with low levels in other tissues, including the germline cells. This can explain why mother-to-offspring transmission of single deletions is rarely observed. The risk for an affected mother to have an affected child is only 4%.[66]

In contrast to single deletions of mtDNA, patients with autosomal inheritance of CPEO demonstrated multiple deletions, indicating that these deletions are not the primary gene defect but secondary changes due to a nuclear gene mutation. Consequently, several nuclear gene defects have been identified during the past years. They are located in genes important in the replication of mtDNA. Those forms of CPEO are therefore classified as defects of intergenomic communication (Fig. 22-15). In some of them, not only multiple deletions, but also depletion of mtDNA can occur. The following nuclear genes can be mutated: polymerase gamma 1 and 2 (*POLG1* and *POLG2*), progressive external ophthalmoplegia 1 (*PEO1*; also called *C10orf1* or *TWINKLE*), adenine nucleotide translocator (*ANT1*), optic atrophy 1 (*OPA1*), and ribonucleotide reductase small subunit of p53 (*RRM2B*). *POLG1* mutations located in the catalytic subunit of the mitochondrial polymerase are detected most frequently. The *PEO1* gene encodes for the mitochondrial helicase. This results in high levels of thymidine that can compromise mtDNA replication and repair, affecting quality (multiple deletions) and quantity (depletion) of mtDNA. Mutations in the *ANT1* gene were found in only some families with CPEO.[30] Patients with mutations in the *OPA1* gene always show optic atrophy in addition to CPEO. Mutations in the thymidine phosphorylase (*TP*) gene have been identified in patients with MNGIE. *ANT1* and *TP* mutations result in an altered nucleotide pool in the mitochondria, which can explain defective replication of mtDNA. Mutations in the *ANT1*, *OPA1*, and *PEO1* gene were identified in autosomal dominant CPEO; mutations in the *POLG1* gene were seen in both autosomal dominant and autosomal recessive CPEO. *TP* mutations are recessive. In sporadic CPEO with multiple mtDNA deletions, nuclear gene defects were not frequently detected.[67]

The gold standard for detection of mtDNA deletions used to be Southern blot analysis of muscle DNA. However, low levels of multiple deletions can be missed by Southern blot analysis. Thus, more sensitive techniques, such as long-range polymerase chain reaction (PCR), are necessary.[64] Nevertheless, due to the highly polymorphic nature of mtDNA there is a risk of false-positive results.[68]

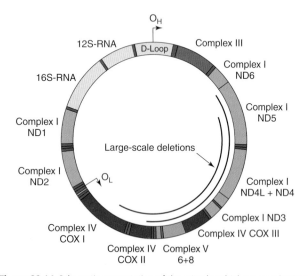

Figure 22-14 Schematic presentation of the mitochondrial genome (mtDNA) and two exemplary large-scale deletions of mtDNA. The genes that encode the subunits of complex I (*ND1–ND6* and *ND4L*) are shown in *light blue*; cytochrome *c* oxidase (*COX I–COX III*) is shown in *red*; cytochrome *b* of complex III is shown in *dark green*; and the subunits 6 and 8 of the ATP synthase (complex V) are shown in *light green*. The two ribosomal ribonucleic acids (rRNAs; 12S and 16S) are shown in *gray* and the 22 tRNAs are shown in *dark blue* (not labeled). The displacement loop (D-loop), or noncoding control region, is shown in *yellow*. It contains sequences that are vital for the initiation of both mtDNA replication and transcription, including the origin of heavy strand replication (shown as O_H). The origin of light strand replication is shown as O_L.

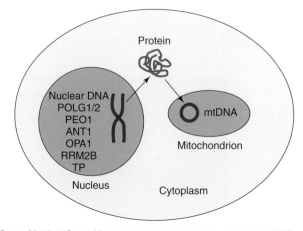

Figure 22-15 Defects of intergenomic communication. Mutations of different nuclear genes result in defective proteins that in turn cause multiple deletions or depletion of mitochondrial genome (mtDNA). *ANT1*, adenine nucleotide translocator gene; DNA, deoxyribonucleic acid; *OPA1*, optic atrophy 1 gene; *PEO1*, progressive external ophthalmoplegia 1 gene; *POLG1/2*, polymerase gamma 1/2 genes; *TP*, thymidine phosphorylase gene.

Moreover, it is important to know that low levels of mtDNA deletions are also observed in normal aging. In general, deletions of mtDNA are detectable only in muscle and not in blood. However, with sensitive PCR techniques it is sometimes possible to detect single deletions in blood. If multiple deletions of mtDNA are detected, analysis of nuclear genes causing intergenomic communication defects should be performed. Analysis should start with *POLG1* because this gene is most often mutated with two common recessive mutations (A467T and W748S).[69] The *OPA1* gene should be sequenced first in patients with CPEO and optic atrophy.

Rarely, point mutations of mtDNA, which are inherited maternally, can be associated with CPEO. A common point mutation of mtDNA is the 3243A>G mutation, which is located in one of the two mitochondrial tRNA genes for leucine. This mutation is typically associated with MELAS, but CPEO was also observed in patients carrying this mutation.[55] Moreover, several very rare point mutations can be associated with CPEO (www.mitomap.org).

Patients with mitochondrial myopathy without CPEO can show different point mutations within mtDNA. Many of them are located in tRNA genes[57–59] but mutations in protein coding genes have also been described.[56]

Defects in different genes of CoQ biosynthesis have been identified (para-hydroxybenzoate-polyprenyl transferase, decaprenyl diphosphate synthase subunit 1 and 2). Also, mutations in the ataxin (*APTX*) gene, first described in patients with ataxia oculomotor apraxia syndrome, can result in severe secondary CoQ deficiency.[61] Secondary CoQ deficiency was also observed in MADD due to a defect of ETF:QO (see section "Muscle Disorders of Lipid Metabolism" in this chapter).[35]

Treatment and Management

There is no curative therapy available except in CoQ deficiency, but symptomatic treatment is important in patients with mitochondrial myopathies because of the various multisystemic symptoms (Table 22-3). Patients should be cared for by an interdisciplinary team.

Supplementation of Vitamins and Cofactors
In general, supplementation with vitamins and cofactors has not been shown to be effective. However, in patients with proven CoQ deficiency, supplementation with CoQ (300 to 500 mg/day) can result in remarkable improvement.[61] In patients with CPEO, improvement after CoQ substitution has been reported only anecdotally; for example, in a patient with Kearns-Sayre syndrome, cachexia, ataxia, and tremor disappeared but ophthalmoplegia and retinopathy remained unchanged.[62] Due to its antioxidant effect, CoQ supplementation might also be helpful in patients with normal CoQ level, because defects of the respiratory chain can result in an increased production of reactive oxygen species. Idebenone, an analogue of CoQ with better penetration of the blood-brain barrier, is thought effective in patients with Leber hereditary optic neuropathy, a mitochondrial disorder, and is being currently tested in a phase III study.

Reduced levels of folinic acid have been measured in CSF in patients with Kearns-Sayre syndrome; improvement after high-dose supplementation with folinic acid was observed in a child with Kearns-Sayre syndrome.[70] Substitution of vitamins and cofactors has virtually no serious side effects, at least in low doses. A therapeutic trial of several months is therefore reasonable.[71]

Symptomatic Treatment
Ptosis not only impairs vision, but can also be a cosmetic problem and a source of embarrassment for younger patients. However,

Table 22-3 Treatment Options for Multisystemic Symptoms in Mitochondrial Myopathies

Symptom/Sign	Treatment
Exercise intolerance	Aerobic endurance training
Ptosis	Surgery using frontalis muscle suspension
Cardiac conduction block	Pacemaker
Diabetes mellitus	Avoid metformin
Strokelike episodes	Steroids, L-arginine
Seizures	Avoid valproic acid; ketogenic diet
Hearing loss	Amplification aids
Cardiomyopathy	Pharmacologically (e.g. beta-blockers), heart transplantation
Hypogonadism	Testosterone
Hypothyroidism	Thyroid hormone
Myalgia	Physical therapy
Neuropathic pain	Pregabalin
Cachexia	High caloric nutrition, tube feeding
Dysphagia due to cricopharyngeal achalasia	Myotomy
Myopathy due to coenzyme Q deficiency	Coenzyme Q substitution

surgery for ptosis should be recommended only if the visual axis is obscured. This is due to the risk of complications of corneal exposure in cases of postoperative lagophthalmus. The preferred surgical technique is frontalis muscle suspension, avoiding levator palpebrae muscle resection, because this ensures better protection of the cornea. Lid height can be adjusted if necessary.

Generally, corneal exposure symptoms are treated with lubricants. Some patients with ptosis do well with "eyelid crutches" mounted on their glasses. Fresnel prisms can be helpful if there is diplopia, especially in patients with poor convergence. However, it is often difficult or impossible to suppress diplopia with prisms in the presence of noncomitant strabismus. When spectacles are prescribed, the motility deficits should be taken into account (e.g., no bifocals in impaired downgaze).[72]

Cardiac conduction blocks should be monitored at frequent intervals (at least once per year) because timely placement of a pacemaker can be lifesaving. Cardiomyopathy can be treated pharmacologically (e.g., beta-blockers) or by heart transplantation in carefully selected cases with no other serious multisystemic symptoms. Physical therapy is important to relieve myalgia and to maintain mobility of joints.

Diabetes mellitus should be treated by standard methods. However, metformin should be avoided because this drug can cause lactic acidosis. Hormone replacement with estrogen or testosterone should be considered in patients with hypogonadism. Thyroid hormone can be given to patients with hypothyroidism, and calcium and vitamin D to patients with hypoparathyroidism. However, growth hormone treatment for children with short stature might be harmful because an increased metabolic demand could be a problem in metabolically impaired patients with mitochondrial disease.

Cachexia should be treated with high-caloric nutrition and tube feeding if dysphagia is present. Myotomy can help in patients with dysphagia due to incomplete opening of the upper esophageal sphincter (cricopharyngeal achalasia).[73] Endurance training to reduce exercise intolerance is safe and efficient. It has been shown that endurance training can increase oxygen uptake, peak work capacity, and activity of citrate synthase in muscle.[74,75]

In several case reports, steroid treatment was effective in reducing focal brain edema in patients with acute strokelike episodes. Infusion of L-arginine 30 minutes after onset mitigated strokelike episodes in a small series. Oral intake of L-arginine reduced the frequency of strokelike episodes.[76]

Dichloracetate is effective to reduce lactic acidosis, but its use is limited by severe neuropathy, a frequent side effect. Bicarbonate can be used in the acute phases of lactic acidosis.

Valproic acid should be avoided in the treatment of seizures because it can trigger hepatic failure in patients with *POLG1* defects.[69] A ketogenic diet is effective in treating seizures. Because of the taste, it is difficult to administer in patients who are not receiving tube feedings. Antiepileptic drugs such as pregabalin can be used in patients with neuropathic pain.

Amplification aids can help overcome hearing loss. If necessary, cochlear implants can be safely and successfully installed.

Allogeneic stem cell transplantation was used in two patients with MNGIE syndrome to restore TP activity and to reduce the thymidine level. One patient improved and the other patient died from disease progression and sepsis 3 months after transplantation.[77] Other possibilities to reduce the thymidine level are dialysis, infusions of platelets that have high TP activity, or carrier erythrocyte entrapped TP enzyme replacement therapy. For these techniques, proof of principle was provided in single patients without analyzing clinical effects.

During surgery and anesthesia, patients with mitochondrial disorders need special care because some drugs (e.g., propofol and midazolam) can inhibit the respiratory chain in vitro. In addition, malignant hyperthermia has been reported in single cases, so trigger agents (e.g., succinylcholine and inhalation anesthetics except nitrous oxide) should be avoided if possible.

Gene Therapy and Prevention of Transmission

Due to the complex genetics of mitochondrial disorders, different strategies to provide gene therapy are under current development, albeit at an early stage. One promising strategy is to reduce the ratio of mutant to wild-type mitochondrial genomes (*gene shifting*) by inhibiting the replication of mutant genomes. Maternal transmission of mtDNA point mutations could be prevented by nuclear transplantation. After in vitro fertilization of an oocyte carrying an mtDNA mutation, the pronucleus is transferred into an enucleated normal donor oocyte. The resulting embryo has the nuclear genomes of the parents but mainly the mitochondrial genome of the donor female, thus showing only very low levels of heteroplasmy, well below the threshold. This approach was successful in mice.[78]

Outcome

Muscle weakness generally develops slowly and progressively in mitochondrial myopathies. Sometimes myopathy results in severe muscle wasting and weakness with severe disability.[58] Exercise intolerance and myalgia can also lead to disability in some patients. Ophthalmoplegia and ptosis usually do not result in major visual impairment; severe ptosis that totally covers the optic axis can be improved by surgery. Optic atrophy frequently results in severe

---

Box 22-3 Causes and Treatment Options in Rhabdomyolysis
Causes
Metabolic myopathies
Exertion
Drugs (e.g., statins)
Toxins (e.g., alcohol)
Crush injury, trauma
Treatment Options
Hospitalization
Intravenous fluid replacement
Alkalinization of the urine
Pain control

---

visual impairment, whereas retinopathy typically leads to moderate impairment only. CNS involvement can result in dementia.

Life-threatening symptoms can occur due to some multisystemic manifestations of the disease. Cardiac disease can be especially problematic. Heart block can result in cardiac arrest, or severe cardiomyopathy can develop. Cachexia can be serious in patients with MNGIE and MELAS. Intractable status epilepticus can occur, especially in patients with *POLG1* mutations.

Patients with mitochondrial disorders do have a reduced life expectancy. However, the variety and the severity of multisystemic involvement seen among these disorders results in very different outcomes. The main causes of death in patients with mitochondrial disorders are cardiopulmonary failure and status epilepticus.[79]

Rhabdomyolysis

Rhabdomyolysis may occur as an acute complication of metabolic myopathies but may also be caused by other conditions affecting muscle membranes, membrane ion channels, and muscle energy supply (e.g., exertion, crush injury and trauma, alcoholism, drugs, and toxins) (Box 22-3). It is characterized by acute damage of the sarcolemma of the skeletal muscle, leading to release of potentially toxic muscle cell components into the circulation, most notably CK and myoglobin. Typical symptoms include muscle pain, weakness, and dark urine. This disorder may result in potentially life-threatening complications, such as acute myoglobinuric renal failure (occurring in 4% to 33% of patients), cardiac arrhythmias via electrolyte abnormalities, disseminated intravascular coagulation, and compartment syndrome. The mainstay of treatment is hospitalization with early aggressive IV fluid replacement to minimize the occurrence of renal failure and correction or prevention of electrolyte abnormalities.[80] Additional adjunctive therapies, such as alkalinization of the urine with sodium bicarbonate, diuretic therapy, and renal protection with mannitol, although commonly recommended, are of unproven benefit. In severe cases, appropriate management may also include continuous venovenous hemofiltration, mechanical ventilatory support, and administration of antibiotics. The overall prognosis for rhabdomyolysis is favorable when treated early and aggressively with proper fluid replacement, and full recovery of renal function is common. Irrespective of the cause of rhabdomyolysis, the mortality rate may still be as high as 8%.

Conclusion

Metabolic disorders are important causes of myopathy. Diagnosis can be difficult because many different enzyme defects are possible. It is important to detect the underlying enzyme defect because this

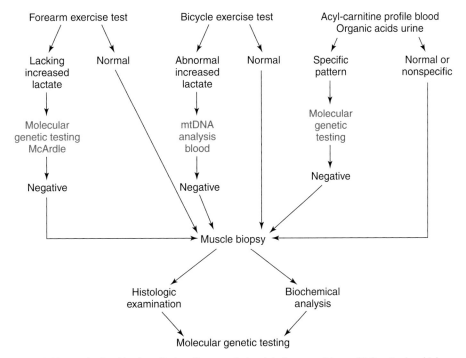

Figure 22-16 Diagnostic algorithm in patients with suspected metabolic myopathies. mtDNA, mitochondrial genome.

may present relevant therapeutic options, although no cure is possible in most disorders. Identification of the molecular genetic defect is important for genetic counseling. Figure 22-16 suggests a diagnostic algorithm in patients with suspected metabolic myopathy.

Suggested Reading

Bruno C, DiMauro S: Lipid storage myopathies, *Curr Opin Neurol* 21:601–606, 2008.

DiMauro S, Hirano M, Schon EA: Approaches to the treatment of mitochondrial diseases, *Muscle Nerve* 34:265–283, 2006.

DiMauro S, Lamperti C: Muscle glycogenoses, *Muscle Nerve* 24:984–999, 2001.

Taylor RW, Schaefer AM, Barrin MJ, et al: The diagnosis of mitochondrial muscle disease, *Neuromuscul Disord* 14:237–245, 2004.

Laforêt P, Vianey-Saban C, Vissing J: 162nd ENMC International Workshop: Disorders of muscle lipid metabolism in adults, 28-30 November 2008, Bussum, The Netherlands, *Neuromuscul Disord* 20:283–289, 2010.

References

1. Joshi PR, Gläser D, Schmidt S, et al: Molecular diagnosis of German patients with late-onset glycogen storage disease type II, *J Inherit Metab Disord* 2008. Epub ahead of print.
2. Rommel O, Kley RA, Dekomien G, et al: Muscle pain in myophosphorylase deficiency (McArdle's disease): the role of gender, genotype, and pain-related coping, *Pain* 124:295–304, 2006.
3. Orngreen MC, Jeppesen TD, Andersen ST, et al: Fat metabolism during exercise in patients with McArdle disease, *Neurology* 72:718–724, 2009.
4. Deschauer M, Morgenroth A, Joshi PR, et al: Analysis of spectrum and frequencies of mutations in McArdle disease: identification of 13 novel mutations, *J Neurol* 254:797–802, 2007.
5. Burwinkel B, Hu B, Schroers A, et al: Muscle glycogenosis with low phosphorylase kinase activity: mutations in *PHKA1, PHKG1* or six other candidate genes explain only a minority of cases, *Eur J Hum Genet* 11:516–526, 2003.
6. Kollberg G, Tulinius M, Gilljam T, et al: Cardiomyopathy and exercise intolerance in muscle glycogen storage disease 0, *N Engl J Med* 375:1507–1514, 2007.
7. Eber SW, Pekrun A, Bardosi A, et al: Triosephosphate isomerase deficiency: haemolytic anaemia, myopathy with altered mitochondria and mental retardation due to a new variant with accelerated enzyme catabolism and diminished specific activity, *Eur J Pediatr* 150:761–766, 1991.
8. Kazemi-Esfarjani P, Skomorowska E, Jensen TD, et al: A nonischemic forearm exercise test for McArdle disease, *Ann Neurol* 52:153–159, 2002.
9. Hanisch F, Joshi PR, Zierz S: AMP deaminase deficiency in skeletal muscle is unlikely to be of clinical relevance, *J Neurol* 255:318–322, 2008.
10. Van den Hout JM, Reuser AJ, Vulto AG, et al: Recombinant human acid alpha-glucosidase from rabbit milk in Pompe patients, *Lancet* 356: 397–398, 2000.
11. Van der Hout JM, Kamphoven JH, Winkel LP, et al: Long-term intravenous treatment of Pompe disease with recombinant human acid alpha-glucosidase from rabbit milk, *Pediatrics* 113:e448–e457, 2004.
12. Amalfitano A, Bengur AR, Morse RP, et al: Recombinant human acid alpha-glucosidase enzyme therapy for infantile glycogen storage disease type II: results of a phase I/II clinical trial, *Genet Med* 3:132–138, 2001.
13. Klinge L, Straub V, Neudorf U, et al: Safety and efficacy of recombinant acid alpha-glucosidase (rhGAA) in patients with classical infantile Pompe disease: results of a phase II clinical trial, *Neuromuscul Disord* 15:24–31, 2005.
14. Klinge L, Straub V, Neudorf U, et al: Enzyme replacement therapy in classical infantile Pompe disease: results of a 10-month follow-up study, *Neuropediatrics* 36:6–11, 2005.
15. Kishnani PS, Nicolino M, Voit T, et al: Chinese hamster ovary cell-derived recombinant human acid alpha-glucosidase in infantile-onset Pompe disease, *J Pediatr* 149:89–97, 2006.
16. Kishnani PS, Corzo D, Nicolino M, et al: Recombinant human acid alpha-glucosidase: major clinical benefits in infantile-onset Pompe disease, *Neurology* 149:89–97, 2007.
17. Quinlivan R, Beynon RJ, Martinuzzi A: Pharmacological and nutritional treatment for McArdle disease (glycogen storage disease type V), *Cochrane Database Syst Rev* 2:CD003458, 2008.
18. Willott CA, Young ME, Leighton B, et al: Creatine uptake in isolated soleus muscle: kinetics and dependence on sodium, but not on insulin, *Acta Physiol Scand* 166:99–104, 1999.

19. Vorgerd M, Grehl T, Jager M, et al: Creatine therapy in myophosphorylase deficiency (McArdle's disease), A placebo controlled crossover trial, *Arch Neurol* 57:956–963, 2000.

20. Vorgerd M, Zange J, Kley R, et al: Effect of high-dose creatine therapy on symptoms of exercise intolerance in McArdle's disease: double-blind, placebo-controlled crossover trial, *Arch Neurol* 59:97–101, 2002.

21. Andersen ST, Vissing J: Carbohydrate- and protein-rich diets in McArdle disease: effect on exercise capacity, *J Neurol Neurosurg Psychiatry* 79(12):1359–1563, 2008.

22. Haller RG, Wyrick MA, Tailvassalo T, et al: Aerobic conditioning: an effective therapy in McArdle's disease, *Ann Neurol* 59:922–928, 2006.

23. Martinuzzi A, Sartori E, Fanin M, et al: Phenoytype modulators in myophosphorylase deficiency, *Ann Neurol* 53:497–502, 2003.

24. Rubio JC, Gómez-Gallego F, Santiago C, et al: Genotype modulators of clinical severity in McArdle disease, *Neurosci Lett* 422:217–222, 2007.

25. Martinuzzi A, Liava A, Trevisi E, et al: Randomized, placebo-controlled, double-blind pilot trial of ramipril in McArdle's disease, *Muscle Nerve* 37:350–357, 2008.

26. Schroers A, Kley RA, Stachon A, et al: Gentamicin treatment in McArdle disease: failure to correct myophosphorylase deficiency, *Neurology* 66:285–286, 2006.

27. Andersen ST, Haller RG, Vissing J: Effect of oral sucrose shortly before exercise on work capacity in McArdle disease, *Arch Neurol* 65:786–789, 2008.

28. Busch V, Gempel K, Hack A, et al: Treatment of glycogenosis type V with ketogenic diet, *Ann Neurol* 58:341, 2005.

29. Phoenix J, Hopkins P, Bartram C, et al: Effect of vitamin B_6 supplementation in McArdle's disease: a strategic case study, *Neuromuscul Disord* 8:210–212, 1998.

30. Deschauer M, Hudson G, Müller T, et al: A novel *ANT1* gene mutation with probable germline mosaicism in autosomal dominant progressive external ophthalmoplegia, *Neuromuscul Disord* 15:311–315, 2005.

31. Longo N, Di San Filippo CA, Pasquali M: Disorders of carnitine transport and the carnitine cycle, *Am J Med Genet Part C Semin Med Genet* 142C:77–85, 2006.

32. Voermanns NC, van Engelen BG, Kluijtmans LA, et al: Rhabdomyolysis caused by an inherited metabolic disease: very long-chain acyl-CoA dehydrogenase deficiency, *Am J Med* 119:176–179, 2006.

33. Shchelochkov O, Wong LJ, Shaibani A, Shinawi M: Atypical presentation of VLCAD deficiency associated with a novel ACADVL splicing mutation, *Muscle Nerve* 39:374–382, 2009.

34. Spiekerkoetter U, Bennett MJ, Ben-Zeev B, et al: Peripheral neuropathy, episodic myoglobinuria, and respiratory failure in deficiency of the mitochondrial trifunctional protein, *Muscle Nerve* 29:66–72, 2004.

35. Gempel K, Topaloglu H, Talim B, et al: The myopathic form of coenzyme Q10 deficiency is caused by mutations in the electron-transferring flavoprotein dehydrogenase (*ETFDH*) gene, *Brain* 130:2037–2044, 2007.

36. Olsen RK, Olpin SE, Andresen BS, et al: *ETFDH* mutations as a major cause of riboflavin-responsive multiple acyl-CoA dehydrogenation deficiency, *Brain* 130:2045–2054, 2007.

37. Hsu HW, Zytkovicz TH, Comeau AM, et al: Spectrum of medium-chain acyl-CoA dehydrogenase deficiency detected by newborn screening, *Pediatrics* 121:e1108–e1114, 2008.

38. van Maldegem BT, Duran M, Wanders RJ, et al: Clinical, biochemical, and genetic heterogeneity in short-chain acyl-coenzyme A dehydrogenase deficiency, *JAMA* 296:943–952, 2006.

39. Bruno C, Bertini E, Di Rocco M, et al: Clinical and genetic characterization of Chanarin-Dorfman syndrome, *Biochem Biophys Res Commun* 369:1125–1128, 2008.

40. Fischer J, Lefèvre C, Morava E, et al: The gene encoding adipose triglyceride lipase (*PNPLA2*) is mutated in neutral lipid storage disease with myopathy, *Nat Genet* 39:28–30, 2007.

41. Gempel K, Kiechl S, Hofmann S, et al: Screening for carnitine palmitoyltransferase II deficiency by tandem mass spectrometry, *J Inherit Metab Dis* 25:17–27, 2002.

42. Ohashi Y, Hasegawa Y, Murayama K, et al: A new diagnostic test for VLCAD deficiency using immunohistochemistry, *Neurology* 62:2209–2213, 2004.

43. Deschauer M, Wieser T, Zierz S: Muscle carnitine palmitoyltransferase II deficiency: Clinical clinical and molecular genetic features and diagnostic aspects, *Arch Neurol* 62:37–41, 2005.

44. Orngreen MC, Ejstrup R, Vissing J: Effect of diet on exercise intolerance in carnitine palmitoyltransferase II deficiency, *Neurology* 61:559–561, 2003.

45. Bonnefont JP, Djouadi F, Prip-Buus C, et al: Carnitine palmitoyltransferases 1 and 2: biochemical, molecular and medical aspects, *Mol Aspects Med* 25:495–520, 2004.

46. Roe CR, Sweetman L, Roe DS, et al: Treatment of cardiomyopathy and rhabdomyolysis in long-chain fat oxidation disorders using an anaplerotic odd-chain triglyceride, *J Clin Invest* 110:259–269, 2002.

47. Roe CR, Yang BZ, Brunengraber H, et al: Carnitine palmitoyltransferase II deficiency: successful anaplerotic diet therapy, *Neurology* 71:260–264, 2008.

48. Djouadi F, Aubey F, Schlemmer D, et al: Peroxisome proliferator activated receptor delta (PPARδ) agonist but not PPARα corrects carnitine palmitoyl transferase 2 deficiency in human muscle cells, *J Clin Endocrinol Metab* 90:1791–1797, 2005.

49. Gobin-Limballe S, Djouadi F, Aubey F, et al: Genetic basis for correction of very-long-chain acyl-coenzyme A dehydrogenase deficiency by bezafibrate in patient fibroblasts: toward a genotype-based therapy, *Am J Hum Genet* 81:1133–1143, 2007.

50. Kelly KJ, Garland JS, Tangl TT, et al: Fatal rhabdomyolysis following influenza infection in a girl with familial carnitine palmitoyltransferase deficiency, *Pediatrics* 84:312–316, 1989.

51. Smolle KH, Kaufmann P, Gasser R: Recurrent rhabdomyolysis and acute respiratory failure due to carnitine palmitoyltransferase deficiency, *Intensive Care Med* 27:1235, 2001.

52. DiMauro S, Bonilla E, Zeviani M, et al: Mitochondrial myopathies, *Ann Neurol* 17:521–528, 1985.

53. Fadic R, Russell JA, Vedanarayanan VV, et al: Sensory ataxic neuropathy as the presenting feature of a novel mitochondrial disease, *Neurology* 49:239–245, 1997.

54. Nishino I, Spinazzola A, Papadimitriou A, et al: Mitochondrial neuro-gastrointestinal encephalomyopathy: an autosomal recessive disorder due to thymidine phosphorylase mutations, *Ann Neurol* 47:792–800, 2000.

55. Deschauer M, Müller T, Wieser T, et al: Hearing impairment is common in various phenotypes of the mitochondrial DNA A3243G mutation, *Arch Neurol* 58:1885–1888, 2001.

56. Andreu AL, Hanna MG, Reichmann H, et al: Exercise intolerance due to mutations in the cytochrome b gene of mitochondrial DNA, *N Engl J Med* 341:1037–1044, 1999.

57. Deschauer M, Swalwell H, Strauss M, et al: Novel mitochondrial tRNA^{Phe} gene mutation associated with late-onset neuromuscular disease, *Arch Neurol* 63:902–905, 2006.

58. Müller T, Deschauer M, Neudecker S, et al: Dystrophic myopathy of late onset associated with a G7497A mutation in the mitochondrial tRNA$^{Ser(UCN)}$ gene, *Acta Neuropathol* 110:426–430, 2005.

59. Swalwell H, Deschauer M, Hartl H, et al: Pure myopathy associated with a novel mitochondrial tRNA gene mutation, *Neurology* 66:447–449, 2006.

60. Bonnefont JP, Bastin J, Behin A, Djouadi F: Bezafibrate for an inborn mitochondrial beta-oxidation defect, *N Engl J Med* 360:838–840, 2009.

61. DiMauro S, Quinzii CM, Hirano M: Mutations in coenzyme Q10 biosynthetic genes, *J Clin Invest* 117:587–589, 2007.

62. Zierz S, Jahns G, Jerusalem F: Coenzyme Q in serum and muscle of 5 patients with Kearns-Sayre syndrome and 12 patients with ophthalmoplegia plus, *J Neurol* 236:97–101, 1989.

63. Hanisch F, Müller T, Muser A, et al: Lactate increase and oxygen desaturation in mitochondrial disorders—evaluation of two diagnostic screening protocols, *J Neurol* 253:417–423, 2006.

64. Deschauer M, Kiefer R, Blakely EL, et al: A novel *Twinkle* gene mutation in autosomal dominant progressive external ophthalmoplegia, 13:568–572, 2003.

65. Gellerich FN, Deschauer M, Müller T, et al: Mitochondrial respiratory rates and activities of respiratory chain complexes correlate linearly with heteroplasmy of deleted mtDNA without threshold and independently of deletion size, *Biochim Biophys Acta* 1556(1):41–52, 2002.

66. Chinnery PF, DiMauro S, Shanske S, et al: The risk of developing a mito-chondrial DNA deletion disorder, *Lancet* 364:592–596, 2004.

67. Hudson G, Deschauer M, Taylor RW, et al: *POLG1, C10ORF2* and *ANT1* mutations are uncommon in sporadic PEO with multiple mtDNA deletions, *Neurology* 66:1439–1441, 2006.

68. Deschauer M, Krasnianski A, Zierz S, et al: False-positive diagnosis of a sin-gle, large-scale mitochondrial DNA deletion by Southern blot analysis: the role of neutral polymorphisms, *Genet Test* 8:395–399, 2004.

69. Horvath R, Hudson G, Ferrari G, et al: Phenotypic spectrum associated with mutations of the mitochondrial polymerase gamma gene, *Brain* 129:1674–1684, 2006.

70. Pineda M, Ormazabal A, Lopez-Gallardo E, et al: Cerebral folate deficiency and leukoencephalopathy caused by a mitochondrial DNA deletion, *Ann Neurol* 59:394–398, 2006.

71. Chinnery PF, Bindoff LA: 116th ENMC International Workshop: the treat-ment of mitochondrial disorders, 14th-16th March 2003, Naarden, The Netherlands, *Neuromuscul Disord* 13:757–764, 2003.

72. Bau V, Zierz S: Update on chronic progressive external ophthalmoplegia, *Strabismus* 13:133–142, 2005.

73. Kornblum C, Broicher CR, Walther E, et al: Cricopharyngeal achalasia is a common cause of dysphagia in patients with mtDNA deletions, *Neurology* 56:1409–1412, 2000.

74. Jeppesen TD, Schwartz M, Olsen DB, et al: Aerobic training is safe and improves exercise capacity in patients with mitochondrial myopathy, *Brain* 129:3402–3412, 2006.

75. Taivassalo T, Gardner JL, Taylor RW, et al: Endurance training and detraining in mitochondrial myopathies due to single large-scale mtDNA deletions, *Brain* 129:3391–3401, 2006.

76. Koga Y, Akita Y, Nishioka J, et al: L-arginine improves the symptoms of strokelike episodes in MELAS, *Neurology* 64:710–712, 2005.

77. Hirano M, Marti R, Casali C, et al: Allogeneic stem cell transplantation cor-rects biochemical derangements in MNGIE, *Neurology* 67:1458–1460, 2006.

78. Gardner JL, Craven L, Turnbull DM, et al: Experimental strategies towards treating mitochondrial DNA disorders, *Biosci Rep* 27:139–150, 2007.

79. Klopstock T, Jaksch M, Gasser T: Age and cause of death in mitochondrial diseases, *Neurology* 53:855–857, 1999.

80. Huerta-Alardin AL, Varon J, Marik PE: Bench-to-bedside review: rhabdomyolysis—an overview for clinicians, *Critical Care* 9:158–169, 2005.

Index